Dimensions
of
Professional
Nursing

Dimensions of Professional Nursing

SEVENTH EDITION

Lucie Young Kelly, R.N., PH.D., F.A.A.N.

Professor Emeritus of Public Health and Nursing
Columbia University
New York, New York

Lucille A. Joel, R.N., ED.D., F.A.A.N.

Professor, College of Nursing
Rutgers, the State University of New Jersey
Newark, New Jersey

McGraw-Hill, Inc.
Health Professions Division

New York St. Louis San Francisco Auckland Bogotá Caracas Lisbon London Madrid Mexico City
Milan Montreal New Delhi San Juan Singapore Sydney Tokyo Toronto

DIMENSIONS OF PROFESSIONAL NURSING, *Seventh Edition*

1 2 3 4 5 6 7 8 9 0 DOCDOC 9 8 7 6 5

ISBN 0-07-105477-4

This book was set in Times Roman by Northeastern Graphic Services, Inc.
The editors were Gail Gavert and Lester A. Sheinis.
The production supervisor was Richard C. Ruzycka.
The text and cover designer was José Fonfrias.
The indexer was Mary Kidd.
R. R. Donnelley & Sons was printer and binder.

This book is printed on acid-free paper.

Library of Congress Cataloging-in-Publication Data

Kelly, Lucie Young.
   Dimensions of professional nursing / Lucie Young Kelly,
Lucille A. Joel. — 7th ed.
     p.   cm.
   Includes bibliographical references.
   ISBN 0-07-105477-4 (alk. paper)
   1. Nursing. 2. Nursing—United States.   I. Joel, Lucille A.
  II. Title
   [DNLM: 1. Nursing   WY 16 K33d 1995]
RT82.K4 1995
610.73—dc20
DNLM/DLC
for Library of Congress   94-36655

Contents

Preface

Dimensions of Professional Nursing has always been written by one author (with, of course, valuable contributions to various chapters by nursing colleagues). Cordelia Kelly wrote the first two editions, beginning in 1962. After her untimely death in 1966, Edith (Pat) Lewis completed the second edition, and some years later I came along and wrote the third edition (1975). From that time on, I have continued to view *Dimensions* as Cordelia Kelly described it: "an overview of the nonclinical aspects of nursing in sufficient detail to be adaptable for use at all stages in all types of preservice programs in professional nursing." Although content has changed greatly with the times, as it must, I have always been proud of the fact that each new edition has kept it one of the most comprehensive and up-to-date books of its type and that readers frequently keep it on their bookshelves after their course to use as a reference.

Now I have one more major change. I have chosen as my coauthor Dr. Lucille Joel, a distinguished nurse, recognized nationally and internationally for her expertise on issues and trends in nursing, indeed in health care. It has been an adventure to work together to produce this edition. As we expected, we have always agreed philosophically about what *Dimensions* should be, and exchanging ideas about approaches and specific content has been an exciting process. I think that it has made the book better than ever. Although we conferred on everything, for the sake of simplicity, the chapters were divided between us. However, there is inevitably a touch of

Kelly in each, since the previous edition was, as usual, the basis for the new one.

Because *Dimensions of Professional Nursing* is intended for use by a diverse readership, the references and bibliography are extensive. Most citations and readings are post–1990, although there are solid classic and otherwise appropriate references with earlier dates. (Some readers also refer back to the previous edition, because many of those references are still pertinent.) Included are references that give opposing views on controversial issues and citations from books and periodicals other than nursing. Both teacher and student will find them valuable for further study.

There are many revisions in this edition because society, health care, and nursing continue to evolve. At the end of the section on history, an epilogue now summarizes the period from 1966 to the present, all of which is presented in more detail throughout the book. Again, a comprehensive review of all major studies affecting nursing is found in Chapter 5, with the addition of the newest studies. Chapters 6, 7, and 8 describe the environment in which nurses learn and practice, including the trends and public sentiment that will inevitably require the health care system to take on a new form and function as we approach the turn of the century. Our predictions continue to be provocative. Chapters 12 and 13 focus on our systems of education for practice, the issues that continue to frustrate and those that have been successfully resolved over the years. There is justifiable pride in the fact that the profession has honored a commitment to provide for the educational mobility of its members and has changed with the times to accommodate an exceedingly diverse constituency.

The chapter on ethics has been expanded but should be read along with Chapter 22 on the rights of patients, since it is almost impossible today to draw the line between ethics and related law. Chapter 10 includes pertinent new information on *do not resuscitate* (DNR) policies and ethics committees. Chapter 22 not only adds new legal cases but also the latest information on advanced directives and professionally assisted suicide. New legal decisions concerning students' rights are also discussed. As might be expected, given the nature of our times, the chapters on credentialing and legal issues required considerable updating. Because of the evolving roles of nurses, such issues and information are of major concern to students. The many new legal cases used as examples of legal principles should be particularly helpful. Another greatly enlarged section is that on the many nursing organizations. This time, information about their publications is included with each organizational overview.

The content that used to be called "Professional Literature" has been integrated into the chapters on organizations as well as into Chapter 30. Chapter 15 again provides considerable depth on nurses' career opportunities, with additional emphasis on the advanced practice nurse. The material on changing practice roles and on nursing supply and demand is particularly pertinent.

Nursing has experienced profound change since the last edition of *Dimensions*. There is stability in the midst of change as we revisit and reconsider our stewardship to the public and the characteristics of today's nurses, discussed in Chapters 9 and 11. These sensitivities to professionalism combined with the content, references, and bibliography of Chapter 16 provide a superb orientation to leadership for uncertain times. Ultimately, students will play out their career lives in the workplace (for some this takes the form of a variety of entrepreneurial choices). Chapter 30 highlights the rights and responsibilities that come with transition to the role of graduate, and then to RN—workplace hazards, legal rights of employees, workplace representation, maintaining competency, and career mapping. Material from earlier editions about professional writing has been retained because no other text includes this basic guidance for sharing your ideas and experiences through publication.

Because cross-referencing from chapter to chapter has always been helpful to readers—enabling them both to get a more complete picture of a topic or issue and to see interrelationships—we have continued this tradition. We believe that the kinds of nurses who will strengthen the profession, change health care for the better, and take influential roles in the nursing community—regardless of the specific positions they select—need and want the kind of in-depth analysis as well as the key information presented here. Nursing is in a period of renaissance. Opportunities abound for nurses with the proper knowledge, courage, confidence, and determination. Our hope is that this book will contribute to their armamentarium and allow them to be leaders in their profession and their times.

Lucie Young Kelly

Acknowledgments

CONSISTENT WITH THE RAPID CHANGES in health care, *Dimensions of Professional Nursing* requires a considerable number of changes with each edition. To be as up-to-date and accurate as possible, we have called on a number of our colleagues to share their expertise. All of them are highly respected, extremely busy, and remarkably generous. Therefore, we would like to acknowledge their valuable contributions. In some cases, the individual updated chapters, and we would like to recognize them first. Sally Cohen, Ph.D., updated Chapter 19, "Major Legislation Affecting Nursing," and Marilyn Chow, D.N.S., Chapter 20, "Licensure and Health Personnel Credentialing."

Shirley Fondiller, Ed. D., organized and edited Chapter 27, and we give special thanks to the executives and staff of all the nursing and other organizations included in that chapter, who provided current material on their respective organizations. Linda Shinn edited Chapter 25 on ANA, and made helpful suggestions for changes in Chapter 23. In addition, Diane Mancino responded with current information on the NSNA, Constance Holleran on ICN, Patricia Moccia, Ph.D., on the NLN, Jo McNeill on APHA, and Linda Brimmer and colleagues on STTI. Donna Richardson added pertinent new information on the legislative process in Chapter 18, and David Price, Ph.D., and Patricia Murphy, Ph.D., contributed some interesting new insights to Chapter 22 on the rights of patients. We additionally took advantage of the expertise of Thelma Schorr on the changing status of women both in the United States and the world at large (Chapter 6) and of Denise Geolot of the Division of Nursing who provided access to the final report of the SCON. Joan Marren of the Visiting Nurse Service of New York contributed new developments on nursing in the community for Chapter 7. Sheila Gorman, Ph.D., was equally expert reporting on health care administration, and Stephen Crane, Ph.D., of the American Academy of Physician Assistants, provided new information on that career.

Because the changes in practice have been quite dramatic even in the brief time between editions, we turned to our practitioner colleagues to whom we are most grateful. We thank Geri Columbraro (staff development and continuing education), Rear Admiral Julia Plotnick (U.S. Public Health Service and international opportunities), Janet Heinrich, D.P.H. (public health/community health nursing), Judith B. Igoe (school health nursing), Bonnie Rogers, D.P.H. (occupational health nursing), Joyce Thompson, D.P.H. (Nurse Midwifery), Cynthia Vlasich (American Red Cross), Brigadier General Irene Trowell-Harris (Air Force Nurse Corps), Nancy Valentine, Ph.D. (Department of Veterans Affairs Nursing Service), Rear Admiral Mariann Stratton and Captain Barbara J. Beeby (Navy Nurse Corps), Brigadier General Nancy R. Adams and Colonel Terris E. Kennedy (Army Nurse Corps), Luis A. Rivera (Nurse Anesthetist), Mary Ann Jones (Office Nursing), Virginia Maroun (CGFNS), Jennifer Bosma, Ph.D. (NCSBN), and Miriam Hirschfeld, Ph.D.

(WHO). Our gratitude to Marla Salmon, Sc.D., for new information on the Division of Nursing.

In addition, we both thank the very capable women who typed portions of the manuscript: Susanne Conyers, Nancy Rispoli, and Rosemarie Britt.

Finally, we owe a great deal to the teachers, students, and colleagues who over the years have used the sixth edition of *Dimensions* and have commented so helpfully. They, like the two of us, agree that nurses, more than ever, need to know about their past as well as their present, in order to influence their future and the future of the profession that continues to endow their lives richly.

Dimensions of Professional Nursing

Part *I*

Development of Modern Nursing

Early
Historical
Influences

Care of the Sick: A Historical Overview

THE CLINICAL PRACTICE of nursing is quite rightly the major focus of most of its practitioners and the prime concern of students. Therefore, there is a tendency to greet nursing history with a "What good is it to me?" attitude. Undoubtedly, nurses can give good nursing care even if they have never heard of Florence Nightingale, Isabel Hampton Robb, Lavinia Dock, or Lillian Wald. But one of the major differences between an occupation and a profession is its practitioners' long-term commitment to the profession, which includes working toward its development. To do so without some understanding of its past is possibly to repeat errors.

Nursing today was formed by its historical antecedents. Its development since ancient times, within the social contexts of those times, explains many things: its power or lack of power, its educational confusion, and the makeup of its practitioners. The changing relationships between nursing and other health care professions, nursing and other disciplines, and nursing and the public can be traced and better understood with the knowledge of past history. The impact of social and scientific changes on nursing and nursing's impact on society are ongoing processes that need to be studied; nursing does not exist in a vacuum. Sometimes there is a repetition of history, with the answer to the problems apparently not much clearer now than at the beginning of professional nursing.

A hundred years ago, there was objection from within and without nursing to nurses having more education; the scenario is repeated today in some instances. Seventy-five years ago, the question of nursing licensure was hotly debated; today, it is again a major concern. These issues affect the practice of every nurse; in some cases, they are a factor in determining whether the nurse even chooses to stay in the profession. An understanding of the past can bring additional clarity to the decisions that shape the future.

This chapter and those that follow in Part I are not intended in any way as a substitute for the many fine texts that are available on nursing history. Instead, they provide an overview to set the stage for the more detailed study of nursing history an individual may undertake for professional reasons or personal satisfaction. In this book's 4th edition, Appendix A presents vignettes of distinguished nurses of the past, which may also be a useful resource.

PRIMITIVE SOCIETIES

Although historians sometimes advance theories and cite an occasional archaeological discovery to prove that prehistoric civilization practiced crude medicine and nursing, the supporting evidence about nursing is somewhat inconclusive. It must be assumed, however, that in most tribes there were some individuals who were more adept than others at caring for the sick and injured and helping the medicine men or witch doctors. It seems reasonable to assume further that some of these men and women taught their sons and daughters and certain members of the tribes to give this care, for these people were able to communicate. They wanted to survive; they were human beings with some ability to think, to recall, and to teach by example, if not by coherent explanation.

Indirect evidence of some of the beliefs and practices of ancient humans concerning illness has evolved from recent studies of primitive cultures. Apparently, many concepts of health and illness were related to belief in the super-natural. Everything in nature was seen as being alive, with invisible forces and supernatural power. There were good spirits and evil spirits that must be placated. Primitive humans believed that a person became sick (1) when an evil spirit entered the body; (2) when a good spirit within the body that was ordinarily able to fend off diseases left, either because someone or something had taken it away or of its own accord; and (3) because witchcraft had been performed upon the affected part of the body, either directly or through some object that had been given to the person.

Thus, although it was probably recognized how heat, cold, certain foods, wounds, and strains were related to health and empirical treatments developed for them, serious illness called for the services of a medicine man (witch doctor, shaman, root doctor). This mysterious figure, sometimes a woman but usually a man, functioned through a ritualistic mystique, frequently a shock or fright technique that was intended to induce evil spirits to leave the body. Included were the use of frightening masks and noises, incantations, vile odors, charms, spells, sacrifices, and fetishes. In a primitive version of modern trephining, the medicine man cut a hole in the skull to let the evil spirit out. Purgatives, emetics, deodorants, applied hot and cold substances, cauterization, massage, cupping, and blistering were frequently used.

A woman in abnormal labor was treated by similarly drastic measures, such as placing a lighted fire between her outstretched legs to hasten delivery. Needless to say, patients did not always survive this treatment, and if they did, there is no evidence that any daily ongoing care was given by the shaman. Probably a relative gave this "nursing" care. Women generally assisted other women in childbearing. But whether treatment of illness and injury by use of herbs and other "natural" means was carried out by all men and/or women, or by specially designated individuals, is not known.

EARLY CIVILIZATIONS

In the written records of the early civilizations (500 B.C. to A.D. 476), there is very little reference to nursing as such. However, if there is evidence of a high standard of living, a good sanitation system, architectural achievement, interest in education and culture and scientific medicine, or even two or three of these, it is reasonably certain that the health of the inhabitants was of paramount importance and that nurses were not only present but were trained in some fashion to prepare them for the work they did.

The Babylonians

Babylonia was the center of ancient Mesopotamian culture, which was in ruins by the time the Christian era began. Located between the eastern Mediterranean Sea and the Persian Gulf and nourished by the Tigris and Euphrates rivers, this land was very fertile, offering a good life to its settlers. Coveted by many people, it was for thousands of years first under the rule of one master and then another who took possession by force. Each influenced the others' development intellectually, socially, and scientifically. Their many wars brought misery and suffering, and, even in that abundant country, there must have been many illnesses and injuries in the normal course of life.

There is evidence that a legalized medical service was instituted and that some type of lay nurse cared for patients. They may have been men, but if they were women, their status was probably quite low, and they must have been subservient to physicians because the women of Babylonia were dominated by men who controlled their every action.

Herodotus, a Greek historian called the "Father of History," recorded that it was customary in Babylon for the sick to go to the marketplace where passersby could see them and stop to inquire into the "nature of their distemper." Those who had knowledge of how to treat a condition (knowledge acquired principally through experience) advised the ill on therapy that had helped them. This was hardly a scientific method of treatment, but it no doubt was effective in many instances.

Excavations made in 1849 of 700 medical tablets show that the Babylonian physician-priest allowed his patients to choose whether they wanted to be treated with medicine or charms. If they selected medicine, the physician had many vegetable and mineral preparations to employ. If they selected charms, the doctor told them which ones to wear for their particular illness and probably uttered a few incantations to accompany them, for they still believed that disease was caused by sin and displeasure of the gods.

However, some of the treatments indicate a realistic attitude toward illness, for they included diet, rest, enemas, bandaging, and massaging, plus emphasis on the importance of good personal hygiene. This care might be given by family or a "nurse."

The first Babylonian Empire was founded by King Hammurabi, who developed a code of laws for the whole empire. The code is engraved on a huge stone, unearthed in 1902, and shows Hammurabi worshipping a sun god from whom he is receiving instructions about the laws. Included are laws concerned with the fees that a physician was allowed to charge for his services and also punishment for the physician who committed "malpractice." Payments were to be made in *shekels* of silver — usually two, five, or ten, depending upon whether the patient was a master or a slave. Punishment for causing a patient to lose his life or an eye was to "cut off the physician's hands if the patient was a noble man." (This kind of punishment was reserved for surgeons, not physician-priests.) Wet nurses were also regulated as to remuneration and responsibility.

The Ancient Hebrews

Much of the story of the ancient Hebrews is told in the Talmud and the Old Testament. The Hebrews, alone of their contemporaries, believed in one God, Yahweh, not many.

Their misfortunes and illnesses they attributed to God's wrath, and they depended upon Him more than on fellow humans to restore them to health when they were sick. One facet of their religion was that it was their duty to be hospitable to strangers as well as to their own people, and they were obliged to give a tithe to augment their personal service in visiting the sick and needy.

The Hebrews brought many hygienic practices from Babylonia, where they had been in captivity, but under the leadership of Moses they also developed principles and practices of hygiene and sanitation. Moses decreed that all meat must be inspected, the selection and preparation of all foods must be carefully supervised, and cleanliness in all areas of living was absolutely essential. This has been called the first sanitary legislation. It represented one of the first public health movements on record.

Their people were taught to help prevent the spread of communicable diseases by burning an infected person's garments and sometimes even his house, and by scrubbing the room in which he was ill and the utensils he used. They were often able to diagnose and control the spread of leprosy and gonorrhea. They performed trephining operations skillfully and humanely, giving the patient a sleeping potion before surgery to dull the pain. They also did cesarean sections, splenectomies, amputations, and circumcisions and set fractures. They dressed wounds with oil, wine, and balsam and used sutures and bandages.

From these operations and careful examination of animals, they developed a body of knowledge about anatomy and physiology, although we know now that some of their information was understandably superficial and inaccurate.

The nurse is mentioned occasionally in the Old Testament and the Talmud, but in what capacity she served, except as wet nurse, is not entirely clear. It does appear that the "nurse" visited and possibly cared for the sick in their homes. She probably also had a role in health teaching.

The Persian Contribution

Between c. 550 and 500 B.C., Cyrus the Great, king of Persia, and his son, Cambyses, acquired a vast empire in the Near East. They adopted many of the medical practices and much of the culture from the great lands they conquered—Asia Minor, Babylonia, Syria, Mesopotamia, Egypt, and several others.

In Egypt, the Emperor Darius, successor of Cambyses, restored a school for training priest-physicians and, in effect, established a government-controlled medical center, the first of its kind recorded in history. It is also known that there were practitioners who healed with holy words, with herbs, and with the knife—in decreasing order of practice.

The Art of Medicine in Egypt

There are references to nurses in accounts of Egyptian medicine as it was practiced in the pre-Christian era. The medical papyri discovered during excavations contain descriptions of such nursing procedures as feeding a tetanus patient and dressing wounds. The extent of the nurse's duties is not clear, however.

Egyptian medicine, on the other hand, is revealed by graven inscriptions, the papyri, and other literature as having been rather far advanced. In spite of the Egyptians' ideas about the origin of life, the journey that humans took after death, the causes of disease, and the catastrophic effects of incurring the wrath of the gods, they also practiced some very good medicine, although it may not have been based on scientific principles. Priests and physicians were identical in early Egyptian civilization, and in healing temples, rest, rituals, and prayer were part of the treatment. Later there emerged physicians who were concerned only with matters of health and hygiene.

Medical specialization became so common that a physician usually spent his entire career in caring for diseases of one particular part of the body. Members of the profession were organized to protect their medical secrets.

It was in ancient Egypt that the great physician Imhotep lived in about 2980 B.C. Skilled in architecture, magic, and priestcraft as well as medicine, he became so famous that he was never forgotten. More than two and a half centuries after his death, he became the god of medicine, identified by the Greeks with their famous god of healing, Asclepios (Latin, Aesculapius).

In Egypt, as in most countries, one of the important areas of concern was the health of the people. The Egyptians formulated regulations about diet, baths, purgatives, and other matters of personal hygiene. They initiated laws of health suited to Egypt's climate and terrain. They developed diagnostic procedures (which differed in some respects from those of other ancient civilizations) for the common illnesses of their people. Examinations of mummies indicate that the Egyptians suffered many bone diseases and injuries. Osteoarthritis was apparently very common, and there must also have been ailments all humans are subject to such as abdominal, gynecological, and genitourinary conditions.

There were medical schools and at least one school of midwifery for women, the graduates of which taught physicians about "women's conditions." They became quite well informed about some aspects of anatomy and physiology. For example, the papyri reveal that Egyptian physicians may have had reasonably accurate knowledge of the circulatory system, which was not described accurately and completely by modern people until the sixteenth century A.D., when William Harvey studied it. Taking the pulse was a common practice, and the quality of both the heartbeat and the pulse was considered important in understanding a patient's condition. Treatments included the use of a kind of adhesive plaster for closing small wounds; swabs, bandages, and tampons made from linen ravelings; sutures; and molded splints. The papyri also contain records of the preparation of pills, ointments, snuffs, gargles, and emollients that have continued, at least in name, until modern times. Drugs included opium, castor oil, hemlock, salts of copper, and many others.

Dentistry was practiced skillfully, if the gold-filled teeth of mummies of wealthy citizens are to be accepted as evidence. Egyptians developed the art of embalming the body to provide a home for the soul as it went on its journey after death.

The Ancient Hindus

The history of pre-Christian India reports the establishment of hospitals, probably the first in the world, and also the first special nursing group of which we have accurate information. These male attendants (perhaps more accurately called physician's assistants instead of nurses) staffed the hospitals to which surgeons with remarkable skills sent their patients for care. The Indian philosophy which assigned women to an inferior role in society would not allow them to work outside the home environment. The qualifications of these "nurses" were stated as follows in the *Charaka Samhita*, a medical manuscript:

> ...there should be secured a body of attendants of good behavior, distinguished for purity or cleanliness of habits, attached to the person for whose services they are engaged, possessed of cleverness and skill, endowed with kindness, skilled in every kind of service that a patient may require...clever in bathing or washing a patient...well skilled in making or cleaning beds...and skillful in waiting upon one that is ailing, and never unwilling to do any act that they be commanded to do.

No one knows who did the "commanding" of these workers—patients or doctors, or both. The

nurse's status is also unclear (it appears that he might have become a physician after training), but we at least know that he performed some nursing functions.

The knowledge about Indian medicine derives principally from several of their books and writings (in contrast to the reliance on archaeological discoveries for data about the Mesopotamian and Egyptian civilizations and others). Of these, the sacred writings called the Vedas, a compendium of surgical works (*Susruta Samhita*), and another of medical works (*Charaka Samhita*) are most informative.

From the Vedas, which are the oldest scriptures of Hinduism, it is learned that the Indian people of ancient times were highly religious and believed in divine control of health and disease. They worshipped many gods, especially the sun god Brahma, until Buddhism originated in the sixth century B.C. They used charms and invocations and other primitive methods to quell the wrath of the gods, but from about 800 B.C. to A.D. 1000, all of India flourished and progressed, and medicine also advanced. It was during this period that the hospitals mentioned earlier were built.

The two outstanding physicians of ancient times were Susruta and Charaka, who in their writings revealed that physicians were members of the upper castes and were required to be pure of mind and body and ethical in every respect. Their knowledge of anatomy and physiology was often inaccurate, but they evolved some theories that persisted for centuries. Among these was the belief that disease might be caused by impurities in the body fluids or humors. They used bloodletting procedures to rid the body of the impure fluids. The theory of humoral pathology was accepted subsequently by Greek physicians and became a basic concept of European medicine. The Indian physician had a great many drugs and other pharmaceutical preparations to help him in his work.

The surgery practiced in India was particularly outstanding for the time. With instruments they designed themselves, under the cleanest conditions possible, without the aid of effective antiseptic or the benefits of anesthesia, the surgeons performed tonsillectomies, herniorrhaphies, tumor excisions, cataract operations, and other forms of surgery.

To help prevent disease, the Hindus formulated religious laws covering particularly matters of hygiene and diet suitable to the tropical climate.

Scientific medicine in India eventually lost its momentum, and during the Mohammedan era beginning about A.D. 622 it began to decline and became almost completely extinguished, a genuine loss to world medicine.

Ceylon (Sri Lanka), an island off India's southeast coast, had an advanced standard of living during the period of India's greatest achievement. History has recorded the establishment of many hospitals in which well prepared physicians and nurses attended the sick. Hospitals for animals also were founded in India as well as Ceylon.

The Chinese

As in other ancient cultures, magic, demons, and evil spirits were part of Chinese medical beliefs. The beginning of a more modern medicine is credited to the emperor Shen Nung (c. 2700 B.C.), who apparently originated drug therapy and acupuncture. These were incorporated into the theory of yang and yin, which still exists. Yang, the male principle, is light, positive, full of life; yin, the female principle, is dark, cold, lifeless. When the two are in harmony, the patient is in good health. Originally, acupuncture consisted of inserting needles into areas called meridians, which controlled the flow of yang and yin. (With new interest in acupuncture, American medicine is trying to determine its anatomic and physiological basis.)

Other Chinese contributions include the use of many still pertinent drugs and further refinement of ancient measures of hydrotherapy, massage, cupping (bloodletting), moxa (a form of counterirritation), cautery, and the promotion of systematic exercise to maintain physical and mental well-being.

Sources of information include a book on medicine written by Shen Nung, and later works, notably the classic *Canon of Medicine*, which is a complete discussion of anatomy and physiology with many details about blood circulation and pulse. Another outstanding book was the *Essay on Typhoid*, written in the first century A.D. by Chang Chung Ching, often regarded as China's greatest physician.

There is little mention of any type of hospital, perhaps because of strong family traditions that would naturally include giving care to the sick within the family circle. Thus, nursing care was probably given in the home.

The Great Achievement of Greece

Whenever ancient Greece is mentioned, one immediately thinks of education, philosophy, and democracy. But Plato, Aristotle, Socrates, Herodotus, Homer, Sophocles, Pericles, Euripides, and other great names of Greece were not typical of its earliest times, for this country too began under primitive conditions in about 2000 B.C.

The ancient Greeks represented many peoples, principally the Achean, Dorian, Aegean, Ionian, Arcadian, and Aeolian, who came from the mountains, from fertile valleys where they had engaged in agriculture, and from the seacoast where seafaring was their occupation. Collectively they called themselves the Hellenes (after their ancestor Hellen, a legendary king of Phthia).

They were barbaric people at first, with the superstitions and practices of primitive people, but gradually there emerged the well-known Grecian character with a thirst for truth and knowledge. Because of their geographical location and the ease of maritime travel, they were able to visit such comparatively advanced countries as Crete and Mesopotamia and to borrow or usurp their cultures.

They were also eager to expand their geographical borders, and were so successful that within a few centuries their culture extended from Geece to India. Gradually they developed their own Hellenic civilization, and by 500 B.C., if not before, they displayed the keen intellect, independence of thought, and democratic action for which they are famous. They also enjoyed religious freedom. Their great center of civilization was Athens, which was at its peak in the fourth century B.C. Athenian culture spread to other beautiful cities, principally along the Mediterranean coast, some of which eventually surpassed Athens in brilliance.

In such a vital society, the art of medicine naturally kept pace with advances in other fields. But, like other ancient cultures, Greece went through centuries of belief in demons and spirits as causes of human ills, but with an element of greater complexity because of its acquisition of other cultures and a divergence of beliefs and practices among them. Here, too, the Greeks gradually evolved their own ideas about the relationships of the gods to health and illness. The famous Greek myths told in story and poem show a mixture of common sense and mysticism in their medical attitudes.

Asclepios, the classical god of medicine, is part of one such myth. Whether he actually lived or not seems uncertain, for his origin is obscure, but it is generally conceded that he did exist in person and that the mystery that surrounds him stems largely from his deification. A parallel is seem in the deification of Imhotep by the Egyptians. Hygieia, the goddess of health, is reputed to have been the daughter of Asclepios.

His contributions, real or imagined, were further recognized by the founding of temples in his honor in localities suitable for rest and restoration to health. Sometimes referred to as hospitals, they were much more like the spas and health resorts of modern times, with mineral springs, baths, gymnasiums, athletic fields, and treatment and consultation rooms.

They differed from modern resorts, however, in that they were controlled by priests and were essentially religious institutions. Prayers, sacrifices, rituals, and thank offerings were part of every patient's regimen in one of these sanitoria. (However, pregnant women and individuals with incurable diseases were not admitted.) The

therapeutic effects of the earthly facilities were considerable, however, and knowledge of them was significant in later medical practice. Priestesses served as attendants and waited upon the sick, but they could not be considered nurses. The best known of these temples was Epidauros, about 30 miles from Athens, the ruins of which can still be seen.

To Asclepios can also be traced the origin of the symbol of the medical profession—a serpent entwined on a staff—known as the caduceus. The staff was the staff of Asclepios; the serpent since primitive times had represented wisdom and knowledge.

The greatest name in Greek medicine—and possibly in all medicine—is Hippocrates. Born in Cos in 460 B.C., he is frequently seen as the epitome of the ideal physician both personally and professionally. Humane, brilliant, progressive, a great physician, teacher, and leader, he is often known as the "Father of Medicine."

Hippocrates' medical achievements can be grouped into four major areas:

1. *Rejection of all beliefs in the supernatural origin of disease.* He divorced medicine from religion, philosophy, and the remaining traces of magic and taught that illness was caused by a breach of natural laws. He did not accept the theories of others who preceded him, but made his diagnosis on the basis of symptoms he observed in his patients. His emphasis was on the whole patient, and he advocated constant and continuous bedside care.

2. *Development of thorough patient assessment and recording.* He thoroughly examined his patients and then made a systematic recording of his findings: general appearance, temperature, pulse, respiration, sputum, excreta, ability to move about, and so on. Never before had physicians prepared good clinical records.

3. *Establishment of the highest ethical standards in medicine.* Hippocrates considered medicine one of the noblest arts and believed that the conduct of the physician

should be above reproach. He must be loyal to his profession and never bring dishonor upon it. He must be equally loyal to his patients and never injure them in any way. The Hippocratic Oath (probably written after his death) is reproduced in part in Chap. 10 and presumably encompasses some of his convictions.

4. *Author of medical books.* Although it is thought that much of the writing was actually done by contemporaries or possibly his students, the information is supposed to be based on Hippocrates' teachings. The works include his case histories, descriptions of techniques such as bathing and bandaging, treatises on fractures and dislocations, diet in acute diseases, ulcers, epidemic diseases, and others. He reported on treatments that did not work, as well as those that did, to avoid repetition of errors.

Little is known of nursing as an occupation in pre-Christian Greece. However, because the Greeks never established hospitals, in spite of nominal advances in surgery, Greek physicians did not need the assistance of nurses to the degree that the surgeons of India did, for example, and that may have been an important factor. Through the ages, the development of nursing seems to have been greatly influenced by the physician's need for assistance, the quality of help that he wanted, and the amount of responsibility he was willing to delegate to others. If there were nurses who worked outside the home in Greece, they must have all been men because women held a very inferior position and were denied education as well as participation in community activities, both civil and humanitarian, except for the few instances in which women became midwives or physicians.

Advances in Alexandria

After Alexander the Great conquered Greece in about 338 B.C., he spread Greek civilization throughout the known world. It reached a par-

ticularly high point in Alexandria, an Egyptian city on the Mediterranean Sea. Here the arts and sciences, including medicine, flourished for about 300 years.

In c. 300 B.C., the first great medical school of this period was established in Alexandria with clinics, laboratories, and a huge library of 500,000 volumes. The physicians were supported by the state and did not have to depend on their practice to make a living. Dissections were permitted, and this resulted in tremendous advances in the knowledge of anatomy and physiology. The studies made by the Alexandrian physicians are considered the first medical research worthy of the name. After Cleopatra was defeated by the Romans in 30 B.C., Alexandria's place in the sun dimmed considerably, and the art of and interest in research declined.

Roman Hospitals and Sanitation

When the Etruscans conquered Rome in about 750 B.C., they brought new arts to this farming community, particularly the use of bronze, skill in building stone edifices, and a written language. In about 500 B.C., the Romans overthrew the Etruscans and became powerful masters of the Western world. Rome soon became a thriving commercial center and, through later conquests, a vast empire. Much emphasis was placed on government administration and related activities, on pleasures for the well-to-do, sometimes at the expense of the less fortunate, and on beautifully constructed public buildings, aqueducts, and roads.

Gradually Rome assimilated what it wanted of the Greek culture, and in some fields that was considerable. Although a temple of Aesculapius was built, Romans were somewhat wary of the Greek methods of treating disease, believing that their own deities, folklore, and magic were functioning well enough. Moreover, they were reluctant to accept advice and direction from the Greek physicians who, they thought, might poison or assassinate them in the name of medicine. They considered them social inferiors and thought them mercenary because they charged fees for their services.

Nevertheless, Greek medicine gradually replaced or supplemented Roman practices, and medicine was soon considered part of the necessary education of upper-class Roman men. Celsus (c. first century A.D.), in his lay work *De Medicina*, reported on, among other things, dietetics, pharmacy, medical conditions (particularly dermatological), surgical conditions (including cataract surgery and the use of ligatures), and mental illness. It might be added that physicians of ancient times had little interest in the care of childbearing women. Soranus, another Greek of this period, did write some treatises on obstetrics and gynecology, which is the first indication of a male physician's interest in these matters. Galen later referred to some of the techniques used by the midwives in delivery and care of the newborn, and it can be assumed that midwives were the key figures in the care of women. Galen (A.D. 130–201), considered one of the greatest of Greek physicians, practiced in Rome after receiving an education in many cities, including Alexandria. He wrote some 100 treatises on medicine, so comprehensive that for 200 years they remained unchallenged. He is seen as the greatest scientific experimentalist before the seventeenth century and perhaps the originator of scientific medicine.

Major Roman contributions to health were in public health sanitation and law. Their aqueducts, sewage systems, and baths were unequaled for centuries, and their city planning included the appointment of both a water commissioner and a public health official. In addition, they may be credited with the development of hospitals. *Valetudinaria* were detached buildings or just a large room designated for the care of valuable slaves on Roman estates. Apparently attendants watched over the sick, possibly with the attention of a physician. There is some indication that, at a later time, individuals other than slaves might have been cared for in *valetudinaria*. Given even more attention was the care of sick and injured soldiers. Originally, they were billeted with local Roman families,

who tried to outdo each other in the quality of care. But as the Roman wars expanded to new frontiers, permanent convalescent camps succeeded temporary mobile hospitals. Modern excavations along the Rhine and Danube show the remains of hospitals that could accommodate 200 patients, with wards, recreation areas, baths, pharmacies, and rooms for attendants. Roman historians report that military discipline prevailed and, although the patients received good care, they were also required to conduct themselves "quietly."

Thus, it appears that the Romans took Greek medicine an additional step to the care of the sick by both male and female attendants.

THE FIRST FIVE CENTURIES OF CHRISTIANITY

After centuries of vilification, Christianity became the official religion of Rome in A.D. 335. The early Christian era brought another dimension to the care of the sick. Christian charity, based to a great extent on the Hebrew model as well as on the teachings of Christ, was reinforced by the persecution suffered by the early followers. Their beliefs included a strong emphasis on the sanctity of human life, and infanticide and abortion were considered murder. In the institutionalization of these ideals, bishops were given responsibility for the sick, the poor, widows, and children, but deacons and deaconesses were designated to carry out the services. (Deaconesses, found almost entirely in the Eastern church until the eighth century and always fewer in number, had almost disappeared in the East by the eleventh century.)

The duties were not the same in all churches, but a deaconess usually assisted with such church services as the baptism of women, visiting sick women of the church in their homes, acting as ushers for women attending church, carrying messages for the clergy, and visiting prisoners when they could be helped through counseling. Not all were ordained by the church fathers, who resisted giving women too much recognition or freedom. Nor were they permitted to form orders with rules until somewhat later in history. The role of women was seen as marriage and the begetting of children. Young widows were encouraged to remarry. Widows over 60 (which in those days of early death must have restricted the number considerably) were designated to, among other things, watch over the sick. Some virgins also chose to take vows of service. It is not certain to what extent the early deaconesses were involved in such care, but it is clear that a group of specially designated women, whether deaconesses, widows, virgins, or matrons, cared for the sick.

Noted Women

Among the fabled women who made noted contributions to the care of the sick were the following:

Phoebe (spelled *Phebe* in the Bible) of Cenchrea in southern Italy, who lived about A.D. 60, was the first deaconess who performed nursing functions that were referred to in records of such early times. St. Paul, in Romans 16:1–2 (King James Version), commends her to authorities in Rome—to which she traveled—as a "succorer of many and to myself, also."

The *Empress Helena*, mother of Constantine the Great of Rome, lived c. 248–328. In c. 312, she converted to Christianity and made a pilgrimage to Jerusalem reportedly to expiate the sins of her son. In the Holy Land, she built two churches and a Christian hospital. An influential personage, she won support for the Christian church and especially for its humanitarian aspects.

Olympias, an aristocratic and beautiful young woman of Constantinople, was born in 368. Widowed at nineteen, she became a deaconess and devoted the rest of her life to work among the sick and poor. She was an excellent organizer, and the 40 deaconesses who worked under her accomplished a great deal in alleviating suffering, caring for orphans and the aged, and converting others to Christianity.

Perhaps unfortunately, Olympias is remembered in history chiefly for her extreme asceticism. She denied herself the luxury of a bath, dressed as the lowliest of beggars, and refused to observe any other rules of hygienic living. Fabiola, Paula, and others (both men and women) of the early Christian era had ascetic tendencies, but none to the degree that Olympias demonstrated. Largely because of her personal neglect, she contracted many illnesses and thus lessened the effectiveness of her work.

Fabiola, a beautiful and wealthy matron of Rome, founded the first free hospital in that city in c. 390. Twice married and twice divorced, she embraced Christianity and spent her fortune and the rest of her life in service to the poor and sick. She personally nursed the sickest and filthiest people who came to her hospital, and was so gentle and kind that she was beloved by all Romans. Following her death, St. Jerome wrote a letter about her, sometimes called "the first literary document in the history of nursing."

Paula, a friend of Fabiola, widowed at twenty-three, learned and wealthy, also became a Christian. In about 385, she sailed from Rome to Palestine, where she built hospitals and inns for pilgrims and travelers along the route to Jerusalem, a monastery in Bethlehem, and a convent for women in Jerusalem. She, like Fabiola, performed nursing duties.

Hospitals

Following the closing of the temples of Aesculapius, in those same early centuries, another form of hospital emerged, the *diakonia*, providing a combination of outpatient and welfare service, managed by the deacons and supervised by the bishop. This was replaced in time by "a house for the sick" as there was a house for the poor and for the old. Generally, only the poor, the destitute, or the traveler, those who could not be cared for in their own homes, chose this alternative, an attitude that persisted to a great extent into the eighteenth and nineteenth centuries. One of these hospitals may have been the Basilias outside Caesarea, built in the third century by St. Basil, one of the Four Fathers of the Greek Church, and his sister Macrina. Huge and apparently magnificent, it had special rooms or areas for patients with different conditions, a separate building for lepers, and a special area where the physically handicapped could learn a new trade. There were homes for physicians and nurses, for convalescent patients, for the elderly, and schools and workshops for foundlings. Presumably, some kind of attendant had to be present. Some of these were the women cited earlier, who probably came from their homes to give care. A brotherhood known as *parabolani*, organized in the third century during a great plague in Alexandria, gave care to the sick and buried the dead.

The most regrettable fact in the history of this period is the negative attitude of the Christians toward science and education—an attitude that stultified progress in all intellectual pursuits, including medicine, and permeated the so-called Dark Ages, which continued for another 500 years.

THE MIDDLE AGES

The term *Middle Ages* usually is applied to the years from approximately A.D. 500 to 1500, of which roughly the first half has been called the *Dark Ages*, to distinguish it from the periods of classical civilization preceding and following it. Some historians acknowledge that the Dark Ages may have been more enlightened than was formerly believed. Certainly there were many areas allied to nursing in which the era might have been termed "light gray" rather than "dark," for progress was made that influenced the later development of nursing as a profession for both women and men.

Politically, the world changed greatly during the Middle Ages. The early centuries brought invasions against the Roman Empire by "barbarians" (to the Roman anyone outside the pale of the Empire), which resulted in the formation of many smaller kingdoms within the empire. By the twelfth century, many kingdoms existed, chiefly England, Scotland, France, Denmark, Poland, Hungary, Sicily, and several in Spain. In

the meantime, the Vikings had settled in the Scandinavian areas and in parts of Russia, and expanded rapidly. Trade routes were established between principal cities, and new occupations developed to meet the needs of a rapidly increasing population and changing economies and goals.

The barbarians were all pagans, and not until the thirteenth and fourteenth centuries were they converted to Christianity. Most of the work of conversion was carried out under the direction of the pope, and Roman Catholicism quite naturally was the principal religion of Europe at that time.

Also significant in the general picture of the known world during medieval times was the rise and fall of feudalism in Central Europe, with its devastating effects on the welfare of the common people. It was a time of famine and pestilence, with accompanying miseries and serious illnesses. Medical and nursing care was needed, but unfortunately was not available in either sufficient quality or quantity. Beginning in the thirteenth century, feudalism gradually disappeared.

During the Middle Ages, the deaconesses, suppressed by the Western churches in particular, gradually declined and became almost extinct. However, a small spark remained that has been fanned into a flame every now and then during history, resulting in the formation of a new order of deaconesses, the most important of which are mentioned later.

As the deaconesses declined, the religious orders grew stronger. Known as *monastic orders* and composed of monks and nuns (though not in the same orders), they controlled the hospitals, running them as institutions concerned more with the patients' religious problems than with their physical ailments. However, monks and some nuns were better educated than most people in those times, and their education may well have included some of the medical writings of Celsus and Galen.

Later, with the coming of the Renaissance in the fourteenth century, separation of hospital and church began, effecting spectacular improvement in the scientific and skillful treatment of the sick and injured. It was within the monasteries, however, that education in general progressed significantly during this earlier period.

Lay citizens banded together to form secular orders. Their work was similar to that of the monastic orders in that it was concerned with the sick and needy, but they lived in their own homes, were allowed to marry, and took no vows of the church. They usually adopted a uniform, or habit. Nursing was often their main work.

The military nursing orders, known as the Knights Hospitallers, were the outcome of the Crusades, the military expeditions undertaken by Christians in the eleventh, twelfth, and thirteenth centuries to recover the Holy Land from the Moslems. The most prominent of these three types of orders—religious, military, and secular—during the Middle Ages are described in the following paragraphs.

The *Order of St. Benedict,* the foremost religious order, was founded by St. Benedict of Nursia (c. 480–543) on the beautiful mountain Monte Cassino, about halfway between Rome and Naples. It became a great and powerful center which sent workers throughout Europe, raising standards of education and culture and providing better care for the sick and poor. St. Benedict's rule placed the care of the sick (in which bathing was stressed, a departure from the ascetic practices of some other orders) above and before every other duty of the monks. He established infirmaries within the monasteries primarily for the care of sick members of the order, but also to help centralize and organize the care of pilgrims, wayfarers, and "refugees." With war, famine, and pestilence common occurrences, such service was sorely needed.

The *Knights Hospitallers,* an outgrowth of the Crusades, was the first military order of nurses. The first Crusade (there were nine in all) originated in 1095 when disorganized hordes of men and women of every age, type, and description answered Pope Urban II's call to march to Jerusalem and recover the Holy Land from the Moslems, who had taken it by force from the Byzantine Empire in the seventh century A.D. Ill

prepared physically and psychologically for such a journey, disorganized and inadequately equipped, the crusaders (whose symbol was an eight-pointed cross) died by the thousands along the way.

The later Crusades were essentially expeditions to assist the earlier crusaders in the Holy Land. It was during the first Crusade that the military order, the Knights Hospitallers, was established for the original purpose of bringing the wounded from the battlefield to the hospitals and caring for them there, which explains the name of the order. Later, two other branches of the Knights were formed, one to defend the wounded from the enemy while they were being brought to the hospital, and the other to defend the pilgrims when they were attacked.

There were three principal orders of the Knights Hospitallers: St. John of Jerusalem; the Teutonic Knights; and the Knights of St. Lazarus, whose principal mission was to care for victims of leprosy, one of the major health problems from the eleventh to the mid-thirteenth century. Women had their own branches of the Knights Hospitallers. They performed their services principally in hospitals to which only women patients were admitted.

The story of the Knights Hospitallers is both colorful and interesting. Wealthy and influential, these orders had their successes and failures for approximately seven centuries.

The *Hospital Brothers of St. Anthony* was a secular order founded about 1095 by a grateful man who had been miraculously cured of St. Anthony's fire, which was probably erysipelas. The men and women who joined the order cared only for patients with this disease in special hospitals to which no other patients were admitted. Thus they succeeded in curtailing the spread of erysipelas and no doubt became specialists of a sort in the treatment of this disease.

The Antonines later became a religious order and, when these orders were suppressed, the character of their contribution to nursing changed. They took care of patients with other illnesses, the special hospitals for St. Anthony's fire closed, and erysipelas became a major problem for several centuries, especially among surgical and obstetric patients in general hospitals.

The *Beguines of Flanders*, believed to have been founded in about 1184 by a priest, was one of the most important secular orders. The widows and unmarried women who comprised its membership (at one time numbering 200,000) devoted their lives to helping others. Their nursing duties included the care of the sick in their homes and in hospitals, serving soldiers and civilians during the Battle of Waterloo, caring for victims of cholera during the dreadful epidemics of the nineteenth century, and responding to calls for assistance in times of disastrous fires, floods, and famines.

These sisterhoods spread to Germany, Switzerland, and France and became so numerous, strong, and popular that they were able to resist attempts to abolish them by monastic orders and religious leaders.

The *Third Order of St. Francis* is one of three orders founded by St. Francis of Assisi (1182–1226), probably the best known of the saints connected with nursing. A compassionate young man who loved people, birds, and animals, he was also a fanatic and ascetic with marked qualities of leadership, attracting the influential and learned as well as the humble and lowly to his orders.

The Third Order of St. Francis, also called the *Franciscan Tertiaries*, worked principally among the lepers. They were assisted by the women of the Order of Poor Clares, the second order formed by St. Francis, whose members were largely young women who had left their noble families for a life of service.

After the death of St. Francis at the age of forty-four, the ideals of the Franciscan friars changed considerably, improving in some respects, degenerating in others. But the friars extended their work to the sick and poor, particularly in the slum areas of Europe's large cities, and rendered remarkable service.

The Order of Poor Clares became an enclosed order, which greatly changed the lives of the sisters. They continued their work in some ways, however. It was the Franciscan sisters who

helped Dr. W. W. Mayo, a Civil War surgeon, to found the famous St. Mary's Hospital in Rochester, Minnesota, in 1889.

The *Order of the Holy Ghost* (Santo Spirito), a secular order, was founded in Montpellier, France, in the late twelfth century. Initiated by a knight known as Guy de Montpellier, its members included both men and women. They nursed the poor in the community and assumed responsibility for all of the nursing at the Santo Spirito Hospital in Rome in 1204. They later extended their service to other large hospitals in Italy, France, and Germany. They cared for lepers in shelters outside the hospitals and for persons with other infectious diseases. The order later became monastic and eventually almost disappeared.

Guy de Montpellier established this order in connection with a medical school which had existed in Montpellier since the eighth century, and which became famous as a center of medical education, reaching its period of greatest achievement in the thirteenth and fourteenth centuries. Patients flocked to Montpellier seeking cures under the care of renowned physicians, one of the most outstanding being the surgeon Guy de Chauliac (1298–1368).

The *Grey Sisters*, an order of uncloistered nuns which originated in about 1222, ministered to the poor and the sick in homes and hospitals for many years. In the fourteenth and fifteenth centuries when the plague invaded Europe, they worked closely with the Alexian Orders in meeting the nursing needs.

The *Alexian Brotherhood* came into being in about 1348 in the Netherlands when the "Black Death" was sweeping Europe. The brothers took no vows, adopted no rule at the time, bending all their efforts to caring for the stricken and burying the victims of plague.

Nearly a century later, in 1431, they organized as a religious order, taking vows of obedience, poverty, and chastity and choosing as their patron saint Alexus, a man of noble birth who in the fifth century had worked in a hospital in Syria. They were among the pioneers of organized nursing in Europe.

There were several outstanding personalities of the Middle Ages who were not members of orders, but who nonetheless made significant contributions to the health and welfare of the masses. Some of these were canonized, notably Elizabeth of Hungary, Catherine of Siena, and Hildegard of Bingen. The most prominent women were abbesses or members of royalty who nursed the sick, established educational programs for nurses, and sometimes wrote books and treatises. Hildegarde of Bingen (1098–1178) was educated in a Benedictine monastery and years later became its abbess. Several of her writings were related to medicine and the care of the sick, including general diseases of the body; their causes, symptoms, and treatment; aspects of anatomy and physiology; and human behavior. Many of these things were unknown to physicians of the time.

Medicine

The Dark Ages on the Continent halted the promising progress of medicine, and except for Galen, who died A.D. 200, no great physician practiced medicine in Europe during this period. The Christian church, obsessed with its belief that man's main purpose on earth was to prepare for a future life, saw little need for the science and philosophy of the Greeks or the hygienic teachings and sanitation systems of the Romans. Plagues swept Europe periodically for centuries. Medical knowledge survived and developed in only three areas.

In the eastern Roman Empire, Byzantine physicians nourished the teachings of Hippocrates and Galen, refusing to let them become obsolete; in Salerno in southern Italy, an educational ideal was fostered for medicine as well as for other areas of learning, a medical school was established, and laymen in Salerno translated many Greek manuscripts of importance in medical history; and vigorous medical activity was carried on in the Moslem empires. Although there was warfare there, as in Europe, the conquerors preserved rather than destroyed the culture they found and encouraged further

development. Within 100 years they had achieved a standard of culture that took the Germanic tribes who invaded the Roman Empire ten times as long to develop.

The Arabs translated the works of Hippocrates, Galen, Aristotle, and others. Physicians adopted the Hippocratic method of careful observation of patients. One of the outstanding physicians was Rhazes (850–932) of Baghdad, who was especially interested in communicable diseases and gave an accurate account of smallpox. Another and far more prominent physician was Avicenna (980–1037), a Persian whose *Canon of Medicine* was studied in the medical schools of Europe from the twelfth to the seventeenth centuries. Moses ben Maimon (Maimonides), born in Moslem-controlled Spain of a Jewish family descended from King David, was an excellent clinician who became the court physician to Sultan Saladin.

Medical centers that included hospitals were founded in Cairo, Alexandria, Damascus, and Baghdad. There the Arabs made advances in physiology, hygiene, chemistry, and particularly pharmacy. Because their religion prohibited human dissection, their knowledge of anatomy changed little during this time. Men probably gave care in these hospitals, because women were kept in seclusion.

Hospitals and Hospital Care

Hospitals in which the sick received care were established as the need increased and the wherewithal became available. At the close of the Middle Ages, there were hospitals all over Europe, particularly in larger cities such as Paris and Rome, and in England, where several hundred had been established. Most of these have long since been eliminated or abandoned, but a few have remained. The oldest of these is the Hotel Dieu of Lyons (House of God's Charity), built in 542, in which both men and women nursed the patients.

The Hotel Dieu of Paris, founded in c. 650, has a less favorable record as far as nursing is concerned. Staffed by Augustinian nuns who did the cooking and laundry as well as the nursing, and who had neither intellectual nor professional stimulation, the hospital was not distinguished for its care of patients. In 1908 the nuns were expelled from the Hotel Dieu. The records of nursing kept by this hospital were well done, however, and have been a source of enlightenment for historians. Still in existence in Rome is the Santo Spirito Hospital, established in 717 by order of the pope, to care only for the sick.

Hospitals in England during the Middle Ages differed from those on the Continent in that they were never completely church controlled, although they were founded on Christian principles and accepted responsibility for the sick and injured. The oldest and best-known English hospitals from a historical point of view are St. Bartholomew's, founded in 1123; St. Thomas's, founded in 1213; and in 1247, Bethlehem Hospital, originally a general hospital that later became famous as a mental institution, referred to frequently as Bedlam.

An interesting sidelight here is the treatment of the mentally ill. In Bedlam, as in similar institutions, the inmates were treated with inhumane cruelty. Beatings and starvation were not uncommon. However, in Gheel, Belgium, reports of miraculous cures at the tomb of St. Dymphna, an Irish princess murdered by her mad father, brought the mentally ill hope of healing. The people of Gheel took in the pilgrims as foster families and gave them care and affection.

The nursing care in most early hospitals was essentially basic: bathing, feeding, giving medicines, making beds, and so on. It was rarely of high quality, however, largely because of the lack of progress of nearly all civilization and the shortsighted attitude toward women that was typical of the Dark Ages.

THE RENAISSANCE

The word *renaissance* as used in history refers to both a movement and a period of time. In years, it is generally conceded to have lasted from 1400 to 1550, the years during which there was a tran-sitional movement toward revival of the arts and sciences in Europe, culminating in the modern age. Also during this period great explorations were made, including the discovery of America. New impetus was given to literature and art, to bookbinding, to the founding of libraries, universities, and medical schools—but not nursing schools. These came more than three centuries later. Merchants made huge fortunes in trade. Bankers likewise became wealthy by making loans, especially to kings and princes.

The Age of Discovery, 1450–1550, a part of this period, brought great increase in geographical knowledge. People became excited about the world around them and about the prospect of finding gold in other lands, particularly America. New passageways were sought to old countries, and the acquisition of new colonies and territories became extremely important to the established kingdoms and empires.

The Renaissance saw the birth and death of Leonardo da Vinci, Michelangelo, and other great artists. And to medicine it gave Paracelsus, Vesalius, and Paré.

Theophrastus Paracelsus (1493–1541), a Swiss physician and exceptional chemist, made contributions chiefly in the area of pharmaceutical chemistry.

Andreas Vesalius (1514–1564), a Belgian, made detailed anatomical studies in universities and hospitals, disproving by his practical methods some of the classical theories of Galen and others. One of his many published works was a voluminous illustrated book, *De Corporis Humani Fabrica Libri Septem (Seven Books on the Structure of the Human Body)*, in which he displayed his great fund of knowledge and also criticized and corrected Galen. For this he was berated by advocates of Galen. He gradually lost his tremendous energy and initiative and settled down to a routine physician's life.

Ambroise Paré (1510–1590), a Frenchman, served as an apprentice to a a barber-surgeon and later became the first surgeon of the Renaissance. A student of Vesalius, he became a great military surgeon who reintroduced the use of the ligature instead of the cautery to occlude blood vessels during surgery, adopted a simple technique of wound dressing to replace the oil-boiling method in wide use, improved obstetrical techniques, designed artificial limbs, and wrote books on surgery.

Barber-surgeons were men in France who not only did barbering but also performed such procedures as bleeding, cupping, leeching, giving enemas, and extracting teeth—procedures that the physicians of medieval times prescribed for their patients but considered undignified to perform. The barber-surgeon was required to wear a short robe, whereas the regular surgeons, of whom there were very few, were entitled to wear a long one.

There was understandable friction among the three groups—physicians, barber-surgeons, and surgeons—and the problems were not completely resolved until the practice of surgery improved greatly and the Royal College of Surgeons was established in 1800. The striped barber pole, symbol of the present-day barber, dates from the time when the patient being bled clung to a staff; the bloody bandage that covered his wound is represented by the red stripe on the barber's pole.

Nursing apparently continued in a way similar to that established in the earlier Middle Ages. The charter of St. Bartholomew's Hospital called for a matron and twelve other women to make beds, wash, and attend the poor patients. They were to receive about two pounds a year and room and board, with the matron receiving more. All slept in one room at the hospital. They cared for about 100 patients. However, whether this arrangement was typical is not known.

FROM REFORMATION TO NIGHTINGALE

The Reformation was a religious movement beginning early in the sixteenth century that resulted in the formation of various Protestant churches under leaders who had revolted against the supremacy of the pope. Monasteries were closed; religious orders were dispersed, even in Catholic countries. Because many of these orders were involved in the care of the sick, nursing and hospital care suffered a severe setback. A startling effect was the almost total disappearance of male nurses. Almost all Catholic nursing orders after 1500 were made up of women. In Protestant countries, too, women and nursing became almost synonymous, for Protestant leaders recognized the vacuum in care of the sick and urged the hiring of nurse deaconesses and other elderly women to nurse the sick. Also out of this era came noted Catholic orders devoted to care of the sick.

The Sisters of Charity were founded by St. Vincent de Paul (1576–1660) of France, a Catholic priest. He was ably assisted by Mlle. Louise La Gras, a woman of noble birth greatly interested in nursing and social work.

Once a prisoner himself, having been captured by pirates, St. Vincent de Paul became vitally interested in lessening the suffering of all slaves and prisoners. This interest expanded to include the sick and poor in his small country parish, and to help him in his work, he organized a society of women. This small group was so successful that similar groups were formed in other localities in France. The most famous of all, the Sisters of Charity, was organized in Paris under the direction of Mlle. La Gras. A younger group, the Daughters of Charity, was formed later. A noncloistered order, the Sisters were free to go wherever they were needed.

The Sisters of Charity were always carefully selected, and from the beginning their ideals and standards were very high. Members of this order took over the nursing service in many European hospitals, and came to Canada and the United States to give similar service during the early history of these countries.

In Spain, the *Brothers Hospitallers of St. John of God* was founded by a man who gave care to the sick, with special attention to the mentally ill. The order spread throughout the world, and its members opened and staffed hospitals wherever they went, including the Americas. The care given in their hospitals in Goa, as described by a sixteenth-century traveler, seemed to be a model of its time, perhaps even ahead of its time.

In Italy, Camillus, also to be canonized, trained and supplied nurses (men) for hospital care and founded an order dedicated to care of the sick and dying.

In the New World, Cortez founded the first hospital (in Mexico City); within 20 years, most major Spanish towns had one. It was 100 years later that a Hotel Dieu was founded in Sillery (Canada) and another at Montreal. In the latter, care was given by a young lay woman and three nursing sisters who came from France, but perhaps the first "nurse" in Canada was Marie Herbert Hobau in Nova Scotia, the widow of the surgeon and apothecary who accompanied Champlain.[1]

Records in Jamestown, Virginia, also tell of the selection of certain men and women to care for the sick. There were numerous health problems in the early American colonies, in part the result of the difficult living conditions. Hospitals of some type existed; one was described as accommodating fifty patients—if they slept two in a bed (not uncommon in Europe either).

The seventeenth and eighteenth centuries were periods of continuing change in Europe, and scientific advances had an enduring influence on medicine and health. Of the creative scientists of those times, the following are key figures:

William Harvey (1578–1657), an English physician generally regarded as the father of modern medicine, was the first to describe completely (except for the capillary system) and accurately the circulatory system, replacing the earlier explanations which, though remarkable at the time, actually were at least partially incorrect.

Thomas Sydenham (1624–1689), an Englishman educated at Oxford and Montpellier, revived the Hippocratic methods of observation and reasoning and in other ways "restored" clinical medicine to a sound basis.

Antonj van Leeuwenhoek (1632–1723), of Holland, improved on Galileo's microscope and produced one that permitted the examination of body cells and bacteria.

William Hunter (1718–1783) and his brother *John* (1728–1793), of Scotland, obstetrician and surgeon, respectively, conducted meticulous anatomical research and thus founded the science of pathology.

William Tuke (1732–1822), an English merchant and philanthropist, instituted long overdue reforms in the care of the mentally ill. Chief founder of the York Retreat (1796), he had important influence on subsequent treatment of the mentally ill.

Edward Jenner (1749–1823), an English physician, friend and pupil of John Hunter, in 1796 originated vaccination against smallpox.

René, Laennec (1781–1826), of France, invented the stethoscope in 1819. Before this, the physician had listened to the patient's heartbeat by placing his ear against the patient's chest wall.

Even with these advances, medical education was still sketchy. Some practicing physicians had no medical education. An MD degree required apprenticeship with a physician, surgeon, or apothecary, some university classes, some dissecting at an anatomical school or hospital—or any variation of these. There were a few noted schools in Italy, Germany, and Scotland; the English colonies had one until 1765. A practical apothecary school started earlier, but most often pharmacists were also physicians.

By the end of the eighteenth century, nurses of some kind functioned in hospitals. Conditions were not attractive, and much has been written about drunken, thieving women who tended patients. However, some hospitals made real efforts to set standards. One set of criteria included such attributes as good health, good sight and hearing (to make pertinent observations), nimbleness, quietness, good temper, diligence, temperance, and "to have no children, or other to come much after her."[2] Already a hierarchy of nursing personnel had begun, with helpers and watchers assigned to help the *sisters*, as the early English nurses were called.

In other parts of Europe, nursing was becoming recognized as an important service. Diderot, whose *Encyclopedia* attempted to sum up all human knowledge, said that nursing "is as important for humanity as its functions are low and repugnant." Urging care in selection, since "all persons are not adapted to it," he described the nurses as "patient, mild, and compassionate. She should console the sick, foresee their needs, and relieve their tedium."[3] Another progressive step was the first nursing textbook, which had been published in Vienna early in the eighteenth century.

Midwifery, too, was gaining new attention. In England in 1739, a small lying-in infirmary was started for the education of medical students and midwives, and soon other lying-in hospitals began to appear. In London, poor women also benefited in home deliveries when a famous physician began to teach medical students midwifery and also taught women to become nurse-midwives at the bedside. (His students had to contribute funds to the care and support of these women.) Nevertheless, it should be remembered that even with the tremendous increase in hospital building at that time, most care was still given in the home by wives and mothers.

The advent of the Industrial Revolution in England saw the development of power-driven machinery to do the spinning, weaving, and metal work that had previously been done manually in the home. Improvement in the steam engine as a source of power improved mining procedures and resulted in the development of factories, which the English called *mills*. The cotton, woolen, and iron industries grew rapidly, and there was a corresponding improvement in agriculture.

The industrialization of Europe did not begin until the mid-nineteenth century, when England had already assumed international leadership, its empire was growing, and British trade was the center of world marketing.

People of means lived a most luxurious life. Graciousness and elegance prevailed, and woman's mission in life was to carry on these traditions. For this she was educated and carefully prepared by her parents.

The common women worked largely as servants in private homes or not at all. With the coming of factories, men, women, and children worked under cruel conditions. Caring for the sick in hospitals and homes were the "uncommon" women—prisoners, prostitutes—unkempt, unsavory, disinterested. Health conditions were still dreadful, with epidemics such as cholera sweeping whole countries. Children orphaned in these epidemics were finally put in almshouses, which provided no improvement in their lot. The situation was no different in America but was probably worst in England, and a number of social reformers began to work for change.

Culturally, great progress was made, particularly on the Continent. The demand for intellectual liberty brought marked advancement in educational facilities for men, but not for women. This was also true in the United States where, for example, Harvard University, established at Cambridge, Massachusetts, in 1636, admitted only men, a policy it steadfastly maintained into the twentieth century. Columbia University in New York City, founded in 1754, followed a similar policy but lowered its ban on women with the founding of Barnard College in 1889. Teachers College was founded as a coeducational institution in 1888.

Out of this confused century came scientists and physicians who made dramatic breakthroughs in medical science:

Oliver Wendell Holmes (1809–1894), a Boston physician, furthered safe obstetric practice, pointing out the dangers of infection. He is author of the famous treatise "The Contagiousness of Puerperal Fever," published in 1843.

Crawford W. Long (1815–1878), an American physician, excised a tumor of the neck under ether anesthesia in 1832 but did not make his discovery public until after Dr. William T. Morton announced his in 1846. This led to one of medicine's most enduring controversies: Who should receive credit for discovering the anesthetic properties of ether?

Ignaz P. Semmelweis (1818–1865), of Vienna, is famous for his advances in the safe practice of obstetrics.

Louis Pasteur (1822–1895), of France, chemist and bacteriologist, became famous for his germ theory of disease, the development of the process known as *pasteurization*, and the discovery of a treatment for rabies. His work overlapped that of Robert Koch.

Lord Joseph Lister (1827–1912), English surgeon, developed and proved, in 1865, his theory of the bacterial infection of wounds on which modern aseptic surgery is based.

Robert Koch (1843–1910), of Germany, founded modern bacteriology. He originated the drying and staining method of examining bacteria. His most important discovery was the identification of the tubercle bacillus, which led eventually to tremendous reductions in loss of life from tuberculosis.

Wilhelm Röntgen (1845–1923), a German physicist, discovered x-rays in 1895 and laid the foundation for the science of roentgenology and radiology.

Sir William Osler (1849–1919), a renowned Canadian teacher and medical historian, was associated with McGill University, the University of Pennsylvania, Johns Hopkins University, and Oxford University, England. He was knighted in 1911.

Pierre Curie (1859–1906), a French chemist, and his Polish wife, *Marie* (1867–1934), discovered radium in 1898.

NURSING IN THE NINETEENTH CENTURY

The dreary picture of secular nursing is not totally unexpected, given the times. Because proper young women did not work outside the home, nursing had no acceptance, much less prestige. Even those nurses not in the Dickens' Sairy Gamp mold or those desiring to nurse found themselves in competition with workhouse inmates, who were cheaper workers for hospital administrations.

It was acceptable to nurse as a member of a religious order, when the motivation was, of course, religious and the cost to the hospital was little or none. During the nineteenth century, several nursing orders were revived or originated that had substantial influence on modern

nursing. In most instances, these orders cared for patients in hospitals that were already established, in contrast to the orders of earlier times, which had founded the hospitals in which they worked. The most influential are the following:

The *Church Order of Deaconesses*, an ancient order, was revived by Theodor Fliedner (1800–1864), pastor of a small parish in Kaiserswerth, Germany, to care for the patients in a hospital he opened in 1836. At first he had only one deaconess, whom he trained in nursing. Although the training was quite superficial, the work expanded, more deaconesses joined the staff, and the deaconess institute at Kaiserswerth became famous. (Florence Nightingale obtained her only "formal" training in nursing there.) Four of the deaconesses and Pastor Fliedner journeyed to Pittsburgh, Pennsylvania, in 1849, to help establish a hospital under the leadership of Pastor William Passavant. Similar assistance was given to the founders of institutions on the Kaiserswerth plan in London, Constantinople, Beirut, Alexandria, Athens, and other localities.

Pastor Fliedner's work began with discharged prisoners (rather than the sick poor), in whom he became greatly interested through the reforms effected in England under Elizabeth Fry. Aided by both his first and second wives, he also established an orphanage and a normal school.

The *Protestant Sisters of Charity* was founded by Elizabeth Fry (1780–1845) of England, whose work among prisoners and the physically and mentally ill was based on reforms that had been instituted by John Howard (1726–1790) a quarter of a century before. Mrs. Fry became interested in the deaconesses at Kaiserswerth and visited the hospital to observe how they functioned. She then organized a small group of "nurses" in London to do similar work among the sick poor. She first called the group the Protestant Sisters of Charity, later changing it to Institute of Nursing Sisters. (Unofficially they often were called the Fry Sisters or Fry Nurses.) The sisters were not affiliated with any church. Their training for nursing was extremely elementary. This group was in no way connected with the Sisters of Charity established earlier by Saint Vincent de Paul.

The *Sisters of Mercy* was a Roman Catholic society formed by Catherine McAuley (1787–1841) in Dublin, which later became an order and adopted a rule. The sisters visited in Dublin hospitals and nursed victims of a cholera epidemic in 1832; their work grew rapidly and spread throughout the world, including the establishment of several Mercy hospitals in the United States.

The *Irish Sisters of Charity*, also a Roman Catholic group, was started by Mary Aikenhead (1787–1858). The sisters visited the sick in their homes and did volunteer nursing in the community during emergencies. They had limited nurses' training and, in 1892, founded a training school for lay persons in St. Vincent's Hospital, in Dublin, in which they previously had assumed all nursing duties. They opened additional St. Vincent's hospitals in other areas of the world, including the United States, to which they had come in 1855 to nurse victims of a cholera epidemic in San Francisco.

Also during this period, several nursing sisterhoods were established under the auspices of the Church of England. One of these, the *Sisters of Mercy in the Church of England,* was organized about 1850. The sisters had little if any formal preparation, but through practical experience acquired in district "nursing" and work in a cholera epidemic, they became quite proficient.

Another Anglican sisterhood, *St. Margaret's of East Grinstead,* was founded by a doctor in 1854. The sisters worked entirely among the sick in the community; they were not associated with hospitals in any way.

The Anglican order that did the most to improve hospital nursing during this period was *St. John's House,* founded in 1848 by the Church of England. Named for the parish in which it was located—St. John the Evangelist in St. Pancras, London—its purpose was to instruct and train members of the Church of England to act as nurses and visitors to the sick and poor. The original plan also stipulated that the order should be connected with "some hospital or hospitals, in which the women under training, or those who had already been educated, might find the opportunity of exercising their calling or of acquiring experience."[4] The first training program was successful, as were the twenty-five subsequent ones developed by St. John's House to meet changing needs, and the graduates were always in great demand.

Progress in medicine and science during these centuries was accompanied by accelerated interest in better nursing service and nurses' training. Neither was achieved to a significant degree, however, despite the fine work of dedicated men and women who belonged to the several nursing orders of the time. Limited in numbers and inadequately prepared for their nursing functions, the members of these orders could not begin to meet the need for their services. Such care as patients received in the majority of institutions was grossly inadequate.

In the mid-nineteenth century, therefore, the time was right—perhaps overdue—for the revolution in nursing education that originated under the leadership of Florence Nightingale and that influenced so greatly and so quickly (from a historical point of view) the nursing care of patients and, indeed, the health of the world.

REFERENCES

1. Dolan JA: *Nursing in Society*, 14th ed. Philadelphia: Saunders, 1978, p 98.
2. Bullough B, Bullough V: *The Care of the Sick: The Emergence of Modern Nursing.* New York: Prodist, 1978, p 57.
3. Ibid, p 6.
4. Moore J: *A Zeal for Responsibility: The Struggle for Professional Nursing in Victorian England, 1868–1883.* Athens, GA: University of Georgia Press, 1983, p 3.

The Influence of Florence Nightingale

IT HAS BEEN SAID that Florence Nightingale, an extraordinary woman in any century, is the most written-about woman in history. Through her own numerous publications, her letters, the writings of her contemporaries, including newspaper reports, and the numerous biographies and studies of her life, there emerges the picture of a sometimes contradictory, frequently controversial, but undeniably powerful woman who probably had a greater influence on the care of the sick than any other single individual.

Called the founder of modern nursing, Nightingale was a strong-willed woman of quick intelligence who used her considerable knowledge of statistics, sanitation, logistics, administration, nutrition, and public health not only to develop a new system of nursing education and health care but also to improve the social welfare systems of the time. The gentle, caring lady of the lamp, full of compassion for the soldiers of the Crimea, is an accurate image, but no more so than that of the hardheaded administrator and planner who forced changes in the intolerable social conditions of the time, including the care of the sick poor. Nightingale knew full well that a tender touch alone would not bring health to the sick or prevent illness, so she set her intelligence, her administrative skills, her political acumen, and her incredible drive to achieve her self-defined missions. In the Victorian age when women were almost totally dominated by men—fathers, husbands, brothers—and it was undesirable for them to show intelligence or profess interest in anything but household arts, this indomitable woman accomplished the following:

1. Improved and reformed laws affecting health, morals, and the poor.
2. Reformed hospitals and improved workhouses and infirmaries.
3. Improved medicine by instituting an army medical school and reorganizing the army medical department.
4. Improved the health of natives and British citizens in India and other colonies.
5. Established nursing as a profession with two missions—sick nursing and health nursing.[1]

The new nurse and the new image of the nurse that she created, in part through the nursing schools she founded, in part through her writings, and in part through her international influence, became the model that persisted for almost 100 years. Today, some of her tenets about the "good" nurse seem terribly restrictive, but it should be remembered that in those times not only the image but also the reality of much of secular nursing was based on the untutored, uncouth workhouse inmates for whom drunkenness and thievery were a way of life. It was small wonder that each Nightingale student had to exemplify a new image.

> **The Nightingale nurse had to establish her character in a profession proverbial for immorality. Neat, lady-like, vestal, above suspicion, she had to be the incarnate denial that a hospital nurse had to be drunken, ignorant, and promiscuous.[2]**

These historical idiosyncrasies should not, and do not, detract from the many Nightingale precepts that are not only pertinent today but remarkably farsighted.

EARLY LIFE

Florence Nightingale was born on May 12, 1820, in Florence, Italy, during her English parents' travels there. She was named for the city in which she was born, as was her older sister, Parthenope, who was born in 1819 in Naples (known in ancient times by the Greek name Parthenope).

The family was wealthy and well educated, with a high social standing and influential friends, all of which would be useful to Nightingale later. Primarily under her father's tutelage, she learned Greek, Latin, French, German, and Italian, and studied history, philosophy, science, music, art, and classical literature. She traveled widely with her family and friends. The breadth of her education, almost unheard of for women of the times, was also considerably more extensive than that of most men, including physicians. Her intelligence and education were recognized by scholars, as indicated in her correspondence with them.

Nightingale was not only bright, but, according to early portraits and descriptions, slender, attractive, and fun-loving, enjoying the social life of her class. She differed from other young women in her determination to do something "toward lifting the load of suffering from the helpless and miserable."[3] Later she said that she had been called by God into His service on four separate occasions, beginning when she was 17. This strong religious commitment remained with her, although she had increasingly little patience with organized religion or with traditional biblical exhortations. At one point she stated, "God's scheme for us was not that He should give us what we asked for, but that mankind should obtain it for mankind."[4] Apparently, the encouragement of Dr. Samuel Gridley Howe and his wife, Julia Ward Howe (who

wrote "The Battle Hymn of the Republic"), during a visit to the Nightingale family home in 1844 helped to crystallize Florence's interest in hospitals and nursing. Nevertheless, her intent to train in a hospital was strongly opposed by her family, and she limited herself to nursing family members. There is some indication that this was the genesis of her firm belief that nursing required more than kindness and cold compresses.

Later, in *Notes on Nursing*, she wrote, "It has been said and written scores of times that every woman makes a good nurse. I believe, on the contrary, that the very elements of nursing are all but unknown."[5] At the same time, she added a few tart remarks about the need for education.

> **It seems a commonly received idea among men and even some women themselves that it requires nothing but a disappointment in love, the want of an object, a general disgust, or incapacity for other things to turn a woman into a good nurse. This reminds one of the parish where a stupid old man was set to be schoolmaster because he was "past keeping the pigs."...The everyday management of a large ward, let alone of a hospital—the knowing what are the laws of life and death for men, and what the laws of health for wards (and wards are healthy or unhealthy, mainly according to the knowledge or ignorance of the nurse)—are not these matters of sufficient importance and difficulty to require learning by experience and careful inquiry, just as much as any other art? They do not come by inspiration to the lady disappointed in love, nor to the poor workhouse drudge hard up for a livelihood.[6]**

Although remaining the obedient daughter, Nightingale found her own way to expand her knowledge of sick care. She studied hospital and sanitary reports and books on public health. Having received information on Kaiserswerth in Germany, she determined to receive training there—more acceptable because of its religious auspices. On one of her trips to the Continent, she made a brief visit and was impressed enough to spend three months in training and observation there in 1851 while her mother and sister went to Carlsbad to "take the cure." (The Nightingales were considered appropriately delicate Victorian ladies, although all lived past eighty.) At the time she wrote positively about Pastor Fliedner's program, but she later described the nursing as "nil" and the hygiene as "horrible."[7] Her later effort to study with the Sisters of Charity in Paris was frustrated, although she got permission to inspect the hospitals there, as she had in other cities during her tours. She examined the general layout of the hospital, as well as ward construction, sanitation, general administration, and the work of the surgeons and physicians. Apparently, these observational techniques and her analytical abilities then and later were the basis of her unrivaled knowledge of hospitals in the next decade. Few of her contemporaries ever had such knowledge.

In 1853 Nightingale assumed the position of superintendent of a charity hospital (probably more of a nursing home) for ill governesses run by titled ladies. Although she had difficulties with her intolerant governing board, she did make changes considered revolutionary for the day and, even with the lack of trained nurses, improved the patients' care. And she continued to visit hospitals. Just as Nightingale was negotiating for a superintendency in the newly reorganized and rebuilt King's College Hospital in London, England and France, in support of Turkey, declared war on Russia in March 1854.

CRIMEA—THE TURNING POINT

The Crimean War was a low point for England. Ill-prepared and disorganized in general, the army and the bureaucracy were even less prepared to care for the thousands of soldiers both wounded in battle and prostrated by the cholera epidemics brought on by the primitive conditions. Not even the most basic equipment or drugs were available, and, as casualties mounted, Turkey turned over the enormous but bare and filthy barracks at Scutari across from Constantinople to be used as a hospital. The conditions remained abominable. The soldiers lay on the floor in filth, untended, frequently

without food or water because there was no equipment to prepare or distribute either. Rats and other vermin came from the sewers underneath the building. There were no beds, furniture, basins, soap, towels, or eating utensils, and few provisions. There were only orderlies, and none of these at night. The death rate was said to be 60 percent.

In previous wars, the situation had not been much different, and there was little interest on the battle sites, for ordinary soldiers were accorded no decencies. But now, for the first time, civilian war correspondents were present and sent back the news of these horrors to an England with a newly aroused social conscience. The reformers were in an uproar; newspapers demanded to know why England did not have nurses like the French Sisters of Charity to care for its soldiers, and Parliament trembled. In October 1854, Sidney Herbert, Secretary of War and an old friend of Florence Nightingale, wrote begging her to lead a group of nurses to the Crimea under government authority and expense. "There is but one person in England that I know of who would be capable of organizing such a scheme…your own personal qualities, your knowledge, and your power of administration, and, among greater things, your rank and position in society give you advantages in such work which no other person possesses."[8] Nightingale had already decided to offer her services, and the two letters crossed. In less than a week, she had assembled 38 nurses, the most she could find that met her standards—Roman Catholic and Anglican sisters and lay nurses from various hospitals—and embarked for Scutari.

Even under the miserable circumstances found there, Nightingale and her contingent were not welcomed by the army doctors and surgeons. Dr. John Hall, chief of the medical staff, and his staff, although privately acknowledging the horrors of the situation, resented outside interference and refused the nurses' services. Hall and Nightingale soon developed a mutual hatred for each other. When Dr. Hall was honored with the KCB—Knight Commander of the Order of the Bath—she referred to him as "Knight of the Crimean Burial Grounds."[9]

Nightingale chose to wait to be asked to help. To the anger of her nurses, she allowed none of them to give care until one week later, when scurvy, starvation, dysentery, exposure, and more fighting almost brought about the collapse of the British army. Then the doctors, desperate for any kind of assistance, turned to the eager nurses.

Modern criticisms of Florence Nightingale frequently refer to her insistence on the physician's overall authority and her own authoritarian approach to nursing. The first criticism may have originated with her situation in the Crimean War. In mid-century England her appointment created a furor; she was the first woman ever to be given such authority. Yet, despite the high-sounding title that Herbert insisted she have—General Superintendent of the Female Nursing Establishment of the Military Hospitals of the Army—her orders required that she have the approval of the Principal Medical Officer "in her exercise of the responsibilities thus vested in her. The Principal Medical Officer will communicate with Miss Nightingale upon all subjects connected with the Female Nursing Establishment, and will give his directions through that lady."[10] Although no "lady, sister, or nurse" could be transferred from one hospital to another without her approval, she had no authority over anyone else, even orderlies and cooks. What she accomplished had to be done through sheer force of will or persuasion. Her overt deference to physicians was probably the beginning of the doctor-nurse game.

Whatever the limitations of her power, Florence Nightingale literally accomplished miracles at Scutari. Even in the "waiting" week, she moved into the kitchen area and began to cook extras from her own supplies to create a diet kitchen, which for five months was the only source of food for the sick. Later, a famous chef came to the Crimea at his own expense and totally reorganized and improved military cooking. Nightingale managed to equip the kitchen and the wards by various means. One report is that when a physician refused to unlock a supply storehouse, she replied, "Well, I would like to have the door opened, or I shall send men to break it down."[11] It was opened, and he was recalled to London.

Miss Nightingale had powerful friends and control over a large amount of contributed funds—a situation that gained her some cooperation from most physicians after a while. Through persuasion and the use of good managerial techniques, she cleaned up the hospital; the orderlies scrubbed and emptied slops regularly; soldiers' wives and camp followers washed clothes; and the vermin were brought under some control. (Wrote Nightingale to Sidney Herbert, "the vermin might, if they had but unity of purpose, carry off the four miles of beds on their backs and march them into the War Office.")[12] Before the end of the war, the mortality rate at Scutari declined to 1 percent. When the hospital care improved, Nightingale began a program of social welfare among the soldiers—among other things, seeing to it that they got sick pay. The patients adored her. She cared about them, and the doctors and officers reproached her for "spoiling the brutes." The soldiers wrote home, "What a comfort it was to see her pass even; she would speak to one and nod and smile to as many more, but she could not do it all, you know. We lay there by hundreds, but we could kiss her shadow as it fell, and lay our heads on the pillow again content." And, "Before she came, there was cussin' and swearin', but after that it was holy as a church." And, "She was all full of life and fun when she talked to us, especially if a man was a bit downhearted."[13] News correspondents wrote reports about the "ministering angel" and "lady with the lamp" making late rounds after the medical officers had retired—which inspired Longfellow later to write his famous poem "Santa Filomena." England and America were enthralled, and she was awarded decorations by Queen Victoria and the Sultan of Turkey.

But all did not go well. The military doctors continued in their resentment and tried to undermine her. There were problems in her own ranks, dissension among the religious and secular nurses, and problems of incompetence and immorality. Later, she wrote:

> **Rebellion among some ladies and some nuns, and drunkenness among some nurses unhappily disgraced our body; minor faults justified *pro tanto* the common opinion that the vanity, the gossip, and the insubordination (which none more despise than those who trade upon them) of women make them unfit for, and mischievous in the Service, however materially useful they may be in it.[14]**

Her problems increased with the unsolicited arrival of another group of nurses under another woman's leadership, although the problem was eventually resolved. No doubt Nightingale was high-handed at times, and despite praise of her leadership, she was also called "quick, violent-tempered, positive, obstinate, and stubborn."[15]

Certainly she drove herself in all she did. When the situation at Scutari was improved, she crossed the Black Sea to the battle sites and worked on the reorganization of the few hospitals there—with no better support from physicians and superior officers. There she contracted Crimean fever (probably typhoid or typhus) and nearly died. However, she refused a leave of absence to recuperate and stayed in Scutari to work until the end of the war. She had supervised 125 nurses and forced the military to recognize the place of nurses.

From her experiences, and to support her recommendations for reform, Nightingale wrote a massive report entitled *Notes on Matters Affecting the Health, Efficiency, and Hospital Administration of the British Army*, crammed with facts, figures, and statistical comparison. On the basis of this and her later well-researched and well-documented papers, she is often credited with being the first nurse researcher. Reforms were slow in coming but extended even to the United States when the Union consulted her about organizing hospitals. In 1859 she wrote a small book, *Notes on Nursing: What It Is and What It Is Not*, intended for the average housewife and printed cheaply so that it would be affordable. These and other Nightingale papers are still amazingly readable today—brisk, down-to-

earth, and laced with many a pithy comment. For instance, in *Notes on Hospitals*, written in the same year, she compared the administration of the various types of hospitals and characterized the management of secular hospitals under the sole command of the male hospital authorities as "all but crazy." And her words were prophetic: "If we were perfect, no doubt an absolute hierarchy would be the best kind of government for all institutions. But, in our imperfect state of conscience and enlightenment, publicity, and the collision resulting from publicity are the best guardians of the interests of the sick."[16]

Her knowledge was certainly respected, and she was consulted by many, including the Royal Sanitary Commission on the Health of the Army in India. When asked by the members of the commission what hospitals she had visited, she listed those in England, Turkey, France, Germany, Belgium, Italy, and Egypt, including all hospitals in some cities, and even Russian military hospitals. Her reforms in India extended beyond the medical and nursing facilities to raising the sanitary level of India.[17] Again, her insights were uncanny. In describing the proper method of analyzing the problem of sanitation and disease, she also suggested checking on "unwholesome trades fouling the water."

What is particularly astonishing is that all of this was done from her own quarters. On her return from the Crimea, she took to her bed or at least to her rooms and emerged only on rare occasions. There is much speculation on this illness—whether it was a result of the Crimea fever, neurasthenia, or a bit of both, or whether she simply found it useful to avoid wasting time with people she did not want to see. For she was famous now and had been given discretion over the so-called Nightingale Fund, to which almost everyone in England had subscribed, including many of the troops.

THE NIGHTINGALE NURSE

In 1860, Nightingale utilized some of the 45,000 pounds of the Nightingale Fund to establish a training school for nurses. She selected St. Thomas's Hospital because of her respect for its matron, Mrs. S. E. Wardroper. The two converted the resident medical officers to their plan, although apparently most other physicians objected to the school. The students were chosen, and the first class in the desired age range of 25 to 35 years and with impeccable character references numbered only 15. It was to be a 1-year training program, and the students were presented with what could be called terminal behavioral objectives that they had to reach satisfactorily. Students could be dismissed by the matron for misconduct, inefficiency, or negligence. However, if they passed the courses of instruction and training satisfactorily, they were entered in the "Register" as certified nurses. The Committee of the Nightingale Fund then recommended them for employment; in the early years, they were obligated to work as hospital nurses for at least 5 years (for which they were paid).

The student's time was carefully structured, beginning at 6 in the morning and ending with a 9 o'clock bedtime, which included a semimandatory 2-hour exercise period (walking abroad must be done in twos and threes, not alone). Within that time there was actually about a 9-hour work and training day (a vast difference from future American schools). This included bedside teaching by a teaching sister or the Resident Medical Officer and elementary instruction in "Chemistry, with reference to air, water, food, etc.; Physiology, with reference to a knowledge of the leading functions of the body, and general instruction on medical and surgical topics,"[18] by professors of the medical school attached to St. Thomas's, given voluntarily and without remuneration. The Nightingale school was not under the control of the hospital and had education as its purpose. The Nightingale Fund paid the medical officers, head nurses, and matron for teaching students, beyond whatever they earned from the hospital in their other duties. Both the head nurses and matron kept records on each student, evaluating how she met the stated objectives of the program. The

students were expected to keep notes from the lectures and records of patient observation and care, all of which were checked by the nurse-teachers. At King's College Hospital, run by the Society of St. John's House, an Anglican religious community, midwifery was taught in similar style and with similar regulations, again under the auspices of the Nightingale Fund Committee. And, at the Royal Liverpool Infirmary, nurses were trained for home nursing of the sick poor under a Nightingale protocol, but were personally funded by a Liverpool merchant-philanthropist. As Nightingale said in 1863, "We have had to introduce an entirely new system to which the older systems of nursing bear but slight resemblance....It exists neither in Scotland nor in Ireland at the present time."[19]

The demand for the Nightingale nurses was overwhelming. In the next few years, requests also came for them to improve the workhouse (poorhouse) infirmaries and to reform both civilian and military nursing in India. In response to these demands, Nightingale wrote many reports, detailing to the last item the system for educating these nurses and for improving patient care, including such points as general hygiene and sanitation, nutrition, equipment, supplies, and the nurses' housing conditions, holidays, salaries, and retirement benefits. (For India, she suggested that they had better pay good salaries and provide satisfactory working and living conditions, or the nurses might opt for marriage, because the opportunities there were even greater than in England.) She constantly reiterated that she could not possibly supply enough nurses but, when possible, she would send a matron and some other nurses, who would train new Nightingale nurses. She warned that one or two could not change the old patterns. "Good nursing does not grow of itself; it is the result of study, teaching, training, practice, ending in sound tradition which can be transferred elsewhere."[20]

Although Nightingale never headed a school herself, she selected the students and observed their progress carefully; with some she carried on correspondence for years. One of her favorites, Agnes Jones, was recommended to reform nursing at the Liverpool Workhouse Infirmary, which, with twelve other nurses, she did admirably, proving to the economy-minded governor that this kind of nursing also saved money. Nightingale often said that conditions there were as bad as those at Scutari; and indeed her young protégé died of typhus there. Nevertheless, reform of this pesthole showed England an example of what nursing care could be.

Despite her reputation and her personal acquaintance with Queen Victoria, her cabinet, and every prime minister during this time, Nightingale and her ideas ran into opposition. Although some doctors who understood what this new nurse could do were supporters, the idea of the nurse as a professional was not commonly accepted. Said one physician, "A nurse is a confidential servant, but still only a servant....She should be middle-aged when she begins nursing, and if somewhat tamed by marriage and the troubles of a family, so much the better."[21] Maintaining standards was a constant struggle; even St. Thomas's Hospital slipped, and Nightingale, who had been immersed in the Indian reforms, had to take time to reorganize the program. What evolved over the years, from the first program, was one of preparation for two kinds of nursing practitioners: the educated middle- and upper-class ladies who paid their own tuition, and the still carefully selected poor women who were subsidized by the Nightingale Fund. The first were given an extra year or two of education to prepare them to become teachers or superintendents; a third choice was district nursing. "This nurse must be of a yet higher class and of a yet fuller training than a hospital nurse, because she has not the doctor always at hand and because she has no hospital appliances at hand."[22] The special probationers were expected to enter the profession permanently. The second group were prepared to be the hospital ward nurses.

In Nightingale's later years, she came into conflict with the very nurses who had been

---

Duties of Probationer under the "Nightingale Fund." St. Thomas's Hospital, 1860.

You are required to be

Sober.	Punctual.
Honest.	Quiet and Orderly.
Truthful.	Cleanly and Neat.
Trustworthy.	Patient, Cheerful, and Kindly.

You are expected to become skillful

1. In the dressing of blisters, burns, sores, wounds and in applying fomentations, poultices, and minor dressings.
2. In the application of leeches, externally and internally.
3. In the administration of enemas for men and women.
4. In the management of trusses, and appliances in uterine complaints.
5. In the best method of friction to the body and extremities.
6. In the management of helpless patients, i.e., moving, changing, personal cleanliness of, feeding, keeping warm, (or cool), preventing and dressing bed sores, managing position of.
7. In bandaging, making bandages, and rollers, lining of splints, etc.
8. In making the beds of the patients, and removal of sheets whilst patient is in bed.
9. You are required to attend at operations.
10. To be competent to cook gruel, arrowroot, egg flip, puddings, drinks, for the sick.
11. To understand ventilation, or keeping the ward fresh by night as well as by day; you are to be careful that great cleanliness is observed in all the utensils; those used for secretions as well as those required for cooking.
12. To make strict observation of the sick in the following particulars: The state of secretions, expectoration, pulse, skin, appetite, intelligence, as delirium or stupor; breathing, sleep, state of wounds, eruptions, formation of matter, effect of diet, or of stimulants, and of medicines.
13. And to learn the management of convalescents.

trained for leadership. In 1886, some of these nurses, now superintendents of other training schools, wanted to establish an organization that would provide a central examination and registration center, the forerunner of licensure. Nightingale opposed this movement for several reasons: nursing was still too young and disorganized; national criteria would not be as high as those of individual schools; and the all-important aspect of "character" could not be tested. She fought the concept with every weapon at her disposal, including her powerful contacts, and succeeded in limiting the fledgling Royal British Nurses' Association to maintaining a "list" instead of a "register." (Nurse licensure came to South Africa before it came to England.) Nevertheless, it was a beginning and, although she was probably right about the standards, recognition of nurses was facilitated with the setting of national standards, however minimal.

Nightingale's prolific writings on nursing have survived, and some of them are still surprisingly apt. Often they reflected her concern about the character of nurses and her own determination that their main focus be on nursing. For instance, in her early writings on hospitals (before the Nightingale schools), she reluctantly conceded that the nurse would have to be permitted visitors on her time off, distracting though that might be, and that spying on the nurse when she went out in her limited free time, although it had some advantages, was "no blessings in the long run and degrading to all concerned." Yet, nurses were to be held strictly to rules that limited their outside excursions to their exercise period, and it was preferred that they live adjacent to the patient wards. Nightingale's views moderated over the years, but her emphasis on morality and other personal qualities never wavered.

It was a time when salaries were low and petty thievery was common, and an accepted, desirable fringe benefit of a job (also recommended by Nightingale for nurses) was a daily allowance of beer, or even wine and brandy. But a Nightingale nurse who was found to be dis-

honest and drunken was dismissed instantly and permanently.

One principle from which Nightingale did not swerve was that nurses were to nurse, not to do heavy cleaning ("if you want a charwoman, hire one"); not to do laundry ("it makes their hands coarse and hard and less able to attend to the delicate manipulation which they may be called on to execute"); and not to fetch ("to save the time of nurses; all diets and ward requisites should be brought into the wards"). Then, as in many places now, status and promotion came through assumption of administrative roles, but Nightingale recognized that "many are valuable as nurses, who are yet unfit for promotion to head nurses." Her alternative, however, would not be greeted favorably today—a raise after ten years of good service!

Nightingale also commented on other issues considered pertinent today. Continuing education was a must, for she saw nursing as a progressive art, in which to stand still was to go back. "A woman who thinks of herself, 'Now I am a full nurse, a skilled nurse. I have learnt all there is to be learned,' take my word for it, she does not know what a nurse is, and she will never know: she has gone back already."[23] Although there is no evidence that she took any action to help end discrimination against women, Nightingale believed that women should be accepted into all the professions, but she warned them, "qualify yourselves for it as a man does for his work." She believed that women should be paid as highly as men, but that equal pay meant equal responsibility. In a profession with as much responsibility as nursing, it was particularly important to have adequate compensation, or intelligent, independent women would not be attracted to it. Until the end, she was firm on the need for nurses to obey physicians in medical matters; however, she stressed the importance of nurse observation and reporting because the physician was not constantly at the patient's bedside, as the nurse was. She was adamant that a nurse (and woman) be in charge of nursing, with no other administrative figure having authority over nurses, in-

What a Nurse Is to Be

A really good nurse must needs be of the highest class of character. It need hardly be said that she must be—(1) Chaste, in the sense of the Sermon on the Mount; a good nurse should be the Sermon on the Mount in herself. It should naturally seem impossible to the most unchaste to utter even an immodest jest in her presence. Remember this great and dangerous peculiarity of nursing, and especially of hospital nursing, namely, that it is the only case, queens not excepted, where a woman is really in charge of men. And a really good trained ward "sister" can keep order in a men's ward better than a military ward-master or sergeant. (2) Sober, in spirit as well as in drink and temperate in all things. (3) Honest, not accepting the most trifling fee or bribe from patients or friends. (4) Truthful—and to be able to tell the truth includes attention and observation, to observe truly—memory, to remember truly—power of expression, to tell truly what one has observed truly—as well as intention to speak the truth, the whole truth, and nothing but the truth. (5) Trustworthy, to carry out directions intelligently and perfectly, unseen as well as seen, "to the Lord" as well as unto men—no mere eye-service. (6) Punctual to a second and orderly to a hair—having everything ready and in order before she begins her dressings or her work about the patient; nothing forgotten. (7) Quiet, yet quick, quick without hurry; gentle without slowness; discreet without self-importance; no gossip. (8) Cheerful, hopeful; not allowing herself to be discouraged by unfavourable symptoms; not given to depress the patient by anticipations of an unfavourable result. (9) Cleanly to the point of exquisiteness, both for the patient's sake and her own; neat and ready. (10) Thinking of her patient and not of herself, "tender over his occasions" or wants, cheerful and kindly, patient, ingenious and feat.

Source: From a Nightingale article on *"Nurses, Training of, and Nursing the Sick,"* in A Dictionary of Medicine, edited by Sir Robert Quain, Bart., M.D., 1882.

cluding physicians. She knew the importance of a work setting that gave job satisfaction. In words that are a far-off echo of nurses' plaints today, she wrote:

> Besides, a thing very little understood, a good nurse has her professional pride in results of her Nursing quite as much as a Medical Officer in the results of his treatment. There are defective buildings, defective administrations, defective appliances, which make all good Nursing impossible. A good Nurse does not like to waste herself, and the better the Nurse, the stronger this feeling in her. Humanity may overrule this feeling in a great emergency like a cholera outbreak; but I don't believe that it is in human nature for a good Nurse to bear up, with an ever-recurring, ever-useless expenditure of activity, against the circumstances which make her nursing activity useless, or all but useless. Her work becomes slovenly like the rest, and it is a far greater pity to have a nurse wasting herself in this way than it would be to have a steam engine running up and down the line all day without a train, wasting coals.
>
> Perhaps I need scarcely add that Nurses must be paid the market price for their labor, like any other worker; and that this is yearly rising.[24]

Obviously, Nightingale is eminently quotable, in matters of health care and nursing today, in part because she was so far ahead of her time, and in part, unfortunately, because the errors of omission and commission in the field have a tendency to reappear or remain uncorrected.

Planner, administrator, educator, researcher, reformer, Florence Nightingale never lost her interest in nursing. As nearly as can be determined, her actual clinical nursing was limited to her early care of sick families, the short period at Kaiserswerth, a briefer interim of caring for victims of a cholera epidemic before the war, and then, of course, her experience in the Crimea. Yet, her perception of patients' needs was uncanny for the time and frequently is still applicable today. In her *Notes on Nursing*, not only is there careful consideration of "Observation of the Sick" and crisp comments on "Minding Baby," but also pertinent directions on hygiene, nutrition, environment, and the mental state of the patient. At age 74, in her last major work on nursing, she differentiated between sick nursing and health nursing, and emphasized the primary need for prevention of illness, for which a lay "Health Missioner" (today's health educator?) would be trained.

When Nightingale died on August 13, 1910, she was to be honored by burial in Westminster Abbey. However, she had chosen instead to be buried in the family plot in Hampshire, with a simple inscription: "F. N. Born 1820, Died 1910."

REFERENCES

1. Barritt ER: Florence Nightingale's values and modern nursing education. *Nurs Forum* 12(4):10, 1973.
2. Ibid, p 34.
3. Bullough V, Bullough B: *The Care of the Sick: The Emergence of Modern Nursing.* New York: Prodist, 1978, p 69.
4. Barritt, op cit, p 10.
5. Seymer LR: *Selected Writings of Florence Nightingale.* New York: Macmillan, 1954, p 124.
6. Ibid, pp 214–215.
7. Bullough and Bullough, op cit, p 86.
8. Dolan JA: *Nursing in Society: A Historical Perspective*, 14th ed. Philadelphia: Saunders, 1978, p 159.
9. Kalisch P, Kalisch B: *The Advance of American Nursing.* Boston: Little, Brown, 1986, p 46.
10. Seymer, op cit, p 28.
11. Dolan, op cit, p 161.
12. Kalisch and Kalisch, op cit, p 46.
13. Ibid, p 47.
14. Seymer, op cit, p 28.
15. Barritt, op cit, p 8.
16. Seymer, op cit, pp 222–223.
17. Hays J: Florence Nightingale and the India sanitary reforms. *Public Health Nurs* 6:152–154, September 1989.
18. Seymer, op cit, p 244.
19. Ibid, p 234.
20. Ibid, p 229.
21. Dolan, op cit, p 169.
22. Monteiro L: Florence Nightingale on public health nursing. *Am J Public Health* 75:181–186, February 1985.
23. Pavey AE: *The Story of the Growth of Nursing.* London: Farber & Farber, 1938, p 296.
24. Seymer, op cit, p 276.

Nursing in the United States

CHAPTER 3

The Evolution of the Trained Nurse, 1873–1903

NURSING IN THE United States between the American Revolution and the Civil War was probably no better or worse than that in Europe. As noted in Chap. 1, nurses from both Catholic and Protestant nursing orders came to America, and their nursing care, although semitrained, was the best offered. But there were not enough of them. Even given the occasional compassionate lady who might have ventured into hospitals to help with care in an epidemic or other emergency, the quality of lay nurses was about the same as that in England.

Early hospitals, privately managed and funded by endowments or public subscription, were modeled after those in Europe, with no improvement in quality; the mentally ill were confined in insane asylums or poorhouses and prisons. Yet, by the time of the Civil War, social reforms had also reached America. One of the key figures was Dorothea Lynde Dix (1802–1887), a gentle New England schoolteacher, who became interested in the conditions under which the mentally ill existed when she went to teach a Sunday school lesson in a jail. She began to survey the needs of those forgotten people, and her descriptive reports and careful documentation eventually resulted in the construction of state psychiatric institutions (the first in Trenton, New Jersey). There was some lessening of inhumane care, even if no improvement in the understanding of the illnesses.

THE CIVIL WAR

When the Civil War began in April 1861, there was no organized system to care for the sick and wounded. There never had been. In the American Revolution, for instance, such basic care as existed was given by camp followers, a few wives, women in the neighborhood, and "surgeons' mates." It is possible that some of these women were employed by the army, for there are female names on the payroll lists as "nursing the sick."[1]

American women, considered by American men to be just as delicate and proper and unsuited for unpleasant service as their European counterparts, nevertheless rushed to volunteer. Within a few weeks, 100 women were given a short training course by physicians and surgeons in New York City, and Dorothea Dix, well known by then, was appointed by the Secretary of War to superintend these new "nurses." Meanwhile, members of religious orders also volunteered, and nursing in some of the larger government hospitals was eventually assigned to them because of the inexperience of the lay volunteers.[2]

Except for that group, almost none of the several thousand women who served as nurses during the war had any kind of training or hospital experience. They can be categorized as follows:

1. The nurses appointed by Miss Dix or other officials as legal employees of the army for 40 cents and one ration a day.

2. The sisters or nuns of the various orders.
3. Those employed for short periods of time for menial chores.
4. Black women employed under general orders of the War Department for $10 a month.
5. Uncompensated volunteers.
6. Women camp followers.
7. Women employed by the various relief organizations.[3]

It is estimated that some 6,000 women performed nursing duties for the Northern armies. The South used only about 1,000 because of the attitude that prevailed for some time that caring for men was unfit for Southern ladies. (Nevertheless, a number of these ladies, such as Kate Cummings, who recorded her experiences, gave distinguished service under severe conditions in Southern hospitals.)[4]

U.S. Army medical officers were no more pleased with the presence of females in their domain than were the British in the Crimea. It was not that Miss Dix didn't try for the serious-minded; her recruiting specified only plainlooking women over 35 who wore gray, brown, or black dresses with no bows, curls, jewelry, or hoop skirts, and who were moral and had common sense. Presumably, those who did not qualify were among the many unofficial and unpaid volunteers. Some of the information on what the Civil War nurses did comes from the writings of Louisa May Alcott and Walt Whitman, both volunteers. In her journal, Alcott described her working day, which began at six. After opening the windows, because of the bad air in the makeshift base hospital, she was "giving out rations, cutting up food for helpless boys, washing faces, teaching my attendants how beds are made or floors are swept, dressing wounds, dusting tables, sewing bandages, keeping my tray tidy, rushing up and down after pillows, bed linens, sponges, and directions...."[5] Volunteers also read to the patients, wrote letters, and comforted them. Apparently, even the hired nurses did little more except, perhaps, give medicines. But so did the volunteers, sometimes giving the medicine and food of their choice to the patient, instead of what the doctor ordered.

By 1862, enormous military hospitals, some with as many as 3,000 beds, were being built, although there were still some makeshift hospitals: former hotels, churches, factories, and almost anything else available. There was even a hospital ship, the *Red Rover*, a former Mississippi steamer captured from the Confederates and staffed by nuns. Other floating hospitals were inaugurated and served as transport units, with nurses attending the wounded.[6] Discipline in the hospitals was rigid for nurses and patients alike, with the latter given strict orders to be respectful to the nurses. According to one Army hospital edict, the nurses, under the supervision of the "Stewards and Chief Wardmaster," were responsible for the administration of the wards, but many of their duties appeared to be related more to keeping the nonmedical records of patients and reporting their misbehavior than to nursing care. If the patient needed medical or surgical attendance, the doctor was to be called.[7]

Georgeanna Woolsey wrote that the surgeons treated the nurses without even common courtesy because they did not want them and tried to make their lives so unbearable that they would leave. The surgeons were often incompetent. As a temporary expedient, contract surgeons were employed with no position, little pay, and only minimal rank. Jane, another Woolsey sister who was also a volunteer nurse, wrote that although some were highly skilled, "faithful, sagacious, tenderhearted," others were drunken, refused to attend the wounded, or injured them more because of their incompetence.[8]

It was surgeons and officers of the latter type that the formidable nurse Mary Ann (Mother) Bickerdyke attacked. She managed to have a number of them dismissed (in part because of her friendship with General Grant and General Sherman). About this tough "Soldier's Friend," one physician stated, "Woe to the surgeon, the commissary, or quartermaster whose neglect of his men and selfish disregard for their interests and needs come under her cognizance."[9]

Another fighter was Clara Barton, who early in the war cared for the wounded of the Sixth Massachusetts Regiment. One story told about her is that while supervising the delivery of a wagonload of supplies for soldiers, she neatly extricated an ox from a herd meant for the Army, so the wounded would have food.[10]

Only in recent years has attention been given to the black nurses of the Civil War. Harriet Tubman, the "Moses of her people," not only led many black slaves to freedom in her underground railroad activities before the war but also nursed the wounded when she joined the Union Army. Similarly, Sojourner Truth, abolitionist speaker and activist in the women's movement, also cared for the sick and wounded. Susie King Taylor, born to slavery and secretly taught to read and write, met and married a Union soldier and served as a battlefront nurse for more than four years, although she received no salary or pension from the Union Army.[11]

There were other heroines, untrained women from the North and South, caring for the sick and wounded with a modicum of skills but much kindness, and, as in the Crimea, the soldiers were sentimentally appreciative, if not discriminating. Even when paid, Civil War nurses had little status and no rank. One exception was Sally Tomkins, a civic-minded Southern woman, who efficiently took charge of a makeshift hospital and was made a captain of the cavalry by Confederate President Jefferson Davis so that she could continue her work. An investigative report by the United States Sanitary Commission noted that nurses had not been well treated or wisely used.

> They have not been placed, as they expected and were fitted to be, in the position of head nurses. On the contrary, with a very inefficient force of male nurses, they have been called on to do every form of service, have been overtaxed and worn down with menial and purely mechanical duties, additional to the more responsible offices and duties of nursing.[12]

Nevertheless, the Civil War opened hospitals to massive numbers of women, well-bred "ladies," who would otherwise probably not even have thought of nursing. Some of these, such as Abby, Jane, and Georgeanna Woolsey, later helped lead the movement to establish training schools for nurses.

THE EARLY TRAINING SCHOOLS

The nursing role of women in the Civil War, however unsophisticated, and probably the fame of Florence Nightingale brought to the attention of the American public the need for nurses and the desirability of some organized programs of training. There had been previous elementary efforts in this direction: an organized school of nursing, founded in 1839 by the Nurse Society of Philadelphia under Dr. Joseph Warrington, awarded a certificate after a stated period of lectures, demonstrations, and experience at a hospital; a school of nursing for a "better type" of woman connected with the Women's Hospital in Philadelphia in 1861 gave a diploma after six months of lectures.

More physicians became interested in the training of nurses and, at a meeting of the American Medical Association in 1869, a committee to study the matter stated that it was "just as necessary to have well-trained, well-instructed nurses as to have intelligent and skillful physicians." The committee recommended that nursing schools be placed under the guardianship of county medical societies, although under the immediate supervision of lady superintendents; that every lay hospital should have a school; and that nurses be trained not only for the hospital but for private duty in the home.[13]

In 1871, the editor of *Godey's Lady's Book*, the most popular woman's magazine of the time, wrote an editorial on "Lady Nurses" that was remarkably farsighted.

> Much has been lately said of the benefits that would follow if the calling of sick nurse were elevated to a profession which an educated lady might adopt without a sense of degradation, either on her own part or in the estimation of others....

There can be no doubt that the duties of sick nurse, to be properly performed, require an education and training little, if at all, inferior to those possessed by members of the medical profession....The manner in which a reform may be effected is easily pointed out. Every medical college should have a course of study and training especially adapted for ladies who desire to qualify themselves for the profession of nurse; and those who had gone through the course, and passed the requisite examination, should receive a degree and a diploma, which would at once establish their position in society. The graduate nurse would in general estimation be as much above the ordinary nurse of the present day as the professional surgeon of our times is above the barber-surgeon of the last century.[14]

Unfortunately, this idea of an educated nurse with professional status was a long time in coming. Nevertheless, in 1872, the New England Hospital for Women and Children, staffed by women physicians who were interested in the development of a school, acted upon a statement in its bylaws of 1863 "to train nurses for the care of the sick." It was a one-year program in which the students provided round-the-clock service for patients; there was no classwork (although a few lectures were given during the winter months), and the duty extended from 5:30 A.M. to 9 P.M., with a free afternoon every second week from 2 to 5 P.M. At the end of the year, one student graduated—Melinda Ann (Linda) Richards, thereafter called America's first trained nurse, probably because of all the nurses who graduated from this primitive early program; she moved on to be a key figure in the development of nursing education. Richards, like some of the other students in the schools that evolved, had been a nurse in a hospital, although some schools would not accept them because they wanted to set a new image. This indicates that despite the frequent descriptions of criminal and thieving women who nursed, some nurses, although untrained in the later sense, must have been at least respectable, intelligent women.

Another outstanding graduate of the New England Hospital for Women and Children (1879) was Mary Mahoney, the first trained black nurse. A tiny, dynamic, charming woman, she worked primarily in private duty in the Boston area but was apparently always present at national nurses meetings. In her honor, the Mary Mahoney Medal was initiated by the National Association of Colored Graduate Nurses, and the award was later continued by the American Nurses Association.

In 1873, three schools supposedly based on the Nightingale model were established.[15] The Bellevue Training School in New York City was founded through the influence of several society ladies who had been involved in Civil War nursing, including Abby Woolsey. Appalled by the conditions—900 patients, 3 to 5 occupying strapped-together beds, tended by ex-convict nurses and night watchmen who stole their food and left them in filth—these women sent a young physician to England to confer with Nightingale. Then they raised funds to set up a nurses' training class for which they were given six wards. The hospital agreed to place these students under the direction of a female superintendent, provided that they also did the scouring and cleaning that had been done by the other "nurses"; they would not hire anyone to clean. Although the school attempted to follow Nightingale principles and reported that it was attracting educated women, its overall purpose was to improve conditions in a great charity hospital, and much of the learning was on a trial-and-error basis. Nevertheless, Bellevue had a lot of interesting firsts: interdisciplinary rounds where nurses reported on the nursing plan of care; patient record-keeping and writing of orders, initiated by Linda Richards, who became night superintendent; and the first uniform, by stylish and aristocratic Euphemia Van Rensselaer, which started a trend. And of course, two of nursing's greatest leaders were Bellevue graduates—Lavinia Dock and Isabel Hampton Robb.

The Connecticut Training School was started through the influence of another Woolsey, Georgeanna, and her husband, Dr. Francis Bacon. Through negotiation with the hospital, the superintendent of nurses was designated as separate from, and not responsible to, the steward (administrator) of the hospital, and teaching outside the wards was permitted. The threatened steward managed to make life so miserable for a series of superintendents that each resigned, but control remained with nursing. Meanwhile, all good intentions notwithstanding, the students soon were sent to give care in the homes of sick families, with the money going to the School Fund—and the school could boast that for thirty-three years it was not financed or directed by the hospital.

The Boston Training School was the last of that first famous triumvirate. Again, a group of women associated with other educational and philanthropic endeavors spearheaded its organization, but this time to offer a desirable occupation for self-supporting women and to provide good private nurses for the community. After prolonged negotiations that allowed the director of the school, instead of the hospital, to maintain control, the Massachusetts General Hospital assigned "The Brick" building to the school because it (The Brick) "stands by itself; represents both medical and surgical departments; and offers the hard labor desirable for the training of nurses."[16] Apparently, there was rather poor leadership, and nurses continued to do dishwashing and other menial tasks, with little attention to training. When Linda Richards became the third director, she reorganized the work, started classes, and set out to prove that trained nurses were better than untrained ones. As an example, she cared for some of the sickest patients herself. By the end of 1876, she had charge of all the nursing in the hospital.

Other major training schools that were to endure into the next century were founded in the next few years, somewhat patterned after Nightingale's precepts. Their success and the popularity of their graduates resulted in a massive proliferation of training schools. In 1880, there were 15; by 1900, 432; by 1909, 1,105 hospital-based diploma schools. Hospitals with as few as 20 beds opened schools, and the students provided almost totally free labor. Usu-

ally the only graduate nurses were the superintendent and perhaps the operating room supervisor and night supervisor. Students earned money for the hospital, for after a short period they were frequently sent to do private nursing in the home, with the money reverting to the hospital, not the school. Except for the few outstanding schools, all Nightingale principles were forgotten: the students were under the control of the hospital and worked from 12 to 15 hours a day—24 if they were on a private case in a home—and lessons, if any, were scheduled for an hour late in the evening when someone was available to teach. (It wasn't necessary for all students to be available.) Moreover, if the "pupils" lost time because of sickness, which was almost always contracted from patients or caused by sheer overwork, the time had to be totally made up before they could graduate. Why then did training schools draw so many applicants? Because the occupational opportunities for untrained women were limited to domestic service, factory work, retail clerking, or prostitution. Even with the strict discipline, hard work, long hours, and almost no time off, after a year or two of training (the second year unabashedly free labor to the hospitals), the trained nurse could do private duty at a salary ranging from $10 a week to the vague possibility of $20 (if she could collect it), a far cry from the $4 to $6 average of other women workers. Of course, on these cases, she was a 24-hour servant to the family and patient, lucky to have time off for a walk, and because there were necessarily months with no employment, even an excellent nurse was lucky to gross $600 a year.[17] Higher education for women was limited to typewriting or teaching, but these were seldom taught in universities. Those colleges and universities that did admit women rarely prepared them for professions. So the more famous hospital schools, particularly, had hundreds and even thousands of applicants a year. On the other hand, there were a multitude of hospitals and sanitoriums of all kinds that were looking for students to meet their staffing needs, and for these, high-quality applicants were frequently lacking. Consequently, application standards were lowered rapidly. Apparently, most schools admitted a class of 30 to 35 (in some cases determined by their staffing and financial needs). Attrition, caused in part by the tremendously high rate of student illness and the unpleasant working and living conditions, was often 75 percent.[18]

Student admission requirements varied, but all nurse applicants were female. Some hospitals accepted men in programs but gave them only a short course and frequently called them *attendants*. In 1888, at Bellevue Hospital, the Mills School was established with a two-year course, but for a long time its graduates were also called attendants. Other early schools admitting men were at Grace Hospital, Detroit; Battle Creek Sanitorium, Battle Creek, Michigan; Boston City Hospital, Carney, and St. Margaret's, Boston; Pennsylvania Hospital in Philadelphia; and the Alexian Brothers hospitals in Chicago and St. Louis.[19] At first, the minimum age for all students was about 25, later lowered to 21, to prevent losing young women to other fields. Eight or fewer years of schooling were common, but usually good health and good character were absolute prerequisites. Obedience in training was essential, and a student could be dismissed as a troublemaker if the overworked girl grumbled, talked too much, was too familiar with men, criticized head nurses or doctors, or could not get along "sweetly" wherever placed. Married women and those over 30 were frequently excluded because they could not "fall in with the life successfully." And, of course, if they were divorced, they were naturally eliminated—"too self-centered with interests elsewhere." Blacks were also generally silently excluded. Over the years, training schools for black nurses were founded, the first organized in 1891 at the Provident Hospital in Chicago.

In the 1890s, only 2 percent of nurse training was theory, containing some anatomy and physiology, materia medica, perhaps some chemistry, bacteriology, hygiene, and lectures on certain diseases. The leading schools developed their own institutional manuals, such as the simply written *Hand-Book of Nursing for Family and General Use*, written by a committee of nurses and physicians at the Connecticut Training School and published in 1878. The other great pioneering texts were *A Textbook of Nursing for the Use of Training Schools, Families, and Private Students*, by Clara Weeks Shaw (1885); *Nursing: Its Principles and Practice for Hospital and Private Use*, by Isabel Hampton (1893); *The Textbook on Materia Medica for Nurses*, by Lavinia Dock (1890); and the first scientific book written by a nurse, a textbook on anatomy, by Diana Kimber (1893).[20] Almost from the beginning, there were physicians who objected to so much education for nurses and devoted considerable medical journal space to their fulminations about the "overtrained nurse."

> **Training, as we understand it, is drilling, and a person who is to carry out the instructions of another cannot be too thoroughly drilled. Pedagogy is another matter. We have never been able to understand what great good was expected from imparting to nurses a smattering of medicine and surgery....To feed their vanity with the notion that they are competent to take any considerable part in ordering the management of the sick is certainly a most erroneous step.**
>
> **The work of a nurse is an honorable "calling" or vocation, and nothing further. It implies the exercise of acquired proficiency in certain more or less mechanical duties, and is not primarily designed to contribute to the sum of human knowledge or the advancement of science....[21]**

One physician even suggested a correspondence course for training nurses to care for the "poor folks,"[22] and a New York newspaper editorial proclaimed, "What we want in nurses is less theory and more practice." But then, this was at a time when a leading Harvard physician held that serious mental exercise would damage a woman's brain or cause other severe trauma, such as the narrowing of the pelvic area, which would make her unable to deliver children.[23]

However, there were also farsighted physicians who supported not "teaching a trade, but preparing for a profession," as Dr. Richard

Cabot noted in 1901. He listed reforms that included the following: (1) nurses should pay for their training and be taught by paid instructors; (2) nursing should be taught by nurses, medicine by physicians; (3) the nurse's training should not be entirely technical. He added, "Subjects like French literature and history, which tend to give us a deeper and truer sympathy with human nature, are surely as much needed in the education of the nurse, who is to deal exclusively with human beings, as in the curriculum of the chemist or engineer, who deals primarily with things and not persons."[24] But, meanwhile, students continued to live a slavelike existence, without outward complaint, poorly housed, overworked, underfed ("rations of a kind and quality only a remove better than what we might place before a beggar," said a popular journal), and unprotected from life-threatening illness (80 percent of the students in the average hospital graduated with positive tuberculin tests).[25] If they survived all this, no wonder they were expected to graduate as "respectful, obedient, cheerful, submissive, hard-working, loyal, pacific, and religious."[26] It was not professional education; it was not even a respectably run apprenticeship, because learning was not derived from skilled masters, but rather from their own peers, who were but a step ahead of them. These principles of sacrifice, service, obedience to the physician, and ethical orientation are embodied in the Nightingale Pledge, written in 1893 by Lystra E. Gretter, superintendent of the school at Harper Hospital in Detroit, a pledge still sometimes recited by students today.

> **I solemnly pledge myself before God and in the presence of this assembly;**
>
> **To pass my life in purity and to practice my profession faithfully;**
>
> **I will abstain from whatever is deleterious and mischievous and will not take or knowingly administer any harmful drug; I will do all in my power to maintain and elevate the standard of my profession, and will hold in confidence all personal matters committed to my keeping and all family affairs coming to my knowledge in the practice of my calling;**

> **With loyalty will I endeavor to aid the physician in his work, and devote myself to the welfare of those committed to my care.[27]**

THE NURSE IN PRACTICE

In the late eighteenth and early nineteenth centuries, the graduate trained nurse had two major career options: she could do private duty in homes or, if she was exceptional (or particularly favored), gain one of the rare positions as head nurse, operating room supervisor, night supervisor, or even superintendent. The latter positions were, of course, much more available before the flood of nurses reached the market. Even so, in private duty, trained nurses often competed with untrained nurses who were not restrained from practicing in many states until the middle of the twentieth century. And, given the long hours and taxing physical work in home nursing, most private nurses found themselves unwanted at 40, with younger, stronger nurses being hired instead. Some of the more ambitious and perhaps braver nurses chose to go west to pioneer in new and sometimes primitive hospitals.

The practice of nursing was scarcely limited to clinical care of the patient. Job descriptions of the time appear to have given major priority to scrubbing floors, dusting, keeping the stove stoked and the kerosene lamps trimmed and filled, controlling insects, washing clothes, making and rolling bandages, and other unskilled housekeeping tasks, as well as edicts for personal behavior. Nursing care responsibilities included "making beds, giving baths, preventing and dressing bedsores, applying friction to the body and extremities, giving enemas, inserting catheters, bandaging, dressing blisters, burns, sores, and wounds, and observing secretions, expectorations, pulse, skin, appetite, body temperature, consciousness, respiration, sleep, condition of wounds, skin eruptions, elimination, and the effect of diet, stimulants, and medications," and carrying out any orders of the physician.[28] One of the more interesting treatments to modern nurses might be the vivid description of leeching, which included placing leeches, removing them from human orifices where they may have disappeared, and emptying them of excess blood.

At the end of the nineteenth century, the growth of large cities was marked in the United States. Although the cities had their beautiful public buildings, parks, and mansions, they also had their seamy sides—the festering slums where the tremendous flow of immigrants huddled. Between 1820 and 1910, nearly 30 million immigrants entered the United States, with a shift in numbers from Northern European to Southern European by the early 1900s. Health and social problems multiplied in the slum areas. In New York, for instance, it was not unusual to house thirty-six families in a six-story walk-up on a narrow 25 × 90 foot lot. Vermin, lack of sanitation, and the fact that many immigrants converted their crowded rooms into sweatshops made it easy for epidemics to rage through the neighborhoods, and death from tuberculosis was common.

Somehow, Americans did not seem to feel a great need to serve the sick poor in their homes; after all, there were public dispensaries and charity hospitals. Nevertheless, in 1877, the Women's Board of the New York City Mission sent nurses, who received their training at Bellevue, into the homes of the poor to give care. In 1886, the Visiting Nurse Society of Philadelphia sent nurses not only to the poor but also to those of moderate means who could pay. In the same year, the nurses of the Boston Instructive District Nursing Association formally included patient teaching in their visits—principles of hygiene, sanitation, and aspects of illness. Other such agencies followed, but by 1900 it was estimated that only 200 nurses were engaged in public health nursing.

One of the key figures in community health nursing was Lilian Wald. After graduating from New York Hospital School of Nursing and working a short time, she decided to enter the Women's Medical College. When she and another nurse, Mary Brewster, were sent to the Lower East Side to lecture to immigrant mothers on the care of the sick, they were shocked at what they saw; neither had known such abject poverty could exist. Wald left medical school, moved with Mary Brewster to a top-floor tenement on Jefferson Street, and began to offer nursing care to the poor. After a short while, the calls came by the hundreds from families, hospitals, and physicians. People were cared for, whether or not they could afford to pay. The concern of these nurses was not just giving nursing care but seeing what other services could be made available to meet the many social needs of the poor. Challenging the entire community to assume responsibility for these conditions of "poverty and misery" was an attitude strongly advocated by Lavinia Dock, who wrote in 1937:

> As I recollect it, this point of view turned rather toward exploration and discovery than simply toward good works alone, when Lillian D. Wald and Mary Brewster went in 1893, free from every form of control, "without benefit of" managers, committees, medical encouragement, or police approval, into Jefferson Street (at first, then later into Henry Street), there to do what they could do; to see what they could see; and to publicize all that was wrong and remediable by making their findings known as widely as possible....
>
> If I am not mistaken, it was Lilian Wald who first used the term *public health nursing*—adding the one word *public* to Florence Nightingale's phrase *health nursing*—in order to picture her inner vision of the possibilities of nursing services as widely and as effectively organized as were state and federal health services, and acting in harmonious cooperation with them, if not a part of them.[29]

After two years of such success, larger facilities, more nurses, and social workers were needed. In 1895, Wald, Brewster, Lavinia Dock, and other nurses moved to what was eventually called the Henry Street Settlement, a house bought by philanthropist Jacob H. Schiff. By 1909, the Henry Street staff had thirty-seven nurses, all but five providing direct nursing service. Each nurse was carefully oriented and was able to demonstrate the value of understanding the family and the environment in giving good nursing care. Each nurse kept two sets of records, one for the physician and another recording the major points of the nurse's work.

The establishment of school nursing was also started by Lillian Wald, who suggested that placing nurses in schools might help to solve the problem of the schools having to send home so many ill children. (Health conditions in New York Schools were so bad that in 1902 10,567 children were sent home from school; local physicians did little in these settings.) Wald sent a Henry Street nurse, Lina L. Rogers, to a school on a one-month demonstration project, which proved so successful that by 1903 the school board began to appoint nurses to the schools. It was not an easy job, and on occasion the schools were the sites of riots because mothers misunderstood the preventive measures that needed to be taken by the nurses. One amusing tale is found in the Children's Bureau records. On being notified that her child needed a bath, a mother wrote, "teacher, Johnny ain't no rose. Learn him, don't smell him."[30]

Industrial nursing also began to provide job opportunities for trained nurses. One of the earliest is generally credited to the president of the Vermont Marble Company in Proctor, Vermont, who in 1895 employed a trained nurse, Ada M. Stewart, to give "district nursing" service to the employees of the company. No public health nursing service was available at that time.

Miss Stewart often traveled about the town on a bicycle, wearing her nurse's uniform and a plain coat and hat, teaching company employees and sometimes other members of the community "habits for healthy living," caring for minor injuries, calling the doctor when indicated, and, at the schoolteacher's request, talking to schoolchildren about hygiene and first aid. Miss Stewart's service was so helpful that in 1895 the marble company employed her sister, Harriet, to give similar service in other Vermont communities in which the company had mills and quarries.

The century ended with another war, in which nurses again proved their worth. The Spanish-American War lasted less than a year, but there was considerable loss of life. The army was completely unprepared for it, and the hospital corpsmen were even less ready to cope with the sick and wounded. The National Society of the Daughters of the American Revolution offered to serve as an examining board for military nurses. The task of separating the fit from the unfit and the trained from the untrained among the 5,000 applicants was overwhelming. Significant questions asked the volunteers were, "Are you strong and healthy?" and "Have you ever had yellow fever?" Although only a small percentage of the soldiers ever left the camps in the South to fight in Cuba, at one point fully 30 percent became ill from malaria, dysentery, and typhoid. Once more, some Army surgeons, particularly the Surgeon General, objected to the presence of trained women nurses, but their efforts to recruit male nurses were unsuccessful because glory, rank, and decent salary were lacking. Consequently, nursing was done by the dregs of the infantry squads. Finally, with serious outbreaks of typhoid killing the enlistees, women nurses from many training schools took over. Wearing their own distinctive school uniforms and caps, they included superintendents of nursing on leave from their noted schools, as well as new, young graduates. Their letters and journals relate the horrible conditions under which they worked. Some literally worked themselves to death in the Army hospitals in the South.

Meanwhile, a hospital ship, the *U.S.S. Relief*, sailed to Cuba with supplies, medicines, and equipment—and Esther Hasson of New London, Connecticut, who would later become the first superintendent of the Navy Nurse Corps. They were just in time to receive the wounded of a naval battle, but again, the greatest problem was disease, including yellow fever, about which little was known. In testing the theory that the disease was caused by a certain type of mosquito, nursing gained its first martyr. Twenty-five-year-old Clara Maas of East Orange, New Jersey, volunteered to be bitten by a carrier mosquito. After being bitten several times, she died of yellow fever and is still considered a heroine in helping to prove the source of the disease.

The conditions under which soldiers and sailors were cared for continued to be horrendous. An investigation after the war indicated that the only redeeming aspect was the quality of the services of the women nurses, even though they were insufficient in number and were forced to work inefficiently. A recommendation was made for "a corps of selected trained women nurses ready to serve when necessity shall arise, but, under ordinary circumstances, owing no duty to the War Department, except to report residence at determined intervals."[31] Still, the attitude of military authorities was hostile. One hospital commander surgeon objected to retaining women nurses, citing their "coddling" of patients, not letting the Army private (orderly) nurse, and the difficulty in preserving "good military discipline with this mixed personnel." So, although the number of women Army nurses had reached 1,158 in September 1898, by the next July there were only 202. Despite this setback, a group of influential women, including some prominent nurses, eventually lobbied through a bill, and the Army Nurse Corps was established on February 2, 1901. Dita H. Kinney, Head Nurse of the U.S. Army Hospital at Fort Bayard, New Mexico, became the first nurse superintendent. It took longer for the Congress to act on a Navy Nurse Corps, although it had the support of the Navy's Surgeon General, but finally it too became a reality in 1908.[32]

THE IMPACT OF NURSING'S EARLY LEADERS

Perhaps it was said best by Isabel Hampton Robb as she spoke to other early nursing leaders. "We are the history makers of trained nurses. Let us see to it that we work so as to leave a fair record as the inheritance of those who come after us, one which may be to them an inspiration to even better efforts."[33]

It was an amazing period of coordinated female leadership in what was barely becoming an accepted, respectable occupation in the last quarter of the nineteenth century. Yet, before the new century was far along, this intrepid coterie of nurses was responsible for setting nursing standards, improving curricula, writing textbooks, starting two enduring professional organizations and a nursing journal, inaugurating a teacher training program in a university, and initiating nursing licensure. They were a mixed group, but with certain commonalities: usually unmarried but, except for Lavinia Dock, not feminist; graduates of the better training schools; later functioning in some teaching and/or administrative capacity, most often as superintendent of a school; and involved in the early nursing organizations. Fortunately, many were also great letter writers and letters savers as well as authors, so that there are many fascinating insights into their lives. (See particularly the Christy series in *Nursing Outlook*, listed in the bibliography.)

Nursing's first trained nurse, Linda Richards, had a continuing impact on the training schools because she spent much of her career moving from hospital to hospital in what seems to have been an improvement campaign. In those earliest days, almost any graduate was considered a prime candidate for starting another program, and some undoubtedly lacked the intellectual and leadership qualities needed, so that the new schools, if not actual disasters, were frequently of poor quality. Linda Richards apparently had the skill and authority to upgrade both the school and the nursing service which were, after all, almost inseparable. However, she seemed willing to accept school management that tied the economics of the hospital to student education, usually to the detriment of the latter.

One of the most noted nursing figures is Isabelle Hampton, who left teaching to enter the Bellevue Training School in 1881. Not only was she attractive and charming, but she was "in every sense of the word a leader, by nature, by capacity, by personal attributes and qualities, by choice, and probably to some extent by inheritance and training; a follower she never was."[34] In her two major superintendencies, she made a number of then radical changes—cutting down the students' workday to 10 hours and eliminating their free private duty services. At Johns Hopkins, which she founded, she recruited fractious Lavinia Dock, who was still at Bellevue, to be her assistant. They must have made an interesting pair, for Lavinia, also a "lady," was outspoken and frequently tactless, particularly with physicians. Later, she was to say:

> **A quite determined movement on the part of our masculine brothers to seize and guide the helm of the new teaching is...most undeniably in progress. Several...have lately openly asserted themselves in printed articles as the founders and leaders of the nursing education, which so far as it has gone, we all know to have been worked out by the brains, bodies and souls of women...who have often had to win their points in clinched opposition to the will of these same brothers and solely by dint of their own personal prestige as women....[35]**

M. Adelaide Nutting graduated in that first Hopkins class, and the three became friends.[36] Nutting followed Hampton as principal of the school when in 1894 Isabel was married to one of her admirers, Dr. Hunter Robb, and, as was the custom, retired from active nursing. (Letters of the time reveal the anger, dismay, and even sadness of her colleagues at her marriage. They were sure Dr. Robb was not nearly good enough for her, and besides, she was betraying nursing by robbing the profession of her talents.) Nevertheless, Isabel Hampton Robb maintained her interest in nursing and continued to be active in the development of the profession. In 1893, she had been appointed chairwoman of a committee to arrange a congress of nurses under the auspices of the International Congress of Charities, Correction, and Philanthropy at the Chicago World's Fair. There, before an international audience of nurses, she voiced her concern about poor nursing education and stated that the term *trained nurse* meant "anything, everything, or next to nothing" in the absence of educational standards. At the same time, Dock pointed out that the teaching, training, and discipline of nurses should not be provided at the discretion of medicine. Simi-

lar themes were reiterated in other papers, as well as the notion that there ought to be an organization of nurses. Shortly after the Congress, eighteen superintendents organized the American Society of Superintendents of Training Schools for Nursing (later to become the National League of Nursing Education) to promote the fellowship of members, establish and maintain a universal standard of training, and further the best interests of the nursing profession. The first convention of the society elected Linda Richards president.

Another attendee at those early meetings was Sophia Palmer, descendant of John and Priscilla Alden and a graduate of the Boston Training School, who, after a variety of experiences, organized a training school in Washington, D.C., over the concerted opposition of local physicians who wanted to control nursing education. She approved the steps that were taken but was impatient with what seemed to be blind acceptance of hospital control of schools. "She had a very intense nature and, like all those who are born crusaders, had little patience with the slower methods of persuasion....She was like a spirited racehorse held by the reins of tradition."[37] Within a short time, she and some of the others in the Society, including Dock and the new Mrs. Robb, recognized the need for another organization for all nurses. Although some of the training schools had alumnae associations, they were restrictive; in some cases, their own graduates could not be members, and any "outsider" could not participate. Therefore, if a nurse left the immediate vicinity of her own school, there was no way in which she had any organized contact with other nurses. In a paper given in 1895, Palmer stressed that the power of the nursing profession was dependent upon its ability to organize individuals who could influence public opinion. Dock also made recommendations for a national organization. In 1896, delegates representing the oldest training school alumnae associations and members of an organizing committee of the Society selected a name for the proposed organization—Nurses' Associated Alumnae of the United States and

Canada (to become the American Nurses Association in 1911), set a time and place for the first meeting (February 1897 in Baltimore), and drafted a constitution. At the end of that February meeting, held in conjunction with the fourth annual Society convention, the constitution and by-laws were adopted and Isabel Hampton Robb was elected president. Among the problems discussed at those early meetings were nursing licensure and the creation of an official nursing publication.

There were a number of nursing journals: the *British Journal of Nursing*, established by one of England's nursing leaders, Ethel Gordon Fenwick; and in the United States, the short-lived *The Nightingale*, started by a Bellevue graduate; *The Nursing Record* and *The Nursing World*, also short-lived; and *The Trained Nurse and Hospital Review*, which Palmer edited for a time, and which continued for seventy years. But the leaders of the new organizations wanted a magazine that would promote nursing, owned and controlled by nursing.

For several years there was discussion but no action, until another committee on the ways and means of producing a magazine was formed. In January 1900, they organized a stock company and sold $100 shares only to nurses and nurses' alumnae associations. By May, they had a promise of $2,400 in shares, and almost 500 nurses had promised to subscribe. Admittedly, they had overstepped their mandate, they reported to the third annual convention of the Nurses' Associated Alumnae, but they were given approval to establish the magazine along the lines formulated. The J. B. Lippincott Company was selected as publisher, and Sophia Palmer became editor, which she did on an unpaid basis for the first nine months. (She had become director of the Rochester City Hospital in New York.) As the first issue went for mailing in October, it was discovered that the post office rules prevented its being mailed because the journal's stockholders were not incorporated. M. E. P. Davis and Sophia Palmer assumed personal responsibilities for all liabilities of the new *American Journal of Nursing*, and it went out. The *Journal*

was considered the official organ of the nursing profession, but the stock was still held by alumnae associations and individual nurses. It was Lavinia Dock who donated the first share of stock to the association, and by 1912 the renamed American Nurses Association had gained ownership of all the stock of the American Journal of Nursing Company, which it still retains.[38]

One other major organization, the American Red Cross, was established by a nurse, Clara Barton, the school teacher who had volunteered as a nurse and directed relief operations during the Civil War. She also served with the German Red Cross during the Franco-Prussian War in 1870. (The establishment of the International Red Cross as a permanent international relief agency that could take immediate action in time of war had occurred in Geneva in 1864 with the signing of the Geneva Convention guidelines.) After her return to the United States, Barton organized the American Red Cross and persuaded Congress in 1882 to ratify the Treaty of Geneva so that the Red Cross could carry on its humanitarian efforts in peacetime. Clara Barton, however, was not an active part of the nursing leadership that was molding the profession.

That group had another immediate goal. The Society recognized that nurses were at a disadvantage because they had no postgraduate training in administration or teaching, so a committee consisting of Robb, Nutting, Richards, Mary Agnes Snively, and Lucy Drown was formed to investigate the possibilities. At the sixth Society convention, they reported their success. James Russell, the farsighted dean of Teachers College, Columbia University, in New York, had agreed to start a course for nurses if they could guarantee the enrollment of twelve nurses, or $1,000 a year. The Society agreed. Members of the Society screened the candidates, contributed $1,000 a year, and taught the course—hospital economics. Later, the students were also allowed to enroll in psychology, science, household economics, and biology. Anna Alline, one of the two graduates of the first class, then took over the total administration of the course.

There was one more major goal to be reached—licensure of nurses. Not only did the 432 hospital-based schools vary greatly in quality, but the market was also flooded with "nurses" who had been dismissed from schools without graduating, "nurses" from six-week private and correspondence courses, and a vast number of those who simply called themselves nurses. It was inevitable that people became confused, for when they hired nurses for private duty in their homes, the "nurse" could present one of the elaborate diplomas from a $13 correspondence course that guaranteed that anyone could become a nurse, a real or forged reference, or a genuine diploma from a top-quality school. How could they judge? Consequently, because of the abysmal care given by individuals representing themselves as nurses, the public was once more disenchanted with the "nurse." Therefore, nursing's leaders were determined that there must be legal regulation, both to protect the public from unscrupulous and incompetent nurses and to protect the young profession by establishing a minimum level of competence, limiting all or some of the professional functions to those who qualified. The idea was not new; medicine already had licensing in some states, and many aspiring professions were also moving in that direction.

In September 1901, at the first meeting of the newly formed International Council of Nurses, which was held in Buffalo, a resolution was passed, stating that "it is the duty of the nursing profession of every country to work for suitable legislative enactment regulating the education of nurses and protecting the interests of the public, by securing State examinations and public registration, with the proper penalties for enforcing the same."[39]

In the United States, such licensing was a state function, so to gain the necessary legislative lobbying power, it was recommended that state or local nurses' associations be formed. In many ways the disagreements that arose in their formation were the forerunners of those that would center on the licensure process. Who should be eligible? In New York, for instance, Sylveen Nye, who became the state association's first president, thought that *all* nurses should be included and that standards could be raised later. Sophia Palmer, another key figure in its formation, believed that only "qualified" nurses should be permitted to belong—those who graduate from certain types of schools. Later, the question was "Who should be eligible for licensure?"

As it was, New York had become the early leader in the licensure drive, for it had in place a Board of Regents that regulated education and licensure. In 1897, Palmer, in a smart political move, had already presented nursing's case to another emerging group of women who were gaining power and prestige—the New York Federation of Women's Clubs. They passed a resolution supporting her licensure concept, which included two major points—the need for a diploma from a school meeting certain standards, and insistence that the examining board consist only of nurses, as in other professions. Immediately Palmer organized a meeting with the secretary of the Board of Regents, who then and later was helpful and supportive, suggesting guidelines for action. (For instance, the licensed nurse needed to be called something. Among the titles suggested by nurses were *graduate nurse, trained nurse, certified nurse, registered nurse*, and *registered graduate nurse*.) The Regents also suggested the formation of a state nurses' association. Once formed, the New York State Nurses' Association developed a licensure bill and embarked on a campaign to gain support for the proposed legislation. Opposition was foreordained. In a circular addressed to the women's clubs, Palmer accurately pinpointed the sources:

The New York State Nurses' Association is preparing to apply for legislative enactments which will place training schools for nurses under the supervision of the Regents of the University of the State, with a view to securing by the authority of the law a minimum basis of education for the nurse, beyond which the safety of the sick and the protection of the public cannot be assured.

> While such a law cannot prevent the public from employing untaught women as nurses, if it so desires, it will prevent such women from imposing themselves upon the public as fully trained nurses.
>
> In this movement the Nurses' Association will meet with opposition: First, from the trained nurses of the State who are afraid to make an independent stand for their own and the public protection. Second, from all of the managers and proprietors of institutions which are not equipped for giving this minimum education, and which now conduct so-called training schools, for commercial advantages, and third, from all the vast army of so-called nurses who, without adequate nursing experience and education, undertake the grave responsibility of a nurse's work.[40]

And there was just that kind of opposition and more, for there were 15,000 untrained nurses in New York at the time, opposed to 2,500 who were trained. In addition, some physicians objected to their lack of representation on the proposed nursing board, as did some nurses, including Nye. Moreover, some physicians did not see the necessity for any fancy standards and worried about overeducation of nurses. Said one, "Nursing is not, strictly speaking, a profession. Any intelligent, not necessarily educated, woman can in a short time acquire the skill to carry out with explicit obedience the physician's directions."

Nevertheless, the bill became law on April 24, 1903. It was pitifully weak by today's standards, but daring for the times. Educational standards were set. A training school for nurses had to give at least a two-year program and be registered by the regents. The board of five nurses was to be chosen by the regents from a list submitted by the New York State Nurses' Association. The regents, on the advice of the board, were to make rules for the examination of nurses and to revoke licensure for cause. The New York State Nurses' Association was given the right to institute proceedings and prosecute those violating the law, a responsibility that was not changed for some years. It should be remembered, though, that this, like all nurse licensure laws in those times, was permissive, not mandatory. That is, only the RN title was pro-

tected. Untrained nurses could continue to work as nurses as long as they did not call themselves RNs.

New York was not the first state to register nurses. On March 3, 1903, North Carolina, and on April 1, 1903, New Jersey, had passed laws. It was said that both were inspired by New York's initiative. (Virginia followed New York on May 14.) However, New York's law was the strongest. For instance, New Jersey's law omitted a board of any kind; North Carolina had a mixed board of nurses and doctors and allowed a nurse to be licensed without attending a training school, if vouched for by a doctor. Partially because New York had the greatest number of trained nurses and because of the experience in regulation of the board of regents, the state's nurses were looked to as leaders in the further developments. The prestige, power, and authority of the board of regents was such that later many training schools in other states and other countries sought and received approval under New York's law—an action that also upgraded schools in those states. In fact, by 1906, more schools were registered outside the state than within it.

The enactment of the first nursing licensure laws was soon followed by like actions in other states; in a sense, it was the end of one era and the beginning of another. Nursing's leaders had shown themselves to be, as a whole, dedicated, strong, and remarkably bold. They set standards for nursing at a time when standards in long-established medicine were still quite weak. Despite internal dissension and the opposition of some powerful hospital administrators and physicians, they had had a licensing law passed—at a time when women had no vote. They literally created a young profession out of a woman's occupation. But the struggle to achieve full professionalism was far from over.

REFERENCES

1. Selavan IC: Nurses in American history: The revolution. *Am J Nurs* 75:592–594, April 1975.

2. Kalisch P, Kalisch B: *The Advance of American Nursing*, 2d ed. Boston: Little, Brown, 1986, p 79.
3. Kalisch P, Kalisch B: Untrained but undaunted: The women nurses of the blue and gray. *Nurs Forum* 15(1):25–26, 1976.
4. Parsons M: Mothers and matrons. *Nurs Outlook* 31:274–278, 1983.
5. Kalisch and Kalisch (1976), op cit, p 5.
6. Austin A: Nurses in American history—wartime volunteers—1861–1865. *Am J Nurs* 75:817, 1975.
7. Kalisch and Kalisch (1976), op cit, pp 15–16.
8. Bullough V, Bullough B: *The Care of the Sick: The Emergence of Modern Nursing*. New York: Prodist, 1978, p 113.
9. Dolan JA et al: *Nursing in Society: A Historical Perspective*, 15th ed. Philadelphia: Saunders, 1983, pp 176–177.
10. Ibid.
11. Carnegie M: *The Path We Tread: Blacks in Nursing 1854–1984*. Philadelphia: Lippincott, 1986, pp 6–11.
12. Kalisch and Kalisch (1976), op cit, p 27.
13. Dolan et al, op cit, p 194.
14. Ibid.
15. Kalisch and Kalisch (1986), op cit, p 88.
16. Dolan et al, op cit, p 206.
17. Kalisch and Kalisch (1986), op cit, pp 167–170.
18. Ibid, pp 135–136.
19. Dolan et al, op cit, pp 308–309.
20. Flaumenhaft E, Flaumenhaft C: American nursing's first text books. *Nurs Outlook* 37:185–188, July–August 1989.
21. Ingles T: The physician's view of the evolving nursing profession—1873–1913. *Nurs Forum* 15(2):123–164, 1976.
22. Ibid, p 148.
23. Bullough B, Bullough V: Sex discrimination in health care. *Nurs Outlook* 23:44, January 1975.
24. Ibid, p 148. Ingles, op cit, pp 139–140.
25. Kalisch B, Kalisch P: Slaves, servants, or saints: An analysis of the system of nurse training in the United States, 1873–1948. *Nurs Forum* 14(3):230–231, 1975.
26. Ibid.
27. Kalisch and Kalisch (1986), op cit, p 171.
28. Ibid, p 174.
29. Our first public health nurse—Lillian D. Wald. *Nurs Outlook* 19:660, 1971.
30. Kalisch and Kalisch (1986), op cit, pp 271–274.
31. Ibid, p 216.
32. Ibid, pp 217–220.
33. Flanagan L: *One Strong Voice: The Story of the American Nurses Association*. Kansas City, MO: American Nurses Association, 1976, p 292.
34. Nutting MA: Isabel Hampton Robb—Her work in organization and education. *Am J Nurs* 10:19, 1910.
35. Ashley JA: Nurses in American history: Nursing and early feminism. *Am J Nurs* 75:1466, September 1975.
36. Poslusny S: Feminist friendship: Isabel Hampton Robb, Lavinia Lloyd Dock and May Adelaide Nutting. *Image* 21:64–68, Summer 1989.
37. Christy T: Portrait of a leader: Sophia F. Palmer. *Nurs Outlook* 23:746–747, December 1975.
38. Flanagan, op cit, pp 35–38.
39. Kalisch and Kalisch (1986), op cit, p 292.
40. Shannon ML: The origin and development of professional licensure examination in nursing. Unpublished Ed.D. dissertation, Teachers College, Columbia University; 1972, pp 57–58.

The Emergence of the Modern Nurse, after 1904

THE PERIOD BETWEEN 1904 and 1965 was a time of multiple changes for nursing, many again precipitated by external forces, including the Depression, two world wars, and various social movements. But the changes were created within nursing by nurses. They included major shifts in education—type, location, curriculum, student body, and alterations in practice—responsibility, economic status, and degree of autonomy. In 1903, the passage of the first nursing licensure laws set standards for nursing education and practice; in 1965, development of new nursing roles and the American Nurses Association (ANA) position paper on nursing education opened the door for major revisions of those licensure laws and the emergence of the modern nurse.

NURSING BEFORE WORLD WAR I

After the licensure breakthrough, the leaders of nursing continued to look toward improvement of nurse training programs and, consequently, the improved practice of graduates of those programs. Most training schools remained under the control of hospitals, and the needs of the hospital superseded those of the school. For instance, it was not until 1912 that an occasional nurse received release time from hospital responsibilities in order to organize and teach basic nursing, and superintendents were warned not to "neglect" patient care in favor of the school or they would face punishment. There

was little support for improvement from physicians. Before the Flexner Report of 1910, the education of the physician, although different, was sometimes less organized than that of the nurse. In the 1870s few of the medical schools required high school diplomas and courses were completed in two years, whereas the nurses' program was being lengthened to three years. For the next 100 years, physicians complained of "overtrained nurses." Moreover, nursing was dominated by and primarily made up of women; it was not considered a profession, in part because it was not situated in an academic, collegiate setting. But to get into that setting as women, much less nurses, was a battle in itself. In essence, then, there were no major changes in the quality of education in the years that followed licensure, once those very limited standards were met. The hours were still long, and the students continued to give free service, with "book learning" as an afterthought.

The public, beginning to be aroused by poor conditions in factory sweatshops, showed surprisingly little interest in the exploitation of nursing students. Only in California, where an Eight-Hour Law for Women was passed in 1911, was there any movement to include student nurses (not even graduate nurses). Yet, when the bill was introduced in 1913, it was fought bitterly not only by hospitals, as might be expected, but also by physicians and nurses. No doubt, some were influenced by a sentiment voiced by physicians who were saying that nursing would be debased by being included in a law enforced by the State Bureau of Labor. Stated one physician to nurses, "The element of sacrifice is always present in true service. The service that costs no pains, no sacrifice, is without virtue, and usually without value." Retorted Lavinia Dock, "I think nurses should stand together solidly and resist the dictation of the medical profession in this as in all other things. Many MD's have a purely commercial spirit toward nurses…and would readily overwork them.…If necessary, do not hesitate to make alliances with the labor vote, for organized labor has quite as much of an 'ideal' as the MD's have, if not more."[1] Although the bill finally passed, thanks to the persistence of Senator Anthony Caminetti, delegations of hospital representatives and physicians went to the governor to ask him to withhold his signature. When he asked where the people were who favored the law, a woman reporter told him that *they* were in the hospitals caring for the sick and unable to plead their own cause; he signed.[2] But, for years, superintendents of nursing complained about the expense of hiring nurses who were now necessary to do the work students had done.

While the Flexner Report was bringing about reform in medical schools, eliminating the correspondence courses and the weaker and poorer schools, Adelaide Nutting and other leaders were agitating for reform in nursing education. In 1911, the American Society of Superintendents of Training Schools for Nurses presented a proposal for a similar survey of nursing schools to the Carnegie Foundation. Then President Pritchitt, stating that the foundation's energies were centered elsewhere and ignoring nursing, directed a considerable amount of the foundation funds in such studies for dental, legal, and teacher education.

Although women were having a little more success in being accepted in colleges and universities, there was only limited movement to make basic nursing programs an option in academic settings. Apparently, before 1900 there was a short-lived program at Howard University, but it was almost immediately taken over by Freedman's Hospital Nursing School. There is also some evidence that the School of Medicine at the University of Texas in 1896 "adopted" a hospital school of nursing to prevent its closing for lack of funds. However, the University of Minnesota program, founded in 1909 by Dr. Richard Olding Beard, a physician who was dedicated to the concept of higher education for nurses, became the first enduring baccalaureate program in nursing. Even this was more similar to good diploma programs than other university programs. Although eventually the students had to meet university admission standards and took some specialized courses, they also worked a 56-hour week in the hospital and were awarded a diploma instead of a degree after three years. Similar programs were started by other universities which took over hospital schools or started new ones, in part to obtain student services for their hospitals. Just prior to World War I, several hospitals and universities, such as Presbyterian Hospital of New York and Teachers College, offered degree options. These developed into 5-year programs with 2 years of college work and 3 years in a diploma school. This became a common pattern that lasted through the 1940s, but in 1916, when Annie Goodrich reported that 16 colleges and universities maintained schools, departments, or courses in nursing education, they were an assortment of educational hybrids.

Nursing practice had also not developed to any extent, with most graduate nurses still doing private duty in homes. A nurse, unless she became the favorite of one or more doctors who liked her work, found her cases through registries, established by alumnae associations, hospitals, medical societies, or commercial agencies. The first two frequently limited the better jobs to their graduates; commercial agencies not only charged the nurse a fee but did not distinguish between trained and untrained nurses. Finally, a county nurses' association gained control of a registry in Minnesota in 1904, and others followed. Nevertheless, private duty was an individual enterprise, with long hours, no benefits, and limited pay. (In 1926, some nurses were still working a 24-hour day at what averaged out to 49 cents an hour, less than cleaning women made.)

However, in 1915, it is estimated, no more than 10 percent of the sick received care in the hospitals, and the majority of people could not afford private duty nurses. From this need, a public health movement emerged that increased the demand for nurses. At first most of these nurses concentrated on bedside care, but others, like those coming from the settlement houses, took broader responsibilities. Nevertheless, there were no recognized standards or requirements for visiting nurses. Therefore, in June 1912, a small group of visiting nurses, representing unofficially some 900 agencies and almost four times that many colleagues, founded the National Organization for Public Health Nursing (NOPHN), with Lillian Wald as the first president. It was an organization of nurses and lay people engaged in public health nursing and in the organization, management, and support of such work. The leaders of the group selected the term *public health nursing* as more inclusive than *visiting nursing*; it was also reminiscent of Nightingale's health nursing, which had focused on prevention. One of its first goals was to extend the services to working and middle-class people as well as to the poor.

Changes had also occurred in the first two nursing organizations. In 1911, the Associated Alumnae changed its name to the American Nurses Association (ANA) and in 1912, the Society of Superintendents adopted the name National League of Nursing Education (NLNE).

The Visiting Nurse Quarterly, the first American publication dealing exclusively with public health nursing, was offered to the NOPHN by its founder, the Cleveland Visiting Nurse Association. It became *Public Health Nursing*, the official journal of NOPHN until 1952–1953, when it was absorbed by *Nursing Outlook*. Also in 1912, the Red Cross established the Rural Nursing Service. Wald, at a major meeting on infant mortality, had cited the horrible health conditions of rural America, the high infant and maternal mortality rates, the preva-

lence of tuberculosis, and other serious health problems, and suggested that the Red Cross operate a national service, similar to that of Great Britain. Later, the name was changed to Town and Country Nursing Service in order to include small towns that had no visiting nurse service, and it was headquartered in Washington. Although the Service provided nurses to care for the sick, do health teaching, and otherwise improve health conditions, it was not wholly successful. Many communities did not choose to call in a national organization for assistance or could not afford the salaries of the nurses. (For a while, a wealthy woman contributed financial support to salaries, but withdrew funds because the rural nurses were not "ladies.") Nevertheless, the rural nurses carried on and proved to be a remarkably resourceful group, coping with an almost total lack of ordinary supplies and equipment. The service survived primarily because the Metropolitan Life Insurance Company decided to use rural nurses for services to their policyholders, for many local Red Cross chapters had no interest in or understanding of the service. (Red Cross involvement gradually decreased until, with increased government involvement in public health, it discontinued the program altogether in 1947.)

By 1916, public health nurses were being called on to be welfare workers, sanitarians, housing inspectors, and health teachers as well. A number of universities began offering courses to help prepare nurses to fulfill this multifaceted role, and Mary Gardner, one of the founders of NOPHN and an interim director of the Rural Nursing Service, authored the first book in the field, *Public Health Nursing*. One of the observations she made was that although broad-minded physicians recognized that public health nurses helped them produce results that would not have been possible alone, the more conservative feared interference by nurses and were resentful of them. She noted that a service had a better chance of success if it was started with the cooperation of the medical profession, and pointed out ways nurses could avoid friction with physicians and still be protected from the incompetents.

Another outstanding public health nurse of that period was Margaret Higgins Sanger. She became interested in the plight of the poorly paid industrial workers, particularly the women. Herself married with three children when she decided to return to work in public health, she was assigned to maternity cases on the Lower East Side of New York, where she found that pregnancy, often unwanted, was a chronic condition among the women. One of her patients died from a repeated self-abortion, after begging doctors and nurses for information on how to avoid pregnancy. That was apparently a turning point for Sanger. After she learned everything she could about contraception, she and her sister, also a nurse, opened the first birth control clinic in America in Brooklyn. She was arrested and spent 30 days in the workhouse, but continued her crusade.[3] She fought the battle for free dissemination of birth control information for decades, against all types of opposition, until today, birth control education is generally accepted as the right of women and one nursing role.

A new specialty for nurses that endured was anesthesia. In 1893, Isabel Robb mentioned this in her textbook, and apparently religious sisters gave anesthesia as early as 1877 in Catholic hospitals. However, the Mayo brothers trained two sisters who were nurses to take over these duties at Mayo Clinic. (Their friend, Alice Magaw, who succeeded them was recognized for her brilliant work and is considered the "Mother of Anesthesia.")[4] The Mayos found a nurse more useful than an intern who was also trying to learn surgery. In 1909, a course for nurse anesthetists was established in Oregon, as were others, and these nurses were promptly as exploited by the hospitals as their sisters. It was not until 1917 that the question was officially raised of whether nurse anesthetists were practicing medicine, and it was ruled then that they were not, if paid and supervised by a physician. However, the legal answer was murky for more than sixty years, and the education of nurse anesthe-

tists remained under the control of hospitals and doctors.

NURSES AT WAR

World War I was different from other wars fought by the United States, because of both its international proportions and the kinds of weapons that were used. Immediately, the demand for nurses was increased. The Army Nurse Corps expanded greatly, as did the Navy Nurse Corps (although to a lesser extent). As the war continued, recruitment standards dropped, and applicants were accepted from nursing schools attached to hospitals with fewer than 100 beds. All nurses needed was certification of moral character and professional qualifications by their superintendent of nurses—and, of course, they had to be unmarried. Once more, untrained society girls were clamoring to be Red Cross volunteer nurses, without knowing what training was required or being willing to accept it. Afraid that Army nursing would fall into untrained hands, as it had in Europe, Nutting, Goodrich, Wald, and others formed a Committee on Nursing to devise "the wisest methods of meeting the present problems connected with the care of the sick and injured in hospitals and homes; the educational problems of nursing; and the extraordinary emergencies as they arise."[5] Some weeks later, the committee was given governmental status and limited financial backing; most funds were contributions from nursing. The committee was able to estimate the number of available nurses and those in training, but, obviously, these were insufficient for both military and civilian needs.

The American Red Cross served as the unofficial reserve corps of the Army Nurse Corps. When these nurses, as well as those who were part of total multidisciplinary base units originating in hospitals, went to Europe, the home situation became desperate. Recruiting efforts were stepped up, first to attract educated women into nursing and then to encourage schools of nursing to somehow increase their capacity, even if it meant the unheard of—having local students live at home for part of their training. Interestingly enough, even though there were male nurses, and they did volunteer, they were usually put in regular fighting units and their skills went unused. Neither, apparently, did the Army choose to use black nurses. Only in mid-1917 would the Red Cross accept them, and then only if the Army Surgeon General agreed. Their eventual acceptance is credited to the efforts of Adah Thom, a black nurse.

Even with the patriotic fervor generated by the war, it was not easy to entice young women into nursing. High school students, queried about their interest in nursing, objected to the life of drudgery, strenuous physical work, poor education, severe discipline, lack of freedom and recreation as a student, and what they saw as limited satisfactory options of employment. However, schools did increase their capacity some 25 percent, and the pressures of the war brought about some educational changes. One of the more daring experiments of the times was the Vassar Training Camp.[6] The idea came from a Vassar alumna and member of the board of trustees, to establish at Vassar in the summer of 1918 a preparatory course in nursing, from which the students would move to selected schools of nursing to complete the program in little more than two additional years. As attested to by graduates of the program, it was the spirit of patriotism that attracted more than 400 young women aged 14 to 40, schooled in many professional fields, and representing more than 100 colleges. They were to be known as Vassar's Rainbow Division because the students wore the various colored student uniforms of the schools they had selected. A large percentage of the women completed the program and entered the nursing schools they had selected, and many of nursing's leaders arose from this group. Soon, five other universities opened similar prenursing courses and also admitted high school students. Because these programs were generally of considerably higher quality than those of the training schools, the movement of nursing education toward an academic setting received another nudge.

Meanwhile, nursing conditions in American military camps were reported as atrocious, and the Committee on Nursing convinced the Surgeon General to appoint Annie Goodrich to evaluate the quality of nursing service. Miss Goodrich, then an assistant professor at Teachers College, had had experience inspecting training schools for New York State. She minced no words in her report—conditions were much worse than in civilian hospitals, because there were not enough nurses to care for the patients, and they found it impossible to deal with a constantly changing group of disinterested corpsmen. Goodrich recommended that nurse training schools be set up in each military hospital, where the students, under careful supervision, would give better care than aides or corpsmen. The suggested Army School of Nursing was to be centralized in the Surgeon General's Office under the supervision of a dean. After some dispute, but with the support of the nursing organizations and influential Frances Payne Bolton of Cleveland, the Army School was approved in May 1918, with Annie Goodrich appointed Dean. The 3-year course was based on the new *Standard Curriculum for Schools of Nursing*, published by the National League of Nursing Education. Unlike civilian hospitals, duty hours did not exceed 6 to 8 hours. The military hospitals provided all medical and surgical experience, and gynecology, obstetrics, diseases of children, and public health were provided through affiliations in the second and third year. The response to the school was overwhelming, and it attracted many more students than it could accommodate.

The service of the nurse in the nightmarish battle conditions of World War I, coping with the mass casualties, dealing with injuries caused by the previously unknown shrapnel and gas, and then battling influenza at home and abroad, is a fascinating and proud piece of nursing history.

BETWEEN THE WARS

In the twenty-three years between World Wars I and II, nursing was affected by the Great Depression and adoption of the Nineteenth Constitutional Amendment in August 1920, granting women the right to vote. Of the two, the latter had less immediate impact. Nurses showed relatively little interest in fighting for women's rights, and only one, Lavinia Dock, can be called an active feminist. "Dockie" was a maverick of the times. A tiny woman who loved music and was an accomplished pianist and organist, she also seemed to take on the whole world in her battle for the underdog. Early on, she decided that nurses could have no power unless they had the vote. Her speeches and writings were brilliant, but she did not move her colleagues. Nevertheless, she devoted a good part of her life to working for women's rights. In England, she joined the Pankhursts and landed in jail. Back in the United States, she picketed the White House, seizing the nearest, if not most appropriate, banner, "Youth to the Colors" (she was almost sixty then). Wrote her colleague, Isabel Stewart, "They all went into the cooler for the night. I think it just pleased her no end."[7]

For all her devotion to women's rights, Dock remained committed to nursing. She was editor of the *Journal*'s Foreign Department from 1900 to 1923, during which she quarreled regularly with Editor Sophia Palmer and managed to ignore World War I because she was a pacifist. She was also involved with the International Council of Nurses and was the author of a number of books, including *Health and Morality* in 1910, in which she discussed venereal disease. She was equally outspoken on the forbidden subject in open meetings. A number of nurses had become infected because physicians frequently refused to tell nurses when patients had the disease. Dock also regularly castigated her profession for withholding its interest, sympathy, and moral support from "the great, urgent throbbing, pressing social claims of our day and generation."[8]

But nursing had problems of its own. Immediately after the war, there was a shortage of nurses, because many who had switched careers "for the duration" returned to their own field, and others appeared not to be attracted. In part,

it was an image problem, one that was to continue to haunt nursing (see Chap. 11), but another quite real aspect was that nursing education was in trouble. As Isabel Stewart said, "The plain facts are that nursing schools are being starved and always have been starved for lack of funds to build up any kind of substantial educational structure."[9] Later, this problem was clearly pinpointed by a prestigious committee. In 1918, Nutting had approached the Rockefeller Foundation to seek endowment for the Johns Hopkins School of Nursing, stressing the need for improvement in the education of public health nurses. The meeting resulted in a committee to investigate the "proper training" of public health nurses, an investigation that quickly concluded that the problem was nursing education in general. The findings of the Goldmark Report (presented in more detail in Chap. 5) concluded that schools of nursing needed to be recognized and supported as separate educational components with not just training in nursing, but also a liberal education. Although the report had little immediate impact, it did result in Rockefeller Foundation support for the founding of the Yale School of Nursing (1924), the first in the world to be established as a separate university department with its own dean, Annie Goodrich. Although a few other such programs followed, progress lagged, for many powerful physicians reached the public media with their notions that nurses needed only technical skills, manual dexterity, and quick obedience to the physician. Charles Mayo, for instance, deciding that city-trained nurses were too difficult to handle, too expensive, and spent too much time getting educated, wanted to recruit 100,000 country girls.[10] But even popular journals recognized that student nurses were being exploited by hospitals and that the kind of student being encouraged into nursing by school principals was one seen as not too bright, not attractive enough to marry, and too poor to be supported at home.

A study following close on the heels of the Goldmark Report soon reaffirmed the inadequacy of nursing schools and practicing nurses.

Nurses, Patients, and Pocketbooks (see Chap. 5) pointed out that the hasty postwar nurse-recruiting efforts had not improved the lot of the patient or nurse; in 1928, problems included an oversupply of nurses, geographic maldistribution, low educational standards, poor working conditions, and some critically unsatisfactory levels of care.

How could education be so poor with licensure in effect? Ten years after the passage of the first acts, 38 states had also passed such laws, but all were permissive, and although the title RN was protected, others could designate themselves nurses and work. The first mandatory law was passed in New York in 1938 and implemented in 1944. At one point, Annie Goodrich cited a correspondence school that had turned out 12,000 "graduates" in ten years. In addition, hospital schools of all sizes felt no need to meet standards that might deprive them of free student labor. Even those schools that chose to follow state board standards found them not too difficult, and follow-up was almost totally absent; most were approved on the basis of paper credentials. The states that did employ nurse "inspectors" ran into problems in withholding approval; members of the boards of nurse examiners were frequently as poorly qualified as the heads of schools, and the political pressures to avoid embarrassing hospitals were overwhelming.

Even in New York State, where the state board was considered a model, the pressures and responsibilities of board members who also held jobs were unbelievable. They not only wrote all licensing examination questions, but corrected all the papers and traveled throughout the state to give the practical exams. Writing about grading the lengthy open-ended questions, one board member complained, "The monotony is horrible; it stultifies the brain and one finds it impossible to work long at a sitting. So tiresome is it that one welcomes the diversion of a stupid answer."[11] By 1940, New York board members were each forced to grade 1,994 tests as well as the practicals. Not until 1943 were exams scored by machine. Aside from grading

fatigue, neither the test-writing skills of the authors nor the state of the art of testing gave any assurance that state boards guaranteed minimum levels of safe and effective practice for the newly licensed practitioner. Many nursing leaders were calling for grading of training schools as a starting point, but the Depression aborted any such action, although there were continued efforts to strengthen the licensing laws.

Unemployment after the stock market crash of 1929 also affected nursing. People who had no jobs could not afford private-duty nurses. It was estimated that 8,000 to 10,000 graduate nurses were out of work, and notices warning nurses not to come to find work in specific areas became frequent in the *Journal*. A 1932 campaign by the ANA to promote an eight-hour day for nurses, hiring of nurses by hospitals, and discontinuance of some nursing schools met a cold reception. Even though they complained of the cost of training students, hospital administrators clung to the schools, perhaps because, despite financial figures to the contrary, students were obviously an economic asset. If one compared what the American Hospital Association said the students gave to hospitals in service—$1,000—with an average of 7,000 hours that the students gave—the hospital seemed to be crediting their contribution at about fourteen cents an hour. This was of questionable accuracy at best.[12] However, even directors of nursing showed a reluctance to hire graduate nurses, and 73 percent of hospitals employed no graduates at all on floor duty. By 1933, the desperate straits of unemployed nurses finally forced many to work in hospitals for room and board. Even then, although some administrators believed this was taking advantage of unfortunate nurses, others thought that they were not worth food and lodging.

Some help finally came with the Roosevelt Administration, when relief funds were allocated for bedside care of the indigent and nurses were employed as visiting nurses under the Federal Relief Administration (FERA). Ten thousand unemployed nurses were put to work in numerous settings under the Civil Work Administration (CWA) in public hospitals, clinics, public health agencies, and other health services. The follow-up Works Progress Administration (WPA) then continued to provide funds for nurses in community health activities. A few nurses also entered a new field that opened— airline stewardess.

By 1936, the number of diploma nursing schools had decreased from more than 2,200 in 1929 to a little less than 1,500 state-accredited programs. There were about 70 "collegiate" programs, most merely of the liberal arts plus hospital school pattern. Many were still floundering. At this point the NLNE presented its third revision of the *Curriculum Guide for Schools of Nursing*, with input from thousands of nurses around the country. A guide that was to endure (probably beyond its optimum usefulness), its major assumptions were that the primary function of the school was to educate the nurse and that the community to be served extended beyond the hospital. Numbers of academic and clinical hours as well as content were suggested.

An obvious problem was the lack of qualified teachers; even in so-called university programs, nurses did not meet the usual requirements for teaching. One outcome was that baccalaureate programs for diploma nurses began to offer specialized degrees in education, administration, or public health nursing. The other was a very slow movement to graduate education. For years, most of the graduate degrees held by nurses were in education, in part because Teachers College and other universities began to accept baccalaureate graduates for graduate preparation in education. In fact, some of the greatest leaders in nursing education either graduated from Teachers College or held teaching positions there. One such was Isabel Stewart, who arrived in 1908 for one semester and stayed for thirty-nine years.[13] She succeeded M. Adelaide Nutting, who was the first nurse ever to receive a professorship in a university (1910) and who remained until 1925.[14] As early as 1932, Catholic University offered graduate courses in nurs-

ing, but that was uncommon. Apparently, the first, or nearly first, nurse to earn a doctoral degree was Edith S. Bryan; it was in psychology and counseling from Johns Hopkins.

Another slow starter in American nursing was nurse-midwifery. In the 1920s, legislation such as the Sheppard-Tanner Act paid for nurses to give maternity and infant care, but nurse-midwives were not included. Still, a considerable amount of maternity care, particularly deliveries, was done by lay midwives, some competent, some dangerously incompetent. When, in 1925, Mary Breckenridge founded the Frontier Nursing Service (FNS) in rural Kentucky, its staff was a mix of British nurse-midwives and American nurses trained in midwifery in Britain. (The rule was that if the husband could reach the nurse, the nurse could make it back to the patient by some means.) The outstanding services of the nurses on horseback (later in jeeps), who gradually increased their services to include other aspects of primary care, is an ongoing success story.[15] The FNS also founded one of the early nurse-midwifery schools (1936); the first was at the maternity center of New York City in 1932. Also formed was a professional association (see Chap. 27).

Of all the entrants into nursing, two groups got particularly short shrift—men and blacks. The prejudice against men was specifically related to nursing and persisted to some extent for some time. As the distorted image of the female nurse evolved, men did not seem to fit the concepts held by powerful figures in and out of nursing. Therefore, although men graduated from acceptable nursing schools, usually totally male, and attempted to become active members of the ANA, even forming a men's section, their numbers and influence remained small until the post-World War II era.

Black nurses, on the other hand, were caught in the overall common prejudice against their race. Individual black nurses, as noted earlier, broke down barriers in various nursing fields. As early as 1908, they organized the National Association of Colored Graduate Nurses (NACGN), both to fight against discriminatory practices and to foster leadership among black nurses. Although the ANA had a nondiscriminatory policy, some state organizations did not and a rule that the nurse must have graduated from a state-approved school to be an ANA member eliminated even more black nurses. Finally, in 1951, the NACGN was absorbed into the ANA, which required nondiscrimination for all state associations as a prerequisite for ANA affiliation. In 1924, it was reported that only 58 state-accredited schools admitted blacks, and most of these were located in black hospitals or in departments caring for black patients in municipal hospitals. Of these schools, 77 percent were located in the South; 28 states offered no opportunities in nursing education for black women. Most of the "schools" that trained black nurses were totally unacceptable, and many of those approved barely met standards. Moreover, there were some 23,000 untrained black midwives in the South, but no one made the effort to combine training in nursing and midwifery, which would have been a distinct service. In 1930, there were fewer than 6,000 graduate black nurses, most of whom worked in black hospitals or public health agencies that served black patients. Opportunities in other fields either were not open to them or could not admit them because they did not, understandably, have the advanced preparation necessary. Middle-class black women were usually not attracted to nursing, because teaching and other available fields offered more prestige and better opportunities. It was not until a 1941 Executive Order, and the corresponding follow-through, that any part of the federal government made any effort to investigate grievances and redress complaints of blacks. The subsidized Cadet Nurse Corps of World War II also proved to be a boon for black nurses. Of the schools participating, 20 were all-black and enrolled 600 black students; the remaining 400 were distributed among 22 integrated schools. However, it was clear that approved black schools were being held to lower standards for a variety of reasons, some political. There were also overt and covert methods in the North and South to pre-

vent the more able black nurses from assuming leadership positions—some as simple as advancing the least aggressive. And for all the desperate need for nurses, the armed forces balked at accepting and integrating black nurses. Not until the end of the war and after some aggressive action by the NACGN and the National Nursing Council for War Service did this change.[16]

THE EFFECTS OF WORLD WAR II

Not just black nurses but nurses in general found that the exigencies of World War II created new opportunities, freedom, and also problems for nurses that proved to be long-lasting. As usual in wartime, nurses were in demand in the armed services. There were not enough nurses for both the home front and the battlefield, even with stepped-up efforts to encourage women to enter nursing programs. Finally, legislation was passed in 1943 establishing the Cadet Nurse Corps. The Bolton Act, the first federal program to subsidize nursing education for school and student, was a forerunner of future federal aid to nursing. For payment of their tuition and a stipend, students committed themselves to engage in essential military or civilian nursing for the duration of the war. The students had to be between 17 and 35 years old, in good health, and with a good academic record in an accredited high school. This new law brought about several changes in nursing. For instance, it forbade discrimination on the basis of race and marital status and set minimum educational standards. The first, theoretically accepted, was not always implemented in good faith. The second, combined with the requirement that nursing programs be reduced from the traditional 36 months to 30, forced nursing schools to reassess and revise their curricula.

Two other major efforts to relieve the nursing shortage had long-range effects in the practice setting. One was the recruitment of inactive nurses back into the field. For the first time, married women and others who could work only on a part-time basis became acceptable to employers and later became a part of the labor pool. The other change was the training of volunteer nurse's aides. Although such training was initiated by the Red Cross in 1919, it was discouraged later by nurses, particularly during the Depression. During World War II, both the Red Cross and the Office of Civilian Defense trained more than 20,000 aides. At first, they were used only for nonnursing tasks, but the increasing nurse shortage forced them to take on basic nursing functions. After the war, with a continued shortage, trained aides were hired as a necessary part of the nursing service department. Their perceived cost-effectiveness stimulated the growth of both aide and practical nurse training programs and eventually increased federal funding for both.[17]

Finally, major changes occurred within the armed forces. Nurses had held only relative rank, meaning that they carried officers' titles but had less power and pay than their male counterparts. In 1947, full commissioned status was granted, giving them the right to manage nursing care. At the same time, as noted previously, discrimination against black nurses ended but, oddly enough, in the male-controlled armed services, it was not until 1954 that male nurses were admitted to full rank as officers.

As in all previous wars, nurses proved themselves able and brave in military situations. Many were in battle zones and some became Japanese prisoners of war. Their stories have been told in films, books, plays, and historical nursing research, and are well worth reading. (See bibliography.)

TOWARD A NEW ERA

The usual postwar nurse shortage occurred after World War II, but this time for different reasons. Only one of six Army nurses planned to return to her civilian job, finding more satisfaction in the service. Poor pay and unpleasant working conditions discouraged civilian nurses as well. In 1946, the salary for a staff nurse was about $36 for a 48-hour work week, less than

that for typists or seamstresses (much less men). Salaries were supposed to be kept secret, and hospitals, particularly, held them at a minimum, with such peculiarities as a staff nurse earning more than a head nurse. Split shifts were common, with nurses scheduled to work from seven to eleven and from three to seven, with time off between the two shifts. The work was especially difficult because staffing was short and nurses worked under rigid discipline. It was small wonder that in one survey only about 12 percent of the nurses queried planned to make nursing a career; more than 75 percent saw it as a pin-money job after marriage, or planned to retire altogether as soon as possible. Unions were beginning to organize nurses, so in 1949 the ANA approved state associations as collective bargaining agents for nurses. However, because the Taft-Hartley Act excluded nonprofit institutions from collective bargaining, hospitals and agencies did not need to deal with nurses. In addition, the ANA no-strike pledge took away another powerful weapon.

As noted previously, one answer that administrators saw was the hiring of nurse's aides. The use of volunteers and auxiliary help—that is, anyone other than licensed or trained nurses, practical nurses, aides, or orderlies—increased tremendously.

One group of workers that proliferated in the postwar era was practical nurses, defined by ANA, NLNE, and NOPHN as those trained to care for subacute, convalescent, and chronic patients under the direction of a physician or nurse. Thousands who designated themselves as practical nurses had no such skills, and their training was simply in caring for their own families, or, at most, aide work. Whereas the first school for training practical nurses appeared in 1897, by 1930 there were only 11, and in 1947, still only 36. With the new demand for nurse substitutes, 260 more practical nurse schools opened by 1954, mostly in hospitals or long-term care institutions, and a few in vocational schools. Aiding the movement was funding from federal vocational education acts. There were, unfortunately, also a number of correspondence courses and other commercialized programs that did little more than expose the student to some books and manuals and present her with a diploma. By 1950, there were 144,000 practical nurses, 95 percent of them women, and, although their educational programs varied, their on-the-job activities expanded greatly—to doing whatever nurses had no time to do. By 1952, some 56 percent of the nursing personnel were nonprofessionals, and some nurses began to fear that they were being replaced by less expensive, minimally trained workers.

Nevertheless, with working and financial conditions not improving, the nursing shortage persisted. Soon a team plan was developed with a nurse as a team leader, primarily responsible for planning patient care, and less prepared workers carrying it out. Although the plan persisted for years, it did little to improve patient care; rather, it kept the nurse mired in paper work, away from the patient or required to make constant medication rounds. Often practical nurses carried the primary responsibilities for patient units on the evening and night shift, with the few nurses available stretched thin, "supervising" these workers.

There were more nurses than ever at mid-century, but there were also tremendously expanded health services, a greater population to be served, growth of various insurance plans that paid for hospital care, a postwar baby boom with in-hospital deliveries, new medical discoveries that kept patients alive longer, and a proliferation of nurses into other areas of health care. Hospitals still weren't the most desirable places to work, and economic benefits were slow in coming. Moreover there were now more married nurses who chose to stay home to raise families. Studies done in 1941, 1944, and 1948 (see Chap. 5), all of which pointed out some of the economic and status problems of nurses, particularly in hospitals, went largely ignored.

When the Korean War broke out in 1950, the Army again drew nurses from civilian hospitals, this time from their reserve corps. War nursing on the battlefront was centered to an extent on the Mobile Army Surgical Hospitals (MASH), located as close to the front lines as possible. Flight nurses, who helped to evacuate the wounded from the battlefront to military hospitals, also achieved recognition. When that war was over and nurse reservists returned to their civilian jobs, it is possible that their experiences increased their discontent with working situations at home.

This was also a period of great medical and scientific discoveries, and physicians became increasingly dependent on hospitals for supportive services. As physicians cured or prolonged the lives of patients, the corollary care required of nurses became more complex. It was not just a matter of patient comfort, but crucial life-and-death judgment. In the 1950s, Frances Reiter began to write about the nurse clinician, a nurse who gave skilled nursing care on an advanced level. This concept developed into the clinical specialist (see Chap. 15), a nurse with a graduate degree and specialized knowledge of nursing care, who worked as a colleague of physicians. At the same time, the development of coronary and other intensive care units called for nurses with equally specialized technical knowledge, formerly the sole province of medical practice. In Colorado in 1965, a physician, in collaboration with a school of nursing, was pioneering another new role for nurses in ambulatory care. As the nurses easily assumed responsibility for well-child care and minor illnesses, they called upon their nursing knowledge and skills as well as a medical component. What emerged was the "nurse practitioner" (see Chap. 15).

Nursing education was also going through a transition period in those decades. In the years immediately after World War II, the quality of nursing education was under severe criticism. There was no question that in the diploma schools, where most nurses were educated, there were frequently poor levels of teaching, inadequately prepared teachers, and a major dependence on students for services; often two-thirds of the hours of care were given by students.

The Brown report in 1948 and a follow-up study in 1950 (see Chap. 5) that attempted to implement that report made it clear that nursing education was anything but professional. It was on the basis of findings of the latter report that national accreditation for nursing by nurses was strengthened. With the reorganization of the nursing organizations, the National League for Nursing (NLN) assumed the responsibility for all accrediting functions in nursing. Dr. Helen Nahm, director of the accrediting service for the first 7 years, saw it as the culmination of all previous efforts to raise education standards—and as a last chance. Those schools that chose to go through the voluntary process and met the standards were placed on a published list, which for the first time gave the public, guidance counselors, and potential students some notion of the quality of one school compared with another. Eventually, accreditation proved a significant force in improving good schools and closing poor ones (although it has also been accused of rigidity throughout the years).

An impetus for collegiate nursing education was an advisory service funded by the Russell Sage Foundation for institutions of higher learning that were interested in enriching and improving their programs. The 1953 report by Dr. Margaret Bridgman, "Collegiate Education for Nursing," helped to stimulate baccalaureate nursing programs to improve academically. In many cases, they were still quite similar to diploma programs, whose quality had improved considerably in the 1950s. The slow rate of growth of collegiate programs resulted in part from the uncertainty of nursing about what these programs should be and how they should differ from diploma education and in part from the anticollegiate faction in nursing that saw no point in higher education—a faction that was cheered and nurtured by a large number of physicians and administrators. At times, it seemed to be a moot question whether any nurses were necessary. A postwar survey of the American College of Surgeons indicated that the vast majority believed, with few exceptions, that the needs of the sick could be met by nurse's aides or, at most, by practical nurses,

and administrators were not averse to the "cheap is best" concept.

Introduction of a different kind of nurse was a startling breakthrough. The development of the nurse technician in community colleges was the most dramatic change in nursing education since its beginning. Based on a study by Dr. Mildred Montag at Teachers College, and funded by the W. K. Kellogg Foundation, pilot programs were established in a number of sites around the country in 1952. It was an idea whose time had come, for not only were community colleges the most rapidly expanding educational entities of the time, but the late bloomer, the mature man and woman, and the less affluent student found this opportunity for a career in nursing and a college degree highly desirable. Follow-up studies showed that these nurses performed well in what they were prepared to do—provide care at the intermediate level in the continuum of nursing functions as defined by Montag. It was probably partially the influence of the associate degree (AD) programs, which were nondiscriminatory and generally nonpaternalistic in their relations with students, that helped loosen the tight restrictions on nursing students' personal lives in both diploma and some baccalaureate programs. Still, even into the late 1960s, some diploma schools excluded married students and men. The growth of AD programs ultimately outran all others in nursing except practical nurse programs.

Graduate education for nurses progressed slowly. Most degrees continued to be in education, in part because of the great shortage of teachers of nursing with graduate degrees and in part because graduate schools of education had part-time programs. In 1953, only 36 percent of nursing faculties had earned master's degrees, and some had no degree at all. In 1954, it was estimated that 20 percent of the positions held by nurses should require master's degrees and at least 30 percent baccalaureate degrees. Yet, only 1 percent of all nurses held master's and about 7 percent baccalaureate degrees, many not in nursing.

Part of the problem, of course, was financial and, although private foundations, such as the Commonwealth Fund, provided some support for graduate education, federal funding made the crucial difference. It also controlled the direction of nursing education. Its funding for the study of public health nursing from 1936 on created more baccalaureate-prepared nurses in public health than in any other field; its support of psychiatric nursing increased the volume of nurses educated in that field. In 1956, the passage of the Federal Nurse Traineeship Act, which authorized funds for financial aid to registered nurses for full-time study to prepare for teaching, supervision, and administration in all fields, opened the door for advanced education for nurses at both the baccalaureate and graduate levels. Short-term traineeships also provided for continuing education programs. Another boost was the 1963 Surgeon General's Report (see Chap. 5) that specifically pointed out differences in the quality and quantity of nurses and their education and recommended both recruitment and advanced education. Following this, there was a new surge of federal aid to nursing. Nurse Traineeship programs continued to be enacted until the present, although the struggle for funds, depending on the administration, was sometimes most difficult (see Chaps. 12 and 19).

Master's programs for nurses still tended to focus on administration or education even in schools of nursing, and not until the 1960s did clinical programs develop. Clinical doctoral programs in nursing were almost nonexistent until the 1960s.

Nursing research also tended to take a slow path. Although there were studies of nursing service, nursing education, and nursing personality, most were done with or by social scientists. When nurses assisted physicians and others in medical research, it was just that—assisting. Nursing leaders realized that nursing could not develop as a profession unless clinical research focusing on nursing evolved. One of the first major steps in that direction was the 1952 publication of *Nursing Research*, a scholarly journal that reported and encouraged nursing research. The other was the ANA's establishment of the American Nurses' Foundation in 1955 for charitable, educational, and scientific purposes. The Foundation conducts studies, surveys, and research, funds nurse researchers and others, and publishes scientific reports. In 1956, the federal government also began to fund nursing research. Federal support in the 1960s provided research training through doctoral programs, including the nurse scientist program, and funding for individual and collaborative research efforts.

In all these changes, it can be seen that the professional organizations of nursing had varied influence. At the same time, as organizations, they too were examining their roles and relationships. A study to consider restructuring, reorganizing, and unifying the various organizations was initiated shortly after World War II. In 1952, the six major nursing organizations—ANA, NLNE, NOPHN, NACGN, the Association of Collegiate Schools of Nursing (ACSN), and the American Association of Industrial Nurses (AAIN)—finally came to a decision about organizational structure. Two major organizations emerged, the ANA, with only nurse members, and the renamed National League for Nursing, with nurse, nonnurse, and agency membership. The AAIN decided to continue, and the National Student Nurses' Association was formed. Practical nurses had their own organization. (See Chaps. 24, 25, 26, and 27 for details of the organizations.) Although there was an apparent realignment of responsibilities, the relationships between the ANA and NLN ebbed and flowed; sometimes they were in agreement and sometimes they were not; sometimes they worked together, and at other times each appeared to make isolated unilateral pronouncements. Some nurses longed for one organization, but there seemed to be mutual organizational reluctance to go in that direction. Yet, it must be said that in those changing times each had some remarkable achievements—NLN in educational accreditation; ANA in its lobbying activities, its development of a model licensure law in the mid-1950s, and its increased action in nurses' economic security.

Then, in 1965, ANA precipitated (or in-flamed) an ongoing controversy. After years of increasingly firm statements on the place of nursing education in the mainstream of American education, ANA issued its first Position Paper on Education for Nursing. It stated, basically, that education for those who work in nursing should be in institutions of higher learning, that minimum education for professional nursing should be at least at the baccalaureate level; for technical nursing, at the associate degree level and for assistants, in vocational education settings.

Although there had been increased complaints by third-party payers about diploma education being hidden in the costs for patient care and diploma schools had declined as associate and baccalaureate degree programs increased, there was an outpouring of anger by diploma and practical nurses and those involved in their education. It was a battle that persisted and became another divisive force in nursing (see Chap. 12). But, then, so was the beginning of the nurse practitioner movement. There were nurses who feared it or saw it as pseudomedicine, detracting from pure nursing professionalism. The issues remained unresolved for years.

Therefore, whether or not 1965 can be considered the gateway to a new era of nursing, it was the beginning of dramatic and inevitable changes in the education and practice of nursing and in the struggle for nursing autonomy.

EPILOGUE

Nursing history, of course, did not end with the year 1965; history is always just our yesterday. Therefore, it may be helpful to reprise the major events of the 30 years that followed, even though they will also be discussed in more depth in the chapters that follow.

The pattern of a nursing shortage followed by a presumed nursing oversupply continued during these years. By the early 1980s, the shortage was seen as acute, but it was followed in 1986 by layoffs and fears of layoffs as the prospective payment system required by the government for Medicare reimbursement resulted in shorter hospital stays for patients. Hospitals that were already overbedded found that they had more empty beds than they could afford and cut back on nursing personnel. Administrators, however, had not reckoned on the fact that because the patients admitted were much sicker during their short stay, more nurses would be required to care for them, especially in intensive care units. Moreover, nurses were being lured from hospitals by other health care opportunities, and soon a "crisis" in the nurse supply was declared. In the attempts to attract and keep nurses, considerable attention was given to the health and welfare of nurses, with funding for higher education made available, flexible scheduling accepted, and salaries dramatically increased. On the other hand, by 1994, as health care facilities became concerned about what a national health care plan might mean to their survival, administrators attempted to cut back on the now well-paid RNs, hiring a variety of assisting personnel to give the less complex care. In some communities, then, new graduates who had been recruited with a high-profile advertising campaign found that they could not necessarily get the jobs they wanted where they preferred to work. This was particularly true of some associate degree and diploma nurses. Nevertheless, predictions continue that in overall terms, a shortage is present and will continue into the new century.

In nursing education, the trends that had been evolving continued: more RNs and LPNs continuing their education toward a baccalaureate, more second career individuals entering nursing; a moderate increase in baccalaureate programs; a spurt in programs that enabled those with a bachelor's degree in another field to move into a shortened master's program that led to licensure; a major increase in associate degree programs, and a gradual loss of diploma programs. Most dramatic was the emphasis on preparing clinical specialists (CNSs) and nurse practitioners (NPs), with or without a master's degree. By 1994, there was some agreement that a master's degree was necessary for this level of practice, although many were still practicing without one, since, in the 1970s, when NPs were gaining a foothold in health care, their background varied from RN with NP training on a continuing education basis to graduate education. An increased need for NPs to give primary health care was seen as part of the Clinton administration's national health care plan, and because enough would not be available, nursing education programs were emphasizing their preparation. Many were developing graduate programs that more or less meshed CNS and NP education to create an advanced practice nurse (APN). (On the baccalaureate level, there was also a move to focus on preparation for primary health care, since the evolving trend toward care in the community as opposed to an institution seemed to be coming to fruition.)

The agreement about the need for a graduate degree for NPs was as heated during the past two decades as the still ongoing quarrel about the baccalaureate for entry into professional practice. Over those years, a few states had moved their basic nursing licensure requirements in that direction, but almost all still granted RN licensure on the basis of the same tests (now computerized) for all graduates. An increasing number of states were requiring a separate license for the APN, often granted after the individual's certification by a voluntary credentialing group, such as the credentialing center of ANA and/or the various nursing specialty organizations' credentialing arms. (The number of specialty organizations had grown tremendously.) Also during these 30 years, there was considerable legislation that granted APNs, including nurse midwives (CNMs) and nurse anesthetists, separate reimbursement for services, and prescription privileges. Some hospitals were also giving NPs and CNMs admitting privileges. However, the AMA continued to object to such nurse practice without physician control, despite the fact that numerous studies showed how effective APNs were in providing

care, and individual physicians accepted them as colleagues.

Nurses also continued to serve their country with distinction in the years after 1965. Their contributions were acknowledged in the Vietnam war and the Persian Gulf war, and a memorial to these nurses was erected in 1994, near the Vietnam memorial in Washington, D.C.—largely through the efforts and fund raising of nurses. Nurses also attained top ranks in the various armed services and were influential in bringing about appropriate changes.

Equally influential were those nurses who were elected to local, state, and national office or held key positions on the staffs of powerful legislators. Other nurses were appointed by U.S. presidents to important offices, such as the heads of the Health Care Financing Administration (HCFA), the Social Security Administration; and the position of National AIDS Policy Coordinator. Nurses, as a whole, also became more active politically, and their input did affect legislation. One stunning result of nursing leadership and political influence as well as acceptance of the validity of nursing research was the establishment of the National Institute of Nursing Research as part of the National Institutes of Health.

As nurses became better educated and assumed more responsibility, they were able to affect positively the care of patients. In the best hospitals, nurse executives with appropriate graduate degrees were more commonly a part of the top decision-making team. Other nurses headed departments in infection control, managed care, quality assurance, staff education, and nursing research. Expert clinical specialists were resources to nurses and others on the health care team. Nurses also participated in major institution-wide committees. They were particularly valuable on ethics committees, since serious ethical problems became more visible because of new technology, the problem of access to care, and the inclination of patients and families to demand participation in health care decision making. Nursing also developed new patterns of patient care, in part to be more cost-effective. Nevertheless, it cannot be said that these patterns of nurse involvement and influence were present everywhere. In some situations nurses and physicians did not function as colleagues, and the administration did not support nurses as professional practitioners.

Most of the changes that emerged in these 30 years could have been predicted by alert professionals, since their roots were in the preceding years. Overall, there is every reason to be optimistic about nursing's role in health care, although progress is likely to be slowed if internal quarrels about education, practice, and research are not resolved. For success, it might be useful to return to the words of a nineteenth century nursing leader, "To advance, we must unite."

REFERENCES

1. Kalisch P, Kalisch B: *The Advance of American Nursing*, 2d ed. Boston: Little, Brown, 1986, p 318.
2. Ibid.
3. Ruffing-Rahal MA: Margaret Sanger: Nurse and feminist. *Nurs Outlook* 34:246–249, September–October 1986.
4. Bankert M: *Watchful Care: A History of America's Nurse Anesthetists*. New York: Continuum, 1989.
5. Kalisch and Kalisch (1986), op cit, p 330.
6. Dreves K: Vassar training camp for nurses. *Am J Nurs* 75:2000–2002, November 1975.
7. Christy TE: Portrait of a leader: Lavinia Lloyd Dock. *Nurs Outlook* 17:74, June 1969.
8. Ibid.
9. Kalisch and Kalisch (1986), op cit, p 372.
10. Bullough V, Bullough B: *The Care of the Sick: The Emergence of Modern Nursing*. New York: Prodist, 1978, p 113.
11. Shannon ML: The origin and development of professional licensure examinations in nursing. Unpublished Ed.D. dissertation, Teachers College, Columbia University, 1972, p 127.
12. Kalisch B, Kalisch P: Slaves, servants, or saints: An analysis of the system of nurse training in the United States, 1873–1948. *Nurs Forum* 14(3):248, 1975.
13. Christy T: Portrait of a leader: Isabel Maitland Stewart. *Nurs Outlook* 17:44–48, October 1969.
14. Christy T: Portrait of a leader: M. Adelaide Nutting. *Nurs Outlook* 17:20–24, January 1969.
15. Tirpak H: The frontier nursing service: Fifty years in the mountains. *Nurs Outlook* 23:308–310, May 1975.
16. Carnegie ME: *The Path We Tread: Blacks in Nursing, 1954–1984*. Philadelphia: Lippincott, 1986.
17. Kalisch B, Kalisch P: The Cadet Nurse Corps in World War II. *Am J Nurs* 76:240–242, February 1976.

Major Studies of the Nursing Profession

DESCRIBED HERE ARE the reports of research and studies that have guided nursing in the past and will always be considered milestones in the development of nursing. The extent to which any of these studies has had a marked effect on the progress of nursing remains questionable. Nonetheless, the studies are noteworthy because they represent the efforts on behalf of nurses and other national health care experts to improve our knowledge of the nursing profession and contribute to its advancement. Detailed descriptions of many of these studies can be found in previous editions of this text.

EARLY STUDIES—1912–1949

The Educational Status of Nursing (1912)

Conducted under the leadership of M. Adelaide Nutting, chairperson of the education committee of the American Society of Superintendents of Training Schools for Nurses, and published by the U.S. Bureau of Education, this report resulted from a questionnaire study of what schools of nursing throughout the country were actually teaching their students at that time and the techniques employed. It also covered the students' working and living conditions. Although this study revealed many appalling practices, it did not create the stir in nursing or in the public that it should have. However, it did begin to establish nursing as a profession and to set a precedent for later studies. It also highlighted

the need for continued investigation of educational practices in nursing, and—even as early as 1912—the need for schools of nursing to be independent from hospitals.

Nursing and Nursing Education in the United States. The Goldmark Report (1923)

Also stimulated by Nutting, the Rockefeller Foundation funded a Committee for the Study of Nursing Education to investigate "the proper training of the public health nurse." It was chaired by Dr. C. E. A. Winslow, professor of public health, Yale University, and included ten physicians (two of whom were hospital superintendents), six nurses (Nutting, Goodrich, Wald, Clayton, Beard, and Ward), and two lay representatives. Secretary and chief investigator was Josephine Goldmark, who had already done a recognized field study. It soon became apparent that the scope of the study needed to be expanded to encompass nursing education in general. Goldmark gathered and synthesized the opinions of leading nurse educators and also surveyed and studied 23 schools of nursing and 49 public health agencies, seeking answers to questions about the preparation of teachers, administrators, and public health nurses, clinical and laboratory experience for students, financing of schools of nursing, licensure for nurses, and the development of university schools.

As the study pointed out, education of nurses was still on an apprenticeship basis, a method abandoned by other professionals. Moreover, the quality of the teachers was poor; formal instruction was erratic, uncoordinated, and frequently sacrificed to the needs of the hospital; and students were often poorly selected. In essence, there was little training and almost no education. The conclusions of this landmark study did not result solely from the survey but also from the firm opinions of its prestigious committee members and the opinions of nursing leaders interviewed. Because some have still not been implemented, they have a remarkably contemporary ring.[1]

Highlights of the recommendations are described here:

1. Prerequisites for employment as a public health nurse in public and private agencies should include basic hospital training followed by a postgraduate course including clinical and classroom components of public health nursing.
2. Every effort should be made to attract young women of high capacity to public health nursing or hospital supervision and nursing education because of the promising career opportunities available in those areas. There was also recognition that the average hospital training school did not offer a sufficiently attractive avenue of entrance to nursing.
3. Patient safety and professional responsibility demand the maintenance of educational standards embodied in the legislation of the more progressive states; and attempts to lower such standards would be fraught with real danger to the public.
4. State legislation should be enacted for the definition and licensure of a subsidiary grade of nursing to serve under physicians and to assist under the direction of trained nurses, depending on the phase of illness.
5. The average hospital training school does not conform to standards accepted in other educational fields; nor are the facilities adequate for the preparation of high-grade nurses required for the care of serious illness or for service in the fields of public health nursing and nursing education.
6. The development and strengthening of university schools of nursing is of fundamental importance in the furtherance of nursing education.
7. The development of adequate nursing services demands as an absolute prerequisite the securing of funds for the endowment of university-based nursing education.

Although the recommendations related to education are usually given the most attention, the Goldmark Report did not neglect its original focus on public health nursing. Among other things, it was concluded that both bedside nursing care and health teaching for preventive care could be combined in one generalized service, as opposed to the separated services and agencies that were more common at the time.

Although the 500-page report was published, it did not have the wide dissemination, interest, or impact of the Flexner Report. Only a few of the recommendations were given serious consideration on a wide scale. This was due, in part, to organized nursing's relatively early stage of development, and nursing education being controlled by hospital administrators and physicians at the time of the Goldmark Report. On the other hand, positive results of the study were the Rockefeller Foundation's endowment of two university schools of nursing—Yale and Vanderbilt—and Frances Payne Bolton's endowment of Western Reserve. These represented significant forward steps in nursing education.[2]

Nurses, Patients, and Pocketbooks (1928)

This study was conducted by the Committee on the Grading of Nursing Schools, composed of twenty-one members representing the American Nurses Association (ANA), National League of Nursing Education (NLNE), National Organization for Public Health Nursing (NOPHN), American Medical Association (AMA) (which later withdrew), American College of Surgeons (ACS), American Hospital Association (AHA), American Public Health Association (APHA), and representatives of general education. Nurses contributed about one-half of the $300,000 needed to finance the study; the remainder came from foundations and friends of nursing, such as Frances Payne Bolton, who also served on the committee. May Ayres Burgess, a statistician, directed the study.

The committee focused on three separate studies: supply of and demand for graduate nurses; job analysis of nurses; and grading of nursing schools. The first report, *Nurses, Patients, and Pocketbooks*, showed that there was an oversupply of nurses, with serious unemployment problems; that there was a geographic maldistribution, with most nurses remaining in large cities; that salaries and working conditions were poor; and that although in general both patients and physicians were satisfied with nurses' services (which were, of course, primarily in the private-duty sector), there was evidence of some serious incompetence.

An Activity Analysis of Nursing (1934)

This was a report of the second study sponsored by the Committee on the Grading of Nursing Schools. The principal purpose of this study, conducted by Ethel Johns and Blanche Pfefferkorn at the committee's request, was to gather facts about nurses' activities that could be used as a basis for improving the curricula in schools of nursing. It represents the first large-scale attempt to find out what nurses were actually doing on the job—in hospitals, in public health agencies, and on private duty—and this focused attention on nursing service as well as on nursing education and encouraged a closer correlation of theory and practice.

Nursing Schools Today and Tomorrow (1934)

This was the final report of the eight-year study conducted under the auspices of the Committee on the Grading of Nursing Schools. It gave statistics on the number of "trained and untrained"

nurses and answered such questions as: What should a professional nurse know and be able to do? How can hospitals provide nursing service? It described the nursing schools of the period and recommended essentials for a basic professional school of nursing.

A number of startling facts were brought to light. For instance, 42 percent of teachers in schools of nursing had not even graduated from high school; only 16 percent had a year or more of college. Again, it was pointed out that nursing was the only profession in which the student essentially provided all the service for her "learning" institution. Moreover, a large number of the existing schools were so small that student education was totally inadequate. The need for consistent evaluation of programs was urgent.

A Study on the Use of the Graduate Nurse for Bedside Nursing in the Hospital (1933)

This was the first study done by the NLNE Department of Studies, which was established in 1932, with Blanche Pfefferkorn as its director. Prompted by previous findings of the Grading Committee, Miss Pfefferkorn and her co-workers made a comparative study of the bedside activities of the graduate and student nurse in the hospital to lend support to the gradually emerging belief (somewhat reluctantly accepted by hospital administrators) that nursing care should be given principally by graduate staff nurses, not by nursing students. The study helped clarify the issues and laid a foundation for further reduction in the number of noneducational assignments given to students of nursing.

A Curriculum Guide for Schools of Nursing (1937)

The guide was prepared under the leadership of Isabel Stewart, chairperson of the NLNE Committee on Curriculum. Intended for students of professional caliber, it placed much emphasis on application of the sciences. The role of the clinical instructor was stressed, and all faculty members were encouraged to use newer and more creative methods of teaching. It was published as a sequel to two previous NLNE publications which proved to be too rigid to meet the changing emphasis on broader education for nurses. Hence, the word "guide" in the 1937 publication was highly significant. The guide was used in many nursing schools for another quarter century.

Study of Incomes, Salaries, and Employment Conditions Affecting Nurses (Exclusive of Those Engaged in Public Health Nursing) (1938)

The ANA initiated this questionnaire survey, which was launched in 1936 and conducted through state studies sponsored by the 23 state nurses' associations that agreed to participate. The data obtained from more than 11,000 private-duty, institutional, and office nurses were presented in the published report as state summaries, national findings, and recommendations. This study undoubtedly had considerable bearing on the development of the ANA's economic security program.

Administrative Cost Analysis for Nursing Service and Nursing Education (1940)

Blanche Pfefferkorn directed this study, which was sponsored jointly by NLNE and AHA in cooperation with ANA. This study, which focused on the purely business side of nursing service and education, produced some interesting and potentially usable data on the cost to the hospital of conducting a school of nursing and the economic value of the service rendered by nursing students, estimated in terms of graduate service.

Hospital administrators and nurse educators were greatly enlightened by this study, although it appears doubtful that many institutions actually adopted cost accounting for nursing education and service at that time.

The General Staff Nurse (1941)

As it became more and more common for hospitals to employ graduate professional nurses to provide bedside nursing care, formerly given almost entirely by students, the organizations most concerned—ANA, NLNE, AHA, and the Catholic Hospital Association (CHA)—felt the need to determine the status of general staff nurses as seen by directors of nursing, the nurses themselves, and others. A joint committee of these organizations was formed to make such a study. The report indicates that general staff nurses had little status at the time. This was reflected in their hours of duty, their salaries, and personnel policies. This study gave impetus to a movement to try to upgrade the status of the general staff nurse.

Hospital Care in the United States (1947)

Conducted by the Commission on Hospital Care, a national group appointed by the AHA representing a wide variety of occupations and professions, this study was primarily concerned with hospitals in this country. It necessarily touched upon nurses and nursing because they are such an integral part of hospitals and the services they render. Its introductory statement noted the outmoded, wasteful, duplicate, and inadequate nature of hospital care in the United States.

The study was far-reaching in scope and recommendations, many of which applied to nursing service and education. The findings were of great interest to legislators, and it is generally agreed that the Hill-Burton Hospital Construction Act was influenced by this study.

Nursing for the Future (1948)

Esther Lucile Brown, a social anthropologist with the Russell Sage Foundation, conducted this study for the National Nursing Council, a large group of representatives of many health organizations and services, which had functioned under other titles before and during

World War II to recruit nursing students and coordinate military and civilian nursing needs.

The study, funded by the Carnegie Foundation for the Advancement of Teaching and the Sage Foundation (which published it), was to analyze the changing needs of the profession. Brown, who had already studied nursing as an emerging profession, gathered data by visiting nursing schools, attending workshops, and consulting with individual physicians and hospital administrators, as well as using both a nursing and a lay advisory committee.

The report of her findings was, ironically, not much different from those of earlier studies, indicating the slow progress of nursing education. At one point, Brown pondered "why young women in any large numbers would want to enter nursing as operated today."[3] Once more, the same inadequacies were pointed out and, once more, the closing of the several thousand small, weak schools was urged. In particular, Brown emphasized the necessity for official examination of all schools, publication and distribution of lists of accredited schools, and public pressure to eliminate the nonaccredited schools.[4]

In addition, she strongly recommended "that effort be directed to building basic schools of nursing in universities and colleges, comparable in number to existing medical schools, that are sound in organizational and financial structure, adequate in facilities and faculty, and well-distributed to serve the needs of the entire country."[5] Noting that many diploma schools still operated for the staffing benefit of the hospital, she found nursing education not professional.

The report was the first to make the point that nursing education as a whole, not just an elite part, should be part of the mainstream of education, and that nurses could be divided into professional and practical groups.

The report received mixed reviews. Many nurses felt threatened, and some physicians and hospital administrators considered it a subversive document, fearing that it had economic security implications for nurses. (Nor did they appreciate the fact that the authoritarianism of hospitals was pinpointed, as was the dilemma of the nurse caught between the demands of physicians and administrators.) In 1970, Lysaught found that many of the recommendations of the Brown Report were still unfulfilled—and still valid.

A Program for the Nursing Profession (1948)

Actually an account of the extended deliberations and thinking of a Committee on the Functions of Nursing rather than a report of study or research, this report was accorded the attention and had the immediate influence of a scientific presentation. Under the direction of Eli Ginzberg, a professor of economics at Columbia University, the committee, which originated in the Division of Nursing Education of Teachers College, Columbia University, with representatives from nursing, medicine, and the social sciences, undertook to identify the problems confronting nursing and to suggest their solutions. The group found the shortage of personnel to be the outstanding problem in nursing at that time and attributed that shortage to minimal economic incentives in nursing, the public's increasing need for health care and more nurses, the apparent financial weakness of voluntary hospitals, and inefficient use of available nursing personnel. The committee recommended a number of broad and specific solutions related to both nursing education and service, encompassing both practical and professional nurses.

Nursing Schools at the Mid-Century (1950)

Current national accreditation procedures for schools of professional nursing were influenced by the findings of this study of practices (in 1949) in more than 1,000 schools of nursing. The study represented one attempt to implement the Brown Report, previously described. Conducted under the auspices of the National Committee for the Improvement of Nursing Services (a committee of the joint board of the six national nursing associations in existence at that time), the study covered such areas as organization of the schools, the cost of nursing education, curriculum content, clinical resources, student health, and others. The report contained statistics, tables, and graphs that schools used to evaluate their own performance as compared with that of others.

Patterns of Patient Care (1955)

This study was conducted under the direction of Frances L. George and Dean Ruth Perkins Kuehn of the University of Pittsburgh. Its main purposes were to determine how much nursing service was needed by a group of nonsegregated medical and surgical patients in a large general hospital and how much of this service could safely be delegated to nursing aides and other nonprofessional personnel. The report, published by the Macmillan Publishing Company, New York, contained much practical information about staffing patterns and the allocation of duties, which was helpful to other nursing service administrators and of interest to all nurses. Variations of these suggested staffing patterns were used in a number of hospitals for years.

Twenty Thousand Nurses Tell Their Story (1958)

This is a report of a five-year sequence of studies of nursing functions, initiated by ANA and the American Nurses' Foundation (ANF), made possible by the financial support of individual nurses throughout the country, and made meaningful by the 20,000 nurses who were "guinea pigs" in one way or another for the study. The report of results, prepared under the direction of Everett C. Hughes, professor of sociology at the University of Chicago, who also helped with some of the 34 studies, was published by the J. B. Lippincott Company, Philadelphia.

These studies, intended to produce better care for patients, revealed what nurses actually were doing on the job, their attitude toward

their role as they saw it, and their satisfaction in their work.

The results formed the basis for the development of stated functions, standards, and qualifications of nurses prepared by each ANA section for its members. The studies also indicated that further research was needed in many rapidly developing areas of nursing practice, both clinical and nonclinical.

Community College Education for Nursing (1959)

Mildred Montag wrote Part I of this report of a five-year Cooperative Research Project in Junior and Community College Education for Nursing. Part II was written by Lasser G. Gotkin. The project was sponsored by the Institute of Research and Service in Nursing Education at Teachers College, Columbia University, New York, and the report was published by McGraw-Hill Book Company, New York.

This was an "action research" project in that a program was developed with methods of evaluating its effectiveness built into the planning. Seven junior and community colleges cooperated in the study by establishing two-year programs leading to an associate degree in nursing. Dr. Montag participated in the planning of all programs.

Part II of the report gives data obtained from 811 graduates of the junior and community colleges, presenting persuasive arguments for the establishment of more associate degree programs to prepare nurses for first-level positions in nursing. (See Chap. 13 for the effect of Montag's dissertation on nursing education.)

Toward Quality in Nursing: Needs and Goals (1963)

The Consultant Group on Nursing, a twenty-five member panel of representatives from nursing, medicine, hospital administration, other areas of the health field, and the public, was appointed in 1961 by the Surgeon General of the U.S. Public Health Service to advise him on nursing needs and to identify what role the federal government should take in assuring adequate nursing services for the nation. The report of this group discussed major problem areas and recommended a number of measures for their solution.

One recommendation urged the nursing profession, with the aid of federal and private funds, to begin a study of the present system of nursing education; the remaining recommendations were directed specifically toward areas requiring federal financial assistance.

An Abstract for Action (1970)

This study was a direct result of a recommendation by the Surgeon General's Consultant Group on Nursing in its 1963 report, *Toward Quality in Nursing*. These experts recommended a national investigation of nursing education with special emphasis on the responsibilities and skills required for high-quality patient care. Although provision of funds for such a study was also recommended, no government funds were forthcoming.

Shortly thereafter, the ANA and National League for Nursing (NLN) established a joint committee to determine ways to conduct and finance such a study. The scope of the proposed study was enlarged to examine not only the changing practices and educational patterns of current nursing, but also probable future requirements. Confident that the problems of nursing ranged beyond the manpower problem, which the President's National Advisory Committee on Health Manpower was about to investigate, the ANF in the fall of 1966 voted to grant up to $50,000 to help launch a study. Impressed by this willingness of nursing to back its conviction that the study was needed, both the Avalon Foundation and the Kellogg Foundation granted $100,000 each to support the investigation. At the same time, an anonymous benefactor contributed $300,000.

In a meeting with the proposed head of the study, W. Allen Wallis, president of the University of Rochester and of the joint committee, it was decided that the study group to be set up would be an independent agency, functioning as a self-directing group with the power to plan and conduct its investigations as it saw fit. By January 1968, the new National Commission for the Study of Nursing and Nursing Education (NCSNNE) was fully established with twelve commissioners (three of whom were nurses); a project director, Jerome P. Lysaught; an associate director, Charles H. Russell; and a small staff. A timetable for the three-year study was set, including the provision for a contingency operation (until January 1971) to initiate implementation of the recommendations.

The commission set as its major objective to "improve the delivery of health care to the American people, particularly through the analysis and improvement of nursing, and nursing education." To meet this objective, two general approaches were used—the analysis of current practices and patterns and the assessment of future needs.

The methods of study included observational and descriptive tasks, combined with collection and analysis of findings from other studies. The findings and recommendations, plus projections for the future, were then subjected to the scrutiny of groups and individuals involved in the delivery of health care. The project staff likened this approach to the work of Flexner in his study of American medicine, refined by the experience of professional studies conducted in the last quarter century. A nursing advisory panel of ten was appointed to advise on plans for the study, suggest locations for site visits, and generally review and criticize each stage of the study. In addition, a health professional advisory panel, consisting of individuals with broad experience and understanding, was selected to ensure a rounded analysis of each content area. The two panels also provided a means for reaching a consensus and a reasonable compromise in terms of the needs of the health field when rival solutions to problems were presented.

Overall, there was an extensive search of the literature, questionnaires and surveys, 100 site visits, and a number of invitational conferences and meetings.[6]

The final report, entitled *An Abstract for Action*, was published in mid-1970 followed by a second volume of *Appendices* in 1971. A total of some 581 specific recommendations and subsumed recommendations emerged from the report.

There were four key recommendations:

1. Government agencies and private agencies should allocate resources to investigate the impact of nursing practice on the quality, effectiveness, and economy of health care.
2. Each state should establish a master planning committee that will take nursing education under its purview…to ensure that nursing education is positioned in the mainstream of American educational patterns.
3. A National Joint Practice Commission with state counterpart committees should be established between medicine and nursing to discuss and make recommendations concerning the congruent roles of the physician and the nurse in providing quality health care.
4. Federal, regional, state, and local governments should adopt measures for the increased support of nursing research and education.[7]

The report was received with mixed reactions, and continued to be controversial. Some stated that the research was poorly done; others that many of the recommendations were not valid; still others that there was little that was new.

Eventually, however, all the major nursing organizations, the AMA, AHA, and other health groups either published a statement of support for the report or endorsed it "in principle." An NLN Task Force studied the National Commission report in depth, and in early 1973 its report was published. Each recommendation had been evaluated and either endorsed or revised and restated, with a rationale for the suggested revision. The greatest concerns were with the concept of "episodic" and "distributive" care and specific recommendations for nursing education.[8]

The determination of the commission and the project staff to begin implementation of the recommendations resulted in a commitment of funds for one year of implementation by ANA and NLN. Thereupon the Kellogg Foundation agreed to underwrite the project for two years and share with nursing the support for a third year. In 1973 the status of the implementation effort was reported in *From Abstract into Action*. The priority items of implementation were set as nursing roles and functions, nursing education, and nursing careers. By the summer of 1971, a newly organized National Joint Practice Commission (NJPC) had been established with 10 nurses and 10 physicians, each a practitioner engaged in direct patient care approximately 50 percent of the time. The group developed a number of specific objectives, focused on the basic charge of the commission's recommendation. Subsequently, NCSNNE attention was given to models of "episodic" and "distributive" care in education and practice, study of new utilization patterns, and progress in nursing research. In terms of educational changes, much interest was focused on open curriculum, preparation of nurses in the expanded role, and some aspects of graduate education. In terms of careers, the commission looked at economic and social satisfactions, new approaches to extend the horizons of nursing, the impact of organizations, and the licensure dilemma.[9]

In summarizing the effect of the National Commission report on nursing and health care, it is necessary to recognize that it is difficult to differentiate between changes that may have occurred through a normal process of evolving trends and those that could have been a direct result of NCSNNE recommendations. For instance, there was an upsurge of action in continuing education, open curriculum programs, and increase in AD and baccalaureate programs. It is entirely possible that the report at least accelerated, if it did not initiate, action.

One specific action that occurred was the formation of the NJPC and its counterparts on the state, local, and institutional levels. Most states began, or continued, formalized nurse-physician dialogue, although many eventually dissolved, frequently because of lack of physician interest or inadequate organization. The national organization, funded in part by the Kellogg Foundation, early on made important statements.[10] It remained active until 1981, when the AMA discontinued participation.

Other NCSNNE interests did not have as long-lasting an impact. Many statewide master planning committees were formed, but actual results of their planning are not as evident. Particularly disappointing was that, after the major increase in federal support to nursing in 1972, there was a totally negative attitude on the part of the administration and a consequent cutback of funds.

In 1977, Lysaught conducted a national survey of nursing service directors to determine how much progress had been made on four selected projections of the final report: joint practice committees, a reward system for increased nursing competence, enhancement of career perspectives through recognition of advanced clinical competence, and increase of ties and joint responsibilities between nursing education and nursing service. The results showed minimum progress toward these goals on the grass-roots level. Perhaps remembering that the commission had repeated some of the recommendations of Brown's report, Lysaught suggested that the next years "should be characterized not by further search but by accomplished fulfillment."[11]

Extending the Scope of Nursing Practice: A Report of the Secretary's Committee to Study Extended Roles for Nurses (1971)

At the request of the Secretary of Health, Education, and Welfare (HEW), a multidisciplinary committee was formed to study potential and actual new roles for nursing. The committee, which was chaired by Dr. Roger O. Egeberg, then Special Assistant for Health Policy at DHEW, consisted of thirteen physicians and thirteen nurses, as well as administrators and trustees of hospitals, administrators of schools of allied health, and knowledgeable DHEW staff. The purpose was to "examine the field of nursing practice, to offer some suggestions on how its scope might be extended, and to clarify the many ambiguous relationships between physicians and nurses."[12] The committee elected to view the subject from the perspective of the consumers of health services. The preface of the report ended with the statement:

> **We believe that the future of nursing must encompass a substantially larger place within the community of the health professions. Moreover, we believe that extending the scope of nursing practice is essential if this nation is to achieve the goal of equal access to health services for all its citizens....[13]**

The report reviewed many current responsibilities of nurses, from simple tasks to expert, considered professional techniques necessary in acute life-threatening situations, and noted the nurse's role on the health team, as leader of the nursing team, and in counseling, teaching, planning, and assessing. Although recognizing that most nurses were not currently educationally prepared to assume extended roles and that some were reluctant to accept these roles, the committee arrived at certain conclusions and recommendations it believed significant in achieving extended roles for nursing. Legal considerations of the role were also reviewed (see Chap. 20).

As with other studies reviewed here, the recommendations are applicable even today. They included the need for:

1. Curricular innovations that demonstrate the physician-nurse team concept in the delivery of health care in a variety of settings.
2. Financial support for continuing education to encourage active and inactive nurses to function in extended roles.
3. Development of a model law of nursing practice suitable for national application through the states.

4. Collaborative efforts between schools of nursing and medicine to demonstrate effective functional interaction between physicians and nurses in the provision of health services.

5. Efforts to attain a high degree of flexibility in the interprofessional relationships of physicians and nurses, without jurisdictional concerns per se interfering with efforts to meet patient needs.

6. Cost benefit and other economic studies to assess the impact of extended nursing practice on the health care delivery system. (An appendix to the paper listed more than 30 locations where nurses were being prepared for or were practicing in extended roles at that time.)

7. Attitudinal surveys of health care providers and consumers to assess acceptance of nurses in extended care roles.

The Study of Credentialing in Nursing: A New Approach (1979)

There were two major considerations that precipitated a study of credentialing in nursing: an ongoing disagreement and/or confusion between ANA and NLN on their respective roles in credentialing nurses, which was becoming somewhat acidulous by the mid-1970s, and increased activity by state and federal governments, presumably indicating public disaffection on the whole matter of health manpower credentialing (see Chap. 20). It was the action of the 1974 ANA House of Delegates "to examine the feasibility of accreditation of basic and graduate education" that stimulated two conferences on credentialing, under the sponsorship of the ANA Commission on Education. The outcome of these conferences, in which NLN and the American Association of Colleges of Nursing (AACN) were also involved, was a recommendation that a feasibility study should encompass more than accreditation, that it should be broadened to include assessment of credentialing mechanisms for organized nursing services, certification, and licensure, and "to formulate a proposal for studying the adequacy of these mechanisms, and to recommend future directions."[14]

In August 1975, ANA contracted with the Center for Health Research, College of Nursing, Wayne State University, to complete a proposal that had been developed in draft form at the second credentialing conference. The proposal that was developed had as its stated purposes (1) to assess the adequacy of current credentialing mechanisms in nursing, including accreditation, certification, and licensure, for providing quality assurance to the public served, and (2) to recommend future directions for credentialing in nursing. The study was to include nursing service and nursing education, but was not to attempt to demonstrate the relationship between credentials and the quality of care.

When the NLN declined to co-sponsor the study, the ANA proceeded to do so alone in August 1976. At that time, the Committee for the Study of Credentialing in Nursing (CSCN) was appointed—ten nurses and five others, with the later addition of Dr. Margretta Styles, a former dean of the Wayne State College of Nursing, as chairperson of the Committee. Inez G. Hinsvark, professor in the School of Nursing, University of Wisconsin, Milwaukee, was selected as project director. The twenty-four-month contract negotiated by ANA specified that the study committee have responsibility for the program, and the university, the administrative responsibility.

The study was a complex task of some magnitude. It began with a comprehensive review of the literature and information, position papers, documents, and laws that were offered by various state agencies, nursing associations, and credentialing agencies.

A model was constructed, composed of three areas identified for analysis: governance, policy, and control of credentialing within nursing; credentialing in the job market; and credentialing in nursing education. In addition, a set of principles appropriate to guide all credentialing endeavors was created, and current issues in credentialing and barriers to change were identified with position statements formulated. The methodologies used in the study included interviews, meetings, a modified Delphi technique, content analysis of written materials, and surveys.

The committee's final recommendations encompassed the following: principles to be applied to credentialing in nursing; position statements concerning definitions of nursing, entry into practice, control and cost of credentialing, accountability, and competence; credentialing definitions and their application to nursing (licensure, registration, certification, educational degrees, accreditation, charter, recognition, approval); the establishment of a national nursing credentialing center; and a statement that "the professional society in nursing, currently called the American Nurses Association, make provision for categories of membership for credentialed nursing personnel and students of nursing."[15] Plans for follow-up were also suggested.

In 1979, an independent task force for implementation of the report was established by the ANA Board of Directors. The task force of fifteen distinguished individuals (including eleven nurses) began its work with funding from ANA, one SNA, and some specialty nursing organizations.

The Task Force on Credentialing in Nursing worked for two and a half years, cooperating with 146 groups that were willing to be "resource groups." These included national, state, and regional nursing associations, nursing certification boards, other health professional associations, educational associations, boards of nursing, the Armed Services Nurse Corps, Veterans Administration Nursing Service, and subgroups of ANA. A small percentage of these groups and some individuals made financial contributions, but ANA bore the major burden of support for the activities of the Task Force. ANF assumed administrative responsibility.

After considerable study of the original report, the major focus of the Task Force was the development of alternative structures and models of a credentialing center. The final recom-

mendations described sixteen design parameters for a center, but the crucial points were that the center should be separately incorporated, established within the private, voluntary sector, with support and involvement of (but not separate control by) current credentialers of nursing, as well as the public and the "community of interests" (such as the American Hospital Association), and that the center must be involved in all aspects of nursing credentialing, including licensure. Specific recommendations were also made on how the center could be implemented immediately through a coalition of nursing organizations.

This report was presented to representatives of national nursing organizations considered potential coalition members and some of the nursing press on April 24, 1982. Although seventy-three resource groups had endorsed the *principle* of a national nursing credentialing center, it was immediately clear that if implementation meant giving up control of their own credentialing activities, the national organizations including ANA were not interested. Although all groups expressed interest in continued dialogue and some still endorsed the concept or principle of a center, a planned meeting of the credentialing organizations to be held later did not occur.

Currently, the nurse credentialing mechanisms continue very much as they did before the original study. As noted in the ANA statement given at the final meeting and later affirmed by the House of Delegates, the ANA moved to the establishment of a separately incorporated credentialing center under the aegis of ANA, but no other organization is participating. The Task Force dissolved itself after the meeting; its final report was distributed through ANF.[16] Nursing credentialing remains in almost the same state of confusion.

Selected Studies Related to Nursing Supply and Demand (1975–1980)

In the late 1970s and early 1980s the number of studies about and important to the nursing profession increased. Some were national studies that were federally funded and included such topics as the career patterns of nurses, trends in RN supply, job availability for new graduates, and the distribution, salaries, and job responsibilities of nurse practitioners. For instance, one major study of this kind, *Analysis and Planning for Improved Distribution of Nursing Personnel and Services*, which was contracted to the Western Interstate Commission for Higher Education (WICHE) by the then Department of Health, Education, and Welfare in 1975, was geared to strengthen nurses' abilities to analyze and plan for improved distribution of nursing personnel and services, explore ways to reduce uneven distribution, and involve nurses in health planning. One of the most complex activities was the development of a state model for planners to project nursing workforce resources and requirements—a major breakthrough in the field.[17] However, just how useful it was or how much it was used is still an open question.

For a number of reasons, the early 1980s produced especially significant nursing studies. Ironically, all began and may have been somewhat influenced by the nursing shortage then at its peak, and almost all the reports were released as the shortage *appeared*, at least, to be subsiding. However, by the mid-1980s, the nursing shortage had once again intensified, and new studies and commissions were called for.

A report released in late 1980, although not directly related to nursing, created a stir in the nursing community because of its implications for the profession. The Graduate Medical Education National Advisory Committee (GMENAC) had been charged by the Secretary of the Department of Health and Human Services (DHHS) to advise on "the number of physicians required in each specialty to bring supply and requirements into balance, methods to improve the geographic distribution of physicians, and mechanisms to finance graduate medical education."[18] The committee consisted primarily of physicians. The overall conclusion was that there would be an oversupply of physi-

cians by the year 2000, and many recommendations were related to this point. As noted by a nurse member in a dissenting opinion, the focus on "non-physician health care practice" centered primarily on the question of physician service substitutability and delegation of medical services as these affect physician workforce requirements, and the attitude was described as skeptical and negative. The recommendations repeatedly stated that the number of physician assistants (PAs), nurse practitioners (NPs), and nurse-midwives being graduated from educational programs each year should not be increased until the need for them could be determined. The desired numbers were those needed to attain the delegation levels which had been deemed desirable by the GMENAC. The "medical" services of NPs and PAs were to be under the supervision of a physician, and third-party reimbursement was to be made only to the employing institution or physician in relation to the physician workforce. While not all the recommendations were so negative, the report was seen by many nurses as one more act of interference by medicine with nursing's professional development.

One study referred to frequently during this time was related to nurse employment in Texas.[19,20] Released in 1980, it was replicated in many other states and helped to stimulate national studies exploring the factors that affected nurses' employment satisfaction, particularly in hospitals. Spurred by the severe nursing shortage, the purpose of *Conditions Associated with Registered Nurse Employment in Texas* was to determine the reasons for nurses' working or not working in nursing and to decide how they might be attracted back into the workforce. By means of a questionnaire and interviews, more than 10,000 Texas nurses were asked to describe their feelings about nursing. In addition, administrators, educators, and nurses participated in a nominal group conference to generate innovative and practical ideas for attracting and keeping nurses.

The findings of the study indicated that the chief component of job dissatisfaction was that structural elements in the job (hospital policies and administration attitudes) kept nurses from providing patients with professional care. These included lack of support for autonomy of practice, professional education, and for participation in patient care policy formation.[21] Major dissatisfactions also included inadequate salaries and benefits, the amount of paper work, and lack of both hospital and nursing administrative support.

Innovative ideas generated by the nominal group included the following: encourage self-scheduling by RNs with appropriate accountability; delineate nursing functions and eliminate nonnursing functions; develop a career ladder; plan recognition and merit awards for high-quality nursing care; establish group peer review; establish a joint practice committee with physicians; provide nursing residencies; give recognition to high-stress areas; provide for flexible schedules; develop pools of part-time nurses; provide child-care facilities; give bonuses to staff nurses who recruit inactive nurses.

One immediate outcome of the study was that a number of hospitals across the country initiated some of these innovative suggestions, with some evidence of success.

Magnet Hospitals: Attraction and Retention of Professional Nurses (1983)

In 1981, the Governing Council of the American Academy of Nursing (AAN) appointed a Task Force on Nursing Practice in Hospitals, charging it "to examine characteristics of systems impeding and/or facilitating professional nursing practice in hospitals." The prestigious nurse administrators who comprised the task force chose to focus on those hospitals across the country that seemed to have created nursing practice organizations that served as "magnets" for professional nurses: that is, they were able to attract and retain a staff of well-qualified nurses and consistently provided high-quality care.

The purpose of the study they developed was basically to identify magnet hospitals in eight regions of the country, to identify, describe, and

analyze the organizational variables that promote job satisfaction, to explicate replicable variables for use by others, and to publish the report. Bureau of Labor Statistics (BLS) regions, combining Regions I and II and Regions VII and VIII, were used, and selected fellows of the academy were asked to nominate and describe potential magnet hospitals in their region. Specific criteria were as follows: nurses considered the hospital a good place to work and practice; the hospital had the ability to recruit and retain professional nurses; and it was in a geographic area in which it had competition for staff. The Center for Health Care Research and Evaluation (CHCRE) at the School of Nursing, the University of Texas at Austin, was selected as the site for data collection, tabulation, and analysis.

A total of 165 institutions was nominated. All the directors of nursing received a letter that explained the project, including a data collection instrument that asked for descriptive personnel and hospital statistics. The letter also delineated what was expected of hospitals and their representatives if selected. The four task force members independently reviewed and evaluated the recruitment and retention records of the 155 hospitals that responded and ranked their ten top choices. At CHCRE, a numerical score was calculated for each, and on the basis of the rankings, 46 institutions were selected as magnet hospitals. The final sample was 41.

The magnet hospitals were primarily private, nonprofit institutions, with the majority in the 201- to 700-bed range. The occupancy rate was 72 to 98 percent. At least 85 percent of their budgeted RN positions were filled throughout the year. There was an average of 1.1 RNs per occupied bed, an RN:LPN ratio of 10:1, RN:aide ratio of 12:1, and RN:unit clerk ratio of 9:1. The educational preparation of the directors of nursing was primarily at the master's level, with about 12 percent holding doctorates and above 7 percent baccalaureates. Associates or clinical directors were also primarily prepared at the master's or doctorate level, although 19 percent held no degree. About one-half of the head nurses and about 43 percent of the area supervisors held no degree.

Interviews were conducted by the task force members in each of the eight areas. The director of nursing and a director-selected staff nurse from each magnet hospital were grouped according to position and interviewed separately. Each group was interviewed in such a way as to assure participation of each individual.

The questions focused on the role and image of nursing at the hospital, sources of nursing staff satisfaction, and inter- and intraprofessional relationships. The participants were also asked to comment on the activities and policies that they believed were effective in contributing to professionalism and staff retention. The staff nurses' responses revealed the importance of high standards, clearly enunciated, with adequate administrative support to ensure that standards can be met. Specifically, they expressed the importance of the visibility, accessibility, and support of the director of nursing; participatory management; decentralized responsibility; and low patient:RN ratios, with qualified staff, and consultation from clinical specialists. Personnel policies that reflect the hospitals' concern with employees' needs and interests were also stressed, as were opportunities for professional practice. These opportunities included involvement in community outreach, development and operation of a career ladder, and opportunities to teach patients and families.

The nurse administrators, while taking more of a conceptual view and being somewhat more abstract in answering the same questions, seemed to agree almost entirely with the staff nurses about what created the positive environment that made their nursing services a magnet for RNs. Although recognizing the importance of their own leadership, they freely acknowledged the importance of supervisors and head nurses in decentralization, especially in the areas of support and communication. They also cited collaboration with schools of nursing, including the beginning of joint appointments, as

adding to the professional milieu. In addition to the areas listed above, the nurse administrators also identified the opportunity to participate in nursing research as a good educational opportunity for the nurses.

The report concluded that change was possible, since some of these hospitals had enjoyed magnet status for some time, while others had changed rather dramatically in a relatively short time prior to the study. This positive change seemed to have followed a change in key leadership people such as the hospital administrator and the director of nursing.

Although the magnet hospitals had certain differences, there were also critical similarities. First, the shared values of administration and staff were clearly evident. Second, both staff and directors recognized their own changing roles, and the continued need to interpret these roles and the needs of patients and to stand up for one's principles. Finally, rather than a voiced concern about power per se, what came through on all sites was a sense of what might be called a lack of powerlessness. Nurses recognized the locus of control in the director and the power held by the physicians in admitting patients to the hospital, but recognized that this could be balanced by the nurses' power as coordinators of care—the care needed by patients. There was also a "fit" of vision and competence between the nurse administrator and the hospital's chief executive officer (and presumably the board of trustees). Without such a balanced power structure, change cannot occur.[22]

Effects of Federal Support for Nursing Education on Admissions, Graduations, and Retention Rates at Schools of Nursing (1982)

In some ways, this report was overshadowed by the congressionally mandated Institute of Medicine (IOM) report. Prepared by Abt, a professional consultant company, for the Health Resources Administration, the study examined federal assistance to nursing education from only one perspective: its impact on the number of students entering, continuing in, and graduating from basic nurse training programs. The authors blamed limitations of available data for their inability to report also on the effect of federal funds on advanced training, educational quality, access of minorities, and other areas of intended impact that were included in the objectives that the legislation of 1964 and subsequent years was intended to achieve.

The study used year-by-year data on the admission, attrition, and graduation of individual nursing schools from 1969 (1968 for associate degree programs) to 1979. Although there were frequent references to lack of data and problems in the statistical analysis of the data, it was clearly stated that federal funds had certain important effects: 47,000 additional admissions and 32,800 to 42,200 additional graduates in basic programs in the ten years studied, and a higher than average retention rate among those entering nursing school as a result of federal funding. It was also noted that although it was unrealistic to expect federal support to produce massive changes in the size of the nursing workforce in a short time, the impact over the decade had been appreciable.

Nursing and Nursing Education: Public Policies and Private Actions (1983)

The findings of this significant study, mandated by Public Law 96-76, the Nurse Training Act Amendments of 1979 (NTA), and contracted to the IOM by DHHS, were presented in 1983. A six-month interim report in July 1981 had raised strong protests in the nursing community, and there were some adjustments in the final report.

The original purpose of this study was in some ways similar to that of the Abt study in that it was prompted by the question of whether further substantial outlays for nursing education were needed to assure an adequate supply of nurses. However, it went further. As expressed in the legislative history, the intent of the mandate was to secure an objective assessment of the need for continued federal support,

to make recommendations for improving the distribution of nurses in medically underserved areas, and to suggest actions to encourage nurses to remain active in their profession.

The study committee was composed of institute members and recognized experts in public policy in disciplines related to nursing. Out of the 26 members, 9 were nurses. Neither the chairperson nor the staff were nurses, but some were included on the ad hoc advisory panels established. Because new data collection was apparently discouraged by a key congressional committee, the study's findings were based primarily on the synthesis and interpretation of data secured from existing sources. This became a controversial point when the interim report was released, since much of the same data, including that garnered from open hearings, was the basis of the Commission on Nursing study, and that interim report, presented only months later, contained very different recommendations. Included in the IOM data were 75 recent state-level studies of nursing, as well as national survey and inventory data about RNs and licensed practical nurses (LPNs). The interim report contained summaries of useful information about nursing in 1981 but raised provocative questions. Frequently, the reports of data analysis were the same as those in other studies. For example, the information on nurses' job dissatisfaction was almost identical to that contained in the Texas study and the commission report. Some of the findings, while not necessarily palatable to organized nursing, were certainly issues already discussed within the profession. Criticism by nursing focused primarily on the fact that, as compared to the GMENAC committee, controlled by physicians, here nurses were in the minority, which could suggest "a view of nursing as an occupation that is not clinically valued and that must have others assume leadership and major input in making recommendations regarding what is best for it."[23]

Moreover, while no actual recommendations were made, certain statements were interpreted to mean that the IOM committee tended to see nursing in relation to resource allocation and cost rather than quality. There was the implication that the minimum baccalaureate degree advocated by nursing might result in increased salaries, fewer nurses, and a lower quality of care. A major concern, of course, was that the IOM report, being mandated by Congress, would also greatly influence legislation affecting nursing, and nursing education and research are both highly dependent on federal funds.

Whether or not these statements were only intended to raise questions for further exploration, or whether nursing's negative attitude toward the report, or the follow-up of additional data from varied sources affected the attitude of some members of the committee, may never be known. Nevertheless, the final report presented some farsighted recommendations. Significantly, the addition of considerable new information received in the interim between the reports was noted.

The recommendations had a major impact on nursing. For instance, within 6 months, legislation was introduced to place a National Institute of Nursing within the National Institutes of Health. The 1985 legislation creating the National Center for Nursing Research and later legislation finally resulting in the National Institute of Nursing Research were the culmination of these initiatives. Most persons traced this unprecedented action directly to the IOM statement that lack of adequate funding for nursing research had inhibited the development of nursing investigations and that the federal government should establish an organizational entity in the mainstream of scientific investigation. The members of the IOM panel recommended that various combinations of public and private support be applied to the following areas:

1. Alleviation of the shortages and maldistribution of nurses in certain geographic and specialty areas, even though the overall supply and demand of RNs was estimated to be in balance for the remainder of the decade.

2. Financial aid for nursing students to assure that generalist nursing education programs graduate a sufficient number of students to maintain aggregate and local supplies of RNs.

3. Recruitment strategies that attract recent high school graduates and nontraditional prospective students, such as minorities and those seeking late entry into a profession.

4. Developing policies and programs to minimize the loss of time and money by students moving from one nursing education program level to another.

5. Grants to nursing education programs that, in association with the nursing services of hospitals and other health care providers, undertake to develop and implement collaborative educational, clinical, and/or research programs.

6. Expansion of the federal government's support of programs at the graduate level to assist in increasing the rate of growth in the number of nurses with master's and doctoral degrees in nursing and relevant disciplines.

7. Federally sponsored competitive programs emphasizing health care delivery to medically underserved populations and better minority representation at all levels of nursing education.

8. More formal instruction and clinical experiences in geriatric nursing to augment the supply of new nurses interested in caring for the elderly.

9. Support to develop programs to upgrade the knowledge and skills of RNs, LPNs, and aides in skilled nursing facilities and other institutions rendering care to the elderly.

10. Restructuring of Medicare and Medicaid payments so as to encourage long-term nursing care at home and in institutions.

11. Support for the education of nurse practitioners to meet the nation's ongoing need; and revisions of public and private policies so as to expand patients' access to and reimbursement for services provided by nurse practitioners and nurse-midwives.

12. Improvement of supply and job tenure of nurses by addressing employment conditions ranging from salaries to child care.
13. Studies and experiments to determine the feasibility and means of creating separate revenue and cost centers for case-mix costing and revenue setting, and for other fiscal management alternatives.
14. Establishment by the federal government of an organizational entity to place nursing research in the mainstream of scientific investigation.
15. Research on the knowledge and competencies of nurses with various levels of education and practice, as well as on the organization and delivery of nursing services, followed by dissemination of research results.
16. Continued federal support for the collection and analysis of timely data on national nursing supply, education, and practice with special attention to filling identified deficits in currently available information.[24]

A surprisingly large number of these recommendations were acted on in the next decade, except that federal funding was not forthcoming to the extent recommended. Yet, the budgetary impact of the committee's recommendations was presented as a modest increase in NTA funding to alleviate certain nurse shortages, holding the line against possible erosion of federal and state funding for higher education, and modifying payment systems of public and third-party payers to permit (nurse) providers of service to the poor and elderly to become financially secure.

The National Commission on Nursing Study (1983)

The National Commission on Nursing was formed as an independent commission sponsored by the American Hospital Association, the Hospital Research and Educational Trust, and the American Hospital Supply Corporation. Composed of thirty leaders in the fields of nursing, hospital management, medicine, government, academia, and business, it was charged, during its three-year charter, with developing and implementing action plans to provide practical solutions for institutions and organizations confronting nursing problems. One-half of the group were nurses. In part because of its sponsorship and because a hospital administrator (distinguished though he was) was chairman, organized nursing at first regarded the National Commission with some suspicion. Once more, there was concern about a nonnursing-sponsored group potentially making decisions about nursing. Yet the commission did, indeed, prove to be an independent entity. With a respected nurse as staff director, the commission began, like the IOM group, to study data about nursing, relying primarily on the literature, policy statements, surveys and studies, and hearings (in this case held in six major cities). A variety of interested people testified. The testimony, published in mid-1981, stressed that nursing, although closely meshed with other health care disciplines, has the professional right and responsibility to define the nature and scope of nursing practice. To be recognized as independent professionals, nurses themselves must understand, value, and promote their professional identity and role in providing high-quality care. Also highlighted was the need for a highly visible, effective nursing leadership promoting a strong, unified image of the profession. There was disagreement on collective bargaining as a mechanism to improve working conditions and control over practice.

The *Initial Report and Preliminary Recommendations*, published in September 1981, was received with considerable enthusiasm and perhaps some astonishment by nursing. The report was seen as much more positive than the IOM report of the same period. Although the National Commission on Nursing recognized that nursing was practiced in a variety of settings, emphasis was on the hospital, where the largest percentage of nurses practice. When viewed from a national perspective, the issues were seen as more similar than different, regardless of settings and geographic areas. Forty different factors were mentioned frequently and consistently as related to the shortage of nursing. Foremost were salaries, flexible scheduling, nurse-physician relationships, the image and status of nurses and their roles in decision making, career mobility, nursing education, and the relationship of nursing education and nursing practice.

All these factors were summarized and discussed in five major categories from which recommendations evolved:

- Status and image of nursing
- Interface of nursing education and practice
- Effective management of the nursing resource, including the mix of organizational factors required for nursing job satisfaction, as well as workforce planning, recruitment, and retention strategies
- Relationships among nursing, medical staff, and hospital administration, including nurses' ability to participate through organizational structures in decision making as it relates to nursing care
- Maturing of nursing as a self-determining profession, including nursing's right and responsibility to define and determine the nature and scope of its practice[25]

In summary, the key recommendations focused on nurses and physicians participating in a collaborative relationship in which nurses are included in clinical decision making and have authority and responsibility for their own practice; administrators establishing a suitable practice environment, including involvement of the nurse administrator as part of the top management team; establishment of salaries, benefits, and educational opportunities for nurses, commensurate with their responsibilities as professionals; the need for diverse nursing constituencies to join together to formulate and support common policies in education, credentialing, and standards of practice; promotion of accessibility and educational mobility in higher education through educational articulation for undergraduate nurses and RNs; continuation of

funding for nursing education; appropriate utilization of nurses related to the competency obtained in the specific educational program; collaboration between educational institutions and practice agencies to provide good clinical experience for students, practice opportunities for faculty, and continuing education for RNs; and implementation and maintenance of nationally accepted standards for licensure. On the controversial issue of baccalaureate education for professional nursing practice, it was seen as a "desirable goal," with consideration given to regional differences in availability of programs, funds, faculty, and students. Specific goals for each set of recommendations were presented, with concomitant demonstration and research projects recommended.

In the interim between the initial and final reports, the National Commission published the results of a survey of innovative nursing programs and projects, and sponsored an invitational conference to learn about evolving trends and innovative approaches to nursing in hospitals, to which chief executive officers, trustees, medical directors, and chief nurses from hospitals with successful models came as a team and discussed strategies and solutions to nursing problems. There were also surveys to discover trends in relationships between nursing education and practice, meetings with various groups, and site visits, as well as review and study of new literature and responses to the *Initial Report*.

Of the major groups interested in the *Initial Report*, it appeared that nursing responded positively (with hesitation by some educators in relation to the educational recommendations). The AMA, with a very positive attitude, bought multiple copies of the document for its most influential members to study. The AHA also distributed copies, but received a less than positive response from some of its constituent organizations and administrators.

When the final report was released, some disappointment by nurses was inevitable since certain recommendations were seen as less strong. For instance, in relation to nursing education, the recommendations were more muted than those in the initial report in advocating the baccalaureate degree for professional nursing practice. As quoted from the final report,

> All types of nursing education programs, which continue to be needed, increasingly operating within the mainstream of higher education and in accordance with local circumstances and statewide planning, should hasten progress toward availability of baccalaureate and higher degrees for those desirous and capable of achieving them. Educational mobility and reentry opportunities should be promoted within the educational system. Accreditation processes should respond to these needs and trends.[26]

Omitted was the statement urging appropriate utilization of nurses according to educational background. On the other hand, a new recommendation strongly urged that a high priority be given to nursing research and to preparation of nurse researchers.[27]

Under "Nursing and the Public," the suggestion for nationally accepted standards of licensure was eliminated, but participation of nurses in community activities and public forums was encouraged.

Why the changes? New data, new analysis, new discussion might be one answer. But another is pragmatic: Nurses alone cannot bring about recommended changes, however desirable they may be; they need the cooperation of physicians and hospital administrators—especially to support changes in the practice setting. The fine art of compromise is necessary to get most plans moving, and the National Commission was certainly concerned that its work not be filed away as simply another report never acted upon, particularly since one of the primary motives for the study was the nursing shortage, which by 1983 was no longer considered serious. (Although a more severe nursing shortage reemerged a few years later.)

Strategies for action concluded the report, and there were tentative plans for assessment of results later, although the commission recognized that many recommended actions had already gained impetus from forward-looking individuals.

The chairman summarized their conclusions:

> ...if we are going to make any progress at all, the first priority would seem to be better educated, more highly qualified nurses; reformed relationships among health professionals; and new types of organizational structures. Action must be long-range. Short-term solutions alone are difficult and costly; they hamper nursing's ability to keep up with the present, let alone prepare for the future.[28]

By the mid-1980s, there was talk of another national nursing shortage. This time, it occurred against the backdrop of turbulent changes in the health care system such as prospective payment for Medicare and Medicaid, a rising number of patients needing high-tech care or treatment of chronic illness, spiraling health care costs, and a federal budget deficit which limited the availability of funds for all federal health care initiatives. As a result, health care providers faced severe financial and resource constraints, and nurses (along with other health care personnel) struggled to meet the demands of a caseload of patients with higher acuity levels than ever before. The supply of nurses seemed unable to meet the quality and quantity of the new types of demand. Some aspects of the nursing shortage stemmed from characteristics of the profession which had always made recruitment difficult, and some originated beyond nursing, within the context of the health care system and society in general.

Thus, in the mid-1980s several public and private agencies launched studies to examine the extent of the nursing shortage, the characteristics of the nurse supply, and recommendations for the future. Many of the studies were based on and often made reference to the earlier landmark studies of the 1980s, especially the reports of the National Commission and the Institute of Medicine. These studies of the late 1980s are reviewed below.

Nursing's Vital Signs: Shaping the Profession for the 1990s (1989)

This publication was intended as an "information collage" based on the 1984–1989 work of the National Commission on Nursing Implementation Project (NCNIP). Four major nursing organizations [ANA, the American Association of Colleges of Nursing (AACN), NLN, and the American Organization of Nurse Executives (AONE)] launched the NCNIP in 1983 when they submitted a proposal to the Kellogg Foundation for funding to implement selected recommendations of the 1983 studies on nursing from the Institute of Medicine and the National Commission on Nursing. In 1984, when the Kellogg Foundation decided to fund the study, Vivien DeBack, Ph.D., RN, was appointed project director. Representatives from other health care, consumer, and business groups joined the nursing organizations to form a 12-member governing body to direct the project.

One of the first actions of the governing board was the designation of three work groups: nursing education, management and practice, and research and development. Phase one of the project involved the work groups' reviews of nursing data and the development of action strategies. Phase two involved the implementation of activities and changes at regional, state, and local levels. The governing board appointed a steering committee to assist organizations to "assume the change process," and a task force for nursing service to guide nurse executives as they worked to improve practice environments for nurses. Activities in phase two included dissemination of information, demonstration of new types of nursing models, and application of innovative ideas into practice.[29]

Although not an "end of the project report," *Nursing's Vital Signs* included descriptions of "innovative approaches and experiences for nurses in practice, education, and research to help them stay in step with change."[30] It depicted the discussions and strategies of the work groups as they wrestled with their long-range goals of planning for nursing at the turn of the century. It also covered the groups' responses to the immediate nursing shortage which prevailed at the time. In that regard, one of the most significant outcomes was the development of the three-year multimedia advertisement campaign to improve the image of nursing. The Advertising Council directed the campaign, which was expected to yield $20 million in donated media time and space.

Additionally, the NCNIP produced and disseminated widely several brochures and documents which offered recommendations for the future of nursing. These included *Features of High Quality, Cost Effective Nursing Care Delivery Systems of the Future; Timeline for Transition into the Future Nursing Education System for Two Categories of Nurse; Characteristics of Professional and Technical Nurses of the Future and Their Educational Programs; Guidelines for Schools of Nursing in Transition*; and *Nursing in Transition: Analyzing Prospective Revenues, Costs, and Benefits from the Educational Provider Perspective.*

Office of Technology Assessment Study of Nurse Practitioners, Physician Assistants, and Certified Nurse-Midwives (1986)

In December 1986, the Office of Technology Assessment (OTA) issued Health Technology Case Study 37, *Nurse Practitioners, Physician Assistants, and Certified Nurse-Midwives: A Policy Analysis*. The study was prepared in response to a request by the Senate Committee on Appropriations to update a previous OTA case study, *The Cost and Effectiveness of Nurse Practitioners*. The committee also requested that OTA address the extent to which various federal health care programs and private third-party payers pay for the services of NPs and CNMs. Issues or payment and reimbursement were controversial because of proposed federal legislation in both houses at that time which provided for the direct reimbursement of nurses under the Federal Health Employees Health Benefit Program (FHEHBP).

An advisory panel of 21 experts with backgrounds in health policy, medical economics, health insurance, medicine, nursing, and consumer advocacy defined the goals for the study and suggested resources and perspectives to consider in presenting the material. The panel based its final report on an extensive review of the literature and consultation with many individuals who were knowledgeable about NP, PA, and CNM practice.

Basically, the panel found that:

> ...**these practitioners have not been used to their fullest potential. Major obstacles to the greater employment and appropriate use of NPs, PAs, and CNMs are that most third-party payers do not cover...the provision by NPs, PAs, and CNMs of many services that are typically and characteristically provided by physicians, and, in those instances where third party payers do cover the services of NPs, PAs, and CNMs, the payments are most often indirect (i.e., to the employing physicians or institutions) rather than direct (i.e., to the NPs or CNMs).**
>
> **Moreover, NPs and CNMs are more adept than physicians at providing services that depend on communication with patients and preventive actions...Patients are generally satisfied with the quality of care provided by NPs, PAs, and CNMs, particularly with the interpersonal aspects of care.**[31]

Although nursing welcomed this report, the AMA was not enthusiastic.[32] However, in the interest of patient welfare, the need to negotiate nursing and medical roles in a rapidly changing health care environment was evident.[33]

Secretary's Commission on Nursing, Final Report (1988)

In 1987, in response to reports of widespread difficulties recruiting registered nurses, Health and Human Services Secretary Otis R. Bowen, MD, established the Secretary's Commission on Nursing. He directed this 25-member panel to advise him on problems related to the recruitment and retention of RNs, and to develop recommendations on how the public and private sectors could work together to implement immediate and long-range solutions for enhancing the adequacy of the supply of RNs.

The report of the Secretary's Commission was important for several reasons. First, it documented the pervasiveness and seriousness of the nursing shortage. It also re-enforced the themes of previous nursing studies in pushing for improvements in the working conditions and status of nurses. However, perhaps because of the seriousness of the nursing shortage at the time, its tone was more emphatic than that of previous studies with regard to the need to actively promote nursing's unique role in the health care delivery system and to ensure the participation of nurses in policy formation and clinical decision making.

Based on its Interim Report of July 1988, the commission concluded that the shortage of RNs was widespread, cutting across all health care delivery settings. Furthermore, the shortage was primarily a result of an increase in demand as opposed to a contraction of supply, with projections into the future indicating a continued imbalance between supply and demand. The commission's final report included 16 specific recommendations with 81 directed strategies designed to alleviate the shortage and assure a healthy nurse labor market in the future.

With regard to utilization of nursing resources, the recommendations called for the provision of adequate support services for nurses, utilization of the most appropriate mix of nursing personnel, and adoption of labor-saving technologies, such as automated information, to increase RN productivity and improve internal management of nurse resources.

In the area of nurse compensation, the commission members urged health care delivery organizations to increase RN compensation by providing a one-time adjustment to increase RN relative wages, implement innovative compensation options for nurses, and expand pay ranges based on experience, performance, education, and demonstrated leadership.

As for nurse decision making, the commission recommended that nurses have greater representation on policy making, regulatory, and accreditation bodies. Such representation would facilitate nurses making unique, critical, and effective contributions to the health care delivery system. Furthermore, the panel members urged employers, as well as the medical profession, to recognize the appropriate clinical decision-making authority of nurses in relationship to other health care professionals.

Noting the downturn in nursing school enrollments during the mid-1980s and its implications for the future supply of nurses, the commission offered recommendations aimed at facilitating the education of nurses. Specifically, these recommendations included increased targeted financial support, improved program accessibility, updating the relevance of nursing curricula, and promoting nursing as a career. Finally, the commission members endorsed the creation of a more permanent body to follow through on their recommendations, monitor the nurse labor market, and conduct research on the supply of and demand for nurses.[34]

In 1990, DHHS Secretary Louis Sullivan, MD, signed a 1-year charter for a new 15-member Commission on the National Nursing Shortage. He appointed a nurse and health researcher, Caroline Bagley Burnett, MSN, ScD, as executive director. In addition to the four ex officio members, the secretary appointed 11 other members as follows: 4 from the nursing community including the president of ANA, 4 from health care providers, 1 from third-party payers, 1 representing economics and data policy fields, and 1 from the general public.

The charter of the Commission on the National Nursing Shortage (CONNS) extended from February 1990 to June 1991.[35] Over that time period CONNS analyzed ongoing public and private sector initiatives related to three focal areas (condensed from the original five) and developed four projects and ten recommendations.

The first initiative related to the focal areas of recruitment, educational pathways, retention, and career was a project to identify long-term-care facilities that participate in career development or have such programs, and to examine their strategies and document their effectiveness in recruiting and retaining personnel. The second was to identify the variables contributing to successful recruitment and retention, somewhat like the AAN's Magnet Hospital study.

The recommendations developed by CONNS for this segment were:

- Federal and state governments, private foundations, and nursing organizations should intensify efforts designed to increase the number of well-prepared nurses from minority populations to better serve the health needs of the nation.
- Support education of faculty and the preparation of nurses for advanced practice, particularly in long-term care, and promote the development of curricula to prepare nurses for practice in settings where long-term care is provided.
- Support legislation that directs Medicaid programs to compensate nursing personnel in long-term facilities and home health agencies at competitive rates.
- Increase nursing representation at the policy-making level in health care organizations, states, and the federal government and increase nurse appointees to the boards of health care organizations.

Two projects related to the second focal area, which encompassed restructuring nursing services, effective use of nursing personnel and information systems, and related technology in nursing. The first was a study of certified nurse midwifery practice arrangements in primary care settings. It involved identifying factors that limit or curtail practice and documenting the cost to consumers and third-party private payers. The second focused on case management as a service that enables nurses to adopt an advocacy role for individuals served, provide quality care, and enhance client quality of life in a cost-effective manner. High-risk groups were to be the target population, and the project was to be in a community setting.

Two recommendations addressed issues relating to this focal area:

- Encourage states and the federal government to assume a leadership role in developing creative financing strategies for nursing practice settings.

- Modify home health care financing mechanisms to reflect evolving patterns of clinical management.

CONNS also made recommendations related to the third focal area, data collection and analysis requirements. These were as follows:

- Support the incorporation of nursing data elements in state, national, and international health care databases.
- Ensure authorization and appropriation within Title VIII of the Public Health Service Act to support data collection and analysis activities of the Division of Nursing, BHPr, on the supply, distribution, and requirements for nursing personnel.
- Support the work of the Interagency Conference on Nursing Statistics as a mechanism to provide coordination for the collection of data on nurses and nursing and to move forward the recommendations of the Project HOPE action plan.

To ensure that the momentum generated by these two commissions would be sustained, CONNS made one final recommendation:

- Charge the Advisory Council on Nurses' Education and the National Center for Nursing Research Advisory Council with the responsibility for monitoring activities in the public and private sectors emanating from the recommendations of SCON and the projects and recommendations identified by CONNS.

Perhaps because the nursing shortage seemed to ease or because it takes time to flesh out such projects and receive government funding, the follow-through on the recommendations was not what CONNS would have wanted. Momentum was indeed lost.

Commonwealth Fund Paper: What to Do About the Nursing Shortage (1989)

Responding to the severe nursing shortage in the mid-1980s, when between 1984 and 1986 the average vacancy rate for nursing positions in hospitals increased from 11 to 20 percent, the Commonwealth Fund conducted a national nursing study. The Commonwealth Fund report explored why the shortage existed when the number of nurses per capita was at an "all-time high" and the number of hospital beds continued to decline.[36]

Although the study's conclusions and recommendations were similar to those of other national studies, the methodology was different. Basically, assuming that nursing "labor markets were highly local and variable" the researchers collected in-depth data for six major metropolitan areas: Boston, Chicago, Houston, Los Angeles, New York, and Pittsburgh. They surveyed 15,000 nurses and 400 hospital administrators, analyzed trends in nursing school enrollments, and came up with a series or recommendations for hospitals, state governments, and nursing schools as to how they could improve the supply of nurses and utilize them more efficiently. The investigators urged hospitals to provide more desirable compensation packages and encouraged organizations involved with education to develop programs which would "make nursing a more available and desirable career."[37]

Health Professions Education for the Future: Schools in Service to the Nation (1993)

This report by the Pew Health Professions Commission, funded by the Pew Charitable Trusts, was a follow-up to their report in 1991 that declared that the education and training of health professions was not adequate to meet the health care needs of the American people. Two years later, the commission was even more convinced that professional education was out of sync with the health care system that was emerging. The president of the trusts noted that there was a need to have vision within the educational institutions, a significant number of leaders accepting new beliefs, a commitment by state and federal governments, and the support of professional organizations and the private sector, before the appropriate changes can be made.

The commission considered the need for change in the allied health professions, dentistry, medicine, nursing, pharmacy, public health, health care administration, and veterinary medicine, and presented both general strategies and recommendations that related to all the health professions and others specific to each profession. Particularly interesting is the Summary of Competencies for 2005:

- Care for the Community's Health—Understand the determinants of health and work with others in the community to integrate a range of activities that promote, protect, and improve the health of the community. Appreciate the growing diversity of the population, and understand health status and health care needs in the context of different cultural values.
- Provide Contemporary Clinical Care—Acquire and retain up-to-date clinical skills and apply them to meet the public's health care needs.
- Participate in the Emerging System and Accommodate Expanded Accountability—Function in new health care settings and interdisciplinary team arrangements designed to meet the primary health care needs of the public, and emphasize high-quality, cost-effective, integrated services. Respond to increasing levels of public, governmental, and third-party participation in, and scrutiny of, the shape and direction of the health care system.
- Ensure Cost-Effective Care and Use Technology Appropriately—Establish cost and quality objectives for the health care process and understand and apply increasingly complex and often costly technology appropriately.
- Practice Prevention and Promote Healthy Lifestyles—Emphasize primary and secondary preventive strategies for all people and help individuals, families, and commu-

nities maintain and promote healthy behaviors.
- Involve Patients and Families in the Decision-Making Process—Expect patients and their families to participate actively both in decisions regarding their personal health care and in evaluating its quality and acceptability.
- Manage Information and Continue to Learn—Manage and continuously use scientific, technological, and patient information to maintain professional competence and relevance throughout practice life.

Achieving these competencies was seen as no easy task. It was pointed out that over the past decade, each of the major professional groups had been studied by a variety of influential bodies. Their recommendations concerning education included many of the themes advanced by the Pew Commission. Yet nothing much happened to implement these recommendations. Why? Among other things, professional identity and territoriality, a stagnant mind-set, the lack of institutional rewards for changed behavior, and the tendency to preserve tradition rather than risk change were all seen as obstacles. "Change is not the natural vocation of most who have selected an academic career."[38]

In relation to nursing, a greater diversity in nursing—racial, ethnic, and gender—was seen as a plus, along with the trend toward higher education. The value of nurse-midwives and nurse practitioners as important sources of primary care was noted, as was the important role of nurses in care of the aging population, in health promotion and disease prevention, in providing cost-effective care, and in management of care. The multiple educational pathways into the professions were seen as an asset to the profession, as was nursing's community orientation in education and practice.

The commission proposed six strategies for nursing education, placing "great emphasis on nursing's proven ability to integrate care by working with a variety of social service providers in the community and linking together teams that effectively meet the health care needs of the public."[39]

Strategy 1: Develop programs at the various levels of nursing education that reflect the contributions that are needed in the changing patient care system. Change licensing and care delivery regulations to ensure that nurses are employed in roles for which they have received appropriate training and that they are rewarded for their contributions. Model new nursing arrangements in the health care delivery system using these differentiated nursing roles, and evaluate their impact on patient and health system outcomes.

Strategy 2: Restructure faculty positions in nursing schools and programs to involve them more directly with the patient care system and nursing practice.

Strategy 3: Develop interdisciplinary teaching, practice, and research programs for the maintenance care of chronic patient populations.

Strategy 4: Redirect a significant part of all nursing programs and schools to the health care needs of community-based patients. This priority will vary greatly from school to school depending upon university mission, tradition of the school, needs of the community, and competition for this role.

Strategy 5: Continue the development of graduate-level clinical training programs for nurses in areas where health care services can reduce cost and improve access and quality.

Strategy 6: Conduct comprehensive and ongoing programs of strategic planning within each nursing school and program.

Finally, there were a number of strong policy recommendations made for consideration by the federal and state governments, the profession, and higher education.

FEDERAL POLICY

1. Review the current policies of funding graduate medical education through the Health Care Financing Administration, and develop a plan to ensure that at least 50 percent of the nation's residency positions are in primary care areas and expanded primary care training in other relevant disciplines. To this end, the Pew Commission supports the continued use of patient revenue to support education.

2. Expand programs funded through the Public Health Services Act to encourage expansion of team delivery and primary care programs.

3. Expand, through the Agency for Health Care Policy and Research, and the National Institutes of Health, research that is focused on evaluating the effectiveness of using different models for the delivery of care.

4. Encourage experimentation of health care delivery models at the state level by streamlining the waiver process for variance from Medicaid and Medicare guidelines.

5. Encourage accrediting bodies to provide leadership for the development of outcomes measures for health professions education as a part of the accreditation process.

6. Enforce faster implementation of efforts to reduce the difference in pay between specialists and generalists.

STATE POLICY

1. Create statewide coalitions to assess the long-term health care needs of the population and relate those needs to the states' investment in health professions education. The coalitions should comprise high-

level representatives drawn from all relevant constituencies. These should be linked to ongoing efforts to reform state health policy.

2. Reformulate the financial arrangements for support of health professions schools to reflect the state's need for primary care providers.

3. Create state- or university-based policy centers to collect and analyze data on health personnel utilization, practice, and education patterns at the state level.

4. Reform the health professional licensing process in a manner that encourages new practitioners to be competent in the areas identified by the Pew Commission. Ensure that these competencies are a part of the ongoing process of relicensing for health professionals.

5. Create opportunities to model and evaluate alternative approaches to health care delivery, finance, and personnel utilization by waiving practice act requirements and using support from Medicaid and other resources.

6. Ensure that planning and financing for higher education is informed by data drawn from the efforts described above.

PROFESSIONAL POLICY

1. Ensure that the accreditation process fully embraces the competencies developed by the Pew Commission as a part of the institutional review of academic programs.

2. Ensure that state affiliates encourage a similar change in the licensing policy in each state.

3. Implement professional certification programs that are aimed at ensuring that practitioners currently in the field understand the changing health care system and develop the necessary skills to remain competent.

4. Assist schools in redirecting their educational programs outside of the walls of the academic health center.

HIGHER EDUCATION POLICY

1. Encourage the health professions schools to develop clear and distinctive strategic directions that are tied to the overall mission of the university.

2. Provide more integration between the academic program of the health professions schools and the rest of the campus.

3. Encourage health professions schools to develop creative organizational structures, partnerships, and financial arrangements in order to meet their strategic directions.

4. Consider the work of the health professions schools in the overall service mission of the university.

5. Insist on routine and timely evaluation of all programs in the context of the mission of the university and school.

The studies described in this chapter provide a rich chronology and resource for understanding the dimensions of nursing and its evolvement over time. They attest to governmental and private sector interest in nursing's professional advancement. Most of these studies were initiated and brought to completion by talented individuals who recognized the importance of acquiring pertinent and timely nursing data. This dedication and interest in studying the profession will take on even more importance as we acquire new technologies and research capabilities and move forward to the twenty-first century.

REFERENCES

1. Goldmark J: *Nursing and Nursing Education in the United States*. New York: Macmillan, 1923.
2. Garling J: Flexner and Goldmark: Why the difference in impact? *Nurs Outlook* 33:26–31, January–February, 1985.
3. Brown EL: *Nursing for the Future*. New York: Russell Sage Foundation, 1948, p 45.
4. Ibid, pp 132–170.
5. Ibid, pp 48, 178.
6. Lysaught J: *An Abstract for Action*. New York: McGraw-Hill, 1970.
7. Ibid, pp 156–161.

8. Report of the task force. *Nurs Outlook* 21:111–118, February 1973.

9. Lysaught J: *From Abstract into Action.* New York: McGraw-Hill, 1973.

10. Nurse and medical practice act must permit flexibility, NJPC says. *Am J Nurs* 74:602, April 1974.

11. Lysaught J et al: Progress in professional service: Nurse leaders queried. *Hospitals* 52:120, August 16, 1978.

12. US Department of Health, Education, and Welfare. *Extending the Scope of Nursing Practice.* Washington, DC: The Department, 1971, p 2.

13. Ibid, p 4.

14. The study of credentialing in nursing: A new approach. A report of the committee. (mimeographed) Milwaukee, January 1979, p 3.

15. Ibid, pp 82–92.

16. de Tornyay R: Report of the meeting convened by the task force on credentials in nursing. Kansas City, MO: American Nurses Foundation, 1983.

17. Lum J: WICHE panel of expert consultants report: Implications for nursing leaders. *J Nurs Admin* 9:11–19, July 1979.

18. Report of the graduate medical education national advisory committee to the secretary, Department of Health and Human Services, vol 7. Washington, DC: DHHS, 1981.

19. Wandelt M et al: Conditions associated with registered nurse employment in Texas. Austin, TX: Center for Research, School of Nursing, University of Texas at Austin, 1980.

20. Wandelt M et al: Why nurses leave nursing and what can be done about it. *Am J Nurs* 81:72–77, January 1981.

21. Ibid.

22. Task force on nursing practice in hospitals. Magnet hospitals: Attraction and retention of professional nurses. Kansas City, MO: American Academy of Nursing, 1983.

23. Jacox A: Significant questions about IOM's study of nursing. *Nurs Outlook* 31:28–33, January–February 1983.

24. *Nursing and Nursing Education: Public Policies and Private Actions.* Washington, DC: National Academy Press, 1983, pp 1–23.

25. Initial report and preliminary recommendation. Chicago, IL: National Commission on Nursing, 1981, p 5.

26. Summary report and recommendations. Chicago, IL: National Commission on Nursing, 1983, p 15.

27. Ibid, p 11.

28. Ibid, p xi.

29. *Nursing's Vital Signs, Shaping the Profession for the 1990s.* Battle Creek, MI: W. K. Kellogg Foundation, 1989, pp 9–13.

30. Ibid, p 9.

31. *Nurse Practitioners, Physician Assistants, and Certified Nurse-Midwives: A Policy Analysis.* Washington, DC: Office of Technology Assessment, 1986, pp 5–7.

32. Ibid, p 6.

33. Jacox, A: The OTA report: A policy analysis. *Nurs Outlook* 35:262–267, November–December 1987.

34. *Secretary's Commission on Nursing, Final Report*, vol I. Washington, DC: DHHS, 1988.

35. *Secretary's Commission on the National Nursing Shortage, Final Report.* Washington, DC: DHHS, 1992.

36. Minnick A et al: What do nurses want? Priorities for action. *Nurs Outlook* 37:214–218, September–October 1989.

37. *What to Do about the Nursing Shortage.* New York: The Commonwealth Fund, 1989, p 20.

38. O'Neil E: *Health Professions Education for the Future: Schools in Service to the Nation.* San Francisco: Pew Health Professions Commission, 1993, p 9.

39. Ibid, p 87.

Contemporary Professional Nursing

The Health Care Setting

6 The Impact of Social and Scientific Changes

AS A PART OF SOCIETY, and as one of the health professions, nursing is affected by the changes, problems, and issues of society in general, as well as those that specifically influence the health care scene. Some of the changes, such as the civil rights of minority groups and women, have been developing for almost 100 years but the issues are still not resolved. Others, such as the new lifestyles and technological and scientific advances, have appeared to emerge on the scene with a suddenness that has created what Toffler called "future shock," the shattering stress and disorientation induced in individuals when they are subjected to too much change in too short a time.[1]

Surrounded by constant change, nurses (and others, for that matter) are tempted to ignore the potential effects on the profession, or at best to cope with the problems only when they become inescapable. Professions that ignore the pervasiveness of social trends find themselves scrambling to catch up, rather than planning to advance; reacting, rather than acting. When the public justifiably accuses the professions of unresponsiveness to their needs, it is, in part, because those professions have not been acute enough to observe patterns of future development or have been too insular to see the necessity to become a part of them. It is a luxury that no profession, least of all nursing with its intimate person-to-person contact, can afford. The purpose of this chapter, therefore, is to review some of the major changes in the last few decades to determine their impact on nursing.

A GLOBAL PERSPECTIVE

For a fifty-year period ending with the 1990s, global military and ideological preoccupation caused the diversion of financial, human, and material resources to essentially unproductive purposes. With the collapse of the former Soviet Union and movement to a more cooperative world order, we can no longer hide from the severest consequences of those years of social neglect. More affluent, industrialized countries can no longer dismiss the problems of less developed countries (LDCs) as belonging to someone else. Modern communications have opened territorial boundaries, challenged old ways, and forced us to realize that as people of this earth, we have some common responsibility for the worldwide human condition. There is a moral imperative to strive for some equitable distribution of the finite and often deteriorating resources at our disposal.

Some modest agreement within the international community exists on the rudimentary ingredients for survival: health, sanitation, shelter, safety. Beyond this there are varied opinions on cause, effect, and relationships. The United Nations Children's Fund (UNICEF) identifies a complex interaction between poverty, population growth, and environmental decline as the principal threat to the world's people and their health.[2] The World Health Organization (WHO) offers another perspective and places blame on governmental inability to reach consensus on priorities.[3] Others challenge the wisdom of separating these problems from one another and call for movement away from a medical or health model to a social model where incremental progress in immunization, housing, prenatal care, screening of high-risk populations for disease, occupational safety, nutrition, family planning, and so on move simultaneously, albeit modestly.

Beyond a host of disparate views, we are left with some grim realities...those truths from which we can run, but cannot hide:

- The economic growth of a country does not guarantee any impact on poverty.[4]
- Increased food output has little effect on nutrition where population growth and unequal income distribution are uncontrolled.[5]
- Malnutrition is as often attributed to disease from environmental conditions, and low birth weight in children, as to actual food shortage.[6]
- A pattern of resource consumption and pollution exists in industrialized nations that cannot be supported without serious damage to the biosphere.... 20 percent of the world's people consume three-quarters of its energy.[7]
- The poor are more numerous in rural areas, but urban poor and urban slums are on an upsurge.[8]
- Programs that target vulnerable populations and specific areas of need, such as immunization or family planning, have greater impact on human welfare than an expansion of the national economy.[9]
- Though its form and function may vary somewhat from culture to culture, the family provides a natural context for safety, protection, and sharing of resources.[10]
- The very young and the very old are both populations who are to some degree dependent on adults of working age.... Birthrates and improved health could create critical dependency ratios.[11]
- Illiteracy, domestic violence, and pandemic AIDS are situations devastating to families and obstacles to developing personal self-reliance.[12]

Clearly, the problem of population growth, a major societal concern for a number of years, is no less urgent now. Between 1985 and 1990, the estimated world population grew from 4.8 to 5.2 billion, or about 9 percent, with over 6 billion expected in 2000 and 8.2 billion by 2025. The greatest rate of growth continues to be in the LDCs. The population in LDCs already outnumbers those in the developed world by three to one.[13] At the same time, these more underdeveloped and overpopulated nations tend to have problems of poverty, with hunger sometimes escalating to starvation.

The attempt of governments to lower the birthrate in many countries has met with varied success. Access to family planning currently ranges from an estimated 95 percent in developing countries like China to less than 10 percent in some parts of Africa. The differences can be attributed to a wide range of circumstances. Where poverty is greatest and education of women is wanting, frequent childbearing is common. Where life is laborious and insecure, large families are seen as a source of support. Short birth intervals and frequent childbearing are also associated with low-birth-weight babies and increased infant mortality.[14]

Because the overpopulation problem is so severe in some countries, the issue will continue to receive government attention. India, with a tremendously high birthrate, is mounting a renewed effort in family planning. China, with a population of over 1.2 billion, already rewards couples limiting their children to one and imposes a fine for those who bear more than one child.

Since more than 1 billion of the 5 billion people in the world are between the ages of ten and nineteen, more attention is being given to their problems. Primarily these relate to education, employment, and health. Worldwide, secondary school enrollment is increasing, but certain groups seldom get beyond primary school: Asians, Africans, and girls. The discrepancy is even greater for girls at the postsecondary level where students are trained for professions. Unemployment is overwhelming in many countries, and the young people migrate to cities where they may find life even more difficult. In 1990, an estimated 2.4 billion, or 45 percent of the world's population, lived in urban areas.[15]

Accidents, alcohol, tobacco, and drugs are seen as major health problems of young people, with accidents the leading cause of death. They are also increasingly susceptible to sexually transmitted diseases, as they become sexually active at an earlier age (even though they may marry later, that is, after age 20). For young women, the health consequences of pregnancy can be serious, especially for those under 17 and without prenatal care, which is not unusual. More than 50 percent of this world's births are unattended by a trained person.[16] The ignorance of young people about fertility and contraception is widespread, and there are ongoing efforts to find the best ways to educate them and others.

Contraceptive practice the world over could be revolutionized in the next decades but current levels of funding for research have been decreasing. Only one major private American company is doing contraceptive research, as compared with thirteen in 1970. The NIH spent only $10 million on applied research in contraceptive development in 1992.[17] This has serious implications for world health. Potential measures under development that could be significant in increasing the use of contraception include a nonsurgical method of female sterilization, several reversible methods for male contraception, an antipregnancy vaccine, and a postpartum sterilization device. Also needed is social service research devoted to understanding the sources of resistance to family planning and methods of overcoming it, particularly in the seriously overpopulated and poverty-stricken countries.

For several decades, problems such as the energy crisis, pollution, housing, crime, illiteracy, hunger, crowding, deforestation, overgrazing, unemployment, endangered species, restrictions on individual freedom, and health threats have been identified as being created by, or related to, overpopulation. In relation to health alone, the World Health Organization (WHO) has reported that four-fifths of the world's population do not have any form of health care, and that almost 1 billion—almost 18 percent of the persons alive—suffer from combined long-term malnutrition and parasitic diseases, and thus are handicapped in their ability to work. Even though smallpox appears to have been conquered, the other infectious diseases are making a comeback, and deaths due to dysentery, diarrhea, and pneumonia, all closely related to malnutrition and poor housing conditions, are rising. In fact, the developing world's progress in combating high death rates may be slowing down, and in some cases reversing.

In 1994, 14 million children under five worldwide die annually from hunger-related causes. The extent to which health could be improved with relatively few resources is impressive. At a cost of $10 per child the world could control the six major childhood diseases (polio, tetanus, measles, diphtheria, pertussis, and tuberculosis) that kill or disable millions of children each year. Tanzania's community-based nutrition program has more than halved the rate of severe nutrition in three years for a current cost of $2.50 per child.[18] Similar small, or even smaller, amounts can control other major killers, but there is less optimism about malaria because of increasing resistance of mosquitoes to insecticides, and sexually transmitted diseases, especially acquired immune deficiency syndrome (AIDS). About one in ten sexually active teenagers and young adults (up to one in five in Africa) contract sexually transmitted diseases. An estimated 5 to 10 million people are now infected with the AIDS virus. On the other hand, WHO noted several major victories, primarily the eradication of smallpox, which, if not wiped out in the later 1970s, would have killed at least 20 million people.

The international conference held in Cairo in September of 1994 was ostensibly about stabilizing world population growth, but in fact it provided the stage for a cultural clash over women's rights. Early in the debate, the interdependence of a range of social concerns became apparent. Literacy, childbearing, childrearing, nutrition, poverty, family planning are a sample of world class concerns that find unity in their special relevance to women. A 113-page proclamation declared a new vision for population stabilization. Earlier conferences (1974, 1984) searched for solutions through quotas and control. In a radical change in philosophy, 150 nations in attendance in Cairo accepted the position that if given adequate information, health care, and access to a wide choice of contraceptive methods, most individuals will choose to have fewer children. Women are being brought to the center of the debate on family planning, and empowered on their own behalf. The discussion turned to family planning as a personal right as never before, and nongovernmental organizations that work with women at the local level are seen to be major allies.[19] Just as the sentiments expressed were unusual, so was the comparative silence of religious authorities, most especially the Vatican and Muslim extremists. This was in sharp contrast to the formidable alliance forged between the Vatican and the pro-life Reagan administration in Mexico City at the 1984 population conference. So imposing was their influence that the term *abortion* was only mentioned once during the entire course of the proceedings and then moved to be excluded from a list of permissible family planning mechanisms. In 1994, although withholding support from conference resolutions on abortion, contraception, and adolescent sexuality, the Vatican broke with tradition and endorsed some aspects of the conference's final declaration. Advocates of the proclamation proposed that national compliance with the intent of the document be a requirement for international aid. Critics caution that these statements on women's rights and family planning establish battle lines between women and the family. They caution that in many cultures the woman belongs to a family, and decisions about family are made in that forum. In contrast, because America is a land of immigrants, many Americans are lucky even to have a family. In many developing countries, the extended family is the only option for survival and personal choices are subordinated to tradition or common practice. This is not offered as a counterargument, but to demonstrate the complexity of the issue and the degree to which it strikes at the heart of culture.

UNITED STATES POPULATION

The 1990 U.S. census counted 250 million people and 105 million housing units. This effort marked the two-hundredth anniversary of the first census taken in 1790 when the United States had just under 4 million residents. The interim since the 1980 census showed some interesting developments besides the 10 percent increase in population.

Changes in age structure reflected past trends in childbearing. By the end of the 1980s the number of those 18 to 24 years old declined 11.2 percent, while baby boomers (ages 25 to 44) grew by almost 26 percent. The median age had risen from 30.0 years in 1980 to 33.1 in 1991. Most dramatic was the increase in the number of elderly to 12.6 percent of the population.[20]

This has great implications for the future but also affects the present. We are an aging country. The drop in the number of young people has created a smaller pool of potential students for higher education, a fact that has some significance for nursing recruitment. It also means that jobs that once were commonly held by teenagers, such as fast food and some clerical positions, are now being advertised at greater than minimum wages because they are not being filled. More elderly are being enticed to return to work with an uncommon amount of flexibility offered. The graying of America is considered the single most significant factor affecting the future of the United States, with special emphasis on health care. This will be discussed more extensively in Chap. 7.

In the year 2000, there are likely to be over 36 million Americans 65 years or older, with about half aged 75 or more. Persons 85 or older are the fastest growing category of the U.S. population. Over one-fifth of the elderly are poor or near-poor; women, blacks, and Hispanics have a higher poverty rate. Social security is the major source of support. Still, the economic level of the elderly varies widely, with income and assets from a variety of sources. Only about 5 percent live in institutions, but of those who do, a disproportionate number are women, generally unmarried or widowed. One major impact that the elderly, better educated than ever, have had is in influencing legislation. With organizations such as the American Association of Retired Persons (AARP) as their lobbyists, and with politicians' appreciation of their voting power, the elderly have clearly influenced legislation affecting them, such as the Catastrophic Illness Law that was both passed and later rescinded because of their pressure. Given that the number of elderly is expected to reach 65 million by 2030, the factors that affect only the elderly must be considered in the context of social and political events that affect all Americans.

Each generation is a product of its times. The aged of the mid-1990s faced the Great Depression as young adults, were patriots of World War II, knew economic deprivation in a period without social welfare programs, and were children of the liberalism and good times of the 1920s. Recent attention has been quick to focus on today's 20-something young adults. They are alternately called the X generation, still defying classification, or the 13ers, being the thirteenth generation in American history.[21] Their relationship with their parents, the boomers, sets the stage for the next generational crisis. They are a generation who inherit the repercussions of the excesses of their elders: a toxic environment, national debt, unemployment, economic recession, AIDS, recurrent TB. The fact that the cold war is over hardly seems an even exchange. Many were raised by grandparents of the silent generation or wartime America; while their parents, the boomers, were caught up in divorce or the super mom phenomenon. Most will suffer a loss in living standards when compared with their parents, a hard blow to Americans who were always expected to better their lot with each ensuing generation. Determined to regain what they have lost, the 13ers will strengthen the family, ask for very little governmental assistance throughout their lifetime, pursue conservative politics and investments, and favor the needs of the very young over the very old (mostly the boomers). Where the boomers were caught up in quick change and episodic relationships, the X generation will look to reestablish our traditional institutions and invest in our traditional social systems. This portends a whole new brand of volunteerism, a movement from adhocracy to a more long-term commitment, but with a no-nonsense attitude about what should be accomplished.

There have also been a number of other changes. The South and West have accounted for the greatest percentage of population growth; over 55 percent of the people reside there. (However, Alaska also saw a 30 percent growth rate.) Almost half the national population lives in 41 metropolitan areas that have populations of over 1 million. New census figures also show greater losses than expected in rural areas. The influx of immigrants to the United States has added to the diversity of America and is responsible for much of the population growth in the last decade. Despite much publicity about illegal aliens, most immigrants enter legally, but if both groups were counted, the numbers in the last decade would surpass even the record 8.8 million admitted in the first decade of this century. Unlike that great European migration, the new immigrants are primarily Hispanic, from the Americas, and Asian (particularly Korean and Filipino). This has affected the population mix in a number of states. The Asian population grew by 70 percent in the 1980s, and the Hispanic population is growing five times as fast as the rest of the population. It is predicted that, if current trends persist, non-Hispanic whites will be a minority in California by 2000. Hispanic-Americans are the youngest population group. One-third are under 18 years old, and half under 26.[22] Most Hispanics now live in Texas and California and other areas of the Southwest, although some cities such as New York and Miami are also favored. The largest number of Asians are in California and Hawaii. Acceptance of the new immigrants has varied. One concern is their assimilation into the community. It has been noted that for the first time in our history, the majority of immigrants speak just one language—Spanish—and tend to live in ethnic enclaves served by media communicating in Spanish. Some Asians have also tended to cluster in ethnic neighborhoods and work in ethnic groups. The fact that foreign-born black and Hispanic people are more likely to have jobs than those native-born has caused resentment (although there is also resentment if the newcomers are receiving public assistance). The same is true of Asians, many of whom have the entire family working long hours to support a small shop or business and often pressure their children to perform well in school. Nevertheless, there is no doubt that the diversity of our population enriches the nation.

Another social factor affecting health care is the size and makeup of American households. These have shrunk to their smallest ever, 2.62 people in 1992, with projections for the year 2000 showing a continued drop, but not as rapid. The decline has slowed because the baby boom generation is getting older and starting families. Women in their thirties and forties are much more inclined to plan for children. The number of individuals living alone is still growing, and the increase of one-parent families has contributed to the decline in family size (defined as two or more people). Only 26 percent of all households with children under 18 include a married couple. The number of families maintained by a woman without a man increased to 11.7 percent of all households; over 46 percent were black, 24

percent Hispanics, and 13 percent white. Many in this group are also likely to be part of the 89 percent of U.S. households receiving at least one noncash benefit such as food stamps and Medicaid. About one out of every four households with children under 19 received such assistance.[23]

In general, there has been an increase in the number of women working; 47 percent of households with children had two parents who were employed. The number of women with children who work outside the home has increased tremendously, with single mothers even more likely to do so.[24] About half of the mothers with infants hold jobs, sometimes because of necessity, sometimes because of career demands. The need for child care arrangements and flexibility is becoming quite evident to employers.

Considered an important social force among these careerists is the baby boom cohort, who, because of their number, have always had an impact in determining social attributes. They are the first group to be college-educated on a mass basis, with at least half attending college. Although this better-educated group is currently most involved in career advancement, buying a home, raising and educating a family, and securing their financial future, by the late 1990s they are seen as showing more interest in public policy, policy that will surely relate to health care and services to the elderly. Their participation in such decision making will influence policy direction.

At the other end of the spectrum are those who have an uncommon share of social and health problems. More than 14 percent of Americans lived below the poverty line. Child poverty, with one in five children under 18 being poor, is of particular concern. Two in five Hispanic children and nearly one out of every two black children are poor.[25]

The fact is that those who are already poor, undernourished, undereducated, and underemployed tend to have the most children. Moreover, the most economically depressed members of the population have converged in the urban areas. As the middle class made a hasty exodus from the deteriorating inner cities, the poor either stayed or moved in. For some, it was merely an exchange of rural poverty with fresh air to urban poverty with polluted air. In an interesting follow-up to the 1968 report of the Kerner Commission that had been convened to investigate the causes of racial riots in cities, it was noted that in the intervening 20 years, three separate black societies had emerged: the middle class, the working class, and the underclass. As the first two moved to better neighborhoods, the inner city, without their influence, deteriorated even more, until what was left was an environment where the greatest cause of death among young men is homicide, where the bitter alienated underclass is especially susceptible to drugs, AIDS, crime, prostitution, and the other ills of that environment. Children, born to young, uneducated, unmarried mothers, little more than children themselves, have poor health, little education, and no positive role models, and the cycle continues. Although some of these observations were made about blacks, the same could be said of any who live in such homes.

If, indeed, they have homes. Advocates of the homeless take objection to the processes and outcomes of the 1990 census. They challenge the manner of counting (shelters, scheduled hours, self-reporting). Based on a seven-day survey in several inner city areas, the Urban Institute estimates that there are two million homeless in this country at any one point in time.[26] Among this group are runaways and homeless youths, many of whom have come from impoverished, chaotic, or violent families. Fifty percent may have lived in foster homes and when they "aged out" of these services were literally left to the streets. Homeless single adults, mostly males, often have a history of alcohol or other drug abuse and, sometimes, mental illness. Families are the fastest growing segment of the homeless, living in shelters, welfare hotels, and campgrounds. Of the 30 percent of the homeless families, 85 percent are single mothers, about age 27, with two or three children. The vast majority receive Aid to Families with Dependent Children (AFDC). Drug use, especially crack, is epidemic among these mothers, who have frequently had chaotic childhoods and abusive adult relationships. The children have difficulty with language skills, motor skills, coordination, and personal and social growth. Many do not attend schools. Their future is questionable. Needless to say, the health problems of all the homeless are horrific, with tuberculosis, AIDS, accidents, drug-related conditions, violence, sexually transmitted diseases, and infections common. Pregnancy occurs at twice the national average and the babies are almost always born with health problems, frequently with AIDS or crack addiction—and abandoned.

The homeless population grew dramatically in the 1980s. Unemployment, lack of affordable housing, urban gentrification, and insufficient federal assistance programs have been cited as reasons for the accelerated growth of the homeless. Although most of the homeless are found in urban settings, there are also some in rural areas. Public and private facilities, often grossly inadequate and sometimes even dangerous, have been opened for temporary housing. Many homeless bypass these shelters to sleep in public facilities like train and bus stations where some also beg and sometimes harass commuters. Homelessness is not a simple phenomenon but is created and complicated by a variety of other social problems: unemployment, parental neglect, poverty, substance abuse, and so on. Where middle America once had a large quotient of sympathy for these people, that goodwill has turned into a backlash. The economic recession, unemployment, problems with health care, and crime on the streets have all tested our patience. Citizens want the streets and public buildings clean and uncluttered. The homeless are a reminder of our shortcomings as a society, and in times of personal stress our tolerance wears thin as our dollars for social welfare programs.

An aspect of poverty made more visible by homelessness was hunger. Soup kitchens, not seen since the Great Depression of the 1930s, were crowded daily. It appeared that not only the Third World had a hunger problem, but also the wealthy United States. Nevertheless, a commission appointed by the Reagan administration, which had been consistently cutting funding for the needs of the poor and near-poor, reported that these cutbacks for food had not harmed the poor. The members asserted that hunger among Americans could not be documented, although it probably "does persist."

Regardless of the accuracy of this report, there is little doubt that the poor not only lack adequate housing, nutrition, and jobs but also have a multitude of health problems for which they may not seek help until there is a serious need. A whole series of specific needs related to health has emerged because of their particular social-ethnic-economic problems. The need is for readily available health services, such as neighborhood family health centers, health workers who understand the problems of the people and are able to communicate with them, understandable health teaching, and coordination of the multiple services required. Some of the more urgent health needs that have been cited are preventive, diagnostic, referral, and counseling services for pregnant women, infants, and preschool children, and community mental health services to alleviate problems or redirect deviant behavior of individuals, families, or groups.

Population control and family planning are also issues in the United States. Although the concept of population control is acceptable to most in the abstract, the specific methods are controversial for various reasons. Use of contraceptive measures may be against the moral, religious, or cultural mores of a group, and there is particular opposition by some to any form of sterilization. Abortion, made legal for the first trimester of pregnancy by a Supreme Court decision (*Roe v. Wade*), has been bitterly opposed by the Catholic Church and various right-to-life groups. Both pro-choice and anti-abortion groups have been active politically. The influence of the two groups seems to wax and wane. In each congressional session and in many state legislatures since the 1973 decision, there have been pressures and subsequent actions related to abortion rights. The current Supreme Court has also chosen to consider and rule on such cases. See Chap. 22 for further discussion of the legal aspects of these issues. In general, while these legal struggles continue, the number of abortions has leveled off, showing no more than 5 percent increase or decrease since 1980.[27]

THE NATION'S HEALTH

The health status of the U.S. population as a whole is, according to health statistics, better than ever. Health status is determined in several ways: using mortality statistics (life expectancy and death rates), which are easily obtained, and morbidity statistics (the incidence and prevalence of illness). The latter are much more difficult to obtain and are less accurate because most diseases are not reportable, and reports, surveys, and research can be interpreted in a number of ways.

Nevertheless, reports on the health of Americans proliferate, and they are usually of a good-news–bad-news nature. The goods news is that life expectancy has reached a new height; infant mortality and the overall death rate has dropped. Mortality from heart disease and cancer (except for smoking-related lung cancer) is down, but there is a slight increase in death from chronic obstructive pulmonary disease. On the other side of the ledger is the fact that the life expectancy of blacks is 71.8 years as opposed to 76.5 for whites (67.8 for black males). The chief causes for the differences, particularly for males, seem to be an increase in homicides, auto accidents, AIDS, tuberculosis and other infectious diseases, and infant mortality as well as lack of medical care. In addition, a report of the National Center for Health Statistics associates health status with income. People with low income had more days in bed because of illness and injury, more visits to the doctor, and more hospital days.[28] And there is disparity of opinion over whether the elderly and our youth are less or more healthy than in past years. Duke University gerontologists noted a significant drop in old age disability.

Perhaps the most discouraging news is that, just as has been true for decades, many of the most common causes for premature death, often due to lifestyle, are preventable. *Healthy People 2000*, published by the U.S. Public Health Service in 1990, summarizes these causes:[29]

1. Abuse of addictive substances: use of tobacco (especially cigarettes) causing degenerative cardiovascular diseases, cancer, and other conditions; alcohol abuse, including deaths from vehicular accidents, falls, suicides, homicides; abuse of other addictive substances such as heroin and cocaine resulting in accidents, homicides, and AIDS.

2. Neglect of preventive care and inappropriate treatment: neglect of high blood pressure resulting in heart disease, stroke, kidney failure; inappropriate medical care, causing complications from unnecessary or inappropriate surgery or drugs; failure to detect and treat treatable cancers; not identifying signs of disease and/or not seeking diagnostic measures or treatment promptly.

3. Hazardous lifestyles: reckless driving, including lack of restraints; promiscuous sexual practices, resulting in sexually transmitted diseases; lack of working smoke detectors and exit plans in the home; poor dietary practices, including too much or too little or the wrong food; lack of regular exercise and sleep.

These points have been made repeatedly over the years by a variety of governmental and private agencies, with mixed results. There is some drop in drug use by teens, except for alcohol, but the greatest increase in AIDS is due to the use of contaminated needles by drug addicts. The smoking rate of the general population has fallen, but for teenagers of both sexes, either black or white, it has risen. Government action, however, has banned smoking in many public places and on public transportation.

There has also been governmental intervention in the use of alcohol; all states are in compliance with the National Uniform Drinking Age Law, raising the drinking age to 21. Adults claim they exercise more, although it is not clear what and how much is meant and, at any rate, this is primarily a phenomenon of the middle and upper-middle classes, particularly young and middle-aged adults. (There is also concern that children are getting very little exercise.) Although Americans, again probably mostly middle class, eat fewer fatty foods, they still eat too much. The improvement in these aspects of lifestyle are credited with the drop in deaths from heart disease. Significant differences in health occur from state to state, with Minnesota the healthiest.[30] This may be due to both lifestyle and environment.

Yet there are other concerns. Tuberculosis (TB) is reemerging as a serious public health threat, particularly in inner cities. This is linked to homelessness, drug and alcohol abuse, and AIDS, whose victims are especially susceptible to TB. In addition, scientists have reported that one in five adults suffer from at least one mental disorder, about the same for men as for women except that more women suffer from depression. More disturbing, the figures are similar for children and young adults. Anxiety disorders, substance abuse, and antisocial personality problems are more common in this young group. It is not known if mental illness, however "mild," might also have a part in the escalating rate of suicide, particularly among young men. (Suicide is also significant among the elderly.) Certainly violence is a major factor in death rates. The Centers of Disease Control reported suicide and homicide as a leading cause of premature death for Americans, after accidents, cancer, and heart disease.

Because cancer is still a major cause of death, 1993 data from the American Cancer Society are pertinent:[31]

1. Lung cancer remains the leading cause of cancer deaths in the United States for both sexes.

2. Breast cancer is still on the rise in all age groups.

3. Prostate cancer is increasing, principally because of the aging population.

4. Colon and rectal cancers are no longer among the four most frequent sites.

5. Skin cancer, especially the highly curable basal cell or squamous cell cancers, has an incidence of over 600,000 cases a year, by far the largest number of any cancer. The potentially fatal melanoma is increasing.

6. The cancer rate for blacks is higher than for whites; the death rate is also higher.

7. Hispanic-Americans are not adequately aware of most of the warning signals of cancer or ways to reduce risk. They tend not to seek early detection or treatment.

8. Millions of Americans are alive in 1994 who have had cancer; those diagnosed over five years ago can be considered "cured," that is, having the same life expectancy as someone without cancer. Two million new cases of cancer will be diagnosed this year.

9. Early detection and treatment is a major factor in survival.

10. Among hazards listed that might lead to cancer are smoking, excess sunlight, excess alcohol, smokeless tobacco, estrogen, radiation, occupational hazards such as industrial agents, and nutritional factors.

11. The greatest number of new cancer cases was found in California and Florida, the fewest in Wyoming and Vermont. (Environmental factors should be considered here.)

Other reports add that one unexplained trend is an increase in the number of deaths of the old-old by brain cancer and multiple myeloma. Cancer mortality for those over 55 appears to be rising both in the United States and in various other developed countries.

Another major issue in the nation's health status focuses on infants and children. According to a 1990 report issued by the House Select Committee on Children, Youth and Families, children in the United States are more likely than children in 11 other industrialized countries to live in poverty, to live with one parent, or to be killed before the age of 25; more are likely to die before their first birthday than in any of the other countries except the Soviet Union. At about the same time, the American Academy of Pediatrics also issued some data about child health, emphasizing such problems as crack babies (375,000 babies a year are born to mothers who use drugs); the effect of environmental hazards on children; the fact that injuries kill six times as many children as cancer, the second leading cause of childhood death; the increase of pediatric AIDS, now the ninth leading cause of death, and poor children's lack of access to care. Equal concern is expressed about the rising toll of child abuse and the resurgence of childhood diseases that could be prevented by routine immunization.

In 1994 adolescent sexuality and pregnancy continued to be major health and social problems. Since 1990, teenage pregnancy and birthrates in the United States have exceeded those in most developed countries. There were one million pregnancies in women ages 15 to 19, over 50 percent resulted in births, and 95 percent of those pregnancies were unintended. Though the number of reported legal induced abortions has remained relatively stable since 1980 (varying within 5 percent), the national rate in 1990 was at its lowest point since 1977. The birthrate among teenagers continued to increase in 1991, as it had in previous years, with 65 percent of those births being out of wedlock (56 percent for whites, 60 percent for Hispanics, 94 percent for blacks). The typical woman selecting abortion is young, white, and unmarried with no previous live births, and having the procedure for the first time.[32] The Children's Defense Fund reported that black teenagers were 2.3 times more likely, and Hispanic teenagers 1.9 times more likely, to give birth than white teenagers, although the level of sexual activity was about the same. Black, white, or Hispanic, one out of every five 16- to 19-year-old women with below-average academic skills, and coming from poor families, was a teenage mother. Generally they dropped out of school and were likely to have a second baby within three years. However, although they opted to have their first child, even when abortion services were available, this was less likely the second time, perhaps suggesting a better understanding of the realities of motherhood. Young teenagers' unrealistic attitudes about childbearing have been seen as reflecting their families' and communities' failure to encourage responsible reproductive behavior (as opposed to other developed societies).

Teens' lack of maturity and sense of responsibility is evident in the fact that many apparently are not concerned about the social, economic, or health consequences of illegitimate births. Yet, studies have shown that young parenthood has adverse effects on the young parents' educational attainment and economic self-sufficiency, and that infants born to young mothers may show deficits in physical health, cognitive development, social and emotional development, and school achievement.

Teenage as well as low-income mothers and their children are also in physical danger. The National Center for Health Statistics (NCHS) claims that maternal deaths related to pregnancy are underreported, with mortality for nonwhite women almost three times greater than for white. Infant deaths (under one year) are particularly high for black babies, many of whom have low birth weight. This is partially due to lack of appropriate prenatal care. The United States infant mortality rate of 8.9 per thousand live births (actually a new low in 1991) is among the highest of industrialized nations.

Frequent teenage pregnancy and the decline of abortions have significant implications for the future health of children and adults, and family structure. As of June 1992, 24 percent of single women aged 18 to 44 had borne children compared with 15 percent in 1982. The proportion of single mothers among women with one or more years of college doubled (4.4 percent in 1982 to 11.3 percent in 1992). There was a similar pattern in those with high school education (17.2 to 32.5 percent) and those without a high

school diploma (35.2 to 48.4 percent). The link between education and childbearing is as true in the United States as in developing countries.

Of all the diseases that affect Americans today, probably the most frightening is AIDS. C. Everett Koop, the former Surgeon General of the United States noted that since AIDS was first identified in 1981, it has spread quickly and irrevocably. By the end of 1990, more than 100,000 people in the United States had died of AIDS, and nearly a third of those deaths occurred in that same year. Currently over 100 people die every day from AIDS in this country, and the rate is increasing. By June 1992, 230,000 cases of AIDS had been reported to the Centers for Disease Control and Prevention (CDCP); and there had been 150,000 deaths. In a one-year period, 1990–1991, reported new cases rose by over 30 percent. Though these statistics are staggering, it has been estimated that only 10 to 15 percent of the total number of people infected with HIV are reported.

Many stereotypes about AIDS have been shattered in recent years. AIDS and HIV are no longer diseases restricted to the largest metropolitan areas. Rather, by 1991, 25 states and 31 metropolitan areas plus Puerto Rico had reported cases in excess of 1,000—and the volume and places continue to expand. AIDS continues to impact gay and bisexual men more than other groups (64 percent). African Americans constitute 28 percent of AIDS cases, and Hispanics 16 percent. The number of women and children infected is growing dramatically. AIDS is currently one of the leading causes of death for women between the ages of 25 and 45.[33] It is sobering to think that worldwide, each woman dying of AIDS will leave behind an average of two children. By the year 2000, nearly 10 million children will have been orphaned by the disease. Grandparents, needing care themselves, bury their children and take on renewed responsibility for child rearing. These are the lucky children. Many will join the ranks of homeless children who are "throwaways," possibly infected themselves, and desperately trying to survive on their own.[34]

AIDS is not curable, but it is highly preventable. Because of the known relation between AIDS and substance abuse, prevention programs have focused on the use of good-quality condoms as protection during sexual intercourse, discouraging needle-sharing practices among substance abusers, and establishing a rigorous standard in processing blood and blood products for transfusion. However, the human element remains. Many individuals are reluctant to demand the use of condoms in their sexual relationships, some religious groups object to publicizing safe sex, and drug users are often ignorant or indifferent. Teenagers continue to feel omnipotent and above harm and pursue risky behaviors. Given the length of time between infection and diagnosis, individuals with AIDS in their mid to late twenties were infected as teens.

AIDS is global in its scope. A 1990 epidemic in an eastern European country could be directly traced to blood transfusions and inadequate sterilization of needles. In 1988, 136 countries reported AIDS cases. Forty-two countries in the Americas had reported 73 percent of the world's total cases.[35] However, in 1990, the most rapid spread was reported in Africa, with a conservative estimate of 5 million adult cases, more than half of an estimated worldwide total of 8 million. All these statistics should be seen as tentative, given the questionable reporting and record-keeping standards.

Even in the midst of this tragedy there has been progress. Though there is no cure, great strides have been made in palliative drug therapy. Individuals with AIDS are living longer and experiencing better quality of life. Persons with AIDS are a protected class under the Americans with Disabilities Act, therefore allowing them to continue in the American mainstream. Compliance with CDCP-approved universal precaution techniques is mandatory for every health care setting and provider. The health care community has held the line to diffuse the public tendency to panic by opposing mandatory testing and disclosure for any group, including health care workers or patients.

Yet, for health care workers, the danger of infection is real. One physician, who claimed infection from a needle-prick, won a large settlement in 1990; other such cases are expected. Some workers, including health professionals, have refused to care for AIDS patients, which can become a legal as well as an ethical problem. However, many nurses have made special efforts to provide psychological as well as physical care to AIDS patients and their significant others, and nursing education programs are including appropriate content in their curriculum.

Environmental conditions as the cause of American morbidity and mortality must also be considered. The point has been made that Americans have a sense of peril, that is, fear of a variety of factors in modern life that are reported as dangerous to health by the media, for instance, chemicals in food, danger in transportation, and inadequately tested drugs. But the fact that, by broad statistical measures, Americans have never been safer should not be cause to underestimate the real hazards. Perhaps one reason the issue of the effect of toxic agents on health has been so controversial in the last several decades is that the morbidity and mortality caused by such agents are often difficult to document. The effect on health may not be seen for decades, and there may not be a clear indication of which of the many interacting factors is clearly responsible for an illness or death. Some occupational illnesses have been identified, and to varying degrees, safety standards have been set and enforced by the Occupational Safety and Health Administration (OSHA) and the Environmental Protection Agency (EPA). Consumer groups and unions have claimed that such protection is generally insufficient, while industry complains that it is so overregulated that expenses for compliance are unreasonable. Some conditions, such as byssinosis (brown lung disease), caused by cotton dust in the textile industries, and silicosis (black lung disease), caused by silica, particularly in mining, are clearly recognized as job-related diseases. It is generally accepted that other occupation-related disabilities are caused by benzine, formaldehyde, waste anesthesia gases, asbestos, ethylene oxide (a sterilizing agent in hospitals and medical products industries), diisocyanate (a chemical used to produce plastic products), vinyl chloride, lead, and radiation, to name a few. Clearly, some of these are particular hazards for nurses, along with the danger of AIDS, hepatitis B, airborne pathogens, and accidents (See bibliography). The Nurses' Environmental Health Watch publishes information on hazards for nurses and how to avoid or minimize them.

Considered a major public health issue is the trend to exclude women, especially those of childbearing age, from positions involving possible exposure to chemical and physical agents with known or suspected teratogenic (birth defect-causing) properties. Men have not been excluded, although there are data suggesting that paternal exposure to these toxic agents may also be teratogenic. It is estimated that 100,000 jobs are closed to women because of these policies. The argument is that instead of such action, the environment could and should be made safe for all workers. This is repeatedly going to the courts with mixed outcomes.

Other environmental hazards are also cited by public health experts and environmentalists. The depletion of the stratospheric ozone layer caused by chlorofluorocarbons (CFC) used in sprays, refrigeration, and air-conditioning systems, industrial blowing agents, insulating foams, metal cleaning and drying, garment cleaning, sterilization of medical supplies, and liquid fast freezing causes skin cancer and potential changes in the world's climate. Limitations have been set by the Clean Air Act for sulfur oxides, suspected particulate matter, nitrogen oxides, carbon monoxides, hydrocarbons, lead, and other pollutants emitted by various industries and automobiles, but there is a constant battle to determine what the limit should be.

Acid rain, resulting from emissions from coal-burning plants and factories—chiefly sulfur dioxide and nitrogen oxides that are chemically changed in the atmosphere—is suspected of destroying freshwater life, damaging forests and crops, and possibly threatening human health. Cited by the EPA as probably the most serious environmental problem in the United States is that of hazardous wastes. These are by-products of the manufacturing process of many products, but the large-scale generators are chemical manufacturers, petroleum refiners, and metal-production companies. Careless dumping of these waters, for instance, in areas where they leak into a water supply or cause an explosion, has resulted in serious danger to whole communities. Scientists contend that it is possible to contain wastes safely if certain caveats are observed, and some manufacturers are making an effort to clean up sites. Meanwhile, dangerous old waste dumps are continually being discovered.

The deadly chemical dioxin, an unwanted by-product of herbicides, pesticides, and other industrial products, has been given considerable attention, particularly since the question was raised as to its effect on soldiers and civilians in Vietnam, where it was a chemical contaminant of the defoliant Agent Orange. There is some belief that others, such as inhabitants of the Love Canal area and those exposed to dioxin in train wrecks or factory explosions, have suffered from a variety of conditions, including kidney and liver ailments, birth defects, and cancer. In other environmental situations, contamination by polybrominated biphenyls (PPBs) and polychlorinated biphenyls (PCBs), now banned, has resulted in the required destruction of food products because of danger to human beings.

Almost daily, there is some report in the media about product or environmental dangers, whether noise, food additives, safety failure of equipment, toys, autos, clothing, hazardous wastes, acid rain, radioactive leaks, unsafe drinking water, or even human destruction from nuclear weapons or plants. Some feel that this is a hysterical reaction to unproven claims. Others ignore the entire issue. Still others feel that with or without more definitive data, a stronger effort must be made to improve the environment. Certainly, the clearly visible smog in so many urban areas is evidence that there is room for improvement.

In part because of rising health care costs and, of course, concern for the public's health, in 1980 the federal government began to publish health objectives for the nation, presumably also putting governmental efforts and funds behind them. In a review of the status of the 1980 objectives, it appeared that the priority areas showing the greatest progress were in the areas of high blood pressure control, immunization, surveillance and control of infectious diseases (except AIDS), and smoking. Showing the least progress were goals related to pregnancy and infant health, family planning, and physical fitness and exercise. The latest publication (1990) is *Healthy People 2000*.[36] The five broad national goals proposed in this document are to

- Reduce infant mortality to no more than 7 per 1000 live births
- Increase life expectancy to at least 78 years
- Reduce disability caused by chronic conditions to a prevalence of no more than 7 percent of all people
- Increase healthy years of life to at least 65 years
- Decrease the disparity in life expectancy between white and minority populations to no more than 4 years

Some of the most important specific objectives were to:

- Improve nutrition
- Improve surveillance and data systems
- Increase physical activity and fitness
- Reduce tobacco use
- Reduce alcohol and other drug problems
- Encourage responsible sexual behavior
- Reduce violent behavior
- Maintain the vitality and independence of older people
- Improve environmental health
- Improve occupational safety and health
- Prevent unintentional injuries
- Improve maternal and infant health

- Improve immunization for infectious diseases
- Reduce HIV infection
- Reduce sexually transmitted diseases
- Reduce high blood cholesterol and high blood pressure
- Reduce the toll from cancer
- Reduce other chronic disorders
- Improve oral health
- Prevent mental and behavioral disorders
- Improve health education and preventive services

A tall order, particularly when health-related organizations promptly began to suggest additions and changes. Nevertheless, it will be interesting to see how much can be accomplished in that decade, particularly since prevention activities have had their ups and downs. With the focus on health promotion and disease prevention, nurses should be especially involved, even taking a leadership position, in working toward achievement of these goals.

TECHNOLOGICAL, SCIENTIFIC, AND MEDICAL ADVANCES

There is little question that the technological advances of the last quarter century have been extraordinary and, combined with scientific-medical advances, the beginnings of a new health care system have been emerging. Some of the most significant technological changes affecting patient care can be categorized as follows:

1. Developments in diagnosis and treatment such as automated clinical laboratory equipment, artificial human organs, improved surgical techniques and equipment, such as microsurgery and laser beams, and the use of computers in diagnosis.

2. Hospital information management— mainly coming from application of the computer for patient billing, accounting, research, record keeping, and diagnostic

applications. These are being developed to control the flow of information so that health practitioners can have ready access to necessary data and can have information transmitted quickly and accurately to all departments.

3. Developments affecting hospital supply and services, such as widespread adoption of plastic, other inexpensive and improved materials, and such equipment as specialized carts, conveyers, and pneumatic tubes.

4. Improvement in the management and structural design of health facilities all aimed at more efficient utilization of personnel, equipment, and space. This involves improved concepts of management and construction of health facilities, putting into effect concepts of patient care and advances in organizing health services.

5. Mass communication, making possible speedy transmission of health information and new knowledge, and exerting a powerful influence in molding public opinion. It can bring about positive results, such as providing information on diseases and ways in which to get help; it can provide knowledge about other social and health problems, and even provide formal educational programs.

Clearly, technology plays an important role in health care. Scientific and medical advances have gone beyond the imagination of science fiction. Almost all have raised many ethical issues, and sometimes legal complications in relation to access, quality of life, and right to life. (Some of these issues are discussed in Chaps. 10 and 22.) The rapidity of technological development has caught almost everyone unprepared. For instance, with the isolation of DNA and the process of cloning (production of genetically identical copies of an individual organism), theoretically, a human being could be created by artificial means.

In 1978, the birth of the first test-tube babies with the ovum fertilized outside the mother's body created worldwide controversy. The re-

placement of nonfunctioning human parts with artificial substitutes or human transplants has the potential of bringing a bionic era to reality. Already there have been implanted or attached titanium and polyethylene thigh bones; cords of woven Dacron for tendons; plastic, steel, and metal-alloy joints; orlon and Dacron blood vessels; plastic and titanium heart valves; artificial voice devices; and even an artificial heart. Moreover, progress has been made in electronic stimulation of the brain for hearing and seeing, and in developing miniaturized versions of the artificial kidney. Versatile lasers can remove the cloudiness from the eyes of the visually impaired, open clogged blood vessels, and break up kidney stones.

New diagnostic techniques are hailed because of both their effectiveness and the fact that they are noninvasive, sometimes eliminating the need for exploratory surgery. Among these are magnetic resonance imaging (MRI), a diagnostic technique utilizing magnetic and radio frequencies to image body tissues and monitor body chemistry. A less recent technique, computed tomography (CT), is still expected to play a major role in medical imaging as is the use of ultrasound with newly developed specialty probes for intracavity applications. Among the newest techniques are monoclonal antibody imaging agents which increase the ability of doctors to detect and diagnose cancer, heart disease, and other conditions. These antibodies are linked to a radioactive isotope and injected into the patient; they flow through the blood and latch onto their targets, e.g., tumors. They show up as hot spots of activity when photographed by the usual means used in nuclear medicine. There is also hope that these might eventually be used as a "magic bullet" to treat disease.

The expense of such equipment and what seems to be a constant need to update equipment is frequently criticized as adding to the cost of health care, but new medical and nonmedical technologies are believed by experts to improve human services. Among the expected impact of technology is the diminishing of genetic and infectious diseases, replacement of blood transfusions by artificial fluids, elimination of chronic pain by electrode implantations, and advances in artificial intelligence and computerization that will allow patients to obtain their diagnoses electronically at home. Computer applications to medicine and health care are particularly significant.

Although there is undeniable progress in health care directly attributable to technology, there is also great fear that the more machines do, the less human interaction there will be. In addition, the fear of loss of privacy becomes particularly acute with revelations of how the government and others could gain access to information about an individual's private life. Some sociologists predicted a few years ago that people would soon carry one card, containing a record of name, age, address, date and place of birth, blood type, IQ, religion, marital status, salary, credit rating, political affiliation, and personality traits, all carefully coded and stored by a computer (accurately, one hopes).

In the United States, the computer is playing a growing role in people's lives. Not only are computers used in almost every phase of business, the professions, and education but they have also become popular in the home for those who can afford them. There they are used for everything from game playing to job- or school-related projects. Children are being taught to work with computers; in some schools computer science is required for high school graduation. Voice-activated computers are used in health care for documentation, particularly in hospital emergency rooms where hands need to be free to minister to patients.

Several immediate problems of current computer usage have alarmed the public. First is the question of security of information. In the last decade computer experts have made headlines with their ability to invade the computers of banks, hospitals, industry, and even the government, in some cases changing or erasing data. While others had already used the computer to commit crimes (and were not always caught and punished), this new danger reinforced earlier

concerns about the confidentiality of computer-stored information. Would an employer, or simply a curious individual, be able to review another individual's credit record or hospital record? For that matter, would the record be accurate? Anyone who has had to deal with the unresponsive computers of businesses and the government knows the difficulty of catching and correcting errors; computer input still has a human component. Confidentiality is precisely the issue that is slowing progress on the electronic transfer of claims information in health care. Though the electronic system that would use a computerized patient record guarantees billions in savings, the confidentiality issues are bigger.

There are some predictions that high-technology computers, microelectronics, satellite communications, and robotics, seen by business and government as the nation's economic solution, will actually have a negative impact on the female workforce. Women already perform most of the low-skilled, high-technology labor at low wages and are even being displaced in their traditional stronghold, the office. It has been noted that job loss for women is high for stenographers, bank tellers, keypunch operators, insurance clerks, and telephone operators when computerization is introduced. On the other hand, there are predictions of increased jobs in specialized areas. Naisbett, in predicting that the 1990s and beyond would be an information-based age, also noted that by 1990 women had already taken two-thirds of the new jobs created in the information era and would continue to do so into the millennium. Naisbett's predictions are discussed later in this chapter.

Computers have had a definite impact on organizational structures such as hospitals. Hospital information systems (HIS) are expected to promote efficiency but have proved in some cases that they can be both disturbing and disruptive to those already employed. If not appropriately selected, introduced, and used, communication can be less effective than expected. The greatest impetus to the development of nursing information systems came about when Medicare-Medicaid coverage required nurses to provide data needed for reimbursement and to document the care given both in hospitals and in community health agencies. Effective use of computer systems in health care organizations requires that nurses be critical of the systems they evaluate and use, which means that they must learn about computers and what they can do. Computers can be deceptive and actually increase the time needed for documentation if software is inadequate and systems are not interactive. Nurses must be involved in planning, design, and standardization of the nursing database.

Over the last several years, there has been a great deal in the nursing literature about the use of computers in education and practice. The variety of uses continually increases, and more nurses are becoming experts.[37] An important point made is that nurses, like others, must find fast, effective ways to turn raw data into useful organized information. Nursing information systems (NIS) can improve both cost-effectiveness and quality of care, helping nurses to use their time in the most effective possible ways. Among the ways health care information systems (HCIS) can be applied are systems that assist in patient assessment and classification, care planning, charting and documenting care, quality assurance, discharge planning, staffing and scheduling and tracking acuity, cost, and quality data. Computer terminals at the patient's bedside, in the examining room, or even the patient's home can ease data entry, improve accuracy, and eliminate duplication of information. If used properly, computers can also improve exchange of information between nurses and other health care professionals and staff. Critical paths are one example of software that promises to enhance interdisciplinary relations, save nursing time, and increase the sophistication of care. Critical paths are the product of interdisciplinary consensus on the preferred course of treatment, the anticipated response of the patient, and the manner in which organizational systems should respond. The path serves as a prompter to clinical decision making and

alerts the provider to instances in which the patient is not responding as anticipated. The existence of the path documents the plan of care and allows the nurse to limit charting to exceptions to the path, thus reducing paperwork.

In addition, computer technology is increasingly being used in nursing education and research. Computer-assisted instruction (CAI) is used in such areas as drill and practice, simulations, and tutorials. Nursing informatics courses are being offered (or required) in many schools of nursing. Much nursing research also depends on competent use of computer technology, whether related to clinical data collection or retrieving information from libraries. The increase in use of electronic media is demonstrated in the new Sigma Theta Tau Center for Nursing Scholarship International Library where just about all information will be in computerized form.

There is no question that the use of computers in health care institutions and agencies will increase. Experts repeatedly identify computer technology as essential to improvement in health care. Particularly named are fully interactive information systems that link patient care with everything from accounting to materials management, computer-assisted clinical prescribing and monitoring drug interactions, and computerized patient records, including bedside information systems. For nurses, this means learning to use the new technology for the benefit of the patient, but continually maintaining the emphasis on individuality and human contact, which no machine can provide, as well as protecting the patient's privacy.

EDUCATION

Trends in education affect nursing in a number of ways: (1) the kind, number, and quality of students entering the nursing programs and the background they bring with them; (2) the development of educational technology, which frequently becomes a part of nursing education;

and (3) the impact of social demands on education, which are eventually extended to education in the professions, including nursing. Usually it is not just one social or economic condition that brings about change in education, nor is there only one kind of change. For instance, overexpansion by most institutions of higher education when the baby boom was at its height created a large pool of unemployed college graduates in the early 1970s. Some of these, as well as college students with a worried eye to the future, looked for educational programs that seemed to promise immediate jobs with a future, among them nursing. Thus, what had once been a trickle of mature, second-degree students into nursing became a steady stream. As the baby boom group diminished, the over-extended institutions of higher education and individual programs found it necessary to use marketing strategies of all kinds to attract enough students. They discovered the working adults in the community, who were a relatively untapped pool.

There were several definitive results. This diversity of age, background, education, and life experience in those seeking (or being sought for) advanced education has been an important factor in both social and political pressures for more flexibility in higher education. At the same time, providing such flexibility is one of the marketing strategies educational institutions are, after considerable resistance, relying on to attract the "older" prospective student. One focus is on liberalizing ways by which individuals can receive academic credit for what they know, regardless of when, where, or how they acquired that knowledge. Credentials are viable currency in the struggle for upward mobility, and those in the health field are as eager as others in society to be a part of this movement. In general education, the concepts of independent study and credit by examination have been explored by an increasing number of colleges, and a variety of testing mechanisms are being used to grant credit, including teacher-made tests and standardized tests, which have wide acceptance. One example of the latter is the College Level Examination

Program (CLEP), which was developed some time ago by the Educational Testing Service and funded by the Carnegie Corporation. It includes tests of general education and numerous examinations in individual courses for which a number of colleges and universities award credit.

Pressure toward a more open curriculum has also been exerted on general and nursing education through recommendations in reports made by prestigious groups and foundations. For example, the Carnegie Commission on Higher Education conducted a series of studies that seemed to voice the complaints of the public about limitations imposed by higher education. Included were recommendations to create alternate routes of entry other than full-time college attendance and to increase opportunities for vertical mobility. Such demands are being repeated in the new decade.

That these pressures have had some results is clear when one sees the increased number of so-called external degree programs. Some are marginally legitimate operations that have given the whole concept a bad name with meaningless mail-order degrees, but more and more respected, accredited educational institutions have established external degree programs using various modes: weekend, evening, summer, or other time periods for concentrated classes; outreach programs for isolated areas or even the workplace; and self-directed study with examinations. A particularly successful example of the last is the Regents College Degrees, previously the New York Regents External Degree Program, which includes both associate and baccalaureate degrees in nursing. (See Chap. 12 for more detailed information on this and other open curriculum practices in nursing.)

It was predicted that an aid to these new educational or flexible patterns was the use of all types of audiovisual media, computers, programmed learning, and other new techniques that can enhance the teaching-learning process. Although these methods appear to be generally successful, they are expensive, and there is some argument as to whether the learning acquired is superior to that gained by more traditional methods. One great asset appears to be that learning can be individualized more easily through use of these techniques and also that satisfactory learning can occur in places other than the classroom and in the teacher's presence—even to the point of checking out these learning tools as books are checked out from the library. The latter is particularly pertinent with a rising demand for continuing education in all professional fields, an aspect of the demand for current competence.

Equally significant are other happenings in higher education. Cost, to student and institution, is an ongoing controversial issue. As government aid declines, the cost to the student for higher education increases. Because there are not as many tax benefits to encourage charitable giving, colleges and universities have a major problem in balancing costs, quality, and service to students. Two-year colleges, which have shown a decline in students in recent years, are under particular pressure because of their very low tuitions. There are also criticisms that relatively few students continue their education in a four-year college and that the drop-out rate is high. On the other hand, despite the cry for higher quality, there is less state interest (and sometimes simply a lack of funds) for improving the public community colleges. Thus, many junior colleges have found it necessary to raise tuition and also to market themselves vigorously to attract more students. Financial problems of some four-year colleges are also serious; many smaller colleges have been forced to close their doors, as have some nursing programs.

Too-high college tuition is also seen as a major problem by the public in various surveys, closely followed by student attitude, drug problems, and poor quality of academic programs, including lack of interest in teaching. The cost of a college education is outpacing inflation. The nontraditional students, although welcomed by institutions of higher learning, have found costs particularly serious since they are often not eligible for funding, primarily reserved for full-time students. In testimony to Congress, the point was made that part-time students who must work often do not have the funds to pay high tuition. This may have had an impact in nursing; in 1989, some nurse traineeship funds were available for the first time for part-time students, although certain restrictions were put on the grant. However, all students who need funding may have problems in the next few years, since federal funding has moved away from grants that do not have to be repaid, to loans. Experts say that this will have a particular impact on the low-income group, since students from poor families are reluctant to go into debt for education. Completing a bachelor's degree in 4 years is no longer the norm. Graduate study is also more drawn out and frequently part-time. Information on nursing students is included in Chap. 13. Retention rates in higher education are also of concern. In private colleges, only 67 percent of entering students remain to graduation, according to the *Chronicle of Higher Education*. In black colleges the rate declines to 22 percent.[38] Some have said that institutional emphasis on research as opposed to teaching is part of the problem, since faculty, especially in universities, tend to be rewarded and promoted largely on the basis of their research productivity. Loudly voiced public discontent has forced such institutions to work on ways to improve teaching.

Today's undergraduate students consist of an equal number of men and women; Asians make up more than half of the foreign students. Most students entered college at age 18 or 19, are white and either Protestant or Catholic; their fathers and mothers had at least a high-school education and generally post-high-school education; fathers are in a business or profession; only 22 percent of mothers are either homemakers or unemployed (about 8 percent are nurses); about half have a family income over $40,000; about 60 percent plan graduate study; about 2 percent are interested in nursing; most drink beer, wine, or liquor, but do not smoke; most are middle-of-the-road politically. They think abortion should be legal; that there should be mandatory testing for

AIDS and drugs; that the chief benefit of college is to increase one's earning power; that a national health care plan is needed. They also support school busing; agree that the courts are too concerned about the rights of criminals; believe the government should do more to protect the consumer, control pollution, promote disarmament, and control the sale of handguns. They consider as very important objectives becoming an authority in one's own field, obtaining recognition from colleagues, raising a family, getting married, and being well off financially. Whether or not students' attitudes change during their college years has never been measured accurately, but it can be assumed that at least some changes will occur. Meanwhile, the data are, at the least, interesting to consider. One basic difference between nursing and non-nursing students is often their age. Many individuals select nursing for a midlife or later-life career change. Consequently, the average age of associate-degree students is almost 40 years old with baccalaureate enrollees in their mid and late twenties.

It is also important to consider the state of general education. Throughout the 1980s, there seemed to be considerable concern about American education. The 1983 report of the National Commission on Excellence in Education, appointed by the Secretary of Education, began with the words, "Our nation is at risk." Warning that the United States was being overtaken by other countries in industry, science, and technological innovation, the report not only listed the indicators of the risk but made a number of strong recommendations. It concluded that the documented decline in education performance was largely a result of "disturbing inadequacies" in the educational process at all levels.[39]

Five years after this declaration that a "rising tide of mediocrity" had eroded the quality of American education, a new Secretary of Education stated that schools had improved, but not enough. He said that students needed more training in the basics and that school officials should restore a sense of "discipline and hard work" to classrooms. He particularly criticized teachers' unions, whereas they criticized the lack of federal funds to improve education. Among the key points made were that national test scores are a little higher, with black and Hispanic students performing better; most 17-year-olds possess at least basic reading skills, but fewer than 5 percent possess the advanced reading skills often needed to "achieve excellence in academic, business, or government environments"; students' writing performance is very bad; math and science knowledge has improved but is far lower than that of students in Japan, for instance; knowledge of history, geography, and civics is abysmal, and rather frightening, since most of the students tested had now reached the voting age. There were also criticisms of the shallowness of much of the curriculum, the minimum amount of homework, and the short academic year. The most serious concerns cited were the drug problems and disruptive behavior in schools and the alarming dropout rate, particularly among blacks and Hispanics. The national average of high school completion rate is 75 percent; for blacks, 65 percent; and Hispanics, 55 percent. Some later return to school or pursue an "equivalency" certificate. Eighty-six percent of Americans between the ages of 25 and 29 have completed 4 years of high school. Recommendations for improvement included recruitment and rewarding of good principals and teachers; ensuring equal intellectual opportunities for all; improving the curriculum; establishing an "ethos of achievement," including helping students develop standards of right and wrong and establishing order and discipline.[40] Unfortunately, follow-up reports on education in the next several years showed no major changes. While this information might seem to be of only general interest, the reality is that such educational issues not only relate to the society in which we find ourselves, but for nurses, it has meaning, as do the college statistics, for the kind of students who may or may not enter nursing as well as the kind of patients they deal with.

THE WOMEN'S MOVEMENT

Nursing, from its beginnings in America, was primarily made up of women, and some nurses have always been involved in the women's movement to some degree. For example, Lavinia Dock was active and prominent in the early struggles for suffrage, and Margaret Sanger fought courageously to bring birth control to the poor. However, feminist women and nurses have historically had an "uneasy alliance." A group of nurse activists describe this relationship as follows:

> **Much of the energy in the women's movement has been directed toward opening up nontraditional fields of study and work for women. Nursing has been seen as one of the ultimate female ghettos from which women should be encouraged to escape…. Feminists have sometimes failed to look beyond the inaccurate sexist stereotypes of nurses and to acknowledge the multiple dimensions of professional nursing.[41]**

Being a suffragette was not easy in the late nineteenth and early twentieth centuries, and often women did not support the movement. That reaction may have been caused, in part, by the negative, even vindictive, portrait newspapers painted of those in the movement, as illustrated by a few typical quotes: "organized by divorced wives, childless women, and sour old maids," "unsexed women," "entirely devoid of personal attractions," "laboring on the heels of strong hatred towards men." Whether the opposition resulted from the fear of overthrowing "the most sacred of our institutions (marriage)"[42] or any other threat to the status quo is a moot point. For despite the success of the women's movement, most notably the passage of women's suffrage in 1921, discrimination against women has not ended. Women still face many formidable economic, social, and political barriers.

Women in all occupations, professions, and walks of life have encountered these barriers, and the success of the women's movement attests to the fervor and commitment with which they have fought to improve women's status. It is no surprise that the women's movement has been considered one of the major phenomena of the mid-twentieth century.

Over the years, there has been a proliferation of women's organizations concerned with women's rights.

Among the most active groups is the National Organization for Women (NOW), founded in 1966 and made up of women and men who support "full equality for women in truly equal partnership with men" and ask for an end to discrimination and prejudice against women in every field of importance in American society.

The founding of NOW offered one of the most politically radical agendas of the twentieth century: Men and women would share equally in public and private responsibilities—in paid work and in the rearing of children.

NOW activities are directed toward legislative action to end discrimination, and it attempts to promote its views through demonstrations, research, litigation, and political pressure. It is interesting that the first president of NOW, Wilma Scott Heide, was a nurse and feminist, demonstrating that nursing and feminism can find common ground.

Another prominent women's organization is the National Women's Political Caucus (NWPC). It was founded in 1971 as the first national political organization to promote women's entry into politics at leadership levels. The main thrust of the NWPC is to ensure that women's issues are given more attention by facilitating the election of women to political office.

Although many of the issues that women have confronted over the past 25 years are slow to be resolved, the women's movement has been the major catalyst in raising awareness and instigating action on sex discrimination and women's rights. The impact of the movement can be observed in both legal and social changes occurring, slowly but surely, in women's roles. But children are still being socialized into stereotyped male and female roles by books, use of toys, and influence of parents, teachers, and others—a problem that feminists and others continue to address. According to NOW, "A feminist is a person who believes women (even as men) are primarily people; that human rights are indivisible by any category of sex, race, class or other designation irrelevant to our common humanity; a feminist is committed to creating the equality (not sameness) of the sexes legally, socially, educationally, psychologically, politically, religiously, economically in all the rights and responsibilities of life."

Certainly these attitudes are not merely American. A 1974 UN report indicated that sexist attitudes were found around the world (and frequently held by UN delegates).

In 1975, the International Women's Year culminated in a UN-sponsored conference in Mexico City, intended to develop a ten-year plan to improve the status of women, particularly stressing education and health care. More than 1,000 UN delegates and 5,000 other feminists and interested spectators attended, but despite a document of official recommendations, the highly politicized meeting was not as successful as had been hoped. Most serious was the division of interests of the women. The caucus of Third World women, for instance, showed little interest in the concerns of Western women. Equal pay and day-care centers were not issues in countries where most women have no voting or property rights. The recommendations that emerged were a mixture and focused on encouraging governments to ensure equality in terms of educational opportunities, training, and employment, to ameliorate the "hard work loads" falling on women in certain economic groups and in certain countries, and to ensure that women have equal rights with men in voting and participating in political life.

In 1979, the United Nations General Assembly adopted "...what is essentially an international bill of rights for women." However, the treaty, known as the United Nations Convention on Elimination of All Forms of Discrimination Against Women, has yet to gain worldwide recognition or acceptance. In 1994, 128 countries had ratified the treaty, and few had made any significant efforts to eliminate discrimination against women. Notably, although the United States was part of the General Assembly consensus in adopting the convention, the Senate has yet to ratify it.

In 1985, a UN conference in Nairobi, Kenya, pulled together the disparate views that had kept women apart in Mexico a decade earlier and focused them into a document called "Nairobi Forward-Looking Strategies for Advancement of Women to the Year 2000." The strategies evolved from three basic objectives: equality, economic and social development, and peace.[43]

In assessing the progress achieved since that Nairobi conference and planning for the next world conference promoting the women's agenda (Beijing, 1995), UN officials decided "the picture is mixed: a greater proportion of women are literate and more of them are visible at high political levels. At the same time, many women are poorer than ever before, and women's human rights are being violated on an unprecedented scale." Despite the progress that has been made during the past 20 years, disparities between men and women, north and south, rural and urban, rich and poor, continue to concern women everywhere.[44]

The UN Commission on the Status of Women, in preparing for the Beijing conference, has enunciated the following critical areas of concern:

- Inequality between men and women in the sharing of power and decision making at all levels
- Insufficient mechanisms at all levels to promote the advancement of women
- Lack of awareness of, and commitment to, internationally and nationally recognized women's human rights
- The persistent and growing burden of poverty on women
- Inequality in women's access to and participation in the definition of economic structures and policies and the productive process itself
- Inequality in access to education, health and related services, and other means of maximizing the use of women's capacities

- Violence against women
- Effects of armed or other kinds of conflict on women
- Insufficient use of mass media to promote women's positive contributions to society
- Lack of adequate recognition and support for women's contribution to managing natural resources and safeguarding the environment[45]

In the United States, resistance to the women's movement was epitomized by the death of the proposed Equal Rights Amendment to the Constitution, 3 states short of the 38 needed for ratification (see Chap. 17). Ten years after it was passed by Congress, and despite an extension of the deadline for ratification from 1979 to 1982, Indiana in 1977 was the last state to ratify. More than 450 national organizations endorsed the amendment, and polls showed that more than two-thirds of U.S. citizens supported it, but to no avail. The conservative opposition, including fundamentalist Christian churches, the so-called Moral Majority, the John Birch Society, the Mormon Church, and the American Farm Bureau, led a well-financed, smoothly organized, and politically astute campaign. Antiamendment forces assured state legislators that the Fourteenth Amendment offered sufficient protection to women, and claimed that the ERA would cause the death of the family by removing a man's obligation to support his wife and children, would legalize homosexual marriages, lead to unisex toilets, and most damaging, lead to the drafting of women for combat duty. Advocates of the ERA were later criticized as lacking political finesse and alienating women who were potential supporters—blacks, pink-collar (office) workers, and housewives. Amendment supporters lay heavy blame on men, particularly in legislature and business.

In the 1980s and early 1990s, feminists determined to concentrate women's new consciousness and resources in building legislative strength to eventually pass the ERA and to mount a campaign for reproductive freedom, including abortion and recognition of all human rights, including gay and lesbian rights, democratization of families, more respect for work done in the home, and comparable pay for the work done outside it. Since 1973, when *Roe v. Wade* was decided by the U.S. Supreme Court, women have had the right to seek an abortion, at least in the first trimester. The basis for this decision was a woman's right to privacy. Efforts to overturn *Roe* have not been successful, but antiabortion forces have succeeded in eliminating Medicaid funding of abortion for poor women (Hyde amendment), requiring a waiting period prior to abortion, and parental consent for minors who seek an abortion.[46]

Three decades after Betty Friedan published *The Feminine Mystique* (called by the futurist Alvin Toffler "the book that pulled the trigger of history") changes can be clearly identified, even though some of the results have varied.

In terms of the ERA, Congress voted down another ERA bill in 1983. The bill was defeated by six votes. Yet, both friends and foes of equal rights note that the campaign for the amendment, along with other social forces, made a definite impact on American life.

For example, labor force participation has become the norm for most women. In 1992, women comprised 45 percent of the workforce, up from 38 percent in 1970, and they are predicted to be 47 percent by the year 2005. More women than ever before are combining responsibilities of raising children, keeping up a household, and working outside of the home. The labor force participation rate of teenage women is 44 percent; of women 20 and older, 57 percent. Seventy-five percent of working women, or a total of 40 million, work full-time; two-thirds of all part-time workers are women, a total of 14 million. These female labor force participation rates seem to be increasing, and projections to the year 2000 call for continued increases and further convergences of male and female labor force patterns over the life cycle. It is interesting to note that the percent of young (20s) mothers in the workforce fell in 1993 to 51.7 percent from 53 percent in 1988.

Although women's wages are still not commensurate with men's, they are improving in that regard. The ratio between what the average woman earns and what the average man earns has risen in recent years to 75 cents on the dollar, up from 62 cents in the late 1960s. In terms of education, young women age 25 to 29 have just about closed the gap in educational attainment between men and women. Nearly the same percentage of women are high school graduates (approximately 85 percent) and college graduates (23 percent) as men. On the downside, many women and men report dissatisfaction with the toll that women working takes on family and personal lives. In a 1989 survey, 48 percent of all women respondents said that they had to sacrifice too much for their gains, especially with regard to time spent with children and family.[47]

The labor force participation of women can be viewed as a further disadvantage when one considers the many single mothers who have no choice but to work outside of the home because they are facing such difficult financial hardships. These problems seem to be intensifying as the proportion of families maintained by women alone increases (see United States Population earlier in this chapter).

Finally, despite the narrowing of the wage gap between women and men, 59 percent of women work in "…low paying 'pink-collar' jobs because they are trained for nothing else, some because such jobs tend to be more compatible with child rearing." It is harder to explain why the higher women advance, the larger the wage gap between men and women. Corporate women at the vice-presidential level and above earn 42 percent less than their male peers.[48]

A growing number of lawsuits and union negotiations have challenged the male-female pay ratio based on the "comparable worth" theory. This theory, going beyond equal pay for equal work, calls for equal pay for different jobs of comparable worth. The intent is to revalue *all* jobs on the basis of the skills and responsibility they require. Neither the Equal Pay Act nor the Civil Rights Act brought about reform at any

level of the workforce. A landmark case resulted in the state of Washington being ordered in 1984 to pay female workers up to $1 billion in back wages and increases because of such pay inequity. However, shortly thereafter, the decision was reversed on appeal.

Generally, federal and state governments, as well as the courts, have not been supportive of comparable worth. For example, in 1985, the U.S. Civil Rights Commission rejected the comparable worth concept. That same year, a Court of Appeals ruling written by Judge Anthony M. Kennedy, who was later appointed to the Supreme Court, approved a state's relying on market rates in setting salaries even if it knowingly paid less to women as a result.

More recently, a federal judge in California ruled that California had not deliberately underpaid thousands of women in state jobs held predominantly by women, a serious blow to the country's largest lawsuit on this issue. Nonetheless, industry and business are becoming more interested in job evaluation studies, with presumably equal pay following.

Just as important are a series of Supreme Court rulings that ban employers from offering retirement plans that provide men and women with unequal benefits. As one justice wrote, "An individual woman may not be paid lower monthly benefits simply because women as a class live longer than men."

Other calls for celebration were the appointment of the first woman to the Supreme Court (Sandra Day O'Connor), who was joined by the second (Ruth Bader Ginsburg) in 1993, the first woman in space (Sally Kristin Ride, with a Ph.D. in physics), the first woman vice presidential candidate of a major political party (Geraldine Ferraro), and, perhaps more prosaically, an increase in the number of women in public and appointed offices at all political levels. In 1986, for the first time, two women ran against each other as major party gubernatorial candidates. The elections in Nebraska featured Kay Orr (Republican) against Helen Bousalis (Democrat). Orr won and became the first woman Republican elected to state governorship. Ella

Grasso was the first woman Democrat elected to the governorship when she won the Connecticut election in 1974. In 1986, Barbara Mikulski (Democrat, Maryland) became the first woman elected to the Senate without previously completing her husband's expired term. In the 103d Congress (1993–1994) women held 47 seats in the House and 7 in the Senate. Furthermore, the growing gender gap (a term used to identify the difference between men's and women's votes) is not being ignored by even the most conservative legislators, since women comprise more than 50 percent of the population.

In 1994, three women were presidents of their nations; four women were prime ministers. Seven of the 184 missions to the United Nations were headed by women ambassadors, including Ambassador Madeline Albright, who headed the U.S. mission. The number of women members in the world's parliaments was 11 in 1994. In the United States, the Clinton cabinet had three women among its 14 members.

Eddie Bernice Johnson (Democrat, Texas) was the first registered nurse to be elected to Congress, taking her seat in the House of Representatives in 1992. Among other prominent nurses who are in powerful positions in Washington are Sheila Burke, chief of staff for Senator and Minority Leader Bob Dole (Republican, Kansas); Shirley Chater, Commissioner of the Social Security Administration; Carolyn Davis, who headed the Health Care Financing Administration in the 1980s; past AIDS czar Kristine Gebbie; and Mary Wakefield, chief of staff for Tom Daschle (Democrat, South Dakota).

Despite the advances women have made over the past 30 years, the burdens of child rearing still fall disproportionately on the shoulders of women. For example, slightly less than 9 out of every 10 one-parent families are maintained by women, and the percentage of single mothers increased from 11.5 percent in 1970 to 23.7 percent in 1988.

Furthermore, the feminization of poverty is a very serious problem facing American society. In 1991, 54 percent of all poor families were maintained by a woman with no spouse present. Among poor black families, 78 percent were headed by a woman; among poor Hispanics, 46 percent; among poor white, 44 percent.[49]

Therefore, political and economic gains women have achieved cannot obscure (in fact they even intensify) the need for a national consensus on family policy. A major step forward was made when President Bill Clinton signed the family leave bill into law, which gives employed parents the right to a leave after the birth or adoption of a child and be ensured of job security. In addition, child-care initiatives from the private and public sector are also important in easing the dual responsibilities of family and career that so many women face. For several years, Congress has wrestled with legislation for both parental leave and child care. Now that parental leave has been enacted, the time seems ripe for day-care legislation as pressure from women's organizations and other groups intensifies. ANA has lobbied for these bills, because of its predominantly female constituency and because of the importance of these bills for the health and welfare of the American people. In the meantime, some state legislatures and private companies have launched programs that assist families, and most often women, with regard to child care and parental leave. None of these initiatives would have evolved without the force and appeal of the women's movement.[50]

In fact, the success of the movement is evidenced by Naisbett and Aburdene, authors of *Megatrends 2000*, who referred to the 1990s as the "Decade of Women in Leadership."[51] They based their prediction on their belief that women were ready to break through the "glass ceiling," the invisible barrier that has kept them from the top, because their talents and abilities are being recognized and because they have already taken two-thirds of jobs in industries of the future. They also pointed out that the tendency to want to balance the top priorities of family and career along with other interests, once attributed to women, is becoming increasingly important to both sexes in these times.

They see the emergence of a new leadership style, which focuses on quick responses to change and the ability to bring out the best in people, as symbolic of women's influence in the workplace. (These are certainly attributes that most nurses have mastered!) They describe a new type of work environment due to the growing numbers of women who work out of the home and the values they bring to their places of employment. In addition to citing the importance of the critical mass that women have reached in the professions, they predict that benefits such as day care and family leave will increasingly be used as recruitment and retention strategies because of their importance to men and women alike, as women continue to increase their labor force participation. (Some companies, including health care institutions, have already decided that this is a major necessity and have provided such services. Funding day care has been a big issue in Congress.)

The issue of women's rights is closely related to the problems, activities, and goals of women working in the health service industry. From 75 to 85 percent of all health service workers are women, and the largest health occupation, nursing, is almost totally female. These women-dominated occupations are also expanding most rapidly, but men continue to dominate the positions of authority within the health care system.

The reasons for so many women in health care are that, first, they are an inexpensive source of labor; second, they are available; and third, they have been safe, no threat to physicians. The rise of nurses as autonomous practitioners certainly is a threat to that traditional power base.

More than any other factor, the absence of professional autonomy for nurses (see Chap. 16) is considered a direct result of sex discrimination in nursing, with the end result that the patient and client ultimately suffer. The movement of nurses toward autonomy is seen partially as the result of the women's movement, and the struggles in achieving autonomy have certainly enhanced interest in the movement.

The fight against sexual discrimination has gained new impetus in nursing, as well as in other segments of society, and has spilled over to include in the consumer movement the entire issue of women's health.

LABOR AND INDUSTRY

As nursing is part of the health care industry and as unions are making new efforts to organize nurses and others in health care, the status of labor unions is an important socioeconomic factor. Labor was said to be at a crossroads in 1978, with membership down to a 41-year low, with loss of bargaining elections at nearly 52 percent in 1977, its legislation repeatedly blocked by newly potent business lobbies and inflationwary legislators, its aging leaders inspiring less public confidence than in any other American institution. In part, this was the result of an inability to adjust to postwar work patterns—a growth switch from industry to white collar, wholesale and retail trade, and service industries. In order to recoup their losses and regain their momentum of the 1940s and 1950s, unions then turned to other potential sources of union activity, such as the health care industries, including both professionals and nonprofessionals.

However, beginning with President Reagan's breaking of the air controllers' illegal strike in August 1981, by firing and subsequently replacing the air controllers, the unions have had special difficulties. Some employers simply threaten to file for bankruptcy, and the courts have supported their right to abrogate any existing union contract under those circumstances. Others find that they can withstand long strikes because they are legally permitted to make permanent job replacements, and the unemployed and workers in lesser paid fields are willing to take the strikers' jobs. On this basis, employers are demanding (and getting) paybacks of benefits and pay in new contracts, citing competition as the reason. Union leadership has been blamed by many for not seeing the economic problems and being greedy in earlier years.

What has also made it easier for management is the growing tendency of people to prefer to work part time, a trend that is predicted to increase. Although this is particularly true of women, including nurses, who have young families or simply need to contribute to the family income, there are also a surprising number of men who make this choice. Both women and men may be attending school, beginning their own business, testing out a different field, working at a second job, or simply looking for more flexibility and independence. Some like the variety and the fact that they need not get involved in the politics and problems of the workplace. On the other hand, wages may be lower (not necessarily true for nurses), there is little opportunity for career advancement, and some temporary workers complain of being "dumped on by regular employees." Industry has found these "contingency workers" economically advantageous. Employers do not usually pay for any benefits, which can be a considerable savings, and they can bring in these workers at busy times, while maintaining a minimum workforce. It provides a way around union work rules and, at times, a way to confront striking unions. The negative side is that part-time or short-term workers may not have the same commitment to the company, and unless they return to the same place frequently, need orientation and perhaps even training. Yet, it is quite possible that the availability of these workers and full-time replacements has made strikes a less popular union tool.

Despite these problems, by the beginning of 1990, there was some optimism in the ranks of labor. For the first time in over a decade, younger, more sophisticated labor leaders had replaced nearly all the old guard. Also, both labor and industry were stressing the need for harmony. The year 1989 had seen union membership grow, although with a greater overall growth in the workforce, the percentage continued to diminish (16.4 percent as opposed to the previous low of 23 percent in 1977). There was considerable growth in governmental unions, but the service industries, accounting for most of the growth in the labor force, had only 6 percent union participation. All seemed to be good candidates for organization. Because women are a large part of the latter group (they are also considered easier to organize), the unions are beginning to tackle "women's issues" such as abortion, and the safety of women on the job. However, their interest has not extended to placing women in the top echelon of the labor federation's hierarchy.

Management, criticized for its authoritarian approach, is trying new techniques to increase worker satisfaction. While far from widespread, there does seem to be growing interest in involving workers in decision making. Most American companies have reform programs in which workers and supervisors discuss operations.[52] In industry these may be called quality circles; in health care they may be shared governance. Some labor experts say that these "reforms" (also known by such names as *job redesign, work humanization, employee participation, workplace democracy*, and *quality of work life*) are more cosmetic than real, since few workers participate in the companies' most important decisions, and that in a difficult situation most managers revert to an authoritarian stance. Others say that this new management style is necessary now that the nation is engaged in vigorous international competition. Similar techniques have been used in Europe and Japan for some time, and production success, particularly in Japan, has concerned American industry. Whether there will be backsliding when economic times are better is the question.

In summary, American unions have been in decline since 1980, with the presence of a federal administration that favored big business and created incentives for the country's financial recovery to occur through the development of small business and industry. This antilabor sentiment was acted out through management-friendly appointments to the Supreme Court and the National Labor Relations Board, the governmental unit critical to facilitating efforts at organizing and unionization. At the same time, more basic employee guarantees were being provided through legislation and regulations, decreasing the need for union protection. A final observation is that the American union tradition had been built on an adversarial relationship between labor and management. This has proved to be inconsistent with the employee-employer relationships that have produced quality outcomes in other countries. American labor is in a state of transition. This transition will be further discussed in Part III of this text under "Transition into Practice."

THE CONSUMER REVOLUTION

The consumer revolution, said to have begun when Theodore Roosevelt signed the first Pure Food and Drug Act in 1906, has been an accelerating phenomenon since the 1950s. Although various interpretations are put on the term, it might be broadly defined as the concerted action of the public in response to a lack of satisfaction with the products and/or services of various groups. The publics are, of course, different, but often overlapping. A woman unhappy about the cost and quality of auto repairs might be just as displeased by the services of her gynecologist, the cost of hospital care, or the use of dangerous food additives.

There have probably always been dissatisfied consumers, but the major difference now is that many are organized in ad hoc or permanent organizations and have the power, through money, numbers, and influence, to force providers to be responsive to at least some of their demands. The methods vary but include lobbying for legislation, legal suits, boycotts, and media campaigns. One of the most noted, albeit highly criticized, consumer activists is Ralph Nader, whose Center for Study of Responsive Law produced a blitz of study group reports in the early 1970s that exposed abuses in a wide range of fields. Currently, his Health Research Group is one of the most influential in health consumerism. There is an increasingly strong force moving in that direction especially with the better educated and more aggressive baby

boomers and elderly. Consumers, who first concentrated their efforts against the shoddy quality of work and indifferent services offered on material goods, have now turned to the quality, quantity, and cost of other services, particularly in health care. Fewer patients and clients are accepting without protest the "I know best" attitudes of health care providers, whether physician, nurse, or any of the many others involved in health care. The self-help phenomenon, in which people learn about health care and help each other ("stroke clubs" and Alcoholics Anonymous, for instance), has extended to self-examination—sometimes through classes sponsored by doctors, nurses, and health agencies. Interest in health promotion and illness prevention has also been manifested by the involvement of consumers in environmental concerns.

The dehumanization of patient care, which is contrary to all the stated beliefs of the professions involved, is repeatedly castigated in studies of health care. Although complaints often are directed at the care of the poor, too often it is a universal health care deficiency. The concerted action of organized minority groups led to the development of the American Hospital Association's Patient Bill of Rights (see Chap. 22), which received widespread attention in 1973, followed by a rash of similar rights statements specifically directed to children, the mentally ill, the elderly, pregnant women, the dying, the handicapped, patients of various religions, and others. In some cases, presidential conferences and legislation have followed. The whole area of the rights of people in health care, which focuses to a great extent on patients' rights to full and accurate information so that they can make decisions about their care, has major implications for nurses.

An excellent example of the rise of a health consumer group is the Women's Health Movement, which emerged from women's disenchantment with their personal and institutional health relationships. Their complaints centered on physicians' attitudes toward women, which seem to be the result of both medical education and professional socialization. The fact that women's complaints of the health care system are neither isolated nor trivial is attested to by the attention given by lay and professional media to such problems as unnecessary hysterectomies and cesarean sections. However, the impetus toward organization is credited to the women's consciousness-raising groups of the 1960s, in which women shared their medical experiences and found support for taking action. Their activities are centered on changing consciousness, providing health-related services, and working to change established health institutions. Specific and well-known (as well as controversial) entities are the various feminist health centers and their know-your-body and self-help courses and books. The organization's scope of functions is increasing to include not only primary care, but nutritional, psychological, gerontologic, and pediatric services. Without doubt, those involved see the need for women to control their own essential femaleness as simultaneously related to the wider issues of female equality and liberation.

Other consumers are also concerned with the power issue and are insisting, with some success, on such rights as participation in governing boards of hospitals and other community health institutions, accrediting boards, health planning groups, and licensing boards. What lies ahead in terms of more regulation, such as an overall federal consumer protection law and state laws that are really enforced, is not yet known. However, the consumer movement continues to gain strength, and some further action is inevitable.

The nursing community has a history of supporting public policy that builds the strength of consumerism. These sentiments are prominent in *Nursing's Agenda for Health Care Reform*, organized nursing's directive for public policy reform.[53] Additionally in 1991, the American Nurses Association and the National Consumers League created a partnership called the "Community-Based Health Care Project." The project is funded by the Kellogg Foundation and supports the establishment of nurse-consumer coalitions in local communities. These coalitions bring pressure to bear for public policy changes and service projects that are responsive to local need.

ANTICIPATING THE FUTURE

This chapter has presented a brief overview of the socioeconomic and technological changes that have occurred and are occurring before our eyes. Nursing and health care must exist within that context. It is incumbent on the professions to identify patterns that allow us a glimpse of the future. There is a story to tell beyond today's reality. Some accurate predictions are possible. They are the product of trending forward the observations we have already made and listening with a sensitive ear to the claims of a host of futurists:

- The shrinking world makes it impossible for any country to exist in a vacuum, monopolizing the use of resources and ignoring the pain of the rest of the planet.
- The complexity of our human problems demands a social model for the delivery of health services, accepting the fact that health care, housing, education, workplace safety, and a host of other concerns interrelate in the search for quality of life and vie for the same resources.
- Health care and its support systems exist within a cultural context and it becomes dangerous to impose an alien value system.
- In the United States, demographics are our destiny; we are faced with an aging and chronically ill population.
- The declining presence of the traditional family in this culture demands the creation of new services, programs, and public policy.
- A fragile environment requires we take every precaution to prevent its further deterioration.
- "High tech" advances will not stop but must be counterbalanced by a conscious

and generous dose of caring and humanism.

- Nurses stand at the center of an information rich environment, the most strategic position for the 1990s.
- Our centralized structures have failed, and we are decentralizing, to rebuild from the bottom up.
- Americans are demanding personal expression in their work, hours that complement a private life, and participation in decisions that impact the quality of their workplace.
- Suspicion of our most basic institutions has moved us to an active consumerism and the demand for more accountability from professionals.
- Americans are returning to self-reliance after a crippling period of dependence on institutions and government to make our decisions and do our bidding.
- The traditional hierarchial model has become flattened, and we are responding to need with networks and ad hoc systems.
- Americans will live with less, they will sacrifice, but they will never give up their right to choose.

The reader is urged to test these predictions in the light of what is said in following chapters.

REFERENCES

1. Toffler A: *Future Shock*. New York: Random House, 1970.
2. UNICEF: *The State of the World's Children 1994*. New York: United Nations Children's Fund, 1994, p 24.
3. WHO: *Implementation of the Global Strategy for Health for All by the Year 2000: Second Evaluation, Eighth Report on the World Situation*. Geneva: World Health Organization, 1993, pp 19–20.
4. Ibid, p 20.
5. Ibid.
6. UNICEF, op cit, p 16.
7. Ibid, pp 23–24.
8. WHO, op cit, pp 24–25.
9. Ibid, p 20.
10. International Council of Nurses: *Healthy Families for Healthy Nations*. Geneva: The Council, 1993, pp 3–4.
11. WHO, loc cit.
12. International Council of Nurses, passim.
13. WHO, op cit, p 22.
14. UNICEF, op cit, pp 24–25.
15. WHO, op cit, p 24.
16. UNICEF, op cit, p 17.
17. *Campaign for Women's Health*. Washington, DC: The Older Women's League, 1993.
18. UNICEF, op cit, p 16.
19. Elliott M, Dickey C: Population wars: Body politics. *Newsweek* 22–27, September 12, 1994.
20. *The World Almanac and Book of Facts 1994*. Mahwah, NJ: Funk & Wagnalls, 1993, pp 358–422.
21. Howe N, Strauss B: *13th Generation: Abort, Retry, Ignore, Fail?* New York: Vintage Books, 1993.
22. Population growth outstrips earlier U.S. census estimates. *The New York Times*, A1, D18, Dec. 4, 1992.
23. *The World Almanac and Book of Facts 1994*, op cit, p 358.
24. Ibid.
25. Ibid, p 371.
26. Foster C et al: *Homeless in America*. Wylie, TX: Information Plus, 1993.
27. *Abortion Surveillance*. Atlanta, GA: CDCP, Dec. 17, 1993.
28. Harrington C et al: *Health Care Access*. Washington, DC: The American Academy of Nursing, 1992, pp 11–16.
29. U.S. Public Health Service: *Healthy People 2000*. Washington, DC: Government Printing Office, 1990.
30. Gordon B: *The Truth about Where You Live*. New York: Times Books, 1991.
31. *Cancer Facts and Figures 1993*. Atlanta, GA: American Cancer Society, 1993.
32. *Abortion Surveillance*, loc cit.
33. The National Commission on AIDS: Americans living with AIDS: Transforming anger, fear and indifference into action, in Lee P et al (eds): *The Nation's Health*. Boston: Jones and Bartlett, 1994, pp 391–397.
34. UNICEF progress report on programme activities in prevention of HIV and in reducing the impact of AIDS on families and communities.

Policy Review, edited advance copy, February 26, 1993.

35. Hurley P, McGriff E: AIDS: Its impact on nursing education and practice. *Imprint* 36:43–44, February–March 1989.

36. U.S. Public Health Service, loc cit.

37. Entire issue. *Nurs Health Care* 9:477–521, November–December 1989.

38. A nation at risk: The imperative for educational reform. *Chron Higher Ed* 26:11–16, May 4, 1983.

39. Ibid.

40. Wilson R: Bennett notes improvement of schools in past 5 years but paints bleak picture of U.S. education in report. *Chron Higher Ed* 31:A29–42, May 4, 1988.

41. Vance C et al: An uneasy alliance: Nursing and the women's movement. *Nurs Outlook* 33:281–285, November–December 1985.

42. Christy T: Liberation movement: Impact on nursing. *AORN* 15:67–68, April 1972.

43. United Nations: The Nairobi forward looking strategies for the advancement of women (as adopted by the World Conference to Review and Appraise the Achievements of the United Nations Decade for Women and Equality) *Development and Peace,* Nairobi, Kenya, 15:26, July 1985.

44. United Nations Department of Public Information: *Conference to Set Women's Agenda into the Next Century.* New York: United Nations, 1993.

45. UN Commission on the Status of Women: Preparations for the fourth world conference on women. *Action for Equality, Development, and Peace.* United Nations: New York, 1994, pp 6–12.

46. Mason D, Talbot S, Leavett S, et al: *Policy and Politics for Nurses,* 2d ed. Philadelphia: Saunders, 1993, pp 415–417.

47. Cowan A: Women's gains on the job: Not without a heavy toll. *New York Times* 1, August 21, 1989.

48. Jones C: Onward, women #1. *Time* 89, December 4, 1989.

49. *World Almanac and Book of Facts,* loc cit.

50. Quinn J: The luck of the Xers. *Newsweek* 73:66–67, June 6, 1994.

51. Naisbett J, Aburdene P: *Megatrends 2000: The New Directions for the 1990s.* New York: Morrow, 1990.

52. Hoerr J: What should unions do? *Harvard Business Review,* 30–45, May–June 1991.

53. American Nurses Association and National League for Nursing: *Nursing's Agenda for Health Care Reform.* Washington, DC: The Association, 1991.

Health Care Delivery: Where?

H EALTH CARE TODAY is given in a variety of settings, such as hospitals, nursing homes, community health centers, state or city clinics, and the homes of patients and clients. Involved in this care are more than 3 million workers. (Depending on who is included in the allied health category, the total may be as high as 8 million.) The majority are employed in hospitals. The size the complexity of the health care system alone create problems in the quality of service provided.

It is generally agreed that some of the essential elements of optimum health services in the community include a unified, cooperative team approach to care; a spectrum of services, including diagnosis, treatment, rehabilitation, education, and prevention; a coordinated community and/or regional system incorporating these services; continuity of care given by the hospital, community, physician, and other health agencies; a continuum of health services; and a program of evaluation and research concerning the adequacy of services in meeting patient and community needs.

This chapter and the next are intended to present an overview of current health care delivery, its organization, and its workers. Specific details on how the nurse may function in these various settings are presented in Chap. 15.

DEFINITIONS

Health care delivery is composed of several levels: self-care, primary care, secondary care, and tertiary care. Another differentiation is primary, acute, and long-term care. Definitions vary, but the following will provide a frame of reference.

Primary care: "(a) a person's first contact in any given episode of illness with the health care system that leads to a decision of what must be done to help resolve his problems; and (b) the responsibility for the continuum of care, i.e., maintenance of health, evaluation and management of symptoms, and appropriate referrals."[1] It is at this level that basic medical and other health care services are provided.

Millis, a layman who has had long-standing relationships with the health professions, puts it this way: "To me, primary care includes all the health services needed by a given population that are not provided by secondary and tertiary care. It includes health services as well as sickness services. It includes response to self-limiting disease, minor disability, and chronic and incurable disease. It includes prevention of disease, health maintenance, and public health. Most important, it includes self-care and thus addresses itself to those health problems that currently account for so much morbidity—automobile accidents, obesity, alcoholism, drug abuse, iatrogenic disease, and environmental hazards."[2]

Secondary care: the point at which consulting specialty and subspecialty services are provided in either an office (group practice) or community hospital inpatient setting.

Tertiary care: the point at which highly sophisticated diagnostic, treatment or rehabilitation services are provided, frequently in university medical centers or equivalent institutions.

Acute care: "those services that treat the acute phase of illness or disability and has as its purpose the restoration of normal life processes and function."[3]

Long-term care: "those services designed to provide symptomatic treatment, maintenance, and rehabilitative services for patients of all age groups in a variety of health care settings."[4]

The definition of self-care, the first level of care, is self-explanatory. Its interpretation varies, chiefly in relation to whether it excludes all physician or other health professional involvement completely, even as a volunteer consultant to a self-help group.

THE HEALTH CARE ENVIRONMENT: ISSUES OF COST AND QUALITY

Before describing the settings in which health care is delivered, it is essential to understand some of the changes that have occurred in the last several decades—changes that relate directly to the public's concern about the cost and quality of health care. As often happens, the public's dissatisfaction with something translates itself into legislation by those they elected. In this case, because the cost of health care was (and is) rising so rapidly, executive branch regulations on both a national and a state level, also began to clamp down on the people (providers) and places delivering health care. (See Chaps. 17 and 19 on how laws are made and how legislation affects health care.) The reason why governmental impact is so great is that most health care facilities and many providers are funded one way or another by government funds. Moreover, others who pay for health care (payers) such as health insurance companies, including the well-known Blue Cross and Blue Shield, tend to follow the patterns of payment set by the government.

Health care in the United States (frequently criticized as more likely to be "sick care"), devours almost 15 percent of the gross national product (GNP), with a steady, sometimes massive, increase in the last decades that exceeds that of any other advanced country.[5] A variety of factors have been blamed. Both Medicare and Medicaid and most health insurance plans traditionally have paid for the "full and reasonable" cost of care on a retrospective basis, that is, whatever the provider said it cost, within certain limits. (Medicare/Medicaid law and its changes are described more fully in Chap. 19.) With the high cost of new technology used for both diagnosis and treatment and the consumer demand for the newest and the best, costs soared. In 1983 federal regulations titled Prospective Payment for Medicare Inpatient Hospital Services, Title VI of the Social Security Act of 1983 were reported in the Federal Register. Because of fear that Medicare funds would run out, a new form of payment was devised. (Actually this approach had been in effect in New Jersey since 1978—including all payers.) Under this prospective payment system (PPS), disorders of the human body were divided into major diagnostic categories with (currently) 477 subgroups called diagnostic related groups (DRGs). Now, the payment for services which hospitals receive per discharge patient is determined based on the patient's principal diagnosis and the predetermined length of hospitalization considered suitable for that diagnosis. Certain other factors are considered, and some hospitals are exempted. One problem for health care institutions, public health agencies, and physicians is that reimbursement can be denied retroactively, after the service has been given, and the amount of documentation needed is both very specific and voluminous. Another concern has been whether patient acuity or intensity is considered, especially in relation to the nursing care needed.[6] On the other hand, if the patient is discharged more rapidly, hospitals may keep the full amount of designated reimbursement. This has resulted in accusations that patients are being discharged "sicker and quicker," with more complex (and new) highly technological care required in the home or nursing home. Hospital utilization has been greatly reduced, and patients are considerably sicker since there are not the grace periods of early admission for tests, now done on an outpatient basis, and leisurely postacuity or postsurgical recovery before discharge.

Since the Reagan administration encouraged competition and introduction of cost-saving approaches, several changes resulted as some hospitals found themselves in a tight financial bind. One was aggressive marketing, aimed particularly at self-paying patients and those with insurance. Although it is sometimes denied, administrators encouraged physicians to admit patients who were likely to be dischargeable early. Some hospitals closed units that were costly and unlikely to be fully reimbursed such as burn units and trauma units. "Patient dumping," transferring certain patients to governmental hospitals, was another cost-saving technique,[7] although in 1989 a law was enacted penalizing hospitals that "dump." Hospitals looked for other ways to fill beds with paying patients, such as those requiring long-term care. As described later, they formed satellite clinics, emergicenters, surgicenters, and home care services. They used helicopters to bring in emergency patients from distant areas and advertised their services and their physicians in media campaigns. Some created profit-making components that included equipment rental, health promotion and teaching classes, and even hotels and contracts with noted fast-food companies. They merged with other hospitals or agencies to share services, sometimes even developing into national chains. In all these activities, they mimicked the more businesslike for-profit hospitals or hospital chains. These had long used those tactics to increase profitability, even to creating health-care malls, which include doctors' offices, a hospital, ambulatory care, laboratory, pharmacy, optometry, physical therapy, and physical fitness services, as well as home care services, restaurants, gift shops, banking, and parking. While "copy-cat economics" was criticized, nonprofit hospitals maintained that these approaches were needed for survival. In fact, in the 1980s, many small hospitals, especially in rural areas, simply went out of business, despite the needs of the population, and more closures are predicted throughout the 1990s.

Even with these limitations on reimbursements, health care costs continued to soar faster than the inflation rate. There were still too many empty beds and too much expensive technology used. To add to the costs, AIDS patients began to fill hospitals beds and draw on complex home care services. In 1992, Medicaid, the largest payer of services for AIDS patients, spent about $2.1 billion, yet this was only 23 percent of the total cost of care. In the same year, Medicare spent $280 million on AIDS care for the disabled and projected an increase to $690 million by 1996. Only care for automobile victims and cardiac patients will be more costly, and it has been said that AIDS will be with us "forever." Another major problem for private hospitals is the care of the uninsured, estimated at more than 37.1 million nationwide. These people are not unemployed but are the working poor, not covered by health insurance or federal programs and unable to afford private health insurance, or those with very limited insurance.[8] Then there are the homeless who come to emergency rooms, also without Medicaid, even though they may be eligible.

Hospitals have always given free care and usually the cost was absorbed by increasing the bills of paying patients. This historic technique, called "cost shifting," has backfired. This strategy has the ultimate consequence of increasing the premiums of private insurance and further increasing the cost of services in settings for care that have a high incidence of "bad debt" or "uncompensated care" (the terminology used for the working poor or the "medically indigent," those neither old enough nor poor enough for entitlement programs). Insurers and employers have not accepted these reforms quietly. The common practice of "cost shifting" is being tested in the courts, and prohibitions against the practice are being sought through legislation.

Many health insurers have put into effect a system, somewhat like that of the government, in which a company employee, reviewing the patient's record and/or a predetermined list, approves or denies payment. In some cases, the approval must be received before treatment. Even so, as the cost of insurance premiums rises, employers, particularly large corporations, are resisting these increases and looking for ways to lower health care costs. Small companies may simply drop this employee benefit. One approach has been managed care. There are a number of versions, but the idea is for the large employer to come to an agreement with one or more hospitals, groups of physicians, or community settings for care in which a certain number of potential patients (the employees) are guaranteed service at a set, discounted price. In some cases, employees choosing not to participate must pay a larger health insurance premium. Freedom of choice is declining. In 1984, 85 percent of all employee coverage was by unmanaged fee-for-service plans allowing free choice; in 1988, only 28 percent had such choices. Some companies are also less likely to simply approve a bill or a procedure since there is a known tendency for some physicians to perform unnecessary surgery; others reward employees who have healthy lifestyles or even pay back those who do not use their health benefits. In addition, employees are being required to pay for a greater part of their health insurance or a greater deductible.

A combination of all these factors has brought back interest in national health insurance (see Chap. 19 for more details), a concept that has not been popular since the Great Society years of the Johnson administration.[9] Except for South Africa, the United States is the only industrialized nation without a form of national health insurance. While there seems to be a trend in those other countries to privatize a portion of their health care, and certainly there are problems, including costs, several national polls of Americans showed that they were interested in governmental guarantees of universal access, and many look to Canada's model as a possibility.[10] Actually, both the ANA and NLN, as well as the American Public Health Association (APHA), have supported the concept of universal access to health care services for years, but the American Medical Association (AMA) and other powerful groups that influence health policy opposed it. Only a few years ago, the predictions were that there would be no national health system in the foreseeable future. Whether such a system will indeed be put in place is not clear. However, given the burden of caring for the uninsured, there is a movement to provide some kind of program. Massachusetts and Hawaii were the first states to put one in place, requiring employers to provide insurance, while providing some state support. Meanwhile, just about everyone agrees that unnecessary use of health care should be curbed, and some of the power figures insist that the way to do that is to shift more of the financial burden on workers. There is some evidence that those who are insured make little effort to limit utilization or search for the best services for the least cost. Of course, such information is not always easy to come by, although consumer advocates are making some progress in having providers or the government present cost and quality information. Meanwhile, the issue of access to care, who gets what, when resources are limited, is becoming a serious ethical problem. (This is explored in more depth in Chaps. 10 and 22.)

Another serious issue is quality of care. Accusations that quality is not commensurate with cost are heard from many sources. Beyond state licensing of hospitals and other health care facilities and agencies, which presumably represents some screening for quality, the Joint Commission on Accreditation of Healthcare Organizations (JCAHO), described later, puts its stamp of approval on institutions and agencies that meet specific criteria of quality. There is some cynicism as to whether this is simply a paper tiger, but the value of accreditation is certainly evident in some circumstances: Federal funding of certain kinds of services requires accreditation. A number of consumer groups, some formal; some loosely organized; some interested in specific kinds of care, such as nursing homes; and some servicing a large group such as the AARP, who see high-quality health care as one of their concerns, are also active in evaluating health care and/or lobbying for improvements. In addition, the federal government has released the names of hospitals with high mortality rates, which some have said is unfair because certain hospitals have more at-risk patients. There are predictions that quality of care will be a major issue in the next decade and that the public expects health practitioners to take responsibility for assuring high-quality care. Although both physicians and nurses have peer review systems in place, to one extent or another, the warning is that unless improvements are made, government oversight, such as the federally funded Peer Review Organizations (PROs) that assess medical necessity, appropriateness, and quality of care provided to Medicare patients to determine if Medicare should pay the hospital, will increase.

Meanwhile, health care experts continue to present varying proposals to change what many call the disarray of the American health care system (although others maintain that it has never been otherwise). These include development of or increased use of alternative systems of delivering care, most of which are discussed in the following sections, to some form of national health insurance, to grouping of health care services on regional levels, with clinical and fiscal accountability established at that level.[11] Even when there is no agreement about which plan is most feasible, almost no one believes that things can go on as they are. The federal government predicts that national health care expenditures will reach $1.5 *trillion* by the year 2000. As one expert stated, U.S. health policy can no longer be set on the basis of "disjointed incrementalism," described as nibbling around the edges of a problem, dealing only with the piece that "has high public visibility, causes the most political discomfort, or both."[12] The task is formidable, especially for a country that prides itself on its autonomy, diversity, and pluralism, as shown in this chapter and the next in relation to health care delivery.

SELF-CARE

Obviously, most people spend most of their lives in a relative state of health or at a level of self-care. The constitution of WHO defines health as a "state of complete physical, mental, and social well-being, and not merely the absence of disease or infirmity," which, although it serves as a broad philosophical declaration, is more an optimum goal than a reality.

On a practical level, the Public Health Service's National Center for Health Statistics defines health implicitly in its use of "disability days," when usual activities cannot be performed.

Self-care can be defined as "a process whereby a lay person can function effectively on his own behalf in health promotion and prevention and in disease detection and treatment at the level of the primary health resource in the health care system."[13] It is not new and ranges from a simple matter of resting when tired to a more careful judgment of selecting or omitting certain foods or activities, or a semiprimary care activity of taking one or more medications self-prescribed or prescribed by a physician at some other point of care. Health care advice comes gratuitously from family, friends, neighbors, and the media (often with a product to sell). People also seek actively, although informally, information or advice from the same groups or a health professional acquaintance, but their self-care often becomes a matter of trial and error. Increasingly, a new consumer mentality has included the help of others with similar conditions or concerns (see Chap. 6), so that the individual has support and reinforcement as needed but can also detect at what point he or she needs professional help.

In some cases, a person may have had some level of professional care previously and may again, but a certain amount of informed self-diagnosis is not only less expensive for the public but may also serve a useful purpose for the individual. For instance, a mother who has been taught to take her child's temperature can give much more accurate information to a doctor or nurse practitioner, or avoid a call altogether if she also knows how temperature relates to a child's well-being. A blood pressure reading taken properly at home is more likely to identify a hypertension problem quickly than is a yearly physical examination. The sale of do-it-yourself medical tests, stethoscopes, blood pressure devices, and other medical devices for home use has become a rapidly growing big business.

Norris has described seven areas of activity in self-care:[14]

1. Monitoring, assessing, diagnosing—breast self-examination, and other monitoring for cancer, and diagnosing minor illnesses and communicable diseases.
2. Supporting life processes—teeth brushing, bathing, and other ritualistic habits.
3. Therapeutic and corrective self-care—care of minor and chronic illnesses, even serious conditions such as kidney disease, which requires dialysis.
4. Prevention of disease and maladjustment states—taking into consideration risk factors for certain illnesses such as cardiac conditions; and methods of maintaining psychological well-being.
5. Specifying health needs and care requirements—youths demanding that their particular health needs be met as they perceive them.
6. Auditing and controlling the treatment program—women and minorities demanding better care.
7. Grass roots or self-initiated health care—using peers as therapists (Weight-watchers; smoking cessation programs).

Besides consumerism, another factor that encourages self-care is the cost of health care. It has been estimated that perhaps 85 percent of all health care could be self-provided and might be quite necessarily self-provided to avoid flooding parts of the health care system. For instance, emergency rooms are frequently filled with patients who have minor conditions that could have been prevented or self-treated at home at an earlier stage.

One interesting approach to encouraging self-care is "holistic" health care, which incorporates a number of precepts of the consumerist ethic. These include providing physical, psychological, and spiritual care, therapeutic approaches that involve the patient and encourage the patient's independence and capacity for self-healing, emphasis on self-care and education, consideration as an individual, and an environment that encompasses other activities besides health care. Centers with this philosophy are often found in churches (where they started) and the nurse is a key figure: teaching, counseling, supporting, making recommendations, organizing support groups, and training volunteers. An important part of self-care that particularly involves nurses is health education and health promotion. As noted in Chap. 6, there is considerable evidence that many of the major causes of illness and death are learned behavior and related to lifestyle.

The role of parents as early models for children's health beliefs and health behavior is undisputed and early experiences structure people's personal beliefs and shape their attitudes.

Because this learned behavior may be deep-seated, it is often resistant to reeducation. Thus, changing undesirable eating patterns, smoking and drinking, and other aspects of lifestyle takes more than simple information. Other determinants influencing health attitudes and behavior are both cultural and socioeconomic. Evaluative research on health education, health promotion, and self-care is being done and is expected to provide helpful information on overcoming some of these obstacles.

Given the choice of continued reliance on costly medical care and preventive care, what will the public decide? Various polls seem to indicate that the public in general believes that the health care system should give more emphasis to preventive rather than curative medicine. The strongest support appears to come from business, the insurance industry, and union leaders (perhaps because of the increasing cost and overuse of health insurance that is often a job benefit). Health care administrators have also voiced strong support for health promotion and disease prevention activities. Reimbursement for these services is becoming more common, and they are regularly included in capitated managed care systems. (In capitated plans, individuals, or employers on their behalf, pay a specified dollar amount for services regardless of the amount used.) Managed care is discussed later in this chapter.

The natural relationship between disease prevention and health promotion and education and counseling has become obvious. These strategies have become linked to a popular interest in healthy lifestyle. Workplace programs have become common, seeing a link between job productivity, satisfaction, and health. Some employers have provided exercise periods and facilities, choices of food with low fat, salt, and cholesterol, and even health education programs. Schools are reemphasizing good health habits and are involving parents. Among the best-selling books are those on diet, exercise, and stress reduction; radio and television have also climbed on this popular bandwagon.

The role of government is equally evident (see Chap. 6), but the degree of governmental follow-through in these proposals fluctuates with the vagaries of political pressures. Though terms are not fully defined, in 1994, the eight major proposals for health care reform before the Congress all specifically guaranteed preventive care. It will be up to the public to assure that these words are present wherever legislative bargains are struck, and to monitor government as the provisions of the law are further defined by the regulatory agencies.

A philosophical point raised frequently is whether a government has the right to legislate individual choice. Attempts to mandate the use of seat belts and motorcycle helmets have not been completely successful. The more complex problems of smoking, drug use, and pollution control have not only personal but also economic ramifications. In the last several years, there has been more governmental intervention on this issue. According to various polls, most of the public approves.

AMBULATORY CARE

It is not practical to discuss the institutions involved in the various types of health care delivery under the headings of primary care and so on, because there is considerable overlap of functions. For instance, hospitals and HMOs may deliver all levels and types of care, even encouraging or sponsoring self-care activities on the part of individuals and community groups. Therefore, institutions and agencies are presented as units.

Ambulatory care is generally defined as that care rendered to patients who come to physicians' offices, outpatient departments, and health centers of various kinds. Because it also includes a number of services in which the provider goes to the consumer such as home care, the terms *community medicine* or *community health care* are also used.

Physician Office Practice

Except for home care and nurse-managed centers (NMCs), most ambulatory services currently involve physician-patient contact. Various sources indicate that the vast majority of care given by physicians is on an ambulatory basis; only about 10 percent of the people seen are admitted to a hospital. Most patient visits for health (or sick) care have been made to health care practitioners in solo, partnership, or private group practice. This is the major mode of organization for physicians and other health care providers generally acknowledged to be licensed to practice independently, such as dentists, chiropractors, podiatrists, and optometrists. Although there is a growing acceptance of nurses practicing independently, most people must be educated to that concept.

Physicians in private practice provide a range of health services and operate on a contractual basis (usually unwritten) with the patient—certain services for a certain fee. When a patient requires hospitalization, he or she pays the hospital for services provided there, except for the physician, who maintains an independent status and is paid directly on a separate fee basis. If a referral is made to specialists (secondary care), those specialists receive their fees, and the primary care physician sees the patient again when specialist services are no longer warranted. For various reasons, including the oversupply of physicians in some localities, more physicians are being employed full time by health care institutions or health care plans, in which case patients do not pay physicians separately, and the office itself may be run and staffed by institutional personnel. On the other hand, anesthesiologists, pathologists, radiologists, and other specialists based in the hospital often bill patients separately, sometimes under contract to the hospital, which gets part of the fee.

Most patient visits to physicians are made in an office. If an emergency arises, the patient may be seen in a hospital emergency room where the physician has staff privileges. Few make house calls. A small percentage of physicians (usually in urban areas) do not have hospital staff privileges, in which case the patient may be seen in the hospital by a referred colleague. From a business and tax viewpoint, private practice may be a corporation or partnership or may have some other designation.

Little is known about how physicians distribute their time in office practice among history taking and examinations, diagnosing, therapy, teaching or counseling, supervising or teaching staff, and paper work; most appear reluctant to have outsiders look into their work. Nor is there much information on how doctors interact, what the doctor-patient relationship consists of, how decisions are made, how quality is monitored, or how much traveling and meeting time is devoted to continuing education.

Patients who can choose their own point of admission into the health care system usually start with a physician office visit, and there is increasing concern that, for all the importance of that choice, people do so on an unsophisticated and relatively uninformed basis—someone's recommendation, proximity to the home, or, at best, a blind choice from a list provided, at request, by the local medical society. Frequently, people do a preliminary diagnosis of their own symptoms and choose a specialist on the basis of the organ that seems to be involved. Because that physician may have no contact with the other specialists the individual has chosen at random, continuity and comprehensiveness of care are generally lacking.

A physician's private practice setting often consists of only the physician (solo practice) and some full-time or part-time clerical help and/or medical assistant, office nurse, and physician's assistant (PA), any of whom may also be a family member. Increasingly popular is group practice with one or more physicians in the same specialty or a multiple-physician specialty conglomerate with all the workers previously cited plus x-ray and laboratory facilities with the appropriate personnel, and other supportive health professionals and services such as health education and physical therapy. More and more of these practice modes also include nurse practitioners (NPs) as employees or as full partners (see Chap. 15). Most private practitioners are paid by the patient or some form of third-party insurance. In recent years, offices serving primarily Medicaid patients in ghetto areas have been labeled "Medicaid mills," in part because of the poor quality of care and physician-encouraged overuse of services.

Nurse Private Practice

Nurses have been in private practice since formal nursing programs were started (see Chaps. 3 and 4). In a manner of speaking, private-duty nursing was and is a professional practice for which the individual has professional and financial responsibility.

In an emerging concept of nurse private practice, the nurse has an office where patients are seen, although he or she may also make house calls. In this form of independent practice, nurses have the same economic and managerial requirements as physicians, with the added concern that reimbursement by third-party payers is still greatly limited. Some insurance companies reimburse, and some laws have been passed to allow for reimbursement of certain practitioners, particularly nurse-midwives and psychiatric clinical specialists. However, because much nurse reimbursement requires a physician's order or supervision, nurses are often dependent on patients' paying their own bills. Although some groups of nurses and a few individuals working in independent practice are managing financially, frequently they also hold other positions, such as teaching posts. There are, of course, nursing faculty who carry a private practice to enhance their faculty role and are not dependent on that income. It should be noted that these nurses do not necessarily do what might be called medical diagnosis and treatment.

In a somewhat hybrid situation are the NPs who practice in an isolated area and are the sole source of health care for that population. These nurses are usually trained as family NPs (see Chap. 15). They may work under specified protocols, are in telephone contact with backup physicians, have arrangements with local pharmacists about prescriptions, have admitting privileges in some hospitals, or any combination of these. The nurses may be paid by the community or state, or by some other special arrangement. The primary care given is whatever is within the scope of that nurse's practice. These entrepreneurial practices are discussed in Chap. 15.

Community Health Centers

Out of the social unrest of the 1960s and early 1970s emerged the *neighborhood health center (NHC)*, an ambulatory facility based on the concepts of full-time, salaried physician staffing, multidisciplinary team health practice, and community involvement in both policy making and facility operations.[15] The NHC movement was stimulated by funding from the Office of Economic Opportunity (OEO) during the Johnson administration. In many ways, NHCs were similar to the early charitable dispensaries, which were established because of the hospitals' lack of interest in ambulatory care and disappeared in the 1920s because of poor financing, poor staffing, and physician disapproval.

Now more commonly called *community health centers* (CHCs), and including migrant health centers, they serve some 6 million Americans, usually poor, in about 2,000 locations nationwide. They may be freestanding, with a backup hospital for special services and hospital admissions, or legally part of a hospital or health department, functioning under that institution's governing board and license, but with a community advisory board.

CHCs are primarily found in medically underserved urban areas, where the minority poor, the homeless, and various ethnic groups rely on hospital ambulatory services for primary care. In many cases, the hospital clinic service and the emergency service, often expensive, overcrowded, fragmented, and disease-oriented, are inappropriately used. Their ineffectiveness is a major reason for the rise of the CHCs, called by some "one-stop health shopping" at acceptable, affordable prices, with interest in providing holistic health care. Often, they are at least partially staffed by the ethnic group served, so that communication is improved, and a real effort is made to provide services when and where patients and clients need them in an atmosphere of care and understanding. Use of nontraditional workers such as family health workers and an emphasis on using a health care team have been characteristic.

Although much of the health care given by CHCs is excellent, their problems have caused a drop in number from the peak development of the 1970s. Problems include tensions between community advisory boards and administrators of the center and/or the backup hospitals, and funding. Maintaining CHCs is extremely expensive, and most patients can pay only through Medicare or Medicaid, if at all. Few centers are self-supporting. When external funds are not available, severe program and personnel cuts are often necessary. The future of CHCs remains uncertain, in part because of a sociological question: Are they perpetuating a separate kind of care for the poor?

Nurse Managed Centers

Nurse managed centers (NMCs) offer "the ultimate autonomous practice opportunities (to nurses) as managers and primary caregivers."[16]

NMCs may also be called community nursing organizations (CNOs), or nurse run clinics. They guarantee direct client access to nursing services, offer services that are reimbursable, place the accountability for both the services and the management of the center with nurses, and allow nurses to practice to the fullest extent of their legal scope of practice.

NMCs are not new creations, but can trace their roots to the turn of the century and the tradition of the visiting nurse and public health nursing. Neither must all NMCs be community based. A modern-day example of an NMC can be observed in the Loeb Center established at Montefiore Hospital in New York by Lydia Hall in the early 1960s. Hall characterized Loeb as a nursing center with the qualities of public health being offered in an institutional setting.[17]

NMCs achieved prominence in the 1970s and 1980s owing to the troublesome gap between nursing service and nursing education, a scarcity of student clinical experiences with a wellness focus, and the continuing resistance to nurse practitioners in the medically dominated delivery system. The NMC movement was aided significantly by philanthropic support and government awards through the Division of Nursing. The Robert Wood Johnson Foundation funded 39 freestanding health clinics based on nurses as principal providers.[18]

The merits of NMCs, especially with underserved populations, were a perfect vehicle to move the reimbursement agenda for nurses forward. In December 1987, legislation was passed to establish Community Nursing Organizations (CNOs) to provide services to Medicare Part B beneficiaries for a single predetermined all-inclusive fee (capitation). A CNO is an NMC; it may also be characterized as a nursing health maintenance organization (HMO). The CNO is required to offer enrollees a package that includes home care, ambulatory services, prosthetics, durable medical equipment and supplies, speech and hearing services, social services, physical therapy, and optionally medical day care and case management. Among the full range of community services only pharmacy, laboratory, and x-ray are excluded from the capitated rate. Though the CNOs were created by legislation in 1987, the difficulties in rate setting and disputes over the right of nurses to practice without physician oversight delayed final implementation. After years of dispute between the profession and the regulatory agencies, four demonstration sites were authorized to go forward in 1991. They are to be evaluated in 1995.

Demonstration sites for CNOs were cautiously selected from among applicants with an existing history of success with the NMC concept. The capitated rates negotiated for the CNOs needed to be counterbalanced by payor groups who represent less at-risk clients. In a 1993 survey of NMCs conducted by the National League for Nursing, 30 percent of NMC clients paid out of pocket, 20 percent were uncompensated care, 14 percent Medicaid, 13 percent private insurance, 10 percent Medicare, and 11 percent undisclosed.[19] The significant presence of out-of-pocket payers and uncompensated care is a response to the resistant reimbursement environment for nurses, and places the NMCs at risk.

NMCs may be freestanding and entrepreneurial, or affiliated with a college of nursing or a health care institution. In any of these relationships, they may become part of a network as we move toward managed care. The services offered by an NMC may be narrow in scope or diverse. Appropriate clusters of services are described by Walker:[20]

- Services for life transitional and developmental changes related to birthing, parenting, puberty and adolescence, midlife, aging, divorce, and death.
- Services for organizations and businesses including expert consultation, clinical case management, education for management and employees, and employee wellness programs.
- Services for those experiencing life altering crises, and for informal caregivers, such as families of Alzheimer's patients.
- Services for longer term continuity of care, designed to enhance quality of life

for individuals and families experiencing chronic illness, physical and developmental disabilities, and the challenges associated with aging.

A 1992 survey estimates 250 NMCs in the United States. A few exemplary programs are summarized here:

- Genesis/Tampa General Health Center for Women and Children is affiliated with Tampa General Hospital and has an annual budget of forty million dollars.
- University of Rochester School of Nursing Community Nursing Center is a vehicle for faculty practice with both education and research goals accomplished through a diversified range of direct and subcontracted services.
- Alcorn State University Division of Nursing, Nursing Center in Natchez, provides care of adolescents and their families living in rural southwest Mississippi.
- The Block Nurse Program in Cleveland is a neighborhood-based home care service for older persons which integrated formal health care and informal support services.
- Community Health Clinic of Lafayette, Indiana, provides comprehensive family focused care to women, children, and male adults to age 65 and concentrates on the uninsured.
- Mercy Mobile Health Program of Atlanta brings primary care, HIV testing, substance abuse counseling, and other services to underserved populations in a fully equipped van.
- UCLA School of Nursing Health Center, Union Rescue Mission, is a large facility bringing primary care to the homeless.
- Community Health Services of Scottsdale provides family health care for individuals of all ages, and at least half are privately insured.

It should be noted that some of our most successful NMCs have been birthing centers established by certified nurse midwives (CNMs).

Models for NMCs have also been developed by clinical nurse specialists within such areas as cardiovascular, oncology, low birth weight babies, patients with chronic obstructive pulmonary disease, diabetics, and so on. Despite these highly focused exceptions, the majority of NMCs pursue primary care as their major agenda.[21]

NMCs have a tradition of serving our most vulnerable populations. Further, RNs employed with NMCs are significantly more educated than the nursing staff complement in other health care settings, with 31 percent holding a baccalaureate degree and 37 percent with a masters.[22]

The future of NMCs will depend on their success as participants in managed care, and in making strategic decisions to diversify or focus their services. Further, our commitment to the underserved is consistent with our history, but to grow and flourish the vast middle class must become our consumers.

Other Health Centers and Clinics

Variations of the CHCs are present in different parts of the country. *Rural health centers*, developed under federal financing such as regional health and the Appalachian projects or funded by communities or foundations, are the rural corollary to CHCs—existing to serve people, usually poor, in medically underserved areas (MUAs). Since few physicians are available, care is often given by NPs and PAs linked to physicians at other sites.

Mental health centers or *community mental health centers* are intended to provide a wide range of mental health services to a particular geographic "catchment area." They may be sponsored by state mental health departments, psychiatric hospitals or departments of hospitals, or the federal government. Staffed by teams of mental health personnel, they may consist of single physical entities or networks, but tend to focus on short-term care, including "crisis intervention." The Community Mental Health Center Act (1963) and its later amendments facilitated the development of comprehensive services and stimulated the community mental health movement. It was intended, in part, to prevent the warehousing of mental patients and assist their reintroduction into the community. Unfortunately, deinstitutionalization moved faster than the available community services, and even today there are mental patients living on the streets (estimated at one-fourth to two-fifths of the homeless population), or in deplorable, but less available, single-room occupancy hotels (SROs). While there are good halfway houses, day-care centers, and semisupervised living services, the services have not caught up with the demand.

There is general agreement that what is needed is a spectrum of services ranging from providing suitable housing to managing serious psychiatric and physical illness, and adequate coordination of these multiple community services. A particular concern is management of the chronically mentally ill, who need psychosocial services of mental health professionals as well as social workers. The noninstitutionalized mentally ill must be reached in many settings, including the streets, shelters, board-and-care facilities, and jails. A recent emphasis is the need for mental health services in rural areas.

Free clinics, often functioning in informal settings and sites, provide health care services to transient youths, minority groups, and students. They are usually staffed by volunteers. Their peak was reached in the early 1970s with the "flower child" generation; many of those that survived became more formally organized.

Women's clinics are usually owned and operated by women concerned about women's health problems and dissatisfied with the quality of care for women and the attitudes of many male health care providers. Most emerged out of the women's movement, along with the consumer and self-care movements. Services may include routine gynecological and maternity care and family planning, as well as some general health care. Emphasis is on self-help, mutual support, and noninstitutional personal care.

Both nurse-midwives and lay midwives are used, as are NPs and supportive physicians, although many staff are lay people. In a number of cities and towns, the clinics have been harassed by conservative groups and medical societies, and some have had to become involved in lengthy and expensive legal suits. These should not be confused with women's health care centers developed and operated by hospitals to target this specific clientele.

Family-planning clinics, of which the clinics of Planned Parenthood are most notable, provide a spectrum of birth control services and information. *Abortion clinics* are sponsored by community and other groups, as well as proprietary organizations, or may be a physician's private practice. However, harassment by antiabortion activists, including picketing and sometimes violent action, as well as some cutbacks in funding by the government and other external funding sources, have resulted in limitation of services and even closings in the last few years. A recent U.S. Supreme Court decision considered the harassment of patients and professionals and came down in favor of the public's right to access these facilities.

Renal dialysis centers were spurred into massive growth by their inclusion in the 1972 Medicare amendment. Once, the treatment of those with chronic kidney disease by using expensive artificial kidneys was a sensitive matter of "who shall live." When Congress decided that all should have that opportunity and funded it, the cost rose to unexpected millions of dollars. Many centers are freestanding, mostly physician owned or developed by proprietary organizations, but they also exist in hospitals. A whole new coterie of specialists at all levels has developed. The desired emphasis now is the less expensive home dialysis.

Another group of burgeoning facilities are those for rehabilitation of drug abusers. Most common are the *methadone maintenance programs* (substituting methadone for heroin, along with certain rehabilitative measures), which have had varying success. *Drug-free* programs include self-help and therapeutic resident programs, halfway houses, counseling centers, and "hot lines."

Adult day-care centers are agencies that provide health, social, psychiatric, and nutritional services to infirm individuals who are sufficiently ambulatory to be transported between home and center. Pyschogeriatric day-care centers were first opened in 1947 under the direction of the Menninger Clinic. Studies ordered by Congress in 1976 showed day-care centers to be cost-effective, but no national policy on reimbursement followed. Funding now comes from uncoordinated disparate sources, and therefore some communities have set priorities as to who can use the services. Yet, day care has been shown to be superior to nursing homes to eligible individuals because of lesser cost, improved health and functional outcomes, and an increased quality of life. Unresolved issues are related to their use for young adults with debilitating diseases, the feasibility of rural centers, and the need for regulation and licensing. Currently governmental distinctions exist between medical and social day care. The former requires some presence of health care personnel or some available health care services.

AMBULATORY CARE ALTERNATIVES TO INSTITUTIONS

The 1980s brought increased complaints about the expense of health care, particularly in hospitals, and ushered in the "competitive model." The core of the model is that consumer choice and market forces rather than regulation should be used to control health care costs.

As a result, alternative health care delivery modes, particularly in ambulatory care, developed and expanded. Among these are the *surgicenters*, independent proprietary facilities for surgery that do not require overnight hospitalization. The first was established in 1970 in Phoenix, Arizona, and their popularity has escalated. Some are specialized, such as the plastic surgery centers, but in general the centers can perform any surgery that does not require prolonged anesthesia. Surgicenters are said to be able to perform up to 40 percent of all surgical procedures, including face lifts, cataract surgery, vasectomy, breast biopsy, dilatation and curettage, knee arthroscopy, and tonsillectomy. Because of low overhead, surgicenters can charge as little as one-third of hospital costs for the same procedure, and patients like being able to return to home, or even work, the same day.[23]

When it was evident that this new delivery mode was not only well accepted (some do as many as 6,000 procedures a year) but reimbursable by insurance plans, many hospitals joined the movement and set up "day surgery" centers. Although greeted enthusiastically by payers at first because of the cost savings, in a few years the unregulated fees soared.

Private, for-profit, freestanding emergency centers or emergicenters designed to treat episodic, nonurgent health problems, are considered among the fastest-growing facets of U.S. health care. Since they first opened their doors in 1976, many more have sprung up around the country. The term *freestanding* may refer either to an independent, physician-owned emergicenter or one that is hospital sponsored or affiliated. The sponsored emergicenter, sometimes referred to as the *hospital satellite emergicenter*, is hospital managed and owned; those affiliated or associated with hospitals have contracts for service. Typically, the emergicenters are in shopping centers or commercial and industrial areas, have a high patient turnover, a short (15 to 20 minutes) waiting period, and a cost that may be 30 to 40 percent lower than that of hospital emergency rooms. Closely related are wound care centers treating chronic nonhealing wounds. Staff may also coordinate access to other needed services. All these centers have the potential to be a lucrative business. Government regulation is still largely nonexistent, and a number of legal issues are bound to arise.

Although some women are again turning to home births attended by midwives, a more popular and growing alternative to hospital births is the *childbearing center*, also called *birth center* or *childbirthing center*. These centers made their appearance in 1973, when the alienated and questioning middle class became disenchanted with hospital maternity care. The demonstration nurse-midwifery model was the Maternity Center of New York. Now an increasing number of out-of-hospital centers are operating. Some are operated by or utilize nurse-midwives; others are sponsored by physicians and/or lay midwives.

There are both freestanding (autonomous) centers and a variation of the concept in hospitals. Both allow for more humane care in a high-quality, homelike setting with the father and other children present—all costing considerably less than hospital care. Lubic, the originator of the modern concept and the first center, estimates that if only one in four pregnant women had access to and used birthing centers, millions and perhaps billions of health care dollars would be saved.[24]

Another humanistically oriented as well as cost-saving mode of care is the *hospice*. The hospice movement was pioneered in Great Britain by Dr. Cicely Saunders at St. Christopher's Hospice in London. The first widely recognized hospice in the United States was Hospice, Inc., established in 1971 in New Haven, Connecticut. Modeled after St. Christopher's, its concentration was on improving the quality of patients' last days or months of life so that they could "live until they die."

The Hospice Association of America estimates that there are between 1,700 and 1,900 hospices in the United States; about 1,158 hospitals have certified hospice services. Medicare classifies hospices into four types: hospital-based; home health-agency-based; skilled-nursing-facility-based; and independent. The first three are part of a larger institution; the independent, of which there are very few, are corporate entities. Hospices may offer inpatient care, home care, or a mix of the two. But whatever the setting, in reality it is a concept, an attitude, a belief that involves support of the family as well as the dying patient. It can be carried out in an ordinary hospital setting, with extraordinary perception. The hospice functions on a 24-hour, 7-day-a-week basis; backup medical, nursing, and counseling services are always available. The typical hospice team consists of a physician and some combination of nurses; medical social workers; psychiatrists; nutritionists; pharmacists; speech, physical, and occupational therapists; and clergy or pastoral counselors. The staff meets regularly both to discuss treatment plans and to provide support to one another. Because they are close to both patient and family, team members may suffer from burnout and stress, so counseling is available for them as well. Hospices frequently rely on well-trained volunteers, who provide respite care, companionship, transportation, patient teaching, and bereavement support. The family is also considered part of the team.

Most hospices serve cancer patients primarily, but many also care for patients with progressive neurological diseases and now AIDS. Except for the latter two groups, the majority of hospice patients are elderly. Any patient whose physician certifies that he or she has a life expectancy of less than six months is eligible for hospice care. Patients must be aware of their diagnosis and prognosis. Most patients die at home, surrounded by their families, and free of technological, life-prolonging devices. Symptom control is a vital step, and pain-relieving medications are dispensed at a level which will ensure that the patient is virtually pain-free at all times. Psychological comfort is considered as important as physical comfort, and the counseling, support, and companionship of hospice staff help relieve fear, depression, and anxiety.

A number of studies have shown that hospice care is less expensive than traditional care, and slowly reimbursement is being offered. Most major private insurance companies and some HMOs reimburse at least partially; however, since this can be an "add-on" benefit, very few patients receive full reimbursement. In 1986, hospice became a permanent Medicare benefit and an optional Medicaid benefit, but at least 80 percent of the care is supposed to be provided in the home.

HOSPITALS

In 1994, there were about 5,916 hospitals in the United States.[25] They are generally classified according to size (number of beds, exclusive of bassinets for newborns); type (general, mental, tuberculosis, or other specialty, such as maternity, orthopedic, eye and ear, rehabilitation, chronic disease, alcoholism, or narcotic addiction); ownership (public or private, including the for-profit, investor-owned proprietary hospital or not-for-profit voluntary hospital, which may be owned by religious, fraternity, or community groups); and length of stay (short-term, with an average stay less than thirty days, or long-term, thirty days or more). Hospitals vary from fewer than 25 to more than 2,000 beds. The most common type of hospital has been the voluntary, general, short-term hospital, followed by the local government, general, short-term hospital. The two major groups in terms of size are short-term general hospitals, averaging 160 beds, and long-term hospitals, averaging 900 beds. Between 1980 and 1990, almost 500 hospitals, mostly small, closed. Causes cited by the American Hospital Association (AHA) included financial cutbacks in federal funding, pressure by insurance companies and business to reduce health expenditures, and changing health care practices (such as those described earlier). If not closed, the small hospitals are likely to become part of a multi-institutional system, a major trend in health care delivery. These may comprise two or more hospitals owned, leased, sponsored, or contract-managed by a central organization. They can be for profit or nonprofit. Advantages can include improved access to capital markets, shared purchasing, technology, economics of scale, and use of technical and management staff. There have been predictions made that by the year 2000 there might be only 10 to 12 megasystems dominating the industry, but in recent years acquisitions have slowed down, perhaps because the chains found it more difficult to find attractive acquisition targets.

The term *teaching hospital* is applied to those hospitals with accredited medical residency programs, in which medical students and/or residents and specialty fellows (house staff) are taught. It does not include those that provide educational programs or experiences for other health professionals or allied health workers. These hospitals (about 9 percent) usually have more than 400 beds and are in medical centers proximate to the medical school (in which case they are often tertiary care centers).

Because of all these variations, it is difficult to draw one picture of the hospital as an entity. Figure 7-1 shows a common organizational pattern of a general hospital, which illustrates both the lines of authority and the kinds of services available. Administrative organization of services varies greatly according to administrative philosophy and types of service. For instance, a hospital that has outreach facilities, home health services, or a long-term care facility differs greatly from a 50-bed community hospital. Smaller hospitals may have fewer diverse clinical services and few, if any, education programs, but almost always there are business and finance departments, physical plant (maintenance of all kinds), laundry, supplies and storeroom, dietary and food services, clinical nursing units (inpatient and outpatient), and the other professional service units, such as laboratories, radiology, other diagnostic and treatment units, pharmacy, and perhaps social service. Some hospitals are now purchasing or sharing laundry and food services in the belief that this is less expensive in the long run. The physical layout of a hospital varies from one-story to high-rise, and may include large or small general or specialized patient units, special intensive-care units, operating rooms, recovery rooms, offices (sometimes including doctors' private offices), space for diagnostic and treatment facilities, storage rooms, kitchens and dining rooms, maintenance equipment, work rooms, meeting rooms, classrooms, chapel, waiting rooms, and

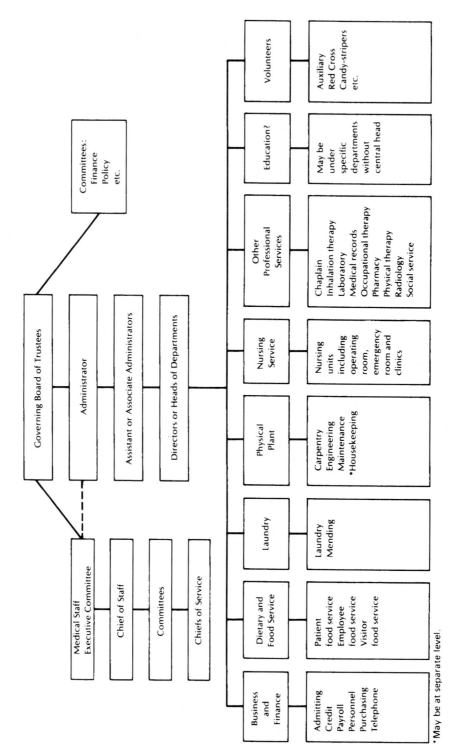

Figure 7-1 One pattern of hospital organization.

*May be at separate level.

gift and snack shops. Most hospitals have some form of emergency service, such as an emergency room, but many no longer maintain their own ambulance services. A great many have outpatient or ambulatory services, and perhaps an extended-care or cooperative-care unit for patients who do not need major nursing service; some provide home care.

The nursing service department has the largest number of personnel in the hospital, in part because of round-the-clock, seven-days-a-week staffing. Other departments, such as radiology and clinic laboratories, may maintain some services on evenings and weekends, and may be on call at nights. There is some trend toward having other clinical services available at least on weekends. For instance, a patient who needs rehabilitation exercises or other treatments in the physical therapy department lacks this necessary care in the evenings and weekends when that department follows the usual nine-to-five, Monday-through-Friday staffing pattern.

The primary purpose of hospitals is to provide patient services. However, many also assume a major responsibility for education of health personnel in basic educational programs or in in-service (staff development) programs, and participate in health research. Frequently, they are associated with schools of health professions and occupations, and provide the setting for health education and research, even though they do not finance such programs.

Hospitals are licensed by the state and presumably are not permitted to function unless they maintain the minimum standards prescribed by the licensing authority. ("Presumably" because the process of closing a hospital due to inadequate facilities and/or staff is long, difficult, and not always successful.) However, to be eligible for many federal grants, such as Medicare, and to be affiliated with educational programs, accreditation is necessary. Accreditation by the JCAHO is voluntary and is intended to indicate excellence in patient care. Specific standards, usually more rigorous than those of the state, are set to measure hospital efficiency, professional performance, and facilities, and

must be met in all facets of health care services (including nursing). By 1992, a new monitoring process was in place, stressing clinical and performance outcomes and continuous quality improvement, as opposed to a one-point-in-time evaluation that focused on structure and process. Visits are made by an inspection team (that may or may not have a multidisciplinary makeup) that reviews various records and minutes of meetings, interviews key people, and generally scrutinizes the hospital. Reports are made that include criticisms and recommendations for action. Accreditation may be postponed, withheld, revoked, granted, or renewed on the basis of the inspection and review of the hospital's report and self-evaluation. Nurses are now usually included on the inspection team, and there is nursing input into the standards for nursing service. To be eligible for an accreditation survey by JCAHO, the hospital must be registered or listed by the AHA, have a current unconditional license to operate as required by the state, and have a governing body, organized medical staff, nursing service, and other supporting services. The JCAHO board of trustees consists of representatives from the American Medical Association, the American Hospital Association, the College of Surgeons, Academy of Medicine, and the American Dental Association. Additionally, since 1992 there have been several consumer representatives, and a seat that is filled by a designated representative of organized nursing. This individual is identified by a coalition of the major nursing organizations. Additionally, a nurse selected by the American Nurses Association sits on the professional-technical advisory group to each of JCAHO's accreditation programs.

JCAHO accreditation is particularly necessary, because it holds "deemed" status with the Health Care Financing Administration (HCFA); that is, if a hospital is accredited by JCAHO, HCFA accepts this credential as verification of quality and allows reimbursement for service to Medicare beneficiaries.

Voluntary hospitals are usually organized under a constitution and bylaws that invest the board of trustees with the responsibility for medical care. This governing board is generally made up of individuals representing various professional and business groups interested in the community. Although unsalaried and volunteer (except for proprietary hospitals, in which members are often stockholders), board members are usually extremely influential citizens and are often self-perpetuating on the board. This type of membership originated because at one time administrators of hospitals did not have a business background, and because of the need to raise money to support hospitals. (Most trustees still see recovery of operating costs as their most crucial hospital problem.) Some consumer groups have complained that most members are businessmen, bankers, brokers, lawyers, and accountants, with almost nonexistent representation of women, minorities, consumers in general, and labor. Physicians also complain of lack of medical representation, although they work closely with the board and are subordinate to it only in certain matters. Because of these pressures, boards are gradually acquiring broader representation.

It is also possible that there will be some lessening of trustee power as hospitals adopt the corporate model, integrating the board of trustees and the administration of the hospital, with the board having full-time and salaried presidents and vice-presidents (see Fig. 7-2). The growth of mergers, consortia, and holding companies that are creating new business-oriented hospital systems may also change the role of trustees.

Public hospitals usually do not have boards of trustees. Hospital administrators are directly responsible to their administrative supervisors in the governmental hierarchy, which may be a state board of health, a commissioner, a department such as the Veterans Administration, or a public corporation with appointed officials. Presumably, all are ultimately responsible to the public.

Although *administrator* is still the generic term for the managerial head of a hospital, in recent years this title has included a variety of designations such as *president* and *chief executive officer* (CEO). The hospital administrator, the direct agent of a governing board, implements its policies, advises on new policies, and is responsible for the day-to-day operations of the hospital. Some years ago, physicians and nurses frequently became hospital administrators, but

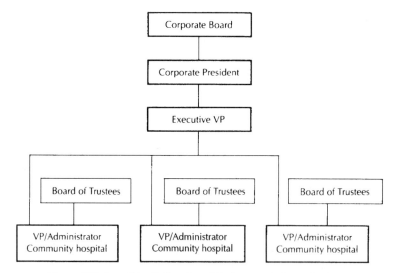

Figure 7-2 A multi-institutional model of corporate-type structure.

increasingly this position is filled by a lay person with a management background and possibly a master's degree in hospital administration or business administration. Hospital or health administration, like any other, encompasses planning, organizing, directing, controlling, and evaluating the resources of an organization. In large institutions, the administrator (the vast majority of whom are men) has a staff of assistants or associates, each responsible for a division or group of departments. Forward-looking hospitals have recognized that the nurse executive should hold one of these positions in order to participate in the policy-making decisions that inevitably affect the largest hospital department. Department heads or supervisors are next in the line of authority; these individuals are also gradually becoming specialists by education and experience in their area of responsibility.

The *medical staff* is an organized entity made up of selected physicians and dentists who are granted the privilege of using the hospital's facilities for their patients. They, in turn, evaluate the credentials of other physicians who wish to join the staff and recommend appointment to the hospital's governing board, which legally makes the appointments. A typical classification of medical staff includes honorary (not active), consulting (specialist), active (attending physicians), courtesy (those not wishing full status but wanting to attend private patients), and resident (house staff of residents and fellows). Through their committees, including the Credentials Committee, the medical staff is an impressive power in the hospital, for it is often in a position to control not only medical practice, but all patient care in the hospital. (The medical staff organization is parallel to and not subordinate to that of the hospital administration.)

Legal pressures, such as the *Darling v. Charleston Community Memorial Hospital* decision (see Chap. 21), increased malpractice suits, community pressures, and governmental pressures, including Medicare amendments (see Chap. 19), are focusing on the responsibility of medical staffs to monitor carefully the medical care given

and to institute immediately necessary improvements.

In hospitals where the medical staff is more progressive, there are nurses and other representatives on medical committees concerned with patient care, and decisions are made jointly. The issue of practice privileges for nurses is discussed in Chap. 15. Though the medical staff is still overwhelmingly physician dominated, it is not unusual for other provider professionals to have practice privileges of some sort. Considered a breakthrough was the 1983 stand of the Federal Trade Commission that medical rules should permit participating hospitals to grant staff membership to nurse-midwives, NPs, and other nonphysician health professionals, and 1984 JCAHO guidelines giving hospitals the option of granting such privileges.

There is some feeling among the nursing leadership, however, that such approval should not come from the medical staff but, if nurses are involved, from nursing administration. Although not widespread, in some hospitals, nursing staff bylaws enable nurses to be self-directed and self-governed, and allow for this orderly change within nursing. With such a mechanism, adjunct nursing staff including community-based NPs could, after having been approved by the nurse credentialing committee, provide care to their hospitalized clients.

The *utilization review committee* reviews records to determine that the patient's admission is valid, treatment is appropriate, and discharge is in a reasonable time. Nurses have been participating in these committees and are even employed full time in many instances.

In the last several years, there have been dramatic changes in hospitals, and even more are expected. Much is due to health economics and the criticism hospitals have received for their part in causing costs to escalate. The precipitating factor was undoubtedly the government-mandated prospective payment system for hospitals, utilizing DRGs to determine payment. Among other things, the PPS is responsible for the drop in length of stay (LOS), which was 7.1

days in 1992 according to AHA,[26] although it varied greatly in individual hospitals. The reactions have also been economically oriented. The "competitive model" advocated by the Reagan administration accelerated the growth of for-profit corporations that bought, built, and leased hospitals and other facilities and operated them under a corporate mantle. Although the type of governance varies, the motive is profit. One executive reported his company's strategy as acquiring hospitals in areas with favorable business factors, creating sophisticated facilities that provide a broad base of services, and involving physicians in profit sharing. The services offered acted as "feeders" to the hospital. Comprehensive long-term care facilities, rehabilitation, and psychiatric hospitals, as well as home care, were cited as increasingly profitable ventures. There has been some criticism that the investor-owned hospitals do not give as good a quality of care as the nonprofit, but these claims have never been substantiated.

This hybridization has led the hospitals down some varied paths. Besides their diversification into areas such as freestanding outpatient surgery programs (the most successful), outpatient diagnostic centers, cardiac rehabilitation services, substance-abuse programs, inpatient rehabilitation units, outpatient surgery satellites, industrial medicine clinics, sports medicine programs, home health services, and women's medicine programs (which have proved to be successful for the vast majority of hospitals developing them), some hospitals have also initiated health information telephone hot lines, medical equipment rentals, weight reduction programs and counseling, fitness programs, TV programs, wellness centers and baby-sitting services in shopping malls, advertising and public relations businesses, cleaning services, catering services, and even a graphics company. Some states have threatened to not only tax these for-profit entities but to cut the subsidies of hospitals so engaged. Oddly enough, among the reported financial losses are wellness- and health-promotion programs, even though the vast majority of hospitals are said to offer such programs.

Certainly, hospitals have had to adjust to many changes and face serious problems, aside from the ongoing issues of cost and quality. Because of heightened public awareness of the dangers of infectious waste, more attention must be given to its safe disposal, which is a costly operation. Inner city hospitals are being drained by bad debt, created in caring for the medically indigent including illegal aliens. Hospital emergency rooms are crowded to capacity, but being used more for primary care than for true emergency care. Hospitals are finally aware of the need to move into ambulatory services, but often find that someone has already captured that market. Malpractice claims made and paid hold a high price tag, as do the environmental improvements and workers' compensation protection that has become critical with the presence of AIDS and drug-resistant TB. The eroding job security and the dangerous working conditions have created a surge of organizing activity from unions.

There is no doubt that hospitals have the opportunity to remain a pivotal component in health care, but the system and consumer preference are changing around them. They will either move with the times or be discarded. The choice falls to each institution. Fewer in-patient beds will be needed. The move is into the community, rather than expecting the community to come to you. Managed care plans will seek out those hospitals that actively manage their patients and curry favor with consumers. Consumer satisfaction and cost are the primary concerns of managed care entities. This is not to cast aside quality; rather there is an assumption that a given baseline standard of quality is assured. Competition will prevail among hospitals. The most potent marketing tool available is to bring to the public assurances of the adequate presence of professional nurses.

GOVERNMENT FACILITIES

In the federal government, at least twenty-five agencies have some involvement in delivering health services. Those with the largest expenditures in direct federal hospital and medical services are the Veterans' Administration, which operates the largest centrally directed hospital and clinic system in the United States, the Department of Defense (members of the military and dependents), and the Health Resources and Services Administration (HRSA) of DHHS. [The Department of Health, Education and Welfare (DHEW) became the Department of Health and Human Services (DHHS) in 1980. See Chap. 27 for details in DHHS.] HRSA operates one Public Health Service (PHS) hospital (devoted to Hansen's disease) and provides care for federal prisoners and Coast Guard personnel. The Indian Health Service (IHS) operates hospitals, health centers, and satellite health clinics for Native Americans and Alaska natives. A variety of DHHS agencies provide indirect funding or contracts for clinics, drug and alcohol rehabilitation centers, maternal-child and family planning, neighborhood health centers, and the National Health Service Corps. In funding for hospital and medical services, DHHS spends the largest amount of money, primarily because of Social Security's Medicare and Medicaid and the Social and Rehabilitation Service.

State and local governments also have multiple functions and multiple services in health care delivery, directly through grants and funding to finance their own programs, and indirectly as third-party payers. Although most states have some version of a state health agency (SHA) or department of public health, health services are often provided through other state agencies, a situation that creates territorial battles, duplication, and gaps. In most states, operation of mental hospitals and the Medicaid program, two of the most important state health functions, is by departments other than the SHA. In direct services, some states operate mental, tuberculosis, or other hospitals and alcohol and drug abuse programs; provide noninstitutional mental health services; fund public health nursing programs and laboratories; and provide services for maternal and child

health, family planning, crippled children, immunization, tuberculosis, chronic respiratory disease control, and venereal disease control. All are considered traditional public health services, in addition to environmental health activities.

On a local level, services offered by a health department depend a great deal on the size, needs, and demands of the constituency. There appears to be little information about local health departments or health officers. Those with considerable visibility are in large urban centers, where health problems are complex and generally unresolved.

Some large municipalities operate hospitals that provide for the indigent or working poor who are not covered by Medicaid or private insurance. Some health departments run school health services and screening programs. Some duplicate services already offered by the state. There are few data on how much state and local agencies coordinate their services to avoid duplication or omission, but lack of coordination or cooperation is not uncommon. Although there is a great deal of criticism of most local health services in relation to high cost, waste, corruption, and poor quality, attempts to terminate any of them, particularly hospitals in medically underserved areas, become political conflicts, with representatives of the poor complaining that no other services are available and that the loss of local jobs will create other hardships. With all the politically sensitive issues involved, most health care experts are pessimistic about reorganization or major improvement of the health systems at any governmental level. One emergent trend that may predict an exception to this statement is the recent tendency to privatize both Medicare and Medicaid. Several states have chosen to give their poor a "voucher" to buy into the managed health care plan of their choice. This in fact forces government health care facilities to rise to the cost-efficiency and attractiveness of the private sector. It substantially reduces the infrastructure that is directly under governmental control. In the same spirit of seeking simplification, talk on Capitol Hill questions whether the existing federal systems should continue to exist as separate entities or should continue to exist at all, the option being to award vouchers for use in the private sector to all individuals having a right to government entitlement programs.

EMERGENCY MEDICAL SERVICES

Ambulance services, originally a profit venture of funeral directors, are a vital link in transporting accident victims or those suffering acute overwhelming illnesses (such as myocardial infarctions) to a medical facility. In most cases, providing for such services, either directly or through contracts, has now become the responsibility of a community, a responsibility that is not consistently assumed. The unnecessary deaths due to delayed and/or inept care have received considerable attention, which was probably responsible for some important federal legislation.

With continued federal and state funding and regulation, the previous diverse ambulance and rescue services of volunteers, firefighters, police, and commercial companies are being coordinated with regional systems. Several hundred are now in place. Criteria include training of appropriate personnel, education of the public; appropriate communication systems, transportation vehicles, and facilities; adequate record-keeping; and some participation by the public in policymaking.

Under these laws, a variety of emergency medical technicians (EMTs) have been trained and staff many ambulance services, including mobile intensive-care units, which have very sophisticated equipment.

HOME HEALTH CARE

Home health care is probably more of a nurse-oriented health service than any other, originating with Florence Nightingale's "health nurses" and the pioneer efforts of such American nurses

as Lillian Wald. (Today the term public health nurse or community health nurse is used.) Nevertheless, what Wald worked for in the late nineteenth century—comprehensive services for the patient and family that extend beyond simple care of the sick—is even more pertinent today.

Home care includes a broad spectrum of services from home birthings to hospice care. One useful definition is:

> **Home health is the provision of health services to individuals and families in their places of residence for the purpose of promoting, maintaining, or restoring health; or to maximize the level of independence, while minimizing the effects of disability and illness, including terminal illness. Individualized services are planned, coordinated and made available by providers organized for the delivery of home health care through the use of employed staff, contractual arrangements, or a combination of the two. Nurses perform, coordinate, or supervise most services delivered in the home. Home care services can alleviate the need for institutional care and help to contain costs. Home care is for persons of all ages of varying health status; persons who experience chronic developmental and handicapping disabilities that require home-based care; and persons with acute needs such as daily ventilator-assisted care, or involved procedures such as enteral and parenteral feedings, and intravenous medications.[27]**

Medical services are primarily provided by the individual's private or clinic physician, although in some instances agencies will employ or contract for a physician's services. In addition, homemaker–home health aide services may be required in conjunction with (or sometimes following) nursing and therapy. These consist of bathing, personal grooming, assistance with self-help skills, meal planning and preparation, and general housekeeping services. Among the other home health services that may be available are medical supplies and equipment (expendable and durable), nutrition, occupational therapy, physical therapy, speech pathology services, and social work. Other services, which may be provided through coordinated efforts of the agency and the community, include audiological services, dental services, home-delivered meals (Meals on Wheels), housekeeping services, information and referral services, laboratory services, ophthalmological services, patient transportation and escort services, podiatry services, prescription drugs, prosthetic and orthotic services, respiratory therapy services, and x-ray services. The National League for Nursing (NLN), describing a model of home health services, also included as highly desirable, environmental and social support services such as barber-cosmetology services, handyman services, heavy cleaning services, legal and protective services, pastoral services, personal contact services, recreation services, and translation services. Some might be developed as volunteer efforts.

Home care in the United States is a varied and rapidly expanding industry. During 1993, nearly 14,000 organizations provided care to approximately 6 million individuals and families, and annual expenditures exceeded 21 billion dollars.[28]

Services are delivered by a number of different types of agencies that have various organizational bases, structures, sponsorship, and auspices. The National Association for Home Care (NAHC) identified a total of 13,951 collective "home care agencies" in the United States as of February 1993. These consisted of 6,497 Medicare-certified home health agencies, 1,223 Medicare-certified hospices, and 6,231 home health agencies, home care aide organizations, and hospices that do not participate in Medicare.[29]

Medicare-certified hospices and home health agencies meet standards set by the federal government for type of services, quality of care, and organizational structure and oversight. Certified home health agencies comprise the largest sector of the home care industry and have various auspices. The major auspice types are Visiting Nurse Associations, public agencies, hospital-based agencies, and proprietary agencies.

Visiting Nurse Associations (VNAs) are free-standing, voluntary, nonprofit organizations governed by a board of directors (volunteers) and supported by contributions as well as by revenues received for care and services delivered. VNAs are the oldest and have been the classic providers of home care service. Depending on the location and resources, the spectrum of services may vary greatly but generally includes at least skilled nursing and other professional services. Many VNAs also operate adult day care centers, wellness clinics, hospices, and Meals on Wheels programs.

The mission of VNAs has always been to provide quality care to all people, regardless of their ability to pay. Volunteers have played a large role in assisting VNAs to accomplish their mission through fundraising, friendly visiting, telephone reassurance, and assistance with clinic and office work.

After a period of decline during the late 1980s, there has been moderate growth in the number of VNAs since 1990. VNAs, numbering 594 nationally, currently represent about 9.3 percent of certified home health agencies.[30]

Public agencies are government agencies operated by a state, county, city, or other unit of local government. In addition to providing home health care services, these agencies have a major responsibility for preventing disease and for community health education. In 1993, there were 1,176 public home health agencies representing 11 percent of the total agencies nationally.[31]

While both VNAs and public agencies have seen modest growth in numbers since 1990, they experienced substantial decline during the 1980s and today represent a much smaller proportion of home health agencies nationally. Their 1993 percentages noted earlier compare with 23 percent (VNAs) and 55 percent (public agencies) of total agencies nationally in 1975.[32] This decrease has been due primarily to financial problems resulting from extensive retroactive Medicare denials in the early 1980s and increased competition from hospital-based and proprietary home health agencies that have grown significantly from 1975 to the present.

Hospital-based agencies are operating units or departments of a hospital. The hospital-based agencies have grown substantially since the initiation of prospective payment for inpatient hospital services in 1983, and most rapidly over the past two years, accounting for more than one-third of new agencies during that period. Currently hospital-based agencies represent 28 percent of total home health agencies, up from only 12 percent in 1975.[33]

Proprietary agencies are freestanding for-profit home health agencies, which now number 2,440 and represent 35 percent of total home health agencies nationally.[34] Proprietary agencies have been characterized by aggressive development of new services, especially in the area of high-tech home care, and by brisk and sophisticated marketing activities. They have often provided the competitive impetus and organizational model for other home health agencies to rethink their service delivery patterns and structures.

Some of the VNAs and other agencies that have survived best now plan on a more businesslike basis, and new organizational patterns have emerged. One includes the development of a holding company or major corporation with both a nonprofit (traditional VNA) and for-profit subsidiary. The for-profit corporation may provide a variety of profitable services, such as home-health aides, chore services for the frail elderly, presurgery counseling before hospital admission, vocational rehabilitation, and more recently, establishing a pharmacy for the home infusion therapy solutions needed. The after-taxes profits from this corporation are then donated to the nonprofit corporation to provide the free services that have sometimes kept VNAs on the point of bankruptcy.

Both voluntary and official (governmental) agencies have been affected by the financial and competitive squeeze, and although total restructuring is not always possible, approaches have been used that were never even considered previously. Computers have become essential for keeping records and statistics and for case management. Seen as the key was marketing of services based on the needs of the consumer.

One of the major factors affecting the expansion of home care has been that it is viewed as both less expensive than institutional care and a more effective, humane approach, especially for the elderly and chronically ill. Whether it is indeed cheaper may depend on what supportive services are needed. Is only health care needed, or a variety of social services? And what of the difficulty of coordinating the physician, agency, and patient, much less other entities? Consideration must also be given to the need for close planning and participation of the family; if the family or significant others are absent in a patient's life or unwilling to take on the necessary responsibility, home care may not be the most desirable approach for dependent individuals. On the other hand, with the participation of health professionals who have a commitment to this aspect of health care, reasonable assurance of quality, and adequate financing, home health care has tremendous potential for filling a health care gap, and has been demonstrated to increase effectiveness and reduce costs of health care for a number of diagnoses.[35]

Another major factor fueling the growth of home care in the United States has been the financial support of Medicare and Medicaid. Medicare is the largest single payer of home care services. In 1992, Medicare spending accounted for 38 percent of total home care expenditures and Medicaid for 25 percent of total.[36] Although home care represents a relatively small percentage of total Medicare and Medicaid expenditures, it has been and is expected to continue to be the fastest-growing category of expenses for both government insurance programs. As a result both federal and state governments are keeping a close watch on continued home care growth and spending. Medicare has initiated several prospective payment demonstrations that may shift home care reimbursement from the current per visit to a per episode system. State Medicaid programs are placing increased emphasis on movement of beneficiaries into managed care systems that will ultimately affect home care utilization and payment.

In fact, the growing emphasis on managed care and the movement toward more efficient health service delivery systems have been and will continue to be the most important changes affecting the home care industry. Managed care companies are pressuring home health agencies to provide fewer visits at lower cost, without compromising quality and at the same time demonstrating positive results (outcomes) of the care provided. In addition, home care agencies will more and more be expected to accept financial risk for their services through per capita payments, regardless of the intensity or variations of services to individual clients. Home health agencies will need to have detailed information about costs and outcomes of care and may need to organize and package services differently in order to succeed in the growing managed care marketplace.

The growth in managed care plans and their desire to bundle payment for acute and postacute services has also influenced a number of freestanding agencies, especially VNAs, to affiliate with or become part of larger integrated health systems. Within these relationships the home health agency often relinquishes at least some autonomy in return for a secure and often expanded referral base.

The focus on managed care and reducing health care costs presents many challenges and uncertainties to the home care industry. Conversely, they also offer a powerful role for home care and for community health nurses in particular. Managed care plans are placing a growing emphasis on preventive care, education, and training as the most cost-effective forms of health care.[37] It is most exciting to anticipate a return to the "roots" of home care through provision of services that community health nurses have always been committed to and are uniquely qualified to render.

LONG-TERM CARE FACILITIES

Long-term care (LTC) services for chronic diseases and conditions comprise one of the fastest-growing components of health care expenditures. In part this is due to the success of medical science in saving those who might have died of their condition at any earlier stage of life, and in part to the fact that the nuclear family has no place for the incapacitated who, years ago, were simply cared for at home with no public help. One comprehensive definition of long-term care presents a good picture of what such care should be.

> **Long-term care should include an integrated mix of health, psycho-social, support and maintenance services provided on a prolonged basis, either continuously or intermittently, to individuals whose functional capacities are chronically impaired or at risk of impairment. Care should be provided in the least restrictive environment possible. Most long-term care is supplied by families and other informal providers. The objective of long-term care is to increase or maintain the level of physical, social and psychological functioning of people to their maximum potential in order to promote functional independence and improve quality of life. The long-term care system should include a network of long-term care services which flow in either direction along the continuum of care between acute and long-term care institutional settings, community-based programs and services and organized services at home. Issues of access, cost, and quality are of concern in all long-term care settings. Populations at risk of requiring long-term care services include the physically disabled, the mentally handicapped and the mentally ill. Across all these populations, the elderly represent the largest group at risk of chronic impairment and functional dependency requiring long-term care services for a sustained period.[38]**

As noted earlier, the use of ambulatory care facilities and a return to home care are being advocated, but the fact remains that such care requires a considerable number of backup services, social and health related, that are not easy to organize or to coordinate and even less likely to be reimbursed. Therefore, despite much rhetoric, institutional care for long-term patients, while considerably more expensive and often lessening the individual's quality of life, still appears to be necessary for part of the population.

There are two major categories of long-term care institutions: long-stay or chronic disease hospitals (for example, psychiatric, rehabilitation, chronic disease, and tuberculosis) and nursing homes. There are about 300 long-term stay hospitals, mostly psychiatric and mostly government owned. According to the American Health Care Association (AHCA), in 1993 there were approximately 16,332 nursing homes that are certified for Medicare and Medicaid, about 75 percent of which were proprietary. There were over 1.7 million persons receiving care in nursing homes in 1990, a 25 percent increase from 1980.[39] This does not refer to residential facilities that may provide some degree of nursing services over and above room, board, and personal care or "custodial" services. About 66 percent have fewer than 100 beds; only 5 percent have more than 200. Although over half are still independently owned and operated, this is decreasing, as chains buy more and more.

Nursing homes can be classified according to the levels of care offered and whether they are certified for the Medicare and/or Medicaid programs. According to these regulations, a skilled nursing facility (SNF) which provides inpatient skilled nursing and restorative and rehabilitative services must provide twenty-four-hour nursing services, have transfer agreements with a hospital, and fulfill other specific requirements. An intermediate-care facility (ICF) provides inpatient health-related care and services to individuals not requiring SNF care. Nursing homes may be certified for either or both levels; about 25 percent are not certified at all. If certified, PROs monitor them; some are also JCAHO-accredited.

The organizational structure of a nursing home is often much like that of a hospital, but there are fewer diagnostic and therapeutic departments, depending on the major purpose of the institution. Usually both short-term and long-term care are offered. The nursing home may or may not be associated with a particular hospital. Some extended-care facilities have expansive services providing a continuum of care from skilled nursing to home care. For those who can afford it, there are complexes in which older people can live in their own apartment for life; health care services, including skilled nursing, are made available when needed. Sometimes a nursing home and even a hospital are on site.

Although about 12 percent of nursing home residents are under 65, the rapid growth of the over-85 population has made the care of the frail elderly and chronically ill a public concern. It has been noted that those over age 85, who are most apt to need long-term care and financial assistance for such services, are increasing seven times as fast as the population as a whole, and elderly Americans who will need some sort of help, now over 6.5 million, will climb to 19 million by 2040. One expert said that actuarially, the odds are nearly one in two that an individual would need LTC between the age of 65 and death, largely because of chronic disabilities.

The cost of nursing home care is quite high on a long-term basis, and often the patient and spouse must "spend down" their assets until the patient is eligible for Medicaid. Not too long ago this could have reduced the spouse to poverty, but now legislation allows the spouse to keep both assets and a monthly income at a more reasonable (but still not generous) level. Some elderly are still often upset that their hard-earned savings, which they had hoped to leave to their children, are almost wiped out when nursing home care is necessary. Whether or not another law like the Catastrophic Coverage Act (enacted in 1988 and repealed in 1989, because some elderly objected to the surcharge all would need to pay) will again cover long-term care is problematic. It is difficult to get agreement on what people need and the government and taxpayers are willing to pay.

Nursing homes are considered good business opportunities for investors, many of whom believe that more elderly will have good investments in years to come and can pay the ever-increasing rates. And these are the kinds of clients they seek—not the Medicaid patients, with relatively low reimbursement and more governmental oversight. There are now some insurance plans (rather expensive) that cover nursing home care, but Medicare covers very little. This may change since now a number of SNFs care for patients that require complex care and technology that was once seen only in hospitals. Giving intravenous (IV) fluids is common, as are tube feedings. Most extended care facilities are moving rapidly to establish sub-acute care units. JCAHO circulated standards for accreditation of this new level of intensity in the summer of 1994. These units will require a greater presence of professional nurses. The variation in care needed by LTC patients has caused the federal government to initiate a refinement of the current classification system.

Aside from the cost, another issue is the quality of nursing homes. The Health Care Financing Administration (HCFA) releases periodic data on the nursing homes that participate in Medicare and Medicaid programs. Among other things, 1989 survey information revealed that 40 percent of these facilities did not meet sanitary standards for food handling, 29 percent incorrectly administered drugs, and almost 30 percent failed to assure personal cleanliness and grooming through personal hygiene. A profile of each nursing home was included. This report echoes previous governmental investigations, although some of these had revealed much more serious problems, such as abuse of patients and theft of their property or money. In all cases, AHCA objected to the wholesale condemnation of the industry, maintaining that the overwhelming majority delivered good to excellent care to their residents. A 1986 study by the Institute of Medicine (IOM) had indeed stated that nursing homes had improved since the early 1970s but still documented the poor care given in many. The ANA commented that one problem in quality was insufficient staffing, especially numbers and availability of skilled nurses—not a new issue. ANA was unsuccessful in its attempt to have 24-hour registered nurse coverage in nursing homes included in a nursing home reform law, the 1987 OBRA, described in Chap. 19.

Some regulations for that law were not published until 1989 and drew fire from almost everyone: nursing homes said they were too tough and expensive, health groups that they were too weak. One key compromise was the requirement for 24-hour "licensed nurse" coverage, with an RN on duty on the day shift. Coupled with a generous waiver clause where

it was difficult to recruit, it was possible that nursing home patients could be entirely without an RN. One happier note was that physicians could designate a nurse practitioner (or PA) to make some of the required visits to nursing home residents, and that nurses' aides must be given a minimum of 75 hours of training. Nurses' aides give up to 85 percent of the care and are often given little or no training.[40] Among other improvements were requirements for a full-time social worker in facilities with more than 120 beds; rehabilitation and dental services; no admissions of mentally ill patients except those with Alzheimer's or related dementia; and residents' guarantee of freedom from abuse, excessive medication, and punitive physical or chemical restraints. Other rights were also spelled out. However, final rules for many parts of the law were not published until 1992.

There will probably still be complaints about the quality of life, if not always the quality of physical care, in nursing homes. In some areas, voluntary ombudsmen regularly make checks to prevent or detect abuses. There are also a few adopt-a-grandparent or similar programs that give the residents caring social contacts outside the home. It has been noted that the factors generally listed by residents as important to quality of care—an adequate, competent, caring staff, a homelike environment, properly prepared and varied food, activities, and medical care—were rated most highly. No doubt if these were present in most nursing homes, people would not be as reluctant, even frightened, to be admitted to them.

Experts disagree on the future of nursing homes. Nursing homes serve the socially isolated woman, a group that is increasing, but no one seems to want to expand the nursing home system because of concerns about cost and quality of care. Yet if all home care and support services were reimbursed, the "latent demand" might cause a financial catastrophe, since almost all of that care is now given without reimbursement by family and friends. As the older population increases, so does the need for a reasonable plan for their long-term care needs.

MANAGED CARE

It is impossible to speak of health care in the mid-1990s without giving significant attention to managed care. What it is. What it is not. What it hopes to accomplish.

Managed care is not a place, but an organizational structure. More correctly, it is a variety of organizational structures that use active risk sharing to provide the best value in health care to a defined group of enrollees or members of a plan. The goal of managed care is to require the decision makers, who are the consumers, payers, and providers, to carefully consider the merit of services, procedures, and treatments in view of the resources available to them.

Managed care includes three basic types of arrangements: the health maintenance organization (HMO), preferred provider organization (PPO), and managed indemnity health insurance plans. In addition, there are growing variations on each of these themes, so that no one definition remains totally pure. Two common features being inserted into managed care systems are the "point-of-service" option and the "single point of entry."[41] The former guarantees the right to select a nonparticipating provider any time you wish without prior approval. This privilege usually includes higher premiums, copayments, or deductibles. The latter requires system entry through a point designated by the entity at risk (the plan) and is usually a primary health care provider. Extensive data collection proves that nurses in advanced practice are especially suitable for this role.[42]

The HMO combines the delivery and financing of services into one system. The HMO assumes an explicit contractual responsibility to provide a stated range of services. There is an enrolled, defined population who agree to a fixed periodic payment (capitation rate) that is established independent of the actual utilization of services by the enrollees. The HMO as-

sumes financial risk but exerts control on the use of services. These services may be provided in facilities which they own, most usually for the ambulatory care component, or at sites where they have contractual arrangements. The name health maintenance organization evolved from the fact that priority is accorded to teaching, counseling, and self-care activities that promote health and independence, therefore reducing the cost to the plan for more complex medical services. It is to the HMO's advantage to avoid hospitalization as the most expensive component of the health care industry.

In comparison, the PPO is somewhat between the HMO and standard indemnity plans in the degree to which it shapes prescribing (the provider) and consumption (the consumer) behaviors. The PPO offers financial incentives for membership by creating a network of providers who agree to reduced fees for enrollees. Because of the lower cost, you are tempted to select from the panel of preferred providers. The providers are assured more rapid cash flow, and business and marketing functions are centralized on their behalf. In most plans, the enrollee maintains the right to go "out of network" for services if desired (point of service option), and on those occasions the indemnity plan "kicks in." In essence, the PPO is an agreement among a limited group of providers to reduce fees for individuals intending exclusive (more or less) use of their services. In a PPO, the actual delivery of service is decentralized, allowing providers to simultaneously continue servicing clients who are not members of the plan.

Indemnity plans (financial protection against the cost associated with covered service) have incorporated some techniques of managed care. Preauthorization, second opinion for surgery, continued stay certification, discharge planning, and even copayment and deductibles are strategies of managed care. The decision lies with the consumer, but the goal is to introduce an incentive to be prudent.

Until very recently, PPOs proved more popular with the public than HMOs by actively managing risk, providing cash incentives, yet allowing a high degree of choice. The latest observations see HMOs gaining in market share among the American public. It should be noted that the entities allowed to become provider partners in a PPO are designated by state law, and in some situations nurses are excluded.

There are four basic types of HMOs: group model, staff model, network model, and individual practice associations (IPAs).

1. In a *group model*, a group of physicians provides care to patients at one or more locations.
2. In a *staff model*, services are delivered at one or more locations through physicians who are employees of the HMO.
3. In a *network*, an HMO contracts with two or more group practices to provide care.
4. In an *IPA*, care is provided through physicians in the community who practice out of their own offices.

A *federally qualified* HMO has been approved by the federal office of Prepaid Health Care for voluntarily complying with a set of quality assurance and financial standards and agreeing to provide a comprehensive benefit package that includes physician and hospital services.

For all their apparent benefits, until the mid-1980s HMO growth was relatively slow. One reason was that physicians were reluctant to change practice modes or opposed HMOs outright; another was that start-up and other costs of the comprehensive services are high, sometimes making HMOs noncompetitive with other forms of health insurance; finally, the original Department of Health, Education and Welfare (DHEW) regulations were so restrictive and complex as to create problems in implementation.

By 1989, the number of HMO plans had peaked, but enrollment continued to climb. In 1988 more than a million Medicare beneficiaries were enrolled in HMOs, although 31 million stayed with traditional fee for service. By 1990, there appeared to be some slowdown of all enrollments.[43] Some HMOs found themselves in financial trouble because of their inability to hold down costs. Their attempts to exert tighter controls over treatments that patients receive angered doctors, who were also unhappy with their salaries. Yet HMOs were either forced to lower costs or raise prices—and lose members, including some large corporations. They also complained that Medicare fees were too low to cover the cost of care for the elderly, who were "high users," and some HMOs chose not to take Medicare contracts. (Some researchers have said that one reason HMOs were cost-effective is that their self-selected enrollees are more conservative users of health services, who are attracted by the HMO philosophy of preventive care and health maintenance.) Nevertheless, forecasters continue to predict growth of HMOs, with an increased number of mergers and conversions to for-profit entities resulting in more cost-effective management. A change in federal legislation also allowed more flexibility in setting premiums: HMOs are expected to continue to offer a viable alternative to fee-for-service health care.[44]

HEALTH CARE REFORM

There is a general public uproar in the United States that our health care delivery system is seriously deficient in access and value and outrageous in cost. In 1993, the cost to the American public was over 800 billion dollars (in excess of 14.1 percent of gross nation product), and over 70 million individuals had inadequate or no health care coverage. Those most frequently denied health care are middle-class Americans caught in low-paying, transient jobs or working for small business.[45] It is difficult or impossible to obtain adequate health care coverage in either of these situations. These are the medically indigent, the most needy, the most vulnerable. Though the cost and access arguments are compelling, quality is of equal concern. Over 35 percent of preschool children in the United States are unimmunized. Maternal-child health in some areas of this country among select ethnic and racial subgroups is no better than that in a third world country.[46] Statistics abound, and the reader is referred to the bibliography to develop a more complete grasp of the immediate need.

The public are well aware of the moral imperative for health care reform, and the search for an equitable and acceptable solution has been the preoccupation of the nation. In 1994, several prominent pieces of legislation and partisan proposals were debated. The most visible was the Health Security Act proposed by the president, and all others were to a greater or lesser degree measured against its provisions. Though no legislative proposal was successful, the tone is set for continuing debate.

Members of the health care industry, including nurses, have been actively involved in shaping the ideas that will eventually characterize change. *Nursing's Agenda for Health Care Reform*,[47] the official platform of organized nursing, was authored and negotiated among the nursing community in the early 1990s and is currently endorsed by over 90 national nursing and allied health associations. It is the only position of a health care group that has been endorsed by the president and publicly acclaimed by the members of the industry. The existence of *Nursing's Agenda*, the American Nurses' Association's powerful presence in Washington, and a well-organized network for grass roots lobbying have been successful in keeping nursing's proposals before our elected officials. As the debate rages, the elements that will characterize a reformed system become clearer.

Although the nurses of America and the president hold firm to the requirement of universal coverage, this remains one of the most controversial aspects of any proposal. Universal coverage has been closely linked with mandatory workplace provision of health care benefits. Given the prevalence of small business on the American scene, and the fact that 25 percent of small businesses claim that they would close if required to assume the burden of health care for all their employees, the future is questionable for this route to universal coverage. The question must be divided, or economic protections must be guaranteed for small business.

Significant sympathy exists for previously disenfranchised groups, pregnant women, and children. In reality, even if sometimes inadequately, the old and the poor have been provided for. Unfortunately what this portends is a fragmented population-based route toward (hopefully) universal access. It also predisposes to a two-tier delivery system. The option should be the creation of programs that serve the rich and the poor, the educated and the uneducated, the young and the old, the aggressive and the passive. This may come to be as more states offer incentives for Medicaid recipients to buy into managed care plans. The same option has been offered to Medicare recipients on an experimental basis, and was included as a permanent provision in the administration's Health Security Act.[48] In fact, these observations add credibility to the suspicion that we may witness a total integration of all public entitlement programs, eliminating counterproductive state and federal and episodic or continuing care distinctions. These trends also capitalize on the tradition of government looking to the private sector for program execution. Precedent has been set by the Medicare program, which is administered through subcontracts to private sector intermediaries at less than 5 cents on the dollar for administrative costs.

Any emergent system of reform will emphasize health and treat managed care plans preferentially. The uncontrollable cost of health care in this country is due to many factors, one being the fee-for-service system which provides no rewards for prudent use of resources and sets no controls on volume. It is also becoming more obvious that many of our most costly health care problems are lifestyle-based and could be significantly impacted by health-promotion and disease-prevention activities. Consumers are being expected to assume more responsibility for their health and self-care.

Much of the cost of health care is defensively generated. Consumers demand more because they fear losing control. Providers readily comply or institute excesses of their own in response to the litigious environment. Empowerment of consumers on their own behalf would shift some of this defensiveness. The final directive requirement discussed in Chap. 22 on the Rights of People is an empowering strategy.

Adequate health care reform would require total infrastructure redesign. To assure the best value, our systems of care would have to be integrated, assuring continuity across a continuum that includes community, long-term, and acute services. Use of the most cost-efficient provider for a clinical situation would be required. Combining this with the prized American right to freedom of choice, consumers must have direct access to a range of providers including advanced practice nurses who can independently resolve over 80 percent of the primary care concerns of the public. The president's Health Security Act included preemptive provisions that would have required every state to provide direct consumer access to nonphysician providers, regardless of state law.[49]

In the interest of thrift and health, every resident of the United States must have access to primary health care services that are community-based. It would be strategic to expand currently existing locations that are convenient, familiar, and friendly. The expansion of school health services into full-fledged family health centers is a proposal that has been well received.[50] Similar models have already been established in the workplace, where both employers and employees see the potential for healthier workers and families, less stress, and fewer total dollars for health care.[51]

In summary, health care reform is inevitable. The characteristics of an emergent system are clear, regardless of the legislation that will bring it into being. Change will be incremental and a combination of both state and federal initiatives. We seem guaranteed of more government involvement in health care through either funding or policy, but the system will be unique to this country, a marriage of public and private sector resources and services. The system will give more attention to health as opposed to an almost exclusive preoccupation with illness. A managed care model will provide increased degrees of freedom of choice and integration of services across settings. For the most part, access to the system will be through a primary provider who is community-based. Advanced practice nurses are an excellent choice to move forward to fill the primary care gap.

The inordinate cost of the current system is largely due to consumer and provider excesses, and bureaucracy and administration. Empowerment of consumers to participate in decisions about their own treatment based on information about outcomes can reduce cost by influencing choice and diminishing defensive practice. Systems modifications such as the electronic transfer of claims and consolidated forms promise savings of over 85 billion dollars.

These observations hold very serious implications for nursing and nursing education, which are discussed at other points in the text.

REFERENCES

1. U.S. Department of Health, Education, and Welfare: *Extending the Scope of Nursing Practice.* Washington, DC: The Department, 1971.
2. Millis J: Primary care: Definitions of and access to. *Nurs Outlook* 25:443, July 1977.
3. U.S. Department of Health Education and Welfare, op cit, p 10.
4. Ibid, p. 11.
5. American Nurses' Association: *Health Care Reform and America's Nurses: Agenda for Change.* Washington, DC: The Association, 1994.
6. Joel L: Reshaping nursing practice. *Am J Nurs* 87:793–795, June 1987.
7. Brider P: Too poor to pay: The scandal of patient dumping. *Am J Nurs* 87:1447–1450, November 1987.
8. *Uninsured in America.* Palo Alto, CA: Kaiser Family Foundation, 1994.
9. Harrington C: A national health care program: Has its time come? *Nurs Outlook* 36:214–216, 255, September–October 1988.
10. Poll shows desire for change in U.S. health system. *The Nation's Health* 19:1,9, March 1989.

11. Shortell S, McNerney W: Criteria and guidelines for reforming the U.S. health care system. *N Engl J Med* 322:463–466, Feb. 15, 1990.

12. Kinzer D: Universal entitlement to health care. *N Engl J Med* 322:467–470, Feb. 15, 1990.

13. Levin L: Self-care: towards fundamental changes in national strategies. *Int J Health Ed* 24:219–228, 1981.

14. Norris C: Selfcare. *Nurs 79* 9:486–489, March 1979.

15. Roemer M: Resistance to innovation: The case of the community health center. *Am J Pub Health* 78:1234–1239, September 1988.

16. Sharp N: Community nursing centers coming of age. *Nurs Manage* 23:18–20, August 1992.

17. Hall L: A center for nursing. *Nurs Outlook* 11:805–806, 1963.

18. Riesch SK: Nursing centers: An analysis of the anecdotal literature. *J Prof Nurs* 8:16–25, January–February 1992.

19. Barger S, Rosenfeld P: Models in community health care. *Nurs Health Care* 14:426–431, October 1993.

20. Walker PH: Comprehensive community nursing center model: Maximizing practice income—a challenge to educators. *J Prof Nurs* 10:131–139, May–June 1994.

21. Phillips DL, Steel JE: Factors influencing scope of practice in nursing centers. *J Prof Nurs* 10:84–90, March–April 1994.

22. Barger S, Rosenfeld P, loc cit.

23. Pica-Furey W: Ambulatory surgery—hospital based versus freestanding: A comparative study of patient satisfaction. *AORN-J* 57:1119–1121, 1123–1127, May 1993.

24. Lubic R: Childbirthing centers: Delivering more for less. *Am J Nurs* 83:1053–1056, July 1983.

25. American Hospital Association: *Hospital Statistics 1993–1994*. Chicago: The Association, 1994, p 7.

26. American Hospital Association, loc cit.

27. Anderson E, McFarlane J: *Community as Client: Application of the Nursing Process*. Philadelphia: Lippincott, 1988.

28. Basic Statistics about Home Care 1993. National Association for Home Care. Fall 1993, p 1.

29. Ibid, p 1.

30. Ibid, p 2.

31. Ibid.

32. Ibid.

33. Ambulatory Care Trendlines 1992. *Growth Trends in Hospital Home Care 1980–90*. Chicago: American Hospital Association, July 1992.

34. Basic Statistics, NAHC 1993, p 2.

35. Ibid, p 8.

36. Ibid, p 3.

37. NAHC Report 511, National Association for Home Care, May 7, 1993, p 6.

38. Infeld D, Kress J: *Crisis of Quality: Management for Long-Term Care*. Arlington: Association of University Programs in Health Administration, 1990, pp 9–10.

39. Nursing home reps draw fire from health groups. *Am J Nurs* 89:551, April 1989.

40. Alfano G: Long-term care, in McCloskey J, Grace H: *Current Issues in Nursing*. St. Louis: Mosby, 1994, pp 501–505.

41. Hicks L et al: *Role of the Nurse in Managed Care*. Kansas City, MO: National Center for Managed Health Care Administration, 1992, pp 5–7.

42. American Nurses' Association: *Nurse Practitioners and Certified Nurse-Midwives: A Meta-Analysis of Process of Care, Clinical Outcomes, and Cost-Effectiveness of Nurses in Primary Care Roles*. Washington, DC: The Association, 1993.

43. Ibid, pp 8–10.

44. Drew J: Health maintenance organizations. *Nurs Health Care* 11:144–149, March 1990.

45. Friedman E: The uninsured: From dilemma to crisis, in Lee P, Estes L: *The Nation's Health*, 4th ed. Boston: Jones and Bartlett, 1994, pp 302–308.

46. American Nurses' Association: *Testimony to the President's Task Force on National Health Care Reform*. Washington, DC: The Association, Mar. 29, 1993.

47. American Nurses' Association and National League for Nursing: *Nursing's Agenda for Health Care Reform*. Washington, DC: The Association, 1991.

48. *The Health Security Act of 1993*. New York: Time Books, 1993.

49. Ibid.

50. American Nurses' Association: *Expanding School Health Services to Serve Families in the 21st Century*. Washington, DC: The Association, 1992.

51. American Nurses' Association: *Innovation at the Work Site: Delivery of Nurse-Managed Primary Health Care Services*. Washington, DC: The Association, 1993.

Health Care Delivery: Who?

A HUNDRED YEARS AGO, the trained health workforce consisted of physicians, dentists, some pharmacists, and nurses. Now there are more than 250 acknowledged health occupations, with more being developed every day. The estimated number of health-related employees is 8.7 million, one of every twelve workers in the United States. This figure includes certain supportive services but not independent practitioners or others who are self-employed. Health care facilities, like other places of business, employ secretaries, clerks, accountants, receptionists, messengers, and others to carry on business operations. In fact, one criticism has been the increased number of highly paid administrators, consultants, lawyers, strategic planners, and marketing people on hospital payrolls. The point is also made that the rapid growth of people covered by government and private health insurance has required more paperwork—and more people to do it. Computer programmers and operators are especially needed for this and for the new medical technology that calls for people to push the buttons and read the printouts.

In addition, some institutions need laundry workers, dietary workers, cooks, plumbers, electricians, carpenters, maids, porters, and similar kinds of employees to function in the hotel-keeping aspect of their services.

Not included in any category are faith healers, root doctors, or certain untrained healers who rely on herbs, meditation, or other semi-self-care techniques of healing. The overwhelm-

ing growth of personnel is in direct health services. Many of the health occupations and suboccupations have emerged because of increased specialization in health care, others on the peculiar assumption that several less-prepared workers can substitute for the scarcer professional. Some of these workers can be employed in almost any health setting—hospitals, nursing homes, clinics, doctors' offices, occupational health, and school health. Some work primarily in one setting. Most of these workers are not licensed; many are trained in on-the-job programs, and even more are trained in a variety of programs with no consistent standards. Others have standardized programs approved by the AMA and/or other health organizations. Generally, this entire group is categorized as *allied health manpower* (AHM); it is described later.

The most recent governmental figures on the health workforce are presented in Tables 8-1 and 8-2. Their accuracy is acknowledged to be somewhat questionable, since the final figures came from a variety of sources, all of which have some problems in data collection. This is particularly true in relation to AHM because of discrepancies in definition, the great variety of work settings, the paucity of licensure data, lack of funding for AHM associations to invest in workforce research, and the fact that most of these workers belong to no association and, indeed, often come and go in the workforce depending on employer demand. Since AHM, defined broadly, could make up as much as 63 percent of the total health workforce, the prob-

Table 8-1 Estimated Active Supply of Selected Health Personnel and Provider-Population Ratios, Selected Years, 1970–1990

Health Occupation	Estimated Active Supply			
	1970	1980	1982	1990
Physicians	326,200	457,500	466,600[1]	600,789
Allopathic (MD)	314,200	440,400	448,660[1]	536,755
Osteopathic (DO)	12,000	17,140	17,970[1]	30,924
Podiatrists	7,100	8,900	9,600	12,500
Dentists	102,220	126,240	132,010	148,800
Optometrists	18,400	22,400	23,300	26,000
Pharmacists	113,700	143,800	151,400	161,900
Veterinarians	25,900	36,000	38,810	51,000
Registered nurses	750,000	1,272,900	1,372,300[2]	2,033,032
Rate per 100,000 population				
Physicians	156.0	197.0	198.8	235.4
Allopathic (MD)	150.0	189.5	191.0	
Osteopathic (DO)	6.0	7.5	7.8	
Podiatrists	3.5	4.0	4.1	4.8
Dentists	49.5	55.2	56.6	60.0
Optometrists	8.9	9.8	10.0	10.7
Pharmacists	54.4	63.0	65.0	64.4
Veterinarians	12.5	15.8	16.7	19.8
Registered nurses	319	560	590[1]	671.0

[1]Data are for 1981.

[2]Data adapted from the *Seventh and Eighth Report to the President and Congress on the Status of Health Personnel in the United States.* Washington, DC: US Department of Health and Human Services, Bureau of Health Professions, 1990, 1991.

lems of accuracy are evident. Nevertheless, it is the periodic report to Congress by DHHS that is considered "official."

When health care is equated with medical care, a functional structure emerges, consisting of independent practitioners, dependent practitioners, and supporting staff. Jonas, although acknowledging that the lines separating the groups are unclear at times, described the independent practitioners as those permitted by law to provide a delimited range of services (physicians, dentists, chiropractors, optometrists, and podiatrists); dependent practitioners as those permitted by law to provide a delimited range of services under the supervision and/or authorization of independent practitioners (nurses, social workers, pharmacists, dental hygienists, physicians' assistants, and various therapists); and supporting staff as those carrying out specific tasks authorized by and under the supervision of independent and dependent practitioners, frequently without specific legal delineation of tasks or authority. Jonas now agrees that in certain situations, many in the "dependent" group can assume the role of independent practitioner.[1] The scope of practice and autonomy of the dependent practitioners are a great source of conflict, particularly because many have an area of expertise not within the knowledge and skills of the independent practitioner. Moreover, the gray areas of overlapping practice are becoming greater; what a particular practitioner does may be legitimately within his or her scope of practice in certain circumstances and just as legitimately within that of another in other circumstances. The legal lines drawn also waver when it comes

Table 8-2 Estimated Active Supply of Selected Allied Health Personnel, Selected Years, 1970–1990[1]

Allied Health Occupation	1970	1978	1982	1990
Total allied health personnel	658,000	1,026,000	1,166,000	1,800,000
Dental hygienists	12,000	34,000	43,000	81,000
Dental assistants	92,000	148,000	163,000	201,000
Dental laboratory technicians	26,000	47,000	55,000	70,000
Dietitians	12,000	28,000	35,000	67,000
Medical records related positions (administrators and technicians)	42,000	80,000	85,000	87,000
Medical laboratory workers	100,000	240,000	265,000	297,000
Occupational therapists	5,000	15,000	23,000	34,000
Physical therapists	11,000	28,000	34,000	71,000
Physician's assistants	—	6,000	13,000	22,000
Radiologic service workers	75,000	108,000	125,000	122,000
Respiratory therapy workers	15,000	52,000	59,000	75,000
Speech pathologists/audiologists	11,000	31,000	36,000	85,000
Other allied health[2]	40,000	200,000	225,000[3]	490,000

Source: Adapted from *Seventh and Eighth Report to the President and Congress on the Status of Health Personnel in the United States,* Washington, DC: US Department of Health and Human Services, Bureau of Health Professions, 1990, 1991.

[1]Because of revisions and independent estimations, some numbers may differ from numbers that appear elsewhere.

[2]Includes such categories as dietetic assistant, genetic assistant, operating room technician, ophthalmic medical assistant, optometric assistant, and technician, orthoptic and prosthetic technologist, pharmacy assistant, occupational and physical therapy assistants, podiatric assistant, vocational rehabilitation counselor, other rehabilitation services, and other social and mental health services.

[3]The figures shown for other allied health personnel are an assumption based on general trends in health manpower employment.

to supportive workers; there are tasks done by nurses' aides or practical nurses that are first of all part of a nurse's responsibility; in times and places of nurse shortage, they are often done with almost no supervision. With a rising acceptance of medical care as a component of health care but not its totality, the independent-dependent status concept of health practitioners will undoubtedly undergo considerable revision.

Credentialing of the health care providers and their educational programs is under a variety of auspices: the state, a single professional organization, or a coalition of professional organizations. The educational programs of some allied health occupations are accredited by the Committee on Allied Health Education and Accreditation (CAHEA), a collaborative effort of some 51 allied health organizations and medical specialty organizations with the AMA.

This accreditation process begins with acceptance of national standards for entry into the occupation, which must be adopted by both the AMA Council on Medical Education and the particular collaborating organizations concerned. Other occupations follow other procedures with their accrediting groups.

Practitioners who are not licensed may become certified or registered on a voluntary basis by the occupation's national organization or a parent medical group. The inconsistency of these various processes is the focus of some of the complaints about health care credentialing. (See Chap. 20 for more details on credentialing controversies.) In 1989, in which the latest report on licensure was published, AHA listed the following as health personnel licensed in every state: nursing home administrators, chiropractors, dentists, dental hygienists, practical nurses, professional nurses, optometrists, pharmacists, physical therapists, physicians (MD and DO), podiatrists, psychologists, and veterinarians. This does not necessarily mean that licensure is required, only that it is available. State regulation seems to be increasing. In the four years preceding the 1989 AHA survey, 29 states and the District of Columbia added new occupations to their statutory rosters. The top four categories were dietitians, occupational therapists, respiratory therapists, and social workers. New Jersey reported a new group for licensure: hemodialysis technicians.

Compared to other nations, the United States has a more than ample supply of health workers, even in terms of the physician-population ratio, which has been estimated by the Department of Health and Human Services to be about 240 to 100,000 by 1995. (In some countries, it is nurses who are in shortest supply.) Types of American health workers are also considerably more diverse; other nations have experimented more with such physician substitutes as the Russian feldsher or Chinese barefoot doctor. The largest categories of health workers, in order, are nurses (all types, as well as aides), physicians, dentists and their allied services, clinical laboratory workers, pharmacists, and radiological technicians. As feminists are the first to point out, *manpower* is a misnomer; from 75 to 85 percent are women. However, they are, or have been, in the lower-paid and less powerful positions. Physicians, dentists, administrators, and others in policy-making positions are overwhelmingly male.

Except for the independent practitioners who are primarily self-employed, the mass of health workers are employed in institutions and agencies, with the greatest number concentrated in hospitals.

It would be unrealistic to attempt to describe all the professional and technical workers with whom nurses work or interact. However, an introduction to the most prevalent health occupations should provide a better understanding of the complex relationships in health care.

The organization of this chapter is primarily alphabetical, although on occasion two closely related groups may be described in logical succession, with general issues and trends discussed at the end of the chapter. The education of RNs and practical nurses is described in Chaps. 12 and 13 and the practice of nursing in Chaps. 15 and 16. A good source of information about health careers is the National Health Council in Washington, D.C.

HEALTH SERVICES MANAGEMENT

Health services administrators or executives manage multiunit systems, health care networks, organizations, agencies, institutions, programs, and services within the health care delivery system. They may work in any setting but are probably more visible in hospitals, managed care plans, nursing homes, neighborhood health centers, and community health agencies. The principles of management can be applied to any setting, and the role of the hospital administrator, described in Chap. 7, is a reasonable example of role and functions. Nurses usually manage nursing services, but a number also hold positions as top executives, particularly in home care agencies and community health centers. Although they may retain their nursing identity, they should be functioning as administrators and have the necessary educational background. Usually, the appropriate credential is a master's degree in health services management, public health, hospital administration, or more recently, business or public administration. Other positions in the operation of health facilities and plants are the usual business positions, financial management, information systems, clinical data systems, human resources, materials management and professional services, with all types of jobs and educational levels.

For many years, controversy in health management education centered on the proper educational credentials. There were those who believed that health services administrators should be prepared in business schools so managers could deal effectively with increasing economic pressure. Others felt that the distinctive nature of health care organizations required managers prepared in programs concentrating in health services administration. As the United States moves into an era of health reform when we will be defining what "health care as a right" means in practice, experts note that

> **The defining challenge of management will be the generation, articulation and realization of a vision of health and medical care organization that recognizes the appropriate level of investment and is responsive to the needs of the community, the patients, and the organization.... A new breed of leaders in administration is needed, a breed that is philosophically committed to and competent to manage the change process.... The knowledge and skills essential for managing the change process are outcomes assessment and continuous quality improvement. As the two concepts converge, it has become clear that a profound change is occurring in the role of management in medical care and health services. They are increasing the validity of quality assessment and changing our concept of management's role in achieving quality improvement. Outcomes assessment and total quality management (TQM) have enormous implications, not only for how medical care is delivered but also for how to achieve improved health status in the community.[2]**

It is apparent that such knowledge and skills will best be acquired in educational settings focusing on health services management. A continuing issue, however, is the proper balance between managerial skills and practical knowledge of the health care delivery environment, because, at the same time that post-master's residencies in health care administration are being recommended, economic pressures in the field are lessening the opportunities for such employer-funded education.

Currently, considerable career opportunities are to be found in managerial roles in the evolving world of managed care. Managed care includes a range of health services delivery organizations such as staff or group model health maintenance organizations, preferred provider organizations, independent practice associations, point-of-service plans, and integrated delivery networks. Although representing a variety of models of prepaid health care, managed

care organizations share three defining features:

1. An agreement by or on behalf of a specific set of health care providers to accept responsibility for the delivery of needed medical services as agreed to in a benefit package to
2. A defined population of enrolled consumers, in exchange for
3. A specific, per-person sum of money agreed upon in advance and paid on a regular basis.[3]

Although there are no managerial functions unique to managed care settings, because of their common features, managed care settings do place a high priority on such managerial activities as strategic planning, marketing sales and services, integrating professionals into the organization, managing costs, controlling utilization, and ensuring quality.

Allied Health Manpower

Allied health manpower (AHM) has been defined by the federal government to include

> **...all those professional, technical, and supportive workers in the fields of patient care, public health, and health research who engage in activities that support, complement, or supplement the professional functions of physicians, dentists, and registered nurses, as well as personnel engaged in organized environmental health activities who are expected to have some expertise in environmental health.[4]**

AHM range from personnel with complex functions and the highest educational degrees, who have always had a great deal of autonomy, to those who function in relatively simple assisting roles and must be supervised, sometimes by others categorized as AHMs. Because of this diversity and changes in health care, there are also many changes occurring within the occupations and professions so identified. Since such a large percentage of health care personnel are AHM (see Table 8-2), it is ironic that there are so few fundamental data, but this is blamed on the elasticity of supply and the constant evaluation of the roles and responsibilities of certain occupations.

Role evaluation can be demonstrated in part by changes in education. At one time, most AHMs were educated in almost apprenticelike programs in hospitals. In the 1960s, with the commitment of federal funds to AHM education, the growth of junior colleges, and increases in educational costs, many AHMs were transferred to a college setting, with the hospital remaining as a clinical practice site. Expansion of both junior and senior college programs was inevitable as the specialization needs grew and as more Americans wanted both a college education and a marketable skill. However, hospitals, vocational schools, and military institutions remained as sites of training programs.

The allied health occupations have moved toward professionalism at various paces. Accreditation, certification, licensing, higher education, and demand for autonomy and increased scope of practice occurred in some; others turned to unionism. Beginning salaries vary a great deal, even for the technically trained, but for some there is lack of opportunity for advancement and increased salary later. Most AHMs are employed by institutions or agencies, or by individual physicians and dentists, who set the qualifications and functions, if the occupation is not licensed or certified, and salaries.

An example of the inconsistency in education and credentialing of the AHM group is that the AHM educational programs accredited by the CAHEA are based in vocational schools, ACHCs, junior and senior colleges, hospitals of all sizes, nonhospital health care facilities, the Veterans' Administration, and the Department of Defense. They range from the relatively new anesthesiologist assistant to the well-established occupational therapist. Only a few of the occupations are regulated by the government in any way.

The great diversity of AHM makes it very difficult to make any firm statement about their future. These occupations are predominantly female, except for EMTs and perfusionists; and

low pay has been common. Some experts say that, with the increasing aging population on the demand side and fewer people interested in health care careers on the supply side, there will be a great need for these workers in a variety of settings, some not yet existing. The U.S. Department of Labor, Bureau of Labor Statistics predicted that by the year 2000, those AHMs most in demand would be occupational therapists (OTs), physical therapists (PTs), OT and PT assistants, medical and dental assistants, radiology technologists and technicians, medical records technicians, and EMTs. Some of these are considered in short supply already. One sign of market response is a rapid rise in salary levels, which may attract more workers. As in the case of nursing, retention is one key to the shortage problem.

Chiropractic

Chiropractic is described by the American Chiropractic Association (ACA) as:

> …**a branch of the healing arts which is concerned with human health and disease processes. Doctors of chiropractic are physicians who consider humans as integrated beings and give special attention to the physiological and biochemical aspects including structural, spinal, musculoskeletal, neurological, vascular, nutritional, emotional, and environmental relationships.**

Chiropractors use standard diagnostic measures, but treatment methods, determined by law, do not include prescription drugs and surgery. Essentially, treatment includes the chiropractic adjustment, necessary dietary advice and nutritional supplementation, necessary physiotherapeutic measures, and necessary professional counsel.

Chiropractic colleges are accredited by the Council on Chiropractic Education (CCE). Successful completion of a minimum of four years of academic study in the sciences, public health, clinical disciplines, and chiropractic principles and practice, preceded by two years of preprofessional college education, results in a Doctor of Chiropractic diploma. The practitioner may be designated *Doctor of Chiropractic, Chiropractic Physician*, or *Chiropractor*. Most are men and are in private practice. They are licensed in all states, the majority of which require continuing education for relicensure. All fifty states and the District of Columbia and Puerto Rico recognize chiropractic as a health profession and authorize chiropractic services as part of their worker's compensation program, as do many federal health benefits programs; services are also reimbursable under Medicare and Medicaid. Virtually all major commercial health insurance carriers include chiropractic in their private policies. Based on their order of size, number of practitioners, and public utilization, chiropractic ranks second after medicine as a primary health care provider.

Clinical Laboratory Sciences

There are a number of technicians or technologists working in the clinical laboratories in such specialties as immunohematology, hematology, clinical chemistry, serology, microbiology, blood banking, and histology. The work involves analysis of human blood, tissues, and fluids to determine the absence, presence, or extent of a disease. The physician in charge is a pathologist, although technologists may have specific responsibilities for technicians. *Medical technologists'* preparation includes three years of college science plus a year of professional course work in a CAHEA-accredited school covering all phases of clinical laboratory work. Certification is granted by the Board of Registry of Medical Technologists of the American Society of Clinical Pathologists, after successful completion of a board examination. The initials *MT (ASCP)* may then be used. Most states do not require licensure. Additional appropriate education and experience qualify a medical technologist for specialist certification in blood banking, chemistry, microbiology, cytotechnology, or nuclear technology.

Certified laboratory technicians, who perform routine laboratory tests, usually complete a two year associate degree in medical laboratory technology. *Histologic technicians*, who prepare body tissues for microscopic examination by pathologists, are usually prepared in one-year programs given by hospitals or laboratory centers, also CAHEA-accredited. Certification is granted after passing an ASCP examination.

Dentistry

Dentists treat oral diseases and disorders. They may fill cavities, extract teeth, and provide dentures for patients. Recognized dental specialties are oral surgery and orthodontics (correction of irregularities of teeth and jaws), which together make up 60 percent of specialist practice; endodontics (root canal therapy); pedodontics (children's dentistry); periodontology or periodontics (treatment of gums, bone, and other surrounding tissue); prosthodontics (replacement of missing teeth); oral pathology (study of diseased oral tissues); and public health dentistry. These specialties usually require two or more additional years of training, and a specialty board examination. Dental school is preceded by two to four years of college with specific science courses; most entering students, however, are college graduates. The dental school curriculum is a three-to four-year course leading to a DDS (Doctor of Dental Surgery) or a DMD (Doctor of Dental Medicine) degree. All dental schools must be approved by the American Dental Association. Dentists are licensed in all states by taking a state board examination or a National Board of Dental Examiners exam. In some states, specialists must pass a special state examination. Most dentists are in private practice; the others practice in institutions, the armed forces, and health agencies, teach, or do research. Most are located in large cities. An increasing number of minorities and women are entering the field.

In recent years, there has been concern about the increasing cost of dental education and a perceived oversupply of dentists. Some dental schools are in severe financial difficulties and are threatened by closure. Legislators maintain that although there are many underserved areas of dental need, the production of more dentists does not solve the problem, since few dentists go to those areas; most prefer a more lucrative practice.

Utilization of comprehensive dental care of elementary school children, and anticipation of the need for more periodontal and endodontic treatment, since more adults are keeping their teeth but are suffering from gum disease, are suggested as directions for future practice.

One overall concern appears to be the fact that there *are* unmet oral health care needs, but that it is almost impossible to project workforce needs for people who don's seek dental care.

Dental hygienists, almost all women, provide dental services under a dentist's supervision. They examine, scale, and polish teeth, give fluoride treatments, take x-rays, monitor patients' medical and oral health, and educate them about proper care of teeth and gums. In many states, hygienists' responsibilities have been expanded to include duties traditionally performed by dentists, such as giving local anesthetics, and it has been said that their training includes much more than they are permitted to do by most dentist employers. Hygienists are licensed in all states and are the only ancillary personnel permitted by law to clean teeth. An RDH (registered dental hygienist) is awarded after passing a written and practical certification examination.

Education may consist of two-, three-, or four-year programs leading to a certificate or an associate or bachelor's degree at vocational-technical institutes, community colleges, and universities. Those dental hygienists with master's degrees may be teachers or administrators. The vast majority of dental hygienists practice with dentists in offices. However, in recent years, a few have set up separate private practices, a move strongly opposed by dentists but approved in some states by court decision or attorney general rulings. A degree of resistance to dentist domination over their practice is emerging. The demand for RDH services is expected to grow by 41 percent by 2005.[5]

Dental assistants maintain supplies, keep dental records, schedule appointments, prepare patients for examinations, process x-rays, and assist the dentist at chairside, but their functions are also expanding.[6] Most assistants complete a 1- or 2-year program at a community college or vocational-technical school. These programs award a certificate, diploma, or associate degree.

Dental technicians or *denturists* make and repair dentures, crowns, bridges, and other appliances, usually according to dentists' prescriptions. Denturists are lobbying to work directly with patients, saying that they not only charge less but are faster and better at fitting dentures. The ADA is fighting this move, insisting that dentists must have total jurisdiction over all oral disorders since they alone are trained to diagnose and treat them. However, several states have already licensed denturists to provide direct service, and the services are proliferating (if illegally) in other states. Most Canadian provinces have had licensed denturists for many years.

The education of denturists usually consists of a 2-year certificate or associate degree program, although some prepare by working for three to four years as trainees in dental laboratories. The military also offers training.[7]

Dietetics and Nutrition

Nutritionist is a general occupational title for health professionals concerned with food science and human nutrition. They include dietitians, home economists, and food technologists. There is no required standard for use of the title, but a bachelor's degree in the area of home economics or nutrition is usual. A master's degree may be required for certain positions, especially in public health. Nutritionists may teach clients and patients, consult, engage in research, or teach in schools of the health professions.

Dietitians may have a general dietary background or preparation in medical dietetics. Medical or therapeutic dietitians are responsible for selection of appropriate foods for special diets, patient counseling, and sometimes management of the dietary service. They may manage a food service, where they are responsible for management of personnel, purchasing, budgeting, and planning menus. With appropriate education, they may also do research or teach students.[8]

Clinical dietitians work with patients not only in the hospital, but in clinics, neighborhood health centers, or in the patient's own home. These patients include pregnant women, diabetics, and those with other nutritional problems.

A baccalaureate program with majors in food, nutrition, and food management is usually basic with the possible addition of a dietetic internship program approved by the American Dietetic Association (ADA). Certification is granted by the ADA, after which the individual may use the RD after her name (most are female). New career opportunities include corporate positions in hotel and other chains with food service, corporate wellness programs, and management companies providing food service in LTC facilities.

Among the actions being considered by the ADA is third-party reimbursement and licensure. The latter is considered important in obtaining third-party reimbursement. In 1983, Texas became the first state to license dietitians, albeit on a voluntary basis. Licensure does not protect the scope of practice of nutrition/dietetics for licensed or registered dietitians; it does protect those titles against unauthorized use.

Another concern is the delegation of functions to assisting personnel. *Dietetic technicians* graduate from one of two kinds of ADA-approved technical programs with an associate degree. A program with food service management emphasis allows the individual to serve as a technical assistant to a food service director and, with experience, to become a director. The program with nutritional care emphasis enables the individual to become a technical assistant to the clinical dietitian. Both programs require clinical practice. Passing the Registration Examination for Dietetic Technicians enables the

technician to use the credentials DTR, dietetic technician, registered.

A *dietetic assistant* is a graduate of a one-year academic program in dietetics requiring classroom instruction coordinated with clinical practice. Included are food preparation, basic nutrition, and menu planning; purchasing; storage, safety, and sanitation; personnel supervision; and cost control. These programs may also be ADA-approved. Most dietetic assistants serve as *food service supervisors* in hospitals, schools of nursing, schools, and nursing homes. However, a number of food service supervisors currently functioning in that position lack such preparation.

Health Educators

Community health educators help identify the health learning needs of the community, particularly in terms of prevention of disease and injury. They may then plan, organize, and implement appropriate programs, for example, screening devices, health fairs, classes, and self-help groups. Some health educators are employed by the state as consultants, others by insurance companies, voluntary health organizations such as the American Heart Association, the school system (school health educators), and, occasionally, industry. Unfortunately, as governmental funding fluctuates, programs may expand or contract, and health educators may be eliminated or spread thin, as has happened in school health. A number of hospitals are employing *patient educators* or health educators to develop and direct programs of both patient education and community health education. Frequently, these people are nurses with or without training in health education and administration. Health educators usually have baccalaureate or master's degrees in health education, public health, or community health education. Master's degrees may include an administration component.

In a few states, health educators are registered and/or certified. Some state health educator groups are working on plans for voluntary certification.

Medical Records

Medical record administrators (MRAs) are responsible for preparation, collation, and organization of patient records, maintaining an efficient filing system, and making records available to those concerned with the patient's subsequent care. Other duties include designing health information systems and providing information for facility reimbursement by third-party payers. They may also classify and compile data for review committees and researchers and must have knowledge and skills in health care databases and systems, medical classification systems, and relationship of financial information to clinical data. CAHEA accredits both four-year baccalaureate programs and one-year hospital-based programs preceded by a baccalaureate degree. After completion of these programs the candidate qualifies for certification administered by the American Association of Medical Record Librarians. Successful completion leads to designation as Registered Record Administrator (RRA).

Medical record technicians assist the physician and the MRA in preparing reports and transcribing histories and physicals, and work closely with others using patient records. In a large institution, they may specialize; in a small one, they may have full responsibility for the department. CAHEA-accredited programs are usually two-year associate degree programs and include theoretical instruction and practical hospital experience. A national exam leads to the title Accredited Record Technician (ART). *Medical record transcriptionists* have specialized courses in terminology in addition to typing and filing. Advances in computerization are creating major changes in the field, and a shortage in the field is predicted. New opportunities are being made available beyond the hospitals because there are a number of alternative delivery systems that require the same medical recordkeeping services.

The entire field of health information management is gaining in importance, and there is already a shortage of prepared personnel. It has been noted that "the health information management professional collects, analyzes, and manages the information that steers the health-care industry."[9] Particularly because of computers, the individual must balance patients' privacy rights with legitimate uses of aggregate data, a basic need for research. Knowledge of medical legal systems, security systems, and the uses and users of health care information is of vital importance.

Medicine

Doctors of medicine and osteopathy practice prevention, diagnosis, and treatment of disease and injury. *Doctor of medicine degrees (MDs)* are awarded in 125 allopathic medical schools in the United States and are considered the first professional degree. Some physicians may later decide to acquire advanced degrees (master's or doctorates) in an advanced science or public health. Admission into medical schools after four, occasionally three, years of preprofessional college work is considered highly selective. Programs are usually four years in length, with required basic sciences and clinical studies. In the last two years students have clinical clerkships, usually in hospitals, but also in clinics or doctor's offices. In this first contact with patients, they are usually supervised and taught by attending physicians or residents as they apply their clinical and scientific knowledge. Generally, physicians and professors of science are the teachers in medical school, although others include ethicists, sociologists, and, occasionally, a nurse (not usually on a full-time basis). In some medical schools, nurse instructors have responsibility for teaching medical students in the clinical clerkship. In most cases, medical education has little interdisciplinary focus, and contacts with other health profession students are seldom formalized, although sometimes students in a multidisciplinary setting develop interactional opportunities of their own.

The number of women entering medicine has gradually been increasing, and there has been a slight increase in underrepresented minorities, particularly women. Because these minority admissions have changed so little, the American Association of Medical Colleges is giving special attention to their recruitment.

The formalized program of education after the MD degree is titled *graduate medical education* (GME) and consists primarily of the residency, which is preparation for specialties, a period of two to five years. At one time, a one-year internship, usually rotating through the various clinical services, was the norm, but after years of debate and two major reports, in the mid-1960s several changes occurred. Family practice was recognized as a specialty, both the rotating and the freestanding internship (almost a general working apprenticeship) were abolished, and residencies in hospitals with at least minimal university affiliations were developed. A 1-year general residency is still required for licensure. Almost all residency programs now are in such hospitals, but there is a dichotomy—education on the one hand and a functional hospital apprenticeship on the other. GME is financed primarily by third-party payers, including Medicare and Medicaid, to hospitals for patient care services. Residencies seem to have three distinct components: acquisition of knowledge, skills, and professional behavior. On completion of the specified years of residency, the physician may take certification exams in the specialty and is board certified; if exams are not taken (or failed), he or she is board eligible. In some cases, continuing medical education is required for recertification.

For a number of years, there were more first-year residency positions than American medical school graduates, and graduates from foreign medical schools, including Americans, filled positions. In some states, the vast majority were foreign medical graduates (FMGs). Because of differences in the quality of education and language and cultural differences, problems often occurred. Legislation has cut drastically the number of FMGs, but since fewer graduates of

U.S. medical schools are entering training directly after graduation, there has been an increase of FMGs in residency programs. Recently the term *international medical graduate* (IMG) is being used and includes Americans graduating from non-U.S. medical schools.

Although most American physicians choose specialties as their field of practice, the need for more general practitioners is being met by designation of the field of family practice (thus the residency) as a specialty and heavy federal funding for those selecting that field. Despite some early concern that soon there may be too many family practitioners, in reality, this is the greatest area of shortage.

Determination of what is too little or too much of a speciality seems to be unresolved whenever the issue arises. One example is the concern that there will not be enough physicians in preventive medicine (including public health), since there seems to be decreasing selection of that field. Yet certain experts say that with an excess of physicians in other specialties, inevitably some physicians will turn to those fields where there are openings, such as geriatrics.

In medical centers, a "fellow" is a postresidency physician who enters even more advanced, highly specialized, or research-oriented programs, although presumably still involved in teaching and patient care. Graduate medical education is under the direction of medical school faculty recognized as specialists or subspecialists. A relatively new issue in graduate education is the unionization of residents (with varied success) in order to obtain better conditions of work, especially reduction of the long hours that may threaten competence. In those states where shorter hours and on-call time are now required, the cause was usually a well-publicized patient's death or injury attributed to decreased competence of exhausted house staff. Many teaching hospitals have developed a residents' hours policy voluntarily.

Physician licensure is mandatory in every state, some of which require continuing education for relicensure. The single licensure exam, called the U.S. Medical Licensure Exam (US-MLE), has three components (steps). The first two are taken in medical school and the third during the GME period. The exam may now be taken anywhere in the world by international medical graduates after graduation from a medical school and successful completion of an English exam. The individual is not fully licensed until after all parts of USMLE are passed; before that, practice is covered by a temporary license or is on a student basis, just as it is with nurses until they have passed state boards. A different aspect of the new USMLE is that the exam may be repeated if failed with no restriction on the number of times. However, although the National Board of Medical Examiners (NBME) suggests a passing score, each state board sets its own score for licensure in that state. Among the physicians not holding a license in any state, besides first-year residents, are the inactive and those engaged in medical teaching, research, or administration.

The major modes of medical practice are described in the preceding chapter, but there are, of course, physicians in every setting where medical care is provided, as well as in medical or public health education, public health practice, and research. Some positions such as that of a medical director are primarily administrative and are beginning to be recognized as such.

In 1994, the AMA found that one-third of physicians in direct care were now involved in group practice (three or more MDs), although another third were still in solo or two-physician practices. Those in group practice were more likely to be board certified and more likely to contract with HMOs.

Although MDs are generally still held in high regard by the public, they have become the target of much criticism, and it appears that they often have difficulty coping with the radical changes in health care and society. For instance, while they have been blamed for the high cost of medical care, they say that one reason for the extensiveness of expensive diagnostic tests is the litigiousness of today's patient, which also drives up their malpractice insurance. At the

same time, there are allegations of peer cover-up of incompetent practitioners instead of peer review and removal from practice. Now there are more deliberate efforts by medicine to identify "impaired" physicians and give them appropriate help until they are qualified to practice. Continuing medical education has also been strongly supported for maintaining competence.

With economic pressures, changes in health care delivery and reimbursement, and oversupply, some physicians are finding it necessary to market their services actively (advertising is now acceptable); others are moving into salaried positions that include bonuses for cost-effective practice. The projected oversupply may also be responsible for increased aggressiveness in trying to prevent nonphysician practitioners such as nurse-midwives and NPs from practicing and receiving direct reimbursement from clients. This can be interpreted as restraint of trade, and the Federal Trade Commission has ruled against the AMA several times on these issues—for example, in relation to advertising and referrals to chiropractors. However, MDs have also had some success in specific states in their attempts to restrain NPs, and the battle continues.

Still another issue is the maldistribution of physicians. National Health Corps physicians do seem to select rural areas for practice more than other physicians (or are assigned there), but these areas, unattractive and isolated places, and big city ghettoes still lack even a minimally satisfactory physician-population ratio, while more affluent areas have unnecessarily high ratios. Even the Health Corps physicians often do not stay after their required time of "payback" for their medical education ends. Given the maldistribution and cost problems, and the new aggressiveness of other health professionals, there is a frequent reiteration of the question, "Why should the physician be the gatekeeper to health care?"

In the last several years, a great deal has been seen in the media and in the professional literature about problems, changes, and predictions concerning the field of medicine; usually referring to allopathic medicine. For instance, with an ongoing prediction of physician over-supply by the end of the century, frequent public criticism of their practice and lack of humanistic qualities, a loss of considerable autonomy and some income because of governmental and insurer programs of cost containment, as well as an increase in malpractice suits, physicians themselves have expressed discontent with their profession. An unusually large number are retiring early, changing to fields such as research and administration, or leaving medicine altogether. Moreover, they are said to discourage potential students from entering the field. College students, whether influenced or not by such attitudes, were choosing the more lucrative business fields, which did not saddle them with immense debt and a lengthy educational and practice period of long hours, much stress, and poor pay. It has been predicted that, as opposed to past trends, the demography of the medical profession would change to a majority of women and nonwhite males (a trend also evident in the overall employment picture in the United States). Some think this may lead to less resistance to radical changes in practice patterns, as those entering the profession have more moderate expectations and a greater commitment to primary care specialties. On the other hand, there has been concern that too many medical students were choosing high-technology specialties over internal medicine, in part because of the potential of a better income that enables them to pay off their enormous educational debt more quickly, and the high status of specialists in the hospital. (Anesthesiologists, surgical specialists, and radiologists have the highest incomes; general practitioners and psychiatrists, the lowest.) Only the escalating malpractice premiums and the fact that in a few years the Medicare payment system might cut down on some surgeon's incomes are likely to be deterrents. However, at least at present, only 23 percent of medical students are opting for the primary care specialties. There is a trend for newly licensed physicians, especially

women, to choose a salaried position in an HMO or other employment setting, instead of private practice. A number of reasons are given for this: the cost of setting up private practice and the struggle for success; the fact that employers often pay for malpractice insurance; and more regular hours and time for self and family and a guaranteed income. Another major reason is that more physicians in solo or group practice are losing their patients, as the latter choose, or are almost forced, to join HMOs because of their employer's health plan. In fact, in some instances, physicians have found that if they did not join an HMO early, they were no longer wanted by the HMO, which had enough physicians. Some experts predict that most physicians will be employees by the end of the century. Such positions, however, are not without problems: Employed physicians in certain HMOs have been seriously considering unionizing because of discontent about their salaries, autonomy, and conditions of work.

There are still major criticisms of physicians by the public, even when those surveyed are generally satisfied with their own physicians, particularly in relation to their lack of communication with patients and their perceived lack of interest in patients as individuals or in the problems of society. Physicians have said that patients are now aggressive consumers, primed to distrust. They maintain that the potential of any patient suing when the health outcome is not as expected (because they expect perfection), even if the physician has made no error, drives a wedge in the physician-patient relationships. A number will not accept patients that they think might create a problem. Yet there is also evidence that the fact that physicians and patients really don't know each other and have not established mutual trust is a major cause for patients suing. (Besides, there really is malpractice.) All of this has had some impact on the medical curriculum and even the entrance examinations. Beginning in 1991, the Medical College Admission Test (MCAT), emphasizes critical thinking, problem solving, and communications, rather than rote learning of scientific facts. Some very distinguished medical schools have revised their curricula so that students will have contact with patients within the first few weeks of their first year, instead of the third. Directed by a preceptor-physician who stays with a particular student throughout the four years, the student learns humanistic values in both patient contact and problem-based tutorials. They also have personal computers for researching the medical literature and working out practice exercises. Whether the approach of emphasizing human values will become widespread remains to be seen.

As the reality of some sort of health care plan coming to fruition became clear to health care providers and institutions, changes in the system began to occur, before any law was ever passed. Physicians realized that their practice would never be the same again and also tried to protect themselves financially. In an AMA survey in 1992, doctors said that they believed that there would be substantial restrictions on their fees. They also believed that a very effective means of controlling costs would be reforming the medical liability system.[10] (Actually, fraud adds more to the cost of health care than malpractice awards.) The actions physicians took included selling their practices to health care corporations or signing long-term contracts with them; investing in companies that provide equipment and medications (raising the specter of conflict of interest); becoming part of "vertically integrated systems," that is, health care systems that provide full service to patients, including hospital, home care, nursing home, pharmacy, and the services of a variety of health care providers; and even forming their own health plan. The profession also realized that something must be done about the uneven balance of specialists and family practice physicians. In 1993, the Association of Academic Medical Centers agreed to establish an independent commission to oversee the supply and specialty mix of physicians, and five medical schools received funds from HRSA to work on changing the curriculum to attempt to graduate

more primary care physicians. More attention was given to family medicine to determine factors affecting the practice.[11] It was recognized that whereas generalists in other developed nations made up 50 to 70 percent of medical practice, the United States had less than 29 percent, and even with the best efforts, a 50-50 ratio would not be met until some time in the 21st century.[12] Ways in which people in rural areas could be given better care was also on the agenda, and telecommunications was considered a likely mode. What seemed to elude everyone, however, was how to overcome the serious maldistribution of physicians. Some experts even suggested using more NPs.

Doctors of osteopathy (DO) are qualified to be licensed as physicians and to practice all branches of medicine and surgery. DOs graduate from colleges of osteopathic medicine (now fifteen), accredited by the Bureau of Professional Education of the American Osteopathic Association (AOA). Admission to the colleges requires at least three years of preprofessional education at an accredited college or university. Applicants also take a qualifying exam. The DO degree usually requires four academic years of education. Required basic sciences, anatomy, physiology, biochemistry, pathology, microbiology, and pharmacology are much the same as those in other medical schools, as are the clinical courses of medicine, surgery, pediatrics, obstetrics, gynecology, radiology, and preventive medicine. The major difference is the integration of osteopathic principles dealing with the interrelationship of all body systems in health and disease and special training in osteopathic palpatory diagnosis and manipulative therapy. Holistic medicine, proper nutrition, and environmental factors are also emphasized. After graduation, almost all DOs serve a 12-month rotating internship, with primary emphasis on medicine, obstetrics/gynecology, and surgery, conducted in an approved osteopathic hospital. Those wishing to specialize must serve an additional three to five years of residency. Continuing education is required by the AOA for all DOs in practice.

Osteopathic physicians are considered separate but equal in American medicine; they are licensed in all states and have the same rights and obligations as allopathic (MD) physicians. The "something extra" they claim is emphasis on biological mechanisms by which the musculoskeletal system interacts with all body organs and systems in both health and disease. They prescribe drugs, use routine diagnostic measures, perform surgery, and selectively utilize accepted scientific modalities of care. DOs comprise about 5 percent of all physicians; they are younger than their allopathic counterparts and are also attracting more women to the field. Most are general practitioners who provide primary care, usually in small towns and rural areas; however, there appears to be a decline in graduates choosing a primary care career. Currently, nearly 40 percent of DOs are in the north central census region. The 190 or so osteopathic hospitals, located in 28 states, usually offer a full range of services. Nursing in osteopathic hospitals is comparable to that in any other hospital.

Physician Assistants

In 1965, Dr. Eugene A. Stead, Jr., inaugurated a program for what was then termed *physician's assistants (PAs)*, designed to assist physicians in their practice, either to enable them to expand that practice or to give them time to pursue continuing education, or to have more time for themselves and their families. The students in the Duke University program came from a variety of backgrounds and included nurses and former military corpsmen. Shortly afterward, a series of programs, called MEDEX, developed specifically for ex-corpsmen, were funded by the federal government.

In the early years of these programs, there was a great deal of confusion about the education, role, legality, and scope of practice of the PA. Educational programs ran the gamut from a few months of on-the-job training to five years. Formalized programs prepared assistants to the primary care physician as well as specialists. Continued federal funding after 1972 not

only encouraged the growth of programs but determined certain directions: training for delivery of primary care in ambulatory settings, placement of graduates in medically underserved areas, and recruitment of residents from these areas as well as minority groups and women. Several changes in programs occurred after that. Since the publication of the AMA Essentials in the early 1970s, all accredited PA programs must meet standardized curriculum requirements. (For a more detailed description of the early developments in PA education and practice, see the fifth edition of this book.)

As defined in HRSA reports, PAs are skilled members of the health care team who, working dependently with physicians and with their supervision, provide diagnostic and therapeutic patient care. They take patient histories, perform physical examinations, and order laboratory tests. When medical problems are diagnosed, PAs develop treatment plans and explain them to patients. They are also permitted to diagnose illnesses. They recommend medications and drug therapies, and in about 40 states, have the authority to write prescriptions without a physician's cosignature. In addition to specific technical procedures which PAs perform, which vary with the practice setting, they carry out a variety of minor surgical procedures. They also may provide pre- and postoperative care. PAs with surgical training often act as first or second assistants in major surgery.

The Association of Physician Assistant Programs (APAP), which represents the PA educational programs in the United States, reports yearly on these programs in order to establish a national data bank. These reports and the surveys of the American Academy of Physician Assistants (AAPA), the only national membership organization to represent all PAs, generally provide much of the PA data in federal manpower reports.

A summary of the current status of PA education and practice follows. PAs perform medical services under physician supervision in all states and in the District of Columbia. Mississippi is the only state without legislation recognizing PA practice, but PAs are employed in federal facilities there. Currently, there are more than 50 PA programs based in a variety of settings: universities, colleges, hospitals, medical schools, and junior colleges. Education may be in programs that end in a certificate, an associate degree, or a baccalaureate, but the trend is to a baccalaureate. Admission requirements usually include two years of college and some health care experience, although a typical student in 1992 already had a baccalaureate or higher degree and over $4\frac{1}{2}$ years of health care experience. The curriculum includes basic and behavioral medical sciences, an introduction to clinical medicine, and a year of supervised clinical expertise. The focus is on broadly based primary care training, but a number of programs now offer a master's degree. Postgraduate programs (PA residencies) offer additional clinical and structured learning experiences in specialties to graduate PAs.

Most states require PA graduates to take the certification exam given by the National Commission on Certification of Physician Assistants (NCCPA), which requires that educational programs be accredited by CAHEA. Although not all PAs are certified, most states (and employers) require certification in order to practice. About 92 percent were certified in 1992. The statutory provisions for utilization of PAs vary from state to state, but because PAs cannot practice without the supervision of a physician, licensure is almost unheard of. This may change; the Federation of State Medical Board's model Medical Practice Act includes PAs. Most of the PAs in the field are white males; 42 percent are female; 9 percent of all practicing PAs are from minority ethnic groups. Typically, PA programs enroll older students, often experienced in some sort of health care, including a large percentage of nurses. In 1992, about 17.5 percent of PA students were from an ethnic minority. However, the attrition rate for minorities is great, particularly unfortunate in that there was supposed to be a focused effort to recruit minorities to serve in their own communities.

Most PAs are employed in one of three specialty areas: family medicine; surgery, including subspecialties; and internal medicine. Surgery is increasingly favored. Although about 35 percent work with physicians in private or group offices and another 30 percent in a variety of clinics, there seems to be a trend in some cities for employment by hospitals. One reason is that medical residents' hours are being limited, and PAs are hired to fill in the gap for patient care, especially in the emergency room and assisting the doctor in the operating room (OR), where they are reimbursed as second assistants. There are still a large percentage practicing in rural areas or small towns (mostly men), but hospital employment in larger cities and suburbs is becoming more common, especially for women. Some say that demand is a major factor; others point out that PAs must go where there is a doctor to supervise them, and doctors prefer urban and suburban areas over rural ones. In reality, though, those in rural clinics are "supervised" from a distance, and now supervision through electronic communication is considered satisfactory. Thirty-eight states grant prescription authority to PAs. Salaries of PAs have increased in the last few years and average about $50,000 to $55,000, differing with specialty, setting, and geographic location. Women consistently make less than men, even when they have the same education and experience. Medicare and Medicaid policies governing coverage for PA services in hospitals and other institutions encourage their being hired. Reimbursement is through either the physician or institutional salaries. PAs are caring for underserved populations in rural areas, inner-city neighborhoods, substance abuse clinics, prison systems, and long-term care facilities. They are also actively involved in the treatment of HIV-infected persons at all levels, from ordering tests to counseling patients.

Unlike the situation a few years ago when demand for PAs was lessening, it is now expected that the demand will exceed the supply (about 28,000, according to new AAPA figures). The federal government is still an important source of funds for PA educational programs, but not as much as before. PA education is not a stepping-stone to medical school, but some PAs enroll in nursing school or receive degrees in public health, which offer additional opportunities.

There are still many unresolved issues related to PA practice, particularly in relation to role and functions. The American Hospital Association has published a statement on PAs in hospitals, which, overall, indicated that the medical staff and administration should formulate guidelines under which the PA can operate, with the request for the PA to be permitted to practice in the hospital being handled by the medical staff credentials committee. Emphasis is on medical supervision; however, current reality has shown that PAs go unsupervised in busy urban hospitals where they handle many emergency and other ambulatory patients. This has created a problem for nurses, for the authority of the PA vis-à-vis the nurse is frequently not clear. Although the nurses' associations, some state boards, some courts, and attorneys general have indicated that nurses do not take PA orders, in about 17 states the rulings are the reverse. Because the PA may function according to a protocol specified by the employer-physician, there may be an operational agreement reached similar to the basis on which a nurse carries out standing orders or some verbal orders from the physician. Nevertheless, there is frequently interdisciplinary conflict when roles are not clarified. Yet, there seems to be an accommodation reached when both work together cooperatively.

Concern about the relative status of nurses and PAs was, and is, an issue in certain situations. Although NPs can offer services to the public beyond any that the PA can offer, frequently nurse and PA may be competing for the same job. For a number of reasons, the PA not only may be the one employed but will also receive a higher salary than that offered to the NP. Despite the fact that most physicians tend to say that they prefer nurses to PAs, the truth is that too often doctors have inadequate or no knowledge about the NP's capabilities. What they are talking about is a nurse as a PA. A number of nurses have made this choice, which is certainly theirs to make, although it has caused some negative reaction from other nurses and nursing associations. It is possible that the situation will be clarified as more NPs are prepared in standardized educational programs, and more physicians work with them in collegial practice.

Other Medical Personnel

Medical assistants (MAs) are usually employed in physicians' offices, where they perform a variety of administrative and clinical tasks to facilitate the work of the doctor; however, some do work in hospitals and clinics. They perform tasks required by the doctor, in accordance with specific state laws, and are supervised by the doctor. The medical assistant, among other things, answers the telephone; greets patients and other callers; makes appointments; handles correspondence and filing; arranges for diagnostic tests, hospital admissions, and surgery; handles patients' accounts and other billings; processes insurance claims, including Medicare; maintains patient records; prepares patients for examinations or treatment; takes temperatures, height, and weight; sterilizes instruments; assists the physician in examining or treating patients; and if trained, performs laboratory procedures. Most medical assistants train in one-year certificate or two-year associate degree programs given by community colleges, universities, and vocational-technical schools. CAHEA accreditation is available.

Emergency Medical Care

Emergency medical technicians-ambulance (EMT-As) respond to medical emergencies and provide immediate care to the critically ill or injured. They may administer cardiac resuscitation, treat shock, provide initial care to poison or burn victims, and transport patients to a health facility.[13] *EMT-As* do not determine the extent of illness, but set priorities in emergency care at the scene of the emergency, and monitor victims on the way to a hospital, often functioning under doctor or nurse voice directions or protocols. They are also responsible for the ambulance and supplies. The basic course of 110 hours and courses for other ratings may be given by hospitals, community colleges, fire, health, and police departments. A few two-year associate degree programs do exist. Those certified may apply to a CAHEA-accredited program for EMT paramedic training of 600 to 1,000 hours plus an internship. *EMT paramedics* are competent in assessing an emergency situation and managing the care, initiating appropriate treatment, and assessing its effect. They are responsible for exercising personal judgment when communication failures interrupt contact with medical direction or in life-threatening situations. EMT-paramedics are employed by community fire and police departments, by private ambulance services, and in hospital emergency departments.

Nursing Support Personnel

Nursing assistants, nurses' aides, orderlies, and *attendants* functioning under the direction of nurses are all part of the group of ancillary workers prepared to assist in nursing care, performing many of the simple nursing tasks, as well as other helping activities besides nursing. Usually training has been on the job and geared to the needs of the particular employing institution, but there has been some increase in public school programs within vocational high school tracks or as outside public education services. The program may vary in length from 6 to 8 weeks or more and costs little or nothing. A high school diploma is often required and generally preferred for employment. Commercial programs usually cost the student an unreasonable amount, make unrealistic promises of jobs, and frequently give no clinical experience; therefore, these "graduates" are seldom employed. Sometimes students who drop out of certain practical nurse programs after 6 weeks receive a certificate as aides. In-service education during employment is relatively common. It should be remembered that the difference in training, patient care assignment, and ability may be enormous on both an individual and an institutional basis. These workers are not licensed or certified as a rule, although there is a move to do so (see Chap. 20).

This is particularly true of nursing assistants in long-term care facilities. Under a change in the Medicare law, assistants employed in LTC nursing facilities participating in Medicare and Medicaid programs must complete 75 hours of training and pass a competency exam. Such programs are being developed. One, introduced by AHCA, uses interactive video, with practice exams (since nursing assistants often are not accustomed to test taking). New Jersey has already regulated LTC ancillary personnel through certification. There is also considerable concern that these "chronic care workers," usually middle-aged, the sole support of a family, and disproportionately minority, are not only undertrained but underpaid, with few benefits available. The turnover is great because of these reasons as well as their low status, few opportunities for advancement, and with sicker patients, a stressful working environment. Consequently, there is an increased tendency to seek union representation.

The major concern about the use of unlicensed assistive personnel (UAP) seems to be focused on the hospital. Since the salaries of professional nurses have increased and, in the wake of the recent shortage, considerable restructuring of nursing care has occurred, UAPs seem to be used more extensively in acute care hospitals. Often, there are no consistent criteria for training or responsibilities nor are there any studies on cost-effectiveness. Issues of competence, motivation, security, and supervision have been raised.[14] Staff nurses say that they need more "help," yet UAPs generate fear, distrust, and a perception of inadequate preparation. Nursing must move to clarify these issues.[15]

Community health aides of various kinds are found in ambulatory care settings. "Indigenous" health aides evolved because not enough physicians or public health nurses were available to help families described as disadvantaged to identify and correct their multiple, related medical and social problems. In addition, professionals do not always communicate effectively with disadvantaged minority clientele. Therefore, in those areas of service, community people are sometimes recruited and trained as health aides. Many are women not previously trained as vocational nurses or hospital aides. There is usually a limited didactic period with ongoing supervision and on-the-job instruction. Certain technical skills are learned, such as auditory and visual screening, but the primary purpose is to identify health problems or deficiencies, including lack of immunization, poor oral hygiene, dermatological problems, and child development problems, and to assist and encourage families to seek and continue necessary medical, nursing, and other services. Although specific changes in the health status of the community are difficult to measure, on an anecdotal basis, evaluation seems to be positive. These workers may be based in a clinic, neighborhood health center, or other ambulatory care facility, and may also go into the community to do case finding rather than wait for the client to appear in the formal health facility.

As more attention is focused on keeping people at home rather than in institutions, the services of *homemaker–home health aides* have become reimbursable by Medicaid, Medicare, and some state or local government agencies, under certain circumstances. The term *home health aide*, introduced in the Medicare Act in 1965, was added to the older term *homemaker*. The first homemaker services were made available in 1923 to substitute for a hospitalized mother. In the Depression, "housekeeping aides" were subsidized by the government to provide work for needy women. They were assigned to assist families with children, the aged, or the chronically ill.

Today's worker is a trained, supervised person who works as a full-fledged member of a team of professional and allied workers providing health and/or social services. The aide is as-

signed to the home of a family or individual when home life is disrupted by illness, disability, or social disadvantage, or if the family unit is in danger of breakdown because of stress. Specific tasks include parenting, performing or helping in household tasks, providing personal care such as bed baths, or helping with prescribed exercises, and providing emotional support. Educational programs are usually developed by the employing agency. An approved program specifies a minimum number of hours of classroom and laboratory instruction to prepare the individual for on-the-job functioning. Most are women who already have housekeeping skills; even so, there is some question as to how effectively they can really be prepared in the limited time suggested. New Jersey was the first state to certify this group (1989), and changes will probably occur.

There is an increasing tendency for proprietary agencies to have homemaker–home health care services, and to contract these workers out to voluntary agencies. Although there is evidence that a well-trained, conscientious home health aide can be extremely helpful to a sick person or disrupted family, there are also some serious problems in the selection of workers, the quality of training, and supervision. There are also some reimbursement problems when the homemaking part of the aide's function is reimbursable and the health part is not, or vice versa. However, the homemaker–home health aide is usually one person doing whichever aspect of the job is needed and is reimbursed in a particular situation. Most often, a combination of the services is needed by the client. Ongoing assessment by health professionals is intended to evaluate the need of the family and client for specific services.

The lack of reimbursement often prevents the use of homemaker–home health aides, for this can cost hundreds of dollars a month. Still, it is less costly health service than institutional care.

Surgical technicians, or *surgical technologists*, function in the operating room and, sometimes, the delivery room. Under the direction of the operating room supervisor, an RN, they perform required tasks, such as setting up for surgery, preparing instruments and other equipment before surgery, "scrubbing in" for surgery (assisting the surgeons by handling instruments, sutures, and so on), and otherwise assisting in the operating room.

Educational programs are most frequently offered by hospitals and some community colleges. If they are accredited by CAHEA, they may vary in length from 9 to 20 months depending on student selection criteria and the program's educational objectives. The curriculum has both didactic and supervised practice components, but does not prepare the student for complicated surgical procedures.

The *psychiatric–mental health technician* works in psychiatric and general hospitals, community mental health centers, and the home, working with the mentally disturbed, disabled, or retarded under the direction of a physician and/or nurse. In hospitals, he or she is concerned with patients' daily life as it affects their physical, mental and emotional well-being, including eating, sleeping, recreation, development of work skills, adjustment, and individual and social relations. In the community, focus is on social relationship and adjustments. In the hospital, psychiatric technicians are expected to give some routine and emergency physical nursing care, but their close contact with patients makes observation and reporting of the patient's behavior particularly important. In some institutions they function almost independently in group therapy and counseling, seeking consultation as necessary. They may be skilled in nursing, communication techniques, counseling, training techniques, and group therapy. The educational program has generally been one year long but an emerging standard seems to be a two-year associate degree program, which includes social and physical sciences, health education, laboratory work in group and interpersonal processes, and clinical experience. In some states psychiatric technicians have the opportunity to become licensed, sometimes under the Nursing Board.

Ward (unit) clerks or *ward (unit) secretaries* are usually trained on the job in an inservice program to assist in the clerical duties involved in the administration of a nursing unit. Ward clerks order supplies, keep certain records, answer telephones, take messages, attend to the massive amount of routine paper work and, in some cases, copy doctors' orders. This relieves the charge nurse to concentrate on administration of patient care instead of paper work. In the more progressive hospitals, unit clerks are on the day and evening shifts and sometimes at night.

Unit managers take even broader responsibilities in the management of a patient unit (usually in a larger institution) and may report directly to hospital administration instead of nursing service administration. Unit clerks often function under the direction of unit managers. In some institutions, unit management is an early step in an administrative career, and managers have full administrative responsibilities.

Pharmacy

Pharmacists are specialists in the science of drugs and require a thorough knowledge of chemistry and physiology. They may dispense prescription and nonprescription drugs, compound special preparations of dosage forms, serve as consultants, and advise physicians on selection and effects of drugs.

With the increase of prepackaged drugs and the use of pharmacy assistants, pharmacists in hospitals and clinics are particularly interested in a more patient-oriented approach to their practice. They may be involved in patient rounds, patient teaching, and consultation with nurses and physicians. Pharmacists working in (or owning) drugstores have also been encouraged to increase their patient or client education efforts in terms of explaining medications. Many keep a "medication profile," which is a computerized record of the customer's drug therapy to ensure that harmful drug interactions do not occur.

The educational program of pharmacists is usually a five-year baccalaureate program including two or more years of professional course work, and some practical experience or internship. There are also 6-year programs for the Pharm D (Doctor of Pharmacy) and here enrollments are increasing. Some schools offer both degrees. The Pharm D is a relatively new development that occurred in part because of the complexity of today's drugs, their potential adverse reaction with each other as multiple drugs are prescribed (or taken), the increased use and abuse of drugs, the fact that physicians often do not have in-depth knowledge of drugs, and the successful implementation of clinical pharmacy services in the 1960s. Besides the traditional responsibilities of pharmacists, the Pharm D or clinical pharmacist provides consultation with the physician, maintains patient drug histories and reviews the total drug regimen of patients, monitors patient charts in LTC facilities, and recommends drug therapy, makes patient rounds, and provides individualized dosage regimens. Pharmacists are also increasingly assuming a role in home care, particularly in relation to infusion therapy. In some states, such as California, clinical pharmacists may also prescribe (as do NPs and PAs), with certain limitations. This new role is well accepted by some physicians, usually those who have worked with Pharm Ds, and is considered an infringement on medical territory by others.

Trends in the field focus on the Pharm D, which the American Council on Pharmaceutical Education sees as the basic degree by the year 2000, but there is also increased interest in postgraduate training such as research fellowships or residencies in a defined area of pharmacy. Three specialties are recognized and certified: nuclear pharmacy, pharmacotherapy, and nutrition support. Enrollment for the first professional degree has been increasing after a period of decline, and there has been an increase in women and a much smaller increase in minorities. Arguments have been advanced that the Pharm D should be the first professional degree, eliminating the baccalaureate. Because

they fear for their economic and professional status, a growing number of pharmacists are taking part-time and off-campus courses toward a Pharm D.[16] Graduate education (Master of Science and Ph.D.) has also increased, although slowly, because of the growing complexity of the field. Continuing education is emphasized for this reason, but also because a number of states require continuing education for relicensure. Pharmacists are licensed in all states and have reciprocity (need not retake licensing exams) in all but California and Florida. Most work in chain or independent pharmacies or hospitals, but one report indicated that pharmacy students have 535 alternatives for career choices.[17] Although projections for future need are seen as rather doubtful as to accuracy, a shortage is anticipated by the year 2000.

The *pharmacy technician*, who will probably be certified, and for whom the pharmacist is responsible, assists with dispensing tasks and is now considered a valuable adjunct to pharmacy practice.[18]

Pharmacologists specialize in research and development of drugs to prevent or treat disease or prolong life. A medical degree or a 4- to 5-year Ph.D. program in pharmacology is usually required.

Podiatry

Podiatrists, doctors of podiatric medicine (DPM) (once called *chiropodists*), are professionally trained foot care specialists who diagnose, treat, and try to prevent diseases, injuries, and deformities of the feet. Treatment may include surgery, medication, physical therapy, setting fractures, and preparing orthoses (supporting devices that mechanically rearrange the weight-bearing structures of the foot). Podiatrists may note symptoms of diseases manifested in the feet and legs and refer the patient to a physician.

Podiatrists complete a 4-year program of classroom and clinical work in a college of podiatry after a minimum of 2 years of college, but the majority have already had 4 years. Although they are permitted to practice immediately after graduation in most states, almost all apply for 1 or 2 years of residency training. The enrollment in the colleges of podiatry has been increasing, owing largely to federal support and the podiatric needs of the aging population. There has been an increase in women and minorities. A unique aspect of podiatric medical education is the attempt to develop a system-wide, competency-based curriculum. The National Board of Podiatry Examiners gives examinations that satisfy the requirements for licensure in more than forty states. Other states use their own examinations; some require a residency, and an increasing number are requiring continuing education.

Most podiatrists are in private practice; others practice in institutions, agencies, the military, education, and research. As a group, they are eager to expand their scope of practice but are being strongly resisted by physicians. Yet podiatrists who have had surgical residencies and the requisite 5 years of practice, and have passed the exacting certification examination of the American Board of Podiatric Surgery, maintain that these physicians are unfamiliar with current podiatric education and practice or are protective of their own economic well-being.

Psychology, Psychotherapy, and Mental Health

Psychology is the scientific study of mental processes and behavior, and *psychotherapy* refers generally to techniques for treating mental illness by psychological means, primarily through establishing communication between the therapist and the patient as a means of understanding and modifying behavior. In the field of mental health, there is a great overlapping of therapists treating patients with various kinds of mental problems. Besides the physician (the psychiatrist), clinical psychologists, psychotherapists, nurses, social workers, and a variety of semiprofessionals trained in mental health participate in individual and group therapy. *Psychologists* may also give and

interpret various personality and behavioral tests, as might a *psychometrician*, who is skilled in the testing and measuring of mental and psychological ability, efficiency, potentials, and functions. An area of dissension in the field is the fact that various mental health therapists are fighting to get prescription privileges and are strongly opposed by psychiatrists. The latter are also complaining that PPOs are demanding that psychiatrists cut their fees considerably because the other practitioners do not charge as much. Education for psychologists and psychotherapists is often at the master's or doctoral level. Clinical psychologists have training in a clinical setting.

Public Health—Environment

Industrial hygienists deal with the effects on workers' health of noise, dust, vapor radiation, and other hazards common to industry. They are usually employed by industry, laboratories, insurance companies, or government to detect and correct these hazards. Their education may include a baccalaureate in environmental health, engineering, or physical or biological science.

Sanitarians, sometimes called *environmentalists*, apply technical knowledge to solve problems of sanitation in a community. They develop and implement methods to control those factors in the environment that affect health and safety, such as rodent control, sanitary conditions in schools, hotels, restaurants, areas of food production and sales. Most work in government, under the direction of a health officer or administrator. Education is generally a BS in environmental health, public health, or the physical or biological sciences. Advanced positions require a master's degree. Registration is required in most states; national certification is also available. In 1992, the federal government declared a crisis in environmental public health education with new graduates not enough to replace annual losses in the workforce, much less the estimated shortage of 120,000 professionals.[19]

Also educated in schools of public health, as well as elsewhere, are *biostatisticians*, who apply mathematics and statistics to research problems related to health, and *epidemiologists*, who study the factors that influence the occurrence and course of human health problems, including not only acute and chronic diseases, but also accidents, addictions, and suicides. Epidemiologists attempt to establish the courses of health problems by focusing on the biological, social, and behavioral factors affecting health, illness, and premature death. They use investigative, analytical, and descriptive techniques. A specialized graduate degree is necessary for both biostatisticians and epidemiologists.

Radiology

Radiologists are physicians dealing with all forms of radiant energy, from x-rays to radioactive isotopes; they interpret radiographic studies and prescribe therapy for diseases, particularly malignancies. A number of technicians work under the direction of a radiologist in radiology departments.

The *radiologic technologist*, sometimes called *x-ray technician, radiology technician*, or *radiographer*, is concerned with the proper operation of x-ray equipment, preparation of patients for x-rays and therapy, developing of film, and some clerical work. Programs are usually two-year CAHEA-accredited hospital certificate programs, sometimes affiliated with a college or university. However, they vary from one to four years depending on the program. The graduate may become registered [RT (R)] after passing an examination given by the American Registry of Radiologic Technicians. A few states license radiology technicians and technologists.

Radiation therapy technicians or *technologists* assist the radiologist in the treatment of disease by exposing affected areas of the patient's body to prescribed doses of radiation, operating and controlling complex equipment and devices, and maintaining records. A one- or two-year program in radiation therapy given by community colleges or hospitals is required. There are some baccalaureate programs.

A *nuclear medicine technologist* works with radioactive isotopes administered to patients for diagnosis and treatment. He or she positions and attends to patients, abstracts data from records, assists in the operation of scanning devices using isotopes, and has responsibility for safe storage of radioactive materials and disposal of wastes. CAHEA accredits both AD programs and baccalaureate programs; the technical portion for each is one year.

Related careers are *sonographers* or *ultrasound technologists* and the *diagnostic medical sonographer*, who assists the physician in gathering sonographic data, records and processes these data, and makes pertinent observations. Programs of 1- to 4-years' duration may be accredited by CAHEA. With advanced training, any of these technologists may work with CAT scans and MRIs. A major trend is to identify this overall group as diagnostic imaging personnel.

Rehabilitation Services

Occupational therapy is concerned with the use of purposeful activity in the promotion and maintenance of health, prevention of disability, evaluation of behavior, and as treatment of persons with physical or psychosocial dysfunction, using a wide spectrum of treatment procedures based on activities of a creative, a social, a self-care, an educational, and a vocational nature. One important responsibility is helping patients with activities of daily living. Adaptive tools such as aids for eating or dressing may also be provided.

Occupational therapists (OTs), the professional workers, and *occupational therapy assistants* and *aides* are usually employed in hospitals. However, OTs may also be in private practice or work for nursing homes or community agencies. They are valuable in working with the elderly. Professional education for the occupational therapists is a baccalaureate program or a two-year master's degree program for those with another type of baccalaureate; the program may be CAHEA-accredited.

The American Occupational Therapy Association certifies for the professional entry-level occupational therapist registered (OTR) or certified occupational therapy assistant (COTA). In some institutions, professional occupational therapists are assisted by OT assistants or aides, who may be trained in a one-year certificate program or in two-year or four-year colleges and vocational-technical institutes. They participate directly in the patient's activities.

Physical therapy is concerned with the restoration of function and the prevention of disability following disease, injury, or loss of body part; sometimes physical therapy is concerned with diagnosis. The goal is to improve circulation, strengthen muscles, encourage return of motion, and train or retrain the patient with the use of prosthetics, crutches, walkers, exercise, heat, cold, electricity, ultrasound, and massage. Most *physical therapists, PT assistants*, and *PT aides* work in hospitals, but PTs may also work in private practice or for other agencies such as VNAs. In home care, they take on a more expanded care role.[20] The physical therapist designs the patient's program of treatment, based on the physician's stated prescription of objectives. He or she may participate in giving the therapy and/or evaluate the patient's needs and capacities and provide psychological support. The aides work directly under the physical therapist's supervision, with limited participation in the therapeutic program. As in occupational therapy, education for the PT is in a baccalaureate or postbaccalaureate program leading to a certificate or master's degree. Registration is possible through the American Registry of Physical Therapists, and all states now license PTs. There has been some limited effort to require licensure of physical therapist assistants, whose education is usually at the associate degree level. This level of PT worker may be certified or registered; aides require no special credential.

Prosthetists make artificial limb substitutes. *Orthotists* make and fit braces. Both work with physicians and other therapists, and have direct patient contact to promote total rehabilitation services. A bachelor's degree in prosthetics or orthotics plus 1900 hours of supervised clinical experience is usual; for those with a bachelor's degree, special 8- to 16-month programs plus 1900 hours of supervised clinical experience is necessary. *Orthotic/prosthetic technicians* make and repair devices but usually have no patient contact. Education is primarily in vocational-technical schools with formal training in orthotics and prosthetics. An alternative is two years of supervised clinical experience, but either way, a high school diploma or GED is required.

Rehabilitation counselors help people with physical, mental, or social disabilities begin or return to satisfying life, including an appropriate job. They may counsel about job opportunities and training, assist in job placement, and help the person to adjust to a new work situation. The usual requirement is a master's degree. Others assisting in patient rehabilitation include *art therapists, dance therapists, horticulture therapists, manual arts therapists, corrective therapists*, and *music therapists* who work primarily with the emotionally disturbed, mentally retarded, or physically handicapped. Their educational requirements are not firmly established and vary a great deal. *Recreation therapists* or *therapeutic recreationists* may plan and supervise recreation programs that include athletics, arts and crafts, parties, gardening, or camping. Professional status usually requires a master's degree, although some therapists have only a bachelor's degree; assistants are generally prepared at the associate degree level. RTs require licensure or certification in a few states.

Respiratory Therapy

Respiratory therapy personnel perform procedures essential in maintaining life in seriously ill patients with respiratory problems and assist in treatment of heart and lung ailments. Under medical supervision, or that of a respiratory therapist, the *respiratory therapy technician* administers various types of gas, aerosol, and breathing treatments, assists with long-term continuous artificial ventilation, cleans, sterilizes, and maintains equipment, and keeps patient records. The *respiratory therapist* may be engaged in similar tasks, but his or her more extensive knowledge of sciences and clinical medicine allows for the exercise of more judgment and acceptance of greater responsibility in performing therapeutic procedures. Respiratory therapy personnel usually work in hospitals and clinics.

A CAHEA-accredited program for technicians is one year long; certification is available. A therapist program, also CAHEA-accredited, may culminate in an associate or baccalaureate degree, with a minimum of two years required. The baccalaureate programs sometimes build on the AD program and prepare for supervision and teaching. Respiratory therapists may be registered, but are not usually licensed. Certification (RRT) may be required for administrative positions.

Social Work

The *social worker* attempts to help individuals and their families resolve their social problems, utilizing community and governmental resources as necessary. Social workers are employed by community and governmental agencies as well as hospitals, clinics, and nursing homes. If the social worker's focus is on patients and families, he or she may be called a *medical* or *psychiatric social worker*. A master's degree is required for advanced and specialized social work. There are also accredited baccalaureate programs. College graduates with degrees in other areas may qualify as social workers by completing the master's degree. Membership in the National Association of Social Workers is open only to social workers graduated from, or students of, accredited schools of social work. Certification is granted by the Academy of Certified Social Workers after other criteria are met. A doctoral degree is usually required for teaching, advanced practice, and administration.

Social workers also have assistants, who sometimes carry a client load in certain agencies. There may be only on-the-job training available for these workers, but in order to move upward they must acquire additional education. Some employers prefer a two-year associate degree in human or social services, even for this assisting level.

One professional issue cited by social workers is related to identity. Since social work was identified as a career only in the 1930s, there is still some preoccupation with defining the field.

Like nurses, social workers are concerned with the distribution, effectiveness, and cost of their service, as well as clarification of responsibilities of each educational level of practitioners. Some also admit to concern for their professional survival, particularly because of role overlap with other health professionals. One particularly competitive area is case management, especially for the elderly. *Case management* is defined as "a systematic process of assessment, planning, service coordination and/or referral, and monitoring through which the multiple service needs of clients are met" (see Chap. 7).[21] Both nurses and social workers, as well as others, perform these activities, but each may claim ownership of the role.

Speech-Language Pathology and Audiology

Speech-language pathologists and *audiologists* are specialists in communication disorders. Speech pathologists or therapists diagnose and treat speech and language disorders that may stem from a variety of causes. Speech therapists are particularly valuable in assisting patients whose speech has been affected by a cerebrovascular accident or patients with laryngectomies. Audiologists often work with children and may detect and assist with the hearing disorder of a child who has been mistakenly labeled retarded. Education for both specialties is at a master's level, after a baccalaureate in human communication science. There has been some attempt to require state licensure. The American Speech and Hearing Association offers a Certificate of Clinical Competence after specific criteria are fulfilled.

Vision Care

Ophthalmologists are physicians who treat diseases of the eye and perform surgery, but they may also examine eyes and prescribe corrective glasses and exercises. *Optometrists*, doctors of optometry (OD),[22] considered independent primary health care providers, are educated and clinically trained to examine, diagnose, and treat conditions of the vision system, but they refer clients with eye diseases and other health problems to physicians. After a variety of diagnostic tests, they may prescribe corrective lenses, contact lenses, and special optical aids as well as corrective eye exercises to provide maximum vision. Some may specialize in such areas as prescribing and fitting contact lenses.

A minimum of 7 years' education is required, with 3 years of college before optometry school and 4 years of specialized professional education and clinical training. The programs are accredited by the American Optometric Association Council. There are also postgraduate clinical residencies for specialization. All states require licensure by state board examinations; most states accept the National Board of Optometry examinations. Continuing education is required for relicensure in most states. One trend is the increase of women and minorities in the field. In addition, optometry is increasingly populated by younger practitioners.

The majority of optometrists are in private office practice; others are in group practice, hospitals, public health agencies, HMOs, research institutions, manufacturing organizations, the military, and other government agencies. Others are teaching and doing research in colleges and universities (which requires a master's or doctorate). About 90 percent are involved in direct patient care activities.

Given the overlap in roles with ophthalmologists in the area of vision analysis, the increasing number of optometrists, and their complaint that their income is below acceptable levels, it is not unexpected to find conflict between the groups on their scope of practice. Optometrists are permitted to prescribe drugs in many states and are authorized to use drugs to diagnose eye problems or disease in all 50 states, but may not perform surgery. These activities are strongly opposed by ophthalmologists. The Federal Trade Commission overturn of bans on professional advertising has also aided optometrists, since it made them more competitive in providing those services that can be rendered by both groups of professionals. However, it is predicted that optometrists will continue to fight for expansion of their scope of practice.

Optometric assistants assist optometrists by performing simple office and patient care duties. *Technicians* may also assist in office tasks, but usually assist in vision training and testing. Assistants complete a one-year certificate or diploma program; technicians, a two-year associate degree offered by two- and four-year colleges, colleges of optometry, hospitals, and the military.

Opticians grind lenses, make eyeglasses, and fit and adjust them. Both AD programs and on-the-job apprenticeship qualify individuals for this job. *Optical laboratory technicians* and *mechanics* may be involved in polishing and grinding lenses.

Orthoptists, working under an ophthalmologist's supervision, correct crossed eyes in adults and children through special exercises. They may also aid with visual field and glaucoma testing. Two years of college or a bachelor's degree plus a 24-month training program given in medical schools, vision clinics, or hospitals is required.[23]

Other Health Workers

There are a number of other health workers not described in this chapter, such as those in science and engineering—anatomists, biologists, biomedical engineers (who design patient care equipment such as dialysis machines, pace-makers, heart-lung machines), and biomedical technicians (who maintain and repair the equipment); technicians dealing with instrumentation—clinical perfusionists (who operate equipment to support or temporarily replace a patient's circulatory or respiratory functions), electrocardiograph (EKG/ECG) technicians, electroencephalographic (EEG) technologists and technicians; specialists in dealing with the visually handicapped; biological photographers, medical illustrators; all of whom have CAHEA-accredited programs, as well as patient advocates, acupuncturists, health science librarians, and computer specialists, to name just a few. In addition, volunteers provide many useful services. That this list is not complete and is expanding may help to explain why, no matter how valuable individual services may be, the public often becomes angered by the fragmentation of services. Even health professionals may be unsure about who does what or when for the client's well-being. Yet, this list is not exaggerated; all these specialties are part of what the federal government calls health manpower and allied health manpower, for which federal funds are often distributed for educational programs. It is clear that if the public is to receive the services it requires, expects, and deserves, there must be direction given through the health care delivery maze.

ISSUES AND PREDICTIONS

Many of the most serious issues in the health workforce—numbers, distribution, proliferation, and especially quality of care—have become issues focused on credentialing. This multifaceted process, which has become a major concern of government, is given full attention in Chap. 20.

However, the problem of health workforce planning transcends or, perhaps, precedes credentialing. The blame for proliferation of workforce is difficult to pinpoint. Is it the practitioners or administrators who see the immediate need for quickly prepared assistants? Or is it the federal government that encourages proliferation through education and reimbursement sup-

port? The health care industry (and it *is* one of the largest industries in the United States) is labor intensive. The health workforce frequently creates its own demands: if a certain type of practitioner is available, the availability of that service to the consumer expands—and, as the critics say, adds to the total cost of care.

Predicting demand and supply is no easy matter: development of health workforce resources may take as little as a few months or as long as ten years; in that time both demand and supply may shift rapidly; decisions on whether to expand or contract either education programs or health services frequently depend on uncontrollable external factors, such as the economy; current workforce data are inexact and usually out of date. Thus, it is not surprising that even the most educated guesses of demand and supply often err. What *is* left behind all too frequently is a mass of undereducated, poorly paid, non-cost-effective workers with little job mobility, poor motivation, and built-in anger. The result is increased union activity, and labor unions are accused of causing escalating costs.

It is true that in the 1960s improved salaries were a major budget item, and the need to move from what were often below-poverty wages to living wages was largely responsible for the jump. Since that catch-up period, the masses of workers have gained a new aggressiveness that affects not only monetary considerations, but power issues. Some are not necessarily in the best interests of the consumer. Nevertheless, one of the trends that was widely predicted is aggressive action by unions to organize every type of health worker—professional, technical, aide, clerical, maintenance, and housekeeping. The likelihood that this will be successful is now in doubt because of the tight economic constraints of health care institutions and their preference for multipurpose workers.

The issue of maldistribution is also not easily resolved. Maldistribution of professionals, toward attractive urban and suburban areas and away from isolated, poor, or ghetto areas, is a major problem. In some cases, nurses, PAs, physician-nurse, or physician PA and/or nurse teams are giving care that is as good as or better than that provided by solo practitioners, but the service gap still exists. Even federal intervention, such as requiring service in medically underserved areas (about 30 percent of the United States) in return for supporting the practitioners' education, has had only short-term results—practitioners leave after their required service.

Health workforce education is a major issue. How many? What kind? Prepared where? Financed by whom? The education for all levels of health service practitioners is under scrutiny. Why is this education so costly? Could institutions develop more economical teaching-learning methods? Are minority groups being actively recruited? Are the types of workers in proper proportion? Should the government continue to subsidize the education of high-earning professionals? How much should any health profession be subsidized, and for whom—the programs or students? Are the practitioners appropriately prepared to give safe and effective care?

Another concern is the workability of the health care team. It is naive to expect that bringing together a highly diverse group of people and calling them a team will cause them to behave like a team. One obvious gap is their lack of communication and "practice" together, either as students or as full practitioners. Sports teams practice together intensively for long periods of time, both to develop a team spirit and to enhance and coordinate their individual skills to produce a functioning unit. Not only do health care teams not have (or take) time to practice together, but often there are serious territorial disputes as areas of responsibility overlap more and more. As for patients, who should be members of the team, unless they are assertive, their only participation is as recipients of care.

Theoretically, legally clear distinctions of each profession would be helpful; practically, it is impossible. Successful coordination depends on collegial behavior, trust, and full, frequent, open communication; otherwise, valuable participants in health care will continue to be un-

derutilized. It has also been said that society can no longer afford, and does not need, to use the physician as gatekeeper to control the flow of patients in and out of the health system. Physician services should be saved to assist patients who need that level of services. In other words, there must be other fully acknowledged practitioners in primary health care. This is slow to happen.

A review of the issues that each occupation sees as vital makes it clear that the struggle between medicine and other health care groups to expand or limit the scope of practice will continue and perhaps escalate. And with the current economic pressures that are not expected to let up, various types and levels of workers may fight even harder to get and keep territory. The trend to increase educational criteria seems to permeate each occupational group, but almost all face the questions asked by the cost-conscious: "Will it cost the consumer more? Will it keep out the poor? Is it really necessary, or is it a status ploy?"

One overriding issue is, who has power or should have power to make these decisions? The consumer? But who advises the consumer? All too often, the power figures in health care make policy, even if indirectly, by their input into legislation or major influential groups like the Institute of Medicine. Legislation or executive action often follows on the heels of IOM committees or task force recommendations, yet the makeup of the committee and staff not infrequently slants a report in one direction or another (see Chap. 5). The AMA and AHA are also influential in issues related to health personnel. Now, with some current or anticipated shortages of RNs, LPNs, PTs, OTs, medical lab personnel, clinical perfusionists, speech pathologists, respiratory therapists, nurse anesthetists, nurses' aides, computer specialists, and according to AHA, fourteen other health care occupations close behind, hospitals particularly are demanding action. (It is interesting that the nonclinical computer specialists are one of the most in demand.) There is concern that patients everywhere will suffer if the needs are not met.

Yet, as discussed in Chap. 6, the shortage of young people available to enter these fields and the strong possibility that those interested may not have an adequate education does not make for a good prognosis.

The nursing shortage (or more accurately, supply and demand) will be discussed in Chap. 15, but solutions proposed by AHA and AMA present a picture of their involvement (not to be seen as always bad). In 1989, the AHA co-sponsored a pilot project with the Illinois Hospital Association to test a new employee group, an all-purpose worker to make beds, empty trash, serve meals, and take over other nonclinical chores to help nurses. The idea was to cross-train staff to handle anything from transport to housekeeping. (How the unions reacted was not reported.) It was expected that other hospitals would replicate this plan, and some did. Meanwhile, some hospitals produced other kinds of assistants called general medical technicians or unit helpers to do all the non-nursing tasks nurses are forced to do. The idea has merit, but will it create one more set of low-paying jobs that go nowhere? And how clear is it to both the public and health care personnel, just what the responsibilities of these unlicensed workers are, how safe they are, and who supervises them?

On the other side of the shortage issue is oversupply, still being predicted for physicians, dentists, and some administrators; given the uncertainties of the health care future, others could be included. The reactions of those concerned follow a pattern: denial or prediction of a later shortage as in medicine; a tendency to warn off potential students; disillusionment with the field; an attempt to hold on to their own territory and resist others' encroachment, but also an attempt to encroach on still others; efforts to expand their services to meet previously unnoted or unattractive needs (serving the elderly); or making some aspect of their services attractive to consumers (cosmetic dentistry). Because real health care needs may begin to be met, there are good aspects to the situation; however, the dissension and the cost to the public are not desirable.

Another major issue is quality of care. This inevitably involves health care personnel. Related to this issue is not only practice but education. Health care personnel, experts say, must develop some special skills to deal with the future and educators should take note. Several have been repeatedly mentioned: care of the elderly; understanding of psychosocial needs; health education; political savvy and the know-how to affect policy; ability to assess individual and community health care needs; and more of a business orientation with an understanding of financial management.[24] Interdisciplinary respect and understanding of health professionals, beginning with some joint educational/clinical experiences is seen as helpful, but most of all, respect for patients' and people's rights is stressed.

All predictions point to tremendous job growth in the health field in the next years, but even more dramatic may be the changes likely with the enactment of some sort of national health plan, presumably covering every American. With the expected emphasis on primary care, health promotion, disease prevention, and, of course, cost containment and quality, the roles of health care providers may overlap, break new ground, expand or contract. Coordination and cooperation to facilitate continuity of care will be expected. Therefore, if some of the concerns cited earlier are not resolved, the periods of mutual tension and disenchantment between consumer and provider will only escalate.

REFERENCES

1. Jonas S: Health manpower, in Kovner A (ed): *Health Care Delivery in the United States*, 4th ed. New York: Springer, 1990, pp 52, 54.
2. Taylor R, Taylor S: *The AUPHA Manual of Health Services Management*. Gaithersburg, MD: Aspen Publishers, 1994, pp 14–15.
3. Ibid, pp 118–119.
4. Pennell M, Hoover D: Health manpower source book 21: Allied health manpower supply and requirements 1950–1980. Bethesda, MD: US De-

partment of Health, Education and Welfare, 1970, p 3.

5. Anderson P: Dentists and hygienists: Is there a crisis? *Dent Econ* 84:30–38, April 1994.

6. Greenblatt F: Expanded-duty dental assistants— The next step in efficient care. *Dent Econ* 84:23–27, February 1994.

7. *200 Ways to Put Your Talent to Work in the Health Field*. Washington, DC: The National Health Council, Inc, 1993, p 4.

8. Ibid, p 5.

9. Ibid, p 7.

10. Beck M et al: Doctors under the knife. *Newsweek* 123:28–33, April 5, 1993.

11. Bowman M: The evolution/revolution of family medicine. *Arch Fam Med* 3:404–406, May 1994.

12. Schroeder S: Training an appropriate mix of physicians to meet the nation's needs. *Acad Med* 68:118–122, February 1993.

13. *200 Ways*, op cit, p 9.

14. Manuel P, Alster K: Unlicensed personnel: No cure for an ailing health care system. *Nurs Health Care* 15:18–21, January 1994.

15. Huber D et al: Use of nursing assistants: Staff nurse opinions. *Nurs Mgt* 25:64–68, May 1994.

16. Bloom M: Getting a "flexible" Pharm D. *Am Pharm* 34:45–49, May 1994.

17. Health Personnel in the United States: Eighth Report to Congress, 1991. U.S. Department of Health and Human Services: DHHS Pub HRS-P-OD-92-1.1992, pp 151–158.

18. Mitchell J: National technician certification program planned. *Am Pharm* 34:27–30, February 1991.

19. Health Personnel, op cit, p 173.

20. Carr M: Physical therapists in home care: Yesterday, today and tomorrow. *Caring* 13:38–40, April 1994.

21. Parker M, Secord L: Private geriatric case management: Providers, services, and fees. *Nurs Econ* 6:165–172, 195, July–August 1988.

22. Health Personnel, op cit, pp 145–150.

23. *200 Ways*, op cit, pp 25–26.

24. Stanfield P: *Introduction to the Health Professions*. Boston: Jones and Bartlett, 1990, pp 64–65.

Nursing in the Health Care Setting

Nursing as a Profession

DEFINITIONS OF NURSING

The word "nurse" has certain cultural connotations and, for most of us, emotional attachment. Further, there are well-established public images of nursing. Add the fact that the discipline of nursing is moving through a period of rapid change, and you can be assured that there exists a range of contradictory and frequently inaccurate perspectives on what nursing is and should be. Schulman, in his historical analysis, sees nursing as rooted in the contradictory roles of mother surrogate and healer, one denoting constancy, affection, intimacy, and physical closeness; the other conveying a spirit of the discontinuous, fragmented, and dynamic.[1] This same dichotomy can be observed in nursing as it is described by many of our contemporary theorists. Lydia Hall spoke of care and cure. Leininger, Benner, and Watson seize the concept of caring, and develop it with a precision that makes it the dynamic equal of curing.[2]

There seems to be a public tendency to equate nursing with illness. Current dictionaries still define *nurse* as someone trained to care for the sick. Moreover, since the proliferation of nurses' aides and practical nurses after World War II, the public is even more confused as to who is the nurse. It is not unusual for patients to call anyone in a uniform who gives them personal care a nurse. Perhaps life was simpler when it was protocol for only the registered nurse to wear a white, long-sleeved uniform, white shoes and stockings, and most important, the starched white cap and special pin of the nursing school, or, as an option, the easily identified navy blue of the public health nurse. It was a symbol, a tradition, an image that came packaged with preconceived notions of what that uniformed figure could do. (Never mind that years ago, one key nursing figure described the uniform as a housedress and the cap as a dust cap.)

It has been pointed out that, in some ways, nurses tend to cherish a traditional image, even as they move into new roles and live uncomfortably with a blurred self-image. Many nursing students enter schools with the concept that "real" nursing is bedside care. Still, surveys indicate that now more people realize that nurses also engage in research, deliver babies, teach health, do psychotherapy, administer anesthesia, hang out a shingle, diagnose patients and treat their illnesses; nurses work not only in hospitals, but in jails, homes, clinics, colleges, schools, industry, and in the most rural as well as the most urban areas. Most of all, with the complexity of nursing care today, it is clear that nurses need intelligence as well as stamina.

There are many interpretations of nursing. Why not? There are many facets to nursing, and perhaps it isn't logical or accurate to settle on one point of view. All nurses must eventually determine their own philosophies of nursing, whether or not these are formalized. The public and others outside nursing will probably continue to adopt a concept or image that is nurtured by contact, hearsay, or education about the profession, and the first may be the most powerful determinant. This chapter seeks to present an overview of the components of nursing, examined in the light of professionalism, legal and other definitions, nursing process, nursing theory, nursing diagnosis, and nursing standards.

PROFESSIONS AND PROFESSIONALISM

Almost everyone talks about the *nursing profession* in the sense of an organized group of persons, all of whom are engaged in nursing (the phrase is used often throughout these pages). But another question discussed both within and without the ranks of nursing is whether or not nursing as a whole is an occupation, rather than a profession in the same sense that medicine, theology, and law have been called professions since the Middle Ages.

Professions have been historically linked with universities or other specialized institutions of learning, implying a certain high level of scholarly learning and study, including research. The specific criteria for a profession vary and are delineated more fully in some of the bibliography for this chapter. There is fairly general agreement, however, that professionalism centers on specialized expertise, autonomy, and service. Based on Flexner's classic criteria,[3] the following delineates the various components in a useful manner:

1. A profession utilizes in its practice a well-defined and well-organized body of knowledge that is on the intellectual level of higher learning.
2. A profession constantly enlarges the body of knowledge it uses and improves its techniques of education and service by the use of the scientific method.
3. A profession entrusts the education of its practitioners to institutions of higher education.
4. A profession applies its body of knowledge in practical services that are vital to human and social welfare.

5. A profession functions autonomously in the formulation of professional policy and in the control of professional activity thereby.
6. A profession attracts individuals of intellectual and personal qualities who exalt service above personal gain and who recognize their chosen occupation as a life work.
7. A profession strives to compensate its practitioners by providing freedom of action, opportunity for continuous professional growth, and economic security.

Looking at these criteria objectively, it is clear that nursing does not totally fulfill all of them. It has been pointed out that nursing's theory base is still developing, that the public does not always see the nurse as a professional, that not all nurses are educated in institutions of higher learning, that not all nurses consider nursing a lifetime career, and that in many practice settings, nursing does not control its own policies and activities. This lack of autonomy is considered the most serious weakness. Sociologists have long contended that an occupation has not become a profession unless the members of that occupation are the ones who make the final decisions about the services they provide.[4]

This issue is addressed in more depth in Chap. 16, and it can be seen that, particularly in recent years, there has been progress in both achieving autonomy and, perhaps more important, nurses' recognition that this is important to both the profession and to themselves in terms of how they practice. This mental turnaround has something to do with the fact that more nurses are seeking higher education and that more are planning nursing careers as opposed to taking nursing jobs. And as intertwined as all these professional threads are bound to be, more of the better educated nurses are also involved in research and theory development (see Chaps. 12 to 14). Nurses are also becoming more aggressive about getting recognition for what they *have* accomplished. Both nurses and others are convinced that the fact that nursing is predominantly female is also a factor in why nurses have had difficulty achieving high professional status. However, with changes in society, including the effect of the women's movement, that have had at least some impact on the stereotyping of women as well as the progress of nurses themselves, this is seen as a time to move the profession forward. If nursing is not considered a profession in the strictest sense of the word, it is well on the way to becoming so. One author commented thoughtfully, "On the continuum of professionalization, qualitatively nursing and many individual nurses excel far beyond contemporary recognized professions in many areas. Quantitatively, the road ahead is very long."[5]

Another way to assess nursing's professional status is to review the manner in which public policy is constructed and applied to our issues. Nursing has had a history of being on the short end of a double standard. In 1992, a new system of Medicare reimbursement was implemented that linked the fee schedule to the service delivered as opposed to the provider. The fee ignored any special rates for specialty preparation. At implementation, the government recanted and proposed that nonphysician providers should receive less compensation because of a lesser investment in education and training. The hypocrisy continues when nurse practitioners are compensated only 85 percent of the physician's customary rate but can receive the full fee if their practice is incidental to the physician and billed through that physician in a supervisory relationship.[6] Since the policy is changing constantly, new opinions will emerge. In the end, whether or not (and when) nursing will become a full profession depends on whether its practitioners choose this demanding status and continue to fight for progress.

It should be pointed out, however, that the term *profession* is essentially a social concept and has no meaning apart from society. Society decides that for its needs to be met in a certain respect, a body undertaking to meet these particular needs will be given special consideration. The contract is that the individuals of that favored group continually use their best endeavor to meet those obligations, constantly reexamining and scrutinizing their functions for appropriateness and maintaining competence. When they fail to honor these obligations and/or slip into demanding status, authority, and privilege that have no connection with carrying out their professional work satisfactorily, society may reconsider. A profession is seen as a body of individuals voluntarily subordinating themselves to a standard of social morality more exacting than that of the community in general. That violation of this code eventually brings retribution from society is evidenced today in the tightening of laws regulating professional practice and reimbursement. Certain behaviors, such as unprofessional conduct, may be specifically punished by removal of the practitioner's legal right to practice—licensure. What comprises unprofessional conduct may, again, vary from state to state, and also in time. This is discussed more fully in Chap. 20.

Flexner's model has remain unchallenged for over 80 years, despite the fact that professionalism is a social concept and is driven by the values and attitudes of the times. Simply put, Flexner depicts the professions as independent, learned, indispensable, committed to a lifetime of service and generously rewarded and esteemed for their dedication. Classically, the public has deferred to the profession to establish its standards and monitor the practice of its members. This is a courtesy given to experts in a complex area of work who exercise unquestioned integrity and respect the client-provider relationship above all others. This tradition of autonomy has seriously eroded in recent years. Surveys tell us that Americans have developed a significant suspicion about professionals. (Nurses have been the exception, as reported in Chap. 11.) Given this discomfort with individuals who provide very essential services, the public has looked to government for more oversight. There are many examples: consumer presence on professional boards, setting of fee schedules for reimbursement, the development of guidelines for the management of certain disease conditions, the governmental requirement to advise patients of their right to execute a living will.

Autonomy and immunity from governmental intrusion has always been the strongest in areas of specialty practice, where consumers feel least qualified to challenge the judgment of professionals. The recent movement to license nurses in advanced or specialty practice is both an example of eroding autonomy and a cue that we are arriving too late.[7] In some instances, physicians have been awarded a limited license when applying to a new state after many years of specialty practice.

Declining autonomy may well be associated with the changing client-provider relationship. For nurses that relationship is further challenged by a U.S. Supreme Court decision of May 1994.[8] In that opinion, the court creates the potential for any nurse who supervises assistive personnel to be considered management. This robs nurses of their employee protections and of the autonomy that has enabled them to be patient advocates first and employees second. These critical incidents provide beginning evidence to cause us to rethink or at least reinterpret our traditional definition of professionalism.

A second point of debate is associated with the uniqueness of the services provided by professionals. The service of any group of providers must be timely, relevant, and offered with an appreciation of what each discipline can contribute. Resistance to change and refusal to move with the times is not only counterproductive but a violation of the public trust. Examples abound as professionals strain to protect their turf. The very public and negative response of the American Medical Association to the role of nurses as primary care providers is one instance.[9] In contrast, the Health Care Financing Administration (HCFA) and the Joint Commission on Accreditation of Health Care Organizations (JCAHO) have issued new definitions of who may belong to the professional staff organization in their accredited or approved sites to allow the membership of a broad range of providers. In another instance, the Canadian government in Ontario has moved to a new

strategy of licensure that is specific about what each provider cannot do, as opposed to what they can do.[10] Such an approach should allow the boundaries between professions to be more flexible, and service to be more responsive to the moment and the needs of the consumer.

The stereotype of idealized professionals who are guaranteed economic security by the public in exchange for a lifetime of dedicated service to their work may also become a rarity. This does not makes these individuals any less, but only a product of their times. First, economic security is a relative term and open to a range of definitions. No group will be guaranteed income, most especially those in the health care field, as we move into models of managed care and providers as employees more commonly than as entrepreneurs. Perhaps even more telling is the trend for members of the American workforce to demand more personal and private time. More Americans are also enjoying the opportunity to change careers or at least enjoy some variety in their work life. Midlife and later-life career changes are not rare, and the professions are not immune to these trends.

Despite the prestige of professionalism, many other myths that were traditionally held are fading. For instance, collective bargaining, unionism, and strikes, once seen as the antithesis of professionalism, have been gradually accepted as legitimate activities by professionals who are employed. Physicians, nurses, teachers, social workers, and others have chosen that route as the only means left to gain certain concessions from employers. Obviously, the very fact that more professionals are employed, and thus lack a degree of autonomy, has precipitated this change.

In addition, there is an increasing tendency to use the term *professional* in another context to describe one who has an assured competence in a particular field or occupation, such as a hairdresser, or someone who participates in an activity for pay as opposed to an amateur—a musician, artist, or baseball player. It is particularly interesting to note the changes in dictionary definitions over the years to include the last two concepts. Looking at it in the "pure" sense, however, the idea of professionalism has been called the most important and powerful in the belief system of nursing. But this ideology does not seem to provide all nurses with universal beliefs and ideals about the profession. Nurses themselves do not hold a common concept of professionalism. The autonomy that lies at the core of professionalism was of little concern to a sizable minority of nurses in a survey of 323 RNs. Those most valuing autonomy completed their initial nursing in college-based programs, held more recent licenses, and verbally committed to long-term career plans.[11]

In a scholarly but personalized treatise on her beliefs about nursing, Margretta Styles introduces new and challenging thoughts about professionalism. One provocative point is that professionalism is not, as perceived, rooted in a two-party arrangement between the professional and the client. Because today professions are practiced predominantly in some type of institutional setting, there are other factors to consider, such as multiple client systems. Faculty members, for instance, may have as clients students, the university, the health care agency, and the patient, to all of whom they have some accountability.[12] (What if their demands conflict?)

Styles' key point is that nurses should not set their sights on an external ideal—professionalism—and on externally applied qualifications, but rather should compete with themselves to be the best they can in accomplishing goals set by themselves—"self-actualized professionals forming an actualized profession." She summarizes the concept that she calls *professionhood:* "Our intent that nursing become its utmost and that we as nurses become our utmost would be better served by a set of internal beliefs about nursing than a set of external criteria about professions."[13]

Professionalism, Styles maintains, emphasizes the *composite character of the profession* and "allows us to lose ourselves in the crowd; it permits the illusion of an 'I-they' relationship; it even encourages a nonproductive or counterproductive range of responses from passivism,

escapism, and blamism. On the other hand, professionhood [focusing on the characteristics of the individual]…forces us to pay attention to our own image as the dominant figure in the mirror of nursing. It recognizes that the professionalism of nursing will be achieved only through the professionhood of its members."[14]

Therefore, we return again to the basic ingredient of professionalism—the individual nurse. A scathing indictment of nurses who "want the name but not the game" unfortunately still has validity today.

> Too small a percentage of nurses have "bought" professionalism as a way of life. The larger segment "mouth" the philosophy, go through the outward rituals, all the while digging deeper ruts from which to be extracted later by another "concerned" generation of truly professional nurses. These are the nurses who find status in the status quo. They are not progressive; they have just transferred their hard-core traditionalism to other settings, and labeled it progress. These are the nurses who demand professional recognition from others, but are reluctant to assume professional responsibilities. They may get caught up in the intellectual ferment around them, but they are not seriously engaged in the professional dialogue. They may be troubled about nursing's professional role, but for self-serving reasons. To the observer, there is serious imbalance between their professional commitment and their personal ambitions. They court professionalism but balk at the price. They command higher salaries, but avoid spending their own money on professional growth…if they can use someone else's, namely, their employer's or the government's. Professionalism as a way of life implies responsibility and commitment.[15]

It should be noted that there are those who feel that, by accepting other American professions as its standard, nursing has deprived itself of its unique identity—that once nurses did not doubt that they were professionals and have since allowed themselves to be intimidated.[16]

The Nature of Nursing: Some Definitions

In *Notes on Nursing: What It Is and What It Is Not,* Florence Nightingale states in the most basic terms that nursing is to "put the patient in the best condition for nature to act upon him."[17]

Since that time, a number of other definitions have evolved, but the emphasis on care has not diminished, even in the scientific era. Definitions of nursing vary according to the philosophy of an individual or group, and interpretations of roles and functions vary accordingly. Many have become classics.

A definition used by nurses internationally is that of Virginia Henderson, a distinguished American nursing educator and writer.

> **The unique function of the nurse is to assist the individual, sick or well, in the performance of those activities contributing to health or its recovery (or to peaceful death) that he would perform unaided if he had the necessary strength, will or knowledge. And to do this in such a way as to help gain independence as rapidly as possible. This aspect of her work, this part of her function, she initiates and controls; of this she is master. In addition she helps the patient to carry out the therapeutic plan as initiated by the physician. She also, as a member of a medical team, helps other members, as they in turn help her, to plan and carry out the total program whether it be for the improvement of health, or the recovery from illness or support in death....[18]**

Many other of today's nursing leaders hold similar concepts, worded somewhat differently or expanded into other configurations. Schlotfeldt states:

> **Nursing is an essential service to all of mankind. That service can be succinctly described in terms of its focus, goal, jurisdiction, and outcomes as that of assessing and enhancing the general health status, health assets, and health potentials of all human beings. It is a service provided for persons who are essentially well, those who are infirm, ill, or disabled, those who are developing, and those who are declining. Nurses serve all people—sometimes individuals and sometimes collectives. They appropriately provide primary, episodic, and long-term care and, as professionals, are independently accountable for the execution and consequences of all nursing services.[19]**

In the ANA position paper of 1965, the terms *care, cure,* and *coordination* were used as part of a definition of *professional practice* (see Chap. 12), and this phrase has been used numerous times, with individual interpretation of the components.

As nurses expanded their functions into the new nurse practitioner role, *cure* acquired a different meaning for some nurses, as management of the patient's care, which includes aspects of what has been medical diagnosis and treatment. Some nurses, like Rogers, feel that such medical (not nursing) diagnosis and treatment diminishes the role of the nurse as a nurse. (The same opponents also usually reject the term *nurse practitioner* or *NP*.) However, Ford, a pioneer of the NP movement, immediately responding, called this "semantic roulette" and added, "I'm not so concerned about the words. I'm convinced that nursing can take on that level of accountability of professional practice that involves the consumer in decision-making in his care and also demands sophisticated clinical judgment to determine levels of illness and wellness and design a plan of management."[20] Indeed the nurse practitioner role represents a very appropriate readjustment of the boundaries between medicine and nursing.

Coordination and integration of the therapeutic regimen have historically been the province of nursing. We did it in the home and in the community within our early models of practice, and took these traditions into hospitals. Our twenty-four-hour presence and holistic philosophy suited us well to this responsibility. Though proposed with new prominence in case management models, active coordination on behalf of our patients has always been a nursing hallmark and is more critical today as nurses are often the only human link between patients and an intimidating experience in the health care delivery system.

Care is also translated in a number of ways, sometimes as a physical activity, such as in giving care, but it is considered by nursing experts as much more. The concept has been given considerable attention in the last several years, with research exploring the meaning and entire curricula based on related theory. Watson, who has written extensively on caring, says: "Caring is a normal ideal that guides and directs human actions, not just as a means but a human end in and of itself that is of intrinsic value to human civilization…human caring values and actions contribute to the health and healing of individuals."[21] Caring is also seen as invisible or hidden, and therefore often undervalued. Says Roberts, "It is necessary that we 'uncover' more of the characteristics of this caring practice, so that it can be recognized, rewarded, and taught to students of nursing."[22] In a much praised book that presents an analysis of expert nursing, based on vivid examples of excellence in actual nursing practice, Benner remarks on "the nature of the power associated with the caring provided by the nurses" and concludes: "One thing is clear: Almost no intervention will work if the nurse-patient relationship is not based on mutual respect and genuine caring."[23]

One concern that has been voiced about emphasizing caring as a major part of nursing is that people will revert to the old notion that nursing does not require intelligence—just love. Therefore, while the NCNIP nursing image campaign of 1990 emphasized caring, posters also carried the tag line, "If caring were enough, anyone could be a nurse." The other side of the coin is presented by a distinguished historian, who contends that nursing's problem is being "ordered to care" in a society that refuses to value caring.[24]

Although, over the years, nursing has been defined according to the functions of nurses or the clinical fields in which they practice, or the specific job titles they may hold, there is a thread running throughout the definitions that indicates that the focus of nursing is the health of whole human beings in interaction with their environment—a wholistic, humanistic focus that is also identified with caring. (The term *wholistic* seems to have been coined to refer to care related to the "whole" patient, physical and psychosocial. *Holistic* once referred to paranormal healing, an aspect of which is described by Dolores Krieger in the nursing literature. However, usage is not consistent and *holistic* is used almost always now in the sense of *wholistic*.)

An extremely significant step in the definition of nursing occurred in 1980 when ANA published *Nursing: A Social Policy Statement.* The work of a task force appointed by its Congress for Nursing Practice, the purpose was to answer the question, "What is nursing?" The introduction stated: "Trends well underway in nursing must now be reflected in a contemporary delineation of the nature and scope of nursing practice and a description of the characteristics of specialization in nursing…. This delineation of the nature and scope of nursing practice is tailored to the diversity, openness, and transition characteristic of the present, actual range of nursing practice."[25]

The definition was intended to maintain the historical orientation of the Nightingale and Henderson definitions, as well as reflecting the influence of nursing theory that is a part of nursing's evolution:

Nursing is the diagnosis and treatment of human responses to actual or potential health problems.

At this writing, *Nursing: A Social Policy Statement* is under revision. It is anticipated that the definition of nursing will be adjusted to reinforce the perspective outlined in ANA's 1987 *Scope of Nursing Practice.*[26] The definition in that document reads:

Nursing is the diagnosis and treatment of human responses to health and illness.

This definition makes it clear that nursing is not limited to a problem-focused orientation. The change is subtle, but significant.

The phenomena or areas of human responses of interest to nurses may be found in individuals, families, groups, or communities. The following examples, included to illustrate the variety of situations, are not intended to be inclusive, or to propose any sort of labels for these situations:

- Self-care processes
- Physiologic and pathophysiologic processes in areas such as sleep, rest, respiration, circulation, reproduction, activity, nutrition, elimination, skin, sexuality, communication

- Comfort, pain, and discomfort
- Emotions related to experiences of health and illness
- Meanings ascribed to health and illness
- Decision making and ability to make choices
- Perceptual orientations such as self-image and control over one's body and environments
- Transition across the life span, such as birth, growth, development, and death
- Affiliation relationships, including freedom from oppression and abuse
- Environmental systems

The nurse can determine where there is a valid indication for nursing intervention through various assessment techniques. Diagnosis is seen as a beginning effort to conceptualize and name a perceived difficulty, and nurses use theory in the form of concepts, principles, and processes to understand these phenomena within the domain of nursing practice. The aims of nursing actions are to ameliorate, improve, or correct the problems and are intended to produce beneficial effects in relation to identified responses.

Another component of the definition was the scope of nursing practice: "the contents of the nursing segment of health care." It was seen as having four defining characteristics:

- Boundary—an external boundary that expands outward in response to changing needs, demands, and capacities of society.
- Intersections—interprofessional interfacings that are meeting points at which nursing extends its practice into the domains of other professions.
- Core—the basis of nursing care—"the phenomena of concern to nurses are human responses to actual or potential health problems."
- Dimensions—characteristics that fall within and further describe the scope of nursing, such as philosophy and ethics that guide nurses; responsibilities, func-

tions, roles, and skills that characterize their work.[27]

It was also noted that all nurses are responsible for including preventive nursing in their practice, that nurses provide care across the life span and in a variety of settings, and that they are ethically and legally accountable for actions taken in practice or delegated.

In 1980, *Nursing: A Social Policy Statement* described what we now call advanced practice as specialty practice. In fact, it is becoming evident that very few nurses, even those with only the first nursing credential and no advanced educational preparation, remain generalists. This is a natural response to a growing knowledge base. So, although specialization still characterizes advanced practice, the more critical characteristic is the complexity of the clinical decisions that are made, leadership, the ability to operate within complex organizations, and expanded practice competencies. Advanced practice is an umbrella term that includes the practice roles of the clinical nurse specialist, nurse practitioner, nurse-midwife, and nurse anesthetist. Advanced practice is characterized by specialization, but specialization is not exclusive to advanced practice.

A separate section on specialization, which was called a mark of the advancement of the nursing profession, stated:

> **Specialization in nursing practice assists in clarifying, revising and strengthening existing practice. It also permits new applications of knowledge and refined nursing practice to flow from the specialist to the generalist in nursing practice and graduate to basic education, thus ensuring progress in the general practice in nursing.[28]**

Criteria for specialists in nursing practice, roles, and functions were delineated.

The social policy statement was intended to "assist nurses in conceptualizing their practice; to provide direction to educators, administrators and researchers within nursing; and to inform other health professionals, legislators, funding bodies, and the public about nursing's contribution to health care."[29]

Despite its somewhat obscure language at certain points (professions do have their own private jargon that, incidentally, can shut out others), which made it less than totally understandable to some nurses, much less nonnurses, the social policy statement is generally considered another major step in defining contemporary nursing and formalizing our contract with the public.

Nursing Functions

Nursing functions can be described in broad or specific terms. For instance, classically, the common elements have included maintaining or restoring normal life function; observing and reporting signs of actual or potential change in a patient's status; assessing his or her physical and emotional state and immediate environment; formulating and carrying out a plan for the provision of nursing care consistent with a medical regimen, including administration of medications and treatments and interpretation of treatment and rehabilitative regimens; counseling families in relation to other health-related services; and teaching. Some of these are referred to in the social policy statement.

Of course, some nurses (and administrators) still see at least some nurses more as managers of nursing care than as face-to-face clinical practitioners—in other words, responsible for nursing care, supervising and coordinating the work of others, but not personally giving care. This issue always emerges with nursing shortages, and now with higher salaries. The idea that nurses are too expensive workers to give bedside care assumes that patients don't need expert care—clearly a fallacy in these times.

In defining functions that should be common to all nurses, Schlotfeldt accurately identifies the following:

1. Interviewing to obtain accurate health histories.
2. Examining, with use of all senses and technological aids, to ascertain the health status of persons served.
3. Evaluating to draw valid inferences concerning individuals' health assets and potentials.
4. Referring to physicians and dentists those persons whose health status indicates the need for differential diagnoses and the institution of therapies.
5. Referring to other helping professionals those persons who need assistance with problems that fall within the province of clergyman, social workers, homemakers, lawyers, and others.
6. Caring for persons during periods of their dependence, to include:
   a. Compensating for deficits of those unable to maintain normal functions and to execute their prescribed therapies
   b. Sustaining and supporting persons while reinforcing the natural, developmental, and reparative processes available to human beings in their quest for wholeness, function, comfort, and self-fulfillment
   c. Teaching and guiding persons in their pursuit of optimal wellness
   d. Motivating persons toward active, knowledgeable involvement in seeking health and in executing their needed therapies
7. Collaborating with other health professionals and with persons served in planning and executing programs of health care and diagnostic and treatment services.
8. Evaluating in concert with consumers, other providers, and policy makers the efficacy of the health care system and planning for its continuous improvement.[30]

The degree of expertise with which a nurse carries out these functions depends on his or her level of knowledge and skills, but the profession has the responsibility of setting standards for its practitioners. In its 1991 *Standards of Clinical Nursing Practice*, the ANA incorporated and ordered standards in a nursing process sequence.[31] These standards serve as the basis for specialty standards as they are developed or updated.

The Nursing Process

Yura and Walsh state that the term *nursing process* was not prevalent in the nursing literature until the mid-1960s, with limited mention in the 1950s.[32] Orlando was one of the earliest authors to use the term, but it was slow to be adopted. In the next few years, models of the activities in which nurses engaged were developed, and in 1967, a faculty group at the Catholic University of America specifically identified the phases of the nursing process as assessing, planning, implementing, and evaluating. The nursing process is described as "an orderly, systematic manner of determining the client's health status, specifying problems defined as alterations in human need fulfillment, making plans to solve them, initiating and implementing the plan, and evaluating the extent to which the plan was effective in promoting optimum wellness and resolving the problems identified."[33] In fact, the nursing process adheres to the steps in logical thinking or problem solving. The fact that it is used in nursing has gained it the label of the nursing process.

At this point, there is considerable information in the nursing literature about the use of the nursing process, and many schools of nursing use it as a framework for teaching. However, there are those who feel that other approaches are more suitable to today's complex care. More specifically, we are not proposing the abandonment of logical thought, but to incorporate in our educational systems and practice the most cutting edge of cognitive techniques. There is promise of great gain from incorporating some recent work on critical thinking, diagnostic reasoning, and skill acquisition.[34, 35]

Nursing Diagnosis

The ability to make a *nursing* diagnosis and to prescribe *nursing* actions is basic to the development of nursing science. Nursing diagnosis is the title given to the act of identifying a problem and labeling it.

A diagnostic taxonomy (a set of classifications that are ordered and arranged on the basis of a single principle or set of principles) has been in the development stage since 1973. It is developing currently under the direction of the North American Nursing Diagnosis Association (NANDA) and may serve as a major communication tool among nurses. It could also facilitate public understanding of what nurses do; just as physicians can pinpoint what they do in relation to treating diseases, nurses can point out nursing diagnosis as the patient problems they try to resolve. However, interesting developments have occurred in recent years, with some argument about the usefulness and appropriateness of nursing diagnosis either as a concept or in practical application.[36]

Others have expressed concern about the need for validation of nursing diagnosis. Nevertheless, there is considerable sophisticated study about its various dimensions.[37]

In the late 1980s, the ANA initiated an era dedicated to recognition of the work nurses do as reflected in their classification systems. A formal appeal to the World Health Organization to incorporate the NANDA system into the next revision of the International Classification of Diseases (ICD) was rejected on the basis that the taxonomy was not internationally useful or relevant. Simultaneously the ANA became responsive to several other classification systems for nursing, and was successful in having all of them accepted for incorporation into the National Library of Medicine's database; these include the NANDA system, Bulechek and McCloskey's classification of nursing interventions, and the Omaha and Saba systems for home care. Work to increase the international usefulness of nursing diagnosis currently continues under the auspices of the International Council of Nurses (ICN).[38]

It will remain to be seen whether the nursing diagnosis movement has been a strategy to bring us to maturity as a profession, or a sign of our maturity. The trends in health care restructuring move us toward interdisciplinary practice. Should our language also reflect a unity of practice?

Nursing Theories, Concepts, and Models

As nursing has developed in professionalism, nursing scholars have developed theories of nursing, and the science of nursing is coming of age. A theoretical base of practice defines nursing's uniqueness; that is, it has a science of its own and is not simply an extension of another profession. In scientific inquiry, observations of seemingly unrelated phenomena are organized into intelligible systems that show relationships among the phenomena and a linking of truths. Nursing research describes, understands, and predicts the life process of humans, supporting the probability that nursing can intervene effectively to promote the maximum health of the well and ill as individuals and social groups. Nursing theory is the umbrella encompassing the concepts. To put it another way, nursing theory is an internally consistent set of interrelated concepts linked to form propositions. These propositions, or relational statements, specify relationships among the variables derived from the concepts and represent a systematic view of phenomena of interest to nursing.

The shift in nursing education from the practice setting of the hospital to the academic setting of the university brought with it a keen interest in identifying and developing a scientific body of knowledge unique to nursing. Theories were sought and formulated that would distinguish nursing, first, from medicine, whose models of disease and dysfunction historically had dominated nursing education and practice; and second, from the common caretaking principles and practices of helping, protecting, and mothering found in the lay public. Without research and theory building, nursing scholars argued, nursing would be unable to carve out a role for itself in the future health care system, and would thus allow itself to be defined, instructed, and controlled by other disciplines.

Although the 1950s and 1960s witnessed a proliferation of nursing concepts and theories, the question of a body of knowledge specific to nursing probably began with Florence Nightingale.[39] Among her other achievements, she identified the relationship between patient and environment as a major focus for nursing intervention and provided "hints" that would guide nurses in providing comfort, speeding recovery, and preventing disease. Like theories, her hints were derived from systematic observation of patients and their responses and, just as theory is used in education today, Nightingale submitted that by using these hints, nurses could teach themselves. While her work was groundbreaking for nursing science, the immaturity and transitional nature of nursing at that point in history is evident in her reference to the importance of precise observations, on the one hand, and to "common sense," for which she had no clarifying definition, on the other. Accordingly, she explicitly distinguished nursing knowledge from medical knowledge "which everyone ought to have." Nevertheless, the seeds were sown for the development of a science of nursing that began to flower over 100 years later.

The question of the uniqueness of nursing knowledge continues to be a thorny issue among nursing theorists, particularly because nursing is said to "borrow" so much of its knowledge from other disciplines. While many nursing scholars find this excessive borrowing troublesome as they seek to identify what is unique to nursing, others argue that the uniqueness of nursing lies in its very reliance on many disciplines—that in fact, *because* it synthesizes knowledge from so many disciplines, nursing provides a more comprehensive, holistic approach to patient care than any of the other health professions.

Theory building in nursing takes several forms and has several purposes. Midlevel theory, for example, has as its major goal the improvement of the technology of nursing, such as the discovery of the most effective procedures for educating clients, managing postsurgical patients, or helping families to deal with death and dying. Middle-range research is highly significant in developing a body of specialized knowledge in nursing. Grand theory, in comparison, takes a more all-encompassing view of nursing, a "world view" that attempts to explain and define nursing—what it is, what it does, why it is important, how if differs from other health professions—and exposes to critical examination such concepts as *patient, nurse, illness, health, support, care*, and *comfort*. A number of grand theories have been proposed to guide nursing research, education, and practice.

The *behavioral system model* is generally credited to Dorothy Johnson. This theory views nursing's client as one or more behavioral systems in interaction with the environment. Nursing's goal of action is to maintain or restore the balance and stability of the person's behavioral system or to help the person achieve a more optimum level of functioning (balance) when this is possible and desirable.

> Starting with nursing's traditional concern for the person who is ill, we have come to conceive of nursing's specific contribution to patient welfare as that of fostering efficient and effective behavioral functioning in the patient to prevent illness, and during and following illness.[40]

The *adaptation model* developed by Sister Callista Roy conceives of the person in constant interaction with a changing environment, to which the person must adapt. The person's adaptation is a function of the stimuli to which one is exposed and the adaptation level: the human adaptation level is such that it comprises a zone that indicates the range of stimulation that will lead to a positive response. (If the stimulus is within the zone, the person responds positively. If, however, the stimulus is outside the zone, the person cannot make a positive response.) Humans have four modes of adaptation: physiological needs, self-concept, role function, and interdependence relations. After plotting the point on the health-illness continuum where the patient currently rests, evaluating the factors that have influence, and judging the effectiveness of coping mechanisms, the nurse changes the person's response potential by bringing the stimuli into a zone where positive response is possible.

> All nursing activity will be aimed at promoting man's adaptation in his physiological needs, his self-concept, his role function and his interdependence relations during health and illness.[41]

Martha Rogers' *Science of Unitary Man* includes a complex series of principles: helicy, resonancy, and complementarity, called *principles of homeodynamics*. Rogers depicts humans holistically, as greater than the sum of their parts and moving through time and space as an integral part of an expanding universe, from the past to the future, which implies human beings' movement toward potential states of maximum well-being.

> Nursing aims to assist people in achieving their maximum health potential. Maintenance and promotion of health, prevention of disease, nursing diagnosis, intervention and rehabilitation encompass the scope of nursing's goals.[42]

The *self-care theory of nursing*, formulated by Dorothea Orem, is constituted from three related theories: self-care, self-care deficit, and nursing systems. Each person has need for the provision and management of self-care actions on a continuous basis in order to sustain life and health or to recover from disease or injury. When individuals' self-care agency (resources) is not adequate to their requirement or the requirements of their dependents (Orem extends the theory to address larger systems as family and community), a self-care deficit is present. The self-care deficit is the target of the nursing system. The nursing role is designed as wholly or partially compensatory, or supportive-educative as dictated by the agency available to the patient.

> Nursing is perhaps best described as giving of direct assistance to a person, as required, because of the person's specific inabilities in self-care resulting from a situation of personal health. Care as required may be continuous or periodic. Self-care means the care which all persons require each day. It is the personal care

which adults give to themselves, including attention to ordinary health requirements, and the following of the medical directive of their physicians.[43]

Myra Levine lists four conservation *principles of nursing* that have as a postulate the unity and integrity of the individual. Nursing intervention is based on the principles of conservation of energy, structural integrity, personal integrity, and social integrity. Levine believes that the holistic approach to nursing care depends upon recognition of the integrated response of the individual arising from the internal environment and the interaction that occurs with the external environment.

> Nursing intervention means that the nurse interposes her skill and knowledge into the course of events that affects the patient…. When nursing intervention influences the adaptation favorably, or toward renewed social well-being, then the nurse is acting in a therapeutic sense. When the nursing intervention cannot alter the course of the adaptation—when her best efforts can only maintain the status quo or fail to halt a downward course—then the nurse is acting in a supportive sense.[44]

Betty Neuman's systems model is influenced by Gestalt theory, stress, and levels of prevention. The model can be visualized as a central core of survival factors surrounded by concentric rings that are bounded by a line of resistance, a normal line of defense, and a flexible line of defense. The work of nursing is to identify stressors and assist individuals to respond by strengthening their normal and flexible lines of defense. Neuman differentiates primary, secondary, and tertiary prevention as it relates to nursing intervention.

> The model is based on an individual's relationship to stress—his reaction to stress and factors of restitution—and is thought of as dynamic in nature…that all parts are intimately interrelated and interdependent (and) emphasis is placed on the total organization of the "field."[45]

There remains a whole school of theorists who contribute a rich and unique philosophical orientation to the science of nursing. Their raison d'être, or reason for being, is "caring." This theme first evolved from the work of Madeleine Leininger and has grown to include Jean Watson and Patricia Benner.[46] These phenomenological theorists sensitize us to the humanistic dimension of caring which can only be effectively practiced interpersonally. Watson has extended her theory and applied it to the teacher-learner relationship. She describes growing competency to the point at which the student becomes colleague to faculty. This progressive growth in some aspects is reminiscent of Benner's concept of skill acquisition where practitioners of nursing move from novice to expert.

Finally, there are two pioneers who have profoundly shaped nursing with their work, but are not usually described as theorists. Virginia Henderson has been internationally credited with providing a major philosophical orientation for nursing. (Her definition has been included at greater length earlier in this chapter.) In a complementary-supplementary approach to practice, Henderson proposes that the nurse acts in the patients' behalf to do those things that they would do for themselves had they the strength, knowledge, or willingness to do so. She focuses on fourteen fundamental needs that correspond closely to Maslow's hierarchy. The influence of her work is clearly seen in the theoretical systems of Orem.[47]

Lydia Hall stressed the autonomous function of nurses, and ultimately seeded the ideas on which primary nursing is based. She contended that illness and rehabilitation are to be viewed as learning experiences in which the nurse's function is to guide and teach the patient through personal care giving. Her targets were adult patients who had passed the acute phase of illness. She identified three interlocking aspects of the nursing role: therapeutic use of self (core), the treatment regimen within the health care team (cure), and nurturing and intimate bodily care (care). Her greatest contribution was the actual implementation of her orientation to nursing in the Loeb Center at Montefiore Hospital in the Bronx, New York.[48]

The main concepts upon which these and other nursing theories are based are *person, nurse, health*, and *environment*. Both Rogers and Levine, for example, use *person* as the organizing principle of their theories: Rogers views person in the entirety interacting with the environment, while Levine focuses on the various components of structural, personal, and social integrity. Nurse-centered theories, on the other hand, take the nurse's actions and roles as their main theme but, like person-centered theories, vary in interpretation of the concept. Thus for Orem, the nurse is a substitute for the patient in the performance of self-care, while for Hall, the nurse is a teacher who assists the patient in making the illness or disability a learning experience. Considerable effort has been made recently in clarifying Orem's concepts, particularly that of self-care agency. The interplay between research and Orem's theory has led to operational measures of Orem's conceptualizations. This will lead to further research and development of nursing knowledge based on her theory.

Johnson's theory typifies those centered on health, which she views as a state of equilibrium that the nurse assists the patient to maintain. Roy also endorses a health-focused model but sees health as a continuum from wellness to illness. Recently an interest has emerged in developing the concept of environment. Few nurse theorists, with the exception of Nightingale, have elaborated on this concept. In developing nursing science and knowledge, nurses may have to be more aware of their client's context and take into account the larger social world in their analysis.

Most grand theories, including the ones presented here, do not begin with observation of empirical phenomena (what nursing is) but rather from a philosophical position on what nursing should be in the best of all possible worlds to be most effective or therapeutic. As such, they contain a significant value component that profoundly influences the development, acceptance, and utility of each theory. But, philosophical unity at some level is essential for the development of the science. Theory is the means to the end but often tells us very little about the end itself. Nursing's diversity demands a wide range of theoretical orientations to allow each of us to choose what is most comfortable. Restated, science builds from the foundation of philosophy. Since philosophy is abstract, it needs the concepts and relations of theory to be operationalized. Under each grand theory there is a philosophy, and midrange theory can be traced to grand theories that lend philosophical underpinnings. Careful analysis convinces us that there is more consensus about what nursing hopes to accomplish than ever before.

As a complement, other theorists develop nursing knowledge through scientific research, hypothesis testing, and empirical observation of what is. Leininger, for example, advocates the cross-cultural comparison of "caring" phenomena in which recurring themes and patterns, which are the essence of nursing as currently practiced, begin to "fall out" and allow us to construct a science of nursing, or, in Leininger's terms, a "science of caring."[49] Benner uses similar techniques to construct her levels of skill acquisition.

Certainly, there is merit to both approaches. From the scientific perspective, nursing is an observational science, sharing with astronomy, zoology, anthropology, medicine, public health, and others a method for formulating its theories by chronicling and analyzing systematic observations. Unlike these other disciplines, however, nursing is still in the early stages of developing its taxonomy. Thus, from medical theory, we have a sophisticated set of classifications for describing disease, but we do not as yet have a very well-developed set of categories for describing *persons* in need of nursing services (the focus of nursing) in terms of their responses to health and illness and developmental processes. The closest nursing has come to a taxonomy for the classification and organization of responses to health and illness of interest to nursing is the classification of nursing diagnoses, as mentioned previously. The purpose of developing such a compilation of diagnostic categories is to assist in clearly defining the body of knowledge for nursing, to provide a framework for research and to aid in the development of nursing science. All health sciences have much to gain by empirical observation of human responses to birth, death, illness, parenting, aging, stress, and other factors. Nursing, perhaps more than any other discipline, is in a position to observe and record these events and develop theories that shift clinical practice from being disease-oriented to patient-oriented.

However, the fact that most of the grand theories are based on the value orientations of the theorist rather than empirical observations does not mean that they are less functional or important for the development of nursing knowledge. Their value in generating new theories and hypotheses that are subsequently tested and refined in the real world of practice cannot be denied. In fact, theory does not even have to be scientific (capable of being refuted) to be useful. Historically, and even for some modern theorists, nursing has been guided by religious knowledge and theories that, while unscientific, may be very successful in providing a framework for effective clinical practice and education.

Debate about philosophies or values underlying nursing theories is currently occurring. The literature is replete with controversy about the two most significant competing philosophies: logical positivism and phenomenology. The arguments frequently center around which of these two approaches is intrinsically better for the progression of nursing knowledge and the development of insights into human responses in a variety of situations. Because different research traditions arise out of each philosophical stance, the debate is more than academic. In truth, both sets of values and many research traditions in nursing can only enhance nursing knowledge, allowing richness and diversity in the developing nursing theory and science.

Indeed, it is becoming increasingly common to hear that in its rigid adherence to the scientific method in generating theory, nursing is trading its birthright of intuitiveness and humanism. Styles specifically called for the reincorporation of human values and personal beliefs into nursing theory. Increasingly, Styles and her ancestor, Nightingale, each make a strong case for nursing knowledge and practice based on *both* ideology and scientific theory, but a comparison of their positions on this issue provides a telling commentary on the direction of nursing theory over the last century. Florence Nightingale stressed that for nurses to best meet the need of patients, they could not solely rely on good intentions: "if you cannot get the habit of observation one way or another, you had better give up being a nurse, for it is not your calling however kind and anxious you may be."[50] Over 100 years later, Styles calls on the nursing community to be guided by ideology as well as science, to work toward what we *should be* and to include in professionalization such themes as commitment, personal motivation, and self-actualization, as well as scientific discovery: "nursing, as a professional community, must have and hold a common, recitable ideology just as nations have their constitutional preambles and pledges of allegiance, fraternal societies have their oaths, religions have their creeds"[51] (unity of science based on philosophy).

Levels of theory such as grand, middle-range, and practice theory are linked together and inform each other. However, because of their level, middle-range theories are more testable and lend themselves to the development of research and eventually the incorporation of research-based changes into practice. The number of variables in middle-range theories is more limited, and the theory itself is more confined in scope. The establishment of the National Institute for Nursing Research (NINR) within the National Institutes of Health has encouraged the progress of middle-range theories to focus research on both the refinement of grand theories and the development of practice innovations grounded in theory-based research.

The growth of nursing diagnosis and nursing theories has been a major development in nursing in the last twenty years. Imperative now is continued and strengthened clinical research to develop and refine nursing theories that can serve as guides for nursing practice and as measurements of the extent to which nursing action attains its goals in terms of patient behavior.

Whether nursing emerges as a mature discipline as well as a profession in the next decade depends to a great extent on the direction that its theory building will take—for instance, constructing explanations of the relationship between nursing phenomena that can be tested against experience; developing its technology, policies, and procedures; clarifying its concepts and categories; and reconfirming its philosophy and ideological base. Ultimately, the most important test of any theory is its applicability and utility in clinical practice.

WHAT IS NURSING?

It can easily be seen that there may not be a single definition of nursing. Perhaps there never will be, since nursing is a multifaceted profession. This is one problem legislators have had in writing a nursing practice act, which is, after all, the legal definition of nursing. (These definitions, along with other aspects of licensure, are discussed in Chap. 20.) Nevertheless, at some point, every nurse has to decide what nursing is to him or her and how to interpret it to others.

This chapter, its references, and its bibliography may provide a basis for working out your own definition, but the final determination is yours.

REFERENCES

1. Schulman S: Basic functional roles in nursing: Mother surrogate and healer, in Jaco EG (ed): *Patients, Physicians and Illness: Behavioral Sciences and Medicine.* Glencoe, IL: Free Press, 1963.
2. National League for Nursing: *Patterns of Nursing Theories in Practice.* New York: The League, 1993.
3. Flexner A: Is social work a profession? *Proceedings of the National Conference of Charities and Correction.* New York: New York School of Philanthropy, 1915.
4. Beletz E: Professionalism—A license is not enough, in Chaska N (ed): *The Nursing Profession: Turning Points.* St Louis: Mosby, 1990.
5. Ibid, p 21.
6. American Nurses' Association: Valuation of nursing services: Payment for non-physician practitioners under Medicare. *A Report to the Board of Directors.* Kansas City: The Association, June 1991.
7. *National Council of State Boards of Nursing Position Paper on the Licensure of Advanced Nursing Practice.* Chicago: The Council, May 18, 1992.
8. ANA Disturbed by Supreme Court Decision on Nurses as Supervisors. *News Release.* Washington, DC: The American Nurses' Association, May 24, 1994.
9. O'Neill SP et al: APNs breaking down the barriers to provide primary care. *The Nursing Spectrum* 4–5, Feb 7, 1994.
10. What LNs and RNAs need to know about the proposed Health Professions Regulation Act. *College Communique* March 1991.
11. Schoen D: Nurses attitudes towards control over nursing practice. *Nurs Forum* 27:27–34, January–March 1992.
12. Styles M: *On nursing: Toward a new endowment.* St Louis: Mosby, 1982, pp 19–20.
13. Ibid, p 76.
14. Ibid, p 8.
15. Clarke A: Candidly speaking: On nursing forum and professionalism. *Nurs Forum* 7:12, 1968.
16. Parsons M: The profession in a class by itself. *Nurs Outlook* 6:270–275, November–December 1986.
17. Nightingale F: *Notes on Nursing.* London: Lippincott, facsimile of 1859 edition.
18. Henderson V: *ICN Basic Principles of Nursing Care.* London: International Council of Nurses, 1961. Expanded in Henderson V: *The Nature of Nursing.* New York: Macmillan, 1967.
19. Schlotfeldt R: The professional doctorate: Rationale and characteristics. *Nurs Outlook* 26:303, May 1978.
20. The nurse practitioner question. *Am J Nurs* 74:2188, December 1974.
21. Watson J: The moral failure of the patriarchy. *Nurs Outlook* 38:62–66, March–April 1990.

22. Roberts J: Uncovering hidden caring. *Nurs Outlook* 38:67–69, March–April 1990.
23. Benner P: Form novice to expert. Menlo Park, CA: Addison-Wesley, 1984.
24. Reverby S: *Ordered to Care: The Dilemma of American Nursing.* New York: Basic Books, 1987.
25. *Nursing: A Social Policy Statement*, Kansas City, MO: American Nurses' Association, 1980, p 1.
26. *The Scope of Nursing Practice.* Kansas City, MO: American Nurses' Association, 1987.
27. *Nursing: A Social Policy Statement*, op cit, pp 13–18.
28. Ibid, p 22.
29. Ibid, p 30.
30. Schlotfeldt, loc cit.
31. *Standards of Clinical Nursing Practice.* Kansas City MO: American Nurses' Association, 1991.
32. Yura H, Walsh M: *The Nursing Process,* 2d ed. New York: Appleton-Century-Crofts, 1973.
33. Yura H, Walsh M: *The Nursing Process: Assessing, Planning, Implementing, Evaluating.* Norwalk, CT: Appleton-Century-Crofts, 1988.
34. Lunney M: Divergent productive thinking and accuracy of nursing diagnoses. *Res Nurs Health Care* 15:303–311, 1992.
35. Miller M et al: Critical thinking in the nursing curriculum. *Nurs Health Care* 11:67–73, February 1990.
36. Bruckhorst B et al: Who's using nursing diagnosis? *Am J Nurs* 89:267–268, February 1989.
37. O'Hearn C: Nursing diagnosis: A phenomenological structural description and multidimensional taxonomy or typological redefinition, in Chaska N (ed): *The Nursing Profession: Turning Points.* St Louis: Mosby, 1990.
38. National Databases/Sets to Support Clinical Nursing Practice. *A Report to the Nursing Organization Liaison Forum.* Kansas City, MO: American Nurses' Association, November 1991.
39. Nightingale, loc cit.
40. Johnson DE: One conceptual model of nursing. Unpublished paper given at Vanderbilt University, 1968.
41. Roy C: *Introduction to Nursing: An Adaptation Model.* Englewood Cliffs, NJ: Prentice-Hall, 1976, p 8.
42. Rogers M: *Educational Revolution in Nursing.* New York: Macmillan, 1961, p 23.
43. Orem D: *Guides for Developing Curricula for the Education of Practical Nurses.* Washington, DC: Government Printing Office, 1959, pp 5–6.
44. Levine ME: *Introduction to Clinical Nursing.* Philadelphia: Davis, 1969, p 10.
45. Neuman B: The Betty Neuman Health Care System Model, in Riehl JP, Roy C: *Conceptual Models for Nursing Practice.* New York: Appleton-Century-Crofts, 1980.
46. Tomey AM: *Nursing Theorists and Their Work.* St. Louis: Mosby, 1989.
47. Henderson, loc cit.
48. Hall L: The Loeb Center for Nursing and Rehabilitation. *Int J Nurs Stud* 6:81–95, 1969.
49. Leininger M: Caring: A central focus of nursing and health care services. *Nurs Health Care* 1:135–143, October 1980.
50. Nightingale, op cit, p 63.
51. Styles, op cit, p 58.

Professional Ethics and the Nurse

CHAPTER 10

THE ETHICS OF ACCESS

Experts in health care and health policy generally agree that ethical decision making will be of increasing concern in the coming years, and access to health care is already a major problem. Most of these experts may look with pride at the new technology, surgery, and drugs that can prolong life, but they are also forced to look at the cost and, sometimes, simple unavailability. For instance, new technology has made possible heart, liver, and kidney transplants and new drugs that fight against organ rejection, but the organs are not readily available and surgery, aftercare, and drugs may run into the hundreds of thousands of dollars during a lifetime, if there even is an extended lifetime. Some people can afford it; health insurance covers others, at least partially, and still others get the attention of the media or powerful figures and receive donations and priority. What of the person who can do none of this? Should the public, through some sort of governmental funding pay for extraordinary treatment an individual can't afford? Or *is* it extraordinary? Under what circumstances should it be paid? Should age, potential quality of life, possibility of good outcome, ability of the individual and significant others to give proper follow-through care, or "worthiness" be considered? What of the simple primary care or any care that vast numbers of Americans cannot access? (See Chap. 7.) If we say everyone should have equal access in an era of limited resources that will probably never change, what other funding should be cut? Education? Environment? Housing? Social service? Transportation? Civil rights enforcement? Drug enforcement? Police? Defense? Not only is the decision not a simple one, it is highly political. Every one of the other areas that exists primarily through public funding is important one way or another to the public's well-being. Every legislator has one or more constituencies that demand attention to their needs or wishes. Therefore, it's not surprising that legislative action is slow in coming, seldom satisfactory, and, unfortunately, hardly in effect before it is evident that the action taken is not enough, too much, or already out of date. Moreover, the cost factor will undoubtedly increase, not decrease, and new, expensive technology continue to develop.

So what happens? Except in rare instances, limits are set by default. In the case of health care, silent or not so silent, rationing is, and has been, in effect. Surveys have been taken to determine how health care power figures feel about the access-to-care issue. In a large 1987 survey of key figures in health care,[1] the majority agreed that there *should* be an adequate quality of care for all citizens and at least a minimum level of access to health care for all, but they also anticipated that what *would be* was that money issues would drive the federal agenda on health care, offering at best minimum access. They also agreed that the most critical medical ethics issues in 1995 would be rationing of health care services, right-to-die issues, and allocation of organs for transplantation. In a later survey of health care administrators, the majority thought all health care recipients should receive the same quality of care, but contradicted themselves in other questions on access and equitable distribution of services. A consumer poll by the Yankelovich group a few years later showed 91 percent felt that *they* should get *maximum* care, but really were not knowledgeable about costs, what contributed to costs, or how maximum care for all could be achieved. In fact, most people now recognize that this would be impossible.

Unequal access to health care is not a new phenomenon, so its current visibility may be due to the unrelenting voices of advocates for the have-nots, the slight possibility of the public having more of a social conscience, or the simple fact that it is quite evident that there are many who do not receive even basic care, particularly children. Nevertheless visibility does not guarantee solutions. What standards should be used to determine who gets what? There has been considerable discussion about age as a criterion, especially in terms of prolonging the life of an elderly patient. In part, this is because a large percentage of Medicare funds is used for life-prolonging care in the last few months of an elderly patient's life. (The fact that such a person may not wish such care, but is given no choice, is another issue.) Clearly it is not easy to use age as an indicator, particularly because of changing demographics of the elderly.[2] However, the director of the Hastings Center suggested some background principles:

1. After a person has lived out a natural life span (late 70s or early 80s), medical care should no longer be oriented to resisting death.
2. Provision of medical care for those who have lived out a natural life span will be limited to the relief of suffering.
3. The existence of medical technologies capable of extending the lives of the elderly who have lived out a natural life span cre-

ates no presumption whatever that the technologies must be used for that purpose.[3]

There was considerable furor about this and similar statements by others, but Callahan argued that the moral problem was to "devise a plan to limit health care for the aged that is fair, humane, and sensitive to the special requirements and dignity of the aged."[4] (No one extended that argument to those who could pay with their own funds.) There were some arguments that probably the majority of the aged preferred such a plan; what they feared was helplessness, pain, disability, loss of mental alertness, that is, a deteriorating quality of life. Actually, there is some evidence that the suicide rate of the elderly is increasing; but also that this kind of rationing is already silently in effect as technology expands.

The entire issue of transplants is another ethical dilemma, even beyond the issue of access and cost. One physician posed some provocative questions:[5]

- Should three organs be used to save three lives or just one?
- When should single organs be kept for use at local centers instead of making clusters available for multiple transplants elsewhere?
- Should doctors, who have long been taught not to abandon a patient, consider the issue of equitable distribution of scarce resources?
- What risks to a living donor are acceptable?
- Under what circumstances should a donor give part of an irreplaceable organ like the liver?
- How old is too old for a donor?
- What are the limits on using a flawed organ as a temporary transplant until a healthy organ is found?

Other questions could be added:

- Should untried animal transplants be used on an infant such as Baby Fae? Or anyone?

- What about mechanical hearts or other such mechanical devices?[6]
- Even if these techniques or devices don't save the patient, is it worth it for the knowledge gained?
- Is it ethical for a mother to get pregnant on the chance that the baby's bone marrow might save its sister who has leukemia? (The baby obviously won't have a choice about being a donor.)
- Should an irrevocably damaged newborn such as an anencephalic be kept alive to "harvest" its organs to save another baby?[7]
- Is there anything wrong with using the tissue of aborted fetuses to implant in an adult with Parkinson's disease to improve his or her condition?[8]

These questions, all relating to real situations, do not necessarily call for a negative response. The point is that there *are* so many questions, seldom a clear-cut answer, and never an easy answer. Overall, putting aside legal ramifications, the health care provider simply acts according to his or her own moral beliefs, or sometimes, the needs or attitude of the health care institution. For instance, in a study on how people were selected for kidney transplants, the most important criteria were reported as medical benefit, prognosis, psychological stability, age, and willingness. Also considered were social value, unique moral duties (whether the life of another person or something equally important depends on the patient's survival), and disproportionate resources (whether the patient would require long or expensive treatment and support of patient's family, friends, and community). A large minority would consider ability to pay, and restrictions would be tighter if resources became scarcer. Neither race nor age was reported as a factor.[9] However, other studies of over 6,000 kidney transplant patients showed that white men were disproportionately receiving kidneys, twice as likely as blacks of either sex and a third more likely than white women. A number of explanations were offered, but physician attitude and cost factors were seen as major reasons for the discrepancy.[10] As is often the case, what is said and what is done is not always the same. Reports in 1993 also indicated that blacks and women had fewer heart bypasses, and that the death rate was higher for poor and poorly educated people regardless of race.[11]

What to do about these access issues? Many suggestions are made, and little agreement is reached. Some ask, "Can we any longer afford the moral price of inequity in health care?"[12] and maintain that although it might prove costly, a universal system of health insurance and government- and employer-based programs are the only answer. Others say we must set limits on new technology, if too costly.[13] Still others have simply concluded that overt, orderly rationing of health care is inevitable. Other aspects of this issue are discussed in Chap. 7: the 37 million uninsured; patient "dumping"; the pressure on employers and insurers to cut back on benefits; the health care institutions' battle to make a profit or even survive; the demands of consumers; and the ever escalating costs. However, still another factor is important: not only are many consumers more sophisticated (or have advocates who are) and insisting on high-quality care, they are also demanding their rightful part in decision making about their care and treatment. In addition, the strong possibility of health care reform will, over the period of its implementation, raise more ethical issues. As one nurse ethicist noted, "The real challenge is to design a reformed health care system that will protect and possibly enhance our most important health values while not ignoring other values important to human dignity and privacy."[14]

These access issues, like all ethical issues, are multifaceted and have no pat solutions, but nurses are finding that they are their business as much as anyone else's. In fact, in a 1994 ANA survey, nurses named rationing of care as the most pressing ethical issue nurses face today.[15] It is impossible to be a student or a nurse in today's health care settings and not be aware that some of these problems exist. Awareness is not enough. Just as it is important to understand the social and economic forces that affect health care, it is even more urgent to know about and think about, and make decisions about, the moral dilemmas to which nurses will inevitably be exposed. Access to care? Nurses have turned patients away from emergency rooms or given them superficial care when they have had no means of paying. Rationing of care? Everytime a unit is understaffed and it is impossible to give all patients all the care they need, within legal limits (usually) nurses decide who gets what when. In another study, nurse executives indicated that *their* most pressing ethical concern was allocation of scarce resources, including use of staff inappropriate to levels of patient acuity.[16] Transplanting organs from anencephalic newborns? Nurses care for those new babies and are often asked for advice by the family.[17] End of life decisions? This was the next highest ethical issue that nurses were concerned about, especially staff nurses, and will be discussed in some detail later and in Chap. 22.

OTHER ETHICAL DILEMMAS

Once, making ethical decisions in health care was probably not as simple as it appears in retrospect. But there were some givens: the physician was known to have the knowledge about the best course of treatment or action and was to be obeyed by the patient, the family, and certainly the nurse; there was a limit to that therapy, and when the heart stopped, the patient died; grossly malformed newborns and tiny prematures died too, with little expectation that they would live. The life span was considerably, shorter, but if someone was dying of "old age," that was considered a natural, unstoppable process, and usually the dying occurred at home. Now, consider some not uncommon examples of ethical dilemmas today:

- A fragile man in his eighties, riddled with cancer, is admitted to the hospital. When his heart stops, he is resuscitated and awakens with tubes in every orifice. He begs to be allowed to die, but is resuscitated again when his heart stops, and then is put on a respirator.

- A twenty-six-year-old quadriplegic woman with cerebral palsy has herself admitted to a hospital and then asks to be kept comfortable, but allowed to die by starvation because she finds life unbearable. The hospital force-feeds her.

- An eighty-five-year-old man with many illnesses has been fasting in a nursing home to hasten his death. His daughter supports his decision, and he dies in a few days.

- Two physicians terminate intravenous feedings on a comatose man, with the consent of the family. They are reported by nurses and criminally prosecuted.

- A baby is born with serious congenital defects, one of which requires immediate surgery in order to save the infant's life. The parents refuse permission because they believe that the child, if she survives, will not have a reasonable quality of life and they will not be able to care for her.

- Another baby with similar defects undergoes surgery, but the mother, an unwed teenager, cannot keep the child. It is in a public institution, requiring total care for all of its five years of life; the mother disappears.

- A depressed patient admitted to a mental hospital refuses electroshock therapy after several treatments because he thinks it will kill him even though he is improving with treatment. He cannot care for himself at home, and his wife cannot manage his erratic behavior. He is committed, under that state's laws, given the treatment, and recovers.

- A retarded fifteen-year-old boy in a county home refuses kidney dialysis because he fears it. No effort is made to relieve his anxiety, and others on the hospital's waiting list are moved forward into therapy. The boy dies.

- Two men on the same hospital unit have a cardiac arrest within several minutes of each other. The first to arrest is an alcoholic street person with various other conditions: the other is a businessman with a wife and four children. There is one cardiopulmonary resuscitation cart. The resident says, "First come, first served" and resuscitates the alcoholic; the businessman dies.

- A young couple with two boys decide that they can only afford one more child and want a girl. If amniocentesis shows a boy, the mother wants an abortion.

- A couple had not been advised that they are carriers of a hereditary disease. Two of their teenage children have it, and one does not. When the mother becomes pregnant again, she decides on an abortion, but both parents decide not to "spoil the children's lives" by telling them that they may later manifest the disease.

- A well-liked nurse with many serious family problems seems to be under the influence of drugs or alcohol when she is on duty. The nurses are concerned that she will injure a patient and assume most of her assignments of very sick patients. They want to give her a chance to "straighten out her life" rather than reporting her and having her lose her job and perhaps her license.

- An older respected physician in a renowned hospital has been making mistakes in surgery. The residents have been able to catch and/or repair them thus far, but the scrub nurse thinks that he ought to be prevented from operating. No physician will report him officially.

- A patient about to undergo surgery clearly does not understand the risks or the available alternatives. The nurse tells the physician, but he replies that he did explain, that patients seldom understand these explanations, and that the patient should be prepared for surgery.

- A patient with cancer is on an experimental drug. Although hospital policy states that the physician must get an informed consent before the drug is administered, the patient's very prestigious physician calls in and tells the nurse to start the drug because it is important to begin at once; he will be in later to get the consent. When the nurse hesitates, her supervisor tells her to go ahead.

If you were the nurse involved in any of these situations, what would you do? Whose rights are or might be violated? The patient's? The family's? The nurse's? The doctor's? Society's? Nobody's? How much would you be affected by your own moral beliefs? If your action was contrary to what the hospital administrators, the physicians involved, or even some of your colleagues thought best (for whatever reason), would you be willing to face the consequences? What if your concept of "right" collided with a legal ruling? What if the patient or family asked you to help them?

All the cases cited are real; a nurse somewhere faced one of these difficult situations (and probably others) and had to make a decision to act or not to act. How that decision was arrived at is the essence of ethics. As you read the sections on morality and the various theories of ethics, as well as the nursing code of ethics, consider the ethical problems given as examples, and note how your decisions depend on your ethical or, perhaps, moral beliefs.

MORALS AND ETHICS: A DIFFERENTIATION

There is a tendency to use the words *moral* and *ethical* interchangeably in the literature of the health professions. However, in the last few years, the need to differentiate between the two terms has become more evident, perhaps because the complexity of modern health care and the always-changing societal mores often create conflicting tensions in those who face a moral-ethical dilemma. (The term *ethics* will be used in this chapter, although *bioethics* is becoming popular in some of the literature. Frequently, *bioethics* seems to be used synonymously with *medical ethics*, and there are experts in the field of ethics who find its meaning unclear.) *Metaethics* "tries to discover reasons given for making a particular moral judgment. Do we say an act is 'right' because our society says so, or do we believe the act is right even if many members of the society do not agree?" What reasons are valid?[18]

Kohlberg, structuring a theory of moral development, used the term *stages* for individual phases of moral thinking. In the O, or Premoral, stage, the individual does not understand the rules or feel a sense of obligation to them, acting only to experience that which is pleasant (good) or avoiding that which is painful (bad). In the Preconventional Level, stages 1 and 2, the individual's moral reasoning is based on reward and punishment from those in authority. In the Conventional Level, stages 3 and 4, the expectations of the social group (family, community, nation) are supported and maintained. In the Postconventional Level, stages 5 and 6, the individual considers universal moral principles, which supersede the authority of groups. Kohlberg believes that most American adults function at stages 3 to 5, but moral maturity is gained at stage 6, when the individual makes up his or her own mind about what is right and wrong. Although the term *moral* is used in this analysis, there are those who interpret stage 6 as a "universal, ethical principle orientation" because:

> At this stage, morality is based on decisions of conscience, made in accordance with self-chosen principles of justice, which are comprehensive, universal, and consistent. These principles are abstract and ethical, rather than concrete moral rules.[19]

Although Kohlberg's theory is still used when discussing moral development, there is some disagreement with his approach, in part because:

1. Actual actions of the subjects in the real world were not studied. They were asked to respond to hypothetical situations.

2. The moral dilemmas presented were very limited, dealing with justice and fairness in terms of competition, property rights, right to life, and obligations.

3. His study was originally based on a sample of 50 males but assumes that both men and women develop in the same way.[20] Women were left at the third or fourth stage; men progressed to higher levels.

Gilligan[21] was particularly disturbed that Kohlberg did not acknowledge the concerns and experience of women in moral development. She carried out a study designed to clarify the nature of women's moral judgment as they faced a real moral dilemma of whether to continue or abort a pregnancy. Results showed that women do progress to the postconventional level, but that their moral judgment differs from that of men. For women, the worst problem was defined in terms of exercising care and avoiding hurt. The infliction of hurt was seen as selfish and immoral. "Women's moral judgment proceeded from initial concern for survival, to a focus on goodness, to a principled understanding of care."[22]

Taking the viewpoint that moral values are usually based on religious beliefs, but also agreeing that an individual's ethics are based on self-examination, Maurice and Warrick state:

> Ethical philosophy is the reflective analysis and evaluation of the goodness or badness of human conduct. Moral theology is the prescription decreed by divine authority regulating human conduct. Both ethics and morals indicate that goodness is that which leads to amity, wholesomeness, ease, peace, and wellbeing. Badness leads to the opposite. In short, goodness leads to happiness and order; badness to unhappiness and chaos. The difference, therefore, is the means to the end. Ethics deals with evaluation and responsibility whereas rules and obedience characterize morals.[23]

Churchill puts it more simply:

> Morality is generally defined as behavior according to custom or tradition. Ethics, by contrast, is the free, rational assessment of courses of action in relation to precepts, rules, conduct.... To be ethical a person must

take the additional step of exercising critical, rational judgment in his decisions.[24]

Noddings'[25] model, building on the work of Gilligan, is more recent, and has been given considerable attention in nursing. She centers her ideas on the value of care and caring, stressing that caring is a relationship, not a unilateral activity. "The choice to enter a relationship as one caring…is grounded in a vision that we hold of our best selves," our "ethical ideal."[26] One author sees Noddings' moral theory as a guide to transforming the nursing curriculum to prepare nurses as more than "applied scientists."[27]

The whole issue of ethics versus morals may seem to be a purely philosophical issue; however, given the differentiation described, the code of ethics of professional nurses may mandate action that goes beyond what their immediate associates see as necessary. It is also possible that individuals must struggle with what seems to be a conflict between ethical behavior and personal religious beliefs.

One Approach to Ethics: Theories

Curtin notes that not all health-care problems are ethical problems and gives the following characteristics of the latter: (1) they do not fall strictly within any one or all of the sciences; (2) they are inherently perplexing; (3) the answer reached will have profound relevance for several areas of human concern. She adds that some ethical problems are dilemmas, choices between equally undesirable alternatives. "A dilemma may not be solvable, but it is resolvable. Even though there is no right or wrong between two *equally* unfavorable actions, taking no action may be even worse than making the choice." However, a true dilemma is relatively rare because often, if there is adequate information and time, there are clearer guidelines for action.[28]

Three levels of decision making are described: (1) the immediate level, in which there is no time for reflection (the first deformed baby); (2) the intermediate level, in which there is some time for explanation and reflection (the individuals who want to die by fasting); and (3) the deliberate level, in which there is enough time to get information and to think and consult in order to make a rational decision (the parents with the hereditary disease). Curtin also indicates that the deliberate level of decision making is probably the most common, although people do not act in that manner because they find that difficult ethical decisions "are personally taxing, entail great responsibility and require a profound sensitivity to the human rights and values of others."[29]

The theories upon which ethical decisions are based are well described by Davis and Aroskar, two other noted nurse ethicists.[30] The *egoism* theory or position says that a decision is "right" because the doer or "agent," in this case the nurse, desires it; it is the most comfortable for that person, without consideration for how the decision might affect others. An example might be that the nurse simply prepares the patient for surgery, accepting the doctor's statement that the patient was given an adequate explanation.

The theory of *deontology* (formalism) asserts that rightness or wrongness must be considered in terms of its moral significance. *Act deontology* considers the agent's own moral values. *Rule deontology* suggests that there are rules or standards for judging morally, often a command by God. Thus, a nurse may oppose abortion because of either personal moral beliefs or religious beliefs. *Utilitarianism* defines right as the greatest good and the least amount of harm for the greatest number of people. For instance, deformed babies might be allowed to die rather than be a burden on society for many years.

More contemporary views have been offered by modern philosophers dissatisfied with the traditional choices. Frankena's *theory of obligation* focuses on the principle of beneficence and the principle of justice as equal treatment. However, the definition of these principles leads to some confusion. For instance, distributive justice is seen as treating people according to their needs. The difficulty of deciding which criterion to use can be illustrated by considering this theory in the case of the two men with cardiac arrest.

Rawl's theory deals with *justice as fairness*—the distribution of benefits (good) or harm (evil) to society. The agents are supposed to function under a "veil of ignorance," not considering or knowing particular facts about themselves or others, such as sex, personal characteristics, or social class. The two principles of justice are equal rights for everyone and the greatest benefit given to the least advantaged. With this reasoning, the retarded boy would take precedence over others for the kidney dialysis, and efforts would be made to persuade him into therapy.

The *ideal observer* theory proposed by Firth requires that a decision be made from a disinterested, dispassionate, consistent viewpoint, with full information available and consideration of future consequences. While this approach can theoretically be applied to any ethical situation, the probable impossibility of any one person being able to do so might necessitate the involvement of other people, perhaps an ethics committee.

These theories, which have been presented very briefly, are often complex and sometimes appear more philosophical than practical. However, they provide a framework for the study of ethical decision making. Such an analysis may help prepare you to deal better with real-life ethical situations.[31, 32]

CODES OF ETHICS

Another guide to ethical behavior is a professional code of ethics. In the last several years, ethical behavior has been increasingly a topic of discussion in almost every field—business, politics, law, and perhaps most of all, the health field. One symbol of this focus might be the new interest in codes of ethics. Codes of ethics, by whatever name, have been common in professions for some time. It is generally conceded that medicine was the first profession in the United States to adopt a code of ethics, but law,

pharmacy, and veterinary medicine were also early comers. However, in the last decade or so, one interesting phenomenon has occurred: ethics has become fashionable, and codes have been newly adopted by organizations representing business and industry.

Both business journals and the popular literature have been commenting on business and industry's burgeoning acceptance of the need for ethical behavior (code or no code). In fact, they are being advised to police themselves, before the government does it for them. Possibly the new outlook is at least partly a reaction to political and other scandals involving "respectable" people. Legislators, stimulated by public pressure, have increasingly incorporated aspects of ethical behavior into legislation, with legal penalties for violations. Indeed, in 1980, the United States Senate itself asked the Hastings Center Institute of Society, Ethics and the Life Sciences to assist them in formulating a new Senate code of ethics. The process and results make fascinating reading.[33] Its utilization in recent years is even more fascinating.

In the history of ethical codes, there is almost no theoretical literature on how they should be written. There are striking differences in both the format and the content of various codes, and even more dramatic changes in the revisions dictated by social changes. Not just the AMA code, but the ANA code, described later, are excellent examples of these contrasts. Moreover in some fields, the codes are a highly important document; in others, the practitioners seem unaware of them.

One ethicist states that there is "no consensus across different fields and professions about the nature, function, and purpose of a code," or on whether there ought to be a code at all. He notes, "There is a fair degree of public and professional cynicism about codes and a wide range of complaints about them—that they are self-serving, pious, or public relation devices."

While he maintains that he has found little evidence to support the very negative charges, he notes that professional codes share a common dilemma: Is there a reasonable balance between hard, tight, narrow, enforceable rules and stimuli to moral ideals, however hard to achieve in practice?[34]

Nevertheless, a code of ethics is considered an essential characteristic of a profession, providing one means whereby professional standards may be established, maintained, and improved. It indicates the profession's acceptance of the trust and responsibility with which society has invested it. The public has granted the professionals certain privileges, with certain expectations in return.

In that context, professionals today need to look at their ethical codes in terms of whether they are focused on the consumer or are more inclined to emphasize professional etiquette—relationships within or across professional lines. For instance, in a previous AMA code, a statement about not associating professionally with anyone who does not practice a method of healing founded on scientific basis was aimed at preventing, among other things, medical referrals to chiropractors. This was deemed restraint of trade by the FTC and no such statement is found in the current code or, as it is called, "Principles of Medical Ethics."

A similar point in the ethics/etiquette debate could be made about the ninth statement in the Code for Nurses, which implies support of collective bargaining actions. Although improved conditions of employment might also improve nursing care, one does not necessarily follow the other in terms of protecting the patient. It *does* protect the nurse from charges of unethical conduct.

It is perhaps because of the influence of changing times that the self-serving aspects of ethical codes have diminished considerably over the last few years and recent revisions of most codes are beginning to show more concern for protecting society than for protecting the profession.

Nursing Codes of Ethics

Although Isabel Hampton Robb wrote a book on ethics and nursing practice at the turn of the century, and although there were columns on ethics in nursing journals, there was no formal code in early American nursing. In the early nursing literature, ethics appears to have been defined as *Christian morality*. There is some feeling that this was due in part to the authoritarian milieu in which nursing existed. Nursing education valued obedience, submission to rules, social etiquette, and loyalty to the physician, instead of judgment, responsibility, and humanitarianism. What might have been a substitute for an ethical code, Lystra Gretter's Florence Nightingale Pledge, quoted in Chap. 3, illustrates the mixture of contemporary morality, ethics, and loyalty expected in 1893. In 1935, Mrs. Gretter revised the last paragraph of the pledge to read, "With loyalty will I aid the physician in his work, and as a 'missioner of health' I will dedicate myself to devoted service to human welfare." The 1935 version is copyrighted by the Alumnae Association, Harper Hospital School of Nursing, Detroit, Mich.; the original is not copyrighted. It also appears to be based on the Hippocratic Oath associated with physicians and supposedly drawn up at the time of Hippocrates to express the commitments of the healing practitioners. You may be familiar with some of that oath's precepts:

> **The regimen that I adopt shall be for the benefit of my patients according to my ability and judgment.... I will give no deadly drug to any.... Whatsoever things I see or hear concerning the life of men, in my attendance on the sick or even apart therefrom, which ought not be noised abroad, I will keep silence thereon, counting such things to be as sacred secrets.**

The Nightingale Pledge is still recited or sung (as the Nightingale Hymn) by some graduating students of nursing, as the Hippocratic Oath is recited by some graduating physicians.

After several years of trying to decide between a pledge of conduct and a statement on the ideals of the nursing profession, in 1926, ANA's relatively new Committee on Ethical Standards presented to the ANA House of Delegates a suggested code of ethics (Exhibit 10-1). The purpose was not to provide specific rules of conduct, but to create an awareness of

<table>
<tr><td>Exhibit
10-1</td><td>First ANA Suggested Code of Ethics (1926)</td></tr>
</table>

The Relation of the Nurse to the Patient

The nurse should bring to the care of the patient all of the knowledge, skill, and devotion which she may possess. To do this, she must appreciate the relationship of the patient to his family and to his community.

Therefore the nurse must broaden her thoughtful consideration of the patient so that it will include his whole family and his friends, for only in surroundings harmonious and peaceful for the patient can the nurse give her utmost of skill, devotion and knowledge, which shall include the safeguarding of the health of those about the patient and the protection of property.

The Relation of the Nurse to the Medical Profession

The term "medicine" should be understood to refer to scientific medicine and the desirable relationship between the two should be one of mutual respect. The nurse should be fully informed on the provisions of the medical practice act of her own state in order that she may not unconsciously support quackery and actual infringement of the law. The key to the situation lies in the mutuality of aim of medicine and nursing; the aims, to cure and prevent disease and promote positive health, are identical; the technics of the two are different and neither profession can secure complete results without the other. The nurse should respect the physician as the person legally and professionally responsible for the medical and surgical treatment of the sick. She should endeavor to give such intelligent and skilled nursing service that she will be looked upon as a co-worker of the doctor in the whole field of health.

Under no circumstances, except in emergency, is the nurse justified in instituting treatment.

The Relation of the Nurse to the Allied Professions

The health of the public has come to demand many services other than nursing. Without the closest interrelation of workers and appreciation of the ethical standards of all groups, and a clear understanding of the limitations of her own group, the best results in building positive health in the community cannot be obtained.

Relation of Nurse to Nurse

The "Golden Rule" embodies all that could be written in many pages on the relation of nurse to nurse. This should be one of fine loyalty, of appreciation for work conscientiously done, and of respect for positions of authority. On the other hand, loyalty to the motive which inspires nursing should make the nurse fearless to bring to light any serious violation to the ideals herein expressed; the larger loyalty is that to the community, for loyalty to an ideal is higher than any personal loyalty.

Relation of the Nurse to Her Profession

The nurse has a definite responsibility to her profession as a whole. The contribution of individual service is not enough. She should, in addition, give a reasonable portion of her time to the furtherance of such advancements of the profession as are only possible through action of the group as a whole. This involves attendance at meetings and the acquisition of information, at least sufficient for intelligent participation in such matters as organization and legislation.

The supreme responsibility of the nurse in relation to her profession is to keep alight that spiritual flame which has illumined the work of the great nurses of all time.

Source: Lyndia Flanagan, *One Strong Voice: The Story of the American Nurses Association.* Kansas City, MO: American Nurses Association, 1976, pp 89–91. Reprinted with permission.

ethical considerations. The code is a realistic reflection of the times, and comparison with succeeding codes illustrates that although certain basic precepts of ethical behavior may persist, codes are altered by the demands of the times and changing concepts of an emerging profession by the professionals. For instance, in the next decade, nurses' ethical concerns encompassed such diverse topics as uniform requirements and outlining diabetic diets to a patient in the absence of a physician.[35] In 1940, a "Tentative Code," published in AJN, was not much different from the 1926 version. Even the more modern and first official Code for Nurses (1950) has been revised a number of times (1956, 1960, 1968, and 1976) and shows the influence of societal changes. For instance, the 1950 Code emphasized respect for the religious beliefs of patients; then, with the civil rights movement, the same statement was broadened to include "race, creed, color, or status"; and currently it stresses human dignity and the "uniqueness of the client unrestricted by considerations of social or economic status, personal attributes, or the nature of health problems." There is also decreasing emphasis on relationships with physicians and professional etiquette. The focus is on protection of the patient/client, and in this sense, represents a change to a real ethical code.

The 1976 version of the code, with interpretive statements, was developed by an ad hoc committee of the ANA's Congress for Nursing Practice and is available from the American Nurses Association (Exhibit 10-2). The interpretive statements are especially valuable because they not only enlarge upon and explain the code in more detail but also provide more focus and direction on how the nurse can carry out the code. These were revised in 1985. Particularly important is the first statement, which sets the tone of the nurse/client relationship as partners:

> **Clients should be as fully involved as possible in the planning and implementation of their own health care. Clients have the moral right to determine what will be done with their own person....**

Key areas in the interpretations deal with the nurse as a patient advocate, nurse participation in political decision making and public affairs, and nurse involvement in advertising. Nurse accountability is a major issue and is considered important enough to require a separate statement.

The code, overall, was intended to express nursing's moral concerns, goals, and values, rather than announcing a set of laws dictating nurses' behavior. However, in 1988 the ANA published *Ethics in Nursing: Position Statements and Guidelines* because "As the context of nursing changes, it becomes necessary to apply those broad principles in the Code for Nurses to very specific practice issues."[36] Therefore, the Committee on Ethics developed some position statements and guidelines for implementing the code, often based on queries from members. Included are "Guideline on Withdrawing or Withholding Food and Fluid," which emphasized the need to respect the competent patient's autonomy, but added many caveats as to when such action was not appropriate. In a statement examining at what point it ceases to be a nurse's duty to undergo risk for the benefit of the patient, probably in response to care of AIDS patients, responsibility to the patient is stressed, but it concludes that there are limits to the moral obligation of the nurse to benefit patients. Examples are given. Other statements emphasize the importance of nurses' participation in institutional ethics committees, a prohibition of nurses' participation in capital punishment, and the "nonnegotiable nature" of the code. A number of ANA resources on ethics are also listed.

The ICN Code for Nurses

In 1933, the International Council of Nurses (ICN) established an Ethics of Nursing Committee to study the method of teaching ethics in nursing, to survey activities by national organizations relative to ethics, and to collect data on ethical problems. From this evolved an ICN Code of Nursing Ethics which, after a long delay partially caused by World War II, was adopted in 1953 at a Grand Council meeting in Brazil. As might be expected, there was major emphasis on nurses, not the nursing profession. Nurses were expected to recognize the limitations as well as the responsibilities of their roles, especially when it came to obeying doctors' orders. With slight revisions in 1965 at Frankfurt, the code was retitled the Code of Ethics as Applied to Nursing, underlining the commonalities in all codes. Finally, at the 1973 meeting in Mexico

Exhibit 10-2	American Nurses Association Code for Nurses

PREAMBLE

The Code for Nurses is based on belief about the nature of individuals, nursing, health, and society. Recipients and providers of nursing services are viewed as individuals and groups who possess basic rights and responsibilities, and whose values and circumstances command respect at all times. Nursing encompasses the promotion and restoration of health, the prevention of illness, and the alleviation of suffering. The statements of the Code and their interpretation provide guidance for conduct and relationships in carrying out nursing responsibilities consistent with the ethical obligations of the profession and quality in nursing care.

1. The nurse provides services with respect for human dignity and the uniqueness of the client unrestricted by considerations of social or economic status, personal attributes, or the nature of health problems.
2. The nurse safeguards the client's right to privacy by judiciously protecting information of a confidential nature.
3. The nurse acts to safeguard the client and the public when health care and safety are affected by the incompetent, unethical, or illegal practice of any person.
4. The nurse assumes responsibility and accountability for individual nursing judgments and actions.
5. The nurse maintains competence in nursing.
6. The nurse exercises informed judgment and uses individual competence and qualifications as criteria in seeking consultation, accepting responsibilities, and delegating nursing activities to others.
7. The nurse participates in activities that contribute to the ongoing development of the profession's body of knowledge.
8. The nurse participates in the profession's efforts to implement and improve standards of nursing.
9. The nurse participates in the profession's efforts to establish and maintain conditions of employment conducive to high quality nursing care.
10. The nurse participates in the profession's effort to protect the public from misinformation and misrepresentation and to maintain the integrity of nursing.
11. The nurse collaborates with members of the health professions and other citizens in promoting community and national efforts to meet the health needs of the public.

Source: Code for Nurses with Interpretive Statements. Reprinted with permission of the American Nurses Association.

City, the Council of National Representatives accepted some drastic revisions (Exhibit 10-3). It was considerably shorter than the 1965 code, and many of the statements appeared to be combined and reworded. It was presented to the ICN congress as an effort to "enunciate concepts that would be clear, concise, universal, broad enough to be useful to nurses in many cultures but able also to stand the tests of time and social change." A striking change is one that makes explicit the nurse's responsibility and accountability for nursing care, deleting statements in the 1965 code that abrogated the nurse's judgment and personal responsibility

and showed dependency on the physician that nurses worldwide no longer see as appropriate. This code was reaffirmed in 1989.

RESEARCH AND ETHICS

When the ANA Code was revised in 1968, the major change was the addition of a statement on the responsibilities of a nurse in research activities. Specific guidelines were delineated in the ANA publication *The Nurse in Research: ANA Guidelines on Ethical Values.*[37] The increasing participation of nurses in medical research as

---

Exhibit 10-3	International Council of Nurses Code for Nurses Ethical Concepts Applied to Nursing (1972)

The fundamental responsibility of the nurse is four-fold: to promote health, to prevent illness, to restore health and to alleviate suffering.

The need for nursing is universal. Inherent in nursing is respect for life, dignity, and rights of man. It is unrestricted by considerations of nationality, race, creed, colour, age, sex, politics or social status.

Nurses render health services to the individual, the family and the community and coordinate their services with those of related groups.

Nurses and People

The nurse's primary responsibility is to those people who require nursing care.

The nurse, in providing care, promotes an environment in which the values, customs and spiritual beliefs of the individual are respected.

The nurse holds in confidence personal information and uses judgment in sharing this information.

Nurses and Practice

The nurse carries personal responsibility for nursing practice and for maintaining competence by continual learning.

The nurse maintains the highest standards of nursing care possible within the reality of a specific situation.

The nurse uses judgment in relation to individual competence when accepting and delegating responsibilities.

The nurse when acting in a professional capacity should at all times maintain standards of personal conduct that would reflect credit upon the profession.

Nurses and Society

The nurse shares with other citizens the responsibility for initiating and supporting action to meet the health and social needs of the public.

Nurses and Co-Workers

The nurse sustains a cooperative relationship with co-workers in nursing and other fields.

The nurse takes appropriate action to safeguard the individual when his care is endangered by a co-worker or any other person.

Nurses and the Profession

The nurse plays the major role in determining and implementing desirable standards of nursing practice and nursing education.

The nurse is active in developing a core of professional knowledge.

The nurse, acting through the professional organization, participates in establishing and maintaining equitable social and economic working conditions in nursing.

Source: Reprinted with permission of the International Council of Nurses.

---

well as nurse-initiated research made this a timely statement. Among the points made, which are still pertinent, are that the nurse is expected to participate in a research or experimental activity only with assurance that the project has the official sanction of a legally constituted research committee or other appropriate authority within the institutional or agency settings, and he or she must have sufficient knowledge of the research design to allow participation in an informed, effective, and ethical fashion. If the nurse sees conflicts or questions related to the well-being and

safety of the patient, this concern must be voiced to the appropriate person in the institution. At all times, nurses remain responsible for their own acts and judgments.

An ANA statement on the ethical issues of research is *Human Rights Guidelines for Nurses in Clinical and Other Research*, developed by two nurse researchers in 1975 and accepted as a position statement on human rights for nurses engaged in various kinds of research, was revised in 1985. This statement focused on nurses' own research activities, which had accelerated considerably in the previous twenty years. Nevertheless, many of the same principles, which are basic to any human research and are based on the 1949 Nuremberg Code and later governmental requirements, were emphasized: protection of the patient's privacy, self-determination, full information, anonymity; freedom from arbitrary hurt and intrinsic risk of injury; and the special rights of minors and incompetent persons. Other nursing organizations such as the American Association of Critical Care Nurses have similar statements. Fry notes that there are two major issues in clinical research: informed consent and determination of benefit-to-risk ratios. The subject must be informed of the procedures to be used, availability of alternative treatments, risks and benefits—with enough time given for adequate comprehension of information and questioning of the researcher. To give voluntary consent, the subject must also be free of any kind of coercion. Determination of benefit to risk is more difficult, but in part, the person most subject to risk must be identified, as well as the types of risk and benefits.[38] The legal and ethical rights of human subjects in research are discussed in more detail in Chap. 22.

There have been a number of scandals that involve universities, physicians, and even governmental agencies concerning research done on prisoners, the military, the mentally retarded, or others who simply weren't properly informed. Some caused serious harm; all violated patients' rights. Therefore, there is special importance in nurses observing the basic principles outlined in the ANA guidelines and elsewhere, since it is possible that nurses are involved, even peripherally, in some of these situations. Moreover, as scientific fraud is revealed, often by the public media, the scientific community loses public confidence, and nursing is becoming more visible as part of that community.[39]

ETHICAL ISSUES AND DILEMMAS IN NURSING

The major ethical issues for those in the health professions today have been identified as the quality of life versus the sanctity of life; the right to live versus the right to die; informed consent; confidentiality; rights of children; unethical behavior of other practitioners; role conflict (who's responsible?); and the allocation of scarce resources (who shall live?). Increasingly, these issues have become subjects of legislation or court decisions (as discussed in Sec. 5), but even this does not lessen potential conflicts in which nurses may find themselves. Not only must they confront the distinct possibility that their personal value systems may be different from that of the profession, but they are also caught in the value systems of their employing institutions.

In the first situation, they must come to terms with their responsibility to the patient or client, regardless of their personal beliefs. For instance, nurses today are faced constantly with the need to make decisions about their roles in euthanasia or abortion. The decision for action may not be easy. When it comes to ending the life of a terminally ill patient, dealing with critically ill newborns,[40] or participating in an abortion, the nurse may choose not to participate if the action is against his or her moral principles. But what about caring for responding, reacting patients? There have been reports of health professionals neglecting or even abusing (mentally if not physically) patients about whom they have moral reservations, such as homosexuals, criminals, alcoholics, or women having abortions. Clearly, this situation is intolerable and violates any professional code of ethics.

These actions, however, are taken on a personal level, and grossly unethical behavior is probably relatively rare. The conflicts nurses face often come from another source. Historically, nurses were seen as servants of physicians and were expected to be obedient and loyal to them. (Note the Nightingale Pledge.) Even as times changed and ethical guides for nurses became less blatant in demanding loyalty at the price of harming the patient, the health care system still fostered the notion of loyalty to the employer and physician first. Thus, in some cases, when the nurse's ethical beliefs and standards conflict with the decisions made by physicians and/or administration, a way must be found to resolve the problem. One example is to provide a liaison between family and care givers to clarify the patient's wishes, possibly in conjunction with a multidisciplinary ethics conference.[41]

Because so many ethical issues in health care have become legal issues, sometimes resulting in precedent-setting court decisions or in state or federal legislation, it is sometimes difficult to differentiate legal from ethical issues. In Chap. 22, the trail from ethics to law is very clear. However, both nurses and physicians are sometimes unclear as to whether certain of their actions are illegal, even if they themselves believe that the actions are ethical. Therefore, they may choose the more conservative path. This is particularly true in so-called right-to-die issues. Vladeck comments:

> **"Beliefs, even beliefs about very important and heavily value-laden issues such as life and death—are not behavior. The two may often conflict with one another."[42]**

He pointed out that contemporary American hospitals are complex institutions and decisions are rarely made by one person. The problem is not that health care professionals are insensitive, unfeeling, or driven by a "technological imperative," at least not most of them. "Rather, those professionals work—perhaps increasingly—in large complex systems that frustrate their ability to be as sensitive and compassionate as they would like to be."[43]

The confusion and difficulties concerning what is "right" and what is legal was illustrated in a survey of 687 physicians in 759 hospitals.[44] Most reported that they were aware of guidelines at their institutions about obtaining informed consent, issuing do-not-resuscitate orders, documenting the reasons for such orders, recording patients' wishes, and determining patients' capacity to make decisions. Yet the majority reported substantial dissatisfaction with the way their patients were actually involved in treatment decisions. Attending physi-

cians seemed most satisfied, but nurses expressed great dissatisfaction, with only 25 percent satisfied that patients' wishes were recorded on the patient chart. The concerns of the house officers were much closer to those of the nurses than to those of the attending physician. Almost half of all the providers reported that they had sometimes acted against their conscience in providing care to the terminally ill. Many more were troubled about providing overly burdensome treatment than about undertreatment. Eighty-seven percent of the total sample agreed that "all competent patients, even if they are not considered terminally ill have the right to refuse life support, even if that refusal may lead to death." (This principle of informed consent is discussed in considerable detail in Chap. 22.) A like number agreed that "to allow patients to die by forgoing or stopping treatment is ethically different from assisting in their suicide." The disparities were clear in relation to specific beliefs. One of the most common was that while it was ethical and legal to withhold treatment, once started, it could not be withdrawn. Both medical and nursing guidelines as well as the opinions of ethicists agree that there is no *ethical* difference. Another involved the difference between "extraordinary" and "ordinary" treatment, which the respondents thought was useful in making termination decisions. In fact, major national ethical guidelines argue that treatment should not hinge on whether it is technologically simple or complex but rather on its potential benefits and burdens to the patient as perceived by the patient or surrogate. A sizable portion of the respondents also felt that "even if life supports such as mechanical ventilation and dialysis are stopped, food and water should always be continued." Yet again, most national and legal guidelines agree that decisions about nutritional support and hydration should be governed by the same principles that guide other kinds of life-sustaining treatments (see Chap. 22). Nurses and attending physicians were more likely to believe food and water should be continued than house officers. (Nurses in long-term-care facilities are particularly concerned about the ethical dimension of long-term tube feeding.)[45] In relation to pain control, the vast majority believed "sometimes it is appropriate to give pain medication to relieve the patient's suffering even if it may hasten a patient's death" and that large quantities of narcotic analgesics may be given when the purpose is not to shorten patients' lives but to alleviate their suffering. Yet 44 percent of nurses felt clinicians gave inadequate pain medications because they feared hastening the patient's death; only one-third of all the physicians thought that. Actually both the medical and nursing literature find that inadequate pain management is a major issue in the care of patients, often because of insufficient knowledge about appropriate pain management and poor communication about pain between patients and providers.[46,47]

Some of these issues that seem to be creating confusion can be clarified when the patient makes a "living will," or as it is more commonly called now, an advance directive, which has legal approval in every state (see Chap. 22). However, most people, including health care providers, still do not have a living will, so if they are not able to speak for themselves, their unwritten wishes about terminating treatment, whatever that may be, could become a legal case, as the institution or physician attempts to get court permission to treat what *they* think is necessary. It's true that sometimes the care provider or institution fears a lawsuit from family or even the patient, if the patient changes his or her mind, but more often, it is simply that years of medical education have trained physicians more to save lives than to consider the quality of life. Physicians, nurses, judges, and others may also have a moral belief that life is sacred, no matter what kind of life, so that fatally deformed newborns, the very old, and those with illnesses or accidents that are totally devastating to them are victims of someone else's moral beliefs. It's possible that, once more, the sheer visibility of such situations, often through the media, is making people more aware of the problems and forcing them to think through the

issue for themselves and their loved ones. This is equally true of health professionals.

The Do Not Resuscitate Order

DNR (do not resuscitate) means that "in event of cardiac or respiratory failure, no resuscitative efforts should be instituted,"[48] but that does not mean that any other care or interventions should be lessened. Presumably, the DNR order should be a shared decision by the patient or surrogate and the physician, with the patient's decision being the ultimate determinant. The order should be written clearly and promptly by the physician, supported in the progress notes, and reviewed as needed.

While this should be clearly understood, nurses cite DNR as a major problem for them. Why? Physicians and others do not like to speak about negative truths, and after all, DNR implies that death will follow. Some patients and families also avoid the topic, although fewer than health providers think. Therefore, a variety of subterfuges are used.

Unwritten orders are a special problem for the nurse. Some physicians believe, wrongly, that their liability is dispelled by not writing a do not resuscitate (DNR) order, or cloaking the intent with words such as "comfort nursing measures only." Sometimes a *slow code* is understood or carried out by nurses when a terminally ill patient is not put on DNR. This means that they do not hurry to alert the emergency team. Again, the fear is that the doctor or hospital would be sued. Yet this is completely unreasonable, since guidelines published by the American Medical Association, the Hastings Center, which deals with ethical issues, and the ANA are clear about what is involved, including the fact that the patient's choices must be given priority or if the patient is not competent, that of the surrogate; that the DNR must be clearly documented, reviewed, and updated periodically (also a JCAHO requirement); that other necessary care must continue to be given; and that there be mechanisms in place, preferably the ethics committee, for resolution of disputes among health care professionals, patients, and/or families. It is also recommended that nurses be educated about various advance directives and educate the family and that they should be involved in developing DNR policies. Nurses who are morally opposed to carrying out DNRs should see about transferring the responsibility for that patient to another nurse.

An important AHA publication makes a similar statement and reiterates that having nurses or other staff solely responsible for making DNR decisions is inappropriate and probably illegal.[49] DNR orders are legally valid, provided that they are in accordance with accepted medical standards. Development of hospital policy on the matter is recommended, including review mechanisms. If there is continuing disagreement about resuscitation, the statement says, the case should be brought to court.

One issue that is receiving considerable attention is the implementation of DNR orders in the operating room. Because CPR was originally developed for the OR, carrying out a DNR order there may present an ethical difficulty. Undergoing surgery may be compatible with having a DNR order when its purpose is the amelioration or palliation of symptoms (for example, treating a pathologic fracture or curing a lesion unrelated to the basic disease). If surgery cannot achieve a beneficial objective, it should not be undertaken. The usual recommendation is that the DNR orders should be suspended during the perioperative period, but reinstated if cardiac arrest occurs during surgery and it is clear that the arrest is due to the underlying condition. Of course, this should be discussed with the patient or surrogate before surgery.[50] Perioperative nurses are urged to review policies related to DNR and to support the surgeon and anesthesia provider in the decisions made in the OR. Again, participation is not required if against the nurse's moral and religious beliefs.[51]

One point that is made consistently is that nurses have a responsibility for reforming deficient DNR policies, putting forth the necessary efforts "to effect improvement in DNR policies and practices in terms of putting the patient first."[52]

Because DNRs are usually intended for direction when an individual is in an institution, problems have arisen when, for instance, an emergency medical team has been called to a home because a person has stopped breathing. It is generally understood that these medics must make an attempt to resuscitate. Therefore, *Choice in Dying* reports a nonhospital DNR has been developed. A physician must complete a form indicating the person does not want to be resuscitated. Presumably, that person wears a bracelet or carries some sort of card that gives the DNR information. A few states have enacted laws to provide for nonhospital DNR orders.

Assisted Suicide

An ethical and legal issue that has received considerable public attention in recent years is euthanasia, now more commonly called assisted suicide, when someone is involved in the killing of another (who may want to die). There are many legal ramifications to this (see Chap. 22), but from an ethical point of view, the question is, "Is it right?" Physicians and others were upset at a published essay written by a "gynecology resident," who related how he helped a suffering young woman with terminal ovarian cancer to die by giving her a large dose of morphine.[53] Many agreed that it was a merciful thing to do, while others maintained that if a doctor (or nurse) was seen as "killing" patients, based on his or her own judgment, people would be terrified. The topic is, and has been, hotly debated.[54,55] On the other hand, right or wrong, this kind of situation has happened before. Even more dramatic was the 1990 case of the physician who developed a mechanism that allowed someone to die peacefully and helped a competent woman with Alzheimer's disease to commit suicide. There are also other publicized (and many quiet) incidents in which family or friends helped an ill person to commit suicide.

Nurses in the ANA survey mentioned previously had mixed opinions about assisted suicide. While 57 percent said that *physician-assisted* suicide should be legalized, 49 percent did not want to see euthanasia legalized. Does that mean that they themselves did not want to participate? The argument that active euthanasia, that is, performing an intervention that directly causes a person's death, is against nursing's code of ethics and morally wrong, is strongly defended,[56] but since other nurses clearly disagree (as does much of the public), the issue is far from closed. In fact, in a study supported by the Agency for Health Care Policy and Research, the researchers found that, regardless of their medical condition, the subjects felt that a number of conditions were "worse than death." Included were permanent coma, severe dementia, loss of essential functions such as being able to feed oneself. They also feared dying in an unfamiliar or institutional setting and did not want to be kept alive artificially. They did not want to be a burden to others, or experience hopelessness, depression, and chronic pain and suffering.[57]

AIDS

AIDS, the modern world's new plague, has brought on new ethical dilemmas. One survey showed that AIDS patients were much more likely to have "do not resuscitate" (DNR) orders than other patients with equally serious diseases. Some health professionals refuse to treat them or even interact with them.[58] Although nurses have been applauded for the quality of personalized care they have given to AIDS patients, a number of studies have shown that the majority of nurses feel that nurses should have a right to refuse to care for AIDS patients, especially if the nurse is pregnant. The majority, also given the choice, would prefer not to care for AIDS patients.[59] However, the reason appears to be fear of infection, not matters of morality or prejudice. (This raises the question of whether all patients should be tested for AIDS.) In addition, the issue of confidentiality is at the forefront. Do families of AIDS patients

have the right to know the patient's diagnosis if the patient doesn't want them to know?[60] Should all newborns be tested for the HIV virus, and if so, should the mother be told if the test is positive? And, of course, the question of assisted suicide is of major concern to many AIDS-infected people.

GUIDANCE IN ETHICAL DECISION MAKING

To make ethical decisions it is sometimes useful to use a structured format. A number of bioethical decision models have been presented over the years, but most include the following steps or variations of them.[61,62]

1. Identify the health problem.
2. List the relevant facts needed to understand the situation.
3. Identify the ethical problem or issues.
4. Determine who's involved in making the decision (the nurse, the doctor, the patient, the patient's family).
5. Identify your own role. (Quite possibly, your role may not require a decision at all.)
6. Define your own moral/ethical position, the profession's (code of ethics), and, as much as possible, that of the key individuals involved.
7. Consider as many possible alternative decisions as you can.
8. Try to identify value conflicts.
9. Consider the long- and short-range consequences of each alternative decision.
10. Reach your decision and act on it.
11. Follow the situation until you can see the actual results of your decision, and evaluate it.
12. Use this information to help in making future decisions.

Referring to the ANA Code of Ethics will help you understand how the philosophical concept is related to the reality situation. No single model is appropriate for everyone, but they can help the decision-maker answer the questions needed for ethical decision making in specific situations. Having some educational background on the issues, including a course in which these frameworks are explained and used, is also important.[63] Other aids in facing ethical dilemmas are consultation with an ethicist, ethical rounds, which allows nurses to routinely review clinical questions and evaluate the presence of ethical concerns, and use of and/or involvement with multidisciplinary ethics committees.[64] These are discussed later.

Using the Nursing Code

The ANA Code of Ethics, like other professional codes, has no legal force, as opposed to the licensure laws promulgated by state boards of nursing (not the nurses' associations). However, the requirements of the Code often exceed, but are never less than, the requirements of the law. Violations of the law may, of course, subject the nurse to civil or criminal penalties. Violations of the code should be reported to constituent associations of ANA, which may reprimand, censure, suspend, or expel members. Most state associations (SNAs) have a procedure for considering reported violations that also gives the accused due process. Even if the nurse is not an SNA member, an ethical violation, at the least, results in the loss of respect of colleagues and the public, which is a serious sanction. All nurses, whether or not they are SNA members, should be familiar with the profession's ethical code, for they have a professional obligation to uphold and adhere to the code and ensure that nursing colleagues do likewise.

Implementation of the code is at two levels. Nurses may be involved in resolving ethical issues on a broad policy level, participating with other groups in decision making to formulate guidelines or laws. But the more common situation is ethical decision making in daily practice, on a one-to-one basis, on issues that are probably not a matter of life and death but must be resolved on the spot by the nurse who faces

them. Still, in clinical areas, such as intensive care units, there *are* life-and-death ethical issues that require decisions.[65]

The code, and particularly its interpretations, are useful as guidelines here, but nurses must recognize that in specific incidents, the reaction will be both intellectual and emotional and strongly influenced by the nurse's cultural background, education, values, cognitive ability, and experience.

Ethics Committees

Ethics committees in one form or another have been in existence for about 20 years. In 1976, a New Jersey Supreme Court judge ordered a sort of internal ethics committee (actually more of a prognosis committee) to help institutions and physicians make decisions about situations such as the Karen Quinlan case, over which he presided. Karen had been in a permanent vegetative state for some years and her family wanted to remove her respirator. (This is discussed more in Chap. 22.) Although it was thought that such a mechanism would be quickly adopted, in 1983, a survey showed that less than 1 percent of all hospitals had established an ethics committee. Today, the majority have one, as well as an increasing number of long-term-care facilities. In 1991, the Joint Commission on the Accreditation of Healthcare Organizations (JCAHO) began to require that institutions have "a mechanism for the consideration of ethical issues arising in the care of patients and to provide education to caregivers and patients on ethical issues in health care." In 1993, JCAHO mandated the same for home health agencies.

The ethics committee may or may not be integrated into the hospital's administrative structure, but the members usually include one or more nurse managers and staff nurses, one or more physicians, a therapist, a social worker, a member of the clergy, an attorney, an ethicist, and one or more representatives from the community. This multidisciplinary group, usually volunteers, form a "community of concern" defined as "that group of persons necessary to grasp all of the essential dimensions of a given issue."[66] The functions of most committees are generally within the framework of those suggested by the President's Commission for the Study of Ethical Problems in Medicine and Biomedical and Behavioral Research in 1983. These are as follows:

- They can review the case to confirm the responsible physician's diagnosis and prognosis of a patient's medical condition.
- They can provide a forum for discussing broader social and ethical concerns raised by a particular case; such bodies may also have an educational role, especially by teaching all professional staff how to identify, frame, and resolve ethical problems.
- They can be a means for formulating policy and guidelines regarding such decisions.
- Finally, they can review decisions made by others (such as physicians and surrogates) about the treatment of specific patients or make such decisions themselves.[67]

The commission noted that ethics committees have an important role in educating professionals about issues relevant to life support, but heads of these committees felt that this was not a particularly successful activity, perhaps because of the difficulty in getting staff, especially physicians, to attend lectures on this topic. The committees were also seen as providing a setting for people within medical institutions to become knowledgeable and comfortable about relating specific ethical principles to specific decisions, especially when real cases in the hospital were used as examples. There was also some concern that the case review function, that is, reviewing certain decisions made by the family of an incapacitated person and his or her practitioner, would be overutilized.[68] However, in 1992, one expert reported that just the opposite had occurred.[69] The reasons were political (infringing upon the authority of the physician), psychological (the difficulty a group might have in making life and death decisions), and cultural

or intellectual (the differences in attitudes about certain ethical dilemmas).[70]

From a practical point of view, the members of the committee, most of whom do not have training in ethics, should be educated themselves, perhaps by the ethicist or external experts. They are then in a better position to recommend or set policies for the institution (depending on what authority the committee is given). They will also be more knowledgeable when called upon for consultation. One role that seems to be helpful is to provide a neutral forum for discussion of difficult cases in which the nurses and others involved can talk out their concerns. The emotional support provided seems to be very helpful in alleviating the stress that usually accompanies difficult ethical situations. One important point is that staff nurses should be on the committee, since they are on the firing line. Unfortunately, there is some indication that this is not a given, and consequently there may be major disagreement between nurses and the committee about issues considered important. Some committees are seen as inadequate to address ethical issues. "Too medically oriented, too theoretical, not knowledgeable, and too inactive" are some of the complaints about them. Nevertheless, nurses are becoming more aggressive about their right to be on ethics committees, and their value as participants is quickly acknowledged when they are members. A good ethics committee has an important role in working out ethical problems.

However, because daily nursing practice problems, which may have ethical components, are not usually suitable for discussion in the institutional ethics committees, nursing ethics committees (NECs) have been established by a number of nursing professionals. The functions of these committees include identifying, explaining, and resolving ethical issues in nursing practice; educating nurses in bioethics and nursing ethics; preparing nurses for interdisciplinary decision making regarding ethical issues; serving as a resource group; reviewing nursing ethics materials; reviewing departmental policies related to ethics; encouraging nursing ethics research; and preparing nurses to serve on institutional ethics committees.[71]

NURSES AS PATIENT ADVOCATES

Over time, it appears that more and more often, nurses themselves, and others, have come to see nurses as natural patient advocates.[72] In a sense, this has been manifested by the fact that long before the American Hospital Association published its Patient's Bill of Rights (see Chap. 22), the National League for Nursing (NLN) had drafted a statement on what the patient might expect from the nurse.[73] (This was done at a time when no one told patients what their care givers should be doing.) The statement coincided closely with the statements in the ANA Code for Nurses.

Then in 1977, the NLN released a new document on patients' rights (Exhibit 10-4). Again, this clearly delineated nursing's support for patients' rights. Many of these statements are now law.

"Patient advocate" could be an employment position or simply individual action. Just what does it mean to be an advocate on an individual basis, officially or nonofficially? In general, it means acting on behalf of a patient/client. It also includes the role of mediator, coordinating services and clarifying communication, trying to resolve conflicting interests of patient and provider. The nurse advocate is also a protector of the patient's right to be actively involved in decision making related to his or her health. This means informing clients adequately so that they can make knowledgeable decisions and supporting their decisions even if you don't

---

Exhibit 10-4	**Nursing's Role in Patients' Rights (1977)**

NLN believes the following are patients' rights which nurses have a responsibility to uphold:

- People have the right to health care that is accessible and that meets professional standards, regardless of the setting.
- Patients have the right to courteous and individualized health care that is equitable, humane, and given without discrimination as to race, color, creed, sex, national origin, source of payment, or ethical or political beliefs.
- Patients have the right to information about their diagnosis, prognosis, and treatment—including alternatives to care and risks involved—in terms they and their families can readily understand, so that they can give their informed consent.
- Patients have the legal right to informed participation in all decisions concerning their health care.
- Patients have the right to information about the qualifications, names, and titles of personnel responsible for providing their health care.

- Patients have the right to refuse observation by those not directly involved in their care.
- Patients have the right to privacy during interview, examination, and treatment.
- Patients have the right to privacy in communicating and visiting with persons of their choice.
- Patients have the right to refuse treatments, medications, or participation in research and experimentation, without punitive action being taken against them.
- Patients have the right to coordination and continuity of health care.
- Patients have the right to appropriate instruction or education from health care personnel so that they can achieve an optimal level of wellness and an understanding of their basic health needs.
- Patients have the right to confidentiality of all records (except as otherwise provided for by law or third-party payer contracts) and all communications, written or oral, between patients and health care providers.

Source: Reprinted with permission of the National League for Nursing.

agree. To do this job well, nurses need to understand the role and competing loyalties (the doctor and the employer),[74] be recognized by others as an advocate (including the patient), have sufficient power, and recognize and be willing to deal with the fact that advocacy in a bureaucracy is bound to be controversial. The "informal, often invisible coercion of the group" is seen as a serious inhibition to "whistle-blowing" that the nurse or other employee faces.[75] It is not likely to be an easy role, and it is not always a matter of another health professional being at fault. Sometimes the nurse advocate must advocate for a patient who is helpless and has a family who is indifferent.[76] Suppose it is the nurses who give inadequate care? Pointing a finger at nursing colleagues is not so simple.

A serious issue is the number of nurses impaired by dependence on drugs or other addictions. In the last few years, both state nurses' associations and individual employers have developed plans for helping these nurses, but also for protecting the public from them.[77] In addition, responsibility is being taken in dealing with incompetent nurses. However, much remains to be done. Nurses surveyed on this issue seemed to agree that they should not turn their backs on colleagues whose performance was deteriorating, for whatever reason, perhaps problems that were family-related or otherwise personal. But "putting patients first is our duty, but being compassionate to colleagues is our honor," seemed to be a common sentiment.[78]

Despite nurses' desire to search for ethical solutions and act accordingly, despite their desire to act as patient advocates, there are still some concerns. Suppose the nurse does carry out his or her ethical and legal responsibilities (see Chap. 20), such as being sure that a patient has given an informed consent before receiving a particular kind of treatment. What if this action comes into conflict with what the doctor or the hospital sees as a limit to the nurse's role? Will the nurse's job be in jeopardy? Will he or she be subtly punished? Whistle-blowers, wrong or right, pay a price, even if they "win."[79] What if the nurse reports unethical or illegal behavior on the part of another practitioner? Again, what happens? Who provides backup support? Nursing administration? Nursing peers? What of dealing with physicians who are incompetents, drug abusers, or alcoholics? Does the profession protect the co-professional or the public? Unlike personal ethical conflicts, these are real dilemmas that may have serious economic repercussions for the nurse, and it is quite possible that a nurse cannot resolve them alone. Instead, nursing must develop a support system for individual nurses who experience conflict in the employment setting with respect to implementation of the Code of Ethics, and the precepts of the code must be widely publicized so that not only nurses, but also the public and others in health care, understand the ethical basis of nursing practice. Nurses may also turn to ANA's Center for Ethics and Human Rights, which provides practical guidance.[80] With the power of the profession behind them, nurses are in a much better position to face and resolve ethical issues.

REFERENCES

1. *The Future of Healthcare: Changes and Choices.* Chicago: Arthur Anderson, 1987.
2. Cohen E: Realism, law and aging. *Law, Med Health Care* 18:183–192, Fall 1990.
3. Callahan D: Terminating treatment: Age as a standard. *Hastings Cent Rep* 17:21–25, October–November 1987.
4. Callahan D: *Setting Limits: Medical Goals in an Aging Society.* New York: Simon and Schuster, 1987.
5. Altman L: The limits of transplantation: How far should surgeons go? *New York Times*, December 19, 1989, p C3.
6. Vaughn-Cole B, Kee H: A heart decision. *Am J Nurs* 85:535–536, May 1985.
7. Fry S: Brave new world: Removing body parts from infants. *Nurs Outlook* 38:152, May–June 1990.
8. Robertson J: Rights, symbolism, and public policy in fetal tissue transplants. *Hastings Cent Rep* 18:5–11, December 1988.

9. Kilner J: Selecting patients when resources are limited: A study of U.S. medical directors of kidney dialysis and transplantation facilities. *Am J Public Health* 78:144–147, February 1988.

10. Blakeslee S: Studies find unequal access to kidney transplants. *New York Times* Jan 24, 1989, pp C1, C9.

11. Pear R: Big health gap, tied to income, is found in U.S. *New York Times*, July 8, 1993, p A1.

12. Bayer R et al: Toward justice in health care. *Am J Public Health* 78:583–588, May 1988.

13. Callahan D: Rationing medical progress. *N Engl J Med* 322:1810–1813, June 21, 1990.

14. Fry S: Ethical implications of health care reform. *Am Nurse* 26:5, March 1994.

15. Health care rationing tops list of pressing ethical issues. *Am Nurse* 26:11, March 1994.

16. Silva M: Nurse executives' responses to ethical concerns and policy formulation for allocation of scarce resources. *Nurs Connections* 7:59–64, Spring 1994.

17. Fries E: The ethical issues of transplanting organs for anencephalic newborns. *MCN* 14:412–414, November–December 1989.

18. Purtilo R: *Ethical Dimensions in the Health Professions.* 2d ed. Philadelphia: Saunders, 1993, p 6.

19. Krowczyk R, Kudzma E: Ethics: A matter of moral development. *Nurs Outlook* 26:255, April 1978.

20. Chally P: Theory derivation in moral development. *Nurs Health Care* 11:302–306, June 1990.

21. Gilligan C: *In a Different Voice.* Cambridge, MA: Harvard University Press, 1982.

22. Chally, op cit, p 304.

23. Maurice S, Warrick L: Ethics and morals in nursing. *MCN* 2:343, November–December 1977.

24. Churchill L: Ethical issues of a profession in transition. *Am J Nurs* 77:873, May 1977.

25. Noddings N: *Caring, A Feminine Approach to Ethics and Moral Development.* Berkeley: University of California Press, 1984.

26. Crowley M: The relevance of Noddings' ethics of care to the moral education of nurses. *J Nurs Ed* 33:74–86, February 1994.

27. Ibid, p 80.

28. Curtin L: Human problems: Human beings. *Nurs Mgt* 25:38, May 1994.

29. Ibid.

30. Davis A, Aroskar M: *Ethical Dilemmas and Nursing Practice.* New York: Appleton-Century-Crofts, 1978.

31. Fry S: *Ethics in Nursing Practice: A Guide to Ethical Decision Making.* Geneva, Switzerland: International Council of Nurses, 1994, pp 19–40.

32. Aiken T: *Legal, Ethical and Political Issues in Nursing.* Philadelphia: Davis, 1994, pp 20–31.

33. Revising the United States Senate code of ethics. Special Supplement, *Hastings Cent Rep* 11:1–28, February 1981.

34. Ibid.

35. Flanagan L: One strong voice. Kansas City, MO: American Nurses Association, 1976, pp 88–91.

36. *Ethics in Nursing: Position Statements and Guidelines.* Kansas City, MO: American Nurses Association, 1988.

37. The nurse in research: ANA guidelines on ethical values. *Am J Nurs* 68:1504–1507, July 1968.

38. Fry, Ethics in nursing practice, op cit, pp 221–225.

39. Abdellah F: Scientific misconduct: Myth or reality. *J Prof Nurs* 6:6, 63, January–February 1990.

40. Smith J: Ethical issues raised by new treatment options. *MCN* 14:183–187, May–June 1989.

41. Meyer C: End-of-life care: Patients' choices, nurses' challenges. *Am J Nurs* 93:40–47, February 1993.

42. Vladeck B: Editorial: Beliefs versus behavior in healthcare decision making. *Am J Public Health* 83:13, January 1993.

43. Ibid.

44. Solomon et al: Decisions near the end of life: Professional views on life-sustaining treatments. *Am J Public Health* 83:14–23, January 1993.

45. Wilson D: Ethical concerns in a long-term tube feeding study. *Image* 24:195–199, Fall 1992.

46. Mitchell J: Administering mercy: The ethics of pain management. *Cancer Invest* 12:343–349, May–June 1994.

47. Henkelman W: Inadequate pain management: Ethical considerations. *Nurs Mgt* 25:48A–48D, January 1994.

48. Price D, Murphy P: DNR: Still crazy after all these years. *J Nurs Law* 1:1, Spring 1994.

49. Read W: *Hospital's Role in Resuscitation Decision.* Chicago: Hospital Research and Educational Fund, 1983.

50. Cohen C, Cohen P: Do-not-resuscitate orders in the operating room. *N Engl J Med* 325:1879–1882, Dec 21, 1991.

51. The do-not-resuscitate order: Moral responsibilities of the perioperative nurse. *AORN J* 59:641–650, March 1994.

52. Price, Murphy, op cit, p 5.

53. It's over, Debbie. JAMA 259:272, January 8, 1988.

54. Special articles: Physician assisted dying. *Trends Health Care, Law Ethics* 7:7–31, Winter, 1992.

55. Dying well? A colloquy on euthanasia and assisted suicide. *Hastings Cent Rep* 22:6–55, March–April 1992.

56. Kowalski S: Assisted suicide: Where do nurses draw the line? *Nurs Health Care* 14:70–76, February 1993.

57. Pearlman R et al: Insights pertaining to patient assessments of states worse than death. *J Clin Ethics* 4:33–41, Summer 1993.

58. Kelly J et al: Stigmatization of AIDS patients by physicians. *Am J Public Health* 77:798–791, July 1987.

59. Wiley K et al: Care of HIV-infected patients: Nurses' concerns, opinions, and precautions. *Appl Nurs Res* 3:27–33, February 1990.

60. Laufman J: AIDS, ethics, and the truth. *Am J Nurs* 89:924–925, July 1989.

61. Curtin L: Doing the right thing. *Nurs Mgt* 24:17–19, December 1993.

62. Thompson J, Thompson H: *Bioethical Decision Making for Nurses.* Norwalk, CT: Appleton-Century-Crofts, 1985, pp 89–208.

63. Fry S: Ethical decision-making Part I: Selecting a framework. *Nurs Outlook* 37:248, September–October 1989.

64. Scanlon C: Developing ethical competence. *Am Nurs* 26:1, 11, March 1994.

65. Baggs J: Collaborative interdisciplinary bioethical decision-making in intensive care units. *Nurs Outlook* 41:108–112, May–June 1993.

66. Haddad A: Developing an organizational ethos. *Caring* 5:10, June 1992.

67. President's Commission for the Study of Ethical Problems in Medicine and Biomedical and Behavioral Research: *Deciding to Forgo Life-Sustaining Treatment.* Washington, DC: The Commission, 1983, pp 160–161.

68. Ibid, pp 162–168.

69. Blake D: The hospital ethics committee: Health care's moral conscience or white elephant? *Hastings Cent Rep* 22:6–11, January–February 1992.

70. Fry-Revere S: Ethics consultation: An update on accountability issues. *Pediatr Nurs* 20:95–98, January–February 1994.

71. Zink M, Titus L: Nursing ethics committees— Where are they? *Nurs Mgt* 25:70–76, June 1994.

72. Nelson M: Advocacy in nursing. *Nurs Outlook* 36:136–141, May–June 1988.

73. National League for Nursing: *What People can Expect of Modern Nursing Service.* New York: National League for Nursing; 1959. Also found in Kelly L: *Dimensions of Professional Nursing,* 4th ed. New York: Macmillan, 1981.

74. Schaefer S: Patient advocacy: An ethical dilemma? *Focus Crit Care* 16:191–192, June 1989.

75. Curtin L: Damage control and the whistle-blower. *Nurs Mgt* 24:33–34, May 1993.

76. Kayser-Jones J et al: An ethical analysis of an elder's treatment. *Nurs Outlook* 37:267–270, November–December 1989.

77. Miller H: Addiction in a coworker—getting past the denial. *Am J Nurs* 90:72–75, May 1990.

78. Haddad A: Acute care decisions: Ethics in action. *RN* 57:22–25, May 1994.

79. Fry S: Whistle-blowing by nurses: A matter of ethics. *Nurs Outlook* 37:56, January–February 1989.

80. Aroskar M: Ethical decision-making in patient care. *Am Nurse* 26:10, March 1994.

Profile of the Modern Nurse

WHO ARE TODAY'S NURSES? Where do they work? How do they differ from the nurses of 10 or 20 years ago? What are their personality characteristics and attitudes? What is the public image of the nurse? Unfortunately, many studies on these topics have been based on small sample sizes, conducted by graduate students, or been limited in scope. Thus, comparisons are difficult. In the late 1980s, the image issue received renewed attention. This was partially due to the concern over the nursing shortage, and the notion that problems in recruitment stemmed from nursing's poor public image.

The oldest continuing study on the characteristics of nursing is the *National Sample Survey of Registered Nurses* conducted by the Division of Nursing of the U.S. Department of Health and Human Services (DHHS). The sample survey was first conducted in September 1977, and repeated in November 1980 and 1984, and in March 1988 and 1992. Nursing is also included in a periodic report to the Congress by DHHS on the status of *Health Personnel in the United States*. In contrast to the sample survey, the report to the Congress deals with supply, distribution, and future projections for health personnel. A final governmental report of interest is the *Survey of Certified Nurse Practitioners and Clinical Nurse Specialists* prepared for the Division of Nursing in 1993 through a contract to the Washington Consulting Group. This report details the supply of advanced practice nurses, who they are, where they work, what

they do, and how much they are compensated for their effort.

Other useful information is provided by national nursing associations. The Division on Research of the National League for Nursing provides comprehensive information on nursing students, faculty, and educational programs. Surveys on the presence of nurses in specific health care settings are regularly conducted by industry interest groups. One example is the *Hospital Nursing Personnel Survey* done annually by the American Hospital Association. A variety of opinion polls and surveys are also initiated around topics such as employment conditions, job satisfaction, wage and salary trends, and attitudes on public policy, most especially health care reform. The authors would be remiss if they did not mention *Facts about Nursing* published by the American Nurses' Association. *Facts* brings together data on nurses and nursing from a broad range of sources, in addition to adding information collected exclusively by ANA to fill gaps. The most recent publication of *Facts* appeared in 1987, and that was its 38th edition.

A very significant trend, beginning in earnest in 1985, has been the effort to identify consumer attitudes toward nurses. Between 1985 and 1994, several well-conceived and well-executed public opinion surveys were conducted. Their purpose has been to determine the public's perception of nurses, and to monitor change in these sentiments over time.

A popular source of information on the attitudes of nurses is the nursing magazine poll. A number of magazines have found the poll to be a way of stimulating reader interest and maybe even attracting new subscribers. There is no question that they *are* usually interesting, but they must be considered with an objective eye (some would say a jaundiced eye). There are, of course, some obvious caveats. First, usually only readers of that magazine are the sample. Second, only those who feel strongly about the particular topic are apt to respond. A more subtle problem may be less apparent to a casual reader. The orientation of a magazine and/or its desire to elicit answers that can be interpreted dramatically or that support a particular viewpoint may result in the wording of questions that could be read several ways. The further interpretation of the author or editor, and the points that are highlighted, can, intentionally or not, mislead the reader.

For demographic data, there is a greater likelihood of obtaining national samples, and in these the difficulty lies in the inconsistency of study components from year to year. Overall, however, the studies and surveys are rather provocative and present an interesting overview of the practitioners of nursing today. The heterogeneity of nursing is quickly evident, for today's nursing workforce includes men and women who might have graduated forty-five years ago, as well as new graduates. Therefore, their attitudes and perhaps their behavior have been affected by concepts that span that time period.

There are also differences between the image and the reality. This has always been true. When Dickens wrote about the slovenly Sairey Gamp, dedicated women were functioning as nurses. Even the British newspapers' glowing reports of Florence Nightingale as the gentle lady with the lamp overlooked her tough and efficient administrative stance, which had a large part in providing better care for soldiers in the Crimea. Indeed, major national nursing organizations found the public image of the nurse so detrimental that in 1989, the National Commission on Nursing Implementation Project (NCNIP) and Advertising Council launched a three-year public-service campaign aimed at improving the image of the nurse.

This chapter, in building a profile of the modern nurse (and student), will deal with four major entities: demographic data, personality characteristics of nurses, nursing attitudes, and the nurse as seen by the public. Comparisons to previous data are made when useful. Obviously, it is necessary to present only a synopsis of the available data, but both the references and the bibliography will provide useful follow-up. Additional data about today's nurses are also incorporated in other chapters, such as 5, 9, 10, 13, and 15.

GENERAL DEMOGRAPHIC DATA

The most current, general, comprehensive demographic data about nurses comes out of the Division of Nursing of the Department of Health and Human Services. The most recent was published in February 1994, and reports 1992 data from the *National Sample Survey of Registered Nurses*. Table 11-1 summarizes data from the 1992 survey and includes comparisons with the 1980 and 1988 surveys. There are easily discernible trends. In March 1992, an estimated 2,239,815 individuals held licenses to practice as registered nurses in the United States. This was a 10 percent increase from March 1988. There was a 4 percent increase in the proportion employed in nursing. This "activity rate" was accompanied by an increase in the numbers of nurses working part-time. In 1988, 26 percent of employed nurses were part-timers, while in 1992 this had increased to 31 percent. All areas of the country, with the exception of New England, showed an increase in the numbers of employed nurses.[1]

The predominant setting for the employment of nurses continued to be the hospital. The overall number of nurses employed in hospitals increased from 1988 to 1992, although they represent a declining proportion of the nursing profession. The number of nurses providing bedside care to inpatients increased only 6 per-

Table 11-1 Who Are the Nurses?

	1992	1988	1980
Total RN population	2.2 million	2.0 million	1.7 million
Employed in nursing[1]	83.2%	79.0%	76.6%
	(about 31% part-time)	(about 26% part-time)	(about 32% part-time)
Sex			
Female	96.0%	96.6%	96.1%
Male	4.0%	3.3%	3.0%
Ethnic-racial background			
White/non-Hispanic	91.1%	91.7%	90.4%
Black	4.0%	3.6%	4.3%
Asian/Islander	3.4%	2.3%	2.4%
Hispanic	1.4%	1.3%	1.4%
American Indian/Alaskan Native	0.4%	0.4%	0.28%
Age			
Under 25	2.1%	3.9%	9.6%
25–34	23.6%	29.8%	36.2%
35–44	34.7%	29.5%	23.3%
45–54	20.6%	19.1%	17.2%
55–64	12.7%	12.3%	15.7%
65 or over	5.6%	5.0%	4.5%
Marital status			
Married	71.5%	70.6%	70.6%
Divorced, separated, widowed	16.5%	15.4%	13.8%
Never married	11.1%	13.0%	14.8%
Places of employment			
Hospital	66.5%	67.9%	65.6%
Nursing home	7.0%	6.6%	8.0%
Community health	9.7%	6.8%	6.6%
Physician's office/ambulatory care	7.8%	7.7%	5.7%[2]
Nursing education	2.0%	1.8%	3.7%
Student health service	2.7%	2.9%	3.5%
Occupational health	1.9%	1.3%	2.3%
Private duty nursing	0.6%	1.2%	1.6%
Other	3.0%	3.6%	1.7%
Type of position			
Staff nurse	61.6%	66.9%	65.0%
Head nurse and supervisor	9.6%	10.9%	13.1%
Administration (service and education)	6.2%	6.6%	4.8%
Instructor	3.5%	3.8%	4.7%
Clinical specialist/clinician	1.9%	2.9%	2.1%
Nurse practitioner/midwife	1.4%	1.5%	1.3%
Nurse anesthetist	1.0%	1.0%	1.1%
Other	6.5%	6.6%	6.8%
Higher educational preparation			
Doctorate	0.5%	0.3%	0.2%
Master's	7.5%	6.2%	5.1%
Baccalaureate in nursing	27.3%	25.1%	20.7%
Other baccalaureate	2.6%	2.3%	2.6%
Diploma	33.7%	40.4%	50.7%
Associate degree	28.2%	25.2%	20.1%

Source: DHHS Division of Nursing, National Sample Survey of Registered Nurses, 1988, 1992.

[1]Data refer to *employed* nurses. Some figures do not total 100% because of no response and rounding of figures.

[2]Refers to physician's office only.

cent, while there was a two-thirds increase of nurses in outpatient departments and a 17 percent increase in the operating room, labor and delivery, and postoperative recovery. Rapid development in less intrusive techniques that decrease the need for major surgery, and the prevalence of managed care programs that often discourage elective surgery will have implications here. There was a 30 percent increased employment of nurses in community settings.[2]

The "aging" of the registered nurse population continues. In 1992, the average age of the registered nurse was 43, compared with 42 in 1988. Put a different way, in 1992, 60.4 percent of the nurse population was under 45 years of age, as compared with 63.3 percent in 1988 and 69.1 in 1980.[3] Not only is the current nursing workforce aging, it is being augmented by RNs who are older. In Knopf's 1962 study, over 86 percent of nurses prepared at the diploma and baccalaureate level started nursing school when they were 19 years old or younger. The average age of a new RN in 1992 was 33.7 years. The average age for an associate degree graduate is 35.7 years, 31.3 years for the diploma graduate, and 29.2 for the baccalaureate.[4] It is obvious how the discipline's appeal to the more mature student or the person looking for a midlife or retirement career change will shape the average age and even the expectations of the incumbents of the role of nurse.

In 1992, the majority of nurses received their basic nursing preparation in an academic as opposed to a service setting. In the first sample survey of 1977, 75 percent of nurses were originally diploma school graduates. In 1992, only 42 percent came from this origin. The greatest growth was among associate degree graduates, who were 11 percent of all nurses in 1977. In 1992, one-third of the universe of registered nurses received their initial nursing preparation in associate degree programs. In total, 30 percent of registered nurses in 1992 had baccalaureate degrees, 8 percent had advanced degrees, 28 percent had associate degrees, and a little over a third had a diploma.[5]

More nurses are married or divorced than in earlier years, and fewer have never been married. Salary gains for registered nurses from 1988 to 1992 were significant, between 28 and 38 percent on a regional basis. The average annual salary in 1992 was $37,738.[6]

The numbers of nurses with master's or doctoral preparation increased to 8 percent in 1992. Also of note is the shifting focus of nurses with advanced degrees. In 1977, 41 percent of such nurses identified education as their primary focus. In 1984, about 46 percent had clinical practice as their emphasis.[7] In 1992, only 14 percent of master's prepared nurses identified education as their primary focus, while less than 66 percent of nurses with doctorates were employed in education.[8] This shift may find its explanation in some very obvious facts. Salaries for nurses in academe have been dramatically outpaced by economic gains in the service setting. Traditionally, schools of medicine and law have retained faculty by basing their salaries on the market for their discipline, rather than faculty salary scales, or by facilitating the maintenance of a practice that could enhance income.

One of the most comprehensive studies of nurses ever conducted was the longitudinal NLN Nursing Career Pattern Study, begun in 1962. It was designed to obtain definitive biographical characteristics of nursing students, their occupational goals, and their reasons for their choice of nursing as a career. Later, the Department of Health, Education and Welfare (DHEW) supported extension of the study to include students who entered associate degree, diploma, and baccalaureate RN programs in 1965 and 1967. The 6,893 students who graduated from the 259 basic nursing programs in the 1962 group became part of the cohort that was surveyed one, five, ten, and fifteen years after graduation. Although declining over that period, from 96 percent the first year, the response rate for the fifteen-year segment was still at 70 percent. The study was completed in 1981[9]

More recently, the NLN has initiated a newly licensed nurse survey. It provides details on the employment, mobility, and demographic characteristics of all newly licensed nurses in the country.

MINORITY GROUPS IN NURSING

Studies on the general population of nursing students and graduates are inevitably influenced by the fact that the majority of nurses are both women and white. There is increasing interest in the minority groups in nursing, such as blacks, Native Americans, and Hispanics, but also including the male minority.

Nursing recruitment for all ethnic minorities has gradually increased, stimulated particularly by federal grants available since 1965. However, despite these efforts, and although there has been an increase in the *numbers* of ethnic minorities, the *proportion* of ethnic minorities among employed RNs has not shown remarkable gain. (See Table 11-1.) Specifically, the proportion of white/non-Hispanic employed nurses was 90.4 percent in 1980, 91.7 percent in 1988, and 9.1 percent in 1992. The percentage of blacks went from 4.3 percent in 1980 to 4 percent in 1992. Hispanic representation stayed at about 1.4 percent over the 12-year period and Asian/Pacific Islanders gained 1 percent. American Indians were less than one-half of a percent. Hence, there are many perceived and real financial and cultural barriers that impede recruitment and retention of ethnic minority nurses.

There is an observable trend of decreasing minority enrollment in basic nursing education programs over the past four years. Minority enrollment accounted for 17.2 percent of students in 1990, 15.8 percent in 1991, and 15.4 percent in 1992. There are other observations when we consider each type of program individually. There has been a decline of minority presence in baccalaureate programs from 19.4 percent in 1990 to 16.3 percent in 1992. Enrollment in associate degree programs has remained stable for 1991 and 1992 at 15.2 percent, and diploma enrollment has increased slightly from 11.7 percent in 1991 to 12.5 percent in 1992.[10] There are serious implications here for a nursing workforce that must be prepared to minister to a population in which the minority presence is rapidly growing. It also perpetuates a vicious circle. How does nursing attract talented minority candidates when there is a deficiency of minority role models? Minority presence among graduate students in nursing is less than in baccalaureate programs at 11.7 percent, with the difference being especially pronounced for blacks at 5.8 percent. This same imbalance is noted among faculty, with 8.7 percent of nursing faculty being ethnic and racial minorities. This is somewhat less than the 13.8 percent minority faculty representation in American medical schools.[11]

Despite low representation in the nursing labor force, ethnic and racial minority nurses have risen to leadership positions in all aspects of the profession, as M. Elizabeth Carnegie, a nurse historian and leader has pointed out.[12] For example, black nurses have held leadership positions as deans and higher at major universities. They have been board members and presidents of major nursing and public health organizations and have been executives in the private and public sector. The Ethnic/Racial Minority Fellowship Program of the American Nurses Association, begun in 1974, has been a major influence in promoting doctoral study among minority nurses. Stipends, tuition, and other forms of support are provided to candidates pursuing doctoral preparation in psychiatric–mental health nursing.

Men have been neglected as potential sources of nurse power, although male nurses have existed almost as long as female nurses in the United States. By 1910, about 7 percent of all student and graduate nurses were men, but in succeeding years the percentage declined, until by 1940 it had dropped to 2 percent. Most men were graduates of hospital schools connected with mental institutions; not many schools (for men) were affiliated with general hospitals, and few coeducational ones existed (see Chap. 3). By 1960, male nurses (not including students) comprised 0.91 percent of the nursing workforce. The current 4.0 percent level reflects a significant increase in the number of male nurses, and a gradual increase in their proportion of the total employed RN population over the past 35 years.[13]

Men suffered the same discrimination in nursing that women encountered in male-dominated fields, although this was not always the fault of nursing. For instance, male nurses were kept in the enlisted ranks in the regular armed services until 1966, when, with the continuous pressure of the ANA, commissions were finally available to them in the Regular Nurse Corps. During World War II, male nursing students were not exempt from the draft, although the need for nurses was critical. Therefore, nursing enrollment for men dropped drastically to fewer than 200. After the war, enrollment began to climb slowly until in the 1971–1972 academic year, a total of 5,170 men, about 6 percent, were admitted to basic RN programs, nearly twice the proportion enrolling over the previous three years. In 1992, the number of men enrolled in basic RN educational programs reached 11.1 percent. There is little variation in this pattern based on the nature of the program (diploma, associate, baccalaureate).[14] This trend has been attributed to a variety of circumstances, including the general economic recession, employment opportunities in nursing, and the good salary gains achieved during the period of the nursing shortage.

Men in nursing have had to tolerate the often insulting and discriminatory behavior that confronts any minority group. Acceptance of their service has sometimes been rejected in obstetrics and gynecology. Many female nurses believe that men in nursing are apt to dominate the upper echelons. These attitudes often create role strain. The response from a preeminently successful male nurse exudes common sense. He described how the fact that nursing is composed of mainly white women "poses both a social and an ethical problem for the profession." He contended that:

> women, when they are in power, are just as reluctant to share power with men as men have been accused of doing in their relationships with women.

He added that:

> The recruitment of men into the profession is not a panacea. Men candidates range from exceptional competence to borderline ability. They bring with them all the positive and negative variables that are indigenous to all humans.[15]

Men in allied health roles or with other health care experience represent a major recruitment pool for nursing. They should not be expected to choose traditional male specialties, such as emergency, anesthesia, or intensive care, but should be urged to consider a whole range of career choices. They should be supported in career mapping to build a future in the profession.[16]

When looking at the issues regarding the role of minorities in nursing, it is important to remember that cultural differences stem from a myriad of components in all our backgrounds— gender, religion, ethnicity, and even geographic locale. The same biases and insensitivities that thwart our attempts to increase the ethnic, racial, gender, and religious diversity among the ranks of nurses hamper our ability to minister to those who are different from ourselves. Thus, it is important to be aware of and sensitive to minority issues in nursing but not to give them greater weight than the human issues that affect all people and are the mainstay of nursing care.

ATTITUDES OF NURSES AND ABOUT NURSES

Studies of the personality characteristics of nurses vary a great deal and therefore are probably more interesting than useful. Most involve only a small sample and are probably not applicable to the total population. Which personality traits are studied depends both on the overall purpose of the researcher and the type of test used.

Small studies have been done on the personalities of nurses in various specialty areas, with inconsistent findings. All these studies, although of interest, should be regarded with some caution. The lack of consistent findings creates some questions of overall usefulness, although the heterogeneity of nurses is undoubtedly a key factor in their diverse results. The variety in nursing guarantees that all nurses can find an area of practice that complements their personality and style. Those that like fast-paced action and the unpredictable may gravitate toward emergency or trauma. Others who prefer healing the mind and can use their own interpersonal and personal skills to advantage may find most satisfaction in psychiatric nursing. Order and precision are constants in operating room or special care units. Work with substance abusers or AIDS patients requires the ability to be nonjudgmental while refusing to accept antisocial behavior. In fact, every personality and style can find satisfaction within the discipline. The danger is to prejudge a person's suitability for an area of practice.

The last nursing shortage, which came to an abrupt halt in the early 1990s, prompted a series of studies about nurses and their job satisfaction. It became obvious that the satisfiers were not the reverse of the dissatisfiers. Nurses were dissatisfied because of low pay and poor working conditions but remained dissatisfied when status, respect, and career mobility were absent. Whether the technique was a summit meeting of nursing organizations, focus groups, or direct mail survey, nurses expressed much the same priorities and motivation. The reason for choosing nursing as a career has not changed over the years. It continues to be a desire to help people and an interest in health care. During career choice, nursing was seen as a route to professionalism, a vehicle for upward mobility, and a provider of good job opportunities. Patient care and professional issues dominate workplace concerns. Examples are fear over quality, safety of patients, adequate staffing, support personnel who relieve nurses of nonnursing duties, nursing representation on committees that make patient care policy, opportunities for maintaining competence in practice, and a safe working en-

vironment. Of far less importance were wages, benefits, time off, opportunities for overtime, and so on. These same priorities as expressed by nurses appear in the report of the 1988 Tri-Council conference on the nursing shortage,[17] Mabel Wandelt's 1981 survey on why nurses leave nursing,[18] and the mail survey conducted by Fleishman-Hillard for the American Nurses' Association in 1991.[19] The sentiment of registered nurses about their work has remained the same. Nurses see their work as stressful, but anticipate the stress and are willing to live with it given a certain modicum of respect and support. The workplace stressors most mentioned by nurses are inadequate staffing, interruptions, paperwork, lack of support from peers, unattractive and disorganized work areas, high noise level, lack of supplies, absence of information or directions, no voice in decisions that affect them, lack of respect, conflict between the business orientation of the industry and the service orientation of the profession, and the death of "my" patient.

Pending health care reform and the proposal that nurses take on increased responsibility within any restructured system prompted a series of consumer surveys to assess the public's receptiveness to nurses as providers. The first public opinion poll was conducted for the American Nurses Association by Ogilvy and Mather in 1985. Some of the important findings were:[20]

- Of those surveyed, 92 percent believed that nurses should expand their areas of responsibility.
- Eighty percent believed that if more services were performed by nurses, health care costs would be lowered.
- Eighty-four percent of respondents favored direct reimbursement to nurses.
- Eighty-three percent expected to hear ideas from nurses on cost containment and health care reform.

A 1990 survey conducted by Peter Hart Associates for the Tri-Council Organizations (American Nurses' Association, National League for Nursing, American Organization of Nurse Executives, and the American Association of Colleges of Nursing), and funded by the Pew Charitable Trusts found similar public sentiment:[21]

- Nurses are far and away the health care provider that the public most respects and supports.
- The public is impressed with nurses, and sees them as competent and caring.
- The public sees nurses as underutilized.
- Americans are receptive to nurses performing more routine health care services such as physical examinations and prescribing medications.

A national sample of 1,000 adults were polled by the Gallup Organization in July 1993. They were polled about their receptiveness to advanced practice nurses assuming some of the role activities currently associated with physicians. They were asked if they would allow nurses to perform physical examinations, deliver prenatal care, immunize, and treat illnesses such as colds and infections. They responded as follows:[22]

- Eighty-six percent were willing to receive everyday primary care services from a nurse.
- Over half of the respondents were very willing.
- One-third, or 34 percent, were somewhat willing.
- Only 12 percent said they would be unwilling to use the advanced practice nurse as their primary health care provider.

A survey conducted by the Kellogg Foundation and completed in April 1994 demonstrates that Americans believe it is important to have nurses involved in their care.[23] Half of the 1,000 respondents had been treated by a nurse practitioner in the last year. In a Gallup poll of the same year, consumers saw reduced RN staffing in hospitals as the most detrimental among cost-cutting strategies commonly used in health care today.[24] To summarize the public attitude, con-

sumers see nurses as an untapped resource for the nation's health and would feel comfortable if they were to assume expanded responsibility.

A word should be said about nurses' attitudes toward certain types of patients. There has been some evidence that nurses do not view all types of patients equally favorably; for example, they tend to be more negative toward the elderly, alcoholic, criminal, mentally ill, or those with certain kinds of conditions. A number of studies, usually small, have been done on these topics. The purpose is primarily to determine what these attitudes are and why, how they affect patient care, and how to encourage or change particular attitudes. Several researchers have explored nurses' attitudes and concerns regarding AIDS. Students with negative attitudes toward intravenous drug users also had stronger intentions to avoid caring for AIDS patients, even with adequate knowledge and perceived control of any occupational risk.[25] Avoidance of AIDS patients was also associated with a negative attitude toward homosexuals.[26] Similar negativism, though less overt, can often be observed in care of the elderly. As originally conceived, the Medicare program included a 10 percent additive to the rate to allow for the increased cost of caring for the elderly as opposed to younger patients. During the development of the DRGs in the state of New Jersey, this assumption was disproved. In fact, nurses actually gave less care to the aged. The amount of nursing care rendered was inversely related to the age of the patient. The government used the occasion of these findings to remove the 10 percent from the rate. Nurses' attitudes toward ethnic minorities and terminally ill patients complicate the picture even more.

Finally, it is necessary for nurses to acknowledge the importance of our attitudes toward each other, especially when such attitudes affect clinical care, the advancement of the profession, and an individual nurse's practice. We need to question if we govern our professional interrelationships with the same guidelines that regulate our performance in patient care. Other areas to consider are attitudes toward nurses who are impaired, handicapped, of different ethnic or national origin, and even nurses of different educational backgrounds.

THE MEDIA IMAGE OF NURSING

Set apart from consumer opinion on nurses as provider professionals is the media image, which often remains as a deadly undercurrent, being laden with all the stereotypes of generations. The thoughtfulness consumers have demonstrated in giving opinion on the value of expanded services delivered by nurses should eventually filter down and reshape the media image. In order to effect that change, a healthy dose of intolerance is necessary from the profession, and vigilance on our behalf, to discourage destructive portrayals of the nurse. Interestingly, a cross-cultural comparison of images of nurses and physicians across 30 cultures found that "cross-culturally, nurses were viewed as positive, active, and kind, but not associated with power, independence and knowledge." This was in contrast to physicians who were viewed as powerful and strong.[27] Clearly, the image problem is not confined to this country.

The rest of this chapter discusses nursing's image by focusing on current and past solutions to the image problem. Topics to be covered include contemporary notions of nursing's image, studies on the public's image of nursing, the role of the media, and collective and individual strategies for improving the professional image of the nurse. While the topic is enormous, only major themes and strategies will be covered. Interested readers can find additional references in the bibliography.

Presently, nurses are at a critical stage in changing this image. The 1980s witnessed a heightened awareness of, and concern with, nursing's image, both within the profession and in the public at large. Much of this awareness and the activities that accompanied it were related to the nursing shortage. Recognizing that nursing's poor image was a hindrance to the recruitment of talented individuals, many organizations and health care professionals were motivated to take a new look at the image issue.

Typically, when many lay people think of a nurse, the crisp white uniform, complete with cap, comes to mind. Nursing's mandate with regard to its image is to educate the public about the intellectual and emotional challenges and rewards that nursing offers.

Several surveys have identified the importance and image of nursing to specific groups. Results show that the image of the nurse is highly variable, depending on the respondent's experiences and impressions. This is to be expected, because if there is no one typical nurse, how can we expect the image of the nurse to be the same across groups?

In one survey of nearly 700 hospital CEOs, nursing was named as the most significant factor in providing high-quality patient care, especially for CEOs at hospitals with 200 to 400 beds.[28] Other studies of the public have shown that the "image of the nurse continues to turn on feminine and nurturant characteristics." One study of college faculty at major universities showed that they held a more positive view of nursing than the one typically presented in the media.[29]

Despite these different images, few would doubt the power of the media in forming the public's image of many professions, not just nurses. Interviews and research articles or programs generally portray the nurse in a reasonably accurate way. As a rule, however, in fiction, the media have not, and still do not, correct a distorted image. Comic strips, novels, and television tend to portray the nurse (almost always female) either as a very sweet and/or sexy young girl, playing obedient handmaiden to the doctors, or as a tough, starched older woman, efficient and brusque. The popularity of medically oriented television series is supposedly a reflection of the public's intense interest in the field. But the images of the nurses portrayed have been no more accurate, and even nursing advisers to the shows seldom get the script changed. On the screen, Nurse Rachet in the award-winning movie *One Flew Over the Cuckoo's Nest*, which was also a book and a play, was probably thoroughly hated by millions of people. An equal number may have leered at the nurses in other popular movies or television series, or even in the various pornographic films where nurses are portrayed primarily as sex objects.

Kalisch and Kalisch have researched extensively the power of the mass media on nursing. They identify six time periods and corresponding nurse stereotypes as follows:

Angel of mercy	1854–1919
Girl Friday	1920–1929
Heroine	1930–1945
Mother	1946–1965
Sex object	1966–1982
Careerist	1983–present[30]

Kalisch and Kalisch view the careerist as the new ideal image for the 1980s and 1990s. The careerist is an "intelligent, logical, progressive, sophisticated, empathic, and assertive woman or man who is committed to attaining higher and higher standards of health care for the American public." They admit that the transition to the careerist image is not easy. However, it is important that nurses strive to communicate this new image, rather than passively accept definitions of ourselves "in which we have had no hand" and to which we have offered "amazingly little resistance." They suggest that perhaps on an unconscious level, nurses have contributed to the maintenance of "dysfunctional stereotypes." In many ways, the image of nursing in the media reflects the image of nursing held by the public. Thus, there are many strong reasons for nurses to persuade the public (as well as many nurses) that the status given to nurses in the media is much lower than what is and ought to be.

Kalisch and Kalisch also describe the implications of the negative image of nursing. One of the most crucial problems, as they see it, is that:

> . . . this poor image affects the quantity and quality of persons who choose nursing as an occupation. A public constantly fed a demeaning image of nursing will not perceive nursing as a desirable profession.[31]

In the late 1980s, nurses did take a proactive stand against the NBC-TV show, *Nightingales*, which portrayed nurses as promiscuous "birdbrains" and tinsel handmaidens.[32] Nursing organizations and individuals offered to provide script consultation and were turned down. Eventually, the surge of protest against the show from nurses across the country led many of its commercial sponsors to back out, and eventually the show was canceled. Nevertheless, in the next season, the same network started a similar program. This is not uncommon, yet not all TV programs portray nurses in a negative manner. *China Beach* managed to depict realistically and sensitively the challenges of nursing during the Vietnam War. Several documentaries on nursing and health care have also been favorable to nurses.

The power of the media and the numerous shows that continue to portray nurses in a negative and unrealistic manner led to the organizing of a group called Nurses of America (NOA) and their publication, *Media Watch*. NOA was sponsored by the Tri-Council organizations (see Chap. 27). It was funded by a grant from the Pew Charitable Trusts and administered by the NLN. NOA described itself as:

> . . . a national, multi-media effort designed to inform the public about the role contemporary nursing plays in the delivery of high quality, cost-effective health care services . . . . NOA's media efforts are designed to demonstrate the real drama of nursing; the vital work that nurses do every day.

NOA worked with a variety of media, ranging from newspapers and magazines to TV and community forums. A large component of their activities included monitoring the media for health-related issues and the portrayal of nurses and nursing practice.[33]

In addition to the image of nursing in the media, another concern of nurses is how physicians perceive them and their profession. Historically, the perception is of an inferior, with some interesting ramifications. If physicians' current image of the nursing *profession* can be equated with their image of the nurse, it is clear that their perceptions are as confused as they were 100 years ago. (See Chaps. 3 and 4.) Now, as then, there are physicians and leaders in organized medicine who see and applaud the changes in nursing toward full professionalism; others find this trend either threatening, incongruent with what they think a nurse's role should be, or not as desirable as the "good old days." As more nurses and physicians engage in collaborative practice, the image of the nurse among physicians should improve.

Other strategies to improve the image of nursing are discussed in articles on how to handle the media and be interviewed. Nurses can also improve their image by being involved in community services and organizations. At the worksite, nurses can improve their image by being more visible and serving on various committees. Most importantly, within the profession, nurses need to educate each other about their own subspecialties. Nurses tend to focus on their own area of practice. But it would benefit the image of the profession if more nurses could converse easily on a wide range of issues, including those of colleagues in areas such as nurse anesthesia, nurse midwifery, occupational health, and critical care.

One of the most widely applauded strategies to improve nursing's image was the advertising campaign launched between 1989 and 1992 by the National Commission on Nursing Implementation Project (NCNIP) and the Advertising Council of New York. The Ad Council guaranteed a minimum of $20 million in creative development and media exposure over a three-year period. Additional commitment of resources depended on public response to the campaign. The idea was to portray nursing as a "discipline that offers excitement, clinical substance, and authority and responsibility, all tied up in the richness of interpersonal closeness with patients."[34]

Obviously, there is no one profile of the modern nurse, particularly in these dynamic times. However, the information obtained from these various studies tells us a great deal about the practitioners of nursing. Resources being allocated to improve the image of nursing have already demonstrated that with work, the image can be changed to one that is more positive and realistic than it has been in the past. Nursing's image has already begun to change in the mass media, among physicians, and most importantly, for members of the profession itself.

REFERENCES

1. Moses EB: *The Registered Nurse Population.* Rockville, MD: U.S. Department of Health and Human Services, February 1994, pp 10, 22.
2. Ibid, p 8.
3. Ibid, p 14.
4. Rosenfeld P: *Profiles of the Newly Licensed Nurse,* 2d ed. New York: National League for Nursing, 1994, p 14.
5. Moses, op cit, pp 17–18.
6. Ibid, p 32.
7. Midwest Alliance in Nursing: Selected findings from the 1988 sample survey of registered nurses. *Main Lines* 10:1–2, April 1989.
8. Moses, op cit, p 52.
9. Knopf L: *From Student to RN.* Bethesda, MD: Department of Health, Education, and Welfare, 1972.
10. National League for Nursing: *Nursing Data Review 1994.* New York: The League, 1994, p 21.
11. Ibid, pp 98–99, 198–200.
12. Carnegie ME: Blacks in nursing: An update. *Am Nurse* 22:6, February 1990.
13. National League for Nursing, op cit, p 20.
14. Ibid.
15. Christman L: Men in nursing. *Imprint* 35:75, September 1988.
16. Perkins J et al: Why men choose nursing. *Nurs Health Care* 14:34–38, January 1993.
17. Tri-Council Nursing Organizations: Implementing nursing's short-term strategies for the management of the nursing shortage: A progress report, in *Proceedings, Invitational Conference on the Nursing Shortage: Issues and Strategies.* Chicago: American Organization of Nurse Executives, 1988.
18. Wandelt MA et al: Why nurses leave nursing and

what can be done about it? *Am J Nurs* 1:72–77, January 1981.

19. Fleishman-Hillard, Inc: *Opportunities for Growth.* A Report to the American Nurses Association, May 1991.

20. American Nurses Association: *National Public Opinion Survey on Nursing.* Kansas City, MO: The Association, 1985.

21. National League for Nursing: *A Nationwide Survey of Attitudes toward Health Care and Nurses.* New York: The League, 1990.

22. American Nurses Association: Consumers willing to see a nurse for routine "doctoring," according to Gallup poll. *News Release*, Sept 7, 1993.

23. Kellogg Foundation: *How People View Their Providers.* Report of a survey, June 24, 1994.

24. American Nurses Association: Consumers believe RN cutbacks hurt quality of care in hospitals according to Gallup survey. *News Release*, June 14, 1994.

25. Jemmott LS et al: Predicting AIDS patient care intentions among nursing students. *Nurs Res* 5:172–177, May 1992.

26. Jemmott JB et al: Perceived risk of infection and attitudes toward risk groups: Determinants of nurses' behavioral intentions regarding AIDS patients. *Res Nurs Health* 15:295–301, 1992.

27. Champion V, Austin J, Tzeng OCS: Cross-cultural comparisons of images of nurses and physicians. *Int Nurs Rev* 34:43–48, 1987.

28. Kaler SR, Levy DA, Schall M: Stereotypes of professional roles. *Image* 21:85–89, Summer 1989.

29. Lippman DT, Ponton KS: Nursing's image on the university campus. *Nurs Outlook* 37:24–27, January 1988.

30. Kalisch PA, Kalisch BJ: *The Changing Image of the Nurse.* Palo Alto: Addison-Wesley, 1987.

31. Ibid.

32. Lone P: TV's Nightingales—or birdbrains? *New York Times.* A31, April 7, 1989.

33. What Nurses of America is all about. *Media Watch* 1:1–2, Winter 1990.

34. Joel L: NCNIP/Advertising Council campaign challenges resistant stereotypes. *Am J Nurs* 22:13, February 1990.

Nursing Education and Research

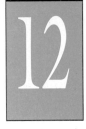

Major Issues and Trends in Nursing Education

UNLIKE MOST PROFESSIONS, nursing has a variety of programs for entry into the profession (also called *basic, preservice*, or *generic education*). This situation confuses the public, some nurses, and employers. The three major educational routes that lead to RN licensure are the diploma programs operated by hospitals, the baccalaureate degree programs offered by four-year colleges and universities, and the associate degree programs usually offered by junior (or community) colleges. Some states have permitted hospital programs to "award" associate degrees or baccalaureate degrees, usually in cooperation with an institution of higher learning and fulfillment of specific criteria, but there are only a few of these. A master's degree program for beginning practitioners is also available at a few universities, as is a professional doctorate (ND). These programs admit students with baccalaureate or higher degrees in fields other than nursing.

Although at one time diploma schools educated the largest number of nurses (more than 72 percent of the total number of schools in 1964 were diploma), the movement of nursing programs into institutions of higher learning has been consistent. Between 1964 and 1992, associate degree (AD) programs expanded from 130 to 848. In this period, BSN programs grew from 187 to 501. At the same time, diploma programs decreased from 833 to 135 for a total of 1,404 basic RN programs. Practical nurse programs, discussed in Chap. 13, number about 1,090. The pattern, then, has been an in-

crease in all collegiate programs and a decrease in diploma programs. A zero growth rate in admissions occurred in 1977; however, by 1992 admissions reached an all-time high of 96,786. This represents a 6.9 percent increase over 1991. There was a 15.9 percent increase for baccalaureate programs, 3.8 percent for associate, and 2.0 percent decrease for diploma. Master's degree programs increased from 154 in 1983 to 243 in 1992, with total enrollment growing from 18,112 to 28,370 in that same decade. There were 7,345 graduates from master's programs in 1992 as compared with 5,039 in 1982. The number of doctoral programs doubled during those years, and the number of graduates expanded by almost 300 percent. This reflects statistics for master's and doctoral programs in nursing, and does not take into consideration nurses who select graduate education in other disciplines.[1]

THE NEW CRISIS

Statistics on admissions, enrollments, and graduations for one date are interesting but provide limited sensitivity to trends without multiple points of comparison along a continuum of time. Recruitment to nursing has been at the mercy of a series of events and circumstances. Some of them were unpredictable, but more often nursing should have been able to predict the sequence of events and consequences.

Nursing education in terms of its students and its programs has been significantly influenced by governmental funding. The Nursing Education Act, as the largest single source of federal dollars for nursing, provided significant support from 1972 to 1980.[2] The years of generous versus meager funding generally paralleled federal administrations who were allies or adversaries of nursing. Some critics question the wisdom of concentrating nursing's governmental agenda in one major piece of legislation. And there are those who oppose becoming so dependent on government funding and would have looked to alternate sources of dollars, such as philanthropy, business, industry, and so on.

A cyclical nursing shortage has also had a significant impact on the decision to choose nursing as a field of work. There was a shortage of nurses in both the late 1970s and 1980s which was preceded by a period of oversupply. Aiken describes this cyclical pattern.[3] Nurses' salaries are held artificially low both because of a perceived oversupply and because they are not usually militant on their own behalf. Salary gains of less sophisticated workers who provide some aspect of nursing service outpace nursing gains. Health care organizations see the value of registered nurses, given their excellent work ethic, potential for cross-training, capacity to expand and contract based on the demands of the moment, and reasonable cost. Consequently, nonprofessionals are replaced by registered nurses, and a nursing shortage ensues. The shortage prompts all sorts of activity aimed at recruitment to educational programs and to the workforce. An essential aspect of enhancing recruitment is securing better salaries and benefits. Once nurses are paid more fairly, they are used more cautiously. The literature documents that nurses spend more than half of their time on nonessential or nonnursing functions.[4] Using nurses (now a costly commodity) more judiciously "kicks in" the oversupply phenomenon. The field becomes less attractive to recruitment for fear that one might not be able to secure employment after a long and expensive period of educational

preparation. The cycle repeats, and market forces produce corrections in a manner that is more or less predictable.

The nursing shortage of the late 1980s was compounded by a simultaneous drop in nursing education program admissions. Some initially blamed this on the reports that, with the inception of prospective payment (see Chap. 7), hospitals were closing units and laying off nurses, so nursing could no longer be seen as an occupation where you could always get a job. Here we see the tragedy of a public view that nurses are more or less exclusively employed in hospitals. However, there were more significant factors relating to social trends. These include a decrease in the number of high school graduates who were traditionally college-bound or at least ready for some occupational training; multiple career options open to women who would once have chosen nursing; young people's interest in more lucrative careers; a poor image of nursing (hard work, little status, poor salary, limited opportunities for advancement, not a profession); and less financial support for nursing education. Whatever the reason, admissions to nursing programs dipped dramatically, beginning in 1983. By 1986, the NLN reported as much as a 30 percent drop in enrollments in all basic RN programs but particularly in baccalaureate programs. Enrollment of first-time nursing students began to pick up in 1987, and increased to a high point of 9.3 percent in 1988. Other years up to and including 1992 have shown good gains. Statistics for 1988 show that the largest admission gains were in associate degree (11.5 percent), and diploma programs (19.3 percent). Baccalaureate programs showed only 1.9 percent gain. In ensuing years, growth has leveled off noticeably in associate and diploma programs and increased in baccalaureate admissions to a 1991–1992 academic year gain of 13.3 percent. Given the years of low admissions and the growing pattern of part-time study, graduation rates are only beginning to approach the numbers of 1985 (82,075 in 1985, and 80,839 in 1992).[5] With the "aging" of the nursing population as described in Chap. 11, this becomes a serious observation.

The 1988 popularity of associate and diploma programs deserves some special analysis. Diploma schools may have profited from good marketing, some hospital subsidization, relatively low cost, and the fact that some of these programs are actually shorter than the AD route. This first-time enrollment surge also occurs at the time of a general economic recession, prominent media attention to the nursing shortage, and anticipated employment after a minimal educational investment. The trend toward selection of nursing as a career and career changes at an older age are also relevant here (see Chap. 11). Though shortsighted in terms of educational mobility (it is possible to complete a bachelor's in the same time), it could hold special appeal to individuals with a preexisting baccalaureate or master's degree to be able to sit for the RN licensing exam after a two-year community college investment.

An increase in the numbers of admissions or first-time enrollments to nursing programs was essential both to swell the total nurses in the workforce and to replace the large numbers of nurses who would drop out of the field due to retirement. However, the nursing shortage was significantly impacted by inactive nurses who returned to work, and the degree to which part-time and full-time employed nurses increased their hours.

One major outcome of the drop in admissions was the participation of schools in the gigantic marketing effort of NCNIP (see Chap. 5) and various nursing and other health care organizations and groups, aimed at attracting prospective students to nursing and generally enhancing the image of nursing. Individual schools also used many new techniques to recruit students to their own particular programs. Among these were establishing relationships with liberal arts programs or schools to funnel students directly into nursing education more easily; "adopting" a high school or even middle school, or "mentoring" specific students in these schools to orient them to nursing careers;

and working with unions to encourage and assist LPNs or aides to move on to RN education. One well-funded program united the forces of over 100 hospitals, long-term care facilities, and nursing programs into consortia to provide educational advancement opportunities for aides and practical nurses, with the expectation that since they had already chosen nursing, they would, as RNs, stay on the job. Included were accelerated training, loan/service payback programs, and support services, remedial help, and counseling.[6] In addition, schools used radio and TV spots, mail campaigns, and booths at shopping malls and health clubs. There were also much discussion and lobbying for more student financial aid from the state and national governments, since there was considerable evidence that this was needed. (Among others, NSNA has reported for years that most nursing students require financial aid.) Launching a new Cadet Nurse Corps, which had increased nursing enrollment so much during World Warr II, was also suggested.[7] Some hospitals provided scholarships or made arrangements with potential students to pay back funding by promising to work in that institution for a specific period of time. One diploma school recruited students in Ireland and other foreign countries, granting them full scholarships and maintenance in return for a promise to work in the hospital for three years after graduation.

As is true of colleges in general, special attention was (and is) given to recruiting the nontraditional pool of potential applicants such as second careerists and older men and women. College graduates were also seen as likely to be attracted to accelerated BSN programs or generic master's. Minorities and men, still not a large percentage of the nursing student population, were also targeted for recruitment. Since 1988, there has been a steady increase in the number of men enrolled in basic RN programs, with very little variation among the program types. The 1992 enrollment level was 11.1 percent as compared with 9.9 percent for 1991. There has been a steady decrease in the number of minority students enrolled in baccalaureate programs from 19.4 percent in 1990 to 16.3 percent in 1992. This is very comparable to the general minority enrollment picture in four-year institutions. Minority enrollment in associate degree programs remained stable at 15.2 percent in 1992, and diploma enrollment increased from 11.7 to 12.5 percent. Baccalaureate nursing programs graduate a greater proportion of their minority students than do baccalaureate programs in general, while minorities are underrepresented among the graduates of associate degree nursing programs as compared to the total percent of minority graduates.[8]

Attrition is a serious problem for many minority students, both for academic and financial reasons and also because they may require considerable support, for which schools are not always prepared or seem unable to provide.[9] One interesting outcome is the speed with which some rather rigid programs have managed to adjust to the need for flexibility in curriculum, class scheduling, and meeting the needs of nontraditional students as well as returning RNs. This is discussed later.

PROGRAM OVERVIEW

There are certain similarities that all basic nursing programs share, in part because all are affected by the same societal changes.

1. Nursing education is becoming more expensive, and financial support is less available for schools and students. The inflationary costs affecting society and education also affect nursing programs and the institutions in which they are located. Moreover, the better the preparation of the teachers and the quality of other resources and facilities, the more costly the program. Both state and federal governments have been tightening the financial reins on programs, apparently indifferent to the effect on quality or student needs. Therefore, although there is verbal encouragement for faculty to develop innovative programs, funds are seldom available for this purpose. Tuition seldom if ever covers the cost of the program, but, even so, it has been rising consistently. Students are finding it more and more difficult to receive scholarships, loans, and grants. The mean annual tuition in public associate degree programs, public and private baccalaureate, and private diploma programs has risen. The most significant increase has been 41 percent in public associate degree programs from 1991 to 1992. The exception has been private associate and public diploma programs, where tuition has actually been reduced.[10]

2. The student population is more heterogeneous. Few, if any, schools refuse admission or matriculation to married students with or without families. Often, leave is granted for childbirth. It is not unusual to have a grandparent in a class, as more mature individuals look for a new or better career. The tight job market in many fields and the target marketing mentioned previously bring to nursing individuals with degrees and sometimes careers in related or unrelated fields. More men are entering nursing.

3. Educational programs are generally more flexible. Educational trends in this direction, plus the admission of a very mixed student body, including aides, LPNs, and RNs seeking advanced education, have required a second look at proficiency and equivalency testing, self-paced learning, and new techniques in teaching. The popularity of the external degree program indicates this trend. Twenty percent of nurses who were newly licensed in 1992 held college degrees prior to nursing school. Baccalaureate graduates were more likely to have had a degree (20.8 percent), as compared with associate (18.8 percent) or diploma graduates (15.6 percent). Further, of 142,494 enrollees

in baccalaureate programs in 1992, over 28 percent were RN students.[11]

The large numbers of RN students and mature adult learners in general predict more dependence on personal earnings and spousal income. This also creates the need for more flexible hours, convenient clinical practice locations, and the ability to extend the educational program beyond the originally planned two, three, or four years.

4. Educational programs copy from each other or are subject to the same waves of educational faddism and jargon. For instance, where once curricula were based on the same standard clinical and supportive courses, the "integrated" curriculum became popular in the 1950s but is fading away to some extent now. Also, today most faculty subscribe to models and theoretical frameworks as the basis for curriculum development.

5. State approval is required and national accreditation is available for all basic programs. Every school of professional nursing, in all three categories as well as practical nurse programs, must meet the standards of the legally constituted body in each state authorized to regulate nursing education and practice within that state. These agencies are usually called *state boards of nursing* or some similar tile. Without the approval of these boards, a school cannot really operate, because the graduates would not be eligible to take the licensing examination. In addition, many schools of nursing also seek accreditation by the National League for Nursing. Accreditation by the League is a voluntary matter, not required by law. Increasing numbers of schools seek it, however, because it represents nationally determined standards of excellence and nonaccreditation may affect the school's eligibility for outside funding or retard the graduates' entrance into BSN or graduate programs.

6. Faculty and clinical facilities are scarce resources. Faculty with the recommended doctoral degree for baccalaureate and graduate programs and the master's degree for other programs are increasing in number, but the total need has not been met. Clinical facilities are at a premium. Most schools, including diploma programs, use a variety of facilities. In large cities, several schools may be using one specialty hospital or clinical area (particularly obstetrics and pediatrics) for student experience. In rural areas, distance, small hospitals, and fewer patients are problems. Community health resources are very limited. Schools are also searching for new types of clinical experiences with various ethnic groups and in new settings such as hospices, community nursing centers, and with nurse entrepreneurs.

7. There is a slow but perceptible trend toward involving students in curriculum development, policy making, and program evaluation. Social trends and the maturity of students, with their demands to have a part in the educational program, are making some inroads on faculty and administrative control of schools.

8. All nursing students have learning experiences in clinical settings. Somewhere a myth arose that only practical nurse and diploma students gave "real" patient care in their educational programs, that AD students barely saw patients, and that baccalaureate students prepared only for teaching and administration. In fact, the time spent in the clinical area differs among programs within a particular credential as much as it does among various types of programs. In all good programs, students care for selected patients in order to gain certain skills and knowledge. Some provide for externships or other additional clinical experience.

9. It is generally agreed that the standards by which nursing education programs are judged should include criteria involving

the organization and administration of the *institution* itself (financial support, other support services, a review process for quality); students (selection, retention, evaluation, participation in identifying and evaluating program goals); *faculty* (preparation, research and publication efforts, development and evaluation of programs, participation in governance); *programs* (objectives, theoretical framework, curriculum of study, satisfactory learning opportunities, relationships with service institutions, and evaluation); *facilities and resources* (funds, support services, library, facilities specific to the program).

EXTERNAL CONSTRAINTS ON NURSING EDUCATION

Nursing education, like other educational fields, is strongly affected by external constraints over which it has limited or no control. To constrain means to compel, oblige, force, or restrain. Nursing education is the object of multiple constraints: those imposed as a part of the system of higher education, those imposed by the responsibilities of a health profession to the public, and those imposed by a more or less cohesive group of practitioners who are, in essence, employers, employees, colleagues, change agents, and even critical consumers. That the constraints imposed by these groups may conflict with each other only adds pressure. Nevertheless, the results of these constraints are not necessarily bad.

The effects of the national economy are not limited to increased costs of the program and increased tuition. Nursing, viewed as a profession "where you can always get a job," as well as challenging work, may be attractive not only to other careerists whose fields are in decline, but to individuals seeking a second or third career change. On the other hand, better financial options in other fields may turn the "best and the brightest" away from nursing. New limitations to federal and state funding for both schools and students put more constraints on expan-

sion, or perhaps more accurately, indicate the direction of new programs. For instance, NP programs increased, in part, because they were funded. Any specialty, such as oncology, psychiatry, even preparation for administration or teaching, seems to expand or contract according to available funding. Moreover, the content of the curriculum may be influenced by the federal guidelines required if federal funds are accepted. And, as shown in Chap. 7, reimbursement policies for health care have resulted in different delivery modes, increasing the need for nurses, and nurses with different types of preparation.

Changing student bodies reflect a changed economy and financial incentives to admit certain students. Federal programs have increased minority representation in schools of nursing, but a cutback in funds to aid their retention has caused problems. Nursing schools have been closed because a board of directors decided that they were not economically feasible to operate. Nevertheless, a tight money market has also resulted in a creative sharing of resources and in regional planning for nursing education.

Naturally, education is influenced by the knowledge explosion and technological advances. For nursing, this demands that practitioners keep up to date and raises multiple questions of curriculum content. Should nurses be educated as generalists or specialists? At what educational level? For primary, secondary, or tertiary care? For acute or long-term care? At what level? If new graduates are expected to practice at a minimum safe and effective level, what is the minimum content that should be in all curricula? If something new is added, should something be deleted, or should less be taught about everything? Are there more effective ways for students to learn, such as independent, self-paced learning? The increase in knowledge also puts more pressure on the profession to create and/or expand a knowledge base for nursing. How then to enlarge the minuscule number of nurses with doctoral education and research interests? These questions are being answered in a variety of ways by nurse educators, and are being raised in the halls of Congress as the various nursing bills are debated.

There are a number of social movements that affect nursing education. One noted previously is the recognition of students' rights. Another is renewed emphasis on the American belief in upward mobility. Moving to advanced education in nursing for either PNs or RNs has generally not been easy; most returning students believe that unnecessary obstacles have been placed in their way. Pressure by organized minority groups and unions, as well as the studies and edicts of national commissions and state and federal governments, and, of course, the nursing shortage, have all been important factors in developing more flexible educational patterns. The public's legitimate demand for competent practitioners has also focused more attention on continuing education. In addition, changes in the delivery of health care services, which may involve both new techniques (space medicine, organ transplants) and new or newly emphasized settings (maternity centers, neighborhood health centers and surgicenters), clients (teenagers, the elderly), health attitudes (prevention, self-care), or other concerns (environmental health, iatrogenic disease), as well as the changing role of other professionals and paraprofessional health workers, all affect nursing education.

Finally, there are the constraints placed on nursing education by the profession, the organizations that represent it, and its various practitioners. These pressures can create more strain than external forces because, unfortunately, there is no common nursing tradition, so the demands often conflict. One key example is the lack of agreement between nursing education and nursing service about the utilization of the graduates of the three major kinds of programs. Another conflict addresses the difference in philosophy as to whether professional nursing education can be a series of steps that build on previous experience and education, or whether professional education is so different from technical education that it requires a fresh start. Nurses also question whether graduate educa-

tion should be primarily clinical. Even though both state board approval and accreditation are fairly well controlled by nurses and affect educational programs, there is no agreement among those who exert that control at the state or national level. Many nursing groups spend time defining the competencies needed for graduates of the various types of programs. Unfortunately they seldom confer and each differs at least slightly from the others. Yet they are all published as definitive and expert. Most devastating of all is the bitter divisiveness caused by the issue of entry into practice.

ENTRY INTO PRACTICE

With five types of basic educational programs in nursing, the uncertainty of both the public and the profession as to the differences among these practitioners has appeared to escalate. To add to the confusion, graduates of all programs are eligible to take the same licensing examination and have the same passing score. There have been arguments that no one could expect the public and employers to differentiate among nursing graduates when all are designated as RNs on licensure. Often, RNs are employed in the same capacity, with the same assignments, same expectations, and same salary. Are they all professional nurses? If so, what justification is there for all these separate educational programs?

An important function of ANA is that of setting standards and policies for nursing education. A major action, taken in 1965, by the Committee on Education, resulted in the ANA position that nursing education should take place within the general educational system. Reaction to "Educational Preparation for Nurse Practitioners and Assistants to Nurses— A Position Paper" was decidedly mixed. Although the concept underlying the paper had been enunciated by leaders in nursing since the profession's inception, reiterated through the years, and accepted as a goal by the 1960 House of Delegates, many nurses misunderstood the paper's intent and considered it a threat. Probably the greatest area of misinterpretation lay in the separation of nursing education and practice into professional, technical, and assisting components. Minimum preparation for professional nursing practice was designated at the baccalaureate level, technical nursing practice at the associate degree level, and education for assistants in health service occupations was to be in short, intensive preservice programs in vocational education settings, rather than in on-the-job training. An obvious omission in the position paper was the place of diploma and practical nurse education. A large number of hospital-based diploma graduates, students, faculty, and hospital administrators were angered by the omission. A major source of resentment was that the term *professional nurse* was to be reserved for the baccalaureate graduate.

Even in this period of confusion, some people realized that the largest system of nursing education, the hospital school, could not be overlooked or eliminated by the writing of a position paper. Later, both the ANA and NLN prepared statements which advocated careful community planning for phasing diploma programs into institutions of higher learning. Others also pointed out that as practical nursing programs improved and increased their course content, their length became close to that of the associate degree program. Nevertheless, the storm raged for more than fifteen years, although repeated attempts were made to clarify the content and intent of the position paper. It was felt that ANA suffered a membership loss through the alienation of some diploma nurses. As expected, social and economic trends gradually brought about many of the changes suggested by the position paper, and the definitions of *professional nurse* and *technical nurse* were widely used in the literature (although there was no major indication that employers were assigning nurses according to technical or professional responsibilities). In June 1973, in what some considered a belated effort to placate diploma nurses, assure them of their importance to ANA, and encourage unity in the profession,

a "Statement on Diploma Graduates" was issued. In essence, the statement asked all units of ANA to give special attention to the needs and interests of diploma graduates, particularly in relation to continuing education and upward mobility. In addition, a task force was appointed to examine the contemporary relevance of the terms *professional* and *technical*, to distinguish basic preparation for nursing practice and to recognize all registered nurses as professionals. Although there appeared to be no major reaction from diploma nurses to this statement, some nurses considered it a step backward, because it seemed to reject the concept that professional nursing was different from technical nursing.

In February 1974, the Commission on Nursing Education approved a report on the contemporary relevance of the terms *professional* and *technical*. Meanwhile, the NLN's associate degree group rejected the term *technical*, but others continued to use it.

In 1976, the New York State Nurses' Association's voting body overwhelmingly approved introduction of a "1985 Proposal" in the 1977 legislative session. Although variations of the proposal evolved over the next years, the basic purpose of the legislation was to establish licensure for two kinds of nursing. The professional nurse would require a baccalaureate degree, and the other, whose title changed with various objections, would require an associate degree. The target date for full implementation was 1985; currently licensed nurses would be covered by the traditional grandfather clause, which would allow them to retain their current title and status (RN). The bill did not pass but was consistently reintroduced during each legislative session. Later, other nurses' associations introduced similar legislation without success. Immediately, the 1985 Proposal became both a term symbolizing baccalaureate education as the entry level into *professional* nursing and a rallying point for nurses who opposed this change. There was, and is, considerable opposition from some diploma and AD nurses and faculty, some hospital administrators, and some physicians. Nursing organizations were formed whose major focus was opposition to such proposals. They were primarily made up of diploma nurses, and supported by hospital organizations and administrators. Nevertheless, an increasing number of ANA's constituent state organizations, primarily made up of diploma nurses, voted in convention to work toward the goal of baccalaureate education for professional nursing. In 1978, the ANA House of Delegates passed such a resolution, as did the National Student Nurses' Association. The ANA resolution had emerged from an ANA-sponsored "Entry into Practice" conference held earlier that year. The 400 or so participants included representatives from various nurses' associations, the federal government, all types of schools of nursing, as well as administrators and staff nurses from all types of employment settings. The major recommendations, supporting the concept of two categories or types of practitioners in nursing (although they could not agree on titles), were that competencies be developed for those levels, statutory distinctions be established, and career mobility opportunities be increased, including the use of innovative and flexible educational programs. All these recommendations were incorporated into resolutions that the ANA House of Delegates also approved in 1978. Where once ANA conventions were consumed with entry into practice debates, gradually the question in education became: how do we facilitate the transition? (See the reports of ANA conventions in *Nursing Outlook*, and the *American Journal of Nursing* in the even years.) The 1980 Social Policy Statement,[12] which clearly stated that baccalaureate education was the basis of professional nursing practice, was accepted, and the Cabinet on Nursing Education continued to work toward this goal.[13] The reader should note that the "entry into practice" controversy consists of three separate issues: the intent of bringing preparation for nursing into the educational mainstream, distinction between two (or more) categories of nurses, and linking these distinctive categories to statutory requirements that

included different competencies and title protection. The idea of establishing licenses for two categories of nurses originated in New York in 1976, was introduced and supported at the ANA House of Delegates in 1978, but was never vigorously pursued until 1983. In 1983, ANA provided grants to several SNAs to implement their plans to establish the baccalaureate as the minimum educational qualification for professional nursing and further set its timetable for implementation in all states before the end of the century. The final report of the interdisciplinary National Commission for Nursing (Chap. 5) saw pursuit of the baccalaureate as an "achievable goal."[14] A three-year project funded by the W. K. Kellogg Foundation in late 1984 to carry out selected Commission recommendations included the objective: "…to outline the common body of knowledge and skills essential for basic nursing practice, the curriculum content that supports it, and a credentialing process that reinforces it." In later meetings, the ANA House of Delegates became involved in trying to agree on how the two types of nurses could be accommodated as members. Eventually, this was more or less resolved by changes in the bylaws (see Chap. 25).

The NLN has played an interesting role in the entry into practice debate. In 1979, it supported all pathways (baccalaureate, associate, diploma, and practical nursing). Given the structure of the NLN and its historic position as the accrediting body for each level of nursing education, this statement is understandable. In 1982, however, the Board of Directors endorsed the baccalaureate degree as the criterion for professional practice. This position was affirmed when the voting body met in June 1983. (See the convention reports published in *Nursing Outlook* in the odd years during those years.)

Later reaffirmations by the board that called for two separate licensing exams infuriated the AD programs and community college presidents, who threatened to pull out of NLN agency membership.[15] There was a demand for clarification and objections that this action downgraded AD nurses for the sake of elevating BSN nurses.[16] (From all this agitation came a number of organizations whose purpose was basically to support AD nursing and to protect AD nurses and programs from ANA and NLN actions they saw as detrimental.) The LPNs were not happy either. What resulted was a compromise statement that seemed reasonably acceptable. An interesting nonaction occurred at the next NLN convention where the issue was tabled and other issues related to a major reorganization were given priority.

Entry into practice and its inevitable corollary, changes in nurse licensure, continue to be a major issue in nursing. Most nursing organizations, at the state and national level, have taken a stand supporting baccalaureate education as the appropriate education for the "professional" nurse. After that, there is still disagreement as to whether the "other" nurse would be the technical nurse with separate licensing and that the PN would remain the same. Some think that AD education should be required for the practical nurse, leaving only two levels of nursing for the time being. Because this means a major change in nurse licensure, which is always a political as well as legal issue, only a few (small) states have taken that big step. As discussed in Chap. 20, the North Dakota Board of Nursing changed its administrative rules to say that after January 1987 the appropriate educational program for those wishing to take the RN licensure exam is the baccalaureate, and that for practical nursing, it is an associate degree. While there was a legal attempt by several hospitals to prevent this from going into effect, the North Dakota attorney general ruled that this decision was within the purview of the board.[17] Also in 1986, the Maine legislature stated their "intent" that there be two levels of nursing (associate degree and baccalaureate) by 1995 or as soon as possible thereafter. In 1985, a number of other state nurses' associations thought that legislation for entry-level changes was possible within a few years. This did not occur, perhaps because a more immediate concern was the nursing shortage. Opponents also seized on the shortage to maintain that this was not the time to make

such changes because all types of nursing education programs were needed. Even when some of the study reports (see Chap. 5) recognized the need for baccalaureate nurses, the approach suggested was often like that of the AHA—encouragement of educational mobility. This refers to articulation of diploma and AD programs with those awarding baccalaureate or higher degrees, as well as more high-quality external degree programs and flexible campus-based instructional programs for nurses who want baccalaureate education.

In the long debate about the nature of education for practice, it is not surprising that there are those who think that the system should stay as it is, others who opt for changing the baccalaureate nurse's title and license to indicate advanced preparation, and a few who are anticipating the time when a professional nurse doctorate, like the MD and DDS of physicians and dentists, will be the entry level to the profession.

Some natural fears of nonbaccalaureate nurses are to be expected: that they will lose status and job opportunities despite the grandfather clause and that those who desire baccalaureate education will find it too expensive, unavailable, or rigidly repetitive. As to the first, there is already some selectiveness and has been; in the latter, there is slow, but definite progress to make BSN completion programs for RNs more accessible. These issues will not be quickly resolved, but inevitable societal and professional changes, such as the decrease in diploma schools and the expectations of professional practice (nursing is the only health profession for which entry is less than a baccalaureate) will be major factors in the final outcome. There are problems that must be resolved and data obtained (for example, will costs limit access to professional nursing? Will such a plan improve patient care?). Because nursing loses power every time its practitioners battle internally it is essential that nurses work together toward a satisfactory conclusion, one that includes appreciation and respect for all competent nurses and focuses on providing the best possible nursing care to the public.

In the meantime, there has been a quiet revolution, one that may end the recurrence of the entry into practice issue that has followed nursing throughout its history. Although many RNs are not convinced that baccalaureate education necessarily means professionalism, others are and back to school they go.[18]

NEW APPROACHES

One of the key developments in nursing education in the early 1970s was the implementation of the "open curriculum" concept, which the NLN defined as a system "which incorporates an educational approach designed to accommodate the learning needs and career goals of students by providing flexible opportunities for entry into and exit from the educational program, and by capitalizing on their previous relevant education and experiences."[19]

This concept emerged only gradually. Nurse educators who were most aware of social and economic trends and sympathetic to the goals of those struggling for upward mobility began to plan and implement programs. Others ignored the signs of disillusionment among those seeking further education in nursing. Both the poor and ethnic minorities, often guided into lower-level nursing positions, and the middle-class nurses who had chosen diploma or associate degree education, as well as service corpsmen returning from active duty, became irritated at the difficulty of moving into other levels of nursing. All became increasingly hostile toward a system that offered no credit for previous study and experience, or, at most, recognized a few liberal arts courses. Unions included in their contracts provisions for organized programs of education for nonprofessionals. Other health workers turned to the legislatures. The result was evident in such states as California, which enacted laws to force schools of nursing to give credit to prospective students with previous health experience, and in recommendations of the federal government.

Soon it became evident that nursing programs were responding to the mandate for more flexibility, perhaps because higher education as a whole was doing so, and by the 1980s, because students were becoming scarcer and costs higher.

Today, almost all programs accept transfer credit as a means of advanced placement. Innovative programs have designed new methods for measurement of knowledge and competency or have developed entirely new programs. There are a variety of approaches for providing flexibility in nursing education. The ladder approach, which provides direct articulation between programs, moves an individual from nursing assistant to practical nurse to AD or diploma nurse to baccalaureate nurse, with any combination in between. For some, this means the ability to begin at a basic level and move one step at a time to the highest achievable level. For others, it means that one can aim at a particular level but be able to exit at distinct points, become licensed, and earn a living if necessity or circumstances dictate. (This exit opportunity is becoming less common.) An increasing number of baccalaureate programs enroll only RNs into an upper division, accepting past nursing education as the lower division to be built on. To attract second-degree candidates, there are a variety of programs that fast-tract these individuals to a master's and specialization.

There are still nurse educators who do not agree that the ladder is a viable concept. They believe that each program in nursing has its own uniqueness and that one cannot be based on the other. Further, they believe that the ladder tends to denigrate the role of workers at each level, implying the necessity to move upward. One solution seems to be the utilization of standardized and teacher-made tests to measure the individual's knowledge, according to a clear delineation of the achievement expectations of the program. There are a number of standardized tests available in both the liberal arts and nursing, but there is still some question as to how to test for clinical competency. Methods used include the use of videotapes, simulated experiences, practicums, and minicourses in the clinical setting. Also being used are the performance assessment centers of the New York State Regent's College External Degree program, as well as their paper-and-pencil exams.

Another approach is to allow students to proceed through a course at their own pace through testing, self-study, the use of media, and computers. A number of schools are experimenting with self-pacing and self-learning, and reports indicate that students find these stimulating and satisfying.

Other ways of giving more opportunities for students are to offer courses more frequently, during evening hours, weekends, and in summer, to allow part-time study, and to have class sessions off the main campus in areas convenient to students living in communities not easily accessible to the main campus.

Regents College (RC), The University of the State of New York (USNY), shares many goals and activities with conventional campus-based programs. However, it differs significantly in the ways students learn and the methods used to recognize and credential that learning. Rather than providing classroom instruction, RC provides the focus for learning through its degree requirements, and related study materials. It provides a comprehensive system of objective assessment of college-level knowledge and skills, using transfer credits from regionally accredited colleges, recognized proficiency examinations, nursing performance examinations, and other specialized evaluation procedures. Sometimes referred to as an external degree program or a university without walls, RC grants credits whenever college-level knowledge is validated through the use of faculty-approved, objective, academic assessment methods.

RC offers the only national total assessment nursing programs and thus it is unique, although there are now other external degree programs. Since 1972, RC has developed associate and baccalaureate programs in nursing, through more than $3.5 million from the Kellogg Foundation, with additional funds from federal capitation grants. [RC is not a state-sup-ported college, and it frequently is confused with the state university system (SUNY).] These external funds made it possible to obtain the essential expertise of nursing and psychometric specialists over an extensive period of time and to use a research orientation to develop, implement, and evaluate the programs and the related cognitive and performance examinations in nursing.

The associate degree nursing program was completed and accredited in 1975. Students must complete 35 credits of general education, six nationally standardized nursing written examinations and a two and one-half day clinical performance examination. The arts and sciences and the nursing content are equivalent to those expected in conventional ADN programs. Graduates are eligible for licensure in all states.

The baccalaureate nursing degree program was completed in 1979, and following a two-year series of meetings and appeals, this most innovative of nursing programs was accredited by the National League for Nursing, retroactively to include all its graduates. The content of degree requirements, in general education and nursing, is consistent with conventional BSN programs. A total of 120 semester credits must be earned, with 72 in the typical categories of arts and sciences, 20 credits in nursing documented by five nationally standardized written examinations, and 28 credits in clinical nursing documented through four criterion-referenced performance examinations.

In June 1994, there were more than 10,000 students enrolled at RC, 7,440 in the ADN and 2,569 in the BSN programs. This represents a 100 percent increase over the past 3 years. Since the inception of the programs, there have been 10,600 ADN and 3,100 BSN graduates. Maintaining students in the program continues to be a problem. Only 45 percent of ADN students return each semester and 35 percent of BSN candidates.

Nearly 80 percent of the BSN candidates are RNs from diploma or associate degree programs, with an average of ten years experience in nursing. Many BSN students have baccalaureate, master's, or doctoral degrees in other fields. Approximately three-fourths of the graduates state intentions of continuing with graduate school.

These external learning assessment programs were developed by a corps of nurse educators who are appointed as long-term consultants and serve on one or more of a complex array of committees, or who are employed as full-time salaried staff in the Albany office. The Overall Faculty Committee for Nursing is the central policy-making and curriculum group. They outline and subsequently approve the detailed work of approximately 20 subcommittees responsible for the examinations for the associate and baccalaureate degree programs and other essential faculty functions. The various faculty committees perform most of the nonteaching functions equivalent to those on campuses.

The performance examinations are administered by some 250 nurse faculty members, all of whom have completed the extensive training developed and administered by RC. Nursing performance examinations are administered on weekends throughout the year at the national network of Regional Performance Assessment Centers created and established by RC. The written nursing examinations are administered by The American College Testing Program (ACT PEP test) at some 160 locations throughout the country and at embassies and military bases throughout the world.

The day-to-day work of coordinating the development, implementation, and evaluation of the degree programs and advising and scheduling students is carried out by a full-time professional staff. The staff and faculty also develop study guides and other program materials to assist students.

Although there are some educators who oppose the external degree on philosophical grounds and others who fear the competition in the tight market for students, studies conducted relative to the program are providing data of significance to other external degree programs that include nursing. The data have also helped educational programs seeking more effective techniques for proficiency and equivalency testing. There is evidence that the examinations to measure clinical proficiency developed in the external degree program are helpful tools in traditional educational settings.[20]

If the trend toward expecting the baccalaureate as the entry to professional practice continues, the necessity for upward mobility becomes even more essential. However, RN students must beware of diploma mills. With nontraditional students comprising a major portion of the nursing education market, there should be plenty of options for RNs and others to continue formal education that is of good quality, and both nursing and society will benefit.

The demand for innovation and fresh approaches, or at least an open mind, has not excluded graduate education. The issues are much the same. The need is to be consumer-friendly yet maintain the integrity of education for advanced practice. Much of the controversy focuses around the term advanced practice. Health care reform promises to catapult nurses with graduate education into prominent roles. The nature of the preparation has become the topic of debate, with slowly growing consensus. One aspect of that debate is whether clinical nurse specialists and nurse practitioners should be educated as advanced practice nurses with the subsequent abandonment of the distinctions between the two roles. A second, with less current controversy, is whether nurse executives require joint degrees in business and nursing to serve the profession, given the complexities of today's health care system, and to claim educational equality with other system executives.[21] Preparation for teaching does not escape scrutiny. Can you, teach it, if you can do it? Or if you can't do it, who should teach clinical nursing in the 1990s? How do you infuse adequate clinical knowledge and skills into a preparation program for teachers? The special challenges of teaching in associate degree programs or the integrated curriculum that may not create assignments according to traditional specialty areas are real. The financial aid problems and need for geographically convenient education at often nontraditional hours are a shared concern for basic, RN, and graduate students.

DOES NURSING EDUCATION PREPARE COMPETENT PRACTITIONERS?

From the time that the last diploma program gave up the apprenticeship approach to nursing education, there have been accusations that the new graduates of modern nursing programs are not competent. Further investigation usually shows that new graduates are not as technically skillful or as able to assume responsibility for a large group of patients as the nurses with whom they are compared—the diploma graduates of yesterday. Nevertheless, the criticisms are understandable. For the director of nursing with fiscal constraints, a lengthy orientation and inservice program is a strain on the budget; for the staff nurse and supervisor, someone who requires extra help or supervision on a usually short-staffed unit is a temporary impediment.

For some unknown reason, useful communication between nursing education and nursing service is erratic at best and nonexistent at worst. In some areas, joint appointments of faculty and clinicians enable each to contribute to the goals of the other, but this practice is largely limited to university programs.

Although there seems to be little disagreement on the qualities, knowledge, and skills nurses need, there is almost no agreement on how much of each and what level of competency is needed at graduation. Graduates from all types of programs are the targets of employer disapproval, but sometimes the diploma graduate, whose program is focused on the hospital and who frequently stays at the same hospital, may find adjustment a little easier. Associate degree graduates who have been practical nurses and have had experience in caring for many patients are also somewhat immune for criticisms about slow adjustment. However, because most graduates today do not have these backgrounds, how justified are the criticisms?

The nursing literature is full of articles on content and methods; nurse educators are most certainly concerned about preparing the best possible practitioner. Everyone agrees that new graduates should be competent to give both physical and psychological/emotional care. Just how much of this is best taught in a clinical setting is a point of controversy.[22] How much of what kind of clinical experience prepares nurses best? It has been suggested that additional emphasis be given to the physical care needed because of patients' pathophysiological problems. There is also some indication that students "need practice in basic technical skills, which some schools deal with by encouraging additional self-study in labs. In others, a concentrated period of time in one or two clinical areas at the end of the program eases students into the work situation and allows them to integrate their clinical knowledge and skills over a continuum of time and to learn to organize the care of larger groups of patients, setting appropriate priorities. Certain programs also have cooperative arrangements with clinical facilities to allow students a paid work-study period in the summer, or specific academic terms in which they work full time while supervised in practice. Field placements, or clinical electives, are other options. There are mixed feelings about whether working as an aide or ward clerk is helpful because of the limited legal scope of practice and the possibility that students are subtly forced into assuming more responsibility than is legal.

Giving the added clinical experience in one mode or another seems to please both students and future employers. There are a number of variations of these methods. A *preceptorship* is usually a one-to-one experience for the student with a staff nurse preceptor guiding the learning in the clinical facility. The carefully selected preceptor, who is often given a clinical faculty appointment (without pay), has an orientation and sometimes classes on clinical teaching strategies. Preceptorships seem to enhance the student's learning, if properly done, but they require careful preparation and monitoring.[23] An *externship*, also often involving preceptors, gives students full-time work experience in a "real-world" environment, often in the summers, for which they are paid. Since the latter involves no academic faculty if it is not a built-in part of the curriculum, both the facility and the student must be careful to adhere to the legal limitations of what the student can do. An *internship* generally occurs after the student has graduated and eases the new graduate into the work setting by providing a variety of supervised experiences. Usually the new nurse is paid less during this time, and if not carefully planned to meet both employee and employer needs, the experience can become nonproductive. Preceptors are often a part of this practice as well.

There is also a question as to whether the various kinds of programs actually prepare different kinds of practitioners. Nurse educators say they do, but often the statements of philosophy and objectives or the NLN competency statements, described in Chap. 13, have obvious areas of overlap. Moreover, some believe that there is a lack of clarity in how heads of AD and BS programs see their type of program as differing from the other. Specifically, most programs do not seem to adhere to the differences spelled out in the literature. For instance, some AD program directors think their graduates have as broad a judgment base as the baccalaureate nurse, and many prepare these nurses for administrative functions without the necessary educational base. On the other hand, this is probably a matter of catching up with reality, because many employers give AD nurses responsibilities for which they are not prepared.[24] But should the teacher then educate the employer instead of reeducating the student?

If success in state boards is considered to be a criterion for competency, the results are no more definitive; differences within each type of program are greater than those among the programs. As to differences in practice among diploma, AD, and BSN nurses, this has been difficult to determine because most studies have been done by graduate students. Not only are the numbers and the studies seldom replicated, but what is being measured is usually different from study to study. Some researchers have concluded that, if properly defined, the leadership/management role could be a viable area of differentiation.[25]

Although the specific competencies of ADN and BSN nurses are discussed in the next chapter, one notable project is mentioned here. Primm's work has differentiated the two and been well received by both nursing education and nursing service. The general approach is categorization in terms of direct care, communication, and management competencies. The BSN competencies include and build on those of the ADN, with BSN nurses also assuming leadership and giving more advanced care in complex situations.[26] The very fact that nursing care is increasingly complex and that the AD nurse will considerably outnumber the baccalaureate nurse if current trends continue has concerned many nursing leaders, who wonder whether very sick patients can be properly cared for.

PREPARATION OF FACULTY AND EDUCATIONAL ADMINISTRATORS

The quality of teachers and the leadership of the program's director are key factors in the overall distinction of any educational program. They develop and implement the curriculum, usually select the students, and provide a milieu in which learning is either a chore or a joy, or something in between.

Teaching a clinical subject is not the same as teaching a course in liberal arts or the nonclinical aspects of nursing. Teachers of clinical nursing must not only know the theoretical concepts but should also be competent practitioners. Should they also know how to teach? These questions are arising in other practice disciplines because for years practicing clinicians have been the teachers, whether or not they were able to communicate their knowledge to students. The problem in nursing is twofold. Because of trends and opportunities in graduate education, there are nursing faculty who have learned curriculum and teaching skills, but shy away from actual patient care because they feel inadequate, and there are newly minted clinicians with graduate degrees who have difficulty communicating their know-how. Expanding knowledge and new nursing roles also combine to create a situation in which experienced teachers who have been competent in their field must continually acquire new skills.

Currently, graduate education provides the student with an area of clinical specialization and a functional role (teaching, management, or advanced practice). The clinical focus can reflect any one of a variety of populations, health problems, or settings, but it is specialized and focused. The term *advanced practice* has come into common usage as opposed to distinguishing between the clinical nurse specialist and the nurse practitioner. This issue is discussed further in Chap. 15. The question now becomes how well are these teachers prepared for an integrated curriculum or for AD programs in which teaching at a specialty level is a luxury? Further, how do you provide both adequate clinical knowledge and skill and the content necessary for the art and science of teaching within a graduate degree? Should we assume that because you can do it, you can teach it? And is there a place for a teacher whose graduate degree is not in nursing? Nonnursing faculty still have a place in schools of nursing teaching in their specialty area, but the trend is toward decreased employment. In 1992, 628 nonnurse faculty were reported among a total of 23,775 faculty. This number reflects all programs and both part-time and full-time appointees.[27] There are those that feel that background from another discipline enriches students' educational experience, but in some states, even nurses who hold a doctorate are not considered acceptable as faculty unless they have a master's in nursing.[28]

A serious problem is that some teachers of nursing do not yet meet the academic requirements for their positions. The preparation of nursing faculty has improved since the 1970s particularly in relation to the number of faculty with master's degrees in nursing. However, the percentages differ greatly within programs. In 1992, baccalaureate and higher degree programs reported about 99 percent, AD 88 percent, diploma about 64 percent, and practical nursing about 80 percent of their faculty with master's degrees in nursing. Over 90 percent of faculty holding doctoral degrees teach in baccalaureate and higher degree programs. Overall, about 41 percent of nursing faculty teaching in those programs have an earned doctorate.

Data on the supply and demand for nurse educators in 1992 do not indicate that a faculty shortage exists. The vacancy rate for faculty across all programs is 4.9 percent. The negative observations are that faculty-to-student ratios have deteriorated somewhat, and declining numbers of full-time faculty are being replaced by part-time positions, particularly in associate degree and diploma programs. Neither can the claims that potential faculty candidates are being attracted to nonacademic positions be substantiated. The movement toward part-time appointments essentially reflects a trend seen in most of the nation's colleges and universities. While reliance on part-time faculty may be an economic expedient, there is a notable difference in academic credentials. In general, 61 percent of full-time university faculty hold doctoral degrees, as compared with only 29 percent of their part-time counterparts.[29]

The lack of appropriate credentials, regardless of the teacher's individual qualifications, puts nursing faculty at a distinct disadvantage in a university setting, where the minimum requirement is the doctorate. Further, often nurse faculty are not considered true colleagues (a problem nurses also have when dealing with physicians in the clinical setting), and they have difficulty in competing for higher rank, tenure, or appointment on committees because of minimum accomplishments in areas of research and scholarship.

Currently, many faculty have doctorates from programs other than nursing, because only recently have there been enough doctoral programs reasonably accessible. However, if faculty also do research in their field, how does such a doctorate prepare one for clinical nursing research? Is a doctorate in a related science preferable? With the scarcity of doctoral nurses, the type of degree has not yet become a serious issue in all but the most selective schools, but it is tending in that direction. On the other hand, even those faculty with doctoral education in nursing face problems they had not anticipated. It appears that nursing doctoral programs are designed to prepare graduates as researchers and scholars rather than as experts in teaching, clinical practice, or even administration. And yet, the reality is that they spend most of their time teaching—probably at the undergraduate level. They complain that heavy clinical loads prevent them from taking time for research. Yet they are chastised for being less scholarly and less productive than their other university colleagues. Deans are advised to give them short-term contracts unless they make scholarly contributions to the program; probably they will not survive in the promotion-tenure race anyhow. They may then seek to concentrate on research and writing, and students have low priority. Students resent it, and in truth, teaching may suffer. But what kind of role model should the teacher be to the student? Scholar? Clinician? Teacher? In a time of economic retrenchment with heavier teaching assignments, can the faculty member be all three—adequately? It should be noted that these are primarily problems of university or college faculty. In AD and diploma programs, there is not yet such an emphasis on scholarly productivity. How these issues affect doctoral education is discussed in Chap. 13.

One trend, particularly in college and university programs is the encouragement, sometimes requirement, that clinical faculty maintain their clinical competence by regular practice beyond their clinical teaching. There are many versions of what is generally called faculty practice.[30] (See the bibliography for an overview of articles on faculty practice.)

The so-called unification model introduced in a number of academic health centers in the 1960s involved much more, often including a complex set of organizational arrangements between nursing education and nursing service. In one model, both the school and the hospital were under one administration; faculty had one appointment and were accountable for both education and service. When the two entities had separate administrations, the faculty had joint appointments. In essence, the teachers in both prototypes performed their usual teaching, research, and other university functions, but, depending on their positions, were responsible for the nursing care given in the hospital and/or gave the nursing care themselves.

While the unification model was hailed as a great breakthrough in uniting practice and teaching, in reality, it was adopted in very few settings. Instead, in some cases of faculty practice, faculty members simply give some lectures, serve on committees, or make themselves generally helpful to a clinical facility in terms of their own expertise.

In others, individual faculty may practice for set periods of time (a day, a week, in the summer, during holiday breaks) in staff nurse, clinical specialist, or nurse practitioner roles, either being permitted to keep the money earned or required to give it to the school toward their salaries. A number of faculty have started a faculty group practice, delivering holistic care in the community to the poor, the homeless, the elderly, children or even college students, faculty, and staff. Some are free, some fee-for-service, but almost all are nonprofit. Some are part of an established health care facility, some independent. It may be an interdisciplinary group that also has other nurses and paid employees. Students usually have part of their clinical experience there.[31] Clearly such practices are not only good experience for the students but enable them to see their teachers as clinical role models. For the teachers, who may find this practice stimulating and rewarding, there is one drawback: they must usually still carry a full teaching load and often find themselves pressed for time to do the necessary research and writing required for promotion. Faculty practice is not considered a scholarly activity by university promotion and tenure committees. Therefore, faculty are being urged to make research a part of this practice. Nurse-managed centers, particularly community nursing centers associated with colleges of nursing, could offer the best of all worlds: teaching students while you are involved in the care of your own patients, and a fertile laboratory for research.[32]

The issue of preparation for the decanal role has received some attention in the last few years. Usually, the dean of a baccalaureate and a higher-degree program is expected to hold a doctoral degree also. However, research-oriented doctoral study does not prepare a person to assume the academic and administrative role that is mandated. Very few deans have had educational programs specifically designed to prepare them for the decanal role; few are available. In recent years, the American Association of Colleges of Nursing (AACN), in concert with the NLN, has presented a continuing education program for deans and a program for prospective deans. Given the political, fiscal, and academic pressures in this position, this may fill only a part of the need. A similar need is related to preparation for the role of nurse executive in the service arena. Are these individuals best served by joint degrees in business and nursing?

ACCREDITATION

The major accrediting organization for all nursing programs is the NLN (The history and process is described in Chap. 26.) The issues involved relate in part to the accrediting process and in part to who should do the accrediting.

Accreditation is defined as the process by which an agency or organization evaluates and recognizes an institution or program of study as meeting certain predetermined criteria or standards. As noted previously, educational accreditation is a voluntary process, but it presumably indicates excellence in program and resources and therefore attracts students and faculty and is often a requirement for external funding.

Perhaps the new manifestation of an old disagreement is the most important issue to be resolved in nursing. Should ANA, NLN, AACN, or a new credentialing center control the accreditation of all nursing education programs? Although most nursing leaders are members of both ANA and NLN, and most deans belong to AACN, there is significant disagreement about this question. There are philosophical and power issues: should the "real" all-nurse professional organization set educational standards and accredit programs, or should the NLN, which was given that responsibility at the reorganization of the major nursing organizations in 1952, continue? Should the AACN, which represents the interests of the academic deans and directors, direct accrediting activities? Should all accreditation activity be handled by a new credentialing center? There is also an obvious matter of control and income. Considerable income (and power) is derived from activities related to accreditation: agency membership, consulting, and the accreditation process. These resources provide attractive incentives to enter the business of accreditation.

Another factor, which is not to be discounted, is the bias or belief system of the accreditation agency. Rejection of programs or denial of accreditation can be attributed to organizational or reviewer bias rather than application of criteria or standards. Negative responses to decisions about accreditation have also stimulated the who-shall-accredit debate.

Other Issues

There are a number of other issues in nursing education, such as those related to continuing education. What kind of continuing education do nurses need? Who decides? Who is best qualified to provide it? Who should pay? Should it be mandatory for relicensure? Who is responsible for seeing that it is available to all nurses? Will it improve practice? (See Chap. 13 for further discussion.)

Recruitment and retention of minority students who may or may not fall into the "disadvantaged" category, legal aspects of admission, and student and faculty rights; what kind and how much preparation is needed for specific clinical areas, such as operating room nursing, public health nursing, and occupational health nursing; the kind of education for RNs entering baccalaureate programs (basically the same as for the generic student? advanced? specialized?), and intradisciplinary education (should PN and various RN students learn together?) are all areas of concern. Interdisciplinary education has also been a point of discussion for some time, with relatively little action taken. There has been minimal experimentation with the concept of core courses from which individual students could move to various health professional programs, as well as certain shared courses when students are already enrolled in separate programs, and occasional joint clinical experiences.

Over the years, certain problems have been consistently identified as important in nursing education. These include:

Financial problems

Insufficient professional leadership, direction, and cohesion

Need for more qualified faculty

Need to produce more competent graduates

Role confusion and changes in nursing

Conflict between nursing education and service

Determination of appropriate competency levels

Adequate clinical facilities

As nursing education, like the society in which it exists, continues to become more complex, new issues will emerge as others are resolved. The danger lies in nonresolution of long-term issues that are professionally divisive and potentially detrimental to the public's welfare.

RISING TO THE OCCASION OF THE FUTURE

The recurrent problems and issues of the profession should not distract us from taking charge of our future in an era of inevitable

health care reform. There are challenges to nursing education that must be addressed from within, even though that has not always been our tradition. Nursing has rather chosen to respond, and often simultaneously, to contradictory messages. Respecting that education prepares for the future and not the past, there is clear direction that has been shaped, in part, by the National League for Nursing's *Vision for Education*.[33]

- Shift our emphasis in education to assure that graduates are prepared to function in a community-based, community-focused health care system.
- Demand from the outset that students are accountable for their practice, including cost and quality implications.
- Include educational experiences to prepare for practice in a multicultural society; realistically this may be no more than becoming aware of one's own biases and accepting others as they are, including their personal definition of health and wellness.
- Establish true interdisciplinary education in the form of required courses and joint practice experiences.
- Socialize students into the tradition of empowering consumers, making consumers the gatekeepers for their own health.
- Realize that you can never teach everything, so make content process. Focus on critical thinking, collaboration, shared decision making, a social epidemiological viewpoint, and analyses at the systems and aggregate level.
- Identify the data bases that hold the information you need and be sure students know how to access them.
- Remember it will be a luxury to just be responsible for your practice; students must be equipped with the skills to delegate and to evaluate the performance of assistive personnel.
- Demand faculty-to-faculty and faculty-to-student relationships that are more egalitarian and characterized by cooperation

and community building . . . . After all, it is the people that make the difference.

- Assure that faculty can teach for a community-based, community-focused health care system.
- Involve employers in curriculum design, so that nursing education is truly preparing individuals suited to the realities of practice.
- Target recruitment and retention efforts toward individuals of diverse racial, cultural, and ethnic backgrounds; especially faculty and graduate students.
- Shift the emphasis for research toward studies concerned with health promotion and disease prevention at the aggregate and community level.
- Seek more balance between the traditional definitions of scholarship and the "scholarship of application," so that faculty can establish their projects within delivery systems as part of their teaching and research.
- Become actively involved in the placement of your graduates, so that nurses will begin to claim their place in new markets.
- Commit to increasing the numbers of advanced practice nurses, so that as a profession we can move forward to fill the primary care gap.

REFERENCES

1. National League for Nursing. *Nursing Data Review*. New York: The League, 1994, pp 29, 37, 87–92.
2. *Fiscal Year Fact Sheet on Nursing*. Washington, DC: American Nurses' Association, 1993.
3. Aiken L, Mullinix C: The nursing shortage: Myth or reality? *N Engl J Med* 317:646–651, 1987.
4. Hendrickson G et al: How do nurses use their time? *J Nurs Adm* 20:31–38, March 1990.
5. National League for Nursing, op cit, pp 37, 49.
6. Dixon A: Project LINC (Ladders in Nursing Careers): An innovative model of educational mobility. *Nurs Health Care* 10:398–402, September 1989.
7. Kalisch P: Why not launch a new Cadet Nurse Corps? *Am J Nurs* 88:316–317, March 1988.
8. Ibid pp 21–24, 74–76.
9. Tucker-Allen S: Losses incurred through minority student nurse attrition. *Nurs Health Care* 10:395–397, September 1989.
10. Ibid, p 18.
11. Ibid, p 47.
12. American Nurses' Association: *Nursing: A Social Policy Statement*. Kansas City, MO: The Association, 1980.
13. American Nurses' Association: *Education for Nursing Practice in the Context of the 1980s*. Kansas City, MO: The Association, 1983.
14. National Commission on Nursing: *Summary Report and Recommendations*. Chicago: The Commission, 1983.
15. Two year colleges prepare for battle over nursing programs. *Chr Higher Ed* Apr 23, 1986.
16. Waters V: Restricting the RN license to BSN graduates could cloud nursing's future. *Nurs Health Care* 7:142–146, March 1986.
17. Wakefield-Fisher M et al: A first for the nation: North Dakota and entry into nursing practice. *Nurs Health Care* 7:135–141, March 1986.
18. National League for Nursing, loc cit.
19. Lenburg C: Preparation for professionalism through regents external degrees. *Nurs Health Care* 5:319, June 1984.
20. Lenburg C: Do external degree programs really work? *Nurs Outlook* 38:234–238, September–October 1990.
21. Minnick A: MSN in nursing administration and the dual degree. *Nurs Health Care* 14:22–26, January 1993.
22. Neighbors M, Eldred E: Technology and nursing education. *Nurs Health Care* 14:96–99, February 1993.
23. Davis L, Barham P: Get the most from your preceptorship. *Nurs Outlook* 37:167–171, July–August 1989.
24. McClure ML: Differentiating nursing practice: Concepts and consideration. *Nurs Outlook* 39:106–110, May–June 1991.
25. Schank MJ, Sollenwerk R: The leadership/management role: A differentiating factor for ADN/BSN programs. *J Nurs Ed* 27:253–257, June 1988.
26. Primm P: Differentiated practice for ADN and BSN prepared nurses. *J Prof Nurs* 3:218–225, April 1987.

27. National League for Nursing, op cit, p 218.
28. Kelly L: Nursing, nothing but nursing. *Nurs Outlook* 36:227, September–October 1988.
29. National League for Nursing, op cit, pp 189–192.
30. Wright DJ: Faculty practice: Criterion for academic advancement. *Nurs Health Care* 14:18–21, January 1993.
31. Gray PA: Can nursing centers provide health care? *Nurs Health Care* 14:414–417, October 1993.
32. Barger S, Rosenfeld P: Models in community health care. *Nurs Health Care* 14:426–431, October 1993.
33. National League for Nursing: *Vision for Nursing Education*. New York: The League, 1993.

Programs in Nursing Education

EDUCATIONAL PREPARATION for licensure as a registered nurse takes place primarily in diploma programs, associate degree (AD) programs, and baccalaureate (BSN) programs. As noted in Chap. 12, the numbers have been shifting, with a decrease in diploma programs and an increase in AD and BSN programs. This chapter gives an overview of these educational modes, as well as graduate education and continuing education. The open curriculum is discussed in Chap. 12.

DIPLOMA PROGRAMS

The diploma or hospital school of nursing was the first type of nursing school in this country. Prior to the opening of the first hospital schools in the late 1800s, there was no formal preparation for nursing. But after Florence Nightingale established the first school of nursing at St. Thomas's Hospital, England, in 1860, the idea spread quickly to the United States.

Hospitals, of course, welcomed the idea of training schools because, in the early years, such schools represented an almost free supply of nursepower. With some outstanding exceptions, the education offered was largely of the apprenticeship type. There was some theory and formal classroom work, but for the most part students learned by doing, providing the bulk of the nursing care for the hospitals' patients in the process.

This is no longer true. Today, in order to meet standards set in each state for operation of a nursing school and to prepare students to pass the licensing examinations, diploma schools must offer their students a true educational program, not just an apprenticeship. Hospitals conducting such schools employ a full-time nurse faculty, offer students a balanced mixture of coursework (in nursing and related subjects in the physical and social sciences) and supervised practice, and look to their nursing staff, not their students, to provide the nursing service needed by patients. The educational program has been generally three years in length, although most diploma schools have now adopted a shortened program. Upon satisfactory completion of the program, the student is awarded a diploma by the school. This diploma is not an academic degree. Because most hospitals operating schools of nursing are not chartered to grant degrees, *no academic credit can be given for courses taught* by the school's faculty. For this and economic and educational reasons, large numbers of diploma schools enter into cooperative relations with colleges or universities for educational courses and/or services. It is not uncommon for diploma students to take physical and social science courses and, occasionally, liberal arts courses at a college. If these courses are part of the general offerings of the college, college credit is granted. Credit is usually transferable if the nursing student decides to transfer to a college or continue in advanced education. (If the course is tailored to nursing only, it is often not transferable to an advanced nursing program, but is sometimes counted as an elective.) Diploma schools usually provide other necessary educational resources, facilities, and services to students and faculty, such as libraries, classrooms, audiovisual materials, and practice laboratories. At one time, it was taken for granted that students would be housed, and the school had dormitory and recreational space, as well as educational facilities, in a separate building. Although the physical setup may still be the same, such housing must now be paid for and may also be used by others educated in or involved with the hospital. The primary clinical facility is the hospital, although the school may contract with other hospitals or agencies for additional educational experiences. Advocates of diploma education usually say that early and substantial experiences with patients seem to foster a strong identification with nursing, particularly hospital nursing, and thus graduates are expected to adjust to the employee role without difficulty.

Admission requirements to diploma schools usually call for a college preparatory curriculum in high school, with standing in the upper half, third, or quarter (depending on the school) of the graduating class. Personal characteristics and health are also assessed.

There are a variety of concepts of what the diploma graduate is or should be. A statement approved by the National League for Nursing (NLN) Council of Diploma Programs is found in Exhibit 13-1.

The diploma school graduates still constitute a large number of practicing nurses. In 1964, more than 88 percent of the 582,000 employed nurses were diploma school graduates. However, with the drop in the number of diploma schools, the percentage of nurses in the workforce with diplomas as their top educational preparation in 1988 was 40.4. In 1992, this had further decreased to 34 percent. And 42.5 percent of the total nurse workforce received their original education for nursing in a diploma program.[1]

Exhibit 13-1	Role and Competencies of Graduates of Diploma Programs in Nursing

Role

The graduate of the diploma program in nursing is eligible to seek licensure as a registered nurse and to function as a beginning practitioner in acute, intermediate, ambulatory, and long-term health care services and settings. The graduate functions within the scope of professional nursing practice as provider, manager, leader, teacher, and advocate and demonstrates the following competencies.

Competencies*

- Provides nursing care for individuals, families, and groups by utilizing the nursing process.
- Provides for the promotion, maintenance, and restoration of health and support and comfort to the suffering and dying.
- Utilizes management skills including collaboration, coordination, and communication with individuals, families, groups, and with other members of the health care team.
- Assumes a leadership role within the health care system.
- Teaches individuals, families, and groups based on identified health needs.
- Functions as an advocate for the consumer and the health care system to improve the quality and delivery of care.
- Practices nursing based on a theoretical body of knowledge, ethical principles, and legal standards.
- Evaluates nursing practice for improvement of nursing care.
- Accepts responsibility and accountability for professional practice.
- Utilizes opportunities for continuing personal and professional development.
- Participates in health-related community services.
- Utilizes critical thinking in professional practice.

*Competency is defined as the ability to apply in practice situations the essential theoretical principles and techniques of nursing.

Source: Reprinted with permission of the National League for Nursing, 1994 (under revision).

The perceptible shift away from diploma school preparation for nursing can be explained (in an oversimplified way) by three factors: (1) some hospitals are terminating their schools, either because of the expense involved in maintaining a quality program and the objections of third-party payers, such as insurance companies and the government, to having the cost of nursing education absorbed in the patient's bill, or because of difficulty in meeting professional standards, particularly in employing qualified faculty; (2) increasing numbers of high school graduates are seeking some kind of collegiate education; and (3) the nursing profession is more and more committed to the belief that preparation for nursing, as for all other professionals, should take place in institutions of higher education. There were 135 diploma programs in 1992.[2]

These social and educational trends will probably continue, but it is expected that diploma programs will be on the scene for some time and that high-quality programs will continue to prepare high-quality graduates. The vast majority of current diploma programs are NLN accredited, and many of the schools that dissolved or were "phased into" associate degree or baccalaureate programs are also accredited. The 1970 National Commission study (described in Chap. 5) recommended that strong, vital schools be encouraged to seek regional accreditation and degree-granting status, but only a few have done so. Another recommendation, that other hospital schools move to effect interinstitutional arrangements with collegiate institutions, has been acted upon more readily.

Although hospitals are less likely to operate schools, they continue as the clinical laboratories for nursing education programs. In the communities where new associate or baccalaureate degree programs are opening, there is often planning for new programs to evolve as diploma programs close—a phasing-in process. This cooperation enables prospective candidates for the diploma program to be directed to the new program, qualified diploma faculty to be employed by the college, and arrangements to be made to use space in the hospital previously occupied by the diploma school. Cooperative planning provides for continuity in the output of nurses to meet the needs of the community.

ASSOCIATE DEGREE PROGRAMS

By far the greatest increase in programs and students has been at the associate degree (AD) level. These programs are two years in length and offered by junior or community colleges, and occassionally by four-year colleges. Associate degree education for nursing is a relative newcomer on the education scene. The first three programs were started in 1952; by 1965 there were more than 130 such programs, and in 1992 there were 848 AD programs.[3] More than half of these schools are NLN accredited, and most of the others are accredited by regional accrediting groups as part of their college's accreditation.

The associate degree program is the first nursing education program to be developed under a systematic plan and with carefully controlled experimentation. In her doctoral dissertation, published as a book in 1951, Mildred Montag conceived of a nursing technician able to perform nursing functions smaller in scope than those of the professional nurse and broader than those of the practical nurse. This nurse was intended to be a "bedside nurse" who was not burdened with administrative responsibilities. Montag listed the functions as (1) assisting in the planning of nursing care for patients, (2) giving general nursing care with supervision, and (3) assisting in the evaluation of the nursing care given.[4] The emerging community college was seen as a suitable setting for this education. Nursing education would be in the mainstream of education, and the burden of cost would be on the public in general, not on patients. The curriculum was to be an integrated one, half general education and half nursing, with careful selection of educational and clinical experiences. An associate degree would be awarded at the end of the two years. The program was considered to be comprehensive and complete in itself (terminal) and not a first step toward the baccalaureate.

At the end of 1951, the five-year Cooperative Research Project in Junior and Community College Education for Nursing was funded, and seven junior colleges and one hospital school were selected to participate in the project; each had complete autonomy in the development and conduct of its pilot program, but had free access to consultation from the project staff (see Chap. 5).

The results of the project showed that AD nursing technicians could carry on the intended nursing functions, that the program could be suitably set up in community colleges, with the use of clinical facilities in the community without charge or student service, and that the program attracted students. The success of the experiment plus the rapid growth of community colleges combined to give impetus to these new programs.

Over the years, as Montag predicted, the AD curricula have varied and changed: for instance, when college policies permit, there is a tendency to put a heavier emphasis and more time on the nursing subjects and clinical experiences, sometimes through the addition of summer sessions or clinical preceptorships. Some programs are also adding team leadership and managerial principles because their graduates are put in positions requiring these skills. A heated area of debate is whether the AD nurse should be able to practice in community health nursing. Obviously many do, but the AD curriculum has traditionally excluded those knowledges and experiences.[5] Today, most AD programs are between eighteen and twenty-four months in length, but some require that all science and general education courses be completed before the nursing program is begun, which may lengthen the AD program to over two years.

The entire concept of the AD nursing program as terminal has changed over the last twenty years, along with general societal and educational concepts of *terminal*. Obviously, no educational program should be terminal in the sense that graduates cannot continue their education toward another degree. Whether or not they get full or only partial credit for their previous education depends on the philosophy and policies of the baccalaureate program they select. Many AD graduates are continuing to a BSN, sometimes through the external degree.

Because AD nursing has been identified for some time as technical nursing practice, the description of technical practice as differentiated from professional practice in the controversial ANA position paper on nursing education may be helpful:

> **Technical nursing practice is carrying out nursing measures as well as medically delegated techniques with a high degree of skill, using principles from an ever-expanding body of science. It is understanding the physics of machines as well as the physiologic reactions of patients. It is using all treatment modalities with knowledge and precision.**
>
> **Technical nursing practice is evaluating patients' immediate physical and emotional reactions to therapy and taking measures to alleviate distress. It is knowing when to act and when to seek more expert guidance.**
>
> **Technical nursing practice involves working with professional nurse practitioners and others in planning the day-to-day care of patients. It is supervising other workers in the technical aspects of care.**
>
> **Technical nursing practice is unlimited in depth but limited in scope. Its complexity and extent are tremendous. It must be rendered under the direction of professional nurse practitioners, by persons who are selected with care and educated within the system of higher education; only thus can the safety of patients be assured. Education for this practice requires attention to scientific laws and principles with emphasis on skill. It is education which is technically oriented and scientifically founded, but not primarily concerned with evolving theory.[6]**

Whether the term *technical* will continue to be used is not clear. The concept of a technical worker, honored in other fields, has not been fully accepted in nursing, possibly because it is considered a step down from the *professional* label that has been attached to all nurses through licensing definitions and common usage over the years. Montag, noting the difficulty of choosing an appropriate term for the new type of proposed nurse, said, "It is also probable that the term 'nursing technician' will not satisfy forever, but it is proposed as one which indicates more accurately the person who has semiprofessional preparation and whose functions are predominantly technical."[7]

The use of the term was rejected by the NLN Council of Associate Degree Programs in a 1976 action and the term *associate degree nurse* (AD nurse) was suggested. This term is frequently used now, although *associate nurse* is also used, especially in terms of licensing.

More important than the name are the role and functions of the associate degree nurse. Because of nursing shortages, lack of understanding of the abilities and preparation of technical nurses, a tendency to use the diploma nurse of previous years as a standard, and general traditionalized concepts of nursing roles, employers have often not assigned AD nurses in the manner that best utilized their preparation. Like nurses through the centuries, AD nurses have been placed quickly as team leaders and charge nurses, positions in which they were not intended to function.

The NLN has published a role and competencies statement for AD nurses, which provides guidelines for identifying their expected level of practice at graduation and six months later. The document is very comprehensive. Exhibit 13-2 presents the role component, which more or less summarizes the scope of the very long list of competencies.

Like other RNs, AD nurses are accountable for their own practice and are expected to function ethically and legally. In addition, the NLN Council has made a point of saying that although these nurses work within the policies of an employing institution, they would also work within the organizational framework to initiate change in policies or nursing protocols.

There have been some complaints that AD nurses are not proficient in some technical skills, cannot handle large patient loads, and are slow to assume full staff nurse responsibilities and activities. Such concerns may be less common as AD nurses increasingly have externships and similar experiences (see Chap. 12). Almost everyone agrees that AD graduates have a good grasp of basic nursing theory, having inquiring minds, and are self-directed in finding out what they don't know. It is also generally agreed that a good orientation program, sometimes combined with internships, can be the key to satisfactory acclimation to the work setting.

Because AD programs are the fastest growing segment of nursing education, AD nurses will be an important part of the nursing scene for years to come.

BACCALAUREATE DEGREE PROGRAMS

The first baccalaureate program in nursing was established in 1909 under the control of the University of Minnesota, through the efforts of Dr. Richard Olding Beard. Since then, these programs have become an increasingly important part of nursing education. Today there are 501 baccalaureate programs.[8]

The individual enrolled in a baccalaureate degree program in nursing obtains both a college education culminating in a bachelor's degree and preparation for licensure and practice as a registered professional nurse.

This program, considered by the ANA as minimum preparation for professional nursing, is usually four academic years in length. Unless the college is tax supported, with minimal tuition fees, baccalaureate nursing education is usually more expensive for students than other basic programs. It is also an expense to the institution. These are serious problems as funding cuts lessen student aid and public funding to higher education in general.

The baccalaureate degree program includes courses in general education and the liberal arts, the sciences germane to and related to nursing, and nursing. In some programs, the student is not admitted to the nursing major (nursing courses) until the conclusion of the first two

| Exhibit 13-2 | Educational Outcomes of Associate Degree Nursing Programs: Roles |

Provider of Care

The practice of a graduate from an associate degree nursing program is characterized by critical thinking, clinical competence, accountability and a commitment to the value of caring. It encompasses clients across the lifespan with emphasis on adult clients who have health needs and require assistance to maintain or restore their optimum state of health or support to die with dignity. Because the aged comprise an increasing proportion of nursing's clients, the nurse with an associate degree is prepared to address acute and chronic health care needs of this population. The nurse is concerned with individual clients with consideration of the person's relationship within a family, group, and community.

The nursing process is used as a basis for decisions. The nurse establishes and analyzes a database, identifies health care needs, selects nursing diagnoses, sets client-centered goals, plans and implements care to achieve the goals, and evaluates client outcomes.

The nurse's commitment to client-centered care is reflected through a collaborative approach involving the client, the family, significant others, and members of the health care team. The provider role of the graduate from an associate degree nursing program encompasses preparation for practice in both acute and long-term care settings where policies and procedures are specified and guidance is available.

Manager of Care

The practice of the graduate from an associate degree nursing program is characterized by collaboration, organization, delegation, accountability, advocacy, and respect for other health care workers. As a manager of care, the nurse with an associate degree provides and coordinates care for a group of clients who have health care needs.

In organizing the nursing care, the nurse may delegate aspects of care to licensed and unlicensed personnel commensurate with their educational background and experience. The nurse is accountable for care delegated to other workers and for knowing legal parameters of their practice as well as their roles and responsibilities. Consultation with other members of the health care team is initiated when the situation encountered is beyond the nurse's knowledge and experience. The nurse participates in evaluation of the client care delivery system, contributes to change, and promotes an environment that fosters team relationships.

The nurse is a manager of care in acute and long-term care settings where policies and procedures are specified and guidance is available.

Member within the Discipline of Nursing

The practice of a graduate from an associate degree nursing program is characterized by a commitment to professional growth, continuous learning, and self-development. The nurse with an associate degree practices within the ethical and legal framework of nursing and is responsible for ensuring high standards of nursing practice.

The nurse contributes to the improvement of nursing and nursing practice through participation on committees of the employing institution, attendance at conferences, and membership in nursing organizations.

Source: Reprinted with permission of the National League for Nursing, 1994 (under revision).

years of college study. In other programs, nursing content is integrated throughout the four years.

As in the other nursing programs, the baccalaureate program has both theoretical content and clinical experience. The baccalaureate student who studies courses in the physical and social sciences will have great depth and breadth, because students majoring in nursing take the college courses in the sciences and humanities with students majoring in biology or English literature. Nursing majors meet the same admission requirements and are held to the same academic standards as all other students. The nursing program is an integral part of the college or university as a whole.

The statement on the "Characteristics of Baccalaureate Education in Nursing" developed by the NLN Council of Baccalaureate and Higher Degree Programs is found in Exhibit 13-3.

The most notable differences between baccalaureate education and that of the other basic nursing programs are related to liberal education, development of intellectual skills, and the addition of public health, community health, teaching, and management concepts, although some of the other programs do include a limited amount of such content. Baccalaureate nurses have the opportunity to become liberally educated. Almost all programs allow free electives in the humanities and the sciences as well as nursing courses. Nursing students are able to participate in the college and university cultural and social activities throughout their whole program and develop relationships with professors and students in other disciplines. Although technical skills are essential to nursing, learning activities that assist students to develop skills in recognizing and solving problems, applying general principles to particular situations, and establishing a basis for making sound clinical judgments are also emphasized. This enables the nurse to function more easily when a familiar situation takes an unexpected turn or when it is necessary to deal with an unfamiliar situation. The baccalaureate program is the only basic program offering both theory and practice in public health and community health nursing. There are also courses in health assessment and administrative and teaching principles. These skills are clearly necessary when the baccalaureate nurse functions as a primary nurse or as team leader, coordinating, planning, and directing the activities of other nursing personnel. It is on the basis of such background that the roles of a baccalaureate nurse are sometimes described as those of a practitioner engaged in direct patient care, teacher, leader, and collaborator.

On completion of the program, most BSN graduates select hospitals as their place of employment, but then often turn to other practice areas. The changing pattern of health care delivery described in Chap. 7 has made home care and ambulatory care centers attractive employ-

---

Exhibit 13-3	**Characteristics of Baccalaureate Graduates in Nursing**

Consistent with the *Criteria for the Evaluation of Baccalaureate and Higher Degree Programs in Nursing*, the following statements characterize the graduate of the baccalaureate program in nursing. Graduates are able to:

- Provide professional nursing care, which includes health promotion and maintenance, illness care, restoration, rehabilitation, health counseling, and education based on knowledge derived from theory and research.
- Synthesize theoretical and empirical knowledge from nursing, scientific, and humanistic disciplines with practice.
- Use the nursing process to provide nursing care for individuals, families, groups, and communities.
- Accept responsibility and accountability for the evaluation of the effectiveness of their own nursing practice.
- Enhance the quality of nursing and health practices within practice settings through the use of leadership skills and a knowledge of the political system.
- Evaluate research for the applicability of its findings to nursing practice.
- Participate with other health care providers and members of the general public in promoting the health and well-being of people.
- Incorporate professional values as well as ethical, moral, and legal aspects of nursing into nursing practice.
- Participate in the implementation of nursing roles designed to meet emerging health needs of the general public in a changing society.

Source: Reprinted with permission of the National League for Nursing, 1994 (under revision).

ment sites for new baccalaureate graduates. However, those hospitals that have primary nursing, which gives nurses individual responsibility for a group of patients, also seem to attract and retain baccalaureate nurses. Graduates with long-term plans for teaching, administration, or clinical specialization continue into graduate study. BSN graduates are more likely to complete a graduate degree than their diploma or AD counterparts.

The number of RNs enrolled in baccalaureate programs has increased steadily, currently being over 28 percent of total enrollees.[9] In most nursing programs, RNs receive some credit and/or advanced standing for their previous education through challenge examinations. Frequently, courses and clinical experiences are individualized to meet RNs' needs and goals. However, RN students have more or less the same baccalaureate curriculum and earn the same degree as generic students. Although many more educational opportunities now exist for RNs (see Chap. 12), some, because of circumstances, desire, or lack of counseling, choose nonnursing majors, which generally precludes their acceptance in a graduate program in nursing and may limit their job options.

As mentioned in Chap. 12, a noticeable trend is admission of students with baccalaureate or advanced degrees in fields other than nursing. These students, of course, receive a second baccalaureate. Depending on how many of their previous courses satisfy the BSN requirements, their program may consist primarily of the upper-division major nursing courses. A growing number of baccalaureate programs are especially designed for the baccalaureate graduate (second-degree student). However, there are other alternatives for these second careerists.

An unusual study that looked at the overall education of a baccalaureate nurse should be of particular interest to those considering this educational route. Although, like other nurse educators, those in baccalaureate programs constantly review (and often revise) their nursing curriculum, relatively little attention has

been given to the liberal arts component, even though this part of the program is supposed to be important in making the baccalaureate nurse an "educated" person as well as a clinical practitioner. However, in 1986, an interdisciplinary "Panel for Essentials of College and University Education for Professional Nursing," reported its recommendations to the American Association of Colleges of Nursing (AACN), its sponsor. Its two-year effort culminated in the distribution of 25,000 copies of a working document to members of the nursing, health care, and higher education communities and followed that by open hearings across the country. The report had two components: one related to nursing knowledge and the other to liberal education. The nursing component delineated knowledge needed to:

- Determine health status and health needs based on the interpretation of health-related data
- Formulate goals and a plan of care in collaboration with patients/clients and other health care professionals
- Implement the plan of care
- Define learning needs of individuals and groups related to health
- Evaluate patient/client responses to therapeutic interventions
- Provide care for multiple patients/clients
- Use an analytical approach as the basis for decision making in practice
- Coordinate human and material resources for provision of care
- Collaborate with patients/clients, coworkers, and others for provision of care
- Refer individuals and their families to appropriate sources of assistance
- Function within the organizational structure of various health care settings
- Demonstrate accountability for own nursing practice
- Serve as a health care advocate in monitoring and ensuring the quality of health care practices
- Promote nursing as a profession

The section on liberal education was particularly interesting. It was based on the reports of three panels recommending improvements for undergraduate education: the National Institute of Education (1984), the National Endowment for the Humanities (1984), and the Association of American Colleges (1985). The AACN group stated, "We recommend that the education of the professional nurse reflect the spirit of these reports so that the graduate will exhibit qualities of mind and character that are necessary to live a free and fulfilling life, act in the public interest locally and globally, and contribute to health care improvements and the nursing profession."

The members noted that a "liberally educated person who is prepared in this manner can responsibly challenge the status quo and anticipate and adapt to change."[10] Their recommendations were that the education of the professional nurse ensure the ability to:

1. Write, read, and speak English clearly and effectively in order to acquire knowledge, convey and discuss ideas, evaluate information, and think critically.
2. Think analytically and reason logically using verifiable information and past experience in order to select or create solutions to problems.
3. Understand a second language, at least at an elementary level, in order to widen access to the diversity of world culture.
4. Understand other cultural traditions in order to gain a perspective on personal values and the similarities and differences among individuals and groups.
5. Use mathematical concepts, interpret quantitative data, and use computers and other information technology in order to analyze problems and develop positions that depend on numbers and statistics.
6. Use concepts from the behavioral and biological sciences in order to understand oneself and one's relationship with other people and to comprehend the nature and function of communities.
7. Understand the physical world and its interrelationship with human activity in order to make decisions based on scientific evidence and responsive to the values and interests of the individual and society.
8. Comprehend life and time from historical and contemporary perspectives and draw from past experiences to influence the present and future.
9. Gain a perspective on social, political, and economic issues for resolving societal and professional problems.
10. Comprehend the meaning of human spirituality in order to recognize the relationship of beliefs to culture, behavior, health, and healing.
11. Appreciate the role of the fine and performing arts in stimulating individual creativity, expressing personal feelings and emotions, and building a sense of the commonality of human experience.
12. Understand the nature of human values and develop a personal philosophy in order to make ethical judgments in both personal and professional life.

Finally, they noted that nursing faculty are responsible for integrating knowledge from the liberal arts and sciences into professional nursing education and practice. "Liberally educated nurses make informed and responsible ethical choices and help shape the future of society as well as the nursing profession."[11]

What long-term action comes from this report remains to be seen. Since its release, there has not been as much discussion of the report as might be expected.

A baccalaureate degree in nursing offers many career opportunities, a fact that is widely acknowledged. Equally important is the fact that when nursing has been under particular scrutiny, experts agree that what is needed to meet the nursing needs in today's complex health care is more baccalaureate nurses. All well-prepared, competent nurses are valuable, but because baccalaureate nurses are still more or less in the minority in the workforce and because the kinds of skills needed now and certainly in the future are those for which the BSN nurse is educated, the recruitment and retention of both generic BSN and RN-completion students is important to the future.

OTHER GENERIC EDUCATIONAL PROGRAMS FOR RN LICENSURE

A number of years ago, several nursing education programs, such as those at Yale and Western Reserve University, admitted only baccalaureate graduates and granted a master's degree in nursing as the basic educational credential. Today, there is a revival of interest in such programs. Some prepare for a generalist role, others for a specialty as clinical specialist or nurse practitioner. Depending on the school's philosophy and state law, the student may take the licensing examination before completion of the master's. There are also "articulation" programs in which a student may get a license after completion of an AD or baccalaureate and then continue directly to the master's degree.

The first program for a professional doctorate (ND) for college graduates was established at Case-Western Reserve in 1979. The program is best suited to universities with health science centers preparing several types of health professionals. Because such universities also offer advanced graduate education, ND students are prepared in an academic climate of scholarship and research. Faculty are prepared at the highest level of scholarship, with some engaged in teaching and research and others, jointly appointed, master's-prepared clinicians engaged in clinical practice, teaching, and some aspect of research. The curriculum prepares the ND graduates to become proficient in the delivery of primary, episodic, and long-term nursing care, and to evaluate their own practices, and that of their assistants, since they are accountable for the outcomes of all nursing practice. Graduates of this program would continue graduate study in a specialization and/or a functional area such

as teaching or administration. As is true of medical students whose professional degree is a doctorate, they might also obtain a master's or Ph.D. concurrently with the first doctorate.[12] This innovative approach, seen as a major step toward the emergence of nursing as a full-fledged profession, has now been adopted by several other universities, but there are still many questions raised as to the functions, role, and job market for the graduates and the best organizational structure for the program.[13]

GRADUATE EDUCATION

Graduate education in nursing, of a kind, can be traced back to the first decades of the twentieth century. However, there was considerable confusion in those early years in that what was called graduate education was actually education for *graduate nurses* beyond their basic diploma program. The first programs concentrated on public health nursing and preparation for teaching and supervision. As late as 1951, it was finally recognized that there was little differentiation between the programs leading to a baccalaureate degree and those leading to a master's; the master's was found to be little more than a symbol that the nurse had previously earned a bachelor's degree. This led to a series of recommendations to place graduate education for nurses on the same basis as that in other disciplines. In the following years, graduate programs for *practice* in public health nursing, teaching, and management were developed. In 1952 only 1,449 nurses had completed a graduate study, and programs reflected a broad range of sophistication. This was aptly described by the League as "microscopic" compared with the nation's needs.[14]

In the years that followed, various reports were issued with recommendations that the public had a dire need for nurses with graduate education (see Chap. 5). Even with the federal funding that followed, the goals specified were not reached. For one thing, only a limited number of master's programs in nursing were available, and even fewer nursing doctoral programs. Therefore, many nurses received their graduate degrees in other disciplines, often education. When federal funding focused on preparing "nurse scientists" in the late 1960s and early 1970s, these nurses who received both master's and doctoral degrees in biological or social science were hailed as fine examples who showed that nurses could indeed compete successfully with others in rigorous nonnursing disciplines. Unfortunately, in another two decades, many found the lack of a nursing master's degree unacceptable for nursing faculty positions. By 1992, there were about 243 nursing master's degree programs and 54 nursing doctoral programs.[15] Although the growth of doctoral programs was extraordinary (from only 18 in 1977), the number of graduates is slow to increase, partially because so many nurses find it necessary to be part-time students and particularly because, as is true for all doctoral students who work and try to write a dissertation, such work is slow going. Many ABD (all but dissertation) nurses may never finish their degree. In 1992, about 8 percent of the nurse population had at least a master's degree. About 13,500 were estimated to have doctoral degrees.[16]

Today, the purpose of master's level education is to prepare professional nursing leaders in the areas of advanced practice, teaching, and administration. Nurses with these special skills and knowledge are desperately required now and will be for the foreseeable future. About 43 percent of RNs with master's degrees have the focus of advanced clinical practice in 1992.[17]

Perhaps because so much of the emphasis in graduate programs over the years had been on attaining functional skills in teaching and management, with little attention given to clinical knowledge and skills, a 1969 ANA statement on graduate education proclaimed that the "major purpose of graduate education should be the preparation of nurse clinicians capable of improving nursing care through the advancement of nursing service and theory."[18]

However, it soon became evident that nurses in education and management/administration did indeed need the functional skills required in these fields. Almost ten years later, a new statement focused on "the preparation of highly competent individuals who can function in diverse roles, such as clinical nurse generalists or specialists, researchers, theoreticians, teachers, administrators, consultants, public policy makers, system managers, and colleagues on multidisciplinary teams...prepared through master's, doctoral, and postdoctoral programs in nursing that subscribe to clearly defined standards of scholarship."[19] Nontraditional graduate programs, such as those previously described, were also encouraged because they "can provide for significant contributions to the advancement of scholarship in nursing."[20] Other nontraditional approaches, such as interinstitutional exchange programs, consortium arrangements, and satellite and off-campus programs, were also cited as innovative and approved "in concert with beliefs about pluralism, diversity, and flexibility in graduate education."[21]

These flexible programs are increasing, with not just the "articulation" model, but also "summers only" and "Friday only" programs, programs for nurses with nonnursing degrees, a program for AD nurse-educators, various offsite programs, some with telecommunications, and a number of accelerated programs.

Graduate programs in nursing vary in admission requirements, organization of curriculum, length of program, and costs. Admission usually requires RN licensure, graduation from an approved (or accredited) baccalaureate program with an upper-division major in nursing, a satisfactory grade point average, achievement on selected tests, and sometimes nursing experience. Some programs will admit a few nurses without BSNs and assist them in making up deficiencies. Part-time study is available in some programs, but often certain courses must be taken in sequence, and at least some full-time study may be required. Reduced federal support and fewer traineeships have stimulated faculty to develop more part-time study options. Swelling part-time enrollment has increased the total number of students. In 1992, of 28,370 students in master's programs, only slightly more than 5,000 were engaged in full-time study.[22] Not all graduate programs offer all possible majors. The degrees granted are usually MS, MSN, M.Ed, MA, or MNSc. Various NLN publications provide information about nursing master's programs, including curricula, clinical and functional majors, and admission requirements, availability of part-time study, length of program, approximate cost, and availability of housing.

Most NLN-accredited master's programs offer study of a clinical area, such as medical-surgical nursing, maternal-child nursing, community health nursing, or psychiatric nursing, based on a theoretical framework developed by that faculty and including relevant advanced courses in the natural and social sciences and supervised clinical experience. The depth of clinical study varies in relation to the functional role selected: teaching, management, or advanced clinical practice. A practicum (planned, guided learning experiences that allow a student to function within the role) is usual for the functional role as well as the area of clinical specialization, and most often they are combined. Practice varies from program to program, from one day a week for a semester to almost a year's full-time residency. Acquisition of research methods is also considered essential. In general, master's education in nursing includes introduction to research methods. Debate continues around whether a thesis or project for the independent study of a nursing problem should be a degree requirement. As the terminal degree becomes the doctorate, the credits for the master's have decreased, and many programs have eliminated the thesis, choosing to reserve any independent research experience for the dissertation.

The NLN states that graduates of nursing master's programs are able to:

- Incorporate theories and advanced knowledge into nursing practice.
- Demonstrate competence in selected role(s).
- Identify researchable nursing problems and participate in research studies in advanced nursing practice.
- Use leadership, management, and teaching knowledge and competencies to influence nursing practice.
- Assume responsibility for contributing to improvement in the delivery of health care and influencing health policy.
- Assume responsibility for contributing to the advancement of the nursing profession.[23]

Although some nurses obtain graduate degrees outside the field of nursing, advanced positions in nursing usually require a nursing degree, preferably with advanced clinical content and experience. The exception may be graduates from schools of public health, who have had programs in public health nursing and/or administration that do not include clinical components per se. With increased emphasis on the need for interdisciplinary collaboration, and new opportunities for nurses, some nursing programs now offer joint or dual degrees with graduate programs in law, business, public health, and other disciplines.

The first American nurse to earn a doctorate received her Ph.D. in psychology and counseling in 1927, although the first doctoral program for nurses opened at Teachers College, Columbia University in 1924, offering an Ed. D. Until 1946, when two of the forty-six colleges and universities offering advanced programs in nursing also initiated doctoral education for nurses, nurses who wanted doctoral studies had to attend programs outside of nursing. By 1969, some twenty-five different doctoral degrees were being awarded to nurses, including the Doctor of Nursing (DN), Doctor of Nursing Science (DNS or DNSc), Doctor of Nursing Education (DNEd), and Doctor of Public Health Nursing (DPHN), as well as Doctor of Philosophy (Ph.D.), and Doctor of Education (Ed.D.).

There is still disagreement, and some confusion, in nursing circles as to the kind of education and degree a nurse should get in a doctoral program. The first definite statement on doctoral education in nursing was made by the NLN in 1955, the same year that the DHEW Division of Nursing activated the Predoctoral and Postdoctoral Nursing Research Fellowship Program in order to assist nurses to qualify for doctoral study in a discipline outside nursing and to encourage the preparation of research personnel. At that time, the NLN committee considering graduate programs made certain assumptions about the doctoral degree:

(1) the doctorate should not be a third professional degree in nursing but should be based upon a second professional degree and constitute new and enlarged experience in relevant intellectual disciplines and scholarly research in the application of such disciplines to nursing; (2) the degree could be interdisciplinary, possibly in the social sciences, biological sciences, and education; (3) in those institutions not permitting interdisciplinary doctorates, the degree should be awarded in a single discipline such as sociology, biology, and the like.[24]

By 1960, the major activity in doctoral education for nurses focused on establishing collaborative arrangements with other disciplines in a university through which nurses could receive doctoral degrees. Only four institutions offered doctoral programs in which an area of nursing, teaching, or administration in nursing was the focus of study.[25] In 1963, the Nurse Scientist Graduate Training Grants Program was initiated by DHEW and new attention was given to doctoral study. The national nursing organizations and universities held a number of programs and conferences to discuss philosophical bases and explore trends affecting doctoral study.

Although many nurses are still enrolled in nonnursing doctoral programs, the pendulum may have swung toward doctoral degrees in nursing in the last few years. However, the "appropriate" doctoral degree for nurses has been a matter of debate. Some nursing leaders favor granting a Ph.D. in nursing with a minor in a relevant discipline. Others have felt that although the nursing Ph.D. is an ultimate goal, nursing science is not sufficiently developed to make this

practical immediately. Instead they suggest either a Ph.D. in some other discipline with a minor in nursing or a strictly professional degree such as the DNS. It is believed that a nurse with an academic degree (Ph.D.) in a cognate discipline could help to generate knowledge, and the nurse with the professional degree (Ed.D. or DNSc) would apply this new knowledge.

The Ph.D. is the degree most commonly held by nurses. As more doctoral programs evolve, the debate becomes more heated. Schools starting doctoral programs must consider what best suits their educational philosophy and the qualifications and interests of their faculty members. Yet, many schools choose a Ph.D. program because it is still considered the most prestigious degree in academia. Sometimes the university denies nursing this option because of the notion that nursing science is not advanced enough; therefore the school chooses a DNS or DNSc instead. What's the difference? Theoretically the Ph.D. is a research degree, and the Ph.D. graduate is expected to develop theory and to do basic research. The person with the professional doctorate (DNS, DNSc, DSN) is supposed to use existing theory and engage in applied research.[26] Both are expected to become researchers, teachers, and administrators. In actuality, the differences blur. Even nurses with a Ph.D. employed in beginning positions in a nursing school may be teaching undergraduate students and have little interest in or time for research. In fact, a doctorate of any kind has been called a "union card" for admission into a teaching position in higher education.[27] Whether or not the person does research of any kind depends on personal inclination or professional pressure (the publish-or-perish syndrome).

In addition, there is some evidence that there is little difference between the research and professional doctorates,[28] which has made some schools try to switch to the Ph.D. Several schools offer both the Ph.D. and the DNS and have identified the differences. (Other disciplines, such as public health and social work, also offer both degrees.) The DSN/DNS/DNSc are often defined as advanced clinical practice-oriented doctorates, which seek to integrate new knowledge into nursing care. However, one noted nurse feels strongly that the DSN should be the preferred doctoral degree, both because it follows logically the MSN degree and "because it is the scientific doctoral degree with nursing as a major as opposed to DNS degrees, which imply that nursing is a science in itself. Nursing is not a science."[29] Andreoli agrees with others that the master's degree programs are not long enough to prepare nursing specialists with the expertise as teachers, role models, researchers, and change agents required in the nursing specialist role. The DNS curriculum is seen as emanating from a common base of knowledge and experience gained in the MNS program and focused on clinical practice, education, research, and administration.

One consistent concern is quality in doctoral programs, particularly as they proliferate, perhaps in schools that do not have an adequate number of faculty properly prepared to guide the education and research of doctoral students. Monitoring of doctoral programs is usually a university prerogative, but it is not clear how well this is done. Meleis has suggested a National Peer Consultant Team,[30] but this idea has not met with any enthusiasm. Yet if inadequate programs are allowed to continue, nursing's doctorates, late on the academic scene as it is, will lose credibility.

The characteristics of high-quality nursing doctoral programs have been described as follows:

1. Well-prepared faculty holding earned doctorates, with the majority holding a doctoral degree in nursing.
2. Evidence of research and scholarly productivity of faculty.
3. Maintenance of a learning climate conducive to intellectual curiosity, advancement of clinical knowledge, and identification of researchable problems.
4. Evidence of continuous, active, productive, quality-based research in the parent institution.
5. Selection of students who are intellectually capable and professionally committed to nursing and the health care of all people.
6. Philosophical and financial accountability of the parent institution to support a doctoral program in nursing and make university resources available for the conduct of the program.
7. Consideration of regional and national resources to enhance program offerings, assure quality, and augment areas of faculty expertise.
8. Provision for evaluation of the doctoral program and the impact of graduates.[31]

Although the role of doctoral nurses is still not clearly understood by many lay people and even some other disciplines, nursing leaders see an urgency in increasing this too-small pool of scholars, because the shortage is expected to remain acute. The fact that a projected need for nurses with master's and doctorates in 1990 (256,000 and 14,000, respectively) was clearly not going to be met was undoubtedly a major factor in the recommendation of the Institute of Medicine (IOM) study of nursing and nursing education (described in Chap. 5) to increase and expand graduate programs. In the eighth *Report to the Congress on Health Personnel in the United States*, predictions appear for 178,100 master's and doctorally prepared nurses by 2020. The report is silent on need or demand, claiming the absence of quantifiable data for justification.[32] Certainly, the availability of federal funds for programs and students will help achieve expansion, but it will be the responsibility of nursing to see that the quality of each program is good and serves the American public. There are currently 59 doctoral programs in nursing, 7 of which award the DNS/DSN, 1 the Ed.D., and the rest the Ph.D.

Continuing Education

Professional practitioners of any kind must continue to learn because they are accountable to the public for a high quality of service—a service impossible to maintain if pertinent aspects of the tremendous flow of new knowledge are not integrated and used. A thought-provoking model of the fleeting hold professionals have on what they learn was described some years ago in a journal:

> Assuming that the professional life of an individual (in this example, a physician) is forty years, the amount of clinically applicable knowledge available in midcareer should be 100 percent. However, the body of knowledge available at the time of the educational program is only about half, leaving 50 percent useful. It is possible to teach only a fraction of this knowledge in any educational program, leaving 20 percent useful. Of this, a small part is erroneous, leaving 19 percent useful. Not all that is taught is learned, leaving 16 percent useful. Much of what is learned is forgotten within a few years, leaving 8 percent useful; some of what is learned is never used because of specialization, leaving 5 percent useful. Much of what is learned becomes obsolete in 20 years, leaving 3 percent of useful knowledge gained in the professional's basic educational program.[33]

While the precision of the figures can obviously be challenged, the message is clear, even in nonquantitative terms: ongoing learning is necessary if a professional is to function effectively.

The American Nurses Association has defined nursing professional development as the "lifelong process of active participation in learning activities to enhance professional practice."[34] Encompassing both continuing education and staff development, "educators in nursing professional development influence the practice environment and the advancement of the profession."[35] When nurses participate in the educational process, through either continuing education activities or staff development activities, they learn to maintain or increase their competency in the ever-changing health care environment.[36]

For nurses, specifically, the need for continuing education is primarily to keep them abreast of changes in nursing roles and functions, acquire new knowledge and skills (and/or renew what has been lost), and modify attitudes and understanding. To achieve these goals, various approaches to continuing education can be used, such as formal academic studies that might lead to a degree; short-term courses or programs given by institutions of higher learning that do not necessarily provide academic credit; and independent or informal study carried on by the practitioner, utilizing opportunities made available through professional organizations and employing agencies. Continuing education does not mean that enrollment in a formal academic, degree-granting program is necessary, although it might be a reasonable route for a nurse who has specific career goals. On the other hand, neither does holding the highest academic degree mean an end to continued learning.

One statement of philosophy, probably not too different from that developed by other groups, is useful in spelling out the scope of continuing education:

> Continuing education refers to those professional learning experiences designed to enrich the nurses' contributions to quality health care and his or her pursuit of professional career goals. Continuing education includes programs, offerings and independent studies that meet specific criteria for contact hours.[37]

In the 1970s, a number of states enacted legislation requiring evidence of continuing education (CE) for relicensure of nurses (and of certain other professional and occupational groups). According to a recent survey, 27 state boards of nursing now have continuing education requirements for renewal of license registration, and 42 state boards of nursing now have continuing education requirements for reentry into active practice.[38] The requirements for renewal generally average about 10 to 15 contact hours annually. The requirements for reentry vary widely from as little as 20 hours over 2 years to as much as a 300-hour approved nurse refresher course. Formalized programs are given under the auspices of educational institutions, professional organizations, and commercial for-profit groups; generally, they must be self-supporting. Most now have accreditation by either the American Nurses Credentialling Center, a national professional nursing organization and certifying board, or the state board of nursing, so that their programs will be acknowledged by licensing boards as legitimate sources of continuing education. Most programs use the contact hour, which is nationally accepted for unit measurement of all kinds of CE programs. A contact is "a unit of measurement that describes 50 minutes of an approved, organized learning experience."[39]

Both ANA and NLN and their constituent organizations have developed a voluntary system of continuing education for nurses. The ICN has also urged its members to take the lead in initiating, promoting, or further developing a national system of continuing nursing education.

More nurses seem to be attending formal programs. How much CE improves practice is still debated; however, many impact evaluation studies appear to confirm what direct effect continuing education has on practice. It has been shown that the motivation of the learner and the opportunity to apply what is learned are key factors. Opportunities and funds to attend programs are often part of some collective bargaining agreements. However, nurses, if they consider themselves professionals, should be prepared to pay for their own CE.

Is CE readily available to most nurses? Despite some justifiable complaints that formal programs are not always available in certain geographic areas, there are many ways for nurses to continue their professional development independently or through home study programs. Examples of self-directed learning activities include self-guided, focused reading, independent learning projects, individual scientific research, informal investigation of a specific nursing problem, correspondence courses, self-contained learning packages using various media, directed reading, computer-assisted instruction, programmed instruction, study tours, and group work projects. Some nursing journals have developed self-learning programs that in-

clude evaluation, for a minimal fee. There are also other innovative ways in which nurses are offered learning opportunities, such as through mobile vans, television, telephone systems, satellites, and other forms of telecommunication, as well as increased regional programs by nursing organizations.

The opportunities for CE in nursing are considerably greater than they were some years ago. What kind of CE a nurse chooses will remain, to a large extent, an individual decision. However, the necessity to be currently competent is a both legal and ethical requirement for any professional. Equally important, nursing cannot advance unless all nurses accept the responsibility of lifelong learning.

PROGRAMS FOR PRACTICAL NURSES

Professional nurses work closely with practical nurses (PNs) in all branches of hospital and public health nursing. Moreover, in the last few years, an increasing number of PNs have been entering RN programs at either a beginning or an advanced level. It is helpful, therefore, to be informed about the educational preparation of a PN, as well as the basic RN programs.

Practical nurses (called *vocational nurses* in Texas and California) fall into four general groups: (1) those whose only teacher has been experience and who are not licensed to practice (this type of PN is gradually disappearing from the scene); (2) those with experience but no formal education who have taken state-approved courses to qualify them to take state board examinations and become licensed; (3) those who have been licensed through a grandfather clause; and (4) those who have graduated from approved schools of practical nursing and, by passing state board examinations, have become licensed in the state or states in which they practice. There are also a few who were enrolled in RN programs and were permitted by their state law to take the PN examination after a certain number of courses. The large majority of licensed practical nurses (LPNs) or licensed vocational nurses (LVNs) are licensed by examination. Although PNs in the third category can be legally employed, employers with a choice usually prefer graduates from an approved school who have been licensed by examination.

PNs are usually educated in one-year programs in vocational, trade, or technical schools, hospitals, or community colleges. Academic credits are awarded by the colleges. In 1992, there were 1,090 PN programs, a 2 percent increase from the previous year. The growth rate of both programs and numbers of students, which had been increasing steadily over the years, leveled off and even decreased between 1983 and 1989. In 1992, there was a 4.1 percent increase in enrollments over 1991.[40] PN education has been heavily supported by the federal government for some time. The desire for LPNs to reach RN status is evident in their increased admission to (and graduation from) RN programs. Almost one quarter (23.7 percent) of newly licensed RNs in 1992 practiced as PNs prior to their RN education.[41] For some years, PN programs have seemed to attract more blacks, more men, and more older students than any other type of nursing program. However, many of these potential students, if qualified, now seem to choose AD or baccalaureate programs. Increasingly available are "ladder" programs in which the student can move from PN to RN status in an organized way. In this approach, a PN program is the first year of a two-year associate degree program. A student may exit at the end of the year, become licensed and work, or become licensed and not work and continue into the second year, becoming eligible for the RN examination. Some RN programs, particularly for the associate degree, give partial or total credit for the PN program[42] (often only if the PN has also passed the licensing examination).

Legitimate PN programs must be approved by the appropriate state nursing authority and may also be accredited, usually by the NLN. Upon graduation, the student is eligible to take the licensing examination (NCLEX-PN) (see Chap. 20) to become a licensed practical nurse (LPN) or a licensed vocational nurse (LVN). The licensing law is now mandatory in all states.

In PN programs, most teachers have a baccalaureate degree or less. PN programs emphasize technical skills and direct patient care, but a (usually) simple background of the physical and social sciences is often integrated in the program. Clinical experience is provided in one or more hospitals and other agencies. The number of skills that are taught increases each year, probably because of employer's demands. Both NLN and the National Association for Practical Nurse Education and Service (NAPNES) have published statements on LPN entry-level competencies. The NLN statement is found in Exhibit 13-4. The NAPNES statement is almost identical.[43]

As in all areas of health care, there is a need for continuing education programs. Employers frequently offer courses, reviews, or in-service programs for giving medications and performing new treatments, but the two PN organizations and NLN have provided programs on care of geriatric patients, psychiatric patients, and others. There are also numerous continuing education programs geared particularly toward the LPN licensed by waiver.

The major employment site for LPNs has shifted again and again, based on the availability and salary expectations of the RN. During the boom years, when RN salaries were significantly depressed and hospitals were proud to claim an all-RN staff, the presence of the LPN declined in acute care. During the nursing shortage of the late 1980s, LPNs were again hired for hospital practice. Within these same years, the American Nurses Association tirelessly lobbied for the 24-hour presence of an RN in nursing homes. As a governmental compromise to the economically strained nursing home industry and given the perceived shortage of RNs, the modifier *registered* was changed to *licensed*, allowing the hiring of either LPNs or RNs. It has become common practice to substitute LPNs for RNs, and often in a very arbitrary manner. A 1993 study conducted by the National Council of State Boards of Nursing shows the largest

Exhibit 13-4	Competencies of Graduates of Educational Programs in Practical Nursing

- Assesses basic physical, emotional, spiritual, and sociocultural needs of the health care client.
- Collects data within established protocols and guidelines from various sources:
  a. client interviews
  b. observations/measurements
  c. health care team members, family, and significant others
  d. health records
- Utilizes knowledge of normal values to identify deviations in health status.
- Documents data collection.
- Communicates findings to appropriate health care personnel.
- Contributes to the development of nursing care plans utilizing established nursing diagnoses for clients with common, well-defined health problems.
- Prioritizes nursing care needs of clients.
- Assists in the review and revision of nursing care plans to meet the changing needs of clients.

- Provides nursing care according to:
  a. accepted standards of practice
  b. priority of client needs
  c. individual and family rights to dignity and privacy
- Utilizes effective communication in:
  a. recording and reporting
  b. establishing and maintaining therapeutic relationships with clients, families, and significant others
- Collaborates with health care team members to coordinate the delivery of nursing care.
- Instructs clients regarding health maintenance based on client needs and nurse's knowledge level.
- Seeks guidance as needed in evaluating nursing care.
- Modifies nursing approaches based on evaluation of nursing care.
- Collaborates with other health team members in the revision of nursing care plans.

Source: Reprinted with permission of the National League for Nursing, 1994 (under revision).

percentage of LPNs were employed in skilled nursing units (30.8 percent) in long-term care facilities, hospital-based medical-surgical units (21.3 percent), and long-term care nursing facilities (17.8 percent).[44]

Recent studies on the role activities of the LPN prove a great deal of state-to-state inconsistency. There is also a tendency for LPNs to expand their practice once they become experienced. This is accomplished through a sequence of events: an educational program appropriate to the activity, supervised practice, documented competency, continued supervision, and state board approvals. However, despite the fact that many of these activities have become a usual part of LPN practice, they are not included in the basic educational program. This may be due to the absence of a national standard on which to base the licensure examination, and the political need to curtail length-

ening the educational program. LPNs report administering IV medications, starting IVs, hemodialysis monitoring, pronouncing death, inserting GI tubes, ventilator care, central line management, management of total parenteral nutrition (TPN), as some examples.[45] These situations are of great concern to the RN, who is not only legally responsible but bound by a code of ethics.

Because LPNs are often pressed to perform functions beyond the level of their education (such as charge nursing and certain specialty practice), there has been an increasing movement of PNs to "be paid for what we do, not what we are." However, health economics, some earlier LPN layoffs, and the continuing trend toward two levels of nursing have brought new concerns. In August 1984, citing "concern for job safety," the National Federation of Licensed Practical Nurses (NFLPN) House of Delegates endorsed two levels of nursing (RN and LPN/LVN) and the expansion of the LPN/LVN curriculum program to at least 18 months. An implementation date of 10 years was set. That target date was not met; however, "ladder" programs are becoming increasingly popular. The number of RN students who are LPNs has already been noted. It has been suggested that this trend may prove to be the key to the entry-into-practice debate as far as practical nurses are concerned.

REFERENCES

1. Moses E: *The Registered Nurse Population.* Washington, DC: U.S. DHHS, 1994, pp 17, 41.
2. National League for Nursing (NLN): *Nursing Data Review 1994.* New York: The League, 1994, p 29.
3. Ibid.
4. Montag M: *The Education of Nursing Technicians.* New York: Putnam's, 1951, pp 94–100.
5. N-OADN perspective on education reform and strategies to position nursing for the future. *National Organization for Associate Degree Nursing Newsletter.* Arlington, VA: The Organization, May–June 1994.
6. American Nurses Association: *Educational Preparation for Nurse Practitioners and Assistants to Nursing: A Position Paper.* New York: The Association, 1965, pp 7–8.
7. Montag, op cit, p 73.
8. NLN, loc cit.
9. Ibid, p 47.
10. *Essentials of College and University Education for Professional Nursing.* Washington, DC: American Association of Colleges of Nursing, 1986, p 4.
11. Ibid, p 5.
12. Watson J, Phillips S: A call for educational reform: Colorado nursing doctorate model as exemplar. *Nurs Outlook* 40:20–26, January–February 1992.
13. Starck PL et al: Developing a nursing doctorate for the 21st century. *J Prof Nurs* 9:212–219, July–August 1993.
14. Roberts M: *American Nursing.* New York: Macmillan, 1954, pp 533–536.
15. NLN, op cit, p 87.
16. Moses, op cit, pp 6, 18.
17. Moses, op cit, p 7.
18. American Nurses' Association: *Statement on Graduate Education in Nursing.* New York: The Association, 1969.
19. American Nurses' Association: *Statement on Graduate Education in Nursing.* Kansas City, MO: The Association, 1978, p 8.
20. Ibid, p 4.
21. Ibid.
22. NLN, op cit, p 88.
23. *Characteristics of Master's Education in Nursing.* New York: National League for Nursing, 1987.
24. Report of the Committee to Formulate Guiding Principles for the Administration and Organization of Master's Programs in Nursing, in *Proceedings of the Meetings of Representatives of Graduate Programs in Nursing,* May 1955 (mimeo).
25. Campbell J: Post-master's education in nursing. *Nurs Outlook* 9:554, September 1961.
26. Meleis A: Doctoral education in nursing: Its present and its future. *J Prof Nurs* 6:436–446, November–December 1988.
27. Brenner M et al: Doctoral preparation of nursing faculty. *Nurs Ed* 15:12–15, March–April 1990.
28. Meleis, op cit, pp 441–442.
29. Andreoli K: Specialization and graduate curricula: Finding the fit. *Nurs Health Care* 8:68, February 1987.
30. Meleis, op cit, pp 444–445.
31. ANA (1978), op cit, pp 3–4.
32. US Department of Health and Human Services, Bureau of Health Professions: *Health Personnel in the US, Eighth Report to the Congress.* Washington, DC: DHHS, 1992, pp 136–141.
33. West K: Influences of the scholar. *Bull Med Libr Assoc* 56:43, January 1968.
34. *Standards for Nursing Professional Development: Continuing Education and Staff Development.* Washington, DC: American Nurses' Association, 1994, p 5.
35. Ibid.
36. Ibid, p 6.
37. Ibid, p 5.
38. Annual CE Survey: State and association/certifying boards CE requirements. *J Cont Ed Nurs* 35:5–8, January–February 1994.
39. Standards, op cit.
40. NLN, op cit, pp 135–141.
41. Rosenfeld P: *Profiles of Newly Licensed Nurse.*

New York: National League for Nursing, 1994, p 34.

42. Pullen C: Are we easing the transition from LPN to ADN? *Am J Nurs* 88:1129, August 1988.

43. National Association for Practical Nurse Education and Service: *Statement of Practical/Vocational Nursing Entry Level Competence*. New York: The Association, 1981.

44. National Council of State Boards of Nursing: *Preliminary Report: Role Delineation Study of Nurses Aides, Licensed Practical/Vocational Nurses, Registered Nurses and Advanced Registered Nurse Practitioners*. Chicago: The Council, 1993, p 30.

45. DeLapp TD et al: Scope of practice for beginning and experienced LPNs: The Alaska experience. *Issues* 13:1, 6–9, 1992.

CHAPTER

14

Nursing Research: Status, Problems, Issues

HISTORICAL OVERVIEW

LIKE SO MANY BEGINNINGS in nursing, research in nursing probably had its start with Florence Nightingale, who made detailed reports on observations of both medical and nursing matters during the Crimean War, documented the evidence, and pointed out significant data, which resulted in reform. After that, there was no other published research by nurses in the early periods of nursing. This was partly because it became an apprenticeship occupation in the United States and because, in the Victorian era, females were encouraged to leave intellectual initiative to males, and nurses often epitomized Victorian females. However, nurses gradually gained more education, moved into universities, and formed a professional organization.

Early studies that might be called a form of research were primarily for the improvement of nursing education and nursing service, because the early leaders were almost always responsible for both of those areas and there were obvious knowledge gaps. At a time when medicine was only semiscientific, it is natural that nurses, scientifically untrained, would not attempt to establish a scientific base for nursing. But there was an attempt to gather data about nursing. One of the first, if not the first, study of American nursing education was Adelaide Nutting's survey of the field, published in 1906. Lillian Wald's school nursing project in New York was probably the first demonstration project reported in the *American Journal of Nursing* (by

Dock in 1902). Wald herself wrote *House on Henry Street* in 1915, about that innovative experiment in public health nursing. (See Chaps. 3 and 4 for further details.) Other studies followed. In 1909, an ANA committee initiated a series of studies of public health. In 1912, Adelaide Nutting's survey of nursing education was published by the U.S. Bureau of Education, followed by the first major study of nursing, the 1923 Goldmark Report. These and succeeding studies by the Committee on the Grading of Nursing Schools, described in Chap. 5, greatly influenced the direction of nursing, and to some degree, nursing research. Although most of these studies focused on the nurse rather than nursing care, some of the nurse-teachers in universities did experiment with nursing techniques. In the late 1920s and 1930s, a few fellowships were granted to nurses in graduate programs who showed aptitude for research, and by 1930, nursing leadership had recognized the value of research and attempted to foster it. However, few were in positions to become involved in problems of patient care, and the nurses closest to the patient did not see themselves in a research role.[1]

Notter,[2] as well as Simmons and Henderson, cites a handful of nurses who did minor studies related to clinical nursing, most often of nursing procedures, in the 1920s and 1930s. But while medical research was plunging ahead and finding new answers to disease, research in nursing and about nursing was still related to the image,

287

role, and functions of the nurse and was done as often as not by social scientists rather than nurses. Still, there was support by nurses of some of this research, such as the five-year ANA-initiated study of nursing functions, which yielded much useful data.[3, 4]

Sigma Theta Tau, the honor society for nursing, awarded the first grant for nursing research in 1936 and since then has awarded research grants to about 300 nurse scientists, often seed money to enable promising researchers to attract larger grants from major funding sources. By 1970, ANA had also established a Commission on Nursing Research, and in 1972 a Council of Nurse Researchers was started.

The growth of the university schools of nursing had a definite effect on nursing research. As better-prepared faculty and students became involved in studies, sometimes a particular school concentrated on particular problems. Some universities also developed research centers, such as the Institute of Research and Service in Nursing Education at Teachers College in 1953 and Wayne State's Center for Health Research in 1969. This trend continued through the 1970s. In addition, the launching of *Nursing Research* in 1952 and the publication of several texts on nursing research at about the same time drew nursing closer to professionalism. The sponsorship of research by national health agencies and services, which emphasized the patient and patient care, may also have been a turning point toward clinical research. The American Nurses' Foundation was established by ANA specifically to further nursing research by conducting and supporting projects, as it still does today.

As might be expected, federal interest in nursing research was highly influential in its development. In 1955, a Research Grants and Fellowship Branch was set up in the Division of Nursing Resources of the U.S. Public Health Service, providing funds that enabled many nurses to complete their doctoral studies, as well as funds for other research, faculty development, workshops, and the nurse scientist programs.[5] In 1960, the Division of Nursing Re-

sources combined with the Division of Public Health Nursing, and the research program became a branch within this new division of nursing. Formal support for nursing research, which had begun in 1955, focused in those years on helping nurses obtain a doctorate in order to prepare leaders needed to facilitate nursing scholarship. Most of these awards went to nurses obtaining doctorates in related biologic, behavioral, or allied fields because of the limited number of doctoral programs in nursing. A Department of Nursing was also established in the Walter Reed Institute (1957), and it was here that much of the early nursing research was done and where prominent nurse researchers received their training.

In 1963, the surgeon general's report noted that research is one of the obligations of society and urged increased government funding because, with the rapidly changing patterns of medical care organization, the need for nursing research had outstripped resources available for studies of nursing care. "The potential contributions of nursing research to better patient care are so impressive that universities, hospitals, and other health agencies should receive all possible encouragement to conduct appropriate studies."[6] Even so, funds were not available in large amounts, and progress in the development of clinical nursing research was slow. Seven years later, the National Commission for the Study of Nursing and Nursing Education (NCSNNE) expressed dismay that so little research had been done on the actual effects of nursing intervention and care; the profession had few definitive guides for the improvement of practice. The kinds of clinical studies done by nurses were cited as major contributions to health, and it was urged that funds for nursing research be increased. Although funds were increased for a time, continued cutbacks in federal funds soon created a major problem in nursing research as well as in education. Still, nurses have been forging ahead in nursing research, particularly clinical research, seeking funds from foundations as well as the government.

WHAT IS NURSING RESEARCH?

Schlotfeldt's definition of the term *research* is classic: all systematic inquiry designed for the purpose of advancing knowledge.[7] Notter makes a useful comparison between problem solving related to patient care (sometimes also described as the *nursing process*) and scientific inquiries.[8] Both go through such steps as (1) identifying a problem, (2) analyzing its various aspects, (3) collecting facts or data, (4) determining action on the basis of analysis of the data, and (5) evaluating the result. In scientific inquiry, step 4 includes developing a hypothesis, as well as setting up a study design or method. After the analysis and evaluation of data in terms of the hypothesis, the findings of the research are reported. These steps may be relatively simple or very complex; they may involve laboratory equipment, human experimentation, or neither. Research may be designed as *basic*, the establishment of new knowledge or theory that is not immediately applicable, or *applied*, the attempt to solve a practical problem. Either way, the same steps are taken.

There are several types of research, and nurses may be involved in any of them, or more than one. *Historical* or *documentary* research provides more than a record of the past; because history tends to repeat itself, its study can prevent mistakes and help point new directions. Real historical research requires study of original records or documents (primary sources) to prevent distortion that comes with interpretation by succeeding historians. Historical research is having a new resurgence in nursing. Not only are the past and its human figures being studied on the basis of new hypotheses, but there is interest in preserving the ideas and attitudes of contemporary nursing leaders—while they are still alive. One good example of a technique being used is the oral history, which involves audiotaped or videotaped interviews that may also be published, such as Gwendolyn Safier's *Contemporary American Leaders in Nursing*.[9] Also available for short-term loan are videocassettes in the Sigma Theta Tau Distinguished Leaders in Nursing Series.

Descriptive research describes what exists and analyzes the findings in terms of their significance. The purpose may be simply to get information, such as the periodic *National Sample Survey of Registered Nurses*, which reports on the nurse population and factors affecting their supply, or to gather facts that might be later used as a basis of a hypothesis of another type of study. Various techniques can be used: interviews, observations, case studies, or literature review. The studies can be both clinical and nonclinical.

In *experimental* research, the researcher manipulates the situation in some way to test a hypothesis. Preferably, one controlled setting or group in which certain factors or variables are held constant, and an experimental setting or group in which one or more variables are manipulated are used and the results compared. Such studies might be done in a laboratory, using animals, chemical or biological substances, or people. If the study involves human beings, whether in a standard laboratory, in a clinical setting, or in the field (the subject's home, school, workplace), the ethical principles and/or laws related to human experimentation must be observed. There are ethical principles that apply to all types of research. All of these kinds of research can also be nursing research, although there might be some argument about some of the examples given, depending on how nursing research is perceived.

The controversy about who should engage in what kind of research seems rather foolish in light of the need. There are proponents of "pure" or basic research, who feel that nursing needs a scientific base before practice can be studied. The separation is artificial. Basic research can be a foundation for applied clinical research but, given the unanswered questions in nursing care, there is no reason that there should not be research of both kinds, the abstract and the pragmatic. Equally pointless is the scientist/practitioner dichotomy. Probably all good nurses should have some configuration of practice, education, and research skills, because all are part of nursing's role. Clinicians who do not know, understand, or care about research are missing a source of knowledge that will enhance their practice; an investigator without sound clinical knowledge is not fully prepared.

One useful definition of nursing research is "research that arises from the practice of nursing for the purpose of solving patient care problems."[10] A noted nurse researcher describes nursing research as a "systematic inquiry into the problems encountered in nursing practice and into the modalities of patient care, such as support and comfort, prevention of trauma, promotion of recovery, health education, health appraisal, and coordination of health care."[11] She emphasizes as key words *patient* and *effect*, calling them the critical nucleus of nursing research. This type of research is also defined as clinical nursing research. However, it has been pointed out that *clinical* can have different meanings to different people: involving a place such as a hospital or clinic; pertaining to some form of disease or symptom; or the testing of an action considered a nursing action. Newman maintains that if the criterion "relevance to practice" is applied, then all nursing research is clinical research, but "the distinguishing factor between basic and clinical research is the purpose of the research: whether it is knowledge for the sake of knowledge or knowledge for a specific purpose."[12] Johnson and others see nursing in a more abstract vein, seeing new concepts developed by the nurse researcher from reformulation of concepts from other sciences, leading to development of "theories of nursing intervention which will yield predictable responses in patients when implemented in nursing care"[13] (see Chap. 9).

There are a number of other variations on the definition of nursing research and how it might be classified, and probably the arguments will persist. One of the most thoughtful nurse researchers (and one with a sense of humor) suggests that perhaps the best answer to "What is nursing research?" is "A good question."[14]

WHY NURSING RESEARCH?

Research of one kind or another has been responsible for the major advances in most fields, has resulted in modern technology, and has had a dramatic effect on medicine. The notion that much of the science of nursing is derived from medicine or the social sciences probably evolved because nursing did borrow many of its concepts and practice patterns from other disciplines. Some nurses began to recognize that many of these concepts had not been tested or tested recently and certainly had not been tested in relation to nursing practice. Others began to wonder what in nursing care made that critical difference in patient outcome. What was the impact of nursing care, how could it affect health care, and how could it affect health care of the future? The NCSNNE believed that the answer lay in nursing research.

> This commission believes it is essential for the future of health care in this country to begin a systematic evaluation of the impact of nursing care. We advocate the development of objective criteria such as measurable improvement in patient conditions, evidence of early discharge or return to employment, reduced incidence of readmission to care facilities, and lowered rates of communicable disease. We do not suggest for a moment that nursing is wholly responsible for these or any other factors in the qualitative measurement of health care. We do believe, however, that nursing represents an important independent variable in our total health system. As such, we must learn how we can utilize nurses—more effectively, more efficiently, and more economically.[15]

More than a decade later, another National Commission said much the same, adding, "Through research, nurses can test, refine, and advance the knowledge base on which improved education and practice must rest"[16] (see Chap. 5).

Thus, it was once more affirmed that research is also necessary to determine just what nurses should be taught—the underlying theory or theories of nursing. Practice disciplines have always needed to develop their own bodies of verified knowledge and to evaluate that knowledge in practice, both for survival as a profession and for the well-being of their clients. This has been constantly reiterated by nursing leaders and scholars in the last few decades: the primary tasks of nursing research as (1) development and refinement of nursing theories that serve as guides to nursing practice and can be organized into a body of scientific nursing knowledge and (2) finding a valid means for measuring the extent to which nursing action attains its goals in terms of patient behavior.

As described in Chaps. 9 and 12, these theories have gained an important place in nursing education, but not nearly as much in nursing practice. In fact, the question is raised, "Does nursing research affect practice?" However, the development of a "scientific community of nurse researchers" characterized by three factors, communality (sharing research ideas and findings), colleagueship (providing a supportive environment within which ideas can be challenged), and constructive competition (providing a strong motivator for creating ideas), is seen as an important cornerstone for building structures and resources for nursing research.[17]

RESEARCH INTO PRACTICE

Over the years, a major issue has been the utilization of nursing research. After all, no matter how critical the findings of research studies may seem, if they are not tested in practice over a period of time, in a variety of settings, the results might still be questioned. If they are not used at all, practice may change, but it will not change as a result of research. The first step is communication. Without communication, there can be no replication, application, utilization, or evaluation by others. In the last few years, means of reporting research and participating in peer review have increased considerably. As late as 1977, *Nursing Research* was the only journal in the United States devoted exclusively to reporting nursing research, but since that time several others have come on the scene. Because they are "refereed" journals, that is, the articles are re-

viewed and approved by a panel of experts before publication, the methodology, content, and analysis have been scrutinized by others in research and found appropriate. This may or may not be true of research articles in other nursing or nonnursing journals, but here, too, peer review is becoming more common, and such articles are increasing in number, although they are not necessarily presented in as much detail.

Other major avenues of reporting research exist: the federal government, state, regional, and national organizations, foundations, universities, and health agencies, all of which might be responsible for publication of newsletters, abstracts, reports, articles, monographs, books, and conferences, seminars, programs (with proceedings), as well as publishing houses that produce various indexes. *Dissertation Abstracts International* carries abstracts of all doctoral dissertations, complete photocopies of which can be purchased through the publisher, University Microfilms, Ann Arbor, Michigan. In addition, there are individual and university libraries, governmental and private networks of health science libraries, and professional association libraries that use computer-based retrieval service techniques to prepare bibliographies on requested topics (see Chap. 29).

Does better communication guarantee utilization? Unfortunately, nursing has a history of ignoring the results or recommendations of research, or at least delaying action. For instance, early recommendations from studies of nursing education about educational preparation of nurses are only now coming to fruition, after about a seventy-five-year time lag. But here, at least, social and economic factors may have been contributors to such slow action. What about utilization of *clinical* findings?

Gortner and others have categorized practice-related research as studies: (1) building a science of practice (systematic identification of health problems and health needs of patients and relationships between nursing and patients), (2) refining the "artistry of practice" (laboratory and field studies of what nurses do), (3) concerned with descriptive, analytical, and experimental studies of physical and social environments in which nurses and their clients interact, (4) aiming to develop methodology or measurement tools, and (5) dealing directly with application of research findings to the field through replication on a small or large scale.[18]

For years, there have been complaints that staff nurses not only did not read research reports but also had no interest in research. Even research results directly applicable to practice probably were not used except in the clinical setting where the research was done, if then. Even today, a number of obstacles to research utilization are still present: lack of perceived value of nursing research; lack of access to resources; lack of preparation; lack of availability of research findings; lack of authority to autonomously change patient care procedures; lack of motivation to change; insufficient methods for implementation and dissemination; and lack of clinician-researcher communication.[19] Or, as another individual put it:

1. They do not know about them.
2. They do not understand them.
3. They do not believe them.
4. They do not know how to apply them.
5. They are not allowed to use them.[20]

Probably in many practice sites this outlook is still prevalent. Most nurses in practice today, including nurse administrators, were not educated at a time when research was considered a part of nursing's responsibility and certainly were not trained to carry out any type of research. Since most hospitals are not affiliated with university programs, where most of the research has been done, and since even in programs of higher education, most nurse faculty do not do substantive research, it is small wonder that research has not been a part of nursing practice.

However, some clear trends are emerging that may turn this situation around. First, some researchers are beginning to realize that they have a responsibility for *translating* the research into terms and concepts understandable to the clinician and disseminating their research results in places other than research conferences. They must make a distinct effort to reach out to nurses who are known as innovators.[21] One editor noted that she doesn't believe practicing nurses want "chewed and well-digested" nursing research, because they would have no reason to change their way of doing things without clear evidence, verified by a scientific publication, that the new way was valid. Instead she gave practical ways to read nursing research and suggested further that "capsules" of nursing research be published in columns clinicians read.[22] There are also suggestions that research findings be brought to the attention of practicing nurses through satellite communication modes and marketing strategies.

Second, more practitioners are being oriented to nursing research in their educational programs. And, perhaps most important, nursing research is being done in clinical sites by nurse researchers and staff.[23] There are several models for clinical nursing research. The most common has been that of the university nurse researcher using a clinical site. The agency-based model calls for either a researcher hired simply to help design and/or conduct a study (and then depart) or, more commonly now, a full-time employed researcher. In the latter case, clinical nurses are actively involved in defining and choosing the research and often participate in gathering the data. It is assumed that the staff would be motivated to use the findings, since the research reflects their concerns and questions. A similar relationship may occur when faculty who are at a clinical site with students or hold joint appointments also involve staff in their clinical research.

For instance, some hospitals with a commitment to nursing research have begun research programs by creating a research committee that helps nurses understand various aspects of research and gives then ongoing support in their efforts. Nurses reporting did not minimize the obstacles that had to be overcome but also stressed the importance of having administrative encouragement and support.[24] Another point is how important the nurses' "curiosity and the yen to discover" is to involvement in nursing research. Educators, supervisors, and clinical specialists are urged to encourage this attitude in students and in staff nurses, even as work pressures tend to discourage these attributes, and to try to identify and reduce curiosity-stifling situations.[25] Two senior hospital-based researchers developed an innovative way to reduce the time and effort necessary to develop a research protocol when the staff had limited knowledge of, and experience in, conducting research. Their "generic research protocol" is a computerized learning package that assists nursing staff in preparing a protocol through step-by-step instruction and guidance.[26]

Research utilization has been described as a "systematic series of activities that can culminate in the change of a specific nursing practice." The activities that comprise research utilization include (1) identification and synthesis of multiple research studies in a common conceptual area (research base); (2) transformation of the knowledge derived from that base into a solution (clinical protocol); (3) transformation of the clinical protocol into specific nursing actions (innovations) that are administered to patients; and (4) a clinical evaluation of the practice to see whether it produced the predicted results.[27] One group of researchers developed seven specific steps to produce "research-based" practice changes: systematically identifying and assessing research-based knowledge to solve those problems; adopting and designing the nursing practice innovation; conducting a clinical trial and evaluation of the innovation; deciding whether to adopt, alter, or reject the innovation; developing the means to extend (or diffuse) the new practice beyond the trial unit; and developing mechanisms to maintain the innovation over time.[28]

Oddly enough, another problem in nursing research is indiscriminate or unthinking application of nursing research findings. Nurses who become aware of research that seems to be pertinent to their field tend to use it without appropriate evaluation or validation. In some cases,

this happens because most nurses currently practicing have not been taught to evaluate the quality of research, although guidelines are available in the literature. Moreover, there is a gap in providing guidelines for applying research to individuals' practice settings. To do so, the consumer (of research) must first make a critical validation of the study, that is, question each step of the author's assumptions, findings, and conclusions. If the conclusions are weak, tentative, or contradicted by others, convincing others to apply the research becomes a problem. If the settings or subjects are too different from the consumer's practice environment, the findings may not make a useful transition. If there are too many constraints in the practice environment, the attempt to implement the findings may require considerable groundwork. Nevertheless, assuming that the study is valid, each indirect application on the cognitive level has useful dimensions in expanding nurses' theory base and making them alert to other studies that might be more directly applicable.[29]

Later, one of the researchers who had developed a model for evaluating the applicability of research findings refined that model and described it as a "prescriptive, practitioner-oriented model designed to mitigate some of the human frailties of decision-making and thus to facilitate appropriate, effective, and pragmatic utilization, raise the consciousness of potential users, and increase the role of critical thinking in professional practice."[30]

Undoubtedly, actually carrying out all these processes in a significant number of hospitals and other health care settings will take time, but the advances that have been made in a relatively short time are impressive. General nursing journals and especially the clinical journals, which staff nurses and other clinicians are most likely to read, are carrying an increasing number of articles or even columns on research findings. Other articles pinpoint the obstacles to applying research in the work setting and make pragmatic suggestions on how to overcome them. There is even some indication that more practicing nurses are aware of, even knowledgeable about, certain kinds of research findings, and most reported using research-based innovations at least some of the time.[31] With the number of nursing research conferences being held locally, regionally, nationally, and even internationally (for example, by Sigma Theta Tau and its chapters), information about current research is much more readily available. It has been found that nurses who read journals and attend conferences are more likely to be interested in research application. Even teaching about research in nursing education programs has improved, especially if the school is research-oriented and students can be involved in the research. Then too it may be useful to consider a broader definition of research utilization: "Research utilization is the process by which research knowledge is moved into the clinical arena, and it can happen in many different ways. Research utilization does not always mean implementing research findings in practice. Research can be used in education to spark additional research or to help nurses better understand clinical situations, even if practice changes do not occur. However, research utilization usually means changing practice or validating that current practice is appropriate and does not require change."[32]

ISSUES AND CHALLENGES

A turning point in nursing research may have been reached with the establishment of the National Center for Nursing Research (NCNR) within the National Institutes of Health (NIH) in 1986. In 1983, two major reports on nursing from the National Commission on Nursing and the Institute of Medicine again reiterated the importance of nursing research (see Chap. 5). Both recommended that a high priority be given to nurse researchers and nursing research. The Institute group specifically commented on the "remarkable dearth of research in nursing practice" and noted that the lack of adequate funding for research and the resulting scarcity of talented nurse researchers have inhibited the development of nursing research. They also made the point that since the government grants were administered at the manpower unit in DHHS (the Division of Nursing), and not at a level of visibility and scientific prestige such as the NIH, there was no encouragement for nurses to devote their careers to nursing research of patient problems. It was recommended, therefore, that the government "establish an organizational entity to place nursing research in the mainstream of scientific investigation."[33]

What is considered a probable follow-up on this recommendation was introduction of legislation in Congress in late 1983 to do just that—in this case, to create a National Institute of Nursing as part of NIH. Although the bill was passed by the House and Senate, it was killed by President Reagan's pocket veto at the end of the 1984 session. He called the creation of a nursing institute "unnecessary and expensive."

Nevertheless, at the end of 1985, Congress managed a compromise by authorizing the NCNR under the Health Research Extension Act of 1985 (P.L. 99-158). In April 1986, the Secretary of DHHS announced the establishment of the NCNR "for the purpose of conducting a program of grants and awards supporting nursing research and research training related to patient care, the promotion of health, the prevention of disease, and the mitigation of the effects of acute and chronic illnesses and disabilities. In support of studies on nursing interventions, procedures, delivery methods, and ethics of patient care, the NCNR programs are expected to complement other biomedical research programs that are primarily concerned with the causes and treatment of disease."[34]

Research funding had originally been one of the responsibilities of the HRSA Division of Nursing and the small staff was moved to NIH as a core of the NCNR. Dr. Doris Merritt, a research physician appointed as acting head, proved to be not only capable as an organizer but also fully supportive of nurses and nursing research. She served until the appointment of the first nurse director, Dr. Ada Sue Hinshaw, a distinguished researcher. Contrary to some expectations, both the head of NIH and the Division of Nursing, who had opposed having a nursing research unit in NIH, were extremely helpful, as were other institute directors.

The NCNR went into action immediately, supporting research, research training, and career development in health promotion and disease prevention, acute and chronic illness, and nursing systems, which included such areas as innovative approaches to delivery of quality nursing services, strategies to improve patient outcome, interventions to assure availability of resources, and bioethics research, a special initiative. The National Nursing Research Agenda (NNRA) was launched in 1987 to provide structure for selecting scientific opportunities and initiatives. Also a number of research training awards were awarded to beginning and advanced nurse researchers through individual and institutional predoctoral, postdoctoral, and senior fellowships. Among the research priorities targeted for the next several years were AIDS and HIV-positive patients, families, and partners; low birth weight infants and their mothers; long-term care; symptom management; information systems; health promotion for adolescents; and technology dependency across the life-span. These were selected by the participants in the first Conference on Nursing Research Priorities (CORP #1) in 1988.

At the request of the Senate Committee on Appropriations, the NIH Task Force on Nursing Research was reconvened in 1989. The Task Force commended the progress of NCNR and made a number of recommendations on how to strengthen nursing research within NIH. Among them were recommendations to foster an awareness of nursing research as an "Area of Inquiry," to foster collaborative and interdisciplinary research in nursing, to assist in the development of nurse researchers, to ensure access to data on nursing research, and to increase the number of nurse reviewers and advisors.[35] As President Bush did recommend an increase in funding following the report, nursing research began to be integrated into the

scientific community, something that had been lacking for a long time.[36]

In the years that followed, the priorities selected were implemented, as awards were given in these areas. Actually, although the NCNR was not an institute in NIH as nursing leaders had wished, its mandate, structure, and activities mirrored those of an NIH institute. Therefore, the various nursing organizations worked together closely to mount a new effort for institute status. They had powerful help from people in Congress and the Executive Branch, and support from the NIH Director Bernadine Healy and other staff, but it still took over two years to achieve because the 1991 NIH reauthorization of which the proposal was a part was stalled because the Bush administration was unhappy with certain components. However, the situation changed with a new administration, and on the evening of June 10, 1993, President Clinton signed the NIH Revitalization Act of 1993, which, among other things, created the National Institute of Nursing Research (NINR).

In its newsletter, *Outreach*, the NINR staff described the NINR mission:

> The *National Institute of Nursing Research* (NINR), part of the National Institutes of Health (NIH), builds a strong scientific base of nursing practice by promoting and supporting nursing research at universities, at clinical sites such as hospitals, and at research centers across the country. NINR also supports predoctoral and postdoctoral research training. Studies supported by NINR include those that lead to health promotion and disease prevention, minimize the effects of acute and chronic illness and disability, and help speed recovery from disease. Additional studies address ways to improve the systems and settings for nursing care and strengthen the effectiveness of nursing practice. The ethics of clinical decisionmaking are also being examined.

It was also noted that NINR had launched a ten-year biological research and research training initiative to ensure that future nursing science increases the link between behavioral and biological research in addressing clinical and other research problems.

The NCNR priorities cited earlier are now called NNRA Phase 1, and except for the last, technology dependence across the lifespan, which was deferred indefinitely, were still considered research priorities. In NNRA Phase 2, CORP #2 was held in November 1992, with the final selection of five research priorities to guide a portion of NINR funding from 1995 through 1999. These follow:

- *Community-based Nursing Models* (1995)
  Develop and test community-based nursing models designed to promote access to, utilization of, and quality of health services by rural and other underserved populations.
- *Effectiveness of Nursing Interventions in HIV/AIDS* (1996)
  Assess the effectiveness of biobehavioral nursing interventions to foster health-promoting behaviors of individuals at risk for HIV/AIDS, and of biobehavioral interventions to ameliorate the effects of illness in individuals who are already infected. The focus is on individuals of different cultural backgrounds—especially women. The need to incorporate biobehavioral markers is noted.
- *Cognitive Impairment* (1997)
  Develop and test biobehavioral and environmental approaches to remediating cognitive impairment.
- *Living with Chronic Illness* (1998)
  Test interventions to strengthen individuals' personal resources in dealing with their chronic illness.
- *Biobehavioral Factors Related to Immuno-competence* (1999)
  Identify biobehavioral factors and test interventions to promote immunocompetence.
  Plans are to implement one priority a year, after refinement of each priority area by a newly constituted multidisciplinary Priority Expert Panel (PEP).

While grants addressing these priorities receive funding emphasis, only about one-third of NINR's total competing grant funds are awarded in this manner. The majority of NINR's funds are for meritorious research proposed by investigators on topics of their choice. Some of those choices may continue to be influenced by the list of research priorities for the twenty-first century, developed by the ANA Cabinet on Nursing Research in 1985.[37] The priorities are:

1. Promote health, well-being, and ability to care for oneself among all age, social, and cultural groups.
2. Minimize or prevent behaviorally and environmentally induced health problems that compromise the quality of life and reduce productivity.
3. Minimize the negative effects of new health technologies on the adaptive abilities of individuals and families experiencing acute or chronic health problems.
4. Ensure that the care needs of particularly vulnerable groups, such as the elderly, children with congenital health problems, individuals from diverse cultures, the mentally ill, and the poor, are met in effective and acceptable ways.
5. Classify nursing practice phenomena.
6. Ensure that principles of ethics guide nursing research.
7. Develop instruments to measure nursing outcomes.
8. Develop integrative methodologies for the holistic study of human beings as they relate to their families and lifestyles.
9. Design and evaluate alternative methods for delivering health care and for administering health care systems so that nurses will be able to balance high quality and cost-effectiveness in meeting the nursing needs of identified populations.
10. Evaluate the effectiveness of alternative approaches to nursing education for the kind of practice that requires broad knowledge and a wide repertoire of skills, and for the kind of practice that requires specialized knowledge and a focused set of skills.

11. Identify and analyze historical and contemporary factors that influence the shaping of nursing professionals' involvement in national health policy development.

There is no question that nursing has made considerable progress in its research endeavors in recent years. The mix of progress and problems may begin to lean toward progress as nursing research becomes more visible. There are university programs and nursing research centers that have an impressive cohort of nurse researchers. Their research is respected not only within the profession but also in other disciplines. Nursing research has been given recognition in the public arena and has been cited in the press. Some examples include research related to incontinence, pain, bed sores, and low birth weight infants. This last study, which determined the safety, efficacy, and cost savings of early hospital discharge of these infants who were provided with follow-up by a nurse clinical specialist, received extraordinary visibility, with articles in major newspapers across the country, in economic and insurance journals here and abroad, and even publication in the prestigious *New England Journal of Medicine*.[38] (The care and follow-up by the clinical nurse specialists not only saved money but was better for the baby and family.) Among the pluses for nursing created by this study were recognition of nursing research and dialogue with medicine and other disciplines about the key role of nurses with advanced preparation in patient care. The authors involved in this research also pointed out other values: "For institutions, research may yield more cost-effective methods of delivering care or teaching, reduce staff or faculty turnover, provide answers for recruitment and publicity for the institution, as well as add income through individual cost recovery."[39] The involvement of both undergraduate and graduate students as well as other faculty, giving them an opportunity to get more experience in research and to publish, was seen as an added benefit. Moreover, in other nursing programs committed to research, both faculty and administrators have developed strategies for integrating research into the faculty workload.[40] Further advances are seen in the clinical settings where nursing research is valued. Both clinical and nonclinical topics may be studied. For instance, nurse practitioners, working with clinical specialists who have research expertise, can develop appropriate research projects that may provide new information on the unique role of nurse practitioners.[41] Such studies have been known to have an impact on public policy.[42]

Despite this good news, there are still a number of problems and issues related to nursing research. In addition to the following discussion, the important issues of ethics and patients' rights in research are presented in Chaps. 10 and 22.

The quality of nursing research is sometimes raised as a problem or issue. Much, probably most, of the research in the past thirty or so years has been done as part of the requirements for a master's or doctoral degree. Although it may be of satisfactory quality, it is almost always limited in scope because of both monetary and time constraints. There are those who say that master's degree research particularly tends to be somewhat superficial, and even shoddy, lacking little more purpose than to complete the degree, with almost no follow-up or replication likely. This may be true, particularly in schools that have an insufficient number of faculty prepared in research techniques. Those qualified may be overextended and others, whose own research experience is limited, may assume some of the responsibilities.

Because education and scholarship are frequently equated, why do so few nursing faculty engage in research, research in which their students might also participate? A number of reasons are given: Most nursing faculty are not educationally qualified for university positions; their high number of student contact hours allows little time for individual research; many are not as clinically competent as they should be or do not have access to clinical facilities that permit clinical research [although with the increase of required faculty practice (Chap. 12), this is changing]; there is little research money available externally and lack of institutional support as well. Nurses have also lacked mentors in research, and research mentors have been shown to make a difference.[43,44] Whatever the reason or combination of reasons, pressure is increasing for nursing faculty to do research, particularly clinical research, in the areas in which they teach. A vital factor in success is the commitment of both faculty and institutions to research.

Another issue related to education is when and how to teach research. Many baccalaureate programs are including more or less research in their curricula, whether as a simple introduction or to involve the students in faculty research, but there is concern as to whether some approaches will actually discourage students' interest in research.

Even more controversial are the rapidly multiplying doctoral programs, which are discussed in more detail in Chap. 13. Besides questions of quality (of faculty and resources particularly), there is considerable debate on what the curriculum should include in order to prepare a scholarly nurse researcher.

Although there are still only a fraction of the doctoral nurses needed and too few pursue research activities after their dissertations are completed, the number is growing, the kind of research done has a rich diversity, and there seems to be collaborative research with other disciplines in which the nurse is an equal partner. Overall, the amount of research has risen considerably, the focus has shifted to clinical problems, and it has become more theoretically oriented and more sophisticated in its methods. There is also reason for optimism about federal funding for nursing research, and, as has been noted, the NINR has set priorities for nursing research, which may also attract other potential funders, such as corporations. Corporations have already funded nursing research through Sigma Theta Tau, as have some individuals. With these advances, the outlook for nursing research is brighter than ever.

REFERENCES

1. Simmons L, Henderson V: *Nursing Research—A Survey and Assessment*. New York: Appleton-Century-Crofts, 1964, pp 7–24.
2. Notter L: *Essentials of Nursing Research*, 2d ed. New York: Springer, 1978, pp 9–10.
3. American Nurses' Association: *Nurses Invest in Patient Care*. New York: The Association, 1956.
4. Hughes E et al: *Twenty Thousand Nurses Tell Their Story*. Philadelphia: Lippincott, 1958.
5. Abdellah F: Overview of nursing research 1955–1968. Part I, *Nurs Res* 19:6–17, January–February 1970; Part II, *Nurs Res* 19:151–162, March–April 1970; Part III, 19:239–252, May–June 1970.
6. Department of Health, Education, and Welfare: *Toward Quality in Nursing*. Report of the Surgeon General's Consultant Group on Nursing. Washington, DC: The Department, 1963, pp 51–53.
7. Schlotfeldt R: Research in nursing and research training for nurses: Retrospect and prospect. *Nurs Res* 24:177, May–June 1975.
8. Notter, op cit, pp 20–23.
9. Safier G: *Contemporary American Leaders in Nursing, An Oral History*. New York: McGraw-Hill, 1977.
10. Larson E: Nursing research outside academia: A panel presentation. *Image* 13:75, October 1981.
11. Gortner S: Research for a practice profession. *Nurs Res* 24:193–196, May–June 1975.
12. Newman M: What differentiates clinical research? *Image* 14:88, October 1982.
13. Johnson D: Development of theory: A requisite for nursing as a primary health profession. *Nurs Res* 23:373, September–October 1974.
14. Downs F, Fleming J (eds): *Issues in Nursing Research*. New York: Appleton-Century-Crofts, 1979, p 15.
15. Lysaught J: *An Abstract for Action*. New York: McGraw-Hill, 1970, p 85.
16. National Commission on Nursing: *Summary Report and Recommendations*. Chicago: The Commission, 1983, p 11.
17. Hinshaw A: Nursing research: Weaving the past and the future, in Aiken L, Fagin C (eds): *Charting Nursing's Future: Agenda for the 1990s*. Philadelphia: Lippincott, 1992, pp 485–503.
18. Gortner S et al: Contribution of nursing research to nursing practice. *J Nurs Adm* 6:23–27, March–April 1976.

19. Lekander BJ et al: Overcoming the obstacles to research-based clinical practice. *AACN Clin Issues* 5:115–123, May 1994.

20. Gennaro S: Research utilization: An overview. *JOGNN* 23:313–319, May 1994.

21. Edwards-Beckert J: Nursing research utilization techniques. *J Nurs Adm* 20:25–30, January 1990.

22. Downs F: Food for thought. *Nurs Res* 35:131, May–June 1986.

23. Weiler K, Buckwalter K: Debate: Is nursing research used in practice? in McCoskey J, Grace H (eds): *Current Issues in Nursing*, 3d ed. St. Louis: Mosby, 1990, pp 45–57.

24. Alley L et al: Attuning staff nurses to clinical research. *Nurs Health Care* 8:77–80, February 1987.

25. Sneed N: Curiosity and the yen to discover. *Nurs Outlook* 38:36–39, January–February 1990.

26. Jairath N, Fitch M: The generic research protocol: An innovative technique to facilitate research skills development and protocol preparation. *J Cont Ed in Nurs* 25:111–114, May–June 1994.

27. Horsley JA et al: *Using Research to Improve Nursing Practice: A Guide*. New York: Grune & Stratton, 1983, p 2.

28. Ibid, pp 7–10.

29. Stetler C, Marram G: Evaluating research findings for applicability in practice. *Nurs Outlook* 24:559–563, September 1976.

30. Stetler C: Refinement of the Stetler/Marram model for application of research findings to practice. *Nurs Outlook* 42:15–25, January–February 1994.

31. Gennaro, op cit, p 317.

32. Ibid, pp 313–314.

33. *Nursing and Nursing Education: Public Policies and Private Actions*. Washington, DC: National Academy Press, 1983, p 217.

34. Merritt D: The National Center for Nursing Research. *Image* 18:84–85, Fall 1986.

35. *Report of the 1989 NIH Task Force on Nursing Research*. Bethesda, MD: DHHS/NIH, 1990.

36. Jacox A: The coming of age of nursing research. *Nurs Outlook* 34:276–281, November–December 1986.

37. *Directions for Nursing Research: Toward the Twenty-first Century*. Kansas City, MO: American Nurses' Association, 1985.

38. Naylor M et al: Institutional yield on research: A case study. *Nurs Outlook* 39:166–169, July–August 1991.

39. Ibid, p 166.

40. Clinton J: Methods for facilitating faculty research, in Chaska N (ed): *The Nursing Profession: Turning Points*. St. Louis: Mosby, 1990.

41. Krywanio M: Integrating research into private practice through consultation. *Nurs Pract* 19:47–50, February 1994.

42. Hinshaw AS: Using research to shape public policy. *Nurs Outlook* 36:21–24, January–February 1988.

43. Sibley P: Mentoring: Implications for the new research investigator. *Sci Nurs* 8:53–54, March–April 1991.

44. Taylor L: A survey of mentor relationships in academe. *J Prof Nurs* 8:48–55, January–February 1992.

The Practice of Nursing

CHAPTER
15
Opportunities in Modern Nursing

ONE OF THE MOST exciting aspects of nursing is the variety of career opportunities available. Nurses, as generalists or specialists, work in almost every place where health care is given, and new types of positions or modes of practice seem to arise yearly. In part, this is in response to external social and scientific changes—for instance, shifts in the makeup of the population, new demands for health care, discovery of new treatments for disease conditions, recognition of health hazards, and health legislation. In part, these roles for nurses have emerged because nurses saw a gap in health care and stepped in (nurse practitioner, nurse epidemiologist) or simply formalized a role that they had always filled (nurse thanatologist).

Usually, further education is required to practice competently in specialized areas. Sometimes, this is part of on-the-job training, but frequently it requires formal or other continuing education. Practice in areas of clinical specialization will vary to some extent according to the site of practice and the level and degree of specialization. For instance, in a small community hospital, a nurse may work comfortably on a maternity unit, giving care to both mothers and babies; in a tertiary care setting, prenatal nurse specialists, psychiatric nurse specialists, and nurses specializing in the care of high-risk mothers may work together; in a neighborhood health center, the nurse-midwife may assume complete care of a normal mother and work with both the pediatric nurse practitioner and hospital nurses.

In addition, nurses hold many positions not directly related to patient care as consultants, administrators, teachers, editors, writers, patient educators, executive directors of professional organizations or state boards, lobbyists, health planners, utilization review coordinators, nurse epidemiologists, sex educators, and even anatomic artists, airline attendants, legislators, and legislative aides.

Therefore, it is difficult to find any one way to present areas of practice. In this chapter, the approach used is first to describe positions and the responsibilities and conditions of employment for each. Certain systems (armed forces, Public Health Service, Veterans Administration) that may have different requirements or opportunities and international nursing are treated separately.

Patterns of employment have changed over the years. The largest number of RNs is still employed in hospitals, but what was once a very popular field, private duty, has dropped considerably. Other changes are described in Chap. 11. One definite trend seems to be toward specialization.[1]

Further information is available from the specialty nursing organizations, educational programs, and career articles published in various nursing journals.

NURSING SUPPLY AND DEMAND

Throughout the history of nursing there have been repeated shortages and, though less frequently, surpluses. Controversy has raged over the causes of these shortages, with less curiosity about how to deal with the periods of oversupply. The consequences to the society of an inadequate number of nurses are appreciated. So, with each shortage there is an outcry, and external pressure is brought to bear on the profession to increase the nursing resources available to the public. That outcry reached a fever pitch in the late 1980s. The shortage became headline news in the *New York Times, Time Magazine*, and the *Wall Street Journal*.

Nurse shortages have always been a response to either public need (as in wartime) or an economic expedient. The relatively low salaries of nurses and their readiness to take on a broad range of responsibilities have continually made them an excellent value. Regardless of the cause, each shortage has prompted organized nursing to rise to the occasion, producing greater and greater numbers, but the demand was never satisfied. Instead demand increased salaries and subsequently economic conditions forced more restraint in how and when the professional nurse was used…and history repeats itself.[2]

The profession's reaction to every shortage in memory has been to respond blindly to external pressures, devising solutions with little thought about the long-term consequences. Nurses were the logical choice to provide continuity and caring as hospitals became commonplace for care of the sick. Inadequate numbers of nurses for both home care (which was the more usual site for the sick) and hospitals inspired the establishment of diploma schools. Nurses for World War I were drawn from the ranks of college-educated women and received further concentrated education for nursing at the Vassar Camp, a program that, if protected and strengthened, would have allowed nursing to resolve its perpetual struggle for educational parity. But non-nurse influentials terminated the Vassar project once wartime need was past. World War II created the licensed practical nurse as a solution to homefront shortages, and the Cadet Corps, which became the prototype for associate degree education.

The nursing community had done its work well and without question. By 1988, RN employment was at an all-time high. There was one employed nurse for every 142 Americans, most of whom were well and self-sufficient.[3] Nursing services were being offered in more varied and diverse settings, but even those new markets had not decreased the concentration of nurses in hospitals. At the peak of the most recent shortage, there were over 90 nurses per 100 hospitalized patients, as opposed to 50 in the late 1970s.[4] The optimist would say that nurses were more central than ever to the care of patients. The pessimist sees that they were an exceptional value, misused, and still unappreciated for their unique role. Nursing salaries had experienced little consistent growth over the years. Nurses willingly expanded and contracted their work, responding to the need of their patients and their employers. Nurses were the ultimate multipurpose worker, easily taking on the work of a variety of other providers. It became the mark of status in hospitals to boast of an all-RN staff. This theory of economic advantage is one explanation for the shortage that should allow us to have more control in future cycles.

The shortage of the late 1980s did provide us with some new challenges and opportunities. Organized nursing was moved to a spirit of solidarity when in 1988, the American Medical Association (AMA) proposed the creation of a new caregiver, the registered care technologist (RCT), to supplement hospital nurses. Hospitals were the hardest hit by the shortage. In some situations 22 percent of nursing positions were vacant (5 percent is considered full employment). The RCT was to follow the orders of the physician but be supervised by the nurse. The proposal was illogical and insulting, and moved nursing to a unity and assertiveness that has since come to characterize its management of issues.[5]

The shortage of the 1980s can be traced to several unique situations. In fact, in some ways it really was a different shortage, a point well established by the Secretary's Commission on

Nursing.[6] An insatiable demand stemming (at least in part) from a more intensely ill hospital patient, the fact that nurses are the most versatile health care worker (and perhaps the most dedicated and docile), and increasing demands for nursing services in what had been secondary markets (home care, nursing homes, ambulatory care) set the stage. A general disenchantment among women with nursing as a career choice (about 90 percent of nurses are women) resulted in enrollment declines of more than 28 percent and 19 percent in baccalaureate and associate degree programs, respectively.[7] So, the demand was high and the future was bleak.

The National Commission on Nursing Implementation Project (NCNIP) (see Chap. 5), jointly sponsored by the leadership of organized nursing and nonnursing groups, spearheaded a major public relations campaign directed at selecting nursing as a career. This initiative, conducted with the Ad Council, in combination with a general economic recession in this country (nurses could always find work), resulted in a dramatic increase in applicants to educational programs. These enrollment trends are discussed in Chaps. 12 and 13, and are characterized by the "aging" of nursing. Nursing has become a preferred choice for the mature learner, such as those making midlife and later life career changes.

During this last nursing shortage, nursing spoke out boldly and detailed what had to be done to recruit and retain nurses. The costliness of the 20 percent annual turnover rate in nursing was graphically depicted. To attract and retain nurses, they needed fair wages and attractive benefits, emancipation from the nonnursing duties that keep them from their patients, status and prestige, and the opportunity to build a career. Salary gains have been substantial, though still not adequate to compensate for years of little or no gain. In 1988, the American Organization of Nurse Executives (AONE) proposed a 100 percent differential between starting salary and the most experienced individual in a job classification. That goal was finally realized in 1993. Nurses represented by the New York State Nurses Association and employed by a Manhattan medical center achieved a starting salary of $40,000 to $43,000 and guaranteed differentials that boost many experienced staff nurses to the $80,000 to $90,000 salary bracket. Several of the most experienced will earn nearly, or over, $100,000.[8] The reader is alerted to the often dramatic variation in salaries based on geography, and among rural, urban, and suburban locations, with the West Coast and the Northeast being the most highly paid markets. The growing range is particularly important. Salary compression, and the fact that in the late 1980s staff nurses would reach their maximum earning capacity in about five years, made it impossible to experience much economic advancement over a lifetime of work. It should also be noted that there are very real salary variations between practice sites and employers; nursing homes pay 15 percent less than hospitals, with government salaries lagging behind private sector.

The health care industry (especially hospitals and nursing homes where the shortage was greatest) took additional steps to resolve their shortage problem. An increasing number recruited nurses abroad, hired contract or "traveling" nurses, employed nurses from supplementary staffing agencies (creating problems of quality and continuity of care), or formed their own pool of nurses who worked per diem (generally with no benefits). The last was sometimes a for-profit venture.[9] Particularly interesting was the variety of techniques used to attract and retain nurses.[10] Most favored were increasing benefit packages, reimbursing for tuition, providing bonuses for referral and retention, seeking new hires, and paying interview expenses. Among the benefits were flexible benefits (giving choices); dental, vision, and malpractice insurance; reimbursement for unused sick time; added vacation days (one hospital offered a nine-month year); free educational seminars; added conference days; child care programs; subsidized housing; a sabbatical after a number of years of service; differentials for shift, weekends, education, and certification; longevity bonuses; paid parking; purchasing discounts; health and fitness center discounts; nonmandatory float policies and frequent-floater bonuses; even maid service and a food purchasing coop.

Although hospital administrators have been advised for decades, through many studies on nursing, on what it takes to retain nurses (see Chap. 5), the advice seemed to fall on deaf ears all too often. By 1990, with a drastic shortage at hand, there was at least some greater inclination to listen. Once salaries, and often benefits, were competitive in most hospitals in a particular commuting area, attention had to turn to improving the environment and the conditions of work where nurses practice.[11, 12] Some changes were elementary and cost little but had been largely ignored, including better communication with accessibility of administrators, attitude surveys, open forums, nurse-relations programs, newsletters, physician-nurse liaison programs, nurse-recognition and nursing image days, positive stories about nurses and ads praising nurses in local newspapers, employee-of-the-month programs, appreciation of nurses by physicians, directors' letters of commendation, and anniversary and recognition teas or receptions. There were also reward systems, including clinical ladders, clinical-excellence-in-nursing awards, promotions from within, liberal transfer policies, and perfect attendance awards.

Most important, the value of the nurse and the nurse's work was demonstrated by involving nurses in various types of planning; shared governance and nurse empowerment,[13] as in one hospital where nurses determine their own schedules, regulate their own staffing needs, and are accountable for their own productivity; employing assistive personnel under the control of nursing who do the fetching, carrying, transporting, message-taking, and other non-nursing tasks often left to nurses; and other reorganizations of staffing (with input from the nurses). Some hospitals have also installed information management systems (computers)

that, while not specifically for nurses, have made their work easier.

Another important recruiting and retention factor was flexibility in scheduling. Some innovations are weekend 12-hour days for a full week's salary; 12-hour shifts and shorter workweeks, and top pay for unpopular shifts. There are also signs of better interprofessional relationships between nursing and medicine. Many physicians recognized the need for more collegial relationships and worked in their own settings toward joint practice committees and patient care activities. The lack of such relationships is considered one aspect of nurses' dissatisfaction. In some cases, looking ahead, medical staffs have funded scholarships for nursing students.

As noted earlier, NCNIP's nationwide campaign for attracting potential students to nursing was in part underwritten by groups other than nursing—a sure sign that the shortage was seen as a national emergency. A second Commission on Nursing (Commission on the National Nursing Shortage), appointed in 1990, set its goal as finding "doable defined projects" that are both "creative and realistic," without duplicating what was already done.[14] The Commission, in its charter, was also urged to seek commitments from private organizations as well as state and local governments to fund some of the specific projects. One example is a Louisiana hospital that provided money to pay nursing faculty in a school that had enough prospective students but not enough faculty. Others have followed.

Clearly, the hospital shortage received most of the publicity, but other areas of nursing such as home care also dealt with shortages. These agencies tried to match the salary and benefit packages of hospitals, as well as many of the communication and service approaches. They also hired per-diem nurses. One practice area of particular concern is long-term care (LTC). Because of fiscal constraints, poor image, and the fact that the federal government mandates only a minimum of RN staff, nurses were even less attracted to nursing homes than they were to hospitals. In various conferences held to consider that problem, it has been recommended (1) that Medicaid, the major payer of long-term care, be restructured so that salaries and benefits can be raised and become competitive with hospitals; (2) that grass roots partnerships between LTC facilities and schools of nursing be developed; (3) that LTC facilities redefine the roles for nurses and restructure staffing and compensation accordingly; and (4) that the image of LTC facilities be improved.[15]

By 1995, the nursing shortage is history, and we may indeed be moving toward a surplus. Nursing enrollments have rebounded, and nursing is seen as a well-paying and desirable career. Nurses are aware the some hospitals are noted for their ability to attract and retain nurses, and others are beginning to emulate them. Today there are new jeopardies. Economic pressures in the health care industry have made it profitable to substitute cheaper workers for the RN.[16] Further, a flurry of activity, under the guise of restructuring systems of care, often compromises the nurses' ability to assure quality or even to guarantee the safety of patients.[17]

Renewed interest in nursing as a career, to some degree based on an assumption that jobs are plentiful, may create a challenge for new graduates. New graduates may have to compromise their choices and exhibit some patience in moving toward their eventual goals. The job market is still rich, but not precisely what you want, when and where you want it. More than ever before there is a need for information on a broad array of practice options as contained in this chapter, and for active participation in career mapping, which is discussed in Part III.

HOSPITAL NURSING

As shown in Exhibit 11-1, most nurses work in hospitals, and almost all new graduates choose staff nursing in a hospital as a starting position. Hospitals differ in size, location, ownership, and kinds of patients. Additionally, there are a variety of other characteristics that are important in predicting the quality of a hospital as a workplace. Some of these qualities were described in the magnet hospital study of the early 1980s (see Chap. 5); our observations have become more sensitive in the intervening years. The shortage motivated us to look more critically; postshortage experiences have verified many of our suspicions. The organization that attracts and retains nurses values the service they bring to patients and expects them to be responsible for their own practice.[18] This sentiment can be detected by the presence of a peer review system, and the fact that peer appraisals are taken seriously in promotion and retention decisions. In some situations this respect results in the decentralization of managerial functions to the unit level. Simply put, autonomy and intrapreneurship are not only tolerated but encouraged. Staff nurses are treated as professionals, responsible for their practice and the environment in which they practice.[19] A salaried model of compensation rather than an hourly wage is more compatible with these expectations, but there is a need to be alert to abuses that become usual.[20] Nurses find respect for the individual in hospitals that provide the mechanisms for career advancement: career ladders, opportunity for internal promotion, financial assistance for both formal and informal education, flexible work scheduling for personal needs, including the pursuit of educational goals. Salary and benefits are important, particularly flexibility within the limits of a total amount: a "cafeteria" approach with buyback of unused portions, and variety tailored to the employee. Elder care is as important as child care to some employees. Beyond a fair compensation and benefit package, the greatest satisfiers to staff nurses are quality of care issues: support personnel to relieve RNs of nonnursing duties, participation in decisions about staffing and patient care policies.[21] Nurses see themselves as part of a health care team, and expect to be treated with the respect accorded to other provider professionals. They see their own status to a large extent determined by the status and respect accorded to the chief nurse executive (CNE). In other words they value strong central leadership with optimum individual practice autonomy.

Three areas of decision making have been discussed: decisions about the environment in which care is given, decisions about systems of nursing care, and decisions about one's personal practice. How each of these systems relates to the other two, and the nature of governance and control is of special interest and will differ from setting to setting. Terms like participative management and shared governance will characterize some models that are unique in the degree to which staff nurses assume responsibility and authority.[22] The terminology may differ. In one model, called collaborative governance, day-to-day decisions take place at the unit level. The process required special education for the head nurse, retitled the clinical coordinator, consisting of budget, team building, performance evaluation, counseling, and so on. In other examples of participatory management, all decision making is centralized, but staff nurses and managers come together to develop policy and decide on aspects of operations, each holding an equal amount of authority (put simply, perhaps too simply). Although not all hospitals require participation of this intensity or share authority to this extent, nurses weighing employment options need to consider the environment in which they would be most comfortable. Some people prefer a more traditional relationship and structure.

These various modes of governance affect all levels of nursing personnel. The sections that follow give a *general* description of the different levels and types of nursing positions. The position responsibilities would differ, of course, if one of the models just described were in operation.

NONGOVERNMENTAL HOSPITALS

Positions described in hospital nursing include all those in which the employing agency is a hospital, whether private or voluntary, general or specialized; and whatever the size. The one element all hospitals have in common is that they are in existence primarily to take care of patients. The greatest differences from an employment point of view are types of responsibility, advancement opportunities, and salaries.

Many hospitals still have fewer than 100 beds, so there may be relatively little separation of specialties with the exception of obstetrics, pediatrics, and, more frequently now, psychiatric care. Even here, when there is a declining census, hospitals are beginning to cooperate by consolidating such specialties or using beds for a variety of patients regardless of clinical diagnosis. In any event, the staff nurse is most often a generalist in these small hospitals. Positions in the emergency room and outpatient department (which are receiving an increasing number of patient visits), operating room, rehabilitation unit, or intensive care unit may require specialized training, but newly developed settings within the hospital, such as an outpatient surgery unit or "overnight" unit, also present new challenges in nursing care without necessarily mandating more formalized education.

Hospitals with home care services usually require nurses to have had community health experience to function in this area. Nursing roles are changing in all of these clinical areas. In the operating room, for instance, many of the technical aspects are carried out by surgical technicians whereas the RN has overall responsibility for the safety of the patient, supervision and education of auxiliary nursing personnel, and sometimes support of the patient through pre- and postoperative visits. The increased utilization of nurse practitioners and clinical specialists, discussed later, adds another dimension to nursing care in these areas. Although students usually do not have extensive experiences in the areas noted, even limited exposure may attract the nurse to certain kinds of practice. The emergency room and intensive care unit, where quick, life-determining decisions must be made, independent judgments are not unusual, and tension is often high, will probably not attract the same kind of individual as the geriatric unit or rehabilitation unit, where long-term planning, teaching, and a slower pace are the norm.

General Duty or Staff Nurse

The first-level position for professional nurses is that of *general duty* or *staff nurse* and is open to graduates of diploma, associate degree, and baccalaureate or other RN programs in nursing education. Individual assignments within this category will depend upon the hospital's needs and policies and the nurse's preferences and ability.

Staff nursing includes planning, implementing, and evaluating nursing care through assessment of patient needs; organizing, directing, supervising, teaching, and evaluating other nursing personnel; and coordinating patient care activities, often in the role of team leader. It involves working closely with the health care team to accomplish the major goal of nursing—to give the best possible care to all patients.

To help attain this goal, the ANA published, in 1991, standards of clinical nursing practice applicable to all nursing situations. Additional, more specific standards, are also available for medical-surgical, maternal-child, geriatric, community health, psychiatric mental health nursing practice, and a number of subspecialties. The standards of clinical nursing practice are generic in nature and apply to all registered nurses engaged in clinical practice, regardless of clinical specialty, practice setting, or educational preparation. These standards consist of "Standards of Care" and "Standards of Professional Performance" and include the following:[23]

STANDARDS OF CARE

- Assessment
- Diagnosis
- Outcome identification
- Planning
- Implementation
- Evaluation

STANDARDS OF PROFESSIONAL PERFORMANCE

- Quality of care
- Performance appraisal
- Education
- Collegiality
- Ethics
- Collaboration
- Research
- Resource utilization

Each of these standards is accompanied by measurement criteria to allow a determination on competence. *Assessment* in Standard I is included here as an example, and the reader is referred to the total document for adequate understanding of other standards.

> **Standard I: Assessment**
> **The nurse collects Client Health Data**
> *Measurement Criteria*
> 1. **The priority of data collection is determined by the client's immediate condition or needs.**
> 2. **Pertinent data are collected using appropriate assessment techniques.**
> 3. **Data collection involves the client, significant others, and health care providers when appropriate.**
> 4. **The data collection process is systematic and ongoing.**
> 5. **Relevant data are documented in a retrievable form.**

Standards should remain stable over time. Criteria must reflect current practice, and so will change with advances in knowledge, practice, and technology.

Involved in meeting these standards are literally hundreds of specific nursing tasks, some of which can be carried out by less prepared workers; it is the degree of nursing judgment needed, as well as knowledge and technical expertise, that determines who can best help any patient.

Because the goals of the various kinds of nursing education programs differ, theoretically the responsibilities of each type of nurse should also differ in the staff nurse position. Unfortunately, the tendency is to assign all to the same kinds of tasks and responsibilities, so that differences are not utilized. This is so common that there is even an inclination to praise as innovative those nursing services that do delineate nursing roles and responsibilities at the staff nurse level according to educational background (differentiated practice).[24]

Three basic methods of assignment for delivering day-to-day care to patients in the hospital are functional, team, and case.[25] In *functional nursing*, the emphasis is on the task; jobs are grouped for expediency and supposedly to save time. For instance, one nurse might give all medications, another all treatments; aides might give all the baths. Obviously, the care of the patient is fragmented, and the nurse soon loses any sense of "real" nursing; patients cannot be treated as individuals or given comprehensive care. Nevertheless, this approach is used in many hospitals, especially on shifts that are understaffed. The work gets done; there is generally little nurse or patient satisfaction.

Team nursing presumes a group of nursing personnel, usually RNs, LPNs, and aides, working together to meet patient needs. It became popular after World War II, when the shortage of nurses was acute. For team leader, a baccalaureate degree had been suggested by the Surgeon General's Consultant Group on Nursing as early as 1963, but there are still not enough baccalaureate graduates to fill these positions, and it is usual to have either a diploma or AD graduate act as team leader. Other team members are under the direction of the team leader, who assigns them to certain duties or patients, according to their knowledge or skill. The team leader has the major responsibility for planning care and coordinating all activities, acting as a resource person to the team (though not always prepared to do so). In addition, if there are few or no other RNs on the team, the team leader may perform nursing procedures requiring RN qualifications. Often, the team leader is the only nurse directly relating to the physician, but, too often, actual patient contact is infrequent or sporadic. The original concept of the team has been diluted. Planning and evaluation are seldom a team effort; conferences to discuss patient needs are irregular; and too frequently, the team leader does mostly functional nursing, doing treatments and giving medications in an endless cycle. Nevertheless, the professional nurse should expect to be part of a nursing team, or, more likely, leader of this team, because most hospitals utilize some version of team nursing, at least to the extent that the registered nurse supervises and directs other nursing personnel in patient care.

"Primary" nursing was instituted in the 1970s and is a somewhat confusing designation for the *case method*, in which total care of the patient is assigned to one nurse. A major difference between primary nursing and other methods of assignment is the accountability of the nurse. The patient has a primary nurse, just as she or he has a primary physician. A nurse is a *primary nurse* when responsible for the care of certain patients throughout their stay and an *associate nurse* when caring for the patients while the primary nurse is off duty. In most places, that nurse is responsible for a group of patients twenty-four hours a day, even though an associate nurse may assist or take over on other shifts. The primary nurse is in direct contact with the patient, family/significant others, and members of the health team, and plans cooperatively with them for total care and continuity. The head nurse then is chiefly in an administrative and teaching (personnel) role. Almost always the primary nurse is an RN, often with a baccalaureate. Sometimes the nursing team involved in primary nursing comprises all RNs, with the exception of aides who are generally limited to "hotel service," dietary tasks, and transportation. There is almost unanimous agreement that the primary nursing pattern is much more satisfying to patients, families, physicians, and nurses and that care is of a highly improved quality.

However, overall, little agreement exists as to which of these methods of assignments is "best," based on patient and nurse satisfaction, quality of patient care, cost, and administrative efficiency. Functional assignment may be the most administratively efficient because of its division of labor according to specific tasks, but almost no one says that either patient or nurse finds it preferable to others. Team nursing, when done according to the original concept, may be satisfying to the team who can give their attention to a small group of patients and also develop an esprit de corps that compensates for the time expended in conference and work coordination. It is often considered expensive because of the need for this additional time spent.[26] Primary nursing, often considered the most "professional" of assignments, also has its detractors; additional stress, role overload, and role ambiguity are cited.[27] The setting and nurses themselves may also have some effect, and the method of assignment could be secondary.

Functional, team, and case methods are distinguished from one another by the extent to which they allow continuity of the provider of care, the use of assistants to the RN and the roles these assistants assume, the degree to which activities as compared with the complexity of the clinical situation drive decisions on the assignment of personnel, and the autonomy or decentralization of authority and accountability. Given these basic categories, there are endless variations on each theme. Modular nursing[28] and district nursing[29] both provide for continuity in provider but make more extensive use of assistive personnel. District nursing is suited to nursing homes and is not proposed for acute care. The ICON (integrated competencies of nurses) system developed at Yale–New Haven Hospital differentiates the practice role based on the educational preparation of the nurse. In this model, which would be considered a case model, the professional nurse is salaried.[30] Another variation on the case method with some unique uses of assistive personnel as environmental supports was created at the Robert Wood Johnson Hospital in New Brunswick, NJ, and is called the PROACT system.[31] The Professional Practice Model of Johns Hopkins builds on primary nursing and decentralizes management functions such as staffing and scheduling.[32] The Primm Model at Sioux Valley Hospital in Sioux Falls, SD, was one of the first systems for differentiated practice.[33] Other noteworthy variations are Manthey's Partners in Practice, which teams different skill mixes of professional, technical, and assistive personnel

on a permanent basis to work in an arm's-length relationship;[34] and the New England Medical Center Case Management Model, which is driven by primary nursing but incorporates a broader view of care coordination and links each primary nurse with a case-specific physician.[35] In models that combine case management with primary nursing, the primary nurse may or may not be the case manager. New graduates should be aware of the differences and of their own comfort zone in practice.

The utilization of clerical and nonnursing personnel to assume nonnursing tasks is increasing. This frees the nurse for the patient contact for which nurses are prepared. Nurses have long complained that they are required to do an endless number of tasks better carried out by assistants (not necessarily nurses' aides). Such work includes finding supplies and equipment, transporting patients and equipment, cleaning equipment, checking the work of other departments, cleaning up after physicians, and moving furniture. Assistive workers are also considerably less expensive than nurses, especially since nurse salaries have escalated. It has been recommended that these people be carefully trained and that staff be oriented to their responsibilities. The employees described here provide what is called environmental support, and do not assist in nursing care.[36] In the best of situations, they are accountable to the head nurse and under the organizational control of the nursing department.

Environmental support staff must be distinguished from unlicensed assistive personnel (UAP) who are trained to assist the RN in providing care. In this situation, the RN delegates specific activities but retains responsibility and provides ongoing supervision of this assistant.[37] The use of UAP has increased dramatically in recent years. This has been a response to the growing array of consumer needs in some cases, and a concession to economics in others. In hospitals, UAP have often been hired instead of RNs as positions become available; or the number of RNs is decreased and UAPs added after "study" and "restructuring" have identified areas for cost efficiency. In 1991, 97 percent of hospital reported the presence of "nurse extenders." This flies in the face of recent reports proving that there is a positive relationship between the proportion of RNs on staff and lower mortality, decreased length of stay and complications, increased patient compliance with the therapeutic regimen, and superior ability to function on discharge.[38] Regardless, it will be rare for the RNs to be responsible solely for themselves, and in fact most professionals accomplish a lot of their work through others. Students should be prepared for this reality within their educational program. The ANA cautions that risk exists:[39]

- When the RN knowingly delegates a nursing care task to a UAP that only a licensed nurse can perform, or when the delegation is contrary to law or involves a substantial risk of harm to a person or client.
- When the RN fails to exercise adequate supervision of the UAPs to whom patient care tasks have been delegated.
- When the RN knowingly delegates a patient care task to a UAP who has not had the appropriate training or orientation.

The issue of UAPs and the registered professional nurse is honeycombed with legal and ethical dilemmas. Can the RN plead ignorance of the extent of the UAP's preparation when a mistake is made and the patient is harmed? How adequate is the degree of supervision provided to assistive personnel in nursing homes? Will the requirement of certifying home health aides and nursing home assistants eventually allow them to become independent of RN supervision? Since these two categories of "nurse extenders" have very little direct supervision and care for the most compromised of our public, how is safety to be assured?

Qualifications and Conditions of Employment. The basic requirement for a staff position is graduation from an approved school of nursing and nursing licensure or eligibility for licensure. The new graduate may be designated as a graduate nurse (GN) and must take and pass the licensure examinations within a specific period of time. Sometimes a lesser salary is offered until the RN is acquired, and the new graduate may be limited to a general nursing unit, that is, not the coronary care unit or another that requires an investment of intensive in-service education. Nevertheless, in the hospital, the variety of experiences is endless. Larger hospitals and those in medical centers may offer a greater variety of specialties, exotic surgery, and rare treatments, and the advantage of being in the center of hospital, medical, and nursing research. Smaller hospitals may be less impersonal, are often in the nurse's own community, and provide the opportunity to be a generalist on smaller patient units (which does not necessarily mean a smaller patient load). A nurse is usually hired for a particular specialty unit (except for very small hospitals), but it is not uncommon to be asked to "float"—replace a nurse on any unit. Floating should not extend to units that require special knowledge and skill unless the nurse is "cross-trained."[40] In some hospitals, there are "float pools" or resource teams—highly skilled nurses who never have a regular unit.

In some cases, hospital nurses will be required to rotate shifts and work on holidays. For this reason, it is possible to work part time in most hospitals. Usually there are salary differentials for working evenings and nights. In recent years, flexible hours and shifts have become popular. Fringe benefits also vary greatly and may include health plans, retirement plans, arrangements for continuing education, holidays, sick time, and vacation time. The amount of autonomy varies considerably. Opportunities for promotion may be through clinical advancement or the managerial ladder.

There are many variations of a clinical career ladder.[41] Most organizations use a committee composed of the CNE, other representatives of management, and staff nurses to develop and implement a career-ladder plan, but other approaches are also used. Criteria are set, usually including educational levels, experience, clinical competencies, certification, continuing education, peer and supervisory evaluation, and seniority. Positions are categorized as I, II, III, and so on based on these criteria. It is important that moving up the ladder not be a form of tokenism and that there be added rights and responsibilities as one progresses.[42] In some settings, the nursing process is the core of the framework, with added expectations in areas such as patient and family education, leadership and coordination, and research. In another, reaching the role expectations and competencies of primary nursing is the second level, and the nurse may choose to stay there. The lateral mobility or horizontal promotion of the career ladder, as opposed to vertical mobility toward managerial positions, broadens a nurse's existing knowledge and skills and allows him or her to stay at the bedside. It may allow for a change in patient population and in job pressures and expectations. In other words, a nurse may move to another type of nursing, if qualified. Salary increases are given with each change in levels. Some nurses may choose realignment (downward mobility), perhaps as they choose to go to school. There are also managerial career ladders. The guiding principle is for nurses to plan and develop their own careers. Through self-assessment, the first step, nurses identify their knowledge, skills, values, and interests in the context of the practice setting.

In preparing for the review that determines one's readiness to progress, the nurse usually prepares a portfolio that contains information demonstrating ability to meet the performance criteria of a particular level of nursing practice. Information may include a case study, a patient-teaching tool, a discharge plan, a nursing database, or other evidence of the nurse's abilities as well as evidence of educational advancement (formal course work or continuing education). The review process should be objective; if it determines the nurse does not meet the criteria, she or he should have a clear idea of what areas of behavior or practice need to be strengthened. Because both increased salary and prestige are

at stake, career ladders must be carefully developed, managed, and explained.

Not everyone likes the clinical career ladder. Some nurses find it time-consuming to develop a portfolio, even with help; some do not want peer evaluation. Others think it really doesn't measure "a good nurse." Still others simply don't care and want to stay where they are. However, if their salaries "top out," nurses may prefer to "ladder" instead of "level."

An employment option is to be placed in a position through a supplemental staffing agency sometimes called a temporary nursing service (TNS). Nurses most commonly using TNSs are some new graduates, nurses enrolled in advanced educational programs, nurses with small children who cannot work full time or all shifts, or nurses who simply prefer the flexibility. The TNS will pay them a salary for the hours worked, with the usual legal deductions, after billing the institution or the patient or client using the worker's services. There are some TNSs who treat the nurse as an independent contractor as opposed to an employee. The distinction is important since you are responsible for your own social security and tax payments as an independent. You also forfeit protections that are legally guaranteed to employees.[43] There are local and national agencies, and selecting a reputable one is extremely important. Job assignments may be made an hour or a week ahead, but the nurse is not obligated to take it; however, a no-show is usually dismissed. As well as a great deal of flexibility and variety, there are also disadvantages, even with a good TNS: no job security, sometimes only the minimum rate paid by the area hospitals with no increases, and of course the constant reorientation to new nursing units and patients, even to new hospitals, although some nurses limit themselves to one particular hospital. The fact that "agency nurses" are sometimes looked down on by regular staff as incompetent (although they may simply be unfamiliar with that hospital's procedure) also creates problems for these nurses.

A variation of temporary nursing is the "flying" nurse, who accepts short-term contracts directly with a hospital anywhere in the country and sometimes abroad. Arrangements are made through an agency. The hospital usually pays only the benefits required by law, but pays for the nurse's travel and sometimes arranges for or provides housing. The nurse must get a temporary license in each state where employed. Although the variety is exciting for many nurses, the place of work is seldom ideal, as there usually is a problem—strikes, extreme shortstaffing, or other poor practice conditions.[44] Because TNSs were being widely used during the nursing shortage, some states are putting regulations in effect, both setting standards and limiting what can be charged. Nursing homes that use TNSs have been particularly concerned by what they consider outrageous costs.

NURSING SERVICE ADMINISTRATION

The administrative hierarchy in hospital nursing usually consists of a head nurse, supervisor, assistant or associate director of nursing, and director of nursing; the titles vary with the times and the philosophy of the hospital concerning nursing service administration.

A clear distinction is maintained between the executive and managerial levels of administration. Managers' strategic planning should be principally focused on the current operations of their program. The executive must have expanded vision, and be able to weigh current decisions in terms of long-term consequences. Much of that sensitivity comes from a positioning that is very much in contact with events outside of the organization.[45] The essential role of the nurse executive should never be minimized. In some organizations, where nursing is seen as secondary, there may be no nurse executive, only nurse managers. This is an important cue to philosophy and values, regardless of lip service.

The nurse executive is complemented by the chief operating officer in nursing (director), middle-manager (supervisor), and front-line manager (head nurse). The middle and front-

line managers are the major securers of resources, facilitators of practice, and bridges for communication to the executive level. They control the environment within which care is given, while the professional at the bedside controls the care.

Realistically, in smaller hospital there may be a less complex administrative hierarchy. The director of nursing may be the chief nurse executive. The important observation is to look for parity with other organizational units within the hospital, and be assured that the executive functions are addressed on behalf of the nursing department.

Head Nurse

Head nurses are first-line managers and in charge of the clinical nursing units of a hospital, including the operating room, outpatient department, and emergency room. Today, head nurses may hold a variety of titles, including *nursing or patient care coordinator*. They are usually also the *charge nurse* when they are present. On shifts where the head nurse (or assistant head nurse) is absent, another nurse is designated as the charge nurse. The deciding factor is who holds managerial authority. In a hospital functioning as a line and staff organization (as most are), head nurses are responsible to the next higher person on the scale, usually the supervisor, or, in a smaller hospital, the assistant director of nursing or the director. The head nurse position is the first administrative position most nurses achieve (or perhaps that of assistant head nurse, who may share some of the head nurse functions and substitute for the head nurse in his or her absence).

It is the head nurse's function to manage the nursing care and assure its quality in a relatively small area of the hospital. How this is done again depends on the philosophy of nursing service and often on the individual's personality. If a democratic philosophy of administration prevails, the staff participates in decision making both on the unit and in the entire setting. The head nurse uses leadership skills in assisting the group to make decisions and coordinates the overall activities.

As the complexity of patient care increased, head nurses found themselves inundated with paper work, which limited their major role in managing nursing care. Hospital administrators began to realize that it was less expensive and more efficient to employ clerical personnel to answer phones and questions, to complete and route forms, to order and check supplies and drugs, and to perform the myriad other necessary clerical tasks that have kept the head nurse away from administration of patient care. *Ward clerks, ward managers, floor managers, unit managers, service assistants*, or whatever the local term is, have a wide variety of responsibilities, with some ward clerks even taught carefully to transcribe doctors' orders. Hospitals utilizing computers have been able not only to cut down on every nurse's paper work but to add greater assurance of accurate, rapid communication interdepartmentally. Since there is now a trend toward decentralization of nursing authority, which means that nurses on individual units may make nursing care and other decisions without going through the nursing hierarchy, the head nurse may be expected to give more attention to acting as a consultant and teacher for staff, to following the clinical progress of the patients, and to maintaining communication with physicians and other health personnel.[46] In other situations, the head nurse has become more administrative and is seen less as a clinical manager. Roles will differ dramatically place to place.

Regardless of the staffing pattern, staff evaluation is a major responsibility of the head nurse. Considered first-line managers, head nurses control the quality of care more than anyone else and often know best how to eliminate waste, improve utilization of personnel and dollars, keep communication systems open, and provide direct leadership.[47]

Qualifications and Conditions of Employment. Qualifications for head nurses are usually evidence of successful nursing experience and preferably a baccalaureate degree. The need for

a master's is predicted, and a few head nurses do have that degree; some have BSNs. Currently, most head nurses have no degree. The successful head nurse should have, besides nursing expertise, administrative ability. Unfortunately, in many hospitals, moving into administrative positions is still the only mode of advancement for RNs. Because a good clinician may not be interested or able in nursing administration, such promotions are not always successful. Employers may offer managerial courses to aid the transition. To some extent, the assistant head nurse position offers this training opportunity, but additional training and education are considered vital for most nurses assuming this position.

Head nurses usually earn more per year than staff nurses; other benefits may vary. Benefits acquired by staff through collective bargaining may or may not apply to the head nurse position. The head nurse is usually considered management and therefore unable to be part of a collective bargaining unit, although benefits awarded to staff are often passed on to managers. In most instances, the head nurse works only the day shift, but may alternate on weekends and holidays with the assistant head nurse.

Supervisor

It has been said that the role of the *nursing supervisor*, called a middle manager, is the most ill-defined in the hospital hierarchy. Because basic management principles for span of control usually specify that no more than six to eight people should report to an administrator, except in small hospitals, the supervisor usually is needed as the middle management person. Some hospitals have eliminated the supervisor,[48] at least on the day tour of duty, putting responsibility directly on the head nurse. In general, however, the supervisor is responsible for several clinical units, delineated by either location or specialty. In a small hospital, the supervisor might be responsible for all the clinical units, and in any hospital, the evening and night supervisors usually have larger areas to supervise. In many hospitals, these supervisors are the only administrative personnel available for any department after 5 P.M. Therefore, they find themselves acting as temporary hospital administrators, devoting more time to overall hospital problems than to their main responsibility, nursing care. At times they dispense drugs because no pharmacist is present, thus violating the Pharmacy Practice Act in most states. Some of the larger and/or more progressive hospitals have now arranged for an assistant administrator to be available for general administration responsibilities, but this is still more likely to be the exception than the rule. Even when limited to nursing, the role of the supervisor often encompasses an enormous amount of responsibility and diversity: many aspects of personnel management, which may include hiring and firing; evaluation and improvement of patient care; and staffing and coordination of nursing systems (policies, procedures, resources).

Qualifications and Conditions of Employment. Generally, supervisors have been employed after showing evidence of ability in a head nurse or other administrative position. Clinical expertise may or may not have been a factor, but an advanced degree was probably a distinct advantage (even if not in administration). Increased emphasis is being put on the combination of clinical expertise, administrative skills, and at least baccalaureate degrees. In larger hospitals, master's degrees are stressed, preferably with experience and/or a nursing administration major in the educational program. Actually, the large majority of supervisors have no degree at all, although there is a trend toward enrollment in both degree programs and in continuing education programs that focus on middle management skills.

Salaries may vary according to education and experience. Some fringe benefits, such as vacation time, may be greater than that of head nurses. Supervisors tend to remain on one work shift although they may also work weekends and holidays. Even more than that of the head nurse, the supervisor position is considered administrative by employers. This has made it dif-

ficult or impossible for these individuals to be included in collective bargaining with other nurses.

Assistant or Associate Director of Nursing

Assistant or *associate directors of nursing* work with the chief nursing executive in any or, occasionally, all aspects of the director's responsibility. Specific areas of responsibility may be assigned, particularly if the institution is large. If there is a diploma program of nursing, its head may also have the title of associate director of nursing. The assistant or associate is generally expected to have at least some of the qualifications of the CNE or to be in the process of acquiring them. As a rule, this individual is hired by the director and thus is expected to share a harmonious philosophical approach and be compatible in the work relationship with the director. Salary is often negotiable on the same basis as that of the director, although it is, of course, usually less. Probably a great majority of the nurses assuming assistant or associate positions do so for the experience and as a step toward becoming a top nurse administrator. They do get that experience, but in a large hospital, many of their day-to-day activities are more likely to be in a direct relationship with staff and somewhat less involved in top-level hospital planning. There are opportunities to represent nursing service on hospital committees and to chair key nursing committees. A good CNE will relate to the associates as peers who will participate in the determination of overall nursing service policies and strategies. It is a highly varied position, with no set routine, but extended hours.

Nurse Executive

The *chief nursing executive* position is the highest in the nursing service hierarchy. (Some are also formally responsible for other departments in the hospital.) The title may also be *director of nursing, director of nursing service, chief nurse, nurse administrator*, or, if this individual is considered part of the top echelon of hospital administration, *assistant or associate administrator for nursing, vice-president for nursing*, or a variation of whatever title the administrator of the hospital carries. For years, nurses and others, including ANA and the American Hospital Association (AHA), have endorsed such a title with the concomitant responsibilities. Nursing service is generally the largest individual department in the hospital, often employing more than half the total number of employees. It affects and is affected by the functions of all other departments.

Unfortunately, a serious problem is that regardless of ANA and AHA recommendations, most nurse executives are not yet part of the upper echelon of hospital administration; the National Commission on Nursing addressed this issue and strongly recommended a change.

Actually, as a matter of two extremes, nurse administrators in very small hospitals or in large medical center hospitals have few similarities in areas of responsibilities. A director of a small hospital may be a jack-of-all-trades, and have no associates or assistants and few managers. Because small hospitals are also usually in rural areas or small towns, management takes on a personalized dimension. On the other hand, in some medical centers, CNEs are also assistant or associate deans or deans of collegiate nursing programs and do little direct management. In larger, more complex systems, you may find layers of hierarchy. As described earlier in this section, the important observation is that the chief nurse executive be on a par with other major department heads. In larger systems, the chief nurse executive may have no day-to-day operations responsibility.

A recent survey of nurse executives and chief executive officers in hospitals revealed the following among the most valuable characteristics of the successful nurse executive:[49]

- Team player
- A strong value system that is modeled through their behavior, and the expectation subordinates emulate them
- Humanistic and respectful of people

- A vision that surpasses what is shared with staff (stretches but does not overwhelm staff)
- Surround themselves with the best staff
- Visible
- Well educated, eclectic, and polished
- Acts, looks, and speaks the part
- Holds a higher standard for self than for others
- No tolerance for detail
- Constantly communicating
- Well-developed business skills
- Risk taker, and will sometimes operate on intuition
- Charismatic
- People skills are without a doubt their forte

Minimum educational qualifications for administrators of nursing services should include completion of a baccalaureate program which has prepared them for professional nursing practice, and completion of a master's degree program with a focus both on clinical nursing and administration of organized nursing services. Completing dual master's degrees, one in nursing and another in business, is also popular. To assume this position in a health science center, academic medical center, or similar sophisticated and complex setting, the doctorate has become essential. Professional experience should have contributed and enhanced the development of role competencies.

There is some agreement, affirmed in a joint 1987 AONE-AACN statement, that the nurse administrator must be clinically knowledgeable, if not proficient, but that it is *essential* to have knowledge and skills in newer management techniques, including labor relations, personnel management, financial theories and skills, systems theory, and organizational theory, as well as knowledge of systems of health care delivery. Postprogram preceptorships are recommended by some. The joint statement also insisted that this education be based in schools of nursing.

Salaries for nurse executives are usually negotiated, but vary a great deal depending on location, size of hospital, responsibilities, and qualifications. This is a difficult, complex position with major responsibilities, frequently great pressure, and no routine 40-hour week, in either time or activities. The director is often expected to be active in community, professional, and other activities, which extend beyond working hours. In some cases, dismissal can be instant and with no reason given (particularly if there is no contract), if the director has not pleased the administration or the hospital board of directors. On the other hand, the leadership of a capable and farsighted director of nursing can create dramatic changes in the quality of nursing care and delivery of health care, and bring immense personal satisfaction and reward.

Staff Development

Although staff development still has a major responsibility for orientation and development of new staff, it is no longer a matter of a few lectures by physicians or demonstration of new equipment. In most hospitals it is an organized, evaluated series of learning experiences based on nurses' needs, and is sometimes done on the basis of self-learning. Staff development refers to "those learning activities designed to facilitate the nurses' job related performance."[50] The three dimensions of staff development include orientation, in-service, and continuing education:[51] "orientation and in-service are components of nursing professional development in the workplace."[52] Occurring at the start of each new employment or position, orientation introduces new nursing staff members to "organizational culture and philosophy, goals, policies, role exceptions, and other factors necessary to function in a specific work setting."[53] "In-service education helps nurses acquire, maintain, and/or increase their competence in fulfilling their assigned responsibilities."[54] This may include how to use new equipment, or changes in policies and procedures, as well as various "mandatory" programs regulated by states or accrediting organizations. Mandatory programs

may include fire and safety, infection control, and blood-borne pathogens.

Some of the current changes are planned programs of CE, based not just on the administration's concept of the learners' needs but also on input from the learners; enlargement of in-service staff for around-the-clock teaching sessions; better-qualified teachers; the employment of knowledgeable outside speakers; the utilization of more sophisticated teaching media; planned teaching on the clinical unit; and self-learning packages.

The responsibilities of the director include the organization, planning, evaluation, and often implementation of orientation, CE, and training programs for the nursing service department, and, increasingly, for other hospital departments. (For instance, all interested hospital personnel might be taught the fundamentals of emergency resuscitation and external cardiac massage.) This educator must be aware of other resources available for the teaching program but is personally responsible for the overall development of courses and programs. If there is a large staff development department, one or more instructors may share with the director responsibility for the teaching programs.

Despite the fact that most staff development departments are still within nursing, a trend to be noted is the move toward hospitalwide training and education departments, which may include CE programs for all health professionals and support staff, and patient education. Nurses who are master's prepared educators still tend to be directors of these departments but may now report to the VP of Patient Care Services, the Director of Professional Development, or the Human Resource Department.

Qualifications and Conditions of Employment. Although some staff development directors and/or instructors have no degrees, it is desirable that they have at least a baccalaureate degree, with some knowledge of teaching principles and techniques (particularly in relation to the adult learner), clinical expertise, and preferably a master's degree (especially as director). They should also be able to work through and with others, with enough self-confidence to assume a staff role with little inherent authority.

Because of the cost of in-service education, there is also a need to develop both strong evaluation tools and programs that meet the goals of the institutions as well as the learner. Salary may depend on the qualifications and the kinds of responsibilities assumed; usually, salary and benefits are at the level of the supervisors for the director, less for the instructor. Some sessions may be held in the evening or at night, but the majority of activities are usually scheduled during the day. This position is particularly attractive to nurses who are stimulated by teaching all levels of nursing personnel and who enjoy remaining in the hospital setting.

Other Positions for Nurses in Hospitals

There are a number of other employment opportunities for nurses in hospitals, although they may have only a tangential relationship to nursing and are often in a department other than nursing service. Nurses on the intravenous (IV) team are especially trained, and responsible, for all the intravenous infusions given to patients (outside of the operating room and delivery room). On the basis of a predetermined protocol, they may bring the appropriate intravenous solution to the bedside or obtain it on the unit, add ordered drugs, and start and/or restart the infusion. In some institutions they are also permitted to start a blood transfusion.

The nurse-epidemiologist or infection control nurse focuses on surveillance, education, and research.[55] The surveillance aspect is designed for the reporting of infections and the establishment, over a period of time, of expected levels of infections for various areas. Patients with infections are checked, and it is determined whether the infection was acquired after admission. Reports are used for epidemiologic research, and staff is educated in prevention of infection. Nurses have also been trained as epidemiologists in public health agencies, where they perform similar but broader duties that involve the total community.

A challenging role is that of ombudsman, or patient advocate, in which a nurse (or a non-nurse) acts as an intermediary between the patient and the hospital in an attempt to alleviate or prevent problems of the patient related to the hospital or hospitalization. Nurses are also being employed as utilization review agents. This role is an outgrowth of the requirement for external monitoring of hospitals by a Professional Review Organization (PRO) to assure that Medicare recipients are admitted and discharged appropriately and that resources are used properly during the hospitalization. To avoid problems, hospitals have established Utilization Review Departments as internal monitors of the progress and utilization practices of all their patients. Improper practices jeopardize reimbursement. It is not unusual to have certain procedures or hospital days decertified (the government or other third party payer refuses to pay for the service, because it was beyond the limits of the policy or program). A selected nurse or nurses check patients and their records at predetermined periods to gather data for the Utilization Review Committee. The aim is to avoid decertification. These positions do not require a nurse, but experience has proven that nurses are the best suited to this work.

A new professional is the director or coordinator of quality assurance (QA), with a variety of titles. Although they may have a medical records background, most are nurses. The primary function of these QA practitioners is to assess and evaluate indicators of outcomes of care. The position arose from the increasing requirements of the JCAHO as well as demands on the part of payers and consumers for accountability. Their numbers are estimated as in the low thousands. Their primary functions are:

1. Planning, with the clinical staff's full input and approval, areas of nursing to be studied and methods to be used.
2. Gathering, analyzing, ordering, and displaying data in useful and appropriate ways (such as practice profiles).

3. Disseminating this information to those who need it, while taking steps to ensure that it is not lost or ignored.
4. Following up on how the information is used to determine that corrective actions really work and that improvements in care are sustained.[56]

The role is still evolving, but in today's climate the numbers are expected to increase.

ADVANCED PRACTICE NURSING

Advanced practice nursing is synonymous with specialization, and specialization is the hallmark of a mature discipline. The advanced practice nurse (APN) is an umbrella term used for nurses who have completed specialized education and experiential requirements beyond their basic nursing program. In the past, those requirements were often satisfied within educational programs that awarded a certificate and there were no admission criteria other than the RN. Many of these nurses continue to practice, and they represent the vanguard of the advanced practice movement. Today, advanced practice nursing requires the knowledge, skills, and supervised practice that can only be obtained through graduate study in nursing (master's or doctorate). The APN includes the roles of the *clinical nurse specialist* (CNS), *nurse practitioner* (NP), *nurse-midwife*, and *nurse anesthetist*.[57]

The roles of the CNS and the NP are in a state of transition. The CNS and NP roles evolved concurrently, the former legitimized expert clinical practice at the graduate level, and the latter pioneered practice autonomy in those border areas of practice that intersect with medicine.[58] NPs were more commonly involved in primary care, and CNSs were mostly secondary and tertiary providers (specialty and subspecialty services with patient access chiefly through referral). The two roles began to overlap to respond to the changing needs of the public, as should be the case. There was a growing need for primary care for many populations with continuing, complex health problems. Further, decreasing dollars for graduate medical education made it very useful for the CNS in acute, critical, and even long-term care to assume a more active role in health assessment and the management of medical problems. The differences were additionally blurred as preparation for both roles moved decisively into graduate education, undergraduate students were expected to develop the skills of physical examinations and history taking, and nurse faculty replaced medical preceptors who were once needed to teach physical assessment and clinical management of illness to NP students.

In 1992, the ANA Councils of NPs and CNSs merged into a single Council of Nurses in Advanced Practice. This was not a step to be taken lightly, and only followed intense debate, testimony from practicing nurses, and a study of the educational programs that prepared for the role.[59] The education for these roles in 1992 was more alike than different. In reality, advanced practice nurses seemed to view the roles interchangeably, and saw the compartmentalization in education as an obstacle to their career options. It should be noted that the ANA had already linked the CNS and the NP in its legislative and regulatory strategy for reimbursement. NPs had become a very consumer-friendly provider, and legislators understood their role and the benefits they brought to the public. No doubt this was because of their primary care focus and ability to substitute for physicians. Linking the less commonly understood CNS with the NP in public policy hastened progress. A convergence of these circumstances allows for more flexibility and a future that is certain but must be developed. The concept of both groups being identified as advanced practitioners is widely accepted, but the use of a single title is still debated.[60] The trend grows as several prominent colleges and universities have merged what had been separate and distinct NP and CNS graduate programs. Being more alike than different, crossover from one role to the other is possible. In selecting a graduate program, an individual should make sure that the faculty are consciously addressing this period of transition, and include the knowledge and skills to compete in a job market that will not always accommodate the subtle distinctions between NPs and CNSs. Assessment skills should be highly developed, and pharmacology should be a major area of study. For the purposes of this presentation, the roles will be presented separately.

Clinical Nurse Specialist

The CNS, who may also be called a *nurse specialist, nurse clinician*, or *clinical specialist*, has become an increasingly important part of the nursing practice scene since the early 1960s. A clinical specialist is an expert practitioner within a specialized field of nursing or even a subspecialty. There are clinical specialists in all the major clinical areas, but also some concentrating on cancer, rehabilitation, and perinatal nursing, tuberculosis, care of patients with ostomies, neurological problems, respiratory conditions, epilepsy, and many other subspecialties.

Stafford and Appleyard identify "expert practice as the sine qua non" of the CNS. Ongoing experience with patients and their support systems directs participation in a range of subroles including direct care research, teaching, consultation, and management.[61] The CNS spends a great amount of time in mediated roles, in other words, working through other people rather than personally laying "hands on." The CNS in institutional practice may be either unit-based or population-based and invests significant effort in the things that have to be done to maintain a quality system on behalf of their patients, such as quality assurance, policy development, and peer review. The basic element in CNS practice is continuing patient involvement with an emphasis on nursing and not a medical care model.[62]

Originally, the intent was to give the CNS staff authority, that is, reporting directly to the chief nurse administrator and acting in an advisory capacity to the nursing staff and supervisors. However, a line position (superior-subordinate or direct vertical relations) gives administrative authority, and there have been some problems when a CNS as a staff member makes recommendations and the supervisor chooses not to accept them, especially in relation to personnel matters (such as disciplining an incompetent nurse), or when the CNS is seen as an outsider. There seems to be a trend now for the CNS to also assume positional authority focused on nursing care.[63] A clinical specialist in the traditional supervisor role of personnel manager is sometimes limited in the amount of time devoted to clinical nursing. The ANA has emphasized the importance of flexibility:

> **When nurse specialists are employed in health care settings, descriptions of their positions and functions ought not to be standardized. The work rules for the specialist must be jointly determined and negotiated by the applicant and the employing institution. The emphasis should be on developing negotiated positions and organizational arrangements that are most likely to result in freedom and responsibility for maximum use of the abilities of the particular specialist in the particular health care setting. In joint practices and partnerships, in which nurse specialists practice on a private basis with other nurses or other professionals, joint determination of working arrangements and shared responsibility also apply.[64]**

Qualifications and Conditions of Employment. Generally, CNSs are expected to have a master's degree in nursing, with emphasis on the specialty area, although some are employed in the position because of experience, clinical expertise, and possibly continuing education without any degree. Certification by ANA or a specialty organization is preferred. In 1993, there were 58,000 CNSs, earning anywhere from $30,000 to $80,000 depending on location and experience.[65] Basic fringe benefits may be the same as those of other nurse employees; sometimes more vacation is offered.

Frequently, there is a great deal of flexibility in the CNSs' time. They may work no specific shift but care for the patients selected according to the patients' needs, which may mean being available evenings or nights or, by choice, even available on call if a problem arises. (Telephone consultations with patients who develop problems or need support at home are not uncommon.) There should be time available for library research and home visits. A CNS usually has office space, preferably near the clinical units.

More than any APN, the CNS is the victim of misunderstanding and ignorance on the part of the health care industry and the general public...and often the recipient of double messages. There was a flurry of hiring CNSs in the early days of DRGs when every sector of health care was caught off guard by rising acuities and the movement of sicker patients into home and community care. Those CNSs who had the data to prove their contribution to the fiscal integrity of the organization flourished; others were eventually sacrificed to the need for economies. CNSs hold the answer to decreasing length of stay, increasing functional ability and self-sufficiency, avoiding complications, optimizing reimbursement, and gaining cooperation from nursing staff to pursue an ambitious clinical agenda. With a new flexibility on the part of both the profession and the industry, CNSs are sought for a variety of role configurations while maintaining a patient-centered focus and continuing their involvement in practice. CNSs can now be found in small as well as large hospitals and medical centers, nursing homes, ambulatory care, and virtually every service setting, including private practice. The presence of a CNS often indicates the seriousness with which an institution views nursing.

Nurse Practitioner

In the emergence of any new role, there is considerable controversy in relation to terminology, function, and education. Not all of these problems have been resolved concerning the nurse practitioner (NP). There is still disagreement as to whether the role is expanded or extended, merely changing, or not new at all. Lillian Wald, pioneer in PHN, made house calls, prescribed and dispensed medications and

treatments, and counseled her client families as needed. In more recent times, the Frontier Nursing Service of Wendover, Kentucky, which was noted for its "nursing on horseback" midwifery services, has been expanding its practice to overall family services. However one views the role, the proliferation of NPs (estimated at about 50,000)[66] reflects the success of the movement and the acceptance of the role among patients and health care providers.

Technically anyone practicing nursing is a nurse practitioner, but the term has come into common usage and conveys to the public a nurse functioning in the expanded role.

The nurse practitioner movement had logical beginnings. The 1960s brought change, reform, Medicare, Medicaid, medical specialization at an accelerated pace, a larger market for primary health care services, and a shortage of primary care physicians. Nursing moved forward to fill the gap. In 1965, the first nurse practitioner program was established by Ford and Silver at the University of Colorado.[67] It is generally agreed that nurse practitioners have acquired additional knowledge and skills, some of which were previously considered the exclusive domain of medicine. Combining these new areas of service with the nursing role creates a comprehensive practice, requiring collaboration and consultation with a range of other provider professionals including physicians. The NP is prepared to assume a primary care role. Though this means many things to many people, the essential definition includes the capacity to serve as the first and continuing contact for the client within the delivery system. Further, the primary provider is concerned with a broad range of interventions including health promotion, disease prevention, the diagnosis and treatment of minor acute illness, and the monitoring and management of stabilized chronic conditions. The NP focuses on broad divisions of practice, as compared with CNS practice, which often takes the form of more highly circumscribed specialties and subspecialties. NPs are prepared for practice in pediatrics, family practice, adult and women's health, geriatrics, school and college health practice, to name a few. Their clients are more usually the well, even if that wellness is a new trajectory with the constant of chronic disease. In comparison, CNS practice areas may be cardiovascular, orthopedics, oncology, geropsychiatry, or medical-surgical or neurological nursing. As mentioned earlier, the distinction has become largely artificial since once-differentiating knowledges and skills have become common to both.

NPs practice in a wide range of settings, such as public or private clinics, HMOs, private offices, schools, occupational health settings; as well as prisons and military facilities. They also provide care in home health, long-term, acute care settings, and many are in private practices of their own. NPs provide health care to many diverse and underserved populations, such as the homeless, migrant families, Native Americans, and other ethnic minorities. The nurse practitioner was a sensitive response to a very real consumer need. The role will continue to evolve in response to a changing health care environment.

A major trend in the education of NPs over the past 25 years has been the shift from certificate programs to the master's degree. Much of this has resulted from positions taken by nursing organizations. For example, in 1984, the ANA House of Delegates adopted a resolution establishing 1990 as the target date by which all programs preparing NPs should be at the graduate level. ANA subsequently extended the date to 1992.[68] Additionally, federal funding has been preferential to graduate as opposed to certificate programs.

No group has been more scrutinized and studied than the NP, probably because of the threat that they pose to the medical establishment and the fact that their success opens the door to a variety of other providers who may be better options than traditional providers. In 1986, a summary of existing studies on the effectiveness of NPs and nurse-midwives was presented in a congressionally mandated Office of Technology Assessment Report.[69] A subsequent meta-analysis of research on nurses in primary care roles as they compared with physicians was funded in 1993 by the ANA.[70] NPs provide more health promotion activities, order more economical tests, achieve higher scores on patient satisfaction and patient compliance, are more successful in maintaining or upgrading the functional status of their clients than physicians. They spent more time with their patients and completed an equal number of visits or encounters, yet the nurse's visit cost 40 percent less than the physician's. Research further shows that NPs can independently diagnose and resolve 80 percent of the primary care complaints of the American public; provide continuity of care where it has been fragmented; are accepted by consumers; save physician time; and are profitable to employers.[71]

Despite the positive aspects of collaboration, competition between MDs and NPs persists on many levels.[72] Although some competition can be considered "healthy," it is not so when it depletes time and energy that could be devoted to clinical practice. It becomes counterproductive given the large numbers of people who lack access to primary care and are in need of both NP and MD services. With the challenges of cutbacks in public health programs and the high cost of health care, collaboration between MDs and NPs could only be in the best interest of the public.

Nurse-Midwife

Nurse-midwives are sometimes categorized as one of the advanced practice roles, but have been in existence for some time. The first school of nurse-midwifery was started in 1931 in New York City by the Maternity Center Association. According to the American College of Nurse-Midwives (ACNM):

> **Nurse-midwifery practice includes services to normal healthy women and their babies in the areas of prenatal care, labor and delivery management, postpartum care, well-woman gynecology, and normal newborn care. Approximately 95% of certified nurse-midwives (CNMs) attend births in hospital, while 11% attend**

births in free standing birth centers, and less than 4% of CNMs attend births in the home (many CNMs attend births in more than one site).[73]

Some 6,000 CNMs are practicing in the United States, earning an average salary of $43,600.[74] They practice in a variety of settings where maternity and gynecological care is given—clinics, private offices, hospitals, birthing centers, or in the woman's home. Their practice may be interdependent within a health care delivery system, for example, a hospital obstetric service largely staffed by nurse-midwives, where a physician might provide consultation or high-risk obstetrical care as needed. They might also have a formal written alliance with an obstetrician or another physician or a group of physicians who have a formal consultative arrangement with an obstetrician-gynecologist. ACNM standards for practice require that CNMs base their care on knowledge, skills, and judgments that are reflected in written policies and practice guidelines.[75] The fact that many mothers now seem to prefer a normal and natural birthing process, when there are no potential complications, has brought a resurgence of interest in nurse-midwifery.

CNMs recently received much support from public and private agencies because of their documented effectiveness in managing the care of pregnant women and infants. Specifically, studies have demonstrated that the care rendered by CNMs resulted in reductions in the rates of premature and low birth-weight newborns. A number of national studies on prenatal care have mentioned the value of CNMs and called for their increased utilization.

CNMs' clinical competence and nursing emphasis has contributed to their acceptance by consumers and professionals. Across the country, CNMs are gaining in recognition and popularity. For example, between 1975 and 1991, the number of hospital births attended by CNMs increased nearly sevenfold, from 19,686 to more than 158,000. This growth is startling when one considers that nearly 15 years ago few states permitted nurse-midwives to practice. New in-terest and political determination on behalf of CNMs has brought about legal changes that permit the nurse-midwife to practice, with a nursing license and ACC certification or whatever else is required under new midwifery laws. However, despite these trends, CNMs still face political battles in the clinical and policy arenas similar to those of NPs.

In the mid-1980s, CNMs faced a crisis in not being able to obtain affordable professional liability insurance. The situation threatened the viability of nurse-midwifery practice across the country and forced many CNMs to give up their practices. Since 1986, insurance has been available to CNMs through a consortium of companies. In addition, many employers offer coverage for the CNMs on their staff. ACNM provides information on insurance and sees it as a key part of nurse-midwifery practice.

The ACNM-approved (accredited) nurse-midwifery programs vary in length from eight months to two years. They include precertification programs, certificate programs, and master's degree programs. There are post-RN certificate programs that do not require a baccalaureate degree, but the trend is toward a master's degree. All programs include theory and practice in prenatal care, care of a woman during labor and birth, attendance of births in hospitals, immediate care of the newborn, care of the postpartum patient, family planning, and well woman health care. After completion of an ACNM-approved program, the nurse-midwife is eligible to take the certification examination. The ACNM, located in Washington, D.C., is the best source of information on careers and issues in nurse-midwifery practice.

Nurse Anesthetist

Certified Registered Nurse Anesthetists (CRNA) are anesthesia specialists who administer more than 65 percent of the 26 million anesthetics given to patients each year in the United States. They have been rendering quality anesthesia services in this country for more than a century. CRNAs practice in a wide variety of settings in which anesthesia services are required, in both urban and rural environments. CRNAs are the sole anesthesia providers in 85 percent of rural hospitals, enabling these medical facilities to provide obstetrical surgical and trauma stabilization services.[76]

CRNAs administer anesthesia and anesthesia-related care in four general categories: (1) preanesthetic preparation and evaluation; (2) anesthesia induction, maintenance, and emergence; (3) postanesthesia care; and (4) perianesthetic and clinical support functions, such as resuscitation services, acute and chronic pain management, respiratory care, and the establishment of arterial lines.

CRNAs provide high-quality, cost-effective anesthesia care. In 1990, the Department of Health and Human Services presented the results of a study of nurse anesthesia manpower needs conducted by the Center for Health Economics Research. This study concluded that a more efficient use of CRNAs to deliver anesthesia could save the nation $1 billion annually by the year 2010.[77]

CRNAs administer anesthesia for all types of surgical procedures, from the simplest to the most complex. Based upon a 1988 study by the Center for Health Economics Research, nurse anesthetists were regularly involved in the same decision-making processes related to anesthesia as were physician providers.[78, 79]

CRNAs have the legal authority to practice anesthesia in all 50 states without anesthesiologist supervision. There is no study that shows that the anesthesia care provided by an anesthesiologist is superior to that provided by a CRNA. In fact, the only studies that exist suggest that the quality of care is not significantly different.

The educational requirements to become a CRNA are as follows:

- Be a graduate of an accredited nurse anesthesia education program. Applicants to a program must have (1) a bachelor of science in nursing or another appropriate baccalaureate degree; (2) a current license as a registered nurse; (3) a minimum of one year's acute care nursing experience.

There are currently 94 accredited nurse anesthesia educational programs nationwide; 85 percent of them offer a master's degree, and all are required to offer a master's degree by 1998. Some programs offer clinical nursing doctorate options for CRNAs.

- Graduates of nurse anesthesia educational programs must pass a national certification exam to become CRNAs.
- CRNAs are required to earn 40 continuing education credits every two years as one of the criteria for recertification.

Reflective of the high level of responsibility, CRNAs are one of the best paid nursing specialties. From 1987 to 1991, their salaries rose 50 percent, with an average annual salary of $80,900. There were about 25,000 CRNAs in 1992.

Depending upon their employment situation, some CRNAs purchase their own professional liability insurance. St. Paul Fire and Marine Insurance Company, the underwriter for the AANA Professional Liability Insurance Program, has steadily decreased CRNA premiums owing to decreased claim losses.

Obstacles to Advanced Practice

The success of advanced practice has come only with much effort and tenacity. The goal has been direct access to patients without the intermediary participation of another provider, namely the physician. Direct access is critically dependent on third party reimbursement, adequate practice acts, prescriptive authority, practice privileges in settings for service delivery, and professional liability insurance.

The history of CNMs and CRNAs predates that of NPs and CNSs, yet the barriers to patient access that frustrate their practice are the same. CNMs were faced with a major challenge in the 1980s. As the malpractice claims history of obstetricians skyrocketed, CNMs were seen as an equal risk by insurers. Their professional liability insurance premiums escalated to a point that could not be supported by their income. Interim coverage was provided through the carrier servicing the American Nurses Association. In time, a more permanent solution was sought. This incident was a repercussion of the interdependent relationship that is required between CNMs and obstetricians. A similar effect is associated with CNSs and NPs as they enter into collaborative relations with physicians to meet the requirements for prescriptive authority. In this case, it has been reported that the physician's malpractice premiums have increased in response to their supervisory role. The additional cost of practice is ultimately passed on to the consumer, frustrating the ability of these advanced practice nurses to offer medical services at a price that is lower than traditional providers. CRNAs, NPs, and CNSs have had no difficulty obtaining coverage. Claims data show that they are an excellent risk and consequently their premiums are very affordable, though more costly than the fee that would apply to a staff nurse. The insurance market has moved to the point where clear distinctions are made between advanced and general practice in policies.

NP and CNS were linked in public policy language by the ANA in the early 1980s. In the early 1990s, the term *advanced practice nurse* was chosen to include the NP, CNS, CNM, and CRNA. Much of this public policy effort has been directed toward the third party reimbursement agenda. All categories of advanced practice nurses are reimbursable in the Federal Employee's Health Benefits Program (FEHB). Similar provisions are included in CHAMPUS, the program for nonuniformed employees and dependents of the military, and military retirees. The one CHAMPUS restriction is that only certified clinical specialists in psychiatric nursing are recognized under the CNS category. Medicaid includes mandatory reimbursement of pediatric and family NPs and CNMs but defers to state discretion for CRNAs and CNSs. Medicare has been the most resistant program. CNMs and CRNAs have been recognized. NPs

and CNSs have the fewest options within Medicare, limited to rural and medically underserved areas, and indirect reimbursement to nursing homes for required periodic medical monitoring, and recertification activities.[80]

Indemnity and commercial insurances are governed by state statutes, and recognize advanced practice to varying degrees. The picture is confusing, and changing from moment to moment. APNs report reimbursement in 34 states.[81] The situation is further confused by the reality that many advanced practice nurses are reimbursed "incident to" the practice of physicians. In that case the fee is equal to that which a physician would be paid. If the advanced practice nurse bills as an independent, the fee is most usually less than 100 percent of the physician's fee.

Some gains were recognized during the deliberations of the Physician's Payment Review Commission (PPRC), charged with proposing policy for Part B of Medicare. The PPRC, in an attempt to increase the attractiveness of general and primary care practice for physicians as compared with specialization, based its fee-setting techniques on the service provided as opposed to the nature of the provider. When it came to applying this same standard to advanced practice nurses, they recanted and proposed that the extent of the educational investment for the role should be built into the reimbursement equation. The detail is tedious, the progress slow and often illogical and unfair. The nursing community has been persistent, and gains are obvious.

As health care reform progresses, and the pressure for cost containment mounts in both public and private programs, we are moving decisively toward managed care. Whoever is recognized in fee-for-service models will have similar recognition and autonomy in managed care systems. Consequently, the struggle for recognition through reimbursement must continue. Chapter 19 includes more detail on legislation enabling reimbursement.

Prescriptive authority provides similar challenges. Studies of medical practice reaffirm the fact that most Americans expect to leave with a prescription when they visit a physician. Without prescriptive authority, advanced practice nurses are unable to provide comprehensive services. Further, with either a joint practice arrangement or referral to a physician for prescription, the fee to the patient is equal to or greater than it would have been for the physician alone. Currently, 45 states award advanced practice nurses some variety of prescriptive authority; in five states this authority is plenary (unassociated with physician supervision, collaboration, or oversight) for all drugs or excluding controlled substances.[82] Prescriptive authority is addressed through state law. The current strategy has been to secure whatever degree of autonomy is possible, and in subsequent public policy to remove restrictions that exist. A good case in point is the success of New Hampshire nurses in the early 1990s. The requirement for physician supervision of prescriptive authority was "carved out" of the existing law through the process of amendment. The American Medical Association has been particularly adversarial over the prescriptive authority of advanced practice nurses. Their attacks have focused on the inconsistent educational standard among advanced practice nurses, and the tendency of the nursing profession to make exceptions by grandfathering current practitioners into a credentialed category as the requirements become more stringent.[83] The economic threat to physicians is not frequently addressed, but it is obvious. An additional point of resistance to advanced practice nurses in prescriptive authority has been the pharmacist. In some cases local pharmacists have refused to fill prescriptions when the order is from an advanced practice nurse. Most of these incidents have been successfully resolved. These occasions may be largely due to incomplete information and inadequate communication, or a reaction associated with pharmacy's own beginning struggle to achieve prescriptive authority.

Advanced practice nurses have also been hampered by confusion over the degree to which they should be recognized in legislation and governmental regulations. CNMs and CRNAs have been recognized as distinct providers for many years, and their status legally codified. In many states, this was accomplished through amendments to medical practice acts. In contrast, the strategy had been to insist that CNSs and NPs need not be named since their practice is included in the scope of practice statements in nursing's licensing laws. This conviction was so strong that in the 1980s grant monies were provided from the ANA to "roll back" state laws that specifically referred to advanced practice nurses. This strategy proved unwise, since as reimbursement moved forward, states required that the advanced practice titles be explicitly included in public policy. An example is helpful here. Mandatory Medicaid reimbursement of pediatric and family nurse practitioners was denied in New Jersey based on the argument that there were no such providers in the state. Organized nursing in New Jersey had vigilantly worked to withhold the NP and CNS titles from public policy. To access reimbursement, these titles had to be subsequently codified. These issues are discussed more fully in Chap. 20. The most current information on reimbursement, prescriptive authority, and licensing is available each year in the January issue of the *Nurse Practitioner*.

Privileging, that is, the right to admit patients to an institution and provide appropriate services (writing orders, consulting, treating, discharging) as part of a professional staff, is an area that has been given less attention but surfaces with prominence as advanced practice nurses become significant in rural and medically underserved areas. The ANA began to do the groundwork for privileging in working to reshape the definitions of professional staff included in public and private sector policy (the Joint Commission on Accreditation of Health Care Organizations and the Health Care Financing Administration). In these instances, professional staffs may include a broad range of provider professionals. However, additional requirements for membership may be imposed at the institutional level. It remains to be tested whether the withholding of privileges is an act of discrimination or restraint of trade. Currently, 19 states report nurses with hospital privileges of some variety.[84] This represents 11 percent of NPs and CNSs.[85] In no case are they inclusive of all advanced practice nurses, but they are limited to a precise category (NP, CRNA, CNM, and so on). In some instances, privileges are associated with joint or collaborative practice with a physician. The privileges themselves may be limited to admission, consultation, treatment (clinical), or some combination.

Another route to institutional access may be the recognition of independent advanced practice nurses by the nursing staff organization in a facility (if one exists). Though admission privileges may not be possible through this route, clinical and consultation options may be. The most current information on progress in this area is available through the ANA.

MUNICIPAL, COUNTY, AND STATE HOSPITALS

Municipal, county, and state hospitals are primarily intended to provide hospital accommodation for indigent people within prescribed political boundaries. In many instances, they operate on a much broader scale and accept patients who pay part or all of their hospital bills. The fact remains, however, that these hospitals are supported principally by city, county, and state funds that come from taxpayers. This means that decisions about the amounts allocated for operating them rest in the hands of a central board, which may also allocate funds for schools, prisons, and many other institutions, all of which invariably want and need more money than they receive. Furthermore, the hospitals are usually obligated to accept all patients who come to them for treatment, even though they may be overcrowded and understaffed. This often spreads money and personnel very thin. It is predicted that, because of the pressures of the health economy, an increasing number of people will be forced to seek care in government hospitals.

Nursing positions in these hospitals usually follow the same general pattern as in other hospitals. Staff nurses rarely need additional qualifications, except possibly for work in a hospital treating such specific diseases as tuberculosis or Hansen's disease. However, in cities where a large part of the poor population comes from an ethnic group that speaks another language, nurses from that ethnic group or speaking that language are particularly welcome. Nurses may find the patient load very heavy at times; however, there may also be more challenges and greater satisfaction here than in a comparable position in any other type of hospital, because of both the learning opportunities and the opportunity to be a change agent in providing quality care for the socially disadvantaged.

Because these hospitals are government operated, nurses and all other staff members are eligible for the benefits given to any employee of the particular governmental entity concerned. These benefits, which are so important to a person's economic security, vary throughout the country, but they often include an early retirement or pension system, not usually offered by nongovernmental institutions.

NURSING WITH THE FEDERAL GOVERNMENT

Professional nurses interested in a career with the federal government will find opportunities in both military and nonmilitary services. The military services include the Army, Navy, and Air Force. The Veterans Administration (VA) is not a military service, although it is closely allied. The other principal nonmilitary federal service employing nurses is the U.S. Public Health Service (PHS).

Many nursing positions in nonmilitary federal services are for specialists in education, administration, research, or clinical areas and therefore require education and experience beyond the basic program. There are many others, however, particularly with the VA, for which newly graduated professional nurses may qualify to practice. Both the PHS and the VA employ new graduates temporarily, pending completion of the state board examinations.

The federal government owns and operates more than 400 hospitals in this country in which many government employees (and sometimes their dependents), veterans of the armed services, Native Americans, and other special groups are eligible for care without charge, regardless of their ability to pay. In addition, the federal government also operates hospitals in other countries for members of the armed services stationed in these countries.

Among the various federal agencies operating hospitals—and sometimes other health services—are the VA, the PHS, the Air Force, the Army, the Navy, and the U.S. Department of Justice (Bureau of Prisons). All these hospitals are supported financially by taxes. These hospitals usually have high standards of service, equipment, and facilities and are able to attract highly qualified personnel. Many are nationally accredited (JCAHO). Many of the country's outstanding physicians and nurses are members of their staffs. Research and teaching are integral parts of the work of many of the larger institutions. Although each branch of the armed services operates hospitals primarily to provide care for its own members, all branches will care for a member of any service in an emergency and until transfer is feasible. Sometimes, because of regional considerations, these patients are kept in the original hospital for the entire period of illness.

All those eligible for care in a government hospital—with the exception of prisoners during wartime—may, if they prefer, go to a non-government hospital for care, but they have to pay their own bills unless authorized to make the change. In some instances it is more economical and practical for the government to pay civilian hospitals to care for members of the armed services and other federal employees than it is to operate federal hospitals in all localities or transport the patients long distances. Exceptions are also sometimes made for cases that would benefit from some special treatment facility not available in a government hospital.

Professional nurses who work in most hospitals operated by the federal government perform essentially the same functions as nurses in a civilian hospital in a comparable position. They give, teach, and direct nursing care. They coordinate the work of various health personnel and plan and implement patient care in cooperation with the health team.

Nurses who work in hospitals connected with federal prisons have somewhat different duties, of course. But their primary concern and responsibility is to keep the prisoners well and give them skilled nursing care when they are ill. In addition, nurses sometimes teach prisoners to care for themselves. (Nursing in state or municipal prisons is generally similar.)

The organization of nursing service within a federal hospital is similar to that of a civilian hospital, and the adaptable professional nurse would find little difficulty in adjusting to its few dissimilarities.

Qualifications and Conditions of Employment. Each branch of the federal government has set up basic qualifications for professional nurses who wish to join its ranks and has established criteria for advancement. The conditions of employment also follow a similar pattern in the several branches of the federal government nursing services.

U.S. PUBLIC HEALTH SERVICE (PHS)

Founded in 1798, the PHS is the principal health agency of the federal government. A component of the Department of Health and Human Services, the PHS is charged with improving and advancing the health of our nation's people. PHS programs are also designed to work with other nations and international agencies on global health problems.

The PHS is a vital force in advancing research in the health sciences, in developing public health programs, in providing therapeutic and preventive services, and in protecting the public health through the regulation of drugs, medical products, and foods. The PHS accomplishes its mission through the following eight agencies: Agency for Health Care Policy and Research, Agency for Toxic Substances and Disease Registry, Centers for Disease Control and Prevention, Food and Drug Administration, Health Resources Services Administration, Indian Health Service, National Institutes of Health and Substance Abuse, and Mental Health Services Administration.

There are opportunities in such fields as clinical care, nursing research, epidemiology, health services research, health promotion, regulatory science, community health, and environmental health. Most of the clinical positions are available in the Indian Health Service (IHS) and the National Institutes of Health (NIH), Clinical Center. Commissioned Corps nurses may be detailed to the Federal Bureau of Prisons, U.S. Coast Guard, Health Care Financing Administration, Immigration and Naturalization Service, and the National Oceanic and Atmospheric Administration.

Nurses may enter the PHS by appointment to either the Federal Civil Service or the Commissioned Corps. Associate degree, diploma, baccalaureate nurses, and nurses with graduate degrees may work in the civil service system. The baccalaureate degree is the entry level for the Commissioned Corps. Other minimum requirements differ. To be considered for appointment into the PHS Commissioned Corps a nurse must be a U.S. citizen, under 44 years of age, have earned a qualifying degree from an accredited program, and must also meet medical, security, and licensure requirements.

The Commissioned Corps is a personnel system composed entirely of health professionals; it is an all-officer corps. It is also one of the seven uniformed services of the United States including the Air Force, Army, Navy, Marine Corps, Coast Guard, and the Commissioned Corps of the National Oceanic and Atmospheric Administration. In the event of a national emergency or war, the President may, by issuing an executive order, declare the PHS Commissioned Corps a military service. Pay, allowances, and other privileges are comparable with those of officers in the armed services. Rank appointments are made depending on the nurse's length of training and experience.

The PHS offers excellent opportunities for students in baccalaureate nursing programs during periods (31 to 120 days) throughout the academic year through the Commissioned Officer Student Training and Extern Program (COSTEP) and Senior COSTEP Program. Both programs are highly competitive and based upon the needs of PHS agencies. (At this time the program has been severely curtailed by budget restraints.) COSTEP allows students to serve in assignments at any time during the year; however, the majority of students are hired for the summer months. Upon completion of their professional education, students may serve an extended active duty assignment with PHS.

In Senior COSTEP, students are assisted financially during their final year of school in return for an agreement to work for PHS after graduation. The student is appointed as an active-duty PHS officer during the senior year and receives monthly pay and allowances as an ensign (01) grade officer. Additional support, in the form of tuition and fees, *may* be paid by the supporting program or agency. Following graduation, the student agrees to work for the agency or program that provided the financial support for twice the time supported.

As mentioned earlier, most of the clinical positions are in the IHS and NIH Clinical Center. Almost half of all the 5,000 PHS nurses work for IHS. IHS is responsible for providing comprehensive care to over 1 million American Indians and Alaska Natives, in hospitals, health centers, and clinics across the United States. Most of the facilities are located west of the Mississippi. The NIH Clinical Center, in Bethesda, MD is a world center for biomedical research. Approximately 900 nurses conduct research, help design experimental treatments, monitor patient responses, analyze data, and educate patients and families. NIH is composed of a number of institutes including the newest institute, the National Institute for Nursing Research. The other PHS agencies employ nurses, though opportunities are more limited than with IHS and NIH.

The National Health Service Corps (NHSC) was authorized in 1970 (and reauthorized in 1990) to recruit health care personnel to urban and rural communities that have critical health manpower shortages. The NHSC recruits primary health care professionals for community-based systems of care throughout the United States and its territories. The greatest needs are for:

- Primary care physicians (allopathic and osteopathic) residency-trained in family medicine, general internal medicine, obstetrics and gynecology, general pediatrics, or general psychiatry
- Primary care nurse practitioners
- Primary care physician assistants
- Certified nurse-midwives
- Dentists
- Mental health professionals

The NHSC offers two forms of federal financial assistance to nurse practitioners and certified nurse-midwives in exchange for service:

- Education loan repayment
- Full scholarships

Both federal financial assistance programs require participants to commit to one year of service in an underserved community for each year of financial support, and both require a minimum two-year commitment.

Health professionals interested in NHSC opportunities are not federal employees; rather, they receive salary and benefits directly from the community-based system of care where they are employed. For additional information about the NHSC, call 1-800-221-9393 (in Virginia, 703-734-6855).

DEPARTMENT OF VETERANS AFFAIRS NURSING SERVICE

The Department of Veterans Affairs (VA) was established in 1930 as a civilian agency of the federal government. Its purpose is to administer national programs that provide benefits for veterans of this country's armed forces. In 1989 the agency was elevated to cabinet status. The VA operates the nation's largest organized health care system, composed of 172 hospitals, over 200 outpatient clinics, more than 100 nursing home care units, and 26 domiciliaries. More than 1.3 million veterans receive inpatient and outpatient care through the VA system yearly. The Veterans Health Services and Research Administration employs more than 35,000 professional nurses.

To accomplish its objective of providing high-quality health care, the VA has developed extensive programs in research and education. A majority of VA medical centers are affiliated with medical schools, schools of nursing, and other health-related schools in a network of health care facilities that cover the entire country. Individual hospitals range in size from approximately 110 to 1,400 beds, most of which provide care for patients with medical, surgical, and psychiatric diagnoses. A few hospitals are predominantly for the care of patients with psychiatric diagnoses. Many VA health care facilities have outpatient clinics and extended-care facilities, such as nursing home care units.

VA medical centers are administered through the Veterans Health Administration, headed by the Under Secretary/Health. The Nursing Service functions within this agency under the leadership of an Assistant Chief Medical Director for Nursing Programs. The National Nursing Service office is located at the Department of Veterans Affairs Central Office, 810 Vermont Avenue NW, Washington, D.C. 20420.

To qualify for an appointment in the VA, a nurse must be a U.S. citizen, a graduate of a state-approved school of professional nursing, currently registered to practice, and meet required physical standards. Graduates from a professional school of nursing may be appointed pending passing of state board examinations.

Nurses employed in VA are covered by a locality pay system (LPS). The LPS is designed to ensure that VA nurses are paid competitive rates within local labor markets. As such, salary ranges vary according to facility location. There are several levels of salary grades for VA nurses.

Qualification standards relating to education, experience, and competencies are specified for appointment or promotion to each grade. The VA salary system recognizes excellence in clinical practice, administration, research, and education. Nurses, including those giving direct patient care, receive salaries commensurate with their qualifications and contributions. A Nurse Professional Standards Board reviews performance and recommends promotion or special salary advancement according to established criteria. A nurse appointed to one VA medical center may transfer to another with continuity of benefits and without loss of salary.

Personnel policies in the VA include a variety of health and life insurance options (partially paid for by the federal government), retirement plans, and liberal annual and sick leave benefits, tuition reimbursement, uniform allowance, annual physical examination, and a smoke-free workplace.

The VA Nursing Service emphasizes continued learning and advanced education. There is a Nursing Career Development Program to provide opportunities within the system. Nurse researchers are employed in some VA medical centers and in the national office. CNSs work in some VA health care settings. Also, NPs function in specific units, clinics, or satellite facilities. Applications and inquiries for full- or part-time employment should be directed to the Personnel Office at the VA Medical Center at the location of interest. A toll-free telephone number (800-368-5629) is available for information about nationwide employment opportunities.

THE ARMED SERVICES

Despite similarities, there are specific differences among the Army Nurse Corps, Navy Nurse Corps, and Air Force Nurse Corps. In recent years there have been a number of changes in qualifications and assignments to meet the changes in society and in the health field. All the armed services have a reserve corps of nurses established by acts of Congress to provide the additional nurses that are needed to care for members of the services and their families in time of war or other national emergency. Nurses may join the reserve without having joined the regular service; the requirements are similar. A certain amount of training (which is paid) is required, usually one weekend a month and two consecutive weeks a year, at local medical units related to that particular service. There are opportunities for promotion, continuing education, and fringe benefits such as low-cost insurance, retirement pay, and PX shopping. More information is available from the reserve recruiter of the particular service. In all the services, nurses have the economic, social, and health care benefits of all officers as well as the opportunity for personal travel. After discharge (or retirement, which is possible in twenty years), veterans' benefits are available.[86]

The Army Nurse Corps

Because it is the oldest of the federal nursing services, the Army Nurse Corps has had considerable influence on the development of nursing and the status of nurses in all of the armed services. When the Army Nurse Corps was established as part of the Army Medical Department in 1901, nurses were appointed in the Regular Army but did not have actual commissions. Their status was basically "no status." Believing that they needed the authority of an officer to assure accountability and responsibility for all nursing care delivered, the ANA, the New York Committee to Secure Rank for Army Nurses, and several other organizations tried to persuade Congress to legislate appropriate military rank and recognition. On June 4, 1920, the Army Reorganization Act authorized relative rank for Army nurses, granting the rank of Second Lieutenant to Major. This act also authorized the wearing of insignia but did not provide for equal pay or privileges such as retirement. During World War II, the federal government gave nurses serving in all branches of the armed services temporary commissions, but it was not until 1947 that women nurses achieved permanent commissioned status. Men in nursing had to wait until 1955 to be so recognized.

Basic qualifications for a commission in the Army Nurse Corps specify that an applicant must:

1. Be a graduate of an educational program accredited by an agency recognized by the U.S. Secretary of Education and acceptable to the Department of the Army. The educational program must prepare the individual for licensure as a registered nurse.
   a. Applicants who enter active duty must possess a minimum of a baccalaureate degree in nursing or nurse anesthesia.
   b. Applicants who desire service in a reserve component must possess a minimum of a diploma in nursing, an associate degree in nursing, or a baccalaureate degree in nursing or nurse anesthesia.
2. Have successfully completed the National Council Licensure Examination for Registered Nurses (NCLEX-RN) and have a valid current license to practice as a registered nurse in the United States, District of Columbia, Commonwealth of Puerto Rico, or a U.S. territory.
3. Be engaged in practice as a registered nurse for a minimum of 20 hours per week for a period of not less than 6 months in the 1-year period immediately preceding the date the application is received.
4. Be the age of 21 to 48.
5. Be a citizen of the United States or lawfully admitted to the United States for permanent residence.
6. Be able to meet the physical standards prescribed for appointment. Applicants can be married or single and have dependents of any age.

A registered nurse just completing a basic nursing program will usually be commissioned as a second lieutenant. Applicants who have acquired professional experience on a full-time basis, received advanced nursing education, or served formerly as a commissioned officer may qualify for an initial appointment at a higher rank. Unless an applicant has previously served in the military, the service obligation is 8 years. For those applicants who enter active duty, at least three of the eight years must be served on active duty. The remainder of the military service obligation may be served in either the active or the reserve components. Army Nurse Corps officers may now advance to the rank of Brigadier General.

Army nurses may give direct patient care in any clinical specialty as staff nurses, head nurses, or nursing consultants. They may teach as directors or instructors for military courses in various hospitals and the Army Medical Department Center and School or be responsible for nursing education and staff development within a Department of Nursing. They may become involved in administration in various clinical services or at Army headquarters. They may also function as nursing methods analysts, nurse researchers, nurse counselors, consultants to the surgeon general, or advisers to military nurses of allied nations. Assignments may be in the United States or various parts of the world. There are numerous educational programs, such as the entry-level clinical nursing specialty courses. Army Nurse Corps officers may also be selected to attend a college or university for advanced degrees with all or part of the costs paid.

Further information may be obtained from the local Army recruiting station (ask for the Army Nurse Corps recruiter) or by writing to Army Opportunities, Army Nurse Corps, Post Office Box 7700, Clifton, New Jersey 07015-4865.

Navy Nurse Corps

Although the Navy Nurse Corps was officially established by Congress in the twentieth century, Navy nurses were recommended by the first chief of the Bureau of Medicine and Surgery in 1811, and sisters of the Order of the Holy Cross served on the Navy ship *Red Rover* as volunteers in 1862. There were the first female nurses to serve aboard the first U.S. Navy hospital ship. The first Navy nurses (called the *Sacred Twenty*) and a superintendent reported to Washington for duty in 1908. By 1910 nurses had expanded their activities to include the Far East, Hawaii, and the Caribbean. In World War I, women nurses were assigned to hospitals in England, Ireland, Scotland, and France. Throughout World War II, Navy nurses also brought nursing care to front-line casualties aboard twelve hospital ships and also to air evacuees. They served in foreign lands where American women had never been seen and some were prisoners of war. In 1944, the *USS Highbee* became the first combat ship to be named for a woman, the second superintendent of the Navy Nurse Corps.

During the Korean and Vietnam conflicts, Navy nurses served in station hospitals and aboard hospital ships caring for ill and wounded soldiers, sailors, and marines. Four Navy nurses received the Purple Heart for injuries received in Saigon, South Vietnam.

Today, Navy nurses provide care for patients; teach patients, corpsmen, and other health care team members; assume administrative positions; and serve as executive and commanding officers of medical facilities. They are assigned to hospitals, clinics, ships, headquarters staff, Officer Indoctrination School, Hospital Corps schools, and other duty stations in the United States and other parts of the world.

Initial appointments are made in grades of ensign to lieutenant, based upon education and other professional qualifications. Nurses may advance to the rank of rear admiral. Basic qualifications for an officer commission state that the candidate must be:

1. A graduate of a nursing education program, approved by a state board of nurs-

ing or accredited by the National League for Nursing, that conferred:
   a. A baccalaureate or an advanced degree.
   b. An associate degree in nursing or a 3-year diploma in nursing of at least 108 academic weeks *and* a baccalaureate degree accredited by a national agency or association in chemistry, biology, physiology, psychology, sociology, zoology, or health sciences.

2. Licensed and in good standing as a registered professional nurse based on a licensing examination provided by the National Council of State Boards of Nursing (NCLEX). Nurse anesthetists must obtain and maintain certification by the Council on Certification of Nurse Anesthetists, nurse-midwives must be certified by the American College of Nurse-Midwives, and nurse practitioners must be certified by their specialty professional organization or the American Nurses Credentialling Center (ANCC).

3. Presently employed in nursing practice.

4. A citizen of United States.

5. Able to attain 20 years of active commissioned service by age 55. Age waivers may be obtained for those in certain specialties.

6. Physically qualified according to Navy standards.

7. Single or married.

8. Able to supply excellent professional, personal, and scholastic references.

9. Of good moral character and of unquestioned loyalty to the United States.

All Navy nurses are encouraged to continue their education through Navy in-service and CE courses, as well as courses leading to academic degrees. Qualified career officers may request assignment to full-time study for an advanced degree in nursing and related health care administration fields.

Further information is available from the local Navy recruiting station or from the Director,

Navy Nurse Corps, Bureau of Medicine and Surgery, Washington, D.C.

The Air Force Nurse Corps

In 1947, with the passage of the National Security Act, the United States Air Force was established as a separate service. The United States Air Force Medical Service, including the nursing component, was established on July 1, 1949. Prior to that date, medical personnel in the Army Medical Service were assigned to duty with the United States Air Force.

The mission of the Medical Service is to provide the medical support necessary for maximum peacetime readiness and combat effectiveness of the Air Force. As an integral part of the mission, the Medical Service will provide, to the greatest extent possible, a peacetime health care system for all eligible beneficiaries. The Air Force Nurse Corps, as one of the five components responsible for medical support of the Air Force, has a vital role in this mission.

Since its establishment, the Nurse Corps has undergone many changes, including increased authorization, increased rank, and new specialty codes. In 1955, male nurses were authorized to receive commissions, and now approximately 25 percent are men. Over 50 percent are married and may have dependents of any age.

Air Force nurses provide quality nursing care in a variety of specialties and settings. They perform duties in one of eleven career fields, such as administration, mental health, operating room, anesthesia, clinical nursing, education, flight nursing, nurse practitioner, and midwifery. They are involved in clinical practice, patient teaching, supervision and teaching of paraprofessional personnel, administration, education, and research.

The majority of the nurses are assigned to medical centers, hospitals, and clinics in the United States and overseas. Most medical treatment facilities are small community hospitals, providing routine and emergency medical, surgical, pediatric, obstetric, and psychoneurological services for beneficiaries. One role unique to

Air Force nursing is that of flight nurse. The Air Force has the Department of Defense responsibility for aeromedical evacuation in peacetime and during conflicts.

Nurses are assigned as flight nurses only after completing an intensive program at the School of Aerospace Medicine at Brooks Air Force Base, Texas. Since the first class graduated in February 1943, the course has been conducted continuously, with over 12,000 graduates. The course includes didactic and practical experiences in aerospace physiology, basic sciences, specialized techniques necessary for the safe and efficient transportation of patients by air, and survival and life support principles, procedures, and equipment. It provides students with the knowledge and skills required for management and nursing care of patients in flight.

Air Force nurses are given every opportunity to grow, both academically and professionally. Nurses are encouraged to continue their formal education at civilian colleges and universities located near Air Force medical treatment facilities. Under a tuition assistance program, the Air Force may pay up to 75 percent of their tuition costs for off-duty courses. Many Air Force nurses compete regularly for undergraduate and graduate study opportunities. A certain number are selected each year to pursue full-time graduate studies in civilian universities. Air Force–sponsored students receive their normal pay during the school terms, plus educational assistance covering tuition and required expenses. Accepting this educational assistance requires an additional active-duty obligation commensurate with the length of the education program.

Tuition assistance is available for generic nursing students via the ROTC programs on most university campuses. Applications are accepted from BSN students who meet certain criteria during their senior year. This program offers an excellent opportunity for a wide variety of clinical experiences to new graduates. Applicants accepted for this program participate in a five-month nurse internship program before reporting to their first assignment. Nurses in the intern program have the opportunity to apply basic nursing knowledge and skills and acquire new, specialized skills. Rotations through several clinical areas help prepare nurses for a variety of nursing duties.

Air Force nurses have two professions; they are professional officers and professional nurses. The ranks of Air Force nurses range from second lieutenant to brigadier general. Most applicants receive their commission as officers in the grade of second lieutenant. Nurses with additional professional experience and education may be appointed at a higher rank after review of records and in accordance with current policy.

To qualify for appointment, the applicant must:

1. Be a graduate of a nursing school acceptable to the Surgeon General of the Air Force.
2. Have a current registration in any state or the District of Columbia.
3. Meet physical and professional requirements.
4. Be at least 18 years old.
5. Be a citizen of the United States.

Additional information may be obtained by contacting a local Air Force recruiter or by writing to HQ USAF Recruiting Service/RSHN, Randolph Air Force Base, Texas 78150. In addition to a full-time career as an Air Force officer, commissions are also available via the Air Force Reserve and Air National Guard Programs. Information on Air Force Reserve Programs may be obtained by writing HQ Air Force Reserve/SG, Robins Air Force Base, Georgia 31098 or HQ ARPC/SG, Denver, Colorado 80280. Information on Air National Guard programs may be obtained by writing National Guard Bureau/SG, Room 2E369, The Pentagon, Washington, D.C. 20310 or ANGRC/DPR, 3500 Fetchet Avenue, Andrews AFB, Maryland 20331-5157.

NURSING IN EXTENDED AND LONG-TERM CARE FACILITIES

Under Medicare and Medicaid, nursing homes that qualify for reimbursement are called *skilled nursing facilities*. The intermediate care facility provides for those who require care beyond room and board but less than that designated as skilled. These include institutions for victims of cerebral palsy or other neurological conditions and mental retardation. The older term *nursing home*, which might apply to either, is still used by most people. More RNs are working in nursing homes than there were even 5 years ago, although the majority of care-givers are practical nurses and aides.

Nurses may have positions in nursing homes similar to those in hospitals, with the additional role of facility administrator being assumed by some nurses. In this case, the nurse must be certified for the position, and although the individual's knowledge of nursing may be extremely helpful in understanding the need for quality care, being a nurse is not a requirement for certification.

The director of nursing, who has the same kinds of responsibilities as any other director of nursing, is sometimes expected to act as the administrator's assistant, whereas some administrators take over some of the director's prerogatives. In small nursing homes, the director might assume both roles. Because most facilities are for-profit, the financial management is extremely important. The administrative nurse should be well prepared in managerial skills; unfortunately, that is rare.

In most nursing homes the pace is slower and the pressure less than in other settings for care. Nurses interested in nursing home care enjoy the opportunity to know the patient better in the relatively long-term stay and to help the patient maintain or attain the best possible health status. This is not the area of practice for someone impatient for quick results. Both rehabilitative and geriatric nursing require a larger amount of patience and understanding. In rehabilitation, nurses work closely as a team with related health disciplines—occupational therapy, physical therapy, speech therapy, and others. In geriatric nursing, the nurse works to a great extent with nonprofessional nursing personnel and acts as team leader, teacher, and supervisor. It may well be that there is only one licensed nurse in a nursing home per shift, with practical nurses as charge nurses and aides giving much of the day-to-day care.

Because the patients are relatively helpless and often have no family or friends who check on them, the nurse must, in a real sense, be a patient advocate. Physicians make infrequent visits and in some cases, where there are limited or no rehabilitative services, the nurse is the only professional with long-term patient contact.

For this reason, geriatric nurse practitioners (GNPs) are considered a tremendous asset in nursing homes. The GNP is responsible for assessing patients and evaluating their progress, sometimes performing certain diagnostic procedures. She or he usually manages medical problems within a general protocol, but a particularly important function is assessing personal and family relationships, patient and staff relationships, and life situations that may affect the patient's health status. In some nursing homes, the GNP is on twenty-four-hour emergency call and also performs the other usual NP functions.[87]

Qualifications and Conditions of Employment. Requirements for employment are similar to those in hospitals for like positions, although often the need for a degree is not emphasized. Conditions of employment and salaries have improved, but are not as good as those in hospitals. Because, under Medicare, orientation and subsequent inservice education are mandatory, the nurse has an excellent opportunity to learn about long-term nursing care and the concepts and techniques of geriatric nursing. Because the increase of older people is one of the trends in society, geriatric care is being given greater attention, and workshops, courses, and programs are available in the field. With an aging population, there are also likely to be good job opportunities for some time to come. It is unfortunate that so few are interested in care of the elderly.

PUBLIC HEALTH (COMMUNITY HEALTH) NURSING

Public health nursing (PHN) synthesizes the knowledge from the nursing and public health sciences to promote and preserve the health of individuals, families, and communities. The goal is to improve the health of the community by identifying subgroups (aggregates) within the community population that are at high risk of illness, disability, or premature death and directing resources toward these groups.[88,89]

Public health nursing practice is a systematic process by which:

1. The health and health care needs of a population are assessed in collaboration with other disciplines in order to identify subpopulations (aggregates), families, and individuals at increased risk of illness, disability, or premature death.
2. A plan for intervention is developed to meet these needs, which includes resources available and those activities that contribute to health and its recovery, the prevention of illness, disability, and premature death.
3. A health care plan is implemented effectively, efficiently, and equitably.
4. An evaluation is made to determine the extent to which these activities have an impact on the health status of the population.[90]

From the very beginning of PHN in 1893, under the inspiration of Lillian Wald and the Henry Street Settlement on New York City's Lower East Side, nurses made visits to people in their homes, schools, or where people and neighbors gathered. Health teaching and care of the sick were intertwined with preventive services and linked with the social and political concerns of the times.

Today, public health nurses (PHNs) practice in many settings. Most are employed by agencies that may carry the title of public health, community health, home health, or visiting nurse. They may be official—governmental and tax supported (such as a city or county health department); nonofficial or voluntary—agencies supported to a great extent by community funds (such as visiting nurse or home health service); or proprietary—for profit. These agencies range in size and services from small, employing only one or two PHNs, to very large, employing a sizable staff of professional nurses, other health professionals, practical nurses, and home health aides and homemakers. Some of the latter may be contracted for from an agency (see Chap. 8).

PHN employment opportunities are not limited, however, to these agencies. Nurses may also be employed by hospitals to conduct home-care programs or to serve as liaison between the hospital and community facilities, or by other institutions and agencies, private and governmental, in need of the kinds of services the PHN is prepared to provide in schools, outpatient clinics, community health centers, free walk-in clinics for drug addiction and sexually transmitted diseases (STD), migrant labor camps, and rural areas.

As part of the official public health services, every state, every United States territory, and many counties, large towns, and cities have a public health department. Health departments may be freestanding departments or combined with hospital and medical care regulatory agencies, environmental health agencies, and welfare and social service agencies. Since the publication of *The Future of Public Health*,[91] there have been heated discussions about the focus of public health and the lack of infrastructure, resources, and appropriately trained public health personnel to honor our commitment to the total community. To accomplish the goal of improving the health status of the total population, official public health agencies balance three core public health functions: assessment of community health status; policy and program development; and assurance of high-quality, safe, and effective services.

Public health services focus on health promotion and disease prevention, community health protection, personal prevention, and assistance in gaining access to care. Examples of such programs and services are:[92]

HEALTH PROMOTION AND DISEASE PREVENTION

Education about risk factors for STD and HIV and AIDS

Promoting seatbelt use

Teaching schoolchildren about the health benefits of good nutrition and physical activity

COMMUNITY HEALTH PROTECTION

Assuring a safe environment through safe housing, workplaces, food, and water

Aiding households and communities exposed to hazardous waste sites or chemical spills

Reducing the occurrence and harmful effects of air pollution

Disaster response preparedness programs

PERSONAL PREVENTION

Early and periodic screening for childhood diseases

Screening and treatment for infectious diseases such as TB, STDs

Behavior change counseling

SERVICES TO IMPROVE ACCESS TO CARE

Coordinating public and private responses to community health needs

Providing outreach services to individuals, families, and groups at risk for communicable diseases

Public health nursing home visits to high-risk pregnant women

Public health offers extraordinary opportunities for the imaginative, competent, and resourceful person to originate and develop ideas that may greatly affect the health of the community. There is a need for collection of data, constant monitoring of trends, and epidemiological surveillance of both communicable and chronic diseases. Public health nurses are constantly collecting data, investigating adverse health conditions, monitoring the outcomes of medical care services in families and communities, and assisting with health policy development at the state or local level. PHNs may also work for various international agencies assisting with the development of public health programs in developing countries. There is growing recognition of the role public health nurses can play in combating serious world health challenges such as AIDS or vaccine-preventable childhood diseases.

Professional nurses make up the largest group of professional public health personnel, and their influence is considerable. However, PHN positions are increasingly threatened, as other nonclinical workers are employed in public health. Funding for PHNs has been cut because of costs; yet no other worker has the vast repertoire of skills. This trend is a major concern and has captured the attention of the nursing community. Workers in the field of public health include physicians, social workers, sanitary engineers, nutritionists, dentists, physical therapists, speech therapists, and others. Members of these groups may work alone or in a team relationship. All public health workers, therefore, need an overview of the entire program to understand their place in the organization and the scope of their own work. An effective public health program requires excellent working relationships with other agencies, both health and nonhealth, because public health activities reach every segment of the community. Although situations differ, nurses in official agencies may make home visits, but their responsibilities are primarily in community health clinics focused on the needs of that agency's population. Traditionally, these have been family planning, maternal child-care, and communicable disease; in a number of communities these agency nurses are also the school nurses and, occasionally, are contracted to do some occupational health nursing. NPs are being employed to care for patients in the areas of their expertise, but all nurses observe and evaluate the patients' physical and emotional conditions and are involved in teaching, therapy, counseling, and prevention; they make referrals as necessary and act in a liaison capacity with other agencies for needed services.

The visiting nurses, or home health nurses, regardless of their place of employment, also carry out these functions and may, in addition, give physical care and treatments. With the advent of much earlier discharge from hospitals, patients are quite a bit sicker when they go home, and nurses are required to know how to care for the acutely ill. If the nurse assessment indicates that the patient's care does not require professional nurse services, home health aides and homemakers may be assigned to a patient family, with nurse supervision and reassessment. Visiting nurses have also set up clinics that they visit periodically in senior citizen centers or apartments, as well as in the single-room occupancy (SRO) hotels commonly used for welfare clients and the homeless in large cities. There are multiple liaison roles with hospitals, HMOs, clinics, geriatric units, and various residences for the long-term disabled and mentally ill or retarded, primarily to assist in admission and discharge planning, as well as coordinating continuing patient care.

Nurses in managerial positions in PHN agencies have responsibilities similar to those in hospitals in terms of general managerial skills. A major difference for the top nurse administrator is that the individual is frequently director of the entire agency, with direct responsibility to the agency board of directors (nonofficial agency) or the health officer (governmental agency).

Some of the major changes that will affect public health nurses, as seen by some public health administrators, are:

1. Health care reform and new requirements for conducting health care quality assurance activities. As leaders in public health redefine what is central to public health as a part of health care reform, there will be renewed emphasis on the linkages between primary clinical services and population outcomes.

2. New health care delivery systems with increased utilization of managed care organizations will require public health nurses to shift the focus from personal services and staffing clinics to emphasis on programs within the core public health services.

3. New types of health and social manpower emerging in the community, placing a greater responsibility on the PHN to coordinate and supervise their activities.

4. Impact of management theory in the health field, requiring nurses to be knowledgeable about these concepts, health care economics, and still remain patient advocates.

5. Changing economics and incentives within the health care system, requiring close surveillance for early hospital discharges and underserved populations, such as families with chronic conditions or children with special needs.

6. Impact of profit-making agencies in competition with governmental and voluntary agencies. All organizations are focused on the cost of services and the ability to compete in changing health care markets.

7. Renewed focus on community-based long-term care as part of efforts to expand needed services for people over 65. Expanded services will be provided outside of nursing homes and may be under the purview of PHNs.

Qualifications and Conditions of Employment. Schools of professional nursing have long recognized that nurses who plan to enter the field of public health need special preparation for it. Most diploma and AD schools give students theoretical instruction in public health nursing, conduct orientation visits to community health agencies, provide several hours of experience in prenatal and well-baby clinics, and integrate public health aspects of nursing wherever possible in all clinical areas. One of the problems in giving experience to students in these schools is the lack of clinical facilities (agencies) for practice. What experience is available is usually reserved for baccalaureate programs, because preparation for PHN is usually a major educational objective of these programs and students have taken a considerable number of courses in preparation. However, their experiences are also not limited to official and nonofficial agencies, as public health is seen in a broader perspective.

Besides state licensure, and for some agencies, prior nursing experience, one major qualification for PHN work is graduation from a baccalaureate nursing program. Many graduates of these schools go on to earn a master's degree and are thus prepared educationally for a lifetime career in this field. Because of the shortage of nurses with the prescribed PHN preparation at the present time, however, graduates of diploma and AD programs can and do find positions in this field, working at the beginning level and under supervision. In some areas they work only in clinics and do not make home visits. Some employers encourage nurses to work toward a baccalaureate degree by providing tuition or scholarship grants.

In March 1992, 66.5 percent of the employed nurses worked in hospitals. Fifteen percent, or 250,004 RNs, worked in community and public health settings, including state or local health departments, non-hospital-based home health agencies, various types of community health centers, student health services, and occupational health services. Over 44 percent of nurses employed in community and public health settings have a baccalaureate or higher degree.[93]

Pay and advancement at all levels are related to educational and other qualifications. Nurses may be promoted as they assume advanced or expanded clinical role functions or administrative positions. Most agencies make available to all staff written personnel policies and conditions of employment. Many official agencies operate within a civil service system.

In the past, PHNs enjoyed standard daytime hours, with most working Monday through Friday. However, with the move toward more care in the community on a twenty-four-hour basis, rather than in institutions, PHNs will be expected to rotate shifts and work weekends, much the same as nurses employed in institutions.

A unique and distinct aspect of PHN practice is the autonomy required when working in a setting "without walls." Clinical judgment and clinical decisions are a central part of the nursing practice that demands a high level of knowledge and clinical versatility.

There is another key point that relates to both the nurse as a practitioner and the conditions of employment. Because PHNs do not generally function in the protected controlling environment of an institution, where there is a degree of implied authority, but rather in the client's setting, where the client determines who will enter his home and whether he will receive or follow the health teaching and counseling given, these nurses should have the personality characteristics to deal with such situations. Even if the setting is a clinic, there is no force that can make a client come to or return to a clinic or, for that matter, follow any regimen given.

Many studies have documented the need for public health nurses to use interventions with clients and families that are specific to ethnic, cultural, and social values. Families may reject health teaching if it is perceived to be judgmental or prejudicial on the part of the health care provider.

Professional nurses who select PHN as a career need outstanding ability to adjust to many types of environments with a variety of living conditions, from the well-to-do in a high-rise apartment house to the most poverty-stricken in a ghetto or rural area, and to appreciate a wide range of interests, attitudes, educational backgrounds, and cultural differences. They must be able to accept these variations, to understand the differences, to communicate well so as to avoid misunderstandings and misinterpretations, and to be able to give equally good nursing care to all. PHNs in any position must use excellent judgment and are expected to use their own initiative. They have the opportunity to work with persons in other disciplines and other social agencies to help provide needed services to the clients, services that may include financial counseling, legal aid, housing problems, family planning, marital counseling, and school difficulties. In some instances, PHNs are not only case finders, but case coordinators—patient advocates in every sense.

SCHOOL HEALTH NURSING

There are approximately 26,000 school nurses employed in public and private schools. This includes RNs with no advanced or specialty preparation, certified school nurses (requirement differs by the state), and school nurse practitioners (SNPs) who are advanced practice nurses qualified to deliver a full range of primary care services. In some cases, school nurses are expected to have the same educational credentials as teachers. The salaries for these positions vary by region but overall are lower than hospital employment when nurses first start out in the field. However, school nurses employed by large urban school districts eventually can compete with and even exceed some hospital salaries for nurses.

School nurses ideally work with and through school health councils to plan and execute their programs. School health councils consist of school and community health administrators, parents, students, senior citizens, teachers, nurses, business people, individuals working for the media, attorneys, and elected officials with an interest in school health. Consequently, community development and coalition-building skills (such as team building, negotiating, needs assessment abilities, and an awareness of how community governance works) are necessary abilities for someone entering the school health field.

School districts vary in size throughout the country. The majority (75 percent) have a total student enrollment of 2,500 students or less. Consequently, school nurses usually work in more than one building. Here, nurses perform a wide range of services including basic screenings for vision, hearing, growth measurements, and risk factors that would interfere with the development of healthy lifestyle habits. Case management services are also provided for students at high risk for health impairments and school failure. Unfortunately, school nurses are often spread too thin to work adequately with students intensively, for example, to develop their consumer health skills.

Almost every school nurse is responsible for activities in the areas of (1) health service, (2) health education, and (3) environmental health and safety. The programs they implement may range from very basic services for students as a whole, such as health risk appraisals, to one-on-one primary health care services provided in a school-based student health center. It just depends on the wishes of the community and the actions of the school health council.

All nurses working in schools must be clinically prepared to work with students with special health needs. With the introduction of the Individuals with Disabilities Education Act (IDEA) in the 1970s, students with complex chronic diseases, emotional disorders, and developmental disabilities as well as those who are dependent on technology (e.g., ventilators) are entitled to a free and appropriate public education. This means nurses must be prepared to do a number of clinical procedures (e.g., gastrostomy feedings, suctioning, dressing changes) to ensure that these students have ready access to school. Additional legislation has since expanded the age range of children with special health needs served by schools from the previous 5 to 18 years of age to birth through adulthood. Consequently, school nurses today must be prepared to work with students of all ages. Furthermore, school nurses in many districts also provide employee health services for school administrators, faculty, and staff, including the processing of workmen's compensation claims.

School nurses function in accordance with the following nationally recognized National Association of School Nurses, Inc., school nursing standards of practice:[94]

1. The school nurse utilizes a distinct knowledge base for decision making in nursing practice.
2. The school nurse uses a systemic approach to problem solving in nursing practice.
3. The school nurse contributes to the education of the client with special health needs by assessing the client, planning and providing appropriate nursing care, and evaluating the identified outcomes of care.
4. The school nurse uses effective written, verbal, and nonverbal communication skills.
5. The school nurse establishes and maintains a comprehensive school health program.
6. The school nurse collaborates with other school professionals, parents, and caregivers to meet the health, developmental, and educational needs of clients.
7. The school nurse collaborates with members of the community in the delivery of health and social services, and utilizes knowledge of community health systems and resources to function as a school-community liaison.
8. The school nurse assists students, families, and the school community to achieve optimal levels of wellness through appropriately designed and delivered health education.
9. The school nurse contributes to nursing and school health through innovations in practice and participation in research or research-related activities.
10. The school nurse identifies, delineates, and clarifies the nursing role, promotes quality of care, pursues continued professional enhancement, and demonstrates professional conduct.

Today, school nurses with other school health personnel are deeply involved in the implementation of the national education goals, two of which are targeted at health. These goals concern early childhood interventions to ensure that students enter school ready to learn and the second goal addresses the need to free schools of substance abuse problems. Because school nurses have ties to both the health and education fields, the following national health objectives related to school health further define their practice for now:[95]

1. Increase to at least 50 percent the proportion of children in grades 1 through 12

who participate in daily physical education activities at school.

2. Increase to at least 90 percent the proportion of school lunch and breakfast programs with menus consistent with nutritional principles contained in *Dietary Guidlines for Americans.*

3. Increase to at least 75 percent the proportion of the nation's schools that provide nutrition education from preschool through 12th grade.

4. Include tobacco use prevention in the curricula of all elementary, middle, and secondary schools.

5. Provide children in all primary and secondary schools with educational programs on alcohol and other drugs.

6. Increase to at least 85 percent the proportion of people aged 10 through 18 who have discussed human sexuality with their parents or received information from parentally endorsed sources such as schools.

7. Increase to at least 50 percent the proportion of elementary and secondary schools that teach nonviolent conflict-resolution skills.

8. Provide academic instruction on injury prevention and control in at least 50 percent of public school systems.

9. Increase to at least 95 percent the proportion of schools that have age-appropriate HIV education curricula for children in grades 4 through 12.

10. Include in all middle and secondary schools instruction on preventing sexually transmitted diseases.

Schools have become an important site for the delivery of primary health care to school-age children and youth. SNPs working as members of interdisciplinary teams are often the primary health care providers. Other advanced practice school health nurses manage and coordinate school-based student health centers and other aspects of the school health program that today are characterized as an integrated comprehensive service package for students. Still other school nurse specialists provide mental health counseling within student assistant programs; serve as active members of the school team responsible for athletic programs, and design, implement, and evaluate health promotion programs for the entire student body.

How successful and satisfying is school nursing? As an example, one nurse practitioner working in a middle school health clinic has made a tremendous difference in the lives of economically deprived children. The NP works in an inner city school on the east coast and provides primary health care to students who otherwise have very limited access to health services. Since the opening of the school-based clinic, this nurse practitioner has been a vital member of a health team that has witnessed a tremendous drop in the teen pregnancy rate, a distinct decrease in suicides, a noticeable increase in the attendance rate, and an increase in the number of mental health problems diagnosed and treated. The health team has been so successful even the school principal and staff are crediting the nurse and school-based clinic facility with keeping the students healthy enough to learn because diagnosis and treatment are provided on site.

Several years ago, a large coalition of nursing organizations cited schools as a key facility for primary care under health care reform.[96] It is likely that nurses who are creative and interested in primary care and prevention will find school nursing a rewarding career. A graduate degree is an essential for the complexity of the role, particularly in the decades to come. Job opportunities now exist in this field for those nurses who have a background in primary health care, public policy, community development, and a commitment to student health.

It is important to recognize that the patterns for school nursing practice vary according to the needs perceived and the limits set by the school boards. In one pattern, the nurse might assume responsibility for the total school health program, assisted by an aide to do clerical work and to triage simple conditions. In a second pattern, the nurse may visit a number of schools, assessing and evaluating children and leaving the follow-up to the regular school nurse. In another, the practice might be limited to doing physical exams or evaluating children with learning difficulties. School-based clinics (SBCs) or school-linked health clinics with SNPs provide comprehensive health care service. There are currently over 150 of these school health centers in the nation. In some, family planning services are included, and this aspect has generated controversy.

Colleges and universities also provide a setting for the nurse interested in student health, although obviously there is considerable adult health involved. Responsibilities vary according to the size of the institution and the types of services offered. College students often pay a health fee that entitles them to specific benefits. Services may include mental health counselling, family planning, and care for minor illnesses or injuries. SNPs also function in these settings.

Many school districts hire their own nurses, but others contract with the local public health agency for school health coverage. School nurse positions are often considered particularly desirable because the time schedule is the same as for teachers, with weekends and summers free. Salaries, particularly in the larger systems, may be equal to those of the teachers if the qualifications are equal. In others, it can be lower than teachers. Schools with SBCs may operate the health centers year-round so that health care services for children are not interrupted.

Opportunities for advancement are found primarily in the larger systems, where the nurse may move to a supervisory position. However, there are many satisfactions to be gained, and there is the possibility of professional growth in systems in which nurses are able to assume a full professional role and have an impact on the health of schoolchildren. School nursing is an evolving field that offers dramatic opportunities for advanced practice.

OCCUPATIONAL HEALTH NURSING

Occupational health nursing (OHN), then called industrial nursing, reportedly began in 1888 with services provided by Betty Moulder to a group of coal miners in Drifton, Pennsylvania. In 1895, the Vermont Marble Company hired Ada Mayo Stewart to care for ill and injured workers and their families. She is generally credited with being the first industrial nurse, as much has been reported about her activities.

Two department stores were the next to provide similar health services for their employees: The John Wanamaker Company of New York in 1897 and the Frederick Loeser Department Store in Brooklyn in 1899. Early in the 1900s more and more industries on both the east and west coasts recognized the economic value of keeping employees healthy and established similar health services. Adding impetus to the trend was the enactment of workers' compensation laws (beginning in 1911), which emphasize accident prevention to employees on the job, and provide for disability compensation for work-related injured or ill workers and encourage immediate and expert attention to injuries received at work. This development brought more industrial nurses into the work sites. World Wars I and II were also strong influences in the growth of OHN nursing because they created a great need to conserve manpower.

For many years nurses employed in these positions called themselves industrial nurses. In 1958, however, the industrial nurses within ANA voted to call their field occupational health nursing, which reflected the broader and changing scope of practice within the specialty. Other organizations also adopted the newer term, including the American Association of Occupational Health Nurses (AAOHN). A key factor in the changes in OHN was the enactment in 1970 of the Occupational Safety and Health Act (see also Chaps. 6 and 19). That act created the National Institute for Occupational Safety and Health (NIOSH) to provide education to occupational health and safety professionals through the establishment of Educational Resource Centers (ERCs) and to research occupational health problems and recommend health and safety standards. With the establishment of the ERCs, specialized education in OHN is now available to prepare nurse practitioners, managers, and specialists to assess workplace hazards, design intervention strategies to minimize risk, and promote worker health and healthy working conditions.

The Occupational Safety and Health Administration (OSHA) was also established to guarantee a "safe and healthful workplace." OSHA inspects the nation's workplaces for health and safety hazards, but its effectiveness has been blunted by lack of funds and the resistance of some employers, who have sometimes sued and won to limit the access of OSHA's inspectors. Nevertheless, unions, environmentalists, and other interested citizens have pressed for more action.

The AAOHN states in its revised 1994 standards of occupational health nursing practice:

> Occupational health nursing is the specialty practice that provides for and delivers health care services to workers and worker populations. The practice focuses on promotion, protection, and restoration of workers' health within the context of a safe and healthy work environment. Occupational health nursing practice is autonomous, and occupational health nurses make independent nursing judgments in providing occupational health services.
>
> The foundation for occupational health nursing practice is research-based with an emphasis on optimizing health, preventing illness and injury, and reducing health hazards. This specialty practice derives its theoretical, conceptual, and factual framework from a multidisciplinary base including, but not limited to:
>
> - Nursing science
> - Medical science
> - Public health sciences such as epidemiology and environmental health
> - Occupational health sciences such as toxicology, safety, industrial hygiene, and ergonomics
> - Social and behavioral sciences
> - Management and administration principles
>
> Guided by an ethical framework made explicit in the AAOHN Code of Ethics, occupational health nurses encourage and enable individuals to make informed decisions about health care concerns. Confidentiality of health information is integral and central to the practice base. Occupational health nurses are advocates for workers, fostering equitable and quality health care services and safe and healthy work environments.[97]

The OHN may work in a multidisciplinary setting or multinurse unit; however, more than 60 percent of OHNs work alone. Physicians are often employed on a contractual basis and provide medical services as needed, but in most cases the OHN is the manager of the unit.

Whether this nurse functions in a sophisticated manner in the delivery of health care depends on his or her education and experience, and the policies of the employer. As a nurse practitioner or nurse clinician, the nurse gives primary care and makes a clinical nursing diagnosis. She or he assesses the worker's condition through health histories, observation, physical examination, and other selected diagnostic measures; reviews and interprets findings to differentiate the normal from the abnormal; selects and carries out the appropriate action and referral as necessary; counsels and teaches. The practitioner must also be concerned with the physical and psychosocial phenomena of the workers and their families, their working environment, community, and even recreation.

When the nurse does not function in an expanded role, standing orders or directions, prepared and signed by the medical director, give the necessary authority to care for conditions that develop while the employee is on the job. In a more conservative environment, where a nurse does not have specialized preparation, activities may be limited. However, these usually include first aid or emergency treatment, assisting the physician, carrying out certain diagnostic tests, and keeping health records. The ability to take and recognize abnormalities in electrocardiograms and to do eye screening, audiometric testing, and certain laboratory tests and x-rays is also important. In addition, the nurse must be vitally concerned with the safety of the employees and often conducts worksite tours with management and the safety engineer to help plan a practical safety program.

The scope of occupational health nursing practice has broadened considerably. More emphasis is being placed on health promotion activities to keep the worker well. There is an increased emphasis of concern on worker health problems that may or may not be directly caused by the job but affect worker performance—alcoholism, emotional problems, stress, drug addiction, and family relations. In many cases, the nurse may be involved in developing employee assistance programs and in counseling and therapy.

In addition, OHNs are assuming the role of manager of the occupational health unit and administration of the overall program. There are a number of legal issues about which the nurse must be knowledgeable. These include the serious and not infrequent responsibility of giving immediate care to workers with serious injuries, often with no physician present, which may have major legal implications. OHNs should be familiar with the laws governing the practice of nursing, medicine, and pharmacy in their own states and discuss them with the physician and management to make sure that they all understand the legal scope of nursing functions. In addition, the nurse must be fully cognizant of laws that govern employee health. This requires interpretation of regulations and the design and implementation of standards to protect worker health. The nurse should be involved in policy decisions affecting worker health and safety.

Qualifications and Conditions of Employment. Graduation from a state-approved school of professional nursing and current state registration are basic requirements for the OHN. More employers are requiring a college degree and many find a graduate degree desirable. A career OHN may seek certification by the American Board for Occupational Health Nurses, an independent nursing specialty board authorized to certify qualified OHNs.

Salaries and fringe benefits vary according to the size of the industry or business and its location. The usual company benefits include vacations, sick leave, pensions, and insurance. Working hours are those of the workers; thus, in an industry with work shifts around the clock, nurses are usually there also. Although some industries carry professional liability insurance that supposedly covers the OHN, it may not apply in all cases of possible litigation. It is advisable, therefore, for the nurses to carry their own professional liability insurance.

OFFICE NURSING

Office nurses are employed by physicians and ambulatory care multispecialty practices and usually see their patients in an office. Office nurses may provide the nursing care needed themselves or assign certain duties to other personnel who work under their direction and supervision. When working for several doctors in a group practice or in a larger multispecialty center employing numerous personnel, the supervising nurse may oversee a staff of registered nurses, licensed practical nurses, medical assistants, clerical, billing, and insurance personnel, receptionists, and other technical personnel.

Nurses may work in a one-doctor (solo) practice with a generalist, internist, or family practitioner. This requires the nurse to have general skills and knowledge. Or they may be employed in a specialist's office, which necessitates skills in the specific specialty. For instance, a surgeon (ophthalmologist, plastic surgeon, orthopedist) may employ a nurse who can also act as a scrub nurse in surgery at the hospital or assist in office surgery. With a current emphasis on primary care, preventive care, and managed care, many physicians are establishing practice groups in which physicians of the same or different specialties provide comprehensive quality medical care for their patients. This means a greater dependence on the office nurse to coordinate the activities in the office and address new problems in the delivery of ambulatory office care. In the larger practice or clinic milieu, several nurses are usually employed as part of a larger staff. Nurses may be employed as part of a team with other technical and professional personnel providing services like x-ray, laboratory, electro-cardiograms and other cardiac procedures, electroencephalograms, physical therapy, pharmacy, nutrition counseling, laser procedures, preventive maintenance, and wellness counseling.

Providing patient education, often of a preventive or rehabilitative nature, is one of the primary functions of office nurses. If nurses are offered the autonomy to initiate programs, they can contribute to the health and welfare of patients, their families, and the community at large. The ability to exercise this initiative in providing ongoing patient education programs may mean developing patient education based on the unique needs of an individual patient or helping to conduct larger-scale office or community programs. Office nurses are involved with teaching patients and/or the public at large about hypertension, diabetes, cholesterol, tobacco cessation, exercise, weight loss, and other topics that promote health or manage existing disease. Obviously, the nurse's ability to exercise this autonomy and initiative is predicated on the philosophy of the individual physician employer or group of employers, the mission of the practice, and the teamwork and cooperation of the physician.

Office nurses must have excellent teaching and communication skills, exhibit organizational and leadership ability, possess good assessment skills, be familiar with community resources, and have good insight in order to anticipate and interpret the needs of their patients. In today's competitive health care climate, they are also called upon to assist the physician in marketing the medical practice, to be a public relations agent to promote the retention of existing patients, and to function as a patient advocate as the patient moves through the medical maze of support services.

While some physicians and larger clinics may employ nurse practitioners with expertise in specific specialty areas to assume responsibility for patient care, most offices depend on the registered nurse to assume these responsibilities along with the accountability for running the office, scheduling patients, hiring, evaluating,

and scheduling staff, and generally overseeing the smooth operation of the office. Today, office nurses are seeking continuing education and collegiate education specific to office practice, office management, and organizational leadership.

Qualifications and Conditions of Employment. All office nurses must be licensed to practice and currently registered in the state in which they work. Although not usually required, education beyond the basic nursing program is desirable. In most cases, nurses have also had previous nursing experience.

Salaries and working conditions in this field, generally speaking, are varied, based on the needs of each specialty practice, the region of the country, and the employer. Salaries may be lower than those offered to acute care nursing counterparts, and benefits are also negotiable with the employer. Office nurses sometimes say that they are willing to make some financial sacrifices because there are other benefits: there are no shift rotations, they often do not work weekends, and they can negotiate their schedules to meet their current needs. There is, however, the possibility of evening or overtime hours based on practice needs.

Some of the most common fringe benefits include paid vacation and holidays, paid sick leave, year-end bonus, and free medical care for the nurse and family. A point of negotiation when seeking employment is medical-surgical or hospitalization insurance, malpractice insurance, pension or retirement plans, and tuition reimbursement and time off to attend continuing education courses and meetings. Although they may be named on the physician's malpractice insurance policy, nurses should carry their own malpractice liability insurance. (This is a point to inquire about at the time of hire.)

Although salary and fringe benefits are likely to be lower than those for the hospital staff nurse, many nurses prefer the field of office nursing because of the professional benefits: they can enjoy being an active and contributing member of the medical team, they can exercise initiative in the delivery of care and patient education, they can be instrumental in the development of office policies and protocols, they can exercise autonomy in suggesting ways to improve the delivery of quality care, and they can exercise their organizational and leadership skills in managing the office.

Those considering a career in office nursing should discuss all aspects of their work and employment conditions in detail with their prospective employer. It is important to make sure that they will be free to function in a nursing capacity and that the employer is in accord with what the nurse expects the role to be. A written job description is critical to mutual understanding of the role and its responsibilities. A written contract setting forth the professional and personal agreements between the nurse and the employer can also be mutually beneficial.

NURSING EDUCATION

Just a few years ago as nursing was straining to control the shortage, there was an outcry for more faculty. The lack of adequate qualified faculty was seen as a major obstacle to educating the numbers of nurses needed. Fewer nurses with advanced degrees were in academia because salaries in health care delivery settings, most particularly hospitals, had increased significantly. Further, the health care industry was beginning to see value in advanced practice nurses. As resources become more constrained in the industry, these APNs are also the first to go unless they have established their value. And so some may have returned to teaching. National League for Nursing 1992 data show no shortage of nurse faculty. There has been substantial growth in part-time faculty in all program types. Further, vacancy rates, the number of unfilled budgeted positions, at the nation's nursing schools remain relatively low (4.1 percent in 1992).[98] But there are other questions that remain unanswered. Are the budgeted positions a proper indicator of need given the economic constraints in higher education? The stu-

dent-faculty ratio has increased during this same period from 12:1 to 13:1 in associate degree programs, and 9:1 to 11:1 in diploma schools, with only baccalaureate programs experiencing a decrease from 10:1 to 8:1.[99] The qualifications of faculty beyond the basic academic credential are another issue.

Master's degrees have been recommended as a minimum for teachers in all nursing programs, and doctorates for deans of collegiate programs and faculty of graduate programs. Because general university standards require a doctorate for teaching positions at almost any level, there is now more pressure for nurses to adhere to this standard (see Chaps. 12 and 13).

The philosophy, objectives, students, and conditions of employment vary in different kinds of nursing education programs. Nurses planning to teach should give thought to the kind of program with which they can identify philosophically and in which they can function effectively. The number and types of positions within each program depend upon the size of the student body, the curriculum content, the faculty organization, and the school's philosophy, aims, and budget. There is a place in some schools for a nurse instructor of sciences, but in most schools, students take courses in physical and social sciences taught by nonnurse instructors at their own or another college or university.

Most nurse teachers are employed to teach nursing in the area of their clinical expertise, but trends toward nursing curriculum "models" may mean the adjustment of the teacher to differing approaches. In associate degree and practical nurse programs, the teacher may be expected to teach a variety of nursing subjects. Other specific differences in settings may also be noted.

Certain aspects of a faculty position are the same regardless of the educational setting. Faculty have certain responsibilities to the total program, usually through committees. Some are development and updating of philosophy, objectives, and conceptual framework, and selecting appropriate courses to meet those objectives; selection, evaluation, and promotion of students; assisting in developing educational and faculty standards, policies, and procedures; participating in promotion and tenure of faculty; developing special projects; and planning for the future. In a university or college setting, the teacher is expected to participate in campus-wide committees of the same nature. In relation to the student, a basic role is teaching in the classroom, laboratory, and clinical setting, individually or in groups, using appropriate and effective techniques with current knowledge and practice in the area of expertise. Advisement and personal and career counseling of students are also important; some teachers are class or student committee advisers and consultants as well. In the college and university settings, research and publication are major expectations; generally the teacher must seek outside funding for research. Almost equally important is service to the profession and the community, as officers of organizations, members of committees, as consultants, or speakers.[100]

Differences in teaching in the various programs relate to both the setting and the level. In universities, particularly medical centers, there is a trend toward joint appointments, with the teacher carrying a patient case load and, occasionally, administrative responsibilities in the clinical setting. In some cases, teachers are reimbursed additionally for this duty. Some set up a group faculty practice in which they deliver direct care to patients.

Graduate faculty are expected to be scholarly and research oriented, for, as well as teaching, they will be directing graduate students' research. They are encouraged to work closely with graduate faculty in other disciplines. They may be expert teachers and practitioners in a particular clinical specialty and/or in nursing administration, nursing education, or other graduate-level studies. Working with graduate students on special projects and guiding or supervising their research may mean spending hours with the student in conference and in committee presentations for the master's thesis or doctoral dissertation, including certain administrative responsibilities. The paper work in most teaching is extensive.

There are students of superior academic and intellectual ability and high motivation in all programs, but certain baccalaureate and almost all graduate programs have a more homogeneous selection, because high admission standards generally screen out those of lesser ability. However, just about all students are much more challenging and demanding than they were ten years ago; they want participation rights, they ask questions, and they don't accept pat answers.

Faculty in college- or university-based programs have the advantage of being in an academic setting with broad interdisciplinary contacts and campus activities. They may have joint appointments in other departments or schools and other responsibilities there. They also have the benefits and problems of being in such a setting; the policies and regulations are less directly controllable. Students in collegiate programs affiliate or rotate through a number of hospitals, agencies, or facilities. Unless the program is in a medical center, or unless the teacher holds a joint appointment, students and teachers maintain somewhat of a guest status and find it more difficult to affect care. If other students are also present, there is competition for good "teaching" patients.

On the other hand, in diploma programs, basic nursing education is significantly influenced by the hospital. Nursing classes and often clinical practice are given in that particular school and hospital, although students may go to other clinical settings. Because of geographic proximity and the fact that hospitals often think of the diploma students as "their" students and future employees, there may be a closer relationship between nurses in the clinical area and the faculty. Often the chief nurse executive has overall responsibility for both nursing service and nursing education, and there are opportunities for both service and education personnel to plan and work together on joint projects related to the hospital in general. Usually there is more national prestige in being affiliated with a university program, but other schools with strong community ties are highly respected.

The teaching opportunities in practical nurse programs offer another type of challenge to the nurse educator. The method of teaching and the philosophy of vocational education differ somewhat from those of professional education. The course of study usually is limited to one year. The setting may be in hospitals, public schools, or community colleges, among which both philosophy and environment vary considerably. It is important that the professional nurse teaching in these programs understand and respect the role of practical nurses in giving patient care and be able to teach accordingly.

Qualifications and Conditions of Employment. Besides the educational requirements, teachers in all nursing programs are expected to have a knowledge of nursing in general and continuously updated knowledge and clinical expertise in the subject area in which they expect to teach. They also need knowledge and skill in curriculum development, the teaching-learning process, and teaching methods and techniques. It is equally important for any prospective teacher to establish rapport with students, and to be open-minded and secure enough to welcome differences in opinion. Evaluation of teacher effectiveness is an ongoing process in a progressive educational setting and includes self-evaluation and evaluation by students, peers, and administrative heads. The quality of teaching is considered in retention and promotion of faculty.

It is also often expected that the teacher will be scholarly and make contributions to nursing through participation in professional activities and/or publications. A teacher in an institution of higher education may be appointed at any level from instructor to full professor, depending on his or her qualifications (and the need of that institution for that individual). Tenure and promotion depend on fulfilling stated requirements.

Tenure in colleges and universities means basically that the individual has a secure place in that institution and cannot be dismissed except under unusual circumstances. Usually there is a span of time (7 years or so) during which the person must be tenured or leave, unless put in some special category outside the tenure track. The more prestigious the institution, the higher the standards for appointment, promotion, and tenure. If university teaching is to be a nurse's career, a plan for doctoral education is a must and a postdoctoral research experience would be wise.

Salaries and fringe benefits vary, and in an institution of higher learning are supposed to be the same as for an individual in another discipline at the same rank. A full professor at the last salary step may earn as much as or more than the administrator of that particular program. Salaries are reported frequently by AACN.

Teaching positions in any educational program usually demand irregular working hours. Except for scheduled classes, the amount of time a teacher will spend at work is unpredictable because there are so many influencing factors, such as class and clinical preparation time, student conferences, student evaluation, participation in school committees and meetings, library study, and participation in student activities.

Teachers are also involved in professional activities, updating their own clinical practice, and advancing their education. Depending on where they teach, they may be able to set their own hours as far as presence in the school is concerned (except for scheduled classes) or may be expected to put in a 40-hour or more week on a regular 8-hour daily basis. It is estimated that the average university nurse teacher spends about 56 hours a week on the job. However, faculty are usually freer than other nurses to attend educational and other meetings. Nurses selecting a career in this field will want to analyze the conditions of each employment opportunity to make sure that it offers them as much as possible of what they want most in both material and professional rewards, and an atmosphere in which they can do their best work.

For a teacher, often the greatest reward is the intellectual and personal stimulation of an educational environment, including interaction with students and peers.

Administration in Nursing Education

At the head of each education program in nursing is a professional nurse who is both administrator and teacher. Nursing education administrators need preparation in administration as well as teaching. Again, it is best, and sometimes required, that the director of the program take graduate courses in educational administration.

Such courses are only rarely available in graduate nursing education programs, so those whose goal is education administration often acquire experience as assistants to a top administrator or in minor administrative positions and apply principles from nonnursing management courses. In some colleges and universities, department chairmen or deans are appointed administratively on recommendation of the faculty for limited terms, after which they return to nonadministrative faculty positions. This approach has advantages and disadvantages. It gives presumably competent faculty members an opportunity in the administrative role, but it may not be considered desirable by the individual whose primary interest is educational administration and who must then relocate to remain in a top administrative position.

Qualifications for nursing administration positions in education usually include experience in nursing and nursing education and frequently in administration of some kind. This nurse should be able to relate well to others in the nursing program, in the profession, in the particular setting of the school, and in the community. The need for leadership qualities is frequently cited. A minimum of a master's degree is usual, and the dean, director, or chairman of a collegiate or university program in nursing is expected to have a doctoral degree. It is also not uncommon to expect these candidates to have achieved national prominence in the nursing field, and to have published and done research.

Frequently, when a top administrative position is open, a search committee, composed according to institutional criteria, looks for, screens, interviews, and recommends an individual after a national search.

The top administrative post of any nursing education program usually requires both long hours of work on the job and active participation in professional activities. If in a college or university, the administrator is expected to be a leader in campus-wide committees and activities. There may be pressure from the faculty, students, administration, and community, all trying to achieve their own ends. Often there are financial problems for the school. There is little time for nurse administrators to keep abreast of their own clinical field, for the demand to keep current on administrative, educational, and general nursing trends is immediate. This is not a position for someone who cannot learn and act quickly and who wilts under pressure. The rewards, however, can be great professionally, in the satisfaction of accomplishments of the nursing program, its faculty, and students, and in the opportunity to be in a leadership position in nursing and in health care. Insights into some desirable attributes for this role may be found in the section on the nurse executive earlier in this chapter.

Salaries, fringe benefits, and sometimes rank and tenure tend to be negotiable and usually depend on a number of factors related to the position, the community, and the qualifications of the nurse.

NURSE RESEARCHER

For some time, nurses have been participating in medical research, often as gatherers of data rather than researchers. They still do, although some are gaining status as researchers in general health research and in nursing research (see Chap. 14 on nursing research and researchers).

Nurses in research may function in a variety of roles, depending on their educational preparation. If the nurse has not had doctoral preparation or research training, working on a research team as a research assistant or associate, collecting data, or doing some data analysis may be a start. Fully prepared nurse researchers are in great demand. They may find employment in universities and health institutions or may choose to freelance as consultants. The need is greater than either the supply of qualified nurses or the funds available for research. The majority of nurses with doctoral degrees have taken positions in universities and colleges, either as professors of nursing or as administrators, where they engage in both research and teaching. This is considered a compatible and necessary combination, because they not only increase knowledge of nursing but train other nurses in research and guide their studies. The need to recruit nursing students early for graduate study and research is important for the development of nursing.

A particularly encouraging trend is the employment of nurse researchers in practice settings, such as medical centers and government. In these positions, nurse researchers may have responsibility for studying patients' nursing needs, defining and evaluating patient care effectiveness, setting up testing situations for development of new nursing techniques, equipment, or procedures, acting as advisers or consultants to nurses developing patient research projects, and planning with other disciplines for the improvement of patient care.[101] Nurse researchers may also become research project directors, directors of research institutes, or be full partners in an interdisciplinary research team.

Qualifications and Conditions of Employment. Nurses engaged in research as described here are expected to have research training and ability that are verified both through their educational credential, the doctorate, and their experience. Personally, they must have the ability both to do creative thinking and to carry through the orderly process of research, which with human beings is seldom static or orderly, and the writing skill to report their findings. Nurses holding university positions earn the same salaries and benefits as other nurse teachers in that setting. Although time may be allotted for research, the funding of this research is often the responsibility of the teacher-researchers, and they must become adept at grantsmanship. There are also nurses hired by universities to head or participate in specific research projects, without teaching responsibilities. These positions are often on a short-term basis and may have been initiated by someone else. Most researchers find that they devote considerable time to their studies, and working hours are often not in a regular forty-hour-a-week framework. This is particularly true if the researcher also has teaching and/or administrative responsibilities.

If employed in a clinical setting, the nurse researcher's salary is probably negotiable, depending on her or his background. Although such positions may be budgeted, there may be very limited budgeting for other personnel and equipment needed for specific research projects. Again, funds must be sought from other sources, such as foundations, individuals, or, most frequently, governmental agencies. The availability of these funds has fluctuated, which has been a detriment to nursing research.

For nurse researchers, however, the satisfactions are great, in terms of both the personal satisfactions of research and the knowledge that they have made meaningful contributions to the nursing field. With all the opportunities available to nurses with doctoral degrees, it is certain that those engaged in research do so because it is their first preference.

NURSE CONSULTANT

There are professional nurse consultants specializing in all areas of nursing—education, administration, and clinical practice, particularly specialties—who provide assistance to individuals and groups. Because the usual purpose of seeking consultation is to bring about change of some kind, which may be a tension-provoking situation for the clients, not just specific knowledge but also the ability to understand and communicate in complex human relations situations is important. Someone who cannot relate to others in a way that is appropriate to the situation will not be successful, regardless of expertise. A good consultant must get a clear and accurate picture of the total situation, attitudes, abilities, and commitment of the people involved, the problems, assets, resources, and other factors that are not always overtly presented or visible, and have the ability to critique and assist. Because consulting is usually done in a limited time span, clients must be stimulated to think productively about what they can and must do to continue the task. There is a difference between giving advice and being a consultant, for the professional role requires the ability to observe, assess, plan, and make accurate judgments and to present them in a way that is workable for the clients. Usually consultants are presented with a problem or a request to help develop a program or service. The consultant collects data, does a preliminary review, and then an analysis, based on information sent and frequently an on-site visit. The client may be given resource materials and a final written report with an analysis of the situation and recommendations for action.

Although many well-prepared nurses in top positions consult apart from their primary jobs (and this kind of prestige is considered desirable by some employers), professional consultants are usually employed in local, state, national, international, private, or governmental agencies and organizations. There are, for instance, consultants with the National League of Nursing (NLN), DHHS, state health departments, the World Health Organization (WHO), and private consulting firms, even private businesses. In the last case, the same aspects of business management apply as for nurses in private practice.[102] Fees may be negotiated or set according to specific criteria.

CASE MANAGER

All nurses manage the care of their patients. The presence of case managers, case coordina-

tors, or discharge planners does not eliminate that responsibility. The case manager as discussed here is a very intense and empowered role that is necessary only for a small number of patients.[103] It is not the case method for organizing the daily care of patients that was discussed earlier in the chapter, although there is a shared philosophy of comprehensiveness. The case manager is best situated in an integrated system of services, although many case managers are hospital-based and terminate their services with discharge and successful community or extended care placement. The benefit of moving with the patient across a continuum of services has resulted in a thriving market for independent case managers, and employment by third party payers or managed care programs. The case manager strives to secure the services that are preferred by the patient within the constraint of available resources. The case manager fosters independence, advocates on the patient's behalf, and supports decisions that are outcome driven and fiscally sensitive. The case manager ideally can authorize the disbursement of resources but does so cautiously in anticipation of the long-term needs of these patients, who are usually very resources-intensive. Practice occurs within an interdisciplinary model, which requires that case managers be secure in their identity as a nurse, and able to command respect from other disciplines.[104]

Although social workers have performed aspects of case management for years, today's more complex patients need a holism and clinical sophistication that makes the nurse the most appropriate case manager. Eighty percent of case managers are nurses. A minimum of a baccalaureate is required with a master's preferred. APNs with a specialty in the target population or community health experience are ideal.

PRIVATE DUTY NURSING

For many years, private duty nursing was second only to hospital nursing in its attraction for professional nurses, but each year has seen a decrease in the total number of nurses in this field of practice, particularly younger nurses.

Private duty nurses are independent practitioners in almost complete control of where they will work, when they will work, the types of patients they will care for, and when they will take vacation or days off. They are limited in what they can charge for services only by the prevailing fee in their community, which is not legally binding.

Private duty nurses make their availability for service known through a nurses' registry, an employment agency, local hospitals, and personal contacts with other nurses, doctors, and members of the community. Individual nurses may build up a list of "clients" composed of families and doctors who always try to engage them whenever they need private duty nurses. Some work only as specialists.

A private duty nurse is usually employed (by the patient or family) to nurse one patient in the hospital or home. Wherever they are, the nurse is responsible for the patient's care while with him or her. When the nurse leaves for any length of time, arrangements must be made for care in the interim. This is also done if the nurse wishes a day or so off after being with a patient continuously for a number of weeks.

Most patients requesting private duty nurses are quite ill, or at least require a great deal of care physically and/or mentally. Some examples may be individuals who have undergone serious surgery or patients with strokes, cancer, and burns. Moreover, there is always a percentage of patients who can afford three nurses around the clock and who simply wish to have someone constantly at hand. These patients may not be in critical condition but require an enormous amount of individualized care. Free from the pressures of time and heavy patient care loads that often harass the staff nurse, private duty nurses have the opportunity to give truly comprehensive professional care to their patients, with limited concern for hospital routines.

Qualifications and Conditions of Employment. For success in private duty nursing and greatest job satisfaction, the private duty nurse must have a genuine liking for people and must be able to adjust well to a wide variety of personalities, establishing and maintaining warm yet professional relationships with both patients and their families, no matter how long a case may last. This nurse must enjoy giving direct comprehensive nursing care to one patient. Naturally, it is necessary to be currently licensed in the state where the nurse practices, with the exception of times when patient and nurse may be traveling and residing temporarily in another state. It is also important to understand the legal implications of the position and use sound judgment to avoid inappropriate involvement or activities. Malpractice insurance is advisable.

As self-employed persons or independent contractors, private duty nurses are almost entirely on their own as far as retirement plans, Social Security payments, and payment of taxes are concerned. They have no sick leave benefits or paid vacations. They are their own business managers in every sense of the word.

The responsibility to keep updated is likely to be the private duty nurse's individual responsibility. Hospital in-service programs are usually available, as are workshops, institutes, and other programs, but no one makes arrangements for the independently practicing nurse. Such CE may be even more important for these nurses than for institutionally employed nurses, because even though theoretically the hospital nursing service is responsible for the overall nursing care of all patients, private duty nurses generally function with little or no supervision. This is obviously even more likely if the nursing care is given in the patient's home.

An 8-hour tour of duty is fairly standard throughout the country, but 12-hour shifts are not uncommon. Fees vary considerably from place to place; they may or may not be higher than those of a staff nurse per diem. Although it is generally agreed that there is sufficient employment available for private duty nurses in most areas, those nurses who limit their practice to the day shift, certain kinds of patients, and limited length of employment may find that they do not have the opportunity to work as much as they would like. Moreover, LPNs are being employed for private duty, particularly in the home, but also in some hospitals. The increased number of well-prepared NPs who are setting up independent private practice may also bring about changes in the private duty picture. Other trends are the tendency for hospitals to set up their own in-house agencies and require patients to hire from that pool. A central issue here is the status as an independent contractor, which was already introduced in the section on temporary nursing service agencies. It is the independent contractor issue that should weigh heavily in considering this practice option.

ENTREPRENEURS AND INTRAPRENEURS

While private duty nurses can be considered one of the first of the entrepreneurs, nurses in private practice seem to be a growing phenomenon. It is estimated that some 20,000 nurses have their own businesses. An entrepreneur is defined as one who organizes and manages a business undertaking, assuming risk for the sake of profit. Most of the studies on the characteristics of entrepreneurs, not thought to be typical of women, have focused on white males. However, Aydelotte, in a study of nurses in private practice, summarized the demographics and characteristics gleaned from a number of studies of female entrepreneurs. In general, these women were 35 to 45 years old, married with two to five children, had a father who was an entrepreneur, were firstborn children, and started their venture because of job frustration, interest, and recognition of an opportunity. They had a need for achievement, described themselves as risk-takers, and scored high on masculine-associated traits such as autonomy, aggression, independence, and leadership but not as high as female managers.[105]

In Aydelotte's own study of nurse entrepreneurs, some new data emerged. The vast majority (96.7 percent) were female; most were between 30 and 50 years old, married, with one to

three children. More than two-thirds had master's or doctoral degrees and 10 to 25 years' experience; they were certified in their specialty and belonged to one or more nursing professional organizations. Experience was a major factor, as only about 9 percent had less than 10 years' experience. Their reasons for initiating the entrepreneurial venture included a wish for independence, the opportunity to do so, and a lack of control and decision making in the workplace. (Unlike nonnurse entrepreneurs, they did not say they were frustrated.) Slightly over half were sole proprietors of their business and worked full time. Their clientele were about 64 percent urban, only about 18 percent earning less than $20,000 a year. The services offered were largely consultation, counseling, direct client and home care service, client education, and nursing continuing education, although a variety of other services were offered and more than one service was usual. Referrals came from clients, nurses, physicians, hospitals, clinics, and public health departments; these nurses also had contracts with agencies. Advertising was done through speaking engagements, flyers, newspapers, magazines, and newsletters. A few used radio and television; almost all were recommended to clients by word of mouth. The income range was tremendous, from less than $10,000 to more than $50,000 per year; most were under $50,000. A number worked in other positions, especially as educator, staff nurse, and manager, in order to supplement their income.[106]

Aydelotte also noted current patterns and future directions of entrepreneurial models, such as an independent professional nurses' association, preferred professional nurse provider organization, and nursing service organization, all somewhat similar to the IPA practices described in Chap. 7. In all cases, the nurse group would contract their nursing services to a hospital or other agency.[107]

For those who would set up a private practice it is essential to understand that setting it up and running it must be a businesslike process. There are basic decisions to be made: what kind of organization should be created (corporation, partnership, for-profit, nonprofit); by whom (nurses and other professionals); for whom; at what fees; what kind and how many employees will be needed; how to get clients (marketing); types of advertising; how to relate to other health professions; where the services will be offered; at what hours; and policies about telephone counseling and/or home visits (house calls). Early expenses include lawyers' and accountants' fees, space, furniture, equipment, supplies, telephone, insurance, stationery, postage, flyers, and brochures. Repeated obstacles or problems to most are the normal business aspects: employee contracts, salaries, benefits, tax deductions, fee preparation and collection, and the multitude of forms and records that must be kept. When federal or other contracts are involved, still more records are necessary.[108]

Intrapreneur is a term coined to describe a person who takes hands-on responsibility for creating innovation of any kind within an organization. As opposed to entrepreneurs, who leave a place of employment to start their own business, intrapreneurs work within the system to create exciting new things.[109]

The reader is referred to Pinchot's early work on intrapreneuring. In analyzing both the system and personal characteristics for the successful intrapreneur, he used the case study technique, interviewing pioneer intrapreneurs from a variety of backgrounds. He calls the intrapreneur the hedge against the "dead wood" syndrome in corporate America. Neither the entrepreneur nor the intrapreneur is taking the safer route; they are not better or worse, just different. The intrapreneur appears as follows:[110]

- Wants freedom, but access to resources …does not want to be totally self-reliant.
- Urgency to meet a timetable to some degree established by the system.
- Cynical about the system, but confident of ability to outwit it.
- An inside-outside orientation, regardless of position in the hierarchy.
- Likes risk, and is unafraid of being fired.
- Hides risky projects until comfortable about their eventual success.
- Mocks traditional status symbols, but plays the game flawlessly…manipulative.
- Values the presence of accessible networks.
- Seeks friends in high places for protection.

Examples of successful intrapreneurial activities are a new type of Kardex, an educational program for certain types of patients, a consultant group, educational materials developed by a nurse educator, and a community nursing center. Depending on the arrangements made, the nurse may receive royalties, direct payments, profits shared with the institution, income for the nursing department to be used in a variety of ways, or nothing extra financially at all, just freedom and excitement. An interesting approach is that of a self-managed group running a unit and being paid by the hospital.[111]

INTERNATIONAL NURSING

The nurse with a taste for adventure and a desire to see the world may enjoy a position with one of the agencies concerned with nursing in areas outside the United States. Such positions are almost invariably challenging and a little off the beaten track. At the same time, the qualifications are usually high, including special preparation in the area in which the nurse will be working.

World Health Organization

One agency to which nurses have turned for international health employment is the World Health Organization (WHO) and its regional office, the Pan American Health Organization (PAHO). Their major concerns currently are in primary care, but related activities in terms of education may also have priority. Because of changing emphasis and varying needs, it is best to contact these agencies for information on the type of positions available, the requirements, and the conditions of employment. However, generally it is necessary to have advanced education, experience, and language capability. The WHO headquarters is in Geneva, but PAHO can be contacted at 525 Twenty-third St. N.W., Washington, D.C. 20037.

Peace Corps

Since the Peace Corps began in 1961, it has employed both volunteer and staff nurses. Staff nurses serve in many of the sixty Peace Corps countries in the preventive and curative program developed to care for the volunteer. Here, too, there are changing priorities and variable funding, depending to an extent on the politics of the moment. Whether interested in a paid or volunteer position, it is best to contact the Peace Corps, P-301, Washington, D.C. 20526 for available opportunities and requirements. As a rule, it has been necessary for the nurse to be an RN, a U.S. citizen, and to have appropriate language skills for the country assigned, good health, stamina, and, of course, the necessary nursing skills.

Project HOPE

The purpose of Project HOPE has traditionally been to bring the skills and techniques developed by the American health professions to other peoples of the world in their own environment, adapted specifically to their needs and their way of life. HOPE is now engaged in a number of projects in the United States, as well as continuing some of its international activities. It is best to get updated information from Project HOPE, Millwood, Virginia 22646. However, as for the WHO positions, advanced education, experience, and language skills are required.

Other International Nursing Opportunities

A number of agencies place nurses internationally.[112] Almost every religious denomination supports some kind of missionary work in foreign countries. Nurses are usually welcomed in such activities because missionary work often includes some form of professional or semiprofessional health care activities. Nurses who select missionary nursing as their life's work must have a strong desire to nurse the sick and underprivileged, often in primitive surroundings; ability to teach religious principles by example, and possibly in religious classes; and knowledge of the language of the people in the regions assigned. They will have many opportunities to teach citizens and health workers of other lands. Missionary nurses must expect to find their rewards principally in personal satisfaction because missionary nurses usually earn a low salary for long hours of hard work. Nurses can obtain specific information about missionary nursing from their own church. Some mission groups accept volunteers who are not of their own religious faith.

Another major possibility in international nursing is occupational nursing for major industries (the multinationals) with overseas branches. On occasion, the governments, universities, hospitals, or industries of foreign countries also seek American nurses with all types of educational preparation. In recent years, Mideastern countries, particularly, have employed recruiters to fill staff and other positions in their hospitals. It is especially important to clarify the job role and functions, as well as personal living conditions, and to learn about the country, for some American women nurses have found it very difficult to adjust in Moslem countries. Limited opportunities are found with the federal government in countries where federal personnel are stationed, but these positions are first filled by transferring career personnel already in the agency.

In all cases, there are usually advertisements in newspapers or professional journals for these positions. If not, the nurse should make inquiries to the private company concerned or the appropriate federal agency.

OTHER CAREER OPPORTUNITIES

It would probably be impossible, or at least extraordinarily lengthy, to give information about every career possibility available for nurses. A list of specific *positions*, directly related to nursing, not even including specialization or subspecialization, runs into the hundreds when the diverse settings in which nursing is practiced are considered. Overall, these are clinical nursing, administration, education, or research (or a combination of all), but the specific setting brings its own particular challenges. They may require knowledge of another culture and the physical/psychosocial needs of these groups, such as nursing on an Indian reservation, or a new orientation to practice such as working in an HMO, or in juvenile court, or the prison system, or a methadone maintenance clinic.

In some cases, specialization or subspecialization, usually requiring additional education and training (because most generic education programs present only a brief exposure), becomes a new career path. There are any number of these and as each becomes recognized as a distinct subspecialty, involved nurses tend to form a new organization or a subgroup within ANA or some related medical organization to develop standards of practice. There are also many articles in journals and papers given at meetings about nursing in these various areas, so that a practicing specialty nurse can keep abreast of current practice; other nurses may also develop interest in new fields.

Specialization and subspecialization are not really new; operating room nurses have been practicing since the beginning of American nursing and coronary care nurses or enterostomal therapists are into their third decade. More recently, there is new emphasis and, consequently, a number of new educational programs in such areas as women's health care, family planning, thanatology, and sex education, all of which have an interdisciplinary context that brings additional dimensions to the practice.

When nurses assume positions such as editors of nursing journals, or nursing editors in publishing companies, they draw not only on their nursing background, but must learn about the publishing field and acquire the necessary skills.

Editing is not the same as writing, and the responsibility for putting out a journal or other publication has financial, administrative, legal, philosophical, and policy-making components. In the same vein, nurses employed as lobbyists, labor relations specialists, executive directors or staff of nursing associations, nurse consultants for drug or supply companies, and staff for legislators or governmental committees all use aspects of their nursing knowledge, but must learn from other disciplines not related to nursing and develop new role concepts. If they choose to maintain a nursing role and orientation as well, nursing is enriched and strengthened; if they abandon all identity with the profession, it may lose valuable input.

As health care and nursing expand, some nurses will develop new positions themselves, for which the need and the qualifications cannot now be determined. It seems safe to say, however, that opportunities and challenges in nursing today are practically unlimited.

REFERENCES

1. American Nurses' Association: *Nursing: A Social Policy Statement*, 2d ed. Washington, DC: The Association, 1994, p 14. (In draft.)
2. Aiken L: Charting the future of hospital nursing, in Lee PR, Estes CL (eds): *The Nation's Health*, 4th ed. Boston: Jones and Bartlett, 1994, pp 177–187.
3. Ibid.
4. Aiken L: The hospital nursing shortage: A paradox of increasing supply and increasing vacancy rates, in Harrington C, Estes: *Health Policy and Nursing*. Boston: Jones and Bartlett, 1994, pp 300–312.
5. Leavitt JK, Herbert-Davis M: Collective strategies for action, in Mason DJ et al (eds): *Policy and Politics for Nurses*, 2d ed. Philadelphia: Saunders, 1993, pp 166–183.
6. *Secretary's Commission on Nursing: Final Report*. vol I. Washington, DC: Government Printing Office, 1988.
7. McKibbon RC, Boston C: An overview: Characteristic impact and solutions, Monograph 1, in *The Nursing Shortage: Opportunities and Solu-*

tions. Chicago: The American Hospital Association and the American Nurses' Association, 1990.

8. Pay levels rise to record highs at NYC hospitals. *Am J Nurs* 93:71, July 1993.

9. Ehrat KS: Administrative issues and approaches. Monograph 2, in *The Nursing Shortage: Opportunities and Solutions*. Chicago: The American Hospital Association and the American Nurses' Association, 1990.

10. McCausland MP: Reward strategies in nursing practice, Monograph 4, in *The Nursing Shortage: Opportunities and Solutions*. Chicago: The American Hospital Association and the American Nurses' Association, 1990.

11. Klem R, Schreiber EJ: Paid and unpaid benefits: Strategies for nurse recruitment and retention. *J Nurs Adm* 22:52–56, March 1992.

12. Havens DS, Mills ME: Professional recognition and compensation for staff RNs: 1990 and 1995. *Nurs Econ* 10:15–20, January–February 1992.

13. Klinefelter G: Role efficacy and job satisfaction of hospital nurses. *J Nurs Staff Dev* 9:179–183, July–August 1993.

14. *Commission on the National Nursing Shortage: Final Report*. Washington, DC: Government Printing Office, 1991.

15. Ibid.

16. Begany T: Layoffs: Targeting RNs. *RN* 57:37–38, July 1994.

17. Healthcare consulting boom fuels cutbacks in RN staff. *Am J Nurs* 94:75, 78–80, April 1994.

18. McDaniel C, Stump L: The organizational culture: Implications for nursing service. *J Nurs Adm* 23:54–60, April 1993.

19. Moreau D: Implementing an expanded role: Rewarding experienced nurses. *Recruit Reten Rep* 5:1–3, June 1992.

20. Kamer M, Schmalenberg C: Job satisfaction and retention: Insights for the 90s, Part 2. *Nursing* 21:51–55, April 1991.

21. Ames A et al: Assessing work retention issues. *J Nurs Adm* 22:37–41, April 19

22. Porter-O'Grady T: *Autonomy in Nursing Practice*, Monograph 6. Chicago: The American Hospital Association and the American Nurses' Association, 1990.

23. American Nurses' Association: *Standards of Clinical Nursing Practice*. Kansas City: The Association, 1991.

24. Koerner JG et al: Implementing differentiated

25. Rowland HS, Rowland BL: *Nursing Administration Handbook*, 3d ed. Gaithersburg, MD: Aspen, 1992, pp 206–216.

26. Rowland, loc cit.

27. Jellinek MS et al: Primary nursing: Psychological implications. *Nurs Mgt* 25:40–42, May 1994.

28. Abts D et al: Redefining care delivery: A modular system. *Nurs Mgt* 25:40–43, 46, February 1994.

29. Joel LA, Patterson JE: Nursing homes can't afford cheap nursing care. *RN* 53:57–59, April 1990.

30. Lenkman S: *Work Re-Design on Nursing Units*, Part I. Hazelwood, MO: Lenkman & Associates, 1994.

31. Brett JL, Tonges MC: Restructured patient care delivery: Evaluation of the ProACT model. *Nurs Econ* 8:36–41, January 1990.

32. Rowland, loc cit.

33. Brubakken KM et al: CNS roles in implementation of a differentiated case management model…Primm's model of differentiated case management. *Clin Nurs Spec* 8:69–73, March 1994.

34. Lenkman, loc cit.

35. Zander K: Managed care and nursing case management, in Mayer GG et al (eds): *Patient Care Delivery Models*. Gaithersburg, MD: Aspen, 1990.

36. Wegner WD: Support services: Contributing to patient care. *Nurs Mgt* 25:64–66, 68, 70, February 1994.

37. Herrick K et al: My license is not on the line: The art of delegation. *Nurs Mgt* 25:48–50, February 1994.

38. Prescott PA: Nursing: An important component of hospital survival under a reformed health care system. *Nurs Econ* 11:192–199, July–August 1993.

39. The American Nurses Association: *Registered Professional Nurses and Unlicensed Assistive Personnel*. Washington, DC: American Nurses Publishing, 1994.

40. Lyons R: Cross training: A richer staff for leaner budgets. *Nurs Mgt* 23:43–44, January 1992.

41. Rowland, op cit, pp 563–568.

42. Sigmon P: Clinical ladders and primary nursing: The wedding of the two, in Brown B (ed): *Operations and the Working Environment*, Gaithersburg, MD: Aspen, 1994, pp 191–194.

43. Flanagan L: *Self-employment in Nursing.* Washington, DC: American Nurses Publishing, 1993.

44. Sanctions against temporary agencies providing service to an employer struck by MNA. *Mich Nurse* 58:11–12, January–February 1994.

45. Rowland HS, Rowland BL, op cit, pp 9–28.

46. Jones NK, Jones TW: The head nurse: A managerial definition of the activity role set, in Brown B (ed): *Dynamics of Administration.* Gaithersburg, MD: Aspen, 1994, pp 77–87.

47. Sovie M: Nurse manager: A key role in clinical outcomes. *Nurs Mgt* 25:30–34, March 1994.

48. Ponte PR, Capodilupo T: Nursing supervisors: Reduction-in-force or redesign. *Nurs Mgt* 23:34–38, January 1992.

49. Dunham J, Fisher E: Nurse executive profile of excellent nurse leadership, in Brown B (ed): *Dynamics of Administration.* Gaithersburg, MD: Aspen, 1994, pp 14–21.

50. American Nurses Association: *Standards for Nursing Professional Development: Continuing Education and Staff Development.* Washington, DC: American Nurses Publishing, 1992, p 5.

51. Ibid.

52. Ibid.

53. Ibid.

54. Ibid.

55. Orcutt MA et al: Associate infection control nurse. *Nurse Mgt* 23:50–51, January 1992.

56. Kibbee P: An emerging professional: The quality assurance nurse. *J Nurs Adm* 18:30–33, April 1988.

57. Advanced practice nursing: A new age in health care. *Nursing Facts.* Washington, DC: American Nurses Association, August 1993.

58. Stafford M, Appleyard J: Clinical nurse specialists and nurse practitioners, in McCloskey J, Grace HK (eds): *Current Issues in Nursing.* St Louis: Mosby, 1994, pp 19–25.

59. Hockenberry EM, Hodgson W: Merging advanced practice roles: The NP and CNS. *J Pediatr Health* 5:158–159, March 1991.

60. Stafford, loc cit.

61. Hamrick AB: History and overview of the CNS role, in Hamrick AB, Spross JA (eds): *The Clinical Nurse Specialist in Theory and Practice.* Philadelphia: Saunders, 1989, pp 6–39.

62. Stafford, loc cit.

63. Joel LA: Master's prepared caregivers in line positions: A case study. *Patterns in Specialization: Challenge to the Curriculum.* New York: National League for Nursing, 1986, pp 235–243.

64. *Nursing: A Social Policy Statement.* Kansas City: American Nurses' Association, 1980.

65. *Nursing Facts,* loc cit.

66. Ibid.

67. Stafford, loc cit.

68. American Nurses Association: *The Scope of Practice of the Primary Health Care Nurse Practitioner.* Kansas City: The Association, 1985.

69. Office of Technology Assessment: *Nurse Practitioners, Physician Assistants, and Certified Nurse Midwives: A Policy Analysis.* Health Technology Case Study 37, Washington, DC: Congress of the United States, 1986.

70. Brown SA, Grimes DE: *Nurse Practitioners and Certified Nurse-Midwives.* Washington, DC: American Nurses Publishing, 1993.

71. *Nursing Facts,* loc cit.

72. American Medical Association Report 35 of the Board of Trustees: Economic and quality of care issues with implications on scope of practice …physicians and nurses, Executive Summary. Interim meeting, 1993.

73. National Center for Health Statistics: *Monthly Vital Statistics Report, 1993,* vol 42 (no 3 suppl).

74. *Nursing Facts,* loc cit.

75. American College of Nurse Midwives: *Standards for the Practice of Nurse-Midwifery.* Standard IV, 1993.

76. *Nursing Facts,* loc cit.

77. *Study of Nurse Anesthetist Manpower Needs.* Washington, DC: DHHS, USPHS, National Center for Nursing Research, February 1990.

78. Rosenbach ML, Cromwell J: Datawatch: A profile of anesthesia practice patterns. *Health Affairs* 7:118–131, April 1988.

79. Rosenbach ML, Cromwell J: *Payment Options for Non-physician Anesthetists under Medicare's Prospective Payment System.* Report prepared under HCFA cooperative agreement No. 18-C-98759/1-02. Needham, MA: Center for Health Economics Research, January 1988.

80. Middelstadt PC: Federal reimbursement of advanced practice nurses' services empowers the profession, in Harrington C, Estes CL (eds): *Health Policy and Nursing.* Boston: Jones and Bartlett, 1994, pp 341–348.

81. Pearson LJ: Annual update of how each state stands on legislative issues affecting advanced nursing practice. *Nurs Pract* 19:11–44, 50, 53, January 1994.

82. Pearson, loc cit.

83. American Medical Association, loc cit.

84. *States with Some Form of Nurse Privileging.* Washington, DC: American Nurses Association, September 1993.
85. Washington Consulting Group: *Survey of Certified Nurse Practitioners and Clinical Nurse Specialists: December 1992 Final Report.* Rockville, MD: Division of Nursing, February 1994.
86. A star-spangled career. *American Journal of Nursing Career Guide,* 1994, pp 238, 240, 242.
87. Mezey M: GNPs on staff. *Geriatric Nurs* 11:145–147, May–June 1990.
88. American Nurses Association: *Standards: Community Health Nursing Practice.* Kansas City, MO: The Association, 1980.
89. American Public Health Association: *The Definition and Role of Public Health Nursing in the Delivery of Health Care.* Washington, DC: The Association, 1981.
90. Ibid.
91. National Academy of Sciences, Institute of Medicine: *The Future Public Health.* Washington, DC: National Academy Press, 1988.
92. Turnock BJ et al: Implementing and assessing organizational practices in local health departments. *Public Health Rep* 109:478–484, July–August 1994.
93. Moses EB: *The Registered Nurse Population, 1992.* Washington, DC: US Department of Health and Human Services, 1994, pp 22, 52.
94. National Association of School Nurses: *School Nursing Practice: Roles and Standards.* Scarborough, ME: The Association, 1993.
95. USDHHS: *Healthy People 2000: National Health Promotion and Disease Prevention Objectives.* Washington, DC: Government Printing Office, 1991.
96. Igoe JB, Giordano BP: *Expanding School Health Services to Serve Families in the 21st Century.* Washington, DC: American Nurses Publishing, 1992.
97. American Association of Occupational Health Nurses: *Standards of Occupational Health Nursing Practice.* Atlanta, GA: The Association, 1994.
98. National League for Nursing: *Nursing Data Review.* New York: National League for Nursing, 1994, pp 189–192.
99. Ibid.
100. Anderson CA: Nursing faculty, in McCloskey J, Grace HK (eds): *Current Issues in Nursing,* 4th ed. St Louis: Mosby, 1994, pp 32–37.
101. Oberst MT: The generalizability and clinical application dilemma. *Res Nurs Health* 14:iii–iv, June 1991.
102. Flanagan, loc cit.
103. Michaels C: A nursing HMO—10 months with Carondelet St. Mary's hospital-based nurse case management. *Aspen Advs Nurse Exec* 6:3–4, January 1991.
104. American Nurses' Association: *Nursing Case Management.* Kansas City, MO: The Association, 1988.
105. Aydelotte M et al: *Nurses in Private Practice.* Kansas City, MO: The Association, 1988, pp 19–20.
106. Ibid, pp 26–35.
107. Ibid, pp 55–60.
108. Carpenito LJ, Neal MC: Nurse entrepreneurs, in McCloskey J, Grace HK (eds): *Current Issues in Nursing,* 4th ed. St Louis, MO: Mosby, 1994, pp 43–48.
109. Pinchot G: *Intrapreneuring.* New York: Harper & Row, 1985.
110. Ibid.
111. Boyar D, Martinson D: Intrapreneurial group practice. *Nurs Health Care* 11:28–33, January 1990.
112. *See the World. AJN Career Guide for 1994.* New York: The Journal, 1994, pp 245–247.

Leadership for an Era of Change

AUTONOMY, LEADERSHIP, and change are presented together in this chapter because of their interdependence. Each is described and the dynamics of each discussed. They are applied to nursing situations to provide a flavor of reality, and so become more personally meaningful to the reader. These are not abstract concepts, but qualities that will distinguish nurses in all their dealings with the public. Professions are expected to change with the times, and nowhere is change more guaranteed and dramatic than in health care. Though human nature may tempt us to drag our feet, nursing will have to change to accommodate the world around it.

The previous chapters in this text have presented a challenging future with discussions of hospital downsizing, a shift of services into community settings, emergent markets for nursing services, industrywide movement into managed care, a focus on disease prevention and health promotion, new consumer rights, and the prominence of advanced practice nurses. If this weren't enough, we are confronted with a variety of models for "restructuring" the way day-to-day services arc provided to our patients and the manner in which nurses are governed or directed in their work. It is necessary for nurses to know when change occurs for the sake of change, and when it is in the best interest of the public. The magnitude of the decisions and the instability of the practice environment can work to our advantage, given that we understand the meaning of autonomy and can lead the way to a preferred future.

AUTONOMY

The public allows professionals a generous amount of freedom as they conduct their affairs. This freedom, better called autonomy, is based on the assumption that professionals are the stewards, not the owners of their fields of service. Because of the complexity of their work, professionals have superior judgment on the internal affairs of their field. However, whatever they do, they do on behalf of the public; and any violation of that contract can result in restrictions on self-governance.

Sociologists have identified autonomy as the most strategic (and cherished) distinction between a profession and an occupation or semi-profession. Components of autonomy which demonstrate our accountability to the public are licensure and certification, control of our educational systems, and a code of ethics. A distinction has been made between "job content" autonomy, the freedom to determine the methods and procedures to be used to deal with a given problem, and "job context" autonomy, the freedom to name and define the boundaries of the problem and role relationships with other providers. The keys to autonomy as applied to nursing are that no other profession or administrative force can control nursing practice, and that the nurse has latitude in making judgments in patient care within the scope of nursing practice as defined by the profession.

There are number of reasons why nursing does not have full autonomy. Early nursing in America did not assume an autonomous stance. In part, this was because most nurses were women, and female status was low at the time. Nurses, usually female, were constantly admonished to obey the physician, usually male, and to abide by his judgment about the patient's condition. Even though nurses were trained to observe, the next step was to report and wait for further direction. Acting on their own judgment of what to do for the patient lay within a very narrow area. Added to this was the nurse's position in the male-dominated hierarchy of the hospital (which, as it became larger, became a male-dominated bureaucracy).

As Ashley reported in her now classic work, nurses have been expected to be mother figures, giving freely (in the financial as well as the social sense) of their time and efforts to meet the needs of all members of the hospital family, from patients to physicians. She attributed nurses' lack of progress and accompanying low status to the fact that they are women and maintained that their work has been virtually ignored and trivialized in comparison to that of physicians. "Nursing's problems, rooted in the tradition of economic exploitation, inadequate education, and long-standing social discrimination, have plagued the profession for the greater part of its history."[1]

The fact that there were some early nurses who struggled free and were able to practice independently, primarily in public health settings, is evidence that there was from the beginning health care practice that was uniquely nursing. It is possible that we may have enjoyed more freedom in the past than in modern-day practice. Current restrictions on autonomy are both experienced in one's personal practice and by the discipline as a whole. The most blatant insult to nursing's autonomy in recent years was the American Medical Association's (AMA) plan to remedy the nursing shortage of the late

1980s by the creation of a new caregiver called the RCT (see Chap. 15). The common practice for government to consult with the AMA on health care legislation has often been presented as proof of the autonomy of American medicine. We can debate whether the interpretation is correct, but given that it is, American nursing has moved closer to that standard through the American Nurses Association's (ANA) prominence on Capitol Hill.

Ashley's theory that economic exploitation is one factor that has retarded the development of autonomy in nursing is well taken. By the 1990s, nurses had realized some significant salary gains. Additionally, as common in the rest of the population, many households were then and still are headed by a woman. This unique set of circumstances allows many women to make autonomous decisions about the use of their money. Case in point: the ANA Political Action Committee (ANA-PAC) raised over one million dollars to direct toward political endorsements in the nonpresidential election year of 1994.[2]

There are other indicators of progress toward autonomy for nurses. Shared governance models that bring staff nurses and nursing service managers together to achieve consensus on clinical management; peer review as a mechanism in retention and promotion; nursing staff organizations and the right to professional staff privileges when JCAHO or Medicare guidelines are applied as they are written; are all intermediate steps toward full autonomy.

Most nurses do not identify with the issues of autonomy as they are played out in the federal or state arenas.[3] They are more concerned with their personal practice.[4] Nurses have gravitated toward roles that hold the promise of autonomy. In advanced practice, this has usually been the NP; and for the staff nurse this has been primary nursing. It is interesting to note that both of these roles are highly focused on the primary relationship between the client and the provider. The autonomy in the NP role is greatly dependent on access to reimbursement in fee-for-service settings; prescriptive authority, and clinical staff privileges. These issues were discussed at greater length in Chap. 15. Primary nursing in its distinguishing features holds promise of autonomy,[5] but that will depend on how these qualities are played out given the presence of an administrative hierarchy. It is consistently agreed that the primary nurse:

- Is responsible for comprehensive and continuous care of the patient from admission to discharge.
- Involves the patient's significant support systems to facilitate smooth transition to discharge.
- Accesses others to the information they need to participate intelligently in care of the patient.
- Decides how nursing care will be administered, and communicates this to those who will share in implementing the plan.
- Participates in a communication triad with the physician and patient.
- Has ready access to peer support and participates in peer review.

Issues of professional autonomy may be particularly frustrating when the professional is an employee. The nature of these conflicts surfaced in a U.S. Supreme Court decision of May 1994. (See Chap. 25.) The decision places in question the distinction between those actions that an employed professional initiates as part of their autonomous practice in contrast to those that are initiated on behalf of the employer. The distinction is important and will be questioned more as professionals are less frequently entrepreneurs.

A LEADER AMONG LEADERS

Hein and Nicholson propose that leadership is "every nurse's domain."[6] In a contrary tone, Marriner reverts to the defeatist interpretation that nurses are overwhelmingly drawn from individuals low on self-esteem and initiative and higher on submissiveness and the need for struc-ture than people in other occupations.[7] While this might have been true of past generations, it is questionable whether nursing in the 1990s is attracting candidates with these characteristics. Those selecting nursing have changed dramatically. Nursing has become the preferred choice for the more mature learners who often choose nursing after an earlier career that in many cases held a variety of leadership successes, and who feel secure in their abilities. They demand state-of-the-art preparation for a challenging future that they are anxious to meet head-on. Personality studies comparing these students with earlier generations would contribute much to nursing's plans for leadership development.

In the ordinary course of events, leadership is often confused with management. In today's prevailing bureaucracy we are most usually overmanaged and underled.[8] The dichotomy between nurse-executives and nurse-managers presented in Chap. 15 is a good point of reference. In many ways, the executive in that comparison was the leader, although a leader does not necessarily have positional status. Managers focus on specific organizational goals and the tasks to accomplish those goals. The manager is assigned to a role. The leader has the interpersonal ability to cause people to respond, because they want to (and sometimes at considerable personal cost and inconvenience). In the best of worlds, managers have leadership ability, but it isn't guaranteed. Leaders are not always managers. As noted in Chap. 15, the most successful executives were endowed with vision, motivated followers to buy into that vision, shared just enough of their vision to motivate people without overwhelming them, and distinguished their relationships with humanism. They lived with human respect and expected no less from their followers.[9] These are only a few of the attributes about successful executives that are also commonly reported of successful leaders.

Theories of leadership are numerous. Most of them emphasize control, competition, power-wielding, and rationality and infer a hierarchy.[10] Most were developed using the scientific method, aiming to describe, understand, predict, and prescribe that elusive quality known as leadership. Aspiring leaders have been encouraged to select an approach most suitable to themselves or the situation at hand. Finding no suitable match, one could always create an eclectic style, borrowing from a variety of orientations. The major theoretical orientations for leadership assume a linear relationship (cause-effect) between a situation, the traits or status of the leader, and the capacity to lead:[11]

- *The great man theory*…Select people are born to leadership. The greatest of leaders possess skill in both instrumental (managerial) and supportive (true leadership) behaviors.
- *Charismatic theory*…The ability to lead is dependent on an emotional commitment from followers. Followers feel secure in the presence of the leader, which is particularly helpful when sacrifices are asked of followers that could only be expected based on personal loyalties. Many of our most successful revolutionary leaders have been described as charismatic. Note that the allegiance is to a specific person. Removal of that person can often result in loss of progress, unless there has been a planned strategy to transfer leadership to a new personality.
- *Trait theory*…Leadership ability can be acquired (or talent identified) given the fact that certain traits have been proved to be most commonly associated with leadership talent: intelligent, emotionally mature, creative and able to see novel solutions for problems, possessing initiative, speaks and writes clearly, listens carefully, able to derive meaning from even clouded communications, skilled at persuasion, a good judge of people, social and socially adaptable.
- *Situational theories*…Leadership depends on the situation. Who will be the most successful leader at any one point in time is relative, depending on the best match

with the circumstances: amount of pressure, task at hand, technical demands, closeness of the working relationship, and on and on.

- *Contingency theory*…A three-dimensional model that aims to create the best fit between leader-follower relations, the task at hand, and the resources or support that can be accessed by the leader due to their position or status.
- *Path-goal theory*…The leader structures work for subordinates and removes obstacles so that they can be successful. Caring and consideration is added to the leadership prescription based on the needs of the group.
- *Life cycle theory*…The most appropriate leadership style is based on the maturity of the followers. With growing maturity there is less need for structure, and a greater need to assume an active role in the work at hand. The leader must be able to adjust to periods of regression if they should occur.

Whereas these varied perspectives on leadership are interesting and provide a useful orientation, it is difficult to control events or predict the nature of any situation. There are new paradigms (models) of leadership that respond to the uncertainty of the times and look to the human relationship to provide stability.[12] This represents the converse of earlier models, where the presumed instability was in the human relationships.

A body of knowledge has begun to take shape around the dynamic of transformational leadership. A transformational model assumes situational instability. In most earlier models, which are transactional, differences between the leader and the follower are seen as the major point of departure for planning and analysis. In a transformational context, the cause-and-effect relationship is not primary; rather the goal is for the leader and the followers to fuse and evolve toward a shared agenda. All parties grow and develop through the process.[13] Transformational leadership is process-oriented. In his discussion of organizations that will thrive in our age of uncertainty (and sometimes chaos), Senge proposes the following strategies[14] (the leadership counterpart is obvious):

- The whole is greater than the sum of its parts...You cannot think of your work as isolated from the larger system. Whereas earlier studies of leadership expected only the designated leader to focus on events external to the primary system, newer thinking expects that all participants will have this broadened view.
- Look internally for solutions to problems. This is actually a by-product of the "tunnel vision" described in the first characteristic. As we become too preoccupied with ourselves, we cease to appreciate that what we do has consequences beyond the boundaries of our system and will come back to compound our problems. As we are exposed to this boomerang effect, it becomes more comfortable to blame external factors that are more usually beyond our control.
- The voguish strategy is to become proactive or to rise to address difficult issues before we are faced with crisis management and forced into a reactive mode. All too often, we are still reacting, though at an earlier stage in the development of the issue. We should look internally for the answers, because it is the only system that we can hope to reform successfully. In other words, "the illusion of taking charge" is just that, an illusion.
- We are hampered by our preoccupation with events and short-term planning. Survival in today's environment of rapid change demands a search for themes, and the identification of trends over time. The events are cues to longer-term patterns of change. DRGs, final directive requirements, and Peer Review Organizations are each events that drew strong reactions from the health care community. Manag-

ing these issues diverted effort from the more basic concerns: the need for cost reduction in acute care, the struggle of consumers to regain control of their choices in the health care system, and consumer suspicion of the industry and provider professionals.

- We tend to adapt to threats to our survival rather than to see them for what they are and respond. The deep penetration of the Japanese into the U.S. car market occurred over a period of many years. Seeing threats for what they are requires us to slow down, compare situations across time, and attempt to forecast.
- Even given the rapid pace of change, it is difficult or impossible today to learn from your mistakes. Decisions made at one time and place will impact people and events in a distant time and place, often generations away. Consequences of many of our actions will be forever hidden from our eyes. The best hedge against doing harm is to assure that leadership for the far-reaching issues cross functional lines. Examples of the application of this strategy can be seen in the Robert Wood Johnson Teaching Nursing Home Program of the 1980s and the current Pew Charitable Trust's project to strengthen hospital nursing.[15,16] In each of these instances, the active participation of the entire executive team from each funded site is required. Leaders must be able to work beyond their primary discipline.
- The traditional image of the team is useless for today's problems. Over time most teams invest more effort maintaining their image of cohesiveness than participating in the process of change. Better suited to the times is a model of collegiality and the mechanism of dialogue. Here everyone has something to contribute and no proposal is dismissed. This decidedly transformational style is inconsistent with the inevitable hierarchy in transactional leadership models. In nursing, the work of

Jean Watson and her proposals for creating a learning environment reflect some of these principles.[17] The role of the leader evolves into one of developing people, actually instigating openness and honesty while removing the threat of reprisals. The leader often assumes the position of consultant on process and facilitator, as opposed to expert and controller…a very difficult transition for those socialized into the traditional mode of leadership.

Transformational leadership focuses on creating the social architecture to sustain a vision, and the attitudes and behaviors that allow progress in these uncertain times. This brand of leadership builds on organizational trust first, because of the organization's likelihood of greater permanence, and then on leaders with positive self-regard and a capacity for humanism.[18]

The trick is to bridge the gap between transactional and transformational leadership. The insights generated by the transactional school of thinking are not to be dismissed but should be enhanced with new assumptions and ways of operating. The autocratic, democratic, and laissez-faire styles of management (often equated with leadership) are naive.[19] Rather, as an intermediate step in transition, the literature supports directive, collaborative, and collegial leadership patterns, each selected to suit the mix of individuals and the challenge at hand.[20] Nurses will be expected to lead as they manage their practice and the care of each of their patients. Broader leadership challenges will find nurses as leaders among leaders. The collegial style is proposed as the natural complement for leadership among peers. In this context, leadership is relative and functional only once it is legitimized by the group. In other words, the claim to leadership must be achieved. Collegial leaders are catalytic, not merely consultative. They don't build teams but integrate the assets of the group. Although the "buck" does stop somewhere, leadership is shared, as is the responsibility and recognition for success. Communication

is authentic and multidimensional, with emphasis on the content and the manner in which it is received rather than the form. Supervision and motivational techniques are nonexistent because these qualities reside in the individual.[21] Shared vision, responsibility, and accountability are more than rhetoric, and prompted several agencies of the federal government to design a pay-for-performance merit system that would properly recognize contributions within a system operating in such a transformational manner, rewarding a group, it being impossible to single out any individual.

Despite any transformations or miracles, the leader still stands out and fulfills some useful role. One such role admittedly smacking of paternalism, but real and valued by followers, is that of buffer or protector. Leaders may advocate or buffer their subordinates from external forces, the organization, other members of the leadership, fellow employees, medical staff, top administration, and even one another. Buffering is accomplished by more closely coordinating work and being clearer on the unity of command (orders come from one person and only one person unless specifically instructed otherwise). Other situations may require conflict resolution, confrontation, or negotiation.[22]

During the late 1970s and 1980s, there was a series of studies of leadership in nursing that used an inductive or case study approach. In chronological order the investigators or authors were Safier, Vance, Kinsey, and Schorr and Zimmerman.[23–27] Each of the influentials who were studied had demonstrated their leadership acumen. They ranked the following qualities as most important to their success (in the order as presented):

- Communication skills
- Intellectual ability
- Willingness to take risks
- Interpersonal skills
- Creativity
- Ability to mobilize people
- Recognition in the profession
- Charisma

An unremarkable and highly predictable list. However, there is one remarkable observation that comes from these biographers. In other professions, leaders are as likely to be drawn from the ranks of practitioners (those who directly do the work of the field) as from individuals who maintain a career identification but do not practice their profession directly (positional leaders), such as teachers, researchers, and administrators. This was not true for nursing in 1983, where most influentials were positional leaders, as opposed to clinicians.[28]

Much is written, in these studies and elsewhere, about the price of leadership: the loneliness at the top, for instance, and it has been said that a good leader must get over the need to be loved and must learn to function without the need for approval of others. No leader can please all of his or her constituents all the time. To lead inevitably requires commitment; at times the leader must sacrifice personal desires, interest, time. The rewards, of course, are to see goals that one believes in met and to know that this might not have happened without one's leadership.

ASPECTS OF POWER

Autonomy and opportunities for leadership do not come to the spineless, the powerless, the indifferent or downtrodden, or those who think they are. As members of a profession who are obliged not only to participate in change but to provide the leadership to make things happen, an understanding of the dynamics of power is essential.

Power is the ability to influence the behavior of others to produce certain intended effects.[29] Power can be actual or potential (indicating power as latent or undeveloped, but still a force to be reckoned with). Power can be directly applied to the point where effect is desired, or indirect so that the nature or source of the power is more discreet or even undetected. Power can be a means to an end, or even an end in itself (the existence of latent power can sometimes achieve

the desired results). Power varies in quantity, scope, legitimacy, its degree of humanism (benevolent vs. destructive), and whether it is situationally unilateral or bilateral.[30]

Power is usually seen as a social relationship. It is given, maintained, or lost within those relationships. Individuals derive power from certain sources or bases, and then use that power according to their personal power orientation. This orientation indicates how an individual perceives or values power. Is power an essential part of one's identity, even if it is never used constructively? "He could do so much good if he only wanted to." Is power interpreted as the exclusive possession, something that is not shared? "You never quite feel that she is telling you everything."

A typology of power bases deriving from the work of many authors is as follows:

- *Coercive power*...real or perceived fear of one person by another.
- *Reward power*...perception of the potential for rewards or favors by honoring the wishes of a powerful person.
- *Legitimate power*...derives from an organizational position rather than personal qualities.
- *Expert power*...knowledge, special talents, or skills held by the person.
- *Referent power*...power flowing from admiration, or charisma, usually rooted in similar backgrounds or some other mutual identification.
- *Information power*...exclusive access to information needed by others.
- *Connection power*...privileged connections with powerful individuals or organizations.
- *Collective power*...ability to mobilize a critical mass or a system on your behalf.

It is well to emphasize that power is given. Further, we often infer that people who claim to have power actually do, but when studied more carefully, they have no claim or legitimacy. Additionally, power invariably fills any vacuum.[31] People generally want peace and order. In situations of stress or chaos, someone will come forward and will be given the power to restore order. Many critical issues return us to the incident of the AMA and the RCT. In 1988, organized nursing had done very little to control the nursing shortage, which was perceived by the public as a crisis. The vacuum was there and the AMA moved forward to fill it with their proposal for a new category of bedside caregiver in hospitals.

The power base of individuals in combination with their power orientation allows prediction on how they will function and provides you with a model to identify your own capacity and style. It can also provide direction for what people expect before they will *give* power. Power may be seen exclusively or in combination as:[32]

- *Good*…power as natural and desirable and used in an open and honest manner. Would probably build on expert, reward, and legitimate power bases.
- *Resource-dependent*…power depending on possession of things, including information, property, wealth. Associated with withholding patterns in the information power base. Greatly diminished in a computer age and the growing presence of transformational leadership.
- *Instinctive drive*…power as a personality attribute, and usually associated with referent power.
- *Charisma*…influence over people through personal magnetism. Power often given to people who are ill prepared or even destructive, and could stifle the growth of those who do the giving.
- *Political*…drawing heavily on referent, connection, and collective bases, power is linked to an ability to negotiate the system.
- *Control and autonomy*…the power broker always calls the shots operating from a base of coercion, information, and connection.

Power and influence are sometimes equated, because both affect or change the behavior of others; however, when they are separated, it is on the theory that power is the potential that must be tapped and converted to the dynamic thrust of influence.[33] Almost all authorities agree that a person or group must be valued on some level in order to have power or influence, again reinforcing the interpersonal dimension of the concept.

Another interesting commentary on power says that no one individual or group necessarily dominates, but that power is diffused in the community. Power may be tied to issues and shift accordingly. Here we see what might be considered nursing power at a national level. Certain influential nurses are usually easily identified, often because of their positions, and may be courted or simply more likely to be heard because they are thought to have influence with nurses (and, of course, they may). On the other hand, there are times when power clearly resides in a group, as when, at the 1982 ANA convention, state nurses' association executives and officers were probably the key actors in moving ANA to adopt a federation model.

Maraldo claims that "power to influence others requires a high level of skill in the strategic manipulation of impressions toward others…. Seekers of power who are skilled at cajoling, flattering, comforting, hedging, exhorting, exploiting, and exciting colleagues and higher-ups alike have an emporium of all the instruments they need to influence others."[34] She adds that manipulation is not always bad and gives an example of how a lobbyist successfully manipulated someone who would not listen to her by having a number of people that that person respected and liked (because of their power, position, or other characteristics) to show support for the quite worthwhile project the lobbyist was promoting. Maraldo also noted that powerful persons have some of the same pain of failure and rejection, the same fears and inadequacies as others, but never let it show. "They always appear to be in command of the situation—even when they are quivering inside."[35]

Does nursing have power? Considering these concepts, it is clear that nursing has the *potential* for power with its overwhelming numbers, its special knowledge and skill, and its place in public trust and has, in fact, already exercised that power successfully. Nursing leaders also have power of various kinds, including positional power in high government policy-making positions. But what of nurses as individuals? They are still complaining of lack of power on the job—the lack of autonomy and of involvement in budget setting and in policy making. Yet nurses do not seem to reach out to fill any vacuum, or mobilize their constituency, or capitalize on their position at the center of health care information networks. Is it a historical pattern of obedience to authority, which has been transmitted by education and practice? Is it their social, cultural, or economic background? Is it because, according to personality tests, nurses have a low power-motive? Is it that they think they don't have what it takes to be powerful and influential—for whatever reason? Groups or individuals "choose" to obey for a number of reasons: habit, fear of sanctions, moral obligation, self-interest, psychological identification with someone in charge, indifference, and lack of self-confidence.[36] No doubt there are nurses who fall into one or more of these categories.

However, those who maintain that lack of self-confidence is the root cause for nurses' apparent lack of interest in gaining power should remember that "both the powerful and the powerless tend to take existing social systems for granted and rarely recognize that it is not *talent*, but rather laws, customs, policies and institutions that, in reality, keep the powerless…powerless."[37]

PARTICIPATING IN CHANGE

Early in the chapter we established the expectation that professionals have a responsibility to change with the times as stewards to the public. Their practice must change, as must the organizational systems that support their practice. Further, in the process of caring patients must be helped to adjust to change, or to change so that they can adjust. The magnitude of change is often measured by the size of the system involved. Whether it is changing the health care practices of the newly diagnosed diabetic, or the body image of the traumatic amputee, a transition from team to primary nursing, or the decentralization of all management decisions to the unit level, the theoretical constructs and strategies are much the same.

Change is any significant departure from the status quo. Change may be planned or accidental. Planned change is a deliberate, conscious effort intended to improve a situation and facilitate acceptance of that improvement by the parties involved. In comparison, accidental change is that minor shift that occurs to maintain balance between a system and its environment.[38] In his classic work on change, Watzlawick describes first- and second-order change. In the former, change occurs but the original system remains unaltered; in the latter, the system itself changes. The difference here is one of accommodation versus assimilation.[39] An example might be a project to increase nurse-physician collaboration, established with all the components of joint practice, integrated patient records, comprehensive critical paths (see Chap. 30), multidisciplinary patient conferences, yet nurse-physician relations remain unchanged. If the supportive systems are held in place long enough, will assimilation or second-order change occur?

Lewin's theory of change is probably the basis for the adaptations of most other theorists. He identifies three basic stages: *unfreezing*, in which the motivation to create change occurs; *moving*, the actual changing, when new responses are developed, based on collected information; and *refreezing*, in which the new changes are integrated and stabilized. A further notion is that in all changes there are *driving forces* that facilitate action and *restraining forces* that impede it. Each must be identified—the first so that they can be capitalized on, and the second so that they can be avoided or modified.[40]

Lippit's theory includes seven phases within Lewin's stages, a delineation that is useful in thinking through action:[41]

Unfreezing:

1. Diagnosis of the problem.
2. Assessment of the motivation and capacity for change.
3. Assessment of the change agent's motivation and resources.

Moving:

4. Selecting progressive change objectives.
5. Choosing the appropriate role of the change agent.

Refreezing:

6. Maintenance of the change once it has been started.
7. Termination of a helping relationship.

A useful nursing-oriented approach based on Lewin's model is summarized as follows:

1. Development of a felt need and desire for the change.
2. Development of a change relationship between the agent and the client system.
3. Clarification or diagnosis of the client system's problem, need, or objective.
4. Examination of alternative routes and tentative goals and intentions of actions.
5. Transformation of intentions into actual change behavior.
6. Stabilization.
7. Termination of the relationship between the change agent and the client system.[42]

The Lewin and Lippit models paint a very simplistic picture of the change process. On the contrary even the most adventuresome participants have trepidation because human nature fears the unknown. The test will be in the day-to-day arduous implementation process. A review of the numerous change strategies and tactics reported in the literature urges the following conditions to make change more acceptable.[43]

- Assure that the need for change is justified, even if there is not agreement. This requires total honesty, exquisite communication, and sensitivity to the cues that you have been heard. Change for the sake of change is never justified.
- Try to safeguard the future security of those who are involved in change.
- Diffuse anxiety by having those involved create the vision for change.
- It is helpful to work from a previously established set of impersonal principles.
- Change is best received when it follows other successes rather than failures.
- It is better to space events so that prior change is assimilated before the system is asked to accommodate another.
- People new to the organization react more comfortably to change than people with longevity in the system targeted for change (vested interest).
- Try to guarantee that there will be personal benefits to those who participate. Things should be better, not worse, after the fact.
- Establish a venturesome environment by making change and improvement a priority.
- Choose the change agent with psychological sensitivity to serve as a bridge to other participants.
- Focus attention on the future, not the past.
- Allow for failure. Nothing is forever. Be ready to compromise once everyone is clear on the "bottom line."
- Provide assurance of administrative support and freedom to act without the constant need for approvals.
- Encourage open expression of concerns.
- Avoid experimentation and never withhold information; be sure people see "the big picture" and know what they are doing.

Conflicts of some kind are probably inevitable. It is important that the change agent develop effective methods of dealing with conflict. Action, rather than reaction, is the better course, but it should be recognized that the emotions associated with change must be dealt with. If not all participants are won over, the decision must be made to stop or go ahead, trying to anticipate the negative aspects of what may become covert resistance if the resister is outvoted. Just how a nurse handles resistance may be a matter of individual style and the particular situation.

Because of their central positioning in systems of care, and their large numbers, nurses often find themselves in the role of "change agent." The change agent guides the change project. The extent to which the change agent is the architect of the process is determined by the strategic approach to change. The manner in which the change agent participates can also vary, but the concept of the role is to provide a catalyst who will disengage from the project after change is complete and transfer continuing aspects of the role to individuals internal to the changed system.[44] Ignoring this need for transition may cause the loss of much that has been accomplished.

The skills necessary to participate in change and even initiate change projects are an integral part of the curriculum for entry into professional practice. The role of change agent is more demanding. Though it may require more highly developed skills or experience, it is a role that can be legitimately and effectively assumed by a nurse at an early stage of career development.

Whether working as an insider or an outsider, each of which has advantages and disadvantages, knowing the process of change, planning carefully and thoroughly, and acting strategically and with an appropriate sense of timing are essential. Because a change agent is a leader in that instance, the leadership role must be assumed and the individual usually must start out by selling herself or himself first before the idea for change is seen as acceptable for consideration.

RELATED STRATEGIES AND RELATIONSHIPS

Nursing does have influence and power. This is particularly evident in areas of politics and public policy. It is evident in the increased status of nursing and in the expansion of nursing practice to every conceivable setting. Hand wringing is not in order. It is probably a healthy sign that so many nurses are saying, "But compared to what we can do and should do, it's not enough." And they're right. The major problems within nursing have been caused by the lack of cohesiveness, the lack of agreement on professional goals, the lack of planned leadership development, the heterogeneity of nurses in background, education, and position, the lack of internal support systems, and the divisiveness of nursing subcultures, all coping with a rapidly changing society. If nursing is to have the full autonomy of a profession, there must be unification of purpose and action on major issues. Leadership is vital, but it must be a transformational leadership, focusing on shared power directed at accomplishing the profession's goals. Those goals must be agreed upon jointly. Although they may indeed be influenced by nurse leaders, the feedback from the grass roots must be a part of the final decision, or achievement of the goals will continue to be an uphill struggle. Therefore, the strategies and relationships that are discussed in the following section are the responsibility not just of nursing leaders, but of all nurses.

Mentors, Networks, Collegiality: The Great Potential

The term *mentoring* is usually defined as a formal or informal relationship between an established older person and a younger one, wherein the older guides, counsels, and critiques the younger, teaching him or her (the protégé) survival and advancement in a particular field. The system has been described as the *patron system*, a continuum of advisory support relationships that facilitate access to positions of leadership, authority, or power.[45] Helping individuals function literally as patrons—protectors, benefactors, sponsors, champions, advocates, supporters, and advisers.

At the far end of the continuum is the mentor, the most powerful, most influential individual, and the relationship with the protégé is the most intense (and perhaps the most stressful). Next is the sponsor—a strong patron, but less powerful than a mentor in shaping or promoting the protégé's career. The guide is next, less able than either of the other two to serve as benefactor or champion, but capable of providing invaluable intelligence and explaining the system, the shortcuts, and the pitfalls.

At the beginning of the continuum are the *peer pals*, peers who help each other to succeed and progress. The Shapiro group, which focused on ways to help women, saw this first step as highly important, more like the feminist concept of women helping women, more egalitarian, less intense and exclusionary, and therefore more democratic, by allowing access to a large number of young professionals. They admitted that it was the mentor relationship, restrictive though it might be, that could give the biggest career boost, whereas the peer pal relationship was often a bootstrap operation. However, mentorships are not democratic. Selection may be very idiosyncratic, as described later, and there are always strings attached—if nothing else, the demand to succeed.

Peer pals can create their own "new-order" networks. There is a male corollary—the "good old boy" networks that, through an informal system of relationships, provide advice, information, guidance, contact, protection, and any other support that helps a member of the group, an insider, to achieve his goals, goals obviously not in conflict with those of the group. The good old boys frequently share the same educational, cultural, or geographic background, but whatever the basis of their commonalities, mutual support is the name of the game. It could be group pressure; it could be a word to the right person at the right time; it could be simply multifaceted information sources, but it exists. You can count on it; you can take risks; you won't be alone. (And you don't necessarily have to like each other or agree on everything.) Could this work for nurses? Why not?

Suppose a system of support could be developed in nursing. Not a good old girl network—no need to duplicate the nearsightedness of the men in their narrow system that so frequently excludes women—but a *good new nurse network* that promotes the support *of* nurses *for* nurses, men or women. A network that provides backup for the risk takers until all can become risk takers for a purpose. A network that shows unified strength on issues that can be generally agreed upon, so that the profession as well as the individual practitioner can put into practice the principles of care to which both voice commitment. A network that avoids destructive self-competition and instead develops new leaders at all levels through peer pals, mentors, and role models. A network that encourages differences of opinion but provides an atmosphere for reasonable compromise. In essence, a network that develops and utilizes the essential abilities of nurses to share, to trust, to depend on one another.

Puetz describes how to start a network in a formal sense, almost like a new organization. It begins with a determination that it is needed and wanted. Then a core of people can decide who else to invite, "doers" and "stars" as well as peer pals. Eventually a meeting is held, goals are set, and the group is formalized. Actually, most networks start and function more informally, although they always require that core of interested people. The rest is almost an analogy of the old chain letter concept, a spreading out of contacts. Puetz also offers an number of practical tips on networking and notes other good advice about networking given by Welch:

- Learn how to ask questions.
- Try to give as much as you get.
- Follow up on contacts.
- Keep in touch with contacts.
- Report back to contacts.
- Be businesslike as you network.
- Don't be afraid to ask for what you need.
- Don't pass up any opportunities.[46]

Because networking is "in" and is sometimes seen as what one writer called a "quick fix for moving up," and because it is also new to many women, it is being abused by some. Besides the warnings noted above, networkers are advised to observe both common and uncommon courtesies: don't make excessive requests; be appreciative; be sensitive to your contacts' situation; and be helpful to others.[47]

There are already nurse networks in operation, often initiated by a nursing organization or subgroup made up of nurses with common interests, clinical or otherwise. The participants help each other make contacts when they relocate, or they supply needed information or suggest someone else who would know. They alert each other to job opportunities and suggest their colleagues for appointments, presentations, or awards. They give visibility to nurses, boost each other, and praise each other, instead of being unnecessarily critical. But they also critique supportively for professional growth.

Could this also be called collegiality? In a sense. A *colleague* is usually defined as an associate, particularly in a profession. Yet, beyond this basic phrase, the term is rich in meaning. In a thesaurus, we also find ally, aider, collaborator, helper, partner, peer, friend, co-operator, co-worker, co-helper, fellow worker, teammate, or even right-hand man and buddy. The implications are even richer. Colleagues may be called upon confidently for advice and assistance, and will give it. Colleagues share knowledge with each other, together rounding out the necessary information to enhance patient care. Colleagues challenge each other to think in new ways and to try new ideas. Colleagues encourage risk taking when the situation requires daring. Colleagues provide a support system when the risk taker needs it. Colleagues are equal, yet different—that is, they may have varying educational preparation, experience, and positions, perhaps even belong to another profession, but when they work together for a particular purpose, that work is bettered by their cooperation. And to take it a step further, a collegium may be formed—a group in which each member has approximately equal power. Clearly, nurse colleagues are part of a nurse network. But developing that spirit of collegiality requires trust, and the trust must be mutually deserved. Then it can also extend beyond

the borders of nursing to include other health professionals.

Now to return to the mentoring continuum. Neither the guide nor the sponsor has been given much attention in the literature, perhaps because of semantics. *Sponsor* is often used interchangeably with *mentor*, and both terms often refer to a relationship that is more at the guide level. For instance, reference is often made to neophytes who are being mentored, when actually those individuals are simply assigned to more experienced people for guidance. Mentors are never assigned; they choose. In most situations, the level of participation is more at the guide level, perhaps progressing to sponsor if a suitable relationship is established. However, most of these senior persons are never mentors; they simply aren't powerful enough, and in the time given and considering the number of "protégés" involved, they probably haven't the interest or commitment to be mentors. Nevertheless, there are mentors that participate in a very intense and deliberate relationship and who have a great impact on their protégés' careers.

Mentorship demands a high degree of involvement between a novice in a discipline and a person knowledgeable and wise in that area. On a cognitive level, the mentor is involved with the novice as a whole person. The mentor-protégé relationship is a "serious, mutual, non-sexual, loving relationship" voluntary on the part of both. The lack of a protégé is a developmental handicap. Mentoring is part of what Erickson calls *generativity*, in which the primary concern is establishing and guiding the next generation. A mentor acts as:[48]

- Teacher to enhance the young person's skills and intellectual development
- Sponsor to case the neophyte's entry and advancement into the workaday world
- Host and guide to welcome the initiate into a new occupational and social world with its unique values, customs, resources, and cast of characters
- Exemplar to serve as a personal example of virtues, achievements, and ways of life

- Counselor to provide advice and moral support
- Most important, the mentor is given the opportunity to leave a legacy in the form of their protégé.

A mentor supports a younger adult's dreams and helps him or her to make them a reality, and is a protector and supporter who provides the extra confidence needed to take on new responsibilities, new tests of competence, and new positions. (Emphasis on competence is of paramount importance; the mentor teaches, supports, advises, and criticizes.)[49] Sometimes the mentor is equated with a role model, preceptor, or the master in a master-apprentice situation. But it is more than that. In other words, the protégé must show that she or he is someone worth investing in, someone who will show a measure of return by success in the field.

Mentors may be or have been role models or preceptors, but role models and preceptors are not necessarily mentors. A role model can be merely that—someone to emulate and admire, even with minimal contact; it is really a passive process. Some preceptorships are carried out with almost total impersonality; preceptors may overtly carry out their responsibilities to their students and yet withhold a vital element of development. Role models, too, have been known to have a negative impact on new graduates, as when they socialize them into a bureaucratic orientation.

Because of the time and effort mentors put forth for their protégés (usually for one at a time), protégés are carefully selected. And they *are* selected. True, someone who wants another for a mentor can bring himself or herself to that person's attention, but the protégé must be seen as worthy. One group of executives cited certain qualities that they looked for in potential protégés: has depth, integrity, a curious mind, good interpersonal skills; wants to impress; has an extra dose of commitment; has a capacity to care; can communicate; understands ideas; can identify problems and help find solutions; ambitious; hard-working; willing to do things beyond the call of duty; someone looking for new avenues and new challenges; someone dedicated to a purpose; and always—someone who would be a good representative of the profession. Usually the individual is also expected to be well-groomed and appropriately dressed. And of utmost importance, the chemistry has to be right between the mentor and protégé.

There is no question that, although protégés get plenty of help, they are expected to produce, to be worth the mentor's time, to make him or her proud. The mentor's rewards are many—seeing someone's potential fulfilled, acquiring a following, and preparing other leaders for the profession. There are dangers to both. The mentor can be overwhelming and try to mold the protégé in his or her image, or the protégé can become too dependent. On the other hand, the protégé can take over the mentor's position; this is one reason that the relationship often ends on a bad note, usually in business, and happens most often when two men are involved. Protégés do outgrow mentors and may move on to another mentor or become mentors themselves. It also happens that a person may be mentor to one person and also give attention to another, although not as intensely.

There is now much literature on mentoring, particularly in business and education and in research studies. A selected list is found in the bibliography. Although almost everyone says that being mentored is a key to success, even quick success, others disagree. After all, there are not enough true mentors for every ambitious person, and yet many succeed with no mentor at all. There is not yet enough research on mentoring to answer all the questions raised. However, almost everyone had help from someone along the way, and everyone can find someone to be helped by and later someone to help, somewhere along the continuum of the patron system.

Interest in mentoring in nursing has been rising in terms of preparation for scholarliness, development of minority nurses, and leadership in general. In relation to this last item, it is particularly important to note several pieces of extensive research, all of which point to the importance of mentors in the development of today's nursing leaders.

In Vance's study, 83 percent of the leaders reported having had mentors, and 93 percent were mentors to others.[50] In Kinsey's replication, the percentages were about the same. In both studies, the mentors were primarily women nurse educators (teachers) or teacher colleagues, advisers, and educational administrators. They, in turn, tended to mentor students and professional colleagues. All cited the importance of mentoring in their success. A more extensive nursing study of 500 women graduates of doctoral programs between 1974 and 1979 also showed the effect of mentoring.[51] Those mentored attributed much of their development to their mentors, and those not mentored often cited the deprivation. Those mentored were slightly more productive and more satisfied with their work and with nursing as a career than the others. Many other details on mentoring are given in this in-depth study. One interesting point is that with the exception of a very few, the mentors and protégés parted amicably and are now friends.

It is generally agreed that mentoring can help develop nurses to resolve the issues that face us. The commitment of nursing leaders to be those mentors is essential.

RISK TAKING AND ROLE BREAKING

Nurses have had to bear up under the constant insult that they are deferential, retiring, prone to suffer in silence, and so on. Their seeming lack of progress toward autonomy has been blamed on internal discord over basic issues. In fact, solidarity has not been so rare. Those who wish to condemn nurses often do so for their own purposes. The speed with which the nursing community can mobilize its critical mass has become evident in a host of recent attacks chronicled elsewhere in this text (the RCT, unlicensed assistant personnel, shortage, wage and salary issues, workplace safety). The fact that

only 12 to 15 percent of RNs belong to a state constituent of ANA is regrettable, but networks have been put in place to reach almost 75 percent of the RNs in the United States through the state nurses associations and specialty nursing organizations. These networks penetrate to the grassroots and have put petty differences aside in favor of winning for the profession and its future generations.

The risk takers and role breakers are there for nursing. And it is no wonder, given nursing's courageous past. The profession has its roots in the early, uncharted territory of community health and in the holism of the social welfare movement. That pioneering spirit was temporarily chilled as cure, hospitals, high tech, and their association with medicine began to dominate. Nurses did not lose their vision but were distracted until leaders and issues surfaced to remind them of the reason they chose nursing.

Nurses have everything it takes for successful risk taking…the issues, the consumer appeal, the strategic position. When we are considering risks, incorporate a healthy dose of Senge's advice:[52]

- Carefully observe patterns over time.
- Be cautious not to waste effort responding to isolated situations.
- Realize that your actions may affect many others unrelated to your target group.
- Try to anticipate the eventual consequences of your actions, even though they may be beyond your time and place…you have some responsibility.
- Adapting to an intolerable situation is not an asset.
- First try to identify how you contribute to your own problems; it should be easier to fix problems internally, and keep them in the family.
- Allow all those potentially affected to participate in problem solving; once anyone feels she or he has an edge on wisdom, that person (or group) is doomed.
- Educate your constituency (or yourself) that some change is only an interim step

toward a grander vision; and perhaps today's wins will have to be purposely undone later.

The doing and undoing process is visible in our movement toward making hospital nursing a separate revenue center with the ability to bill patients for their variability in nursing resource use. The logic is indisputable; the amount and sophistication of nursing vary on a patient-to-patient basis. Unbundling nursing from room and board and billing for these variations has been identified as a significant step toward independence. But now everything is being bundled, whether through negotiated rates, DRGs, or managed care systems. Were the few successes a necessary intermediate step toward more parity in the next generation of modeling?

An area of role breaking worthy of attention can be found in interdisciplinary relationships, especially those with physician colleagues. Nursing's ill-defined service, central role in delivery systems, and critical mass have allowed nurses to demand special treatment and avoid the need of becoming a full partner in interdisciplinary practice. Regardless of the rhetoric, physicians still resist recognizing the RN as an equal and autonomous professional. Some have conjectured that the true level of professional parity with medicine is advanced practice. Recent MD–CNS/NP turf battles would put that proposal into debate (Chap. 15). The National Joint Practice Commission of the 1980s, created by ANA and AMA, generated realistic proposals for cementing the relationship, which were dismissed as foolishness (integrated patient records, joint practice committees, interdisciplinary conferences).[53] There are those, including the recent Pew Health Professions Commission, who believe that true collaboration will come only with interdisciplinary education.[54]

Nurses have also been criticized because many RNs seem to have a tenuous commitment to a field that demands professional intensity. Nursing is no different from other disciplines. Regardless of the rigor of preparation, each field has those who see the work as an interlude

in their lives, draw firm lines between work time and private time, and care very little about the politics of the discipline. In fact, most RNs continue to nurse for a lifetime, moving in and out of full and part-time status. In unprecedented numbers, nurses are returning to school as discussed in Chap. 12. Further, all RNs may not be professionals in the classic sense of the term, setting aside the educational distinctions that have fueled internal warfare for generations. Chapter 9 also alerted us to the changing nature of professionalism including autonomy. There is no doubt about the basically decent and proud work we do as nurses; we believe it and so does the public. Proceed with caution in risk taking and role breaking. The times will take care of some of the reshuffling.

Political Action

Politics may be defined as the art or science of influencing policy. There is a legitimate tendency to think of politics in the context of government, but affecting policy and operations at the institutional level is often just as important in the work life of a nurse. The term *in-house law* has been used to describe the power nurses can have if they can determine policies and procedures that affect daily practice. An example is policy stating that nurses may (or should or must) develop and implement teaching plans for patients or arrange for referrals to the visiting nurse, all of which have been blocked by physicians or administrators in some hospitals.

It is vital that nurses participate actively in the agencies or community groups where decisions are being made, such as local or state planning agencies. The strategy used to gain input may vary. A basic principle is applicable: before, during, and after gaining entrée, nurses must show that they are knowledgeable, that they have something to offer, and that they can put it all together into an action package. There are many places to start, for most community groups are looking for members who work and are willing to hold office (for example, church groups, societies, and PTAs). These activities may be seen as (1) a way of getting experience on boards, using parliamentary procedure to advantage, politicking, gaining some sophistication in participating and guiding decisions, and (2) being visible to other groups and the public. Many community groups interlock, and, by being active in some, nurses come in contact with others. It also helps to gain support of women other than nurses. Organized women are becoming more successful in getting representation on policymaking groups. It pays for them to have someone who is ready and able to assume such responsibilities. But participating nurses must be capable; there is nothing worse than having an incompetent as the first nurse on a major board or committee. At this stage of nurses' reach for influence, it could do the profession more damage than having a nonnurse, for it appears that women (and nurses) still have to be better than those already in power to gain initial respect.

Another aspect to consider and use is the potential economic power of nurses. A nurse executive who controls a multimillion-dollar budget wields power in how that money is spent. On the other hand, those nurses who have major responsibility for patient care and have no budgeting control are at an immediate disadvantage. Budgetary control (and administrative control), which may include workers other than nurses, increases nurse executives' circle of power, but they must act on it. The aura of status enables these nurses to move in power circles where they can cultivate individuals who influence public and private decision making. Community nurses are also particularly good resources, because most make strong community contacts. Today, the participation of the consumer in health care decisions is increasing. An activated consumer who supports nursing has impact on local decision making as well as on state and national legislation. A legislator is more inclined to hear the consumer who presumably is a neutral participant, as opposed to an obvious interest group. But nursing must sell that consumer the profession's point of view and balance consumer needs and nursing goals.

Although it is often through the influence of consumer groups and the community's traditional power figures that nurses get on decision-making committees, boards, and similar groups, after that, they're on their own and must be prepared, perceptive, articulate, and under control. In meetings, at coffee breaks, the politicking and the formation of coalitions may well determine which way a decision goes. Nurses who haven't learned to play that game had better take lessons: using role play, assertiveness training, group therapy, group process, speech lessons—whatever is necessary.

On the level of governmental politics, nurses can and have influenced not only such issues as Social Security, quality assurance, patient rights, care of the long-term patient, and Medicare, but have a vital interest in such issues as reimbursement for nursing services, nurse licensure, use of technology, children's services, funds for nursing education, and workplace safety. The specifics of the legislative process and guidelines for action are described in Chap. 18. However, there is no reason that nurses should not run for office. They are intelligent, well educated, and know a lot about human relations. In 1992, the first nurse was elected to the House of Representatives. Those holding state offices are not only effective, but often offer extraordinary insight into health issues. Some have been responsible for major legislative breakthroughs for nurses and for health care. This is equally true of the dynamic group in regulatory agencies and congressional offices. These influentials always point out the importance of nurse involvement in health policy formation.

Regardless of the setting, there are some basic guidelines for effective political action. First is to know the social and technical aspects of professional practice; second, to know the current professional issues and the implications for various alternative actions; third, to be aware of emerging social and political issues and trends that will affect health care and nursing; fourth, to learn others' points of view (those of potential supporters or opponents) and come to terms with what policy changes are possible, as well as desirable; and fifth, to seek allies who can espouse or at least see the desirability of a particular course of action.

FEMINISM AND SEXIST STEREOTYPING

A point frequently made, when it is asked why nurses, with so much potential for influence, do not seem to be able to or want to use it, is that nursing is still about 96 percent a woman's profession, and, even with changing legislation and attitudes, women as a whole are still subject to discrimination and harassment (see Chaps. 6 and 17) and still often victims of female socialization.

For many years, most women nurses looked at nursing as a useful way to earn a living until they were married, a job to which they could return if circumstances required. Most nurses did marry and most married nurses did drop out to raise families, working only part-time, if at all. Unmarried nurses (like male nurses) were more inclined to stay in nursing but, unlike men, frequently did not plot an orderly path to positions of authority and influence. This is similar to the career patterns of other women. In business, most women have traditionally been in their thirties or forties before they realized that they either wanted to or would be forced to continue working, and by then they were often frozen in dead-end, low-prestige (but productive) jobs. When they decided to compete for power positions in management, they were up against an "old boy" network that prevented or deterred their progress. Moreover, they had to overcome their own reluctance to be aggressive and to reject traditional female social goals.

Nurses have tended to move into the administrative hierarchy more through default than intent, perhaps gathering credentials on the way. But until the last few decades, relatively few had attained power *outside* nursing, either as recognized expert practitioners within a practice setting or as representatives of nursing in health policy determination.

Has the women's movement had an impact on this situation? As noted in Chap. 6, despite many obstacles still in the path of women on the way up (and even of those who aren't interested in this path) the women's movement has had a tremendous influence in improving many aspects of women's lives. Yet, nurses have had an uneasy relationship with feminists as a group, in part because many feminists have incorrect knowledge about nursing and were more interested early on in encouraging women to move into the powerful male bastions of law, medicine, and business. On the other hand, many of the issues concerning nurses such as comparable worth and child care are also feminist issues.

Feminism can be defined as a world view that values women and confronts systematic injustices based on gender. There are a number of feminist theories and ideologies, but none are antimale, they are simply opposed to the male-defined systems and ideologies that oppress women. These feminists point out that, even now, women believe that they must choose between the male-defined feminine role and the more interesting male role. Overall, they feel that nursing, with its largely female component, follows oppressed group behavior and also tries to emulate what they see as powerful, that is, male.[55]

Shea agrees that nursing tends to identify with the oppressor (administration? medicine?) and is sometimes self-aggressive. An example of this self-aggression is given in relation to the long-standing entry-into-practice battle. It is pointed out that the debate is largely taking place on the professional organization level, to which most nurses don't belong, ignoring the fears of those without a baccalaureate and the means or motivation to get one. The fact that nurses blame themselves and each other for failure to solve the complex dilemmas of the profession is seen as another form of antifeminist self-aggression.[56]

Women nurses now entering the field are generally more comfortable with the tenets of feminism and see no need to take an inferior role in a profession they have chosen to make a career. Instead, they demand equality, for which they are still often castigated by women as well as by men.

One danger in feminism is the temptation to adopt an antimale attitude, for which some feminists are adjudged guilty. Although men in nursing may not suffer gender discrimination as such from other men, they do from some women nurses. In certain instances they may even suffer wage discrimination. There are reports that the salaries of some male nurse executives, for instance, are not comparable with those of other men with equal status and responsibilities in the same institution. Being a nurse counts for less than being a male. If nursing is to become stronger, both men and women in the field need to work together toward that common cause.

The winds of change blow constantly. As we approach the turn of the century, there is a decided change in the feminist perspective. Feminists today choose a more low-key and gentler approach to their issues. They emphasize the differences between men and women as opposed to their similarities. This shift in ideology comes on the scene as nursing is more influenced to define its own uniqueness as caring. The works of Watson and Benner have already been noted. The emergent "soft feminism" is comfortable and persuasive to nursing. You could well see these constituencies converge on the issue of women's health.[57]

Physician-Nurse Relationships

Physician-nurse relationships are a large, if not major, factor in nurse autonomy and deserve special consideration (a variety of issues and incidents on this topic are included elsewhere in the text). There is necessarily a fine line between overstating or understating the problems, or, as some would have it, between paranoia and servility. Physicians' recognition of nurses as co-professionals and colleagues has been present almost since the beginning of nursing, but a hard core of physicians who see and prefer a nurse-handmaiden role, although less common than even a decade ago, still exists. Some individual physicians and, to some extent, a part of organized medicine seem to have limited, stereotypic images of nurses and resist nurse autonomy—either because they honestly doubt nurses' ability to cope with certain problems (bolstered, unfortunately, by the behavior of some nurses they work with) or because they are threatened by the expansion of nursing roles. More serious is the periodic action of certain medical societies and boards to restrict expanded nursing practice by lobbying against the newer expanded definitions of practice in nurse practice acts, by opposing reimbursement for nursing services unless there is physician supervision, or by using their power to limit nursing practice in a particular community or health care setting.

The reasons for problems in nurse-physician relationships have been examined repeatedly. One reason given is that physician education tends to impress on the medical student a captain-of-the-ship mentality and a need for both omniscience and omnipotence (Aesculapian authority), whereas nursing education often has not developed nurses as independent and fearless thinkers. This is also seen as one cause of the doctor-nurse game in which the nurse must communicate information and advice to the physician without seeming to do so and the physician acts on it without acknowledging the source.[58] This "game" has an inhibitory effect on open dialogue both stifling and anti-intellectual.

Other reasons include the different socioeconomic and educational status of doctors and nurses; the MDs' lack of accurate knowledge about nursing education and practice, and vice versa, which enables nurses and doctors to work side by side without really understanding each other or communicating adequately (prompting some authors to compare their behavior to the parallel play of toddlers); different orientations to practice, including physician disapproval of the nursing emphasis on psychosocial aspects of patient care; the difference in attitudes about their professions as a long-term career commitment; nurses' lack of control over their practice, particularly in hospitals; physician exploitation of nurses; and general male misogyny (although some find that female physicians may not act much differently).

With many nurses looking toward expanded practice, the fact that many physicians surveyed do not seem comfortable in having nurses carry out responsibilities that were traditionally medicine has caused considerable misunderstanding. This is particularly true when nurses feel that they must prove themselves to be accepted in new roles and that there is a "role-challenge" thrown out by physicians. Again, apparently interrelated is the male-female role, the dominance-deference pattern that has had such strong historical roots that as someone stated, the nurse/woman must "feel like a girl, act like a lady, think like a man, and work like a dog."

On the other hand, an increasing number of physicians encourage and promote nurse-physician collegial relationships and see them as inevitable and necessary for good health care. Joint practice and other collaboration, both at the unit level and in various manifestations of physician-NP practice, are evidence of this cooperation. (The NJPC was not a success, as was mentioned earlier.)

That doctors and nurses are willing to work together, that is, to collaborate, has a more serious meaning than symbolism. Over the years, an impressive amount of data has been gathered to show that nurse-physician collaboration has a significant outcome for patient well-being. Collaboration had positive results by improving the conditions of geriatric patients in several settings, including lowering mortality; lowering costs; increasing patient satisfaction; improving professional nurse-physician relationships; and decreasing the hospital stay of patients. The most dramatic instance of the importance of collaboration was reported by a study team headed by a physician. Thirteen hospitals were ranked according to their ratio of actual to predicted deaths of 5,030 patients in intensive care units. The differences, considering all factors, were clearly due to physician-nurse relationships. In the "best" hospital, excellent communication between physicians and nursing staff was ongoing to ensure that all patient needs were met. Major elective surgery could be canceled by the charge nurse if not enough nursing staff

were available. A similar degree of respect extended to other physician-nurse interactions. In the "worst" hospital there was an atmosphere of distrust between doctors and nurses and poor communication. The pattern matching collaboration with good results and vice versa was consistent throughout the study.

Stein, who named the "doctor-nurse game" and restudied this phenomenon after 20 years, notes major changes. He admits that in some places the game still functions as described 20 years ago, but he predicts that the changes visible elsewhere will spread. One factor is that "the image of nurses as handmaidens is giving way to that of specialty-trained and certified advanced practitioners with independent duties and responsibilities to their patients.[59] Physicians depend on this special expertise. Interdisciplinary models have also been shown to improve care in specialty areas. Stein adds that the many other influential roles nurses take in utilization review and quality assurance may threaten doctors' authority in clinical decision making. In explaining how and why the physician-nurse interaction has changed, he stresses the nurses' goal of becoming autonomous practitioners; changes such as the civil rights and women's movements and the nursing shortage; nurses' education, in terms of both content and socialization of nursing students to relate to physicians differently than in the past; and the improved environment of some hospitals. The effect on those physicians who still see the RN as primarily carrying out their orders is bewilderment; they often turn to LPNs who "cheerfully" do what they're told. While Stein reiterates the positive aspects of a collegial relationship, he also suggests that both participants might be a little uncomfortable with the new roles. Yet, "When a subordinate becomes liberated, there is potential for the dominant one to become liberated, too."[60] Is Stein too optimistic? Given his caveats that the doctor-nurse game still exists and realizing that everything takes time, probably not. In recent years, there have been many more reports of health care settings where the new interdependent mode prevails. Resolving the overall issue is a part of the challenge that both medicine and nursing must face.

REFERENCES

1. Ashley JA: *Hospitals, Paternalism, and the Role of the Nurse.* New York: Teachers College Press, 1976.
2. American Nurses Association–Political Action Committee (ANA-PAC): Internal correspondence, August 1994.
3. Blegen MA et al: Preferences for decision-making autonomy. *Image* 25:339–343, Winter 1993.
4. Supples JM: Self-regulation in the nursing profession: Response to substandard practice. *Nurs Outlook* 41:20–24, January–February 1993.
5. Villaire M: Marie Manthey on the evolution of primary nursing. *Crit Care Nurse* 13:100–107, December 1993.
6. Hein EC, Nicholson MJ: *Contemporary Leadership Behavior*, 4th ed. Philadelphia: Lippincott, 1994, p 53.
7. Marriner A: Theories of leadership, in Hein EC, Nicholson MJ (eds): *Contemporary Leadership Behavior*. Philadelphia: Lippincott, 1994, pp 55–61.
8. Bennis W: *Why Leaders Can't Lead.* San Francisco: Jossey-Bass, 1990.
9. Dunham J, Fisher E: Nurse executive profile of excellent nursing leadership, in Brown B (ed): *Dynamics of Administration*. Gaithersburg, MD: Aspen, 1994, pp 14–21.
10. Barker AM: An emerging leadership paradigm: Transformational leadership. *Nurs Health Care* 12:81–86, April 1991.
11. Marriner, loc cit.
12. Barker, loc cit.
13. Porter-O'Grady TP: Transformational leadership in an age of chaos. *Nurs Adm Q* 17:17–24, January 1992.
14. Senge P: *The Fifth Discipline.* New York: Doubleday, 1990, pp 17–26.
15. Small N, Walsh M: *Teaching Nursing Homes: The Nursing Perspective*. Maryland: National Health Publishing, 1988.
16. The Pew Charitable Trusts, The Robert Wood Johnson Foundation: *Strengthening Hospital Nursing, A Progress Report*. St Petersburg, FL: The Authors, 1992.
17. Watson J: The moral failure of the patriarchy. *Nurs Outlook* 38:62–69, April 1990.
18. Barker, loc cit.
19. Zerwekh J, Claborn JC: *Nursing Today*. Philadelphia: Saunders, 1994, pp 107–110.
20. Cribbins JJ: *Leadership*. New York: AMACOM, 1981, p 105.
21. Block P: *The Empowering Manager*. San Francisco: Jossey-Bass, 1991.
22. Smith HL, Mitry NW: Nursing leadership: A buffering perspective, in Hein EC, Nicholson MJ (eds): *Contemporary Leadership Behavior*. Philadelphia: Lippincott, 1994, pp 63–70.
23. Safier G: Leaders among contemporary U.S. nurses: An oral history, in Chaska N: *The Nursing Profession: Views Through the Mist*. New York: McGraw-Hill, 1978.
24. Safier G: *Contemporary American Leaders in Nursing: An Oral History*. New York: McGraw-Hill, 1977.
25. Schorr T, Zimmerman A: *Making Choices, Taking Chances*. St Louis: Mosby, 1988.
26. Vance C: *A Group Profile of Contemporary Influentials in American Nursing*. Unpublished Ed. D. dissertation, Teachers College, Columbia University, 1977.
27. Kinsey D: The new nurse influentials. *Nurs Outlook* 34:238–240, September–October 1986.
28. O'Connor A: Continuing education for nursing's leaders, in Chaska N (ed): *The Nursing Profession: A Time to Speak*. New York: McGraw-Hill, 1983.
29. Gillies DA: *Nursing Management: A Systems Approach*, 2d ed. Philadelphia: Saunders, 1994, pp 407–420.
30. Ibid.
31. Zerwekh and Claborn, op cit, pp 238–243.
32. Ferguson VD: Perspectives on power, in Mason DJ et al (eds): *Policy and Politics for Nurses*. Philadelphia: Saunders, 1993, pp 118–128.
33. Syrett M, Hogg C: *Frontiers of Leadership*. Cambridge: Blackwell, 1992.
34. Maraldo P: The illusion of power, in Wieczorek R (ed): *Power Politics and Policy in Nursing*. New York: Springer, 1985, pp 64–70.
35. Ibid.
36. Sweeney S: Traditions, transitions and transformations of power in nursing, in McCloskey J, Grace HK (eds): *Current Issues in Nursing*, 3d ed. St Louis: Mosby, 1990, pp 460–464.
37. Ibid.

38. Gillies, op cit, pp 457–478.
39. Watzlawick P et al: *Change*. New York: W.W. Norton, 1974.
40. Welch LB: Planned change in nursing: The theory, in Hein EC, Nicholson MJ (eds): *Contemporary Leadership Behavior*. Philadelphia: Lippincott, 1994, pp 313–324.
41. Ibid.
42. Olson E: Strategies and techniques for the nurse change agent. *Nurs Clin North Am* 14:323–329, June 1979.
43. Rowland HS, Rowland BL: *Nursing Administration Handbook*, 3d ed. Gaithersburg, MD: Aspen, 1992, pp 34–35.
44. Welch, op cit, p 323.
45. Shapiro E et al: Moving up: Role models, mentors, and the patron system. *Sloan Mgt Rev* 19:51, Spring 1978.
46. Puetz B: *Networking for Nurses*. Rockville, MD: Aspen, 1983, pp 63–80.
47. Puetz BE: Networking: Making it work for you. *Health Care Trends Transition* 20–22, 24, 26, 28.
48. Yoder L: Mentoring: A concept analysis. *Nurs Adm Q* 15:9–19, 1990.
49. Prestholdt C: Modern mentoring: Strategies for developing contemporary leaders. *Nurs Adm Q* 15:20–27, 1990.
50. Vance C: Mentorship, in Fitzpatrick JJ et al (eds): *Ann Rev Nurs Res* 9:175–200, 1991.
51. Spengler C: Mentor-protégé relationships: A study of career development among female nurse doctorates. Unpublished Ph.D. dissertation. University of Missouri–Columbia, 1982.
52. Senge, loc cit.
53. The National Joint Practice Commission: *Together*. Chicago: The Commission, 1977.
54. *Report of the Pew Health Professions Commission*. San Francisco: The Commission, February 1993.
55. Reverby SM: Other tales of the nursing-feminism connection. *Nurs Health Care* 14:295–301, June 1993.
56. Shea CA: Feminism, in McCloskey J, Grace HK (eds): *Current Issues in Nursing*. St Louis: Mosby, 1994, pp 572–579.
57. Ibid.
58. Pillitteri A, Ackerman M: The "doctor-nurse game": A comparison of 100 years—1888–1990. *Nurs Outlook* 41:113–116, May–June 1993.
59. Stein L et al: The doctor-nurse game revisited. *N Engl J Med* 322:546–549, Feb 22, 1990.
60. Ibid.

Legal Rights and Responsibilities

17

An Introduction to Law

L AW HAS BEEN DEFINED as "the sum total of rules and regulations by which society is governed. It is man-made and regulates social conduct in a formal and binding way. It reflects society's needs, attitudes, and mores."[1] The more complex the society is, the more complicated the legal system that governs it and also the more likely that the law will be in a state of change. Everyone dealing with law knows that there is no final or absolute answer—something that is quite frustrating for those who want to know exactly what they can or cannot do. Yet, there are certain principles that may serve as guidelines and as a basis of understanding American law.

ORIGINS OF MODERN LAW

The first "laws" were probably set up by the leaders of primitive peoples who found they could not live successfully in groups without rules or codes to govern them. Certain leaders, known as *lawgivers*, sometimes had prevailing customs and traditions set down as the basic law of the land. One of their early tasks was to distinguish between sensible laws and those that were merely taboos or superstitions.

The most illustrious lawgiver of ancient history was Hammurabi, king of Babylon (2067–2025 B.C.), who developed a detailed code of laws to be used by the courts throughout the empire. Known as the *Code of Hammurabi*, the text was inscribed on stone columns, the ruins of which are now in the Louvre in Paris.

The laws governing Greece remained unwritten until about 621 B.C., when Draco, an Athenian statesman and lawgiver, codified them. Although the code was a marked advance toward equal justice under the law for all people, it was so stern (demanding the death penalty for nearly all crimes) that the word *Draconian* is still used to describe an unduly cruel person or action. Draco's code was replaced by a milder one prepared under the direction of Solon (c. 638–558 B.C.) and was later revised by Plato (c. 428–c. 348 B.C.).

In Rome, Emperor Justinian I (A.D. 483–565) appointed a commission of legal experts to prepare a revision—actually a consolidation—of Rome's inefficient set of laws, which had developed over a period of approximately 1,000 years. This revision, the *Corpus Juris Civilis*, issued in four parts, served as a basis for civil law in most European countries and in England. Later it had considerable influence on the structure of laws in the United States. The third part of the document, the *Digest* (A.D. 533), intended for use by judges and practitioners of the law, contained the law in concrete form and was by far the most important section, influencing jurists and scholars for many years, possibly even to this day.

Another famous code of laws, parts of which are still in effect in France, was prepared under the leadership of Emperor Napoleon of France (1769–1821). The legal system of the state of

Louisiana, once a French colony, was originally based on the Napoleonic Code; all other colonies based their laws on the English system of common law.

In England, centuries ago, the king reigned supreme, but because of great distances and limited communication facilities, he found it necessary to enlist the help of lords and barons in settling disputes in their geographic areas. He, however, retained the privilege of overriding or vetoing their decisions if he deemed it to the crown's or the kingdom's advantage to do so.

The lords and barons, in turn, passed on authority for settling certain disputes to persons of lesser standing, retaining the power of veto over their decisions. To achieve a degree of order and uniformity, the same persons traveled from place to place in the manner of circuit judges to hear arguments pro and con and serve as mediators in settling controversies. It was quite natural for these "judges" to make similar decisions when cases presented similar sets of circumstances.

As so often happens, the administrative official (in this case, the king of England) became concerned lest some of his power be stripped from him, and he took steps to regain and centralize control over the dispensation of justice throughout his land. This he did by assuming responsibility for the appointment of judges to preside over hearings of disputes to be held in designated places called the *king's courts*. To help them in their duties and serve as guides for future deliberations, the judges often kept written records of their decisions for their personal use. Later, the keeping of such records became mandatory. These records and the principles found therein were the foundation of common law.

With the introduction of written decisions, one of the most important principles known in the law was born, the principle of *stare decisis*, which means to stand as decided or "let the decision stand."

When a previous case involving similar facts has been decided in the jurisdiction, the court will be strongly inclined to follow the principles of law laid down in that prior adjudication. Unless precedents are carefully regarded and adhered to, uncertainty would be both perplexing and prejudicial to the public. However, when the precedent is out of date or inapplicable to the case before the court, the principle of *stare decisis* will not be followed and the court will announce a new rule.[2]

Courts of law presided over by competent lawyers quickly gained the confidence and respect of the English people. As a result, common law achieved extraordinary power, at times claimed to be even greater than that of the reigning monarch, whose arbitrary despotism remained almost unquestioned until the barons forced King John to sign the Magna Carta in 1215 at Runnymede. The following excerpts from the Magna Carta are applicable to some of the current issues in our society:

No freeman shall be taken, or imprisoned, or outlawed, or exiled, or in any way harmed, nor will we go upon or send upon him, save by the lawful judgment of his peers or by the law of the land. [Article 39]

To none will we sell, to none deny or delay, right or justice. [Article 40]

These clauses were the antecedents of due process of law and the guarantee of trial by jury. The charter also provided for a committee of twenty-five barons to enforce it. This was the beginning in England of a government that provided a system of checks and balances that would keep the monarchy strong but prevent its perversion by a tyrannic or inept king or queen. Though severely tested at times, government in England from then on meant more than the despotic rule of one person; custom and law stood even above the king.

The British Parliament, the supreme national legislative body, established in 1295 and actually an outgrowth of the Magna Carta, marked the beginning of self-government in England. It took its name from the French *parlement* (derived from *parler*, "to speak"), which in France was originally used to describe any meeting for discussion or debate. The English form *parlia-*

ment was first used to designate a debate, later a formal conference only. The laws enacted by this body were termed *statutory law*, as contrasted to *common law*. The rules and regulations developed to guide the deliberations of Parliament, and now widely used in other countries, are often called *parliamentary law*. They are not laws, however, and are more correctly termed *parliamentary procedure*.

THE UNITED STATES LEGAL SYSTEM

As the American colonies were founded one by one, the manner in which they would be governed was a vital and primary consideration. The edicts of the governments in the homelands of the settlers were a persuasive force, of course; in addition, the colonists were influenced greatly by their own previous experience and knowledge. From the beginning, self-government became their goal, a goal that seemed more attainable in the English colonies than in those originally settled by the Spanish and French.

One of the early problems was to establish methods of dealing with disputes over property and personal injuries. To handle such disputes, the Pilgrim Fathers adopted a system similar to that of the common law then in effect in England. Judges were appointed and courts established, but because the life and customs were so different here from those in England, it often proved impractical and unfair to apply decisions that had been made in the mother country. Furthermore, the problems within the colonies varied so widely that a judge's decision regarding a dispute in one colony was not necessarily applied by another judge to a similar set of circumstances in another. Each colony, therefore, developed its own procedures and laws, both common and statutory, based on its own peculiar needs.

From this evolved the concept of *states' rights*, which has played such an important role in the history of the United States. For many years, any infringement of these rights either from the federal government or from other states was vigorously opposed, although over the years there was less resistance to the initiation of federal programs that assume or share responsibilities that for years were carried by the individual states alone. Nevertheless, the concept of states' rights has been increasingly invoked concerning major federal legislation such as welfare reform and health care, when the state government felt that specific pending legislation was not in the state's best interest.

It is not unusual, of course, for several states to adopt in their separate legislatures an identical law, such as that governing the age at which people may vote if they meet other qualifications. The fact remains, however, that a state that enacts its own laws can retain, revise, or repeal them without interference from other states or the federal government. Relinquishment of this right is a serious matter in a democracy, because doing so sets a precedent that may be difficult to overcome. On the other hand, variance in state laws also gives rise to a great deal of confusion, misunderstanding, and red tape. How much simpler it would be, for example, if the laws governing the licensure of nurses and the practice of nursing were uniform throughout the country—provided they were adequate laws, of course.

The founders of the United States did not depend on common law alone to govern the colonies; neither did they give unlimited power to the governors and councils appointed by the governments of their homelands. To establish and maintain a degree of control, each of the original thirteen colonies early in its history established legislative bodies elected by the voters. The first was the House of Burgesses, which met in Jamestown, Virginia, in 1619 and which was attended by two burgesses (citizens) from each of twenty-seven plantations.

Such localized government was considered adequate as well as advisable until 1774, when the colonies felt the need to unite to voice their collective grievances against England's colonial policies. In that year, the First Continental Congress, attended by representatives of all colonies except Georgia, met in Philadelphia from September 5 to October 26. The Congress did more than express grievances; it also created an association to impose extensive boycotts against British trade, thus firmly establishing the tradition of pooling strengths and resources in time of national stress and emergency.

By the next year, war had begun and the Second Continental Congress, meeting in session from May 10, 1775, until December 12, 1776, created a Continental Army under the direction of George Washington to oppose the British. With the Declaration of Independence, formalized on July 4, 1776, the colonies were launched on a course of liberty from which they—and the states that were later formed—never retreated, although discussions, disagreements, financial difficulties, jealousies, and friction hampered progress time after time.

The Continental Congress continued to meet annually for varying periods of time in several different cities. With limited funds and little experience in affairs of state, the representatives retained the will and courage to continue to advance toward full independence. In 1778, the Congress submitted the Articles of Confederation to the legislatures of the states for ratification; this was accomplished in 1781. The states considered themselves practically as separate countries, however, delegating to the central government only those powers which they could not handle individually, such as the authority to wage war, establish a uniform currency, and make treaties with other nations. They made no provision for an executive head of the central government.

The Articles of Confederation proved to be too weak to hold the colonies together, giving rise to fears that foreign powers might reconquer part or all of the country. Under the leadership of farsighted patriots such as George Washington and Alexander Hamilton, a movement toward nationalization was given impetus. As a result, in 1787 a Constitutional Convention met in Philadelphia to draw up the Constitution of the United States, the idea for which had originated in English and earlier colonial his-

tory. Ratification of the Constitution by a majority of the thirteen colonies established the permanent structure of the Congress of the United States, which held its first meeting in New York, March 4, 1789. Its first meeting in our present capital, Washington, D.C., was held in 1800. The Constitution also designated that a president, elected by the people, should be at the head of the government.

Since then, the volume and complexity of problems facing the legislature have increased tremendously. Numerous departments and councils have been set up to assist in the work of making laws. But at the hub of the work, guiding the action, is always the Constitution of the United States—the law of the land—which, although amended twenty-six times (to 1995), could scarcely be improved upon were it rewritten from the start today. Its basic principles are as pertinent now as they were in 1789.

Constitutional Amendments

Shortly after the adoption of the Constitution, it became apparent that the government's police power, that is, the power to provide for the health, safety, and welfare of the people,[3] needed to be limited by spelling out the rights of the states and the individual citizen. Congress, therefore, submitted to the states twelve amendments to the Constitution intended to clarify these rights, ten of which were ratified by the states in 1791, thus establishing the Bill of Rights. Social and political developments in the last few decades have placed renewed emphasis on these. It may be well, therefore, to review these amendments here to help form a basis for later discussion of the legal rights and responsibilities of citizens, including nurses.

The *First Amendment* guarantees United States citizens freedom of religion, speech, press, and the right "peaceably to assemble and to petition the Government for a redress of grievances." This amendment is often the center of controversy in disputes related to the freedom guaranteed herein. In the last few years, it has been invoked and upheld, even when related to situations most Americans abhor, such as the marches of neo-Nazis, or about which there is public disagreement, such as the anti-abortion picketing of clinics.

The *Second Amendment* gives the people the right to keep and bear arms, because a well-regulated militia is necessary to the security of a free state. Even with recent federal and state restrictions on what kind of arms and the procedures for obtaining them, this amendment, too, is firmly defended, particularly by some groups and certain states, although others argue about its interpretation for modern times. The *Third* refers to the quartering of soldiers in a private home in time of peace or war.

The last seven amendments included in the Bill of Rights have direct or indirect bearing on crimes, trials, and other legal matters in which nurses might become involved. They are therefore reproduced here in full. Given the increasing media coverage of many high-profile criminal trials, where these amendments are frequently invoked, it is possible that more of the public is becoming aware of just what constitutes the Bill of Rights.

Article IV [Fourth Amendment] Protection Against Search

The right of the people to be secure in their persons, houses, papers, and effects, against unreasonable searches and seizures, shall not be violated, and no warrants shall issue, but upon probable cause, supported by oath or affirmation, and particularly describing the place to be searched, and the persons or things to be seized.

Article V [Fifth Amendment] Due Process of Law Assured

No person shall be held to answer for a capital, or otherwise infamous crime, unless on a presentment or indictment of a Grand Jury, except in cases arising in the land or naval forces, or in the militia, when in actual service in time of war or public danger; nor shall any person be subject for the same offense to be twice put in jeopardy of life or limb; nor shall be compelled in any criminal case to be witness against himself, nor be deprived of life, liberty, or property without due process of law; nor shall private property be taken for public use, without just compensation.

Article VI [Sixth Amendment] Rights of Accused in Criminal Cases

In all criminal prosecutions, the accused shall enjoy the right to a speedy and public trial, by an impartial jury of the State and district wherein the crime shall have been committed, which district shall have been previously ascertained by law, and to be informed of the nature and cause of the accusation; to be confronted with the witnesses against him; to have compulsory process for obtaining witnesses in his favor, and to have the assistance of counsel for his defense.

Article VII [Seventh Amendment] Jury Trial in Civil Cases

In suits at common law, where the value in controversy shall exceed twenty dollars, the right of trial by jury shall be preserved, and no fact tried by jury shall be otherwise reexamined in any court of the United States, than according to the rules of the common law.

Article VIII [Eighth Amendment] Excessive Punishment Forbidden

Excessive bail shall not be required, nor excessive fines imposed, nor cruel and unusual punishments inflicted.

Article IX [Ninth Amendment] Unenumerated Rights of the People

The enumeration in the Constitution, of certain rights, shall not be construed to deny or disparage others retained by the people.

Article X [Tenth Amendment] The Rights of States

The powers not delegated to the United States by the Constitution, nor prohibited by it to the States, are reserved to the States respectively, or to the people.

Later Amendments. The *Eleventh Amendment* (1798) is concerned with judicial powers; the *Twelfth* (1804), with the method of electing a president and vice-president; the *Thirteenth* (1865) abolished slavery. The *Fourteenth Amendment*, added in 1868 during the Reconstruction period following the Civil War, states, in part:

No state shall make or enforce any law which shall abridge the privileges or immunities of citizens of the United States; nor shall any State deprive any person of life, liberty, or property, without due process of law; nor deny to any person within its jurisdiction the equal protection of the laws.

The *Fifteenth Amendment*, ratified in 1870, reads:

1. **The right of the citizens of the United States to vote shall not be denied or abridged by the United States or by any State on account of race, color, or previous condition of servitude.**
2. **The Congress shall have power to enforce this article by appropriate legislation.**

The *Sixteenth Amendment* (1913) authorized Congress to "lay and collect taxes on income"; the *Seventeenth* (1913) refers to the election of United States senators; the *Eighteenth*, adopted in 1920 and repealed in 1933, prohibited the manufacture, sale, or transportation of intoxicating liquors for beverages within the United States and all territories subject to its jurisdiction.

The *Nineteenth Amendment*, known as the Women's Suffrage Amendment, went into effect August 26, 1920. It reads as follows:

1. **The right of citizens of the United States to vote shall not be denied or abridged by the United States or by any State on account of sex.**
2. **Congress shall have power to enforce this article by appropriate legislation.**

The *Twentieth Amendment* (1933) specifies the dates on which the terms of the president, vice-president, senators, and representatives shall assume office.

The *Twenty-first Amendment* (1933) repealed the *Eighteenth Amendment*; the *Twenty-second* (1951) limited the presidential terms of office to two; the *Twenty-third* (1961) gave citizens of the District of Columbia the right to vote for presidential and vice-presidential candidates.

The *Twenty-fourth Amendment* (1964), which was enacted because of the laws passed by certain states to make it impossible, or at least very difficult, for black citizens to vote, states:

The right of citizens of the United States to vote in any primary or other election for President or Vice President, for electors for President or Vice President, or for Senator or Representative in Congress shall not be denied or abridged by the United States or any State by reason of failure to pay any poll tax or other tax.

The *Twenty-fifth Amendment* (1965) deals with the disability of a president or a vacancy in the office of vice-president and stipulates how the offices shall be filled in event of an emergency.

The *Twenty-sixth Amendment* (1971) reduced the voting age to eighteen.

For a while, there was great hope that the Twenty-seventh Amendment would be passed, barring legal discrimination against women based on sex. The bill, passed by Congress (1971–1972) and sent to the states for ratification, read, "Equality of rights under the law shall not be denied or abridged by the United States or any State on account of sex." To be adopted, two-thirds of the states (thirty-eight) needed to ratify the amendment by a specific time. When it was apparent that this goal would not be reached by the legal deadline of March 22, 1979 (three votes were still needed by mid-1978), both the House and Senate voted to extend the deadline to June 30, 1982. At the same time, a proposal to allow states that had already ratified the amendment to rescind their decisions was defeated, but the final decision on whether rescinding was possible remained open. Most of the states in which the Equal Rights Amendment (ERA) was defeated were in the South (Florida, Georgia, Alabama, Mississippi, Louisiana, North Carolina, South Carolina, Virginia, Oklahoma, Arkansas), but the legislators of Nevada, Utah, Arizona, Missouri, and Illinois also voted not to ratify. The required number of states was never won, so the bill was defeated in 1982 by lack of ratification. What is rather amazing is that more than a decade later, no new bill has been passed in Congress.

The Constitution and its amendments encompass some of the provisions made by the federal government to ensure the rights of individuals to protection under the law and to fair and just practices in the application of laws at any political level. Guards against usurpation of the privileges and authority of individuals, as well as state and local jurisdictions, are also provided. Beyond this, it is up to the states, counties, townships, and municipalities to develop laws and legal procedures to protect their citizens. It is the individual's responsibility to be well informed about the laws governing his or her geographic area and especially those that are applicable to his or her status and vocation. This will help avoid legal infractions and provide some protection against miscarriage of justice should an individual become involved in litigation.

LEGAL STRUCTURE OF THE UNITED STATES

Under the United States government, the law is carried out at a number of levels. The Constitution is the highest law of the land. Whatever the Constitution (federal law) does not spell out, the states retain for themselves (Tenth Amendment). Because they can create political subdivisions, units of local government—counties, cities, towns, townships, boroughs, and villages—all have certain legal powers within their geographic boundaries. On all levels, but most obviously on the federal and state levels, there is a separation of power: legislative, executive, and judicial. The first makes the laws, the second carries them out, and the third reviews them, a system which the founders of the United States believed would create a balance of power.

Besides constitutional law, there are three basic sources of law: statutory law; executive, administrative, or regulatory law; and judicial, or common law.

Statutory law refers to statutes that are enacted (codified) by legislative bodies, declaring, commanding, or prohibiting something. Statutes are always written, are firmly established, and can be altered only by amendment or repeal. The federal government's explicit powers come from the Constitution; the states have broader inherent power. Both have broad powers to legislate for the general welfare, for instance, health and safety. The Nurse Education Act that, over the years, has provided funding for nursing education is one example of a federal law. A state law requiring professional nurses to be licensed before they can legally practice nursing is another example. In the federal system, the laws are published in the United States Code; state laws are published in that particular state's code. (The legislative process is described in Chap. 18.)

Executive, administrative, or regulatory law refers to the rules, regulations, and decisions of administrative bodies, delegated by the statutes. For example, the DHHS Division of Nursing develops the regulations that determine the requirements for the various programs in the Nurse Education Act; the State Board of Nursing spells out the requirements for a nursing school; a city health code may adopt a patient's bill of rights as a requirement for all hospitals in the city. All have the effect of law. The state's "police power" to provide for and protect the public health, a basic, inherent power of the government, is also delegated to lower levels of government (county, municipal, etc.). This includes "promulgation of health and sanitary codes, hospital and nursing home codes, and housing and plumbing codes, as well as health services such as municipal hospital systems and school health services."[4]

Judicial law, also called *decisional, case,* or *common law,* as distinguished from law created by the enactment of legislatures, comprises a body of legal principles and rules of action that derive their authority from usage and custom or from judgments and decrees of courts based on these usages and customs. Courts are agencies established by the government to decide disputes. (The term *court* is also sometimes used to refer to the person or persons hearing a case.) There is usually only one judge for a trial (with or without a jury) and two or more to hear the appeals (with no jury). The kind of court in which a case is brought depends upon the offense or complaint.

There are also various classifications of law.

Criminal or penal law deals with action harmful to the public and the individual and designates punishment for offenders. Three gradations of criminal acts are recognized by the law: (1) *offenses,* such as traffic violations or disorderly conduct; (2) *misdemeanors*, such as small thefts, perjury, conspiracies, and assaults without the use of weapons; and (3) *felonies*, which include major robberies, assault with a dangerous weapon, arson, rape, and murder.

Civil law states the rights of persons and stipulates methods of maintaining or regaining them. The word *civil* means "citizen"; civil laws, therefore, pertain to the individual citizen. Many acts of negligence, libel and slander, and commercial disputes are examples of cases that are subject to the application of civil law. It is distinct from criminal law.

There are many subdivisions of civil law. One of particular interest to nurses is *contract law*. Laws of contract govern all legal actions related to the making, keeping, or breaking of legal contracts of any type—for example, employment contracts, marriage contracts, and contracts for the sale of property. Contract law also deals with fraudulent contracts. No fraudulent contract against an innocent person is binding unless that person wants to make it so.

Laws are additionally classified by subject matter, such as labor laws, maritime laws, mercantile laws, tax laws, motor vehicle laws, and others. Two other major categories of law are martial and military law.

Martial law means the suspension of civil law in time of emergency and the enforcement of military law on the civilian population.

Military law is a branch of national (or state) law which governs the conduct of national (or state) military organizations in peace or war. The rules or laws are enacted by the legislative body and administered in courtmartial—a court consisting of military officers where personnel are tried for breaches of military law or discipline. Nurses enrolled in the armed forces as commissioned officers are subject to military law, which applies to all branches of the military services.

Enforcement of Laws

Besides generally adhering to the principle of *stare decisis*, courts also abide by another basic legal principle—that the court must have juris-

diction over the person or thing involved, that is, that the proceeding commences in a court located where the defendant lives or is served a subpoena or where the property in dispute is located. An exception occurs when, because of extraordinary publicity or emotionalism about a situation, the defendant claims that she or he cannot get a fair trial in that place and requests a change of venue—to be tried in some other jurisdiction.

The Constitution of the United States provides for the enforcement of federal laws by establishing a system of courts (sometimes called *constitutional courts* because they hear cases about matters mentioned in the Constitution), headed by the Supreme Court, the only one specifically mentioned in the Constitution. Other federal courts—courts of appeal, district courts, and others—have been established in all states and territories on either a permanent or a temporary basis. Staffed by judges, lawyers, and other personnel employed by the federal government, they try all cases arising under the Constitution and laws of the United States except those over which the Supreme Court has original jurisdiction. For example, cases involving violations of federal income tax laws, civil rights, and the passing of counterfeit money are tried in federal courts. These courts have no jurisdiction over state and local courts.

Most citizens are not involved in legal action handled by a federal court. Misdemeanors are usually dealt with on a local level, often by a justice-of-the-peace court, common in rural areas and small towns, or, in urban areas, a magistrates court, sometimes called a *municipal* or *police court*. A district court, often called a *county court*, may hear cases in one county or in several. Matters related to estates and wills often are handled at the county level in surrogate courts (sometimes called *probate courts*) under the direction of surrogate, or probate, judges.

At the state level, no two states have court systems that are identical. They may differ in the names of the courts, their methods of selecting and removing judges, the number of jurors needed to convict the defendant in criminal cases, and in other ways. They do not differ widely, however, on fundamental principles or in their conduct of judicial affairs.

State courts have jurisdiction over all cases arising under common law and statutory laws in their respective states, except in Louisiana, which still operates partially under the Code of Napoleon, which makes other provisions. All states have a high court for the trial of cases, usually called a *supreme court.*

To meet changing times in general, and advances in the legal profession particularly, reform of the courts at all levels is almost constantly under consideration by the state legislatures. It is a slow process, however, because it involves a change in the law and possibly the enactment of a new one; in some states a constitutional amendment is necessary.

Juries

A **petit jury** is a group of persons, usually twelve, but now often six, sworn to listen to the evidence of a trial and pronounce a verdict. The right to trial by jury is guaranteed by the Constitution of the United States and by the constitutions of the individual states.

A juror must have the qualifications specified by the statute that applies in a particular situation and be free from any bias because of personal relationships or interests. A person cannot serve as a juror on a criminal case if she or he has formed an opinion beforehand on the guilt or innocence of the accused (which is, of course, difficult to determine and may be based on what the prospective juror says).

Jurors are supposed to be selected impartially. Jury duty is one of the privileges of a citizen in a democratic society, and many persons find it challenging, educational, and enjoyable. It may also be boring. Some jurors never participate in a trial because they are not the type of person wanted by one or the other of the lawyers, who have a certain number of peremptory challenges, which require no explanation. Prospective jurors may spend their entire time

of service in a jury room. There is a definite technique to jury selection, intended to be most favorable to a lawyer's client. For instance, in malpractice or accident cases, nurses are sometimes not selected to serve; they know too much and may be unsympathetic, say some lawyers.

Blacks and woman have been particularly affected by the use of peremptory challenges. It was common for prosecutors, assuming that black jurors would be sympathetic to black defendants, to use their challenges to create an all-white jury. In a 1986 landmark decision (*Batson v. Kentucky*), the Supreme Court barred prosecutors from using their peremptory challenges to remove black jurors from black criminal cases, ruling that the Constitution's equal protection guarantee did not permit assumptions about group behavior to determine a person's ability to serve on a jury. In subsequent rulings, the court expanded that ruling to relate to civil trials and to private litigants as well as government prosecutors.

Over the years, a woman was often excused from jury duty if she had home and family responsibilities that would suffer because of her absence, or if she was pregnant. In some states, nurses, or women in general, were not called or were quickly excused. Because this violates the woman's right to serve if she so chooses and is able, women's rights groups have fought those restrictive laws. In 1975, the Supreme Court ruled that it is constitutionally unacceptable for states to deny women equal opportunity to serve on juries. The decision was based on the Sixth Amendment guarantee of a jury trial from a cross-sectional representation of the community. Women comprise over 50 percent of the population; therefore, systematically excluding them would deny those rights. In 1994, the high court barred sex as a standard for picking jurors. Harry Blackmun, who retired later that year, said, "Discrimination in jury selection, whether based on race or on gender, causes harm to the litigants, the community and the individual jurors who are wrongfully excluded from participation in the judicial process." A warning note was sounded by Justice Sandra Day O'Connor, however, although she concurred with the majority. She wrote, "We know that like race, gender matters," citing research that showed that in rape cases, female jurors are more likely to convict than male jurors. She added, "moreover, though there have been no similarly definitive studies regarding, for example, sexual harassment, child custody or spousal or child abuse, one need not be sexist to share the intuition that in certain cases, a person's gender and resulting life experience will be relevant to his or her view of the case....Individuals are not expected to ignore as jurors what they know as men or women. Today's decision severely limits a litigant's ability to act on this intuition."

A person must have a very good reason to be excused, although those with pressing duties, such as doctors, lawyers, members of a fire or police department, and the armed forces, are usually exempt. Various reasons for requesting release from a call to jury duty are accepted in all states, although these people may be called later. A juror receives a modest daily fee. Many employers keep an employee on full salary while he or she is on jury duty, usually for two weeks or a month, although the individual may be expected to report for work when not actually in court. The length of an increasing number of trials today, extending into months, is creating new problems for jurors and employers, especially when the jurors are sequestered.

A **grand jury** is a group of persons, usually numbering from 12 to 23, whose principal function is to examine the accusations against someone charged with a crime and to determine whether or not she or he should be indicted, that is, brought to trial before a petit jury. The grand jury system is based on the English system dating from the thirteenth century, intended to prevent a citizen from being imposed on by a despotic government and charged with a crime based on insufficient evidence. Some states rarely use a grand jury, although indictment by grand jury is provided for in all states. Members of the grand jury are selected even more carefully than members of a petit jury; they are called for a month of duty at more or less regular intervals and are paid more for their services.

LEGAL STATUS OF YOUNG PEOPLE

United States citizens of any age are endowed with the rights of freedom of religion, speech, press, petition, and others as set forth in the Bill of Rights. Furthermore most people agree that all are entitled morally (at least until they forfeit the privilege through their own actions) to respect, tolerance, and understanding from their fellow man. Children born into citizenship in the United States have certain civil rights and responsibilities, some of which are in effect all of their lives; others they relinquish when they become adults and take on new ones. In general, parents' duties to their children include support, protection, education, and control, the last allowing parents to make rules by which their children will live. The children's duties are to obey (reasonable orders and rules), to render reasonable services (chores), and to live with parents until majority.[5]

In the last few years that point of legal adulthood or majority has been in a state of flux, but even more so has been the question of the rights of young people in the nebulous state between minority and the age of majority. Legislation has begun to deal with the rights of children in relation to privacy, informed consent, and many health-related matters. Some of the major legal decisions concerning health care and youth are discussed in Chap. 22, but a few basic facts on the legal status of young people should provide useful background.

Infant, minor, child, and *juvenile* are terms, usually used interchangeably, for someone who has not yet attained majority. The *age of majority* is the age designated by state law at which a citizen of the United States becomes legally adult and is entitled, therefore, to assume full civil rights and responsibilities. This term, sometimes abbreviated to *majority*, is synonymous with *full* or *legal age*. Each state adopts its own law setting the age of majority. In most states, this had been 21; however, since the passage of the Twenty-sixth Amendment, most states have changed to 18, the voting age. On attaining legal age, individuals are permitted by statutory state law to perform certain acts with or without the consent of parents or guardian. Nevertheless, even within a particular state, the law varies with respect to the activities or purposes involved. The state has the right to set the age of qualification for such activities as serving on a jury, marrying without parental consent, buying, possessing, and drinking alcoholic beverages, making a contract, drawing a will, inheriting money, working for wages, obtaining a license to drive a motor vehicle, attending school, receiving juvenile court treatment for illegal or criminal conduct, using the court to sue another person or one's parents, and receiving medical care without parental consent. Most laws have a bias toward parental authority.

In 1975, the United States Supreme Court forbade setting separate ages of majority for males and females, but some state laws have retained sexual differentiation in setting majority status. Moreover, young people under the age of majority are not only denied certain rights enjoyed by adults but are denied others by their parents as well, although they also have certain protections.

Emancipation describes the condition whereby children are released from some or all of the restrictions of childhood and receive the rights and duties of adulthood before the age of majority. Emancipation may be partial or complete. Theoretically, only the court or a specific state law can determine emancipation except under certain classic circumstances such as the young person's marriage or membership in the armed services. Parents can petition the court for a declaration of emancipation, which releases them from their legal obligation to the child—the duty to support, maintain, protect, and educate. They give up the custody and control of their child and the right to receive services and earnings. When parents abandon their parental duties, it implies consent, even when formal action is not taken. On the other hand, when young people leave home, and/or earn an independent living, and are otherwise free from the authority and control of parents, this may be grounds for emancipation. Usually the petition for emancipation requires the consent of both the parents and the child, but the reality is that unless there is a serious problem, an individual in those circumstances is considered emancipated for all general purposes. Minors can also be emancipated with the "express consent" of their parents, even without formal permission.

In cases involving consent for medical treatment, the term *mature minor* may be used, indicating that the child is sufficiently intelligent to understand the nature and consequences of treatment.

Right of Sustenance and Shelter

Besides the constitutional rights cited earlier, minors have additional legal rights. From the moment of birth until legal age, children are entitled by state law to such food, shelter, medical care, and clothing (legally termed *necessities*) as the parents can reasonably afford. State laws are changing from the traditional focus on "father" to include the mother or the term *parent*.

Wherever minors may be—in school, recreation camp, hospital—they always have the right to food, clothing, and shelter as provided by their parents, either directly or through written or unwritten contract with the agency or individual under whose care any children have been placed temporarily. Failure to provide for a child in this way (including medical care) is termed *child neglect*.

In case of extreme parental neglect or abandonment, the state is obligated to intervene and either see that the parents resume their responsibility for the child's care or take the child from them, temporarily or permanently, and place the child in the custody of a guardian, foster family, or institution. The state also must assume financial responsibility for the child until or unless other means of support is available. The concept that the state has an interest in the welfare of children is expressed in the doctrine of *parens patriae* or the state as guardian.[6]

Although many young people are earning money—sometimes enough to live on—before they are eighteen or twenty-one, they theoretically are entitled by law to continue receiving sustenance and shelter as provided by their parents or a legally appointed guardian. Also theoretically, the parents are entitled to that minor's earnings. It is unlikely, however, that a court would require a parent to support a wage-earning child under circumstances of hardship without requiring the child to contribute at least part of his or her earnings. Neither is it likely to require the child to turn over a full paycheck to the parent.

When a person reaches legal age, parents no longer are liable for child support; neither are they permitted to confiscate the child's earnings. If the child is mentally or physically incapable of assuming the responsibilities of adulthood, however, the law will usually require the parents or legal guardian to continue to provide the necessities.

Right of Protection

The law requires parents to protect their children from danger and harmful exposures of all kinds. Failure to do so constitutes *negligence*. A parent who in a fit of rage or as a means of inflicting punishment seriously injures a child is guilty of *assault*, which is unlawful beating or other physical violence inflicted upon a person without his consent. On the other hand, physical punishment *is* permissible "for the purpose of punishment"; it must be "reasonable and never excessive," not resulting in "great physical injury or mental distress."[7] Differentiating between what is "reasonable" and what is abuse is not always easy, and the determination may end in the courts, where decisions are often inconsistent.

Child abuse is reportable in every state, although defined differently. Hospitals, all health professionals (including nurses), and sometimes schoolteachers are required to report reasonable suspicion of child abuse. Failure to do so may expose the individual to civil and, perhaps, criminal charges. In most states, those reporting in good faith are rendered free from civil liability (lawsuits) for having made the report.[8]

Nurses should ask three questions about a child's injury. Has the child suffered injury or harm? Does the injury appear nonaccidental or inconsistent with the history given? Did the parent or caretaker cause the injury or fail to prevent it? If yes, the nurse should report a case of suspected child abuse and carefully gather and report specific information.[9]

Sexual abuse is usually part of the statutory definitions of child abuse even if no physical injury has occurred. Among the specific forms of sexual assault identified are rape, incest, sodomy, lewd or lascivious acts upon a child under 14, oral copulation, penetration of a genital or anal opening by a foreign object, and child molestation.[10]

The entire issue of identification and reporting has become particularly sensitive since sexual abuse of children has become more visible, and children have died. The question has been raised as to whether it is always in the best interest of the child and family to report the situation, if changes are being made. On the other hand, health professionals, teachers, and social agencies have been sued for *not* reporting or following through on these cases. The minor's right of protection extends to her or his school where, in most states, the law stipulates what punishment a teacher can employ to maintain discipline in a classroom or school. Private schools are not always subject to the same legal restrictions as public schools in this respect.

The law requires the administrative officers of schools, hospitals, places of amusement, all public buildings and vehicles, transportation systems, health and beauty salons, and others to observe specific rules of safety for the protection of all citizens, minors and adults alike. Such establishments must have and enforce regulations intended especially to protect the young child or else risk getting into legal difficulties of various degrees of seriousness. Furthermore, they must employ persons capable of providing the services they offer safely and competently.

Right to Give Consent

Under the law, *consent* means that a person gives permission in writing or orally for the performance of a certain act. In many cases, minors have not been able to consent to health care, but many changes are occurring (see Chap. 22).

Female minors are protected against sex crimes to a certain extent by penal laws that state at what age a girl can legally consent to sexual intercourse. The age varies in different states—from ten to eighteen. A person who violates the law is guilty of rape and subject to the punishment prescribed by law. The law is frequently inadequate in its handling of sex offenses against both young boys and girls, but the issue is getting increased attention legally and socially in terms of child abuse legislation.

Right to an Education

Children are legally entitled to an education until they complete elementary school, without cost, except indirectly in the form of taxes, transportation charges, and the like. This right makes it mandatory for parents or legal guardians to see that they attend school regularly. Children cannot legally be deprived of their rights, even if they are needed at home, without special permission from school authorities. A recent development concerns the rights of AIDS children in the classroom. Children linked with AIDS have been excluded, but courts have generally ruled that exclusion is not permitted under the Rehabilitation Act of 1973.[11]

Rights of Marriage and Parenthood

Every state has its own statutory laws governing the right of a couple to marry with or without the consent of their parents, guardian, or a superior court, and with or without reputable witnesses. The majority of states permit a couple to marry without the consent of their parents or anyone else at age 18. The ages at which a couple can marry with the consent of their parents or other responsible person are also stipulated by state laws. They are usually lower than the ages required for marriage without consent. Minors who marry declare their independence by so doing and, therefore, assume the same legal responsibilities as adults who marry. Minors in general have the right of custody over their children, but whether or not the mother can consent to adoption of her child without parental consent or notifying the father, varies from state to state. This inconsistency has caused problems for adopting parents in recent years. Children born when their parents are not married have most of the legal rights of children born in wedlock, particularly within the last few years, as courts and legislation have overturned old statutes discriminating against these individuals.

Right to Make Contracts and Wills, Inherit Property, and Sue

Most states do not consider a contract binding if one of the parties is a minor. This does not mean that the contract cannot be carried out but that the child may disaffirm it. Therefore, many adults do not enter into contracts with minors unless there is a parental signature; the parent, as an adult, cannot repudiate legal contractual obligation. Contracts that cannot be voided by minors are those for "necessaries" (food, clothing, shelter, and medical care), marriage, enlistment in the armed forces, and, in some states, educational loans and automobile and motorcycle insurance.

A contractual agreement to work, written or unwritten, can be legal, subject to the laws of the state that delineate the kinds of jobs that children can hold, at what age, and under what circumstances (hours, hazards, and so on). Most states require work permits, which, in turn, require parental consent and proof of age. Acquisition of a Social Security card is also necessary. Generally, salaries and fringe benefits should be the same for adult and child, male and female. Exceptions may be in the areas of babysitting, housework, and agricultural work.

In most states, the law does not recognize a will made by a minor as a legal document. Exceptions are sometimes made, however, particularly if a minor is married. A minor may inherit money or property, but usually does not have control over it until a specific age or the age of majority, on the assumption that the minor cannot manage an estate. Therefore, the court or an adult designated in the will acts as a guardian of the minor. The guardian or trustee has the legal responsibility of safeguarding the estate. Sometimes the disbursement of money inherited by an infant is subject to the discretion of an orphans' court, which might release money to pay for the minor's education or medical expenses or for other purposes.

There appears to be no hard-and-fast rule that states at exactly what age a person may witness a will or other legal document or serve as a witness in legal action, or as a legal witness at marriages and other ceremonies. The courts have permitted testimony of children as young as seven years old. It is not so much a question of age as of intelligence and understanding. Some children have more ability and demonstrate better judgment than persons of considerably older age. A witness must be mentally capable of knowing what he or she is doing. This obviously excludes the mentally deficient witness and the child who is too young to realize the import of his or her acts. The issue of children testifying is quite controversial in cases of sexual abuse. Questions have arisen as to whether the children had been coached or might be intimidated by the perpetrator. Some courts have allowed videotaped testimony; others have not. More decisions are pending.

A minor can sue or be sued to enforce any civil right or obligation. Before any action against the child can be taken, however, if there is no parent or legal guardian, a court of law must be asked to appoint a guardian to institute the action on behalf of the minor or to act for the minor. This person is generally referred to as a guardian *ad litem*, that is, the capacity as guardian ceases when the action or claim is settled.

If the child is suing, an adult—a lawyer, parent, guardian, or "next friend"—must bring the suit for him or her. In a few states, a child may bring suit against parents or other family members for negligent or injurious harm; other states have an *intrafamily tort immunity* law. Even in the latter circumstances, a child can often sue for damage to personal property or *willful* personal injury.

Other legal action against juveniles in relation to arrest, detention, trial, and punishment has been in a constant state of change in recent years, in terms of both protecting the minor and protecting the public from the minor.

THE LEGAL RIGHTS OF WOMEN

There was a time when adult women were considerably restricted by the law, simply because they were females (see Chaps. 3, 4, and 16). Married women were even more limited than single women, because husbands were entitled to the wife's worldly goods and usually represented them in the execution of all legal procedures. Even if the woman was not married, she was usually under the control of a male family member. The history of women's struggle for equal rights precedes the Constitution, at which time Abigail Adams warned her husband that if the new legal codes did not give attention to women, they would foment a rebellion. Two hundred years later, women are still at a legal disadvantage.

The women's suffrage amendment drafted by Susan B. Anthony was introduced into the Senate in 1875, but ratification was not certified until 1920. Efforts toward an equal rights amendment have been under way for more than fifty years.

Between 1920 and 1963, little legislation useful in securing women equal rights was passed, but, probably because of the civil rights, black power, and women's rights movements that gained strength in the 1960s, new energies seemed to be released. Dumas cites and describes forty-three pieces of legislation related to women's rights or of special interest to women that were enacted into law between 1963 and 1978.[12]

All of the laws cited by Dumas specifically prohibit sex discrimination in employment, military service, or education. However, even with legal protection, women are not necessarily granted equal work opportunities and equal pay for equal work, even in state and federal agencies. This is testified to in the number of court cases won (and lost) since these laws were passed, as well as the thousands of complaints of sex discrimination filed under the 1964 Civil Rights Act. As discussed in Chap. 19, the erosion of that law by Supreme Court decisions has resulted in introduction of new civil rights legislation to restore those rights. Over 300 cases, many involving women, have been dismissed because of those decisions.[13] A few Supreme Court decisions have supported affirmative action for women. One was considered particularly important because it affirmed that an employer could take sex and race into account when making employment decisions.[14] Another, which found that sex stereotyping had been a major factor in denying a woman partnership in a large firm (the employer thought she did not dress or act feminine enough), was seen as applicable to other settings, such as in higher education where covert sexism and racism affects employment and promotion decisions.[15] Another action (1988) backed a New York law ending sex bias in large private clubs that play an important role in business and professional life. Nevertheless, much discrimination is still evident, overtly or covertly.

Comparable Worth

Comparable worth (equal pay for different jobs that require similar levels of training, education, and responsibility) is an issue in which nursing is particularly involved because, in many situations, nurses are still paid less than men in jobs requiring much less training, education, and responsibility. In 1984, when the state of Washington was ordered to pay its female workers up to $1 billion in back wages because of pay inequities, women thought that they had moved a giant step. However, the U.S. Court of Appeals for the Ninth Circuit overturned that lower-court decision in 1985. Earlier that year, the Federal Civil Rights Commission chairman contended that comparable worth amounted to "middle-class white women's reparations" and referred to the concept as "the looniest idea since Looney Tunes."[16] The comparable-worth concept was officially rejected. However, the Washington State legislature mandated that a comparable-worth system be put in place by 1993, and in 1986 signed a $482 million accord with its largest employee union, increasing the salary of workers, mostly women. The state also agreed to measure the worth of different jobs in terms of skill, effort, training, education, responsibility, and working conditions. While many court decisions still rule against comparable worth and others are dismissed, the National Committee on Pay Equity, a nonprofit coalition in Washington, D.C., notes that there appears to be a grass-roots movement to recognize and act on such inequities. Some 20 states, led by Minnesota in 1982, began to reassess the public workforce, which is filtering down to municipalities. Not surprisingly, it has been found that women, and often minorities, start and stay at lower pay levels. In 1986, when Minnesota instituted pay equity for state employees, clerical workers and health care workers, almost all women, reportedly accounted for 90 percent of the employees who received raises. No one thinks the battle is over. In 1990, Washington state officials reported that men were shunning government jobs for private industry because now the salaries were not high enough. However, in 1994, women were still earning 75 cents compared with men's one dollar. Clearly, there is still much ground to be covered. Besides legislation, legal suits, and union action, which have their ups and downs, job evaluation and focused research activities will also be useful in resolving the comparable-worth issue.[17]

Sexual Harassment

The problem of sexual harassment of women by their employers or professors has also had some visibility, with limited positive legislation but some judicial response and EEOC action. In 1980, EEOC ruled that sexual harassment was a violation of the 1964 Civil Rights Act. Then, in 1986, the U.S. Supreme Court affirmed that sexual harassment is a violation of Title VII of the Civil Rights Act (*Meritor Savings Bank v. Vinson*). The court recognized two forms of actionable harassment: quid pro quo and hostile environment. With each, the underlying premise is that unwelcome sexual conduct is proscribed by Title VII. *Quid pro quo* sexual harassment is the more blatant and explicit form—the demand for sexual favors for favorable job benefits or continuation of employment.[18] These are actually the minority of complaints made or cases filed, perhaps because the plaintiff must be able to prove that the advances were unwelcome and that job benefits and/or retention actually depended on submission to these demands. Since such situations usually occur in places and at times in which only the two participants are present, a case may be hard to prove. It is also said by opponents that while such a threat may not have occurred, a woman who was not capable in her job might use a sexual harassment complaint as a way to retain her job or receive promotion, without concern for the reputation of the supervisor (with a similar corollary in an academic setting). The *hostile environment* allegations are much more common, but also more difficult to quantify. The complainant must show "that the harassment was based on his or her gender; that he or she was subjected to unwelcome sexual conduct; that the harassment either affected a term or condition of employment; or the conduct was so serious or pervasive as to have created a hostile or offensive working environment (*Meritor Savings Bank v. Vinson*)."[19] In its 1993–1994 term, the Supreme

Court also ruled unanimously that if the environment "would reasonably be perceived, and is perceived, as hostile or abusive," Title VII was violated and the plaintiff need not show that the harassment had caused them "severe psychological injury," which lower courts had required (*Harris v. Forklift Systems*). This ruling makes it easier for employees or ex-employees to bring suits against their employer, and more such legal action is expected.

Why all the attention to sexual harassment issues now, when most women, even if they have themselves not been victims, acknowledge that sexual harassment in the workplace has been going on for a long time, perhaps as long as women have been employed in male-controlled environments? One reason is the visibility that the subject has received in recent years. This includes the accusations leveled against a Supreme Court nominee and a well-known senator and the sexual harassment by Naval officers at the infamous 1991 Tailhook Convention which was followed by cover-up and limited punishment. The resignation by a noted female physician from a distinguished university medical school because she was tired of the sexual harassment by some of her male colleagues was followed by an AMA survey in which 41 percent of women physicians indicated that they had been sexually harassed in their practice, primarily by management staff or a colleague. (Another survey revealed that 75 percent had been sexually harassed by patients.) These and other incidents are receiving considerable media attention. Therefore, because an employer is not only potentially liable for the acts of nonemployees as well as those of management and employees,[20] and because the new court and EEOC rulings make great the possibility of increased legal suits that can result in major costs,[21] employers are beginning to recognize that prevention and training are necessary. Many employers are now making greater efforts to sensitize employees to the kinds of behavior that might be seen as "hostile environment" sexual harassment. Although some behavior, whether verbal or physical, would seem to be clearly identified as such, in reality, what some might find offensive and unwelcome, others would not. It is seen as important that both male and female executives be trained to recognize behavior that might prompt a complaint, that they communicate that this is not acceptable, investigate and resolve the complaints promptly, and educate, counsel, and discipline the offender as appropriate.

Sexual harassment is certainly present in the nurse's workplace, and both men and women nurses are victims. (For instance, in an environment that is dominated by women, some men nurses have been on the receiving end of sexual jokes that, if the role were reversed, women would find offensive, but in this case may be seen as only "good-natured fun" with a female executive also not sensitive to the situation.) In high-profile cases, positive action may follow. For example, the medical school made changes and the woman physician returned. All resolutions are not that neat, but there is evidence that women are not as likely to tolerate sexual harassment in the workplace: the EEOC reported that charges of sexual harassment had increased from 6,892 to more than 12,500 in 1993. No doubt, later years will see even more.

Other Areas of Discrimination

Other concerns about women's rights are common. Many, if not most, insurance companies and retirement plans are reluctant to give women the same retirement benefits as men. They may also discriminate in the availability and amount of disability insurance on the grounds that women are more inclined to fake illness. Legislation was introduced, but not passed, on the insurance and retirement questions. The argument was that women lived longer than men and therefore should not get as much as men. However, a series of Supreme Court rulings now ban employers from offering retirement plans with unequal male and female benefits.

Women's rights issues that have resulted in legislation include rape prevention and control, but in the very important area of abortion rights and family planning, the judicial and legislative action changes with the political climate (see Chap. 22).

The fact that action on women's rights has been so fragmented, frequently contradictory, and not always implemented is a major reason that the ERA is still considered so important. The misunderstanding about what it will or won't do has been widespread, particularly in relation to support and protection of women. (It is important to remember that the ERA prohibits discrimination against either sex.) Some of the projections of what ratification of ERA would mean in relation to some controversial issues are:

1. Decisions about the support obligation of each spouse and about alimony after divorce would be based on individual circumstances and resources, instead of on sex. It is unclear what would happen in the distribution and control of marital property.
2. Women would be permitted to volunteer for military service, or be drafted, if necessary, with appropriate exemption. They would be assigned to duty compatible with their physical and other qualifications and service needs.
3. In school, enrollment in certain kinds of courses could not be limited to a particular sex; only legitimate, activity-related physical qualifications could be used to set restrictions.
4. Labor laws that provide real protection for women would probably remain and be extended to men also, but those barring women from certain occupations would be invalidated.
5. The constitutional right to privacy is expected to permit continued segregation of public toilets and sleeping quarters in dormitories, prisons, and so on.
6. Homosexual marriages would not automatically be permitted or prevented; this is generally a state decision.

7. Private or business relationships between men and women would not be affected in any legal sense.

Because some of these changes are already occurring as a result of the action of individual states, courts, or a lack of objection, there are attorneys and others who say that ratification of the ERA is not necessary and that the trend toward equality between women and men is so strong that lack of a constitutional amendment will not stop it. Nevertheless, because trends do not take care of the problems of here-and-now and equal rights decisions, as noted in Chap. 6, and because laws are so inconsistent, grossly unjust treatments for thousands have resulted. The fight for passage of the ERA is expected to continue.

REFERENCES

1. Hemelt M, Mackert ME: *Dynamics of Law in Nursing and Health Care*. Reston, VA: Reston Publishing Company, 1978, p 3.
2. Creighton H: *Law Every Nurse Should Know*, 5th ed. Philadelphia: Saunders, 1986, p 7.
3. Grad F: *The Public Health Law Manual*, 2d ed. Washington: American Public Health Association, 1990, p 10.
4. Ibid, p 10.
5. Schetina E: *Human Rights as a Child: Safeguarding Children's Rights*. Vero Beach, FL: Rourke Corporation, 1992, pp 13–17.
6. Rhodes AM: Children and the law. *MCN* 13:171, May–June 1988.
7. Schetina, op cit, p 19.
8. Switzer J: Reporting child abuse. *Am J Nurs* 86:663–664, June 1986.
9. Rhodes AM: Identifying and reporting child abuse. *MCN* 12:399, November–December 1987.
10. Switzer, op cit, p 663.
11. Equal opportunities: Protecting the rights of AIDS-linked children in the classroom. *Am J Law Med* 376–430, 4, 1989.
12. Dumas R: Women and power: Historical perspective, in *Nursing's Influence in Health Policy for the Eighties*. Kansas City, MO: American Academy of Nursing, 1979, pp 68–73.
13. de Vries C: It's time for new civil rights act. *Am Nurse* April 1990, p 40.
14. Balancing Act. *Time*, April 1987, pp 18–20.
15. Fiske S: Court's ruling against sex stereotyping in employment decisions will make it easier for professors to win discrimination law suits. *Chron Higher Ed* May 31, 1989, pp B1, B2.
16. Washington State settles dispute over pay equity. *New York Times* Jan 2, 1986, p A15.
17. Bennett S: Comparable worth: The sex and salary debate. *Nurs Health Care* 9:245–247, May 1988.
18. Outwater L: Sexual harassment issues in home care: What employers should do about it. *Caring* 13:54–60, May 1994.
19. Ibid, p 55.
20. Cournoyer C: *The Nurse Manager and the Law*. Rockville, MD: Aspen, 1989, p 78.
21. Outwater, op cit, pp 56–60.

18

The Legislative Process

IMPORTANCE OF ACTION

THE SUCCESSFUL FUNCTIONING OF a democracy depends on the willingness of its citizens to participate in their government. Perhaps the most important activity involved in a successful democracy is exercising the right to vote, with understanding of the issues concerned and the potential impact of election of the candidates. Further involvement might include participating actively in campaigns or in organizations that promote or oppose certain legislative issues; contacting legislators about issues; giving testimony at hearings; and even helping to originate and encourage the enactment of specific legislation.

Nurses, particularly, need to take on these responsibilities of citizenship, not only on general principles, but because so much of their professional lives are, and will continue to be, affected by legislation. The nursing practice act of each state controls nursing education and practice and can be eliminated, amended, or totally rewritten in the legislative process. Laws authorizing expanded nursing practice and reimbursement for nursing services can only be enacted if nurses excel in the political arena. Furthermore, any law involving health care, general education, or almost any other social issue might well have an impact on nursing. For example, at the end of one session of a state legislature, there were 149 bills of interest to nurses in some way. Included were bills for changes in the practice acts of professional nurses, practical nurses, phy-

sicians, physical therapists, pharmacists, dentists, and chiropractors; practice of other paramedical workers; treatment of drug addiction; funds for nursing education; funds for scholarships; funds for health facilities; abortion; birth control; malpractice; and matters related to consumer protection. On the national level, existing or pending legislation for Medicare, Medicaid, Social Security, health programs, the Nurse Education Act, development of health maintenance organizations, health care reform, health research, mental health grants, public health services, and labor relations all have an impact on nursing practice.

There has been an increasing recognition that nurses must become involved or find that someone else has made the legislative decisions on health care and workplace issues that affect nurses' practice, economic security, and their patients. Serving in state legislatures has been an effective training ground for many of these nurses who have gone on to serve in elected and appointed positions nationally. An interesting development is that a number of nurses have successfully run for office. In fact, over half of the states report nurses holding political office, usually on a local level. In 1991, nine nurses entered primaries for congressional office and three successfully made it to the general election. Eddie Bernice Johnson, a Democrat from Texas, became the first nurse elected to Congress.

Many students with political know-how are taking a part in influencing legislation at all levels. Nursing students, in their heterogeneous groups of the young and the not so young, with their variety of backgrounds, have become increasingly active, and their impact has been felt. In one state they were a powerful influence in the enactment of child-abuse legislation. Their influence has also been felt at the national level. Although they initially began giving testimony on federal funding for nursing education, along with their licensed nurse colleagues, they have expanded into other public policy issues. Among these are pay equity, family and medical leave, patient self-determination, organ transplantation, gun control, and HIV disease.

As a group, nurses have become more sophisticated in the legislative process and political action. They have achieved significant steps in developing influence as individuals, as members of a profession that numbers over 2 million, and as members of other power groups. In part this results from a knowledge of the process itself, the ways in which they can make their power felt, and the best time to take action. This chapter presents a pragmatic view of the legislative process, strategies for enhancing nurses' political savvy, and action to ensure nurses' full participation.

BECOMING KNOWLEDGEABLE IN THE LEGISLATIVE PROCESS

There are a number of ways in which nurses can become more knowledgeable in the legislative arena. To begin with, ANA and its state and local constituent groups take an active part in shaping legislation. Because ANA represents a profession, it may take part in developing a bill, testifying, and lobbying in behalf of its members, and has the responsibility to do so. For example, ANA tries (usually succeeding) to influence policies pertaining to nursing under the Social Security and Public Health Acts, and state nurses' associations are involved in actions pertaining to nurse practice acts.

The major legislative activities of the nursing organizations are discussed in the chapters on these organizations and in Chap. 19. Pertinent at this point is the means by which members are kept informed about legislation. All major nursing journals, particularly the *American Journal of Nursing*, report key legislative movements on the national level, and, if particularly significant, those on the state level. The *Capital Update*, written by the ANA governmental affairs staff, who are also the ANA lobbyists and the political action–education staff, is sent biweekly to state and district nursing associations, individual and corporate subscribers, and selected others. It is an informative summary of current policy-related issues that ANA is actively pursuing and is an excellent resource for nurses, covering a wide range of social policy issues. ANA also uses its newsletter for action alerts, urging nurses to contact their legislators, the administration, or regulators about a particular issue. States publish legislative newsletters or have legislative sections that describe legislation on national, state, or local levels in their journals or other means of communicating with members. Directors of nursing or heads of nursing education programs often post these legislative newsletters so that all nursing personnel have access to them. (And if not, they can certainly be requested to do so.)

Some institutions have special legislative groups who keep abreast of pertinent legislation and see that the other nurses are informed. Students may be involved in these groups on their own. The National Student Nurses' Association, with its various communications, is also a means of gaining current information about legislation important to nursing. NLN's newsletters and legislative reports in its journal are excellent, and many specialty organization publications feature legislative updates on topics relevant to their area of practice.

The kind of legislative information available in the newspapers depends on their editorial policies. Feature articles, news stories, and editorials on particular legislation are usually published, and many of them are relevant to nurses and their patients. Some newspapers list the major bills in the state legislature and/or in the Congress and report action taken and current status. They may also report the vote of the legislators of that particular region on major bills. This enables readers not only to follow the action of a particular bill, but also to see how their own legislators vote in general. The League of Women Voters and various political action groups often publish some sort of legislative roundup for varying subscription prices. Legislators may also send newsletters to voters.

There are several ways for individuals to find out the names of their legislators, the numbers of their legislative districts, and where they are supposed to vote. Calling the local Board of Elections is the most reliable way to obtain this information. A local or state League of Women Voters branch will also usually give this information and for a minimum fee will often send pamphlets or more detailed and useful information, such as the committees on which the legislators serve. Similar detailed information might be available from the district and state nurses' association. Another possible source is local political clubs. It might even be educational to see whether family, friends, or neighbors know the names of their legislators. In addition to knowing the national legislators, it is useful to become acquainted with state and local legislators, because of the growing number of health-related issues that the federal government has delegated to state and local authorities.

THE LEGISLATIVE SETTING

It is not possible to influence legislation unless there is a clear understanding of how a bill becomes a law and the setting in which this happens. Presumably, legislators, whether state or national, are elected on platforms of their own and/or their party's which set their goals, and on certain promises for action that they make to their constituents. Fulfillment of these goals and promises, of course, means successful passage of appropriate legislation, but also voting on other, perhaps unforeseen, legislation to the general satisfaction of the "folks back home." *It is important to remember that most legislators want to be reelected at the same or a higher level, and many of their actions reflect this desire.* It is equally important to know that it is not unusual to have hundreds or even thousands of bills introduced in a state assembly (or house) and senate. On the national level, over 25,000 bills may be introduced in the two-year course of a congressional session. Although not all of these are voted on finally, and not all are of interest to nurses, a legislator must have pertinent information on at least those that are likely to be of importance to his areas of interest and his constituents. (In order to avoid constant reiteration of the phrase "his or her," the masculine pronoun is used in this chapter when referring to legislators; most legislators in the Congress are men.) For this, legislators have staffs of varying size, depending on seniority and other factors. The staff total for both houses is well over 19,000 and rising. Some perform secretarial and other similar duties, but others act as aides, assistants, and/or researchers. These are individuals who gather, sort out, and sum up background material on key bills and brief the legislator on specific issues and on his constituents' feedback. The legislator generally uses this information to decide how he will vote. The men and women who are administrative assistants share the power of the legislators, if not the glory. Committee staff do the preparatory work that comes before committees and subcommittees, drafting bills, writing amendments to bills, arranging and preparing for public hearings, consulting with people in the areas about which the committee is concerned, providing information, and frequently writing speeches for the chairman.

Because these assistants get information from numerous sources, representatives of organizations, individuals, and lobbyists find it wise to become acquainted with them, maintain good relations, educate them, and provide accurate, pertinent information about the issues with which that particular legislator must deal and about his constituents. When representatives of nursing have not done so, they have found that the information about nursing that a legislator gets may be inaccurate, incomplete, out of date, or simply skewed in the direction another informant favors.

A measure of the influence a legislator has is his placement on committees, where most of the preliminary action on bills occurs. Appointments are influenced or made by party leaders in the House or Senate. It is customary that the chairmanships of committees, extremely powerful positions, are awarded to members of the majority party, usually senior members of the House or Senate, although this is changing as more aggressive younger members have begun to demand a chance to compete for these positions. Some committee assignments are more prestigious than others and are eagerly sought. There are cases in which the chairmen of some of these committees, particularly on the national level, have remained for years, but the makeup of a committee may change with each new session. The legislator's performance on his assigned committees may be a means of gaining attention and prestige with his colleagues and his constituents, particularly if major issues arise

and there is attendant news media coverage. It is, however, not unknown for him to lose a favorable position because of clashes with his party heads. It is vital to know on which committee your legislators sit, because the action of committees affects the future of a bill. It is also important to know who chairs the major congressional committees with jurisdiction over health care and whether your legislator sits on any of those committees. See Table 18-1 for a listing of congressional committees for health issues.

Other useful people to know are the party "whip" at both the state and national levels. They are selected by their party or delegation and have the job of "whipping in" the vote, seeing that all party members are present for a particular vote, and/or persuading the recalcitrant to vote a certain way. In times of stress, the whips can offer all kinds of political favors. If they fail, the party leaders take over. The func-

Table 18-1 Key Congressional Committees and Subcommittees with Health Legislation Responsibilities

Committee or Subcommittee	Area of health involvement
House of Representatives:	
Committee on Energy and Commerce	Most health programs in DHHS, including Medicaid
Subcommittee on Health and Environment	and Part B of Medicare
Committee on Ways and Means	Taxes, Social Security
Subcommittee on Health	Medicare, Part A
Committee on Appropriations	Allocation of tax funds in the budget, for DHHS health
Subcommittee on Labor, Health and Human Services, and Education	programs, except for Medicare and Medicaid.
Committee on Budget	Budget resolutions: overall priority setting
No health subcommittee	
Veterans Affairs Subcommittee on Hospitals and Health Care	
Senate:	
Committee on Labor and Human Resources	Most health legislation, jurisdiction over the Public
No health subcommittee	Health Service Act (most programs in DHHS)
Committee on Finance	Taxes, Social Security
Subcommittee on Health	Medicare, Medicaid
Committee on Appropriations	Allocation of tax funds in the budget, for DHHS health
Subcommittee on Labor, Health and Human Services, and Education	programs, except Medicare and Medicaid
Committee on Budget	Budget resolutions: overall priority setting
No health subcommittee	
Veterans Affairs	
(No subcommittee on health)	

tion of the whip goes back to 1769, when the British parliamentarian Edmund Burke, in a historic debate in the House of Commons, used the term to describe the ministers who had sent for their friends as "whipping them in"—derived from the term *whipper-in*, the man who keeps the hounds from leaving the pack.

Influencing the Legislative Process

There are many elements to be considered before a legislative body or even individual legislators make a final decision on how to vote on a piece of legislation. Some are undoubtedly personal—how the legislator feels about an issue. Some are internally political—support of the party leadership or a favor owed to a colleague. But likely to be most influential is the voice of the legislator's constituency—"the folks back home."

In other words, if the constituents do not see that legislator, whether national or local, voting as they wish, the intractable or insensitive legislator is replaced. Of course, what is important to them may not be the great national or international issues, but those that affect their own lives and livelihood. But just who are these powerful constituents—the ordinary householder or a power conglomerate? Actually both, as interested individuals or interest groups.

The purpose of interest groups is basically to represent and promote the policy preferences of their constituents and use the power of the group to influence public decisions that affect them. Interest groups have been categorized as economically motivated, such as business and labor; professionally motivated, with emphasis on service rather than economic gain, such as ANA and AMA; and public interest groups that claim to speak for the public (even if they do not always seem to express popular views), such as Common Cause and Nader's Raiders. The reality is that such categorization does not hold in the rough-and-tumble of politics and in today's environment of overlapping interests.

Professional groups may be at odds with each other as they lobby for the interests of their constituents. ANA has been steadfast in the fight to ensure that labor protections apply to nurses. This has been vehemently opposed by the American Hospital Association (AHA). The AMA's attempt to exempt physicians from the Federal Trade Commission's authority is unacceptable to ANA where assuring marketplace competition for the advanced practice nurse is a priority. However, since success in influencing legislation is so often a matter of power through numbers, there is a tendency for a variety of interest groups to form coalitions to support or oppose an issue, sometimes on a very short-term basis. Lee and Benjamin describe this process of building intricate networks as "pluralism." These coalitions penetrate every socioeconomic stratum and include a variety of "strange bedfellows" who come together around a mutually important issue.[1] Nursing has been creative and successful in network building, with success in financing research, education, and prevention of HIV, civil rights, pay equity, pension reform, women's health, nursing home reform, and so on. ANA has long been the convenor of women's groups in Washington, a seemingly disparate but powerful coalition of liberals and conservatives, one-issue and broad-based interest groups.

One method used to influence legislation is support of a legislator, either for election or for reelection. For many decades, making political contributions had been illegal for certain incorporated groups such as ANA. Because the law requires that campaign contributions be kept as a separate fund and that no organization money may be used for this purpose, many groups have created separate organizations for political activity. These are known as *political action committees*, or *PACs*.[2] They may be located in the same office as an organization, such as ANA, but funding activities are carefully separated, if not unrelated. PACs are powerful determinants of legislative action since the first priority of any legislator is to get elected, and campaigning is becoming extraordinarily expensive. Recently, tighter constraints have been placed on contributions and spending. While limits are set by law on the amounts that can be given to candidates, there are ways of manipulating the system. For instance, AMA, often identified as one of the largest contributors in congressional races, has in some years contributed some $3 million to various campaigns.

In 1994, ANA-PAC (see Chap. 25) could boast of a "war chest" of $1 million, significant growth from $300,000 in contributions during 1988. The PAC has also demonstrated an over 85 percent success rate in its endorsements for many years. Dollars contributed to campaigns are substantial, and complemented by a functional grass-roots network with a rich spirit of volunteerism where nurses believe in the candidate.

The ANA-PAC's congressional district and senatorial coordinator's network (CDC/SC) provides a vehicle for identifying and organizing nurses at the local level. A CDC or SC is a nurse designated by the state nurses association as the liaison with a specific federal legislator. They build a relationship with the legislator, supply information on health care issues, educate him to nursing's positions, recommend to the PAC Board of Trustees regarding candidate endorsement for reelection, and participate in campaign activities if this legislator proves to be an advocate for nursing. ANA-PAC endorsements of state candidates for the U.S. Congress are always reviewed by the state nurses association.

In 1993, ANA established a second grass-roots network, Nurses Strategic Action Team (NStat) to ensure the passage of legislation for health care reform. The network was initiated to augment the work of the CDC/SC. State nurses association members were recruited to participate in NStat. Within six months over 20,000 SNA members were participating in NStat's rapid response system and media efforts. Whereas the CDC/SC is linked to the legislator, NStat is linked to the issue. Those 20,000 NStat nurses generated over 20,000 letters, faxes, and phone calls during a period of intense committee votes on health care reform.

In addition to PACs, other ways of assisting candidates have been identified, such as using union dues (or company funds) and resources to provide computers, telephone banks, printing, mailing, sound equipment, and the salaries of union or company people assigned to specific campaigns. The legality and ethical nature of these practices has been questioned, but variations continue and people find loopholes in the law. The 1989 resignations of the Speaker of the House and the Majority Leader over their questionable campaign financing, as well as accusations that other legislators had unlawful financing practices, brought the issue under congressional and public scrutiny.

In 1992, 19 incumbent House members spent at least $1 million each for reelection campaigns. In 1990, a U.S. senate race cost $2.5 million,[3] and figures for later campaigns are even more startling. While the public may be poised to demand some type of campaign financing reform, frustration is common. Despite the considerable congressional rhetoric, the campaign finance reform bill failed at the end of the 103d Congress (1994).

What, then, is the ultimate effect of PAC support? Periodically, a consumer group will publish a legislator's voting record, matching it to the source of his campaign contributions—and they do match more often than not. Moreover, when a particular interest group such as the Moral Majority targets a legislator for defeat and pours money and people into that effort, that candidate is often defeated. That is not to say that there is anything illegal or necessarily unethical about these activities. However, there are unethical aspects, as when distortion, false information, scandal, and a variety of other "dirty tricks," some quite serious, are used to destroy a candidate's reputation. Many examples of this can be found in some of the issues in which nurses have been involved, such as ERA and family planning. On the other hand, PAC leaders will tell you their endorsement dollars and volunteer effort do not buy votes on legislation. Instead, they assure access, and support candidates who share a political philosophy.[4]

Another important component of lawmaking is lobbying. *Lobbying* is generally defined as an attempt to influence a decision of a legislature or other governmental body. Since it is a type of petition for redress of grievances, lobbying is constitutionally guaranteed. Lobbying exists at several levels, from a single individual who contacts a legislator about a particular issue of personal importance to the interest groups that carefully (and often expensively) organize systems for monitoring legislation, initiating action, or blocking action on matters that concern them.

Professional lobbyists must be registered with the Clerk of the House and the Secretary of the Senate. They spend all or part of their time representing the interests of a particular group or groups. A good lobbyist makes it his or her business to "know everyone" and to cultivate such friendships. There are numerous ways in which lobbyists attempt to influence legislators; much lobbying is done on a personal level, sometimes in the semisocial setting of a lunch, dinner, cocktail party, golf date, or other such activity. Lobbyists provide information to legislators and their staff (not necessarily objectively) and introduce resource people to them. Lobbyists are knowledgeable in the ways of legislation and are often familiar with legislators' personalities and idiosyncracies. They are invaluable in keeping their interest group informed about any pertinent legislation and the problems involved, and in aiding the group in taking effective action. It has been said that the skill with which a lobbyist monitors, analyzes, and participates in the political process is a major influence on success, but one should never minimize the ability of an interest group with its passion over an issue and its unique blend of resources to sway opinion among those who are neutral and opposed, as well as to hold the allegiance of allies.

A skilled lobbyist can have great influence on lawmakers, and many times this is all to the good. When it is done properly and is controlled, lobbying is a desirable and accepted way of bringing important information and sound arguments to the attention of legislators. In this sense, lobbyists act as ombudsmen. Unfortu-nately, some lobbyists present biased information in order to influence opinions and decisions in a group's favor. Lobbying may lead to bribery, which has already created state and national scandals and caused great public concern, as mentioned earlier in this chapter. Legal measures have been taken to curb dishonest lobbying, rarely with complete success. The Congressional Reform Act of 1946 requires lobbyists to register and file statements of expenses incurred to influence legislation.

This organized approach to lobbying, effective though it is, should not overshadow the efforts of the individual who, in effect, lobbies when she or he contacts the appropriate legislator about an issue. Groups such as nurses, who do not necessarily have millions of dollars to spend, have proved to be very effective in lobbying by coordinating the efforts of individuals for unified action on an issue important to nursing. Therefore, how well and how much the individual citizen lobbies can be crucial in political action.

The most effective influence comes from the constituency of a legislator. Commonly called grass-roots lobbying, it may take the form of telephone calls, telegrams, and letter-writing campaigns, as well as letters to the editor, press conferences, and various other media activities. It is often most effective if it includes not only the group most involved, but also other influential people. The aim is to educate and/or mobilize at the local level to influence a policy decision. This is often referred to as *outside lobbying*.

Inside lobbying attempts to influence in a more direct manner through submission of testimony, drafting of legislation, amendments, or regulations, and face-to-face visits with legislators and their staff. A good lobbyist can "count heads" to determine which legislator should be targeted, especially the uncommitted swing vote, and can coordinate inside and outside lobbying efforts to the best advantage.

To influence the legislative process requires, first of all, information and, second, lobbying strategies. Later in the chapter, some sources of information are listed, as well as effective techniques for grass-roots lobbying.

HOW A BILL BECOMES A LAW

Anyone can initiate a bill. Legislation is basically a citizen's demand for action because of discontentment with an existing situation or because of an emerging need. A vocal group is more likely to get action than one that is silent. A citizen who takes his or her complaints to a legislator is more likely to get a response than one who just complains. And the larger and more politically active the complainer group, the better the chance of being heard. There have been instances of legislation based on the concerns of one individual, but most commonly ideas for a bill are suggested by groups, which may or may not be organized. Some common originators of bills are organizations representing various interest groups, a governmental administrator, agency, or department, a delegation of citizens in a legislator's district, a legislative committee, or the legislator himself. A prolific source of legislation is the executive communication—a letter from the President, a member of his Cabinet, or the head of an independent agency transmitting a draft of a proposed bill to the Speaker of the House and the President of the Senate. This communication is then referred to the standing committee that has jurisdiction over that particular subject matter. The chairman of that committee usually introduces the bill promptly, either in the form received or with changes he considers necessary or desirable.

In general, the enactment of a law follows the same procedure in all states and the federal government (see Fig. 18-1). The differences are slight and do not have an effect on the citizen's participation in the legislative process.

Basically, there are two types of bills, authorizations and appropriations. An authorization bill is a legislative prerequisite for an appropriations bill. Congress passes authorizing legislation to initiate or continue a federal agency or program, establish program policies, and put a ceiling on monies that can be used to finance programs. Once an authorization bill is passed, the appropriations process determines the actual amount of funds that will be available for that particular piece of legislation.

To keep the explanation of the process as simple as possible, introduction of a bill in the House of Representatives will be used as an illustration. Only the major steps are given, but the details, which can be quite complex, are both useful and interesting, and can be found in a variety of basic books on the legislative process.

A bill may be sponsored or introduced by one or more legislators. The legislator whose name appears first on the bill is often known as the *author* and has the responsibility for the procedural handling of the bill. Although a legislator may be requested to sponsor a bill simply because he is from an interested citizen's district, sophisticates in legislation choose more carefully. The more senior, more prestigious a legislator is, the better the chance for a bill's enactment. Bipartisan sponsorship is desirable, but on occasion a key member of the majority party alone can be just as effective. To have one or more sponsors who are members of the committees to which the bill will be sent is also a highly positive factor. Junior members of Congress often seek senior co-sponsors to enhance the opportunity for their bills to succeed.

Before a bill can be introduced, it must be couched in legal language. Although an organization may have its own knowledgeable attorney to do this, the bill is always put in its final form by a government legislative counsel; drafting of statutes is an art requiring considerable skill and experience.

After introduction in the House (which is commonly called *putting the bill in the hopper*), the bill is assigned a number by the Speaker. (The Speaker of the House is a member selected by the House membership to preside. He is usually of the majority party.) Numbers are given consecutively as bills are introduced in each session; if the bill is reintroduced in the next session, it is unlikely to have the same

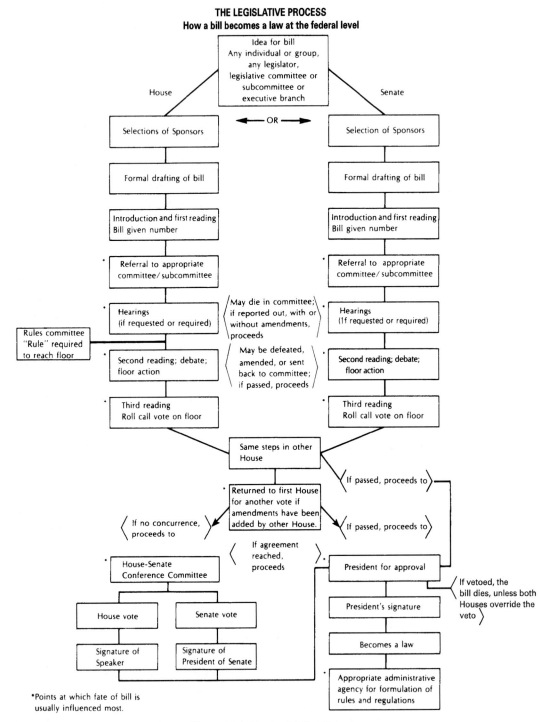

Figure 18-1 The Legislative Process.

number. The number is preceded by an HR in the House (an A or AB for Assembly in some states) or an S in the Senate. When the bill is "read" in the House by its number only, that is known as the *first reading*. (In a Senate the sponsor introduces the bill more fully.) The Speaker then refers the bill to an appropriate committee or subcommittee (health, education, judiciary, and so on), and the bill is released for printing. Usually the printed bill includes the branch of Congress, the legislative session, bill number, by whom introduced, date, reference committee, and amendment to particular law (if pertinent). Consecutive numbers precede each line of the bill for easy reference. Definitions of key words may be given. Amendments to existing law may be shown by having deleted words or phrases crossed out or put in parentheses and having new words or phrases put in italics or underlined.

Copies of bills may be obtained from the sponsor or from one's own senator or representative. However, it is preferable to obtain them personally or by mail from House Documents Room, U.S. Capitol H226, Washington, D.C. 20515. (For Senate bills: Senate Documents Room SH-B04, U.S. Capitol, Washington, D.C. 20510. States also have document or bill rooms.) The bill title and number should be given, if possible, or at least the subject of the bill and approximate date of introduction. Free copies are limited to one of each bill requested, and a self-addressed mailing label should be included.

A great deal of a legislator's time is spent in committee. Some committees may go on simultaneously with the House session, and when the bell rings to indicate a roll call, members quickly go to vote, presumably having made their decisions previously. The committee to which the bill is referred is the first place where its fate can be influenced. If the bill is never put on the committee agenda or is not approved, it will generally proceed no further. The chairman has the power to keep the bill off the agenda or, conversely, to introduce it early or at a favorable time.

Open or public hearings may be held, at which any interested person may present testimony. The date and time of public hearings are published. The committee then considers the bill—sometimes in executive (closed) session, if it is so agreed by open roll-call vote—and either kills it or approves it (reports it out) with or without amendments, or drafts a new bill. This activity is called *mark-up*.

Committee action is determined by a voice vote or roll call, but no record is kept of individual votes. (For this reason, there is some pressure toward having open committee meetings and voting.) For favorable action, the majority of the total committee must vote affirmatively. To get the desired vote, interested persons begin their legislative action at the committee level. Letters, phone calls, telegrams, faxes, and personal contact are used in reaching the chairman and other committee members. This is usually most effective if done by the legislator's own constituents, by whom he is understandably more influenced. Here, also, written testimony and/or oral statements can be given.

ANA and other nursing groups often testify at congressional hearings. Their expert witnesses have helped win passage of several key pieces of legislation, such as annual appropriations for nursing education and research and the 1985 authorization of the National Center for Nursing Research (NCNR). This was followed by successful lobbying to redesignate NCNR to the National Institute for Nursing Research, increasing its funding capabilities and status among researchers. (See Chaps. 14 and 19.) (Techniques for testifying, which are highly important, are presented later in this chapter.)

In Congress, the Director of the Congressional Budget Office submits a financial estimate of the cost of the measure if enacted. This is included in the Committee Report written by a member of the committee. If the bill is recommended for passage, it is listed on the calendar and is sent to the Rules Committee (House only). In the House, the Rules Committee, with more majority than minority members, is most powerful; it can block the bill or clear it for debate. Presumably, the purpose is to provide some degree of selectivity in the consideration of measures by the House. The Rules Committee may also limit debate on the bill at the second reading. If a bill is blocked (no rule obtained), the discharge petition signed by a certain percentage of the House members can clear it, but this seldom succeeds.

A bill that survives all committee action is then scheduled for action "on the floor," meaning the total membership of the House. When the bill and number are read, that becomes the second reading. Amendments may be proposed at this stage and are approved or rejected by the majority.

Debate is cut off by moving the previous question. If it is carried, the Speaker asks, "Shall the bill be engrossed and read a third time?" If approved, first the amendments and then the bill are voted on; but if the required number of objections exist, action may be postponed. If a group whose bill of interest seems to be in danger of defeat (or the reverse, if the aim is defeat) can influence at least the minimum number of congressmen to object, they can buy time to try some other approach to achieve their goals. Delay may also be desired if the amendments appended in committee or in the House are undesirable to concerned individuals. Locking on amendments to a bill that seems sure to pass is a technique for putting through some action that might not succeed on its own and that may be only remotely or not at all connected to the content of the original bill. For instance, in one year in which the administration wanted to authorize only $12.2 million for the Nurse Training Act, the congressionally approved appropriation of $52.5 million was tagged on to another appropriations bill that the President could not veto for political reasons. Nursing also achieved many successes through amendments to the Omnibus Budget Reconciliation Acts, traditionally one of the last bills to be brought to the Congress at the close of a session, with a positive vote necessary to comply with budget requirements. Nursing was successful in nursing home reform, creating community nursing or-

ganizations, and a variety of reimbursement options for nurses. On the other hand, amendments that are totally unacceptable to the bill's sponsors may be added as a mechanism to force withdrawal or defeat of the bill. In general, amendments are introduced to strengthen, broaden, or curtail the intent of the original bill or law. If passed, they may change its character considerably. When debate is closed, the vote is taken by roll call and recorded. Passage requires a majority vote of the total House or a two-thirds vote for certain types of legislation. (Some legislators who, for some reason, do not wish to commit themselves to a vote find it convenient to be absent at the roll call.)

If the bill is passed, it goes to the Senate for a complete repetition of the process it went through in the House, and with the same opportunities to influence its passage. A bill introduced in the Senate follows the same general route with certain procedural differences. Also, the President of the Senate is the Vice-President of the United States.

A major difference between the House and Senate is that bills that are not objected to are taken up in their order and debated. Filibustering is also a unique senatorial process—a motion to consider a bill that has been objected to is debatable, and senators opposed to it may speak to it as long as they please, thus preventing or defeating action by long delays. It takes a three-fifths vote to invoke cloture (closing debate and taking an immediate vote). This is quite difficult to achieve for political reasons of senatorial courtesy. At times, the same or a similar bill is introduced in both houses on certain important issues. The introduction of bills for nursing funding is an example. If these bills are not the same when passed by each house, or if another single bill has been amended by the second house after passing the first and the first does not concur on the amendments, the bill is sent to a conference committee consisting of an equal number of members of each house. The conference committee tries to work out a compromise that will be accepted by both houses. Sometimes the two houses are not able to arrive at a compromise and the bill dies, but usually an agreement is reached and the compromise version of the bill is returned to each house for approval.

After passing both houses and being signed by each presider, the bill goes to the President, who may obtain opinions from federal agencies, the Cabinet, and other sources. If he signs it or fails to take action within ten days, the bill becomes law. The President may choose the latter route if he does not approve of the bill but for political reasons, such as a big margin of votes, cannot afford to veto it. He may also veto the bill and return it to the house of origin with his objections. A two-thirds affirmative vote in both houses for repassage is necessary to override the veto. Because voting on a veto is often along party lines, overriding a veto in both houses is difficult. Nursing lost a critical provision that would have required reimbursement of nurses who provided covered services to federal employees because it was in a federal employees' compensation package vetoed by President Reagan. The National Center for Nursing Research was established in 1985 through a veto override of a National Institutes of Health authorization bill, demonstrating the political strength of nurses and others who lobbied for the bill. If the Congress adjourns before the ten days in which the President should sign the bill, it does not become law. This is known as a *pocket veto*. All bills that become law are assigned numbers, not the same as their original number, are printed, and attached to the proper volume of statutes.

Another type of legislation is a resolution. Joint resolutions originating in either house are, for all practical purposes, treated as a bill but have the whereas-resolved format. Concurrent resolutions usually relate to matters affecting both houses. They are not considered law but are used to express facts, principles, opinions, and purposes of the two houses. They do not require the President's signature if passed. These are identified as *H. Con. Res.* or *S. Con. Res.* with a number. Simple resolutions concern the operation of one house alone and are con-

sidered only by the body in which they are introduced. They are designated as *H. Res.* or *S. Res.* with a number. State legislatures use similar procedures.

One of the criticisms of the legislative process is that action is slow at the beginning of a session and relatively few bills are introduced, debated, and voted on. Many bills may be introduced near the end of a session and receive inadequate attention. It is not unusual for a tremendous number of bills to be acted on in the last weeks of a session (often passed), with some question as to whether they have been studied carefully. A technique used by some state legislatures is "stopping the clock"; the clock is figuratively stopped before midnight of the last day of the session (which has been predetermined), and all-night legislative action goes on until the necessary bills, frequently budgetary in nature, are acted on.

With so many checks and balances provided by "due process of law" in this democratic government, often accompanied by extreme political pressure from within the government and the influence of lobbyists, one can readily understand why it is so difficult and time-consuming to translate an idea for legislation into statutory law, urgent though the need may seem to those who originated and promoted it. Some policy makers contend that this type of deliberating safeguards Congress against acting in an impulsive manner.

A particularly good illustration of the time-consuming nature of policy making is the federal budget process. It is important to keep in mind that the federal government's fiscal year is designated by the calendar year in which it ends. Thus, the period from October 1, 1993, to September 30, 1994, is fiscal year 1994. Also, the budget process originates in the Executive Branch, wherein each agency submits its budget requests two years in advance of the intended fiscal year.

The president (Executive Branch) submits his budget to Congress for the next fiscal year in approximately January or February. The Congressional Budget Office (CBO) completes its analysis and forwards the budget to the House and Senate Budget Committees where hearings are held, and a congressional budget plan is drafted for each respective legislative chamber. By May a budget resolution is developed which is a compromise between the two houses. While this process is occurring, appropriations committees in the Congress are considering the dollar amounts that should be allocated to new and continuing programs. These amounts are then incorporated into the budget as proposed. Subsequently, the Office of Management and Budget (Executive Branch) and CBO independently estimate the deficit (a deficit seems to be usual). Once their analysis of the budget has been reconciled, final action is taken on the appropriation bills. In a final action, the President reviews the budget and issues an Executive Order for line item reductions to comply with a predetermined goal, if necessary. This last step in the process has varied in previous years, giving more or less control to the Congress for mandatory or discretionary reductions. If final action has not occurred by the beginning of the new fiscal year, Congress passes a "continuing resolution," which provides access to dollars to run the government until final approval of a complete budget. The reader is also alerted that each bill, as it is presented, includes a financial analysis. In passing legislation, the Congress authorizes a set amount of dollars for the programs in the legislation. In effect, this authorization sets a "ceiling" on the amount. Program amounts are then considered again during the budget process, and specific amounts are appropriated. In other words, a piece of legislation with a three-year program commitment cannot be included in the budget until an appropriation amount is determined, and this is not always the amount authorized.[5] Figure 18-2 depicts the budget process, from its beginning in the Division of Nursing to presentation to Congress, where it takes yet another nine months for completion.

However, action on a law does not end with its enactment. Laws are usually general; too much specificity makes them obsolete too rapidly and requires another trip through the legislative process to add amendments. Therefore, rules and regulations are developed by the governmental agency or department within whose purview the law falls. For instance, amendments to the Nursing Practice Act are the responsibility of the department under which the state board of nurse examiners falls, and this group will develop the regulations. On the national level, health legislation is sent to DHHS. Advisory committees of citizens are usually appointed, as spelled out by the law or the department. There is public notice of hearings for the proposed rules so that interested individuals may respond. These are published in the *Federal Register*. (States have counterparts.) Regulations are as important as the law itself, because they have the force of law and spell out the specifics of how it is to be carried out. ANA and other nursing organizations follow regulations that DHHS promulgates such as standards for nursing home care, Medicare, or family planning and respond accordingly. It is also possible to influence legislation at this point and to strengthen or weaken the intent of the law. For example, rules and regulations that delineate a particular piece of legislation such as nursing home reform may be flexible, rigid, or extremely loose, and a facility must adhere to them to become and remain approved. The opportunity to contribute to the development of regulations is available to interested organizations, which may make recommendations for individual appointments on advisory committees or offer informal participation and cooperation. They may also testify at the hearings on regulations. Regulations have been changed after hearings because of major protests by interested groups, the presentation of well-thought-out alternative regulations, or letters written in response to proposed rules.

NURSES AND POLITICAL ACTION

As noted in Chap. 16, nurses as individuals and as a group are becoming more active for a variety

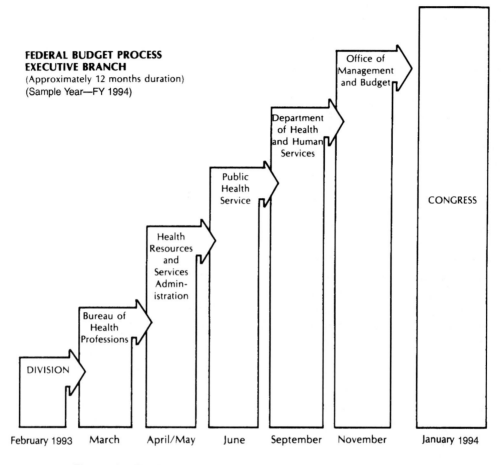

Figure 18-2 The Federal Budget Process. Adapted from DHHS, FMB, BHPr.

of reasons. On the political scene, momentum has been building for a number of years, and organizations such as the ANA, NLN, American Association of Colleges of Nursing (AACN), and AONE, have taken leadership roles in mobilizing nurses in grass-roots lobbying. Among the approaches are educational programs and political consciousness-raising sessions both to teach nurses techniques and strategies and to make them aware of issues. ANA and other nursing organizations have set up networks, where the lobbyist or a monitoring group in the state or national capital alerts the organization about the status of a bill at a crucial time and an action plan begins. Usually not all members are mobilized,

only certain volunteer activists. The network is activated through a state legislative committee and a "telephone tree" that passes on the "act now" directive, or simply by mailgram, first-class mail, or fax. If, as is often true, mass action is not needed, the difficult part is to select the nurses who are best suited for that situation. For instance, if the legislator is particularly sensitive to a constituency such as the elderly, or an influential citizen, or a particular part of his district, the members fitting that category are called on to act. Another type of categorization is by expertise. Using but not overusing the network is essential to success, as is follow-through to determine its success.

While various techniques are used for lobbying, selection of one or a combination is part of the strategy. Such strategies, an active PAC, and a well-developed grass-roots network have made nursing increasingly influential, particularly in Washington. A 1993 *Washington Post* article referred to the "Nightingale Network" as being a major player and potential winner in the discussion on health care reform. Similar accolades have come from other provider professionals.[6]

This simply points out once more the importance of skilled participation in the political process. Nurses and students of nursing have a large stake in legislation. Acting as individuals or part of a group, they can make an impact on public policy. However, learning how to communicate effectively with legislators is essential. Legislators want to hear from their constituents, but because they are extremely busy, carefully planned and organized contacts are most effective.

Personal Contact

It is sensible for nurses to become acquainted with their legislators before a legislative crisis occurs. This gives them the advantage of having made personal contact and shown general interest, and gives the legislator or staff member the advantage of a reference point. In small communities, legislators often know many of their constituents on a first-name basis through frequent contacts. This personal relationship may be more difficult to achieve in large areas, but the effort to meet and talk with legislators is never wasted.

Having identified and located the legislator, the nurse may call for an appointment or check when the legislator is available in his local office (or in his capital office if this is convenient for both). Before the visit, it is helpful to know:

1. The geography of his legislative district and district number.
2. His present or past leadership in civic, cultural, or other community affairs.
3. How he voted on major controversial issues recently under consideration.
4. How he has voted in the past on major bills of concern to nurses.
5. The subject areas of his special interest such as health, consumer affairs, and so on.
6. His political party affiliation.
7. His previous occupation or profession with which he may still have some involvement.
8. What bills of major importance he has authored or coauthored.
9. Previous contacts with nursing organizations in the area.
10. Nursing organizations' endorsements of him or his opponents in past elections.

This information may be available from the state nurses' association, political action groups (of which a partial list is included in this chapter), or literature about him from his own office.

No one can say how such a visit should be conducted—it is obviously a matter of personal style—but generally it is wise to be dressed appropriately, to be friendly, to keep the visit short, to identify yourself as a nurse and, depending on your own level of expertise, to offer to be a resource. It is always thoughtful to comment on any of his bills or votes of which you approve. If the first visit coincides with pending health legislation, it is suitable to ask whether he has taken a stand and perhaps add a few pertinent comments. Not more than three major issues should probably be discussed, and it is useful to recommend specific solutions to problems if at all possible. A *brief* written account of the key points and/or documentation of facts can be left, along with an offer to provide additional information if he wants it. Legislators respond best if what is discussed is within the context of what his other constituents might want. In other words, is it good for the public and not just for nursing?

It is important to be prompt for the visit, but you must be ready to accept the fact that the legislator may be late or not able to keep the appointment. Administrative assistants who substitute are usually attentive and often know more about the details than the legislator. They are people with whom nurses should be well acquainted because they make recommendations to the legislator as to how to vote. If distance and time make visiting difficult, a telephone call is a good approach. The same general guidelines can be followed, and here also, speaking to the legislator's administrative assistant serves almost as good a purpose as speaking to the legislator.

Although personal visits and calls are considered useful in trying to influence a legislator, especially if an initial introductory visit has already been made, letter writing is also effective and is the most frequent way to communicate. Legislators are particularly sensitive to communications from their constituents. They give far less attention to correspondence from outside their state or district and are often annoyed by it. If a local address is not known, addressing the letter to the state or federal house or senate is satisfactory. However, addresses should be on hand before the need arises, and some say that mail received in the local office is apt to get

more attention, since the letters don't compete with other mail at the capital.

Accepted ways of addressing public officials are found in Table 18-2.

After the proper salutation, you should identify yourself as a nurse and a constituent and state the reason for the letter. A good letter persuades not by emotionalism, vague opinion, threats, or hostility, but by reason, good sense, and facts. The letter should be brief, to the point, specific, and without trivia. In developing arguments to support a position, it is best, when possible, to cite specific local situations that will be affected by the legislation of concern. It is vital that the information about the bill be complete and accurate and the reasons for a particular stand honest and reasonable. A simple objection without reason may have some influence on the legislator, if he tends to count letters, but has little value in educating him on the issues. The writer should include in the letter the bill number, author or authors, or at least its popular title, its status, the general purpose or interest of the bill, the specific recommendation to the legisla-

Table 18-2 How to Address Public Officials			
Official	Address	Official	Address
President	The President of the United States The White House Washington, D.C. 20500 Dear Mr. President:	Assemblyman	The Hon. Mary Doe *The State House Trenton, N.J. 08625 Dear Ms. Doe:
Governor	The Hon. John Doe Executive Chamber Albany, N.Y. 12224 Dear Governor Doe:	Mayor	The Hon. John Doe City Hall New York, N.Y. 10007 Dear Mayor Doe:
U.S. Senator	Senator John Doe *Senate Office Building Washington, D.C. 20510 Dear Senator Doe:	City Councilman	The Hon. John Doe City Council New York, N.Y. 10007 Dear Mr. Doe:
Congressman	The Hon. John Doe *House Office Building Washington, D.C. 20515 Dear Mr. Doe: or Dear Congressman:	Judge	The Hon. Mary Doe (Address of Court) Dear Judge Doe:
State Senator	The Hon. John Doe *Senate Chambers Albany, N.Y. 12224 Dear Senator:	Other officials	(not included above) The Hon. John Doe Dear Mr. Doe:

*The local office, or if none, the home address may be used. *Note:* Addresses at state capitals vary.

tor regarding the bill, how this stand is justified in terms of public interest, not just the profession, and what other organizations or groups have a parallel stand. If the legislator is the bill's sponsor or is on the committee considering it, the content of the letter is altered to take this into consideration.

Berating or threatening the congressman, pretending to wield vast political influence, making promises, or demanding a commitment are all counterproductive. Writing too often or too lengthily on nothing much is just as bad. For professional nurses, incorrect grammar or spelling reinforce a negative image and are inexcusable.

A letter requesting support on an issue is obviously more effective if letters are also written by other nurses and especially by nonnurses in the community. Nurses who can persuade family, friends, neighbors, or groups to support their viewpoints may supply guidelines for writing, if desired, but a form letter should *never* be written. Mimeographed letters and petitions could end up in the legislator's wastebasket, although again there are the letter counters.

The amount of mail reaching the capital on a sensitive issue has been known to bog down the congressional mail system for days, and it was reported that with the periodic flood of mass-produced mail, congressmen and senators were never sure how much seriousness to attach to a campaign. What does catch the eye is an example or an anecdote about how a particular bill would affect people. Some politicians have framed whole speeches around constituent anecdotes.

Some information can best be communicated to a legislator by telephone or telegram, particularly if speed is important, as when a vote is pending. A twenty-word "public opinion message" can be sent to any congressman, President, or Vice-President for a minimal cost. A fax might also be used, but if too many clutter the recipient's machine, the impact could be negative.

Nurses using these methods should find that they have an increasing amount of influence with their legislators. Over a period of time, the legislators will come to recognize these nurses as persons of integrity and reliability who are accurate and confident about their facts and who are interested in the legislators' positions, attitudes, and problems.[7] Nurses who generally agree with their legislator's approach will find that it is also politically astute to contribute to his reelection campaign and/or offer their services in the campaign. These might include house-to-house canvassing to check voter registration or to register voters, supplying transportation to the polls, making telephone calls to stimulate registration and voting, acting as registration clerk and watcher, poll clerk and watcher, block leader, or precinct captain, raising funds, preparing mailing pieces, planning publicity, writing and distributing news releases, making speeches, answering telephones and staffing information booths, planning campaign events, or having "coffees" to meet the candidate. Groups or organizations can become more extensively involved if they are able to do so legally and financially. Most nurses who have participated in political action have found it stimulating and educational.

Testifying at Hearings

Committee hearings are intended to get the opinions of citizens on particular bills or issues. Student nurses and nurses can be effective speakers for health care but, if poorly prepared, can cause just as negative an impact.

Attending public hearings of the committee to which health issues are referred is both an educational experience and a good preliminary before testifying yourself. It provides an opportunity to become more familiar with the atmosphere and setting of hearings, as well as the attitudes and personalities of the committee members, and to become acquainted with them individually.

It may be disconcerting for someone testifying to find only the chairman present at a hearing or, on the other hand, to find a full committee and hundreds in the audience. A nurse or organization may or may not be specifically invited to give testimony. Either way, it is a courtesy (and may be mandatory) to notify the committee in writing of the intent to appear or to request placement on the agenda and to provide a copy of the testimony if possible. Prior presentation of testimony does not exclude the possibility of adding appropriate remarks verbally or in answer to committee questions.

It can have a negative effect to request the opportunity to present testimony if the bill is of marginal interest or if a written statement inserted in the record would serve as well. Testimony should be prepared well in advance, or as much as possible, because hearings may be called on short notice and sloppy testimony is worse than none. The ground rules applicable to the hearing (time limitations, length of testimony, number of copies to be submitted, deadline for submitting advance copies) should be requested from the committee staff and be followed.

Legislators, lobbyists, and others interested in legislative action have suggested some guidelines for giving testimony before legislative bodies:

1. Be prepared to adjust your schedule so that you can participate as the committee schedule permits. Hearings may start late, be cut short, run late into the night, be recessed and reconvened later, or otherwise changed.

2. Learn about your audience in advance, with accurate names and titles. Pronounce names correctly.

3. Although you have the right to disagree with your professional organization, totally independent action confuses the issues for legislators. It is better to work within the organization, ironing out differences. A collective voice usually carries more weight than isolated testimony.

4. Pay attention to protocol; be sure to thank the committee for the opportunity to address it.

5. Introduce yourself with a very brief biographical sketch; state the issue on which you are testifying, and note whether you represent a group or only yourself.

6. If the testimony is in writing and has been given to the committee, they may prefer that the information be briefly recapitulated rather than read completely. Be prepared with both a long and a short text.

7. Be brief and concise (about ten to fifteen minutes); discuss only the specific bill or issue concerned, refrain from irrelevant comments, and speak plainly and without professional jargon. Relate your arguments to people, not abstractions.

8. Be secure in your knowledge of the facts, totally honest, and comfortable in speaking to a group. Have additional data available to help in answering questions accurately. It is disastrous to present false information or a dishonest interpretation. If possible, know the data on which your testimony is based and do not simply read a statement prepared by someone else.

9. When being questioned, it helps to be able to think under pressure, remain cool, not become angry, and have a sense of humor. (Some legislators use committee hearings as stages; some may not be friendly to the nurse's cause; others have predetermined ideas and prefer to keep them.) Never try to bluff; if you do not know the answer, it is best to say so and perhaps volunteer to provide the answer to the committee before the vote or have it placed in the record.

10. As in any other situation, appearance is important. Be appropriately dressed; a uniform is not appropriate except in unusual circumstances.

11. Be aware that appearing at a hearing is often all that is necessary. Testifying may not be the best action for various reasons and should not be forced. The appearance of a large number of nurses and students at a hearing indicates that it is of major concern to them. Behavior should be courteous. This is also no time for intraprofessional quarreling.

12. Be aware that everyone appearing before a committee represents a special interest

group; legislators weigh conflicting views to make their own decision.

13. Don't be shocked or disillusioned if the vote goes against you at the hearing. Votes may have been promised to colleagues at this initial stage, even before the hearing, but may be reversed on the floor. If the bill is filed, a new version may be introduced, with changes made to minimize the opposition.

14. Always be courteous, whether in the audience or testifying. Catcalls, boos, or similar noises from the audience are not taken well. Even certain kinds of body language can have a negative effect. In one televised hearing, a Senator actually on the side of those testifying chastised them for rolling their eyes and making other gestures at the words of another committee member.

Politics is often a matter of compromise. Adherents of a bill must be prepared to yield on some issues as necessary, meanwhile holding firm on the most vital issues and allowing opponents to compromise on these points. Most of all, it is essential that nurses continue to be involved in political action, becoming ever more knowledgeable, sophisticated, and effective.

Other Means of Influencing Legislation

There are times when individual nurses are selected to participate in legislative and governmental advisory committees on the local, state, and national levels. Most often such a nurse comes to the attention of the appointing individual through professional achievements, political or professional activities, or recommendation by organizations. Organizations such as the ANA and NLN keep alert for the inception of pertinent committees and exert pressure to have nurses included. More and more nurses and students are being appointed to such multi-disciplinary and advisory groups. The contributions of thoughtful and informed nurses to committee deliberations, actions, and recommendations can

change the course of health care. Nurses have shown that they can be a positive force in legislation, and have found, in addition, personal and professional satisfaction in participation in what Woodrow Wilson called the dance of legislation: "Once begin the dance of legislation, and you must struggle through its mazes as best you can to the breathless end—if any end there be."

REFERENCE SOURCES FOR POLITICAL ACTION AND/OR LEGISLATION

Primary sources of information in Washington, D.C., are:

1. Government agency staff experts
2. Congressional committee and subcommittee staff members
3. Staff members of senators and congressmen
4. The Library of Congress
5. Private research organizations.
6. Professional, trade, and labor organizations
7. Directories
8. Publications

Many government publications and directories are available from the Government Printing Office, Washington, D.C. 20402. Federal government bookstores throughout the country sell government publications and can help individuals locate appropriate resources.

For vacation, adjournments and recess, or scheduling of bills for a floor debate or vote, phone the Senate or House majority whips' offices. For committee hearings and schedule, see the *Congressional Record* for the next day (the last issue of the week lists the following week's schedule) or the *Washington Post*, "Today's Activities in the Senate and House." To check if the President has signed a particular bill passed by the Congress, contact the White House Records Office (give bill number) or Archives.

The *Grassroots Lobbying Handbook* is an excellent resource for nurses of all degrees of political expertise. It includes strategies for communicating with legislators and committee staff, testifying, and organizing nurses in the workplace and community.[9] Another useful resource is ANA's *Legislative and Regulatory Initiatives for the 103d Congress* (published biennially to coincide with the current Congress). The publication details the association's legislative priorities including the underlying issue, background, and ANA's position.

REFERENCES

1. Lee R, Benjamin A: Health policy and the politics of health care, in Lee P, Estes C (eds): *The Nation's Health*, Boston: Jones and Bartlett, 1994, p 125.
2. Curtis B, Lumpkin B: Political action committees, in Mason D et al (eds): *Policy and Politics for Nurses*, 2d ed, Philadelphia: Saunders, 1993, pp 562–576.
3. Ibid.
4. Ibid.
5. The federal budget process is given in detail in *The Congressional Budget Process, An Explanation*, Washington, DC: Government Printing Office, 1993.
6. Sardella S: Nurses are a model in health reform. *APA Monitor* 35, March 1994.
7. Talbott SW: Political analysis: Structure and process, in Mason D et al (eds): *Policy and Politics for Nurses*, 2d ed. Philadelphia: Saunders, 1993, pp 129–148.
8. ANA: *Grassroots Lobbying Handbook: Empowering Nurses Through Legislative and Political Action*. Washington, DC: The Association, 1993.

19 *Major Legislation Affecting Nursing*

Sally S. Cohen, R.N., Ph.D., F.A.A.N.

FEDERAL AND STATE LAWS have a major impact on nursing practice and education. At the state level, nurses need to know about their own nursing practice acts and should be acquainted with the licensure laws of other health practitioners. These are discussed in Chap. 20. Other state legislation affecting the health and welfare of nurses may be equally important, and nurses should keep abreast of both proposed and enacted legislation. One of the best ways to keep informed is to be an active member of a nursing association. Such organizations provide leadership and information that is invaluable for nurses who want to have input into health care policy.

This chapter focuses on federal legislation that affects the practice of nursing and the rights of nurses. State laws will be discussed only as they pertain to federal issues. Obviously, there are a plethora of health bills and laws that are relevant to nursing, but only those that have particular significance will be highlighted here.

OVERVIEW OF FEDERAL GOVERNMENT

The federal agencies with responsibility for health care are primarily within the Depart-

ment of Health and Human Services (HHS), although certain health-related programs are administered by other departments. An example is the Food Stamps Program, which the Department of Agriculture administers. Within HHS, there are several major agencies: the Public Health Service (PHS), Health Care Financing Administration (HCFA), and Administration for Children and Families (see Fig. 19-1). Other divisions, such as the Administration on Aging and the Office for Civil Rights, also lie within HHS. Most of the programs discussed in this chapter are under the auspices of the HCFA or the PHS. In 1994, Congress passed legislation that authorized a separate Social Security Administration, effective March 31, 1995. Until then, the Social Security Administration was an agency within HHS, but legislators figured that making it a separate entity might help increase its visibility, accountability, and administrative efficiency.[1]

The HCFA administers the Medicare and Medicaid programs. The PHS includes the Agency for Health Care Policy and Research (AHCPR), Agency for Toxic Substances and Disease Registry, Centers for Disease Control and Prevention, Food and Drug Administration (FDA), Health Resources and Services Admini-

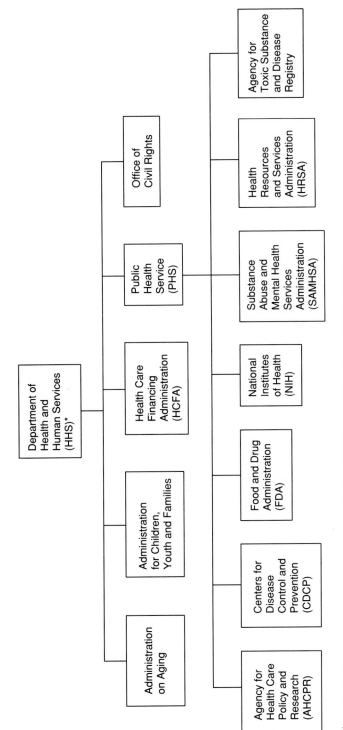

Figure 19-1 Department of Health and Human Services.

*The Social Security Administration was part of HHS until 1994, when it became a separate agency.

stration (HRSA), Indian Health Service, National Institutes of Health (NIH), and the Substance Abuse and Mental Health Services Administration (SAMHSA). The Division of Nursing within the HRSA and the National Institute of Nursing Research (NINR) at the NIH are focal points for nursing initiatives at the federal level and are discussed later in this chapter. However, nurses are involved in every agency listed, and the activities of each agency have an impact on nursing practice. It behooves nursing students and faculty to be knowledgeable about them and provide input whenever possible. It is also important to note that the organization of federal programs for health and social services often undergoes revisions, especially at the beginning of a new presidential administration. Thus the structures depicted in Fig. 19-1 are subject to change at any point in the near future.

Follow-up of federal legislation requires close attention. In addition to the law itself, regulations implementing the law are also important. On one hand, some legislators have charged that regulations circumvent the intent of the law. On the other hand, especially with controversial issues, lawmakers have been known to omit details in legislation and leave them to the regulatory agency to finalize. Federal agencies—such as the FDA and Federal Trade Commission (FTC)—are created by law and responsible for particular issues. Agency decisions can affect nursing practice, as illustrated by various examples throughout this chapter.

SOCIAL POLICY AS A CONTEXT FOR HEALTH CARE

Health care is one facet of America's complex social policy scheme. Compared with other industrialized nations, the United States has been reluctant to establish a government-sponsored social policy system. This is largely because of the traditional American belief that individuals should be self-sufficient, the strong emphasis that Americans have traditionally placed on in-

dividualism and market economics, and political trends and factors that produced a patchwork of social policies over the course of the twentieth century.

One of the earliest social insurance programs developed in the United States was for what is known as social security. The origin, funding, authorization, and development of social security are relevant to those of other social and health programs.

Social Security

Beginning in the mid-1920s there was a growing sense that federal and state governments should play a larger role in helping meet people's unmet needs and that certain risks of a growing industrialized nation could best be met through the development of social insurance programs. By the late 1920s, almost every state had enacted some type of workers' compensation program. But these programs could hardly meet the growing need of individuals and families under an industrialized state. The economic depression of the 1930s intensified the urgency for some type of government intervention in social policies, and culminated in the *Social Security Act of 1935*. The lawmakers who produced the original act based it on the conviction that a program of economic security must "have as its primary aim the assurance of an adequate income to each human being in childhood, youth, middle age, or old age—in sickness or in health" and that it must "provide safeguards against all of the hazards leading to destitution and dependency."

The Social Security Act (SSA) is the origin of most health and social welfare in this country. Each title (or component) covers a specific social program. The act is far broader than the Social Security program. Its later amendments provide many benefits: federal old-age and survivors' insurance (OASI); unemployment compensation; federal grants-in-aid to states to promote special health and welfare services for children; and matching funds to help finance state-administered relief programs for dependent children and other needy persons who are aged, blind, or permanently disabled. Disability insurance programs were enacted in 1956. And since 1965, the Medicare program (Title XVIII of the SSA) has financed a large share of the medical and hospital costs of persons over sixty-five. Title XIX, Medicaid, passed at the same time, was a hasty compromise on the part of the Congress and can probably be best described as a cooperative federal-state medical assistance program for the poor or near-poor. Medicare and Medicaid are discussed in detail later in this chapter.

Old-Age and Survivor's Insurance. The average citizen who talks about Social Security is typically referring to the federal Old-Age, Survivors' and Disability Insurance (OASDI) program. OASDI provides a monthly payment from the federal government to replace, in part, the income that is lost to a worker and his or her family when the wage earner retires, becomes disabled, or dies. OASDI has two components: social security and disability. While the funding mechanisms are similar, the administration of the two programs is somewhat different.

Contributions to OASDI are made under the Federal Insurance Contributions Act (FICA) of the Internal Revenue Code. In most cases, coverage is universal and compulsory for all employees. Approximately 95 percent of all jobs in this country are covered through contributions made by employees, even if self-employed, and matching taxes paid by employers. Employee contributions are withheld from wage and salary payments. They are based on wages and earnings up to the annual maximum taxable wage base. (In 1994, it was $60,600, with adjustments as wages increase.) In 1994, employers and employees were each taxed at a rate of approximately 6.2 percent for social security and disability, combined. The majority—approximately 5.6 percent—was for social security. These rates are not likely to fluctuate much in years to come. Deductions for OASDI appear on employees' paycheck stubs under FICA.[2] As discussed later in this chapter, a similar but separate mechanism exists for financing Medicare.

Monthly cash benefits under social security are paid to workers who are insured for benefits and to their eligible dependents and survivors. The amount of these benefits is based on the individual's average earnings and length of employment during his or her working life. Retirement age is officially 62 for both men and women. If she or he prefers, however, an individual may wait until 65 to start drawing benefits; if so, monthly checks will be larger than if begun at 62. If a person continues to work for a salary after retirement age, the amount of annual earnings affects the Social Security benefits. For example, in 1994, a beneficiary aged 65 to 69 may earn $11,160 before benefits are reduced $1 for each additional $3 of earnings.[3] Beginning in the next century, the retirement age will gradually be increased until it reaches 66 in 2009 and 67 in 2027. Meanwhile, delayed retirements (beyond 65) will gain higher benefits for people with incomes above certain base amounts.

The Social Security Advisory Council, a group of prominent private citizens established by the law, has periodically made suggestions (with no guarantee of acceptance) to Congress and the President. One of the council's recommendations was that all Social Security credits and benefits be shared equally by husbands and wives, and that every retired person have minimal Social Security benefits at age 65 plus whatever benefits may be earned as workers. Based on the reports of the Advisory Council, as well as pressure from interest groups representing the elderly, Congress has periodically made changes in the Social Security program. For example, since 1984, all federal employees and those in nonprofit organizations must be covered by Social Security. Also, under the Omnibus Budget Reconciliation Act (OBRA) of 1986, Social Security is exempt from automatic spending cuts required to reduce the federal budget deficit. (See Chap. 18 for a discussion of the federal budget process.) In 1990, congress enacted legislation requiring the SSA, upon request, to provide individuals with statements of their contributions and estimates of their future benefits.

To a great extent, Social Security was originally and still is slanted toward the male wage earner, with the assumption that most couples would remain married, that the husband would be the main breadwinner, and that the wife would stay home. These trends have been offset by the longer lifespan of most women compared with men, and the rising labor force participation rates of women of all ages, even those with young children. Thus "the social security system has not kept pace with the changing roles of men and women." For example, women's wages remain lower than men's, resulting in lower benefits paid to women when they retire. Furthermore, women are still likely to spend less time in the workforce than men because they also carry the major responsibilities for home and children.[4] Future changes in social security might include adjustments to correct these imbalances.

Disability Insurance. Contributions to the Disability Insurance Trust Fund from employers and employees are made in the same manner as those for social security. However, unlike social security, which is solely under the jurisdiction of the federal government, disability insurance is administered through both federal Social Security offices and state disability determination services. Nearly 5 million individuals are receiving disability insurance, and the numbers have been increasing since the mid-1980s.

An insured worker of any age, male or female, who becomes totally disabled can begin receiving benefits after a five-month waiting period. Benefits are also paid to dependent spouses, widows (or widowers), and children of those who are disabled. To be eligible for these benefits, the worker must (1) have been covered by social security for a specified number of years (five to ten); (2) have a physical or mental disability of indefinite duration; and (3) be so badly disabled that she or he cannot work at gainful employment.

In recent years, payments and benefits for disability have expanded and shifted in several notable ways. For example, there has been an increase in the proportion of women receiving disability benefits, reflecting the surge of women in the paid labor force. In addition, compared with 1970, the percentage of disabled who have a mental, psychoneurotic, or personality disorder has grown from 11 to 25 percent in 1992, while those with circulatory conditions have decreased commensurably.[5]

In 1989, Congress took action to alleviate the burden of health insurance on the disabled by passing a law extending the period in which employers must let former workers who are disabled keep the group rate. The period was extended from 18 to 29 months, and the law is expected to protect 40,000 disabled, including 12,000 infected with HIV.[6]

In sum, Congress periodically revises OASDI policies, based on shifts in the target population and lobbying efforts in behalf of those involved with the programs. The over 41 million social security and disability beneficiaries comprise a formidable interest group for politicians. The size and success of the social security system in protecting many elderly and disabled against poverty means that it will continue to hold a prominent place on the legislative agenda for years to come.

Unemployment Insurance. Another major provision of the Social Security Act of 1935 is a system of unemployment insurance to protect workers who are unemployed through no fault of their own. Unemployment insurance is administered by state governments. Federal law specifies a maximum and minimum benefit, and the states must remain within these limits. Each state has its own law governing the amount of weekly benefits allowed the unemployed person and the number of weeks for which it will be continued. This is because the cost of living and employment conditions vary so widely in different sections of the country. Thus unemployment policies are very much dependent on state laws.

Changes in federal and state unemployment laws usually parallel trends in the economy, in particular, unemployment rates. For example, during the economic recession of the early

1990s, Congress enacted several Emergency Unemployment Compensation laws to assist the long-term unemployed. These laws supplement standing unemployment policies, to assist those who have been out of work for an extended period of time. In some cases, the laws allowed for an additional 26 weeks of unemployment payments. Emergency unemployment laws are often of limited duration, and in addition to requiring states to offer particular benefits, they also establish funding mechanisms for the extended unemployment payments.

As health care agencies respond to changes in the health care delivery system by restructuring and perhaps laying off registered professional nurses, these nurses will find that unemployment policies are more germane to their practice than in the past. Furthermore, the emotional stress of unemployment for an individual or family warrants that nurses be attuned to unemployment laws.

Information pertaining to state eligibility requirements and administration of benefits is available from local unemployment offices. To collect unemployment insurance, a person must have been out of work for at least a week; be able to work and willing to take a job in his or her line of work at the prevailing rate; must not have left the previous job without good cause or have been asked to resign because of misconduct. In some states, marriage, pregnancy, and further education do not qualify one to claim unemployment insurance, and a mother cannot collect unemployment benefits for a certain period after childbirth.

Medicare-Medicaid

When enacted into law in 1965, Medicare (Title XVIII of the Social Security Act) provided hospitalization for Social Security recipients, as well as allowing purchase of insurance for physicians' services at a nominal monthly fee. Medicare, when originally proposed, was extremely controversial, with some citizens and legislators not completely committed to the idea and the AMA rigorously and uncompromisingly op-

posed to it. ANA, however, supported it. Passed in 1965, Medicare went into effect on July 1, 1966.[7,8]

Medicare Benefits and Coverage

Medicare is a nationwide health insurance program for the aged and certain disabled persons. In both of the two parts (A and B) of Medicare, the benefits are limited to those who are sixty-five years of age or older and some disabled under sixty-five. Parts A and B are separate but coordinated health insurance programs. Medicare is the largest payer of health care costs in the U.S. medical system, paying for approximately 20 percent of all personal health services, with sizable increases in costs expected in future years.[9]

Most Americans, upon turning 65, are automatically enrolled in part A, which consists of Hospital Insurance (HI). Others, who qualify as disabled or are in need of kidney dialysis, are eligible for part A regardless of age. Part A is financed out of payroll taxes collected under the Social Security system in a manner similar to the funding for OASDI. That is, employees and employers each contribute 1.45 percent of an employee's earnings to the HI Trust Fund. All HI benefits and administrative costs are paid for out of this trust fund.

Approximately 31 million aged and 3.7 million disabled are covered under part A, and nearly 7 million and 1 million, respectively, receive reimbursed services. Given trends of increased longevity and the aging "baby-boom" generation, the number of beneficiaries covered under Medicare part A will inevitably increase in the near future.

Under part A, the patient pays a deductible, which has been increasing, for hospital care, and the government pays the rest for a given period. In 1994, the deductible was $696. Part A also covers skilled nursing facility (SNF) care, home health care, and hospice care, with certain limits on the number of days or visits in each category. For example, part A covers up to 100 days in a skilled nursing facility, following hospitalization. Hospice care for those with a life expectancy of six months or less is covered for 210 days. Reimbursement for home care under Medicare requires that certain criteria be met, such as the client being referred to a Medicare certified agency, and being homebound. Although home health comprises only about 5 percent of Medicare outlays, it is expected to soar in years ahead.[10, 11]

Part B of Medicare is an optional Supplemental Medical Insurance (SMI) program available to those over 65 upon payment of a monthly premium. The monthly premium, as of January 1994, was $41, with increases planned for ensuing years. SMI is financed through these premiums along with general government revenues. Approximately 31 million aged and 3.5 million disabled are enrolled in part B. Most part A beneficiaries are also enrolled in part B.

Part B pays 80 percent of the individual's cost for physicians' services in excess of an annual deductible. Specific services covered are physician's care in the hospital, home, or office; laboratory and other diagnostic tests; outpatient services at a hospital; therapeutic equipment such as braces and artificial limbs; home health services for those not covered under part A; mammography; and respite care consisting of in-home personal services that allow homebound enrollees' usual caretakers to take respite. In recent years, Medicare has covered the services of certain nonphysician providers, such as certified registered nurse anesthetists, nurse practitioners, and clinical nurse specialists (in collaboration with physicians), clinical psychologists, and physician assistants.

The Medicare program is the responsibility of the Health Care Financing Administration (HCFA) within HHS. However, much of the daily operational work of Medicare is under the auspices of *intermediaries*, who handle claims from hospitals, home health agencies, and skilled nursing facilities. HCFA assigns intermediaries on a regional basis, and their responsibilities include conducting reviews and audits, determining costs and reimbursement amounts, and monitoring for fraud and abuse. Subject to

HCFA approval, a hospital or other provider under part A can contract with national, state, or other public or private agencies as intermediaries.[12] Similarly, HCFA contracts with *carriers*—typically Blue Cross Blue Shield plans and commercial insurance companies insurance organizations—to handle claims from doctors and other suppliers of services under part B. The use of intermediaries and carriers is considered by some not only as adding another layer of bureaucracy but also as increasing costs. However, the administrative costs of Medicare are approximately 2.5 percent of total outlays, which is less than those for private insurance.

Over the past decade, the federal government has promoted coordinated care plans under Medicare, which are prepaid, managed care plans, usually administered by health maintenance organizations or competitive medical plans. These entities contract with Medicare to provide all of the services for Medicare beneficiaries, at a fixed premium and small copayment. Coordinated care plans may also offer benefits—such as preventive care, dental care, and eyeglasses—not covered under Medicare. As the health care delivery system moves toward managed care plans for all consumers of care, these arrangements will be increasingly prevalent under Medicare.

Long-term care is likely to be an area to which Congress and health policy experts will devote more attention in the near future as the demand for such services increases and the costs remain prohibitive. During the 1980s, costs for long-term care (skilled nursing facilities and home health care) more than doubled from 2.9 to 6.1 percent of total Medicare payments. Despite the increase in costs, long-term care is only one of several services that the elderly often need, but for which they are not adequately covered under Medicare. Preventive care and prescription drugs are other examples. Given the gaps in Medicare coverage, many private insurance companies sell Medigap policies for services not covered under Medicare. In 1990, Congress enacted legislation that established standards for Medigap and limited the number of standard benefit plans that could be available in any state or jurisdiction to no more than 10.[13]

Many discussions regarding health care reform call for ways to expand coverage for Medicare beneficiaries, while keeping costs in line. Financing these expansions would require placing a greater financial burden on beneficiaries, lowering provider reimbursement rates, or raising taxes on employers and employees (or some combination of these alternatives). The political stakes involved in any of these options create fierce competition and turmoil in the legislative arena. Regardless of what route federal lawmakers take to pursue health care reform, Medicare will probably endure, given its large constituency. However, this does not make it immune from changes in reimbursement, benefits, payments, and other policies.

Medicaid Benefits and Coverage

Medicaid was authorized in 1965 as Title XIX of the Social Security Act to pay for medical services in behalf of certain groups of low-income persons. It is a federal-state means-tested entitlement program, also administered by the HCFA. Certain groups of persons (i.e., the aged, blind, disabled, members of families with dependent children, and certain other children and pregnant women) qualify for coverage if their incomes and resources are sufficiently low. Each state designs and administers its own Medicaid program, setting eligibility and coverage standards within broad federal guidelines. As a result, substantial variation exists among the states in terms of persons covered, types and scope of benefits offered, and amount of payments for services. On the average, the federal government pays 56 percent of the benefit costs and states pay the rest. Approximately 36 million people are enrolled in Medicaid. The rapid rise in Medicaid costs is of concern to state and federal lawmakers. From 1991 to 1992, total Medicaid outlays increased from $90.5 billion to almost $115 billion.

Until 1986, Medicaid eligibility was tied to welfare. In that year, Medicaid was extended to include certain women and children with low incomes who were not covered by the Aid to Families with Dependent Children (AFDC) program. This change was important because state poverty levels are considerably lower than the federal poverty level and were used as AFDC eligibility criteria, thus keeping many poor women and children from receiving necessary health care.

It is important to note that Medicaid does not cover all poor people. In addition to income, assets and resources are considered in determining eligibility on a state-by-state basis. Furthermore, besides the poor, other medically needy individuals can be eligible, based on federal and state criteria.

The Medicaid program also provides services to a diverse elderly population, mostly in terms of nursing home care. Medicaid remains the nation's major program of financial support for persons needing nursing home care. Approximately 68 percent of Medicaid payments for the aged is for nursing home care, 11 percent is for inpatient hospital care, and 21 percent is for other services (such as outpatient hospital, home health, and laboratory services).

Another notable aspect of Medicaid is that the proportion of beneficiaries in a particular category does not necessarily correspond to the percentage of funds that are allocated to that group. For example, in 1992 children in AFDC families comprised approximately 49 percent of Medicaid recipients, but received 16 percent of total Medicaid payments. The historically low proportion of payments going to families with children, especially given the number of children and pregnant women lacking adequate health care, spurred Congress to enact a number of laws expanding Medicaid coverage and eligibility for children and pregnant women. These laws are discussed in later sections.

Major Amendments Affecting Medicare and Medicaid

In the years following enactment, much criticism was directed toward Medicare and Medicaid. As a result, frequent amendments were enacted, with the intent of controlling soaring costs and eliminating fraud and abuse of funds. There are now rigid regulations about the length of institutional stay that will be reimbursed, level of care requirements for skilled nursing home services, payment for specific services, and coverage of particular groups. Another major concern, quality of care, also resulted in legislative amendments. Although any institutions participating in Medicare must be certified by HHS and those participating in Medicaid must abide by standards set by each state, the quality of care Medicare beneficiaries receive has often wavered.

One legislative initiative aimed at improving the quality of care under Medicare was the Professional Standards Review Organization (PSRO) amendment in 1972, which mandated the establishment of PSROs within all states to improve the quality of health care and make it more cost-effective. The intent was to involve local practicing physicians in the ongoing reviews and evaluation of health care service rendered under Medicare and Medicaid. PSROs were primarily the responsibility of and under the control of physicians.

Despite the activities that PSROs generated in quality assurance and utilization review, they still presented several problems: lack of adequate funding, lack of uniformity among PSROs, difficulty in changing physician practice behavior, and lack of agreed-upon measures of success. In 1982, P.L. 97-248 changed PSROs to PROs (Peer Review Organizations) and permitted quality assurance by private entities in a competitive market. PROs review only Medicare services. Medicaid and other reviews are left entirely to the states. There is only one PRO per state, with some subcontracting with regional units in larger states. In addition, PROs have had much more input from nurses and consumers than PSROs, some of which has been required by law.

In 1986, as part of another effort to improve quality under Medicare, Congress enacted the Health Care Quality Improvement Act (P.L. 99-

660). Among its provisions was the establishment of a National Practitioner Data Bank (NPDB), "to encourage health care practitioners to identify and discipline practitioners who engage in unprofessional behavior and restrict the ability of incompetent practitioners to move from state to state without disclosure of discovery of the practitioner's previous performance."[14]

The NPDB pertains to physicians and other practitioners, such as registered nurses. The Medicare and Medicaid Patient and Program Protection Act of 1987 clarified the responsibilities of the NPDB, and of registered nurses in relation to the NPDB. In short, nurses may be reported to the board for adverse licensure actions or adverse professional actions. They also may be reported for medical malpractice claims paid with certain stipulations.[15] The NPDB has generated concern among many physicians and nurses that the federal government is monitoring their practice too closely and infringing on their rights. However, the potential for the NPDB to safeguard the public from the dangers of unqualified health professionals seems to outweigh its drawbacks, as long as professional organizations, such as ANA, continue to work to protect the rights of the practitioners with regard to NPDB activities.

Another important development in 1990 was the Institute of Medicine (IOM) study on Medicare and quality of care. The report covered methods and research strategies for assessing quality and implementing quality assurance programs. It called for a redirection of quality assurance programs under Medicare toward clinical evaluations and patient outcomes, and emphasized the importance of conducting assessments in settings other than hospitals. The report also criticized PROs for not devoting enough attention to quality, and for creating excessive burdens for providers.[16]

In addition to concerns about quality, the problem of funding Medicare reached panic proportions by the 1980s. The system's trustees reported that even under the most optimistic conditions, either disbursements would have to be reduced by 30 percent or financing would have to be increased by 43 percent to prevent exhaustion of the Hospital Insurance Trust Fund by 1996. Two ongoing problems were the escalating growth of the over-sixty-five population, which the Census Bureau projected would comprise 13.1 percent of the population by the year 2000, and the shrinking tax base. The 116 million workers and their employers each paid a portion of workers' wages into the Trust Fund, but this was dwarfed by the rising cost of hospital care.

At the same time, the newly elected Reagan administration clearly stated that they were not interested in large-scale federal subsidies of health care. Costs had escalated tremendously but had been grudgingly absorbed in each new funding year. Medicare was a political "hot potato," especially with an active "graying America" lobbying force (and after all, everyone will someday grow old and may be threatened by serious illness). Medicaid had always stirred controversy among federal and state politicians. Thus, cuts were inevitable—in fact, had been creeping up since the end of Johnson's Great Society. Legislation affecting the Medicare-Medicaid program came in various guises, some directly aimed at resolving its problems, some as part of other laws. Some actually increased benefits.

The *Omnibus Budget Reconciliation Act of 1981* (P.L. 97-35) (OBRA 81) was one of the first major legislative reforms with far-reaching results. The new law made many changes. About $1 billion of the cuts in health care spending for fiscal year (FY) 1982 were from Medicaid. Federal payments were cut progressively for each year through 1984. Medicare funding too was cut, and all but one public health hospital were closed.

Even more dramatic were the provisions of the *Tax Equity and Fiscal Responsibility Act of 1982* (TEFRA) (P.L. 97-248). It required the Secretary of HHS and certain congressional committees to develop Medicare prospective reimbursement legislative proposals for hospitals, SNFs, and, to the extent feasible, other providers. Other cost-cutting mechanisms affecting health care facilities and providers were also included.

The work on the prospective payment mechanisms resulted in enactment of P.L. 98-21, variously called the *Social Security Amendments of 1983*, the *Social Security Rescue Plan*, or simply the *DRG law*. This legislation established a "prospective payment system based on 467 Diagnostic Related Groups (DRGs) that allow pretreatment diagnosis billing categories for almost all United State hospitals reimbursed by Medicare."[17] Separate payment rates applied to urban and rural areas. Psychiatric, long-term care, children's, and rehabilitation hospitals continued to be reimbursed under the cost-based system. But over time, the feasibility of prospective payment for these types of facilities (as well as home care) was also explored, and implemented, with various degrees of success. The DRG category to which a patient is assigned is determined by their principal diagnosis (reason for entering the delivery system), age, the presence or absence of surgery or major procedure, and complications or secondary diagnosis (comorbidity).

The DRG system was phased in over 3 years. The Secretary of HHS was required to collect data and report to Congress on the advisability and feasibility of including physician payments under prospective payment. What DRGs mean to a hospital is that if a patient is kept more than the number of days designated by the patient's DRG category, the extra costs must be absorbed. If the patient goes home early, the amount designated for the scheduled days is the hospital's clear profit. Some predicted that hospitals would encourage doctors to admit more patients who were not potential "problems" or those who were self-paying or insured.

Needless to say, the DRG system had a direct impact on nursing. In some cases, hospitals, desperate to cut costs, chose to retain lower-paid nursing personnel, rather than RNs. Others chose to turn to all-RN staffs that could actually save money by teaching patients or by anticipating potential complications, so that the patient would be discharged before the DRG designated days. As noted in Chap. 15, the job market for nurses also became tighter. However, some nurses felt that this was also a good time to identify nursing services, so that they could be separated from general daily charges. Others identified ways of determining the acuity of nursing care so that these could be considered in the DRG system.[18,19]

Since the enactment of prospective payment in 1983, there have been a series of revisions in Medicare through legislation and regulation. Many of the new laws deal with prospective payment rates, based on recommendations of the Prospective Payment Assessment Commission (ProPAC) and the Physician Payment Review Commission. Nursing has had an impact on these deliberations through its nurse representatives on the Commissions, studies of costing out of nursing services under DRGs, and the lobbying of major nursing organizations.

One of the most fascinating episodes in Medicare history was the enactment and one year later repeal of the Medicare Catastrophic Coverage Act of 1988. The legislation was to provide a new part B drug program to cover prescription drugs; to extend coverage for SNF, hospice, and respite care; and to cover other services, such as mammography. In 1989, in response to protests from beneficiaries over the rising costs they were forced to incur, Congress repealed the act, eliminating all of these Medicare benefits. (Medicaid and other components of the bill were maintained.)

Many policy makers thought that the repeal of catastrophic coverage would hit states the most, as state Medicaid programs would have to pick up the burden of health care for the elderly. Once the mood in Congress subsided after the stormy sessions over the catastrophic repeal, some legislators expressed interest in restoring a few of the benefits the act had provided (and adding some new ones). Biennial mammography screening and elimination of a limit on hospice care were reinstated by Congress in the Omnibus Budget Reconciliation Act of 1990.

It is difficult to ascertain what the exact effect of prospective payment has been on quality of care, primarily because no study has uncovered a systematic pattern of diminished quality as a result of DRGs. Nonetheless, certain trends are discernible. Average hospital stays dropped 18 percent (1.8 days) between 1981 and 1990. Hospital patients are more acutely ill, requiring more nursing resources. Nursing home admissions increased nearly threefold over approximately the same period. Medicare and other patients are discharged in more clinically unstable conditions than in previous years, placing greater demands on family members, community resources, and providers.

As we move past the midpoint in the decade, there are more recent observations that begin to contradict our earlier statements. We now have empty nursing home beds, the average hospital length of stay has leveled off, and managed care will decrease the overall acuity of hospital patients (stressing prevention and early intervention). The movement toward community services continues, and health care resources are being moved in that direction, with infrastructure redesign in hospitals echoing these patterns.

All of these issues reinforced the need for standardized data regarding billing and services. Standardized definitions can enhance data collection and analysis with regard to cost and quality, and streamline what are now burdensome administrative costs due to the plethora of forms generated by various providers and insurers. To that end, Medicare's Current Procedural Terminology (CPT) codes for classifying services are used by all Blue Cross Blue Shield plans, and by most commercial insurers. Similarly, most providers use the International Classification of Disease, Ninth Revision, Clinical Modification (ICD-9-CM) coding system to classify diagnoses. Despite the problems associated with this system, it does allow for comparisons within and across payers and providers.

The trend is for greater standardization of forms used by all hospitals and institutions, and to include data regarding severity of illness, multiple diagnoses and procedures, and other conditions. Since October 1993, all hospitals and institutional providers have been required to use the same Medicare billing forms. Professional and community-based providers will also be subject to uniform billing and data collection systems in the near future.[20]

Medicare policies have also expanded reimbursement for specific health care practitioners. In recent years, nurses have successfully lobbied for Medicare reimbursement of various types of nursing services. For example, in 1987, Congress approved Community Nursing Organizations (CNOs) under Medicare as a way of providing the continuum of care that beneficiaries often require in a cost-effective manner (see Chap. 7). As another example, the 1987 Budget Reconciliation Act of 1987 (P.L. 100-203) included a provision for Medicare payment of services of certified nurse-midwives working in HMOs.

The reconciliation bill of 1989 (P.L. 99-509) included major revisions in reimbursement for physician services under Medicare part B, prompted by the dramatically rising costs of Medicare part B. The bill revamped the system of paying doctors on the basis of customary, prevailing, and reasonable fees, and replaced it with a Medicare fee schedule (MFS) that based payments on the resource costs involved in providing care. The resource costs included physician work, practice expense, and malpractice insurance expenses. The MFS also included the costs of a doctor's training and the relative value of the technical skills needed.[21,22]

The new system, which went into effect in January 1992, is based on a resource-based relative value schedule (RBRVS), which compensates based on the service rendered as opposed to the person rendering the service.[23]

These changes in physician reimbursement under Medicare provided incentives for review of nonphysician and noninstitutional reimbursement, which affected nursing practice and reimbursement, too. For example, in 1989, nurses made headway in Medicare reimbursement of their services. First, certified registered nurse anesthetists (CRNAs) succeeded in obtaining direct reimbursement under Medicare for anesthesia services that they are legally authorized to perform in a state. In previous years, CRNAs lobbied successfully to ensure

that the cost of their services was not included in hospitals' DRG rates but would be "passed through" on the basis of reasonable cost.

Second, the 1989 reconciliation bill authorized nurse practitioners (NPs) and clinical nurse specialists (CNSs) working in collaboration with a physician to certify and recertify the need for skilled nursing facility care under Medicare. It also included indirect reimbursement to institutions for NP services as part of nursing home reform.[24]

Third, the reconciliation bill mandated a Physician Payment Review Commission (PPRC) study of nonphysician providers, to be submitted to Congress by July 1, 1991. Nurses had input into the call for this study through their representatives on the PPRC and the lobbying of ANA and other nursing organizations. In 1992, the PPRC made recommendations to Congress based on this study. The PPRC found a tremendous amount of variation in how nurses were paid for their services under Medicare, especially with regard to services "incident to" those of physicians. (Services "incident to" a physician's are those provided by nonphysicians that are an integral, although incidental, part of the visit, and necessary for diagnosing or treating an injury or illness.) The PPRC recommended that all services provided by nonphysicians should be identified as such on the claims forms. In 1993, HCFA issued rules allowing nonphysician providers to be eligible for "incident to" compensation at the full physician reimbursement rate, under physician supervision, even if a physician did not provide care to the patient at the time of the visit.[25]

The PPRC also recommended that nonphysician providers (including nurse practitioners, nurse-midwives, and CRNAs) be reimbursed at rates less than those for physicians, to reflect differences in educational investment. This was in direct contrast to the position of nursing organizations, such as the ANA and the National Alliance of Nurse Practitioners, who argued that the services provided by nurse practitioners should be reimbursed at the same rate of comparable services provided by physicians. By

1994, payment of advanced practice nurses under Medicare varied, depending on the location of the service and the setting. For example, nurse practitioners in rural areas were eligible for direct payment for their services (though at a percent of the physician rate if not "incident to"), while those practicing in nursing homes could receive no more than 85 percent of the physician's payment, payable to the employer.

As of 1994, the PPRC still endorsed percentage differentials for nonphysician practitioner fees, contending that the services provided by nonphysician practitioners are not the same as those rendered by physicians.[26] Organized nursing continues to claim otherwise and is committed to fighting to increase the reimbursement of nurses under Medicare, and other insurers. As an example, ANA and other nursing groups worked to ensure that under President Clinton's reform proposals, all services that advanced practice nurses are allowed to perform under state law would be reimbursable under Medicare, as well as other programs. The fee schedule would be determined by the particular plan or alliance.

Medicaid reforms for the elderly have focused largely on quality of care in long-term care facilities. In 1987, Congress enacted legislation addressing various quality issues in nursing home care under Medicaid. The legislation (P.L. 100-203) included changes in the standards of care nursing homes must meet. The law included a minimum data set for resident assessment, new nurse staffing requirements of one RN 8 hours a day and 24-hour licensed nurse coverage, guidelines for nursing assistant training, and rigorous standards for the use of chemical or physical restraints. Much of this legislation was in response to the findings of a 1986 Institute of Medicine (IOM) report, *Improving the Quality of Care in Nursing Homes* (see also Chap. 7).

In 1990, the HHS issued a report on resident abuse in nursing homes. The major findings showed that abuse is a significant problem, with aides and orderlies as the primary abusers. Recommendations for training and educational programs and research on staff-patient ratios were included in the report. The legislation,

regulations, and reports on nursing home care are of major importance to the nursing profession because of the prominent role nurses play in the continuity, provision, and supervision of nursing home care.

As with Medicare, nurses also improved their reimbursement under Medicaid, reaching an important milestone in 1989 when Congress enacted legislation providing for coverage of FNP and PNP services under Medicaid (as long as they are practicing within the scope of state law). This was deemed important in improving access to care for many pregnant women and children. Since July 1990, states have been required to cover the services of PNPs and FNPs for Medicaid patients, regardless of whether the NPs are under the supervision of, or associated with, a physician. Payment rates are determined by individual states, and vary considerably.

Surveys of state Medicaid programs revealed that more than half of the states allow other types of nurse practitioners to participate in Medicaid, even though only PNPs and FNPs are required. In addition, unlike Medicare, state Medicaid policies do not limit coverage to rural settings. Nurse practitioners are covered in all types of locales. The status of reimbursement for nurses in advanced practice by state is reported in several sources and treated with more detail in Chaps. 15 and 20.[27] The contributions of nurse practitioners to improving access to and patient satisfaction with care bode well for future expansions of their role and reimbursement under Medicaid, as well as under private insurance.

Other very significant changes in Medicaid were enacted throughout the 1980s. When President Ronald Reagan came into office, he and his staff were intent on removing many of the working poor from the Medicaid program, as well as reducing AFDC eligibility levels. Decreases in funding and eligibility criteria for Medicaid ensued. Between 1981 and 1984, Medicaid's average annual growth rate slowed to 7.5 percent, down from an average of 15 percent between 1975 and 1981. In response to lobbying from many maternal and child health interest groups, most notably the Children's Defense Fund, the end of the 1980s brought expansion of Medicaid eligibility criteria and renewed interest in maternal and child health initiatives in Congress and the Reagan and Bush administrations. Three factors were mostly responsible for the prompt legislative action in these areas: (1) the high rate of poverty among children (approximately 25 percent); (2) the large proportion of the uninsured who are individuals under 18 (approximate 66 percent); and (3) the nation's embarrassingly high infant mortality rate and large number of unimmunized preschool children.

The expansion of Medicaid in recent years has occurred incrementally, with intense deliberations at state and federal levels of government. The discussions focused on what states were required and had the option to provide under Medicaid. The changes have had a significant impact on access to and financing of health care for American's women and children.

Most significantly, the Sixth Omnibus Reconciliation Act of 1986 (SOBRA) gave states the option of extending automatic Medicaid coverage to pregnant women and children younger than 5 years of age, with family incomes below the federal poverty level but above state AFDC eligibility levels. This option represented a major shift toward ending the dependency between AFDC and Medicaid programs.

Through federal legislation enacted in the late 1980s and early 1990s, Medicaid is required to cover all pregnant women and children under age six who are eligible for AFDC in a particular state, or whose family income is at or below 133 percent of the federal poverty level. In addition, Medicaid must cover all children born after September 30, 1993, in families with incomes at or below the federal poverty level. This phased-in coverage will ensure that by the year 2002, all children under age 19 from poor families have benefits.

Despite these incremental changes, many children still lack health coverage. Thus many legislators and advocacy groups prefer a mandated Medicaid eligibility level of at least 185 percent of poverty and continue to push for enactment of such a law. In the meantime, states have the option of extending Medicaid coverage to infants and pregnant women with family income up to 185 percent of poverty, certain poor children under age 21, and other categories of individuals deemed medically needy, such as the disabled. The extent to which these options become implemented remains linked to the status of federal and state budgets. Moreover, some proposals for health care reform give children and pregnant women priority. However, even if more children receive health insurance, barriers to care unfortunately will persist, making public health measures all the more important.

PUBLIC HEALTH PROGRAMS RELEVANT TO NURSING PRACTICE

Block Grants

In addition to Medicare and Medicaid, there are several important public health initiatives relevant to nursing practice. Block grants have been in existence for many years, but they became increasingly popular under President Reagan, who favored block grants over categorical funding for separate programs. Block grants, funded through federal and state matched funds, shift much of the political and administrative accountability to the states, without subsequent increases in state funding. The result is often inequities among states in terms of populations covered by the programs, and competition among the various programs funded under a block grant in a particular state. The major advantage to block grants is the streamlining they provide at the federal level by consolidating programs into clusters for legislative and programmatic purposes.

In 1981, several health block grants were formed: maternal and child health, preventive services, and mental health (including alcohol and drug abuse). Congress originally designated a primary care block grant that consisted of community and migrant health center programs, but it was never officially made a block grant, and today these remain categorical programs.

In 1992, under P.L. 102-321, which reorganized the administration of mental health treatment and research services at the federal level and created the new SAMHSA, the mental health block grant was divided into two components. First, the Substance Abuse Prevention and Treatment Block Grant was formed, in recognition of the scope and costs of substance abuse and that more attention was needed in that area. It became the largest specialized form of support for substance abuse, funded at approximately $1.2 billion in 1994. Each state must spend at least 35 percent of this block grant for prevention and treatment of alcohol addiction, and at least another 35 percent for drug abuse and treatment services. Another sign of the importance of this block grant is that for fiscal year 1995, President Clinton proposed $345 million additional funding for treatment of hard core addictions. The second mental health block grant is the Community Mental Health and Services Block Grant, which provided support to states to develop community mental health services, emphasizing networks of families, providers, and other community resources. It was funded at approximately $280 million in 1994.

By the mid-1990s, Congress appropriated approximately $670,000 for the Maternal and Child Health Block Grant. This includes programs for children with special health care needs, immunizations, school health, prenatal care, and other child health services. The Prevention Block Grant was funded at approximately $160 million by the mid-1990s and covers activities as diverse as health education, rape crisis intervention, fluoridation, hypertension prevention, and funding for tuberculosis and immunizations. Since the late 1980s, federal funding for the public health block grants has increased, albeit very incrementally. They still lack the support needed to reach members of the populations they are intended to serve, and their future will depend on budget resources and the extent to which their advocates can successfully compete for political support.

Health Planning Legislation

One of the early health services laws that provided funds (on a matching grant basis) for constructing and expanding health care facilities was the *Hospital Survey and Construction Act of 1946*, popularly known as the *Hill-Burton Act*. It was highly successful, providing funds for more than 30 percent of the hospital beds in this country in its first twenty years, and funding was renewed several times.

Under Hill-Burton, states received money for developing a planning program, supposedly based on need. As might be expected, however, politics was a more important factor than any rational basis for planning. This resulted in a substantial oversupply of hospital beds and contributed to inflation of health care costs as it became imperative to keep those beds filled.

After the enactment of several unsuccessful health planning laws in the 1960s, Congress passed the *National Health Planning and Resources Development Act of 1974*. It was designed to set up a new system of state and local health planning agencies and to integrate into those agencies a program for the support of certain kinds of health facility construction. Under the act, each state was required to establish a state health planning and development agency (SHPDA) and a state health coordinating council (SHCC) to advise the agency. Health Systems Agencies (HSAs) were responsible for collecting and analyzing data concerning the health care status of the residents in their designated health service area, the state of the area's health care delivery system, and its utilization, among other things. Most HSAs were private, nonprofit organizations with governing boards of 10 to 30 persons, the majority consumers. Nurses served on a number of these boards. Their power lay in their ability to review and approve or disapprove use of certain federal funds in their areas. HSAs were always accused of "playing politics." Moreover, there was often poor communication and coordination among HSAs, state, and national agencies.

In 1979, the Health Planning and Resources

Development Amendments were signed into law. Agreement on the amendments was delayed for three years because of the various conflicts about the effectiveness of the law. Too much provider influence was one accusation. Another was related to the "certificate of need" (CON) power of the HSAs, without which existing health facilities cannot buy certain expensive equipment or expand.

Health planning provisions squeaked through under the budget reconciliation act of 1981 but lost its authorization in 1986. This was in part because they failed to do enough to keep costs down (even though the original intent of health planning was not cost control). In addition, the political and administrative burdens they imposed often outweighed any type of planning effectiveness.[28] Since then, most states continue health planning efforts on their own without a federal mandate. They continue to operate CON programs, even if they have liberalized requirements, exempt certain types or projects, or expand CON purview.[29]

Although no longer mandated under federal law, HSAs left a legacy on the health planning landscape that is not easily erased. In particular, they demonstrated how even the best-laid plans for consumer and provider collaboration can fall prey to political maneuvers, and they left many government and health professionals leery of trying such a structured, bureaucratic route for regulating health care. In the wake of health care reform, states have developed new options for health planning. Many have initiated studies or commissions to determine the state's health needs or to focus on particular populations. These projects are often coordinated with public health initiatives while making the most efficient use of state dollars and resources.

Health Services Legislation and Programs

Various other laws providing health care programs and services of interest to nurses include the following:

The *Health Maintenance Organization Act of 1973* authorized funding over five years to help set up and evaluate HMOs in communities throughout the country. HMOs are a prepaid group health plan, for which subscribers pay a predetermined flat fee monthly or yearly that entitles them to basic health care services as needed (Chap. 7). The 1973 law encouraged employers to offer HMOs as an option of health coverage for their employees, and it provided grants and loans to encourage HMO growth. Emphasis is on preventive care and health teaching. In the 1970s and 1980s, Congress extended and amended the 1973 HMO law and relaxed some of its rigid requirements. Throughout the 1970s and 1980s, HMOs continued to receive federal support, primarily because of the cost-effective and competitive incentives they build into the delivery system.

The popularity of HMOs in the private sector prompted several federal initiatives for increasing their use among Medicare and Medicaid populations. For example, the Medicare risk program passed under the reconciliation act of 1982 allowed the federal government to develop contracts with HMOs for Medicare beneficiaries, with the intent of saving dollars. Similar arrangements have been made for Medicaid recipients, following the easing of federal restrictions in 1981. Although these arrangements have proliferated, largely because of federal laws and rules that encourage their development, it is unclear if HMOs either save dollars or improve access to care. HMOs present the same disadvantages and advantages for Medicare and Medicaid recipients as they do for groups who use them under private insurance (i.e., lack of flexibility in choosing a provider and restrictions on selection and usage of specialists). Their potential for aggregating costs, emphasizing health promotion, and streamlining the delivery of services gives them a prominent role under health care reform.

Human Immunodeficiency Virus/Acquired Immune Deficiency Syndrome. During the 1980s, federal funding for acquired immunodeficiency syndrome (AIDS) became a hot topic. Federal policies for AIDS remain extremely fragmented, lacking well-coordinated programs in health care or education. Nonetheless, the government supports a wide range of programs, which many AIDS advocates believe is still insufficient given the needs for research, community-based alternatives, and support for health professionals.

The AIDS Commission appointed by President Reagan urged broad and comprehensive plans to fight the epidemic. Issuing one of its first reports in September 1991, it criticized the Reagan administration for its lack of leadership on AIDS, especially with regard to prevention, and providing a continuum of care. One of the most controversial issues pertaining to AIDS is whether the federal government should be allowed to limit immigration to this country of people who are infected with HIV. AIDS activists, and many members of the AIDS commission, are against such measures, arguing that it violates human rights. Other more conservative players and government officials, even within the Clinton administration, have taken a different stand. They claim that AIDS is a public health threat, that neither the federal government nor the American taxpayer can afford to care for these individuals, and that lenient immigration policies with regard to AIDS increase the public's risk of HIV/AIDS transmission. This policy was enacted into law under the 1993 NIH reauthorization bill (P.L. 103-43). However, the U.S. attorney general has the right to grant waivers from the exclusion. Nurses, public health professionals, and other civil rights groups continue to challenge this exclusionary policy, because HIV is not spread by casual contact, and the policy restricts the freedom of many individuals—in particular, refugees seeking political asylum here. Under the same 1993 NIH law, the federal government created an Office of AIDS Research within NIH, the director of which would be the leading federal official responsible for AIDS research. This was an important move for centralizing AIDS research and planning and advancing AIDS research at NIH. Other funding and planning provisions for AIDS research were also enacted at that time.[30]

Across the federal government, HIV and AIDS programs are also are funded through various initiatives at the Centers for Disease Control and Prevention (CDCP), and research on new treatments to prevent and treat AIDS at the FDA. At the CDCP, approximately $550 million is allocated annually for HIV/AIDS prevention. This includes grants to states, in addition to CDCP funding for nationwide prevention programs.

One of the ongoing concerns of AIDS activists has been the lack of funding for the Ryan White Comprehensive AIDS Resource Emergency (CARE) Act, enacted in 1990. The bill authorized economic assistance to cities with the highest rates of AIDS to help absorb the costs of caring for people with AIDS. In addition, it established funding for community-based services to promote care for children, families, and minorities affected by the disease. President Clinton proposed increases in funding for the Ryan White CARE Act, but it was unclear how much, if at all, Congress would appropriate. In the meantime, the bill is due to be reauthorized in 1995, and its future remains uncertain with health care reform on the horizon.

President Clinton, attempting to improve policies for AIDS, appointed a National AIDS Policy Coordinator, known colloquially as the "AIDS Czar." The first one to fill the position was a nurse, Kristine Gebbie, RN, MPH. She resigned in August 1994, criticizing Congress and the Clinton administration for lack of sufficient funding to implement important AIDS programs, especially in the area of HIV prevention. Thus, although the federal government had allocated millions of dollars for research to prevent and treat AIDS, given the challenges that AIDS presents to health care providers and practitioners, the consensus among those in the field is that services for people with AIDS remain underfunded. AIDS-related policies continue to be hampered by lack of steady leadership and coordination, and a reluctance on the part of the federal government to fund many AIDS initiatives. Nurses have been in the forefront of efforts to reverse these trends.

Agency for Health Care Policy Research. In the 1980s, one of Congress's attempts to combine concerns about the costs and quality of health care was the establishment of the Agency for Health Care Policy and Research (AHCPR) within the PHS. The agency was authorized under OBRA 1989 (P.L. 101-239), replacing what had been the National Center for Health Services Research and Health Care Technology Assessment. The mission of the AHCPR includes conducting research on the quality and effectiveness of health care services, developing practice guidelines, and assessing technology. The agency has the primary responsibility for implementing the Medical Treatment Effectiveness Program (MEDTEP) within the HHS. The purpose of the medical effectiveness initiative is to improve the effectiveness and appropriateness of health care services through better understanding of the effects of health care practices—including nursing—on patient outcomes. The effectiveness initiatives are of particular importance because many policy makers look to effectiveness research as a way of controlling health care costs and streamlining medical practice. The AHCPR convened a Nursing Advisory Panel on Guideline Development to provide input to effectiveness research as it pertains to nursing. It is important for nurses to understand and contribute to the agency's programs as much as possible, because its recommendations will affect nursing practice.[31]

In many ways, MEDTEP is a back-door approach to stemming the litigious environment by empowering consumers. Providers have been directed to reach consensus around the preferred treatment for select disease conditions that are highly variable in their treatment despite a substantial body of scientific evidence on clinical management, challenging to quality of life and costly to the federal government (Medicare). This consensus process yields guidelines for consumer use. The guidelines are not meant to drive reimbursement, nor do they limit the provider's ability to propose alternate treatment. It does place the burden on providers to justify their alternate recommendations. In seeking legal opinion on MEDTEP, the ANA has determined that these guidelines potentially have the force of law and establish the standard for clinical management in these specific situations.

In 1992, AHCPR released its first clinical practice guidelines. They were for postoperative pain management, urinary incontinence in adults, and the prevention of decubiti. Since then, AHCPR has been issuing several other guidelines in areas of otitis media in children, depression, strokes, and managing patients with unstable angina. Many nurses have high-level positions at the AHCPR and have provided input and leadership to the committees on clinical practice guidelines, as well as directing several of the AHCPR research activities. Three of the consensus panels were chaired or cochaired by nurses. The publications, resources, and information that AHCPR provides are useful for nurses engaged in many aspects of research relevant to advancing health care policy.

Occupational Health and Safety. In recent years, health professionals and policy experts have placed growing attention on the importance of occupational health and safety, largely because of the increases in rates of many infectious diseases, such as tuberculosis, hepatitis, and HIV/AIDS. In December 1991, the Occupational Safety and Health Administration (OSHA) released standards on prevention of bloodborne diseases, requiring nurses and other health workers to receive protection. The standards require all employers to provide hepatitis B immunizations, as well as protective equipment and procedures, to prevent transmission of hepatitis B, HIV, and other infectious diseases.[32] More information on HIV/AIDS and the workplace is included in Chap. 30.

Another occupational safety and health development occurred in May 1993, when a new Office of Occupational Health Nursing was established at OSHA "to underscore the major role such nurses play in striving for safe and healthful workplaces." The office will increase the visibility of nurses within OSHA and in related activities across the country. The nurses working in the office will be responsible for developing standards and surveillance policies. They also will be educating, training, and working with employers to improve care to employees at worksites and minimize work-related illnesses. When the office was established, nursing faced the challenge of keeping it a separate entity, not combined with occupational medicine.[33]

Finally, nurses have joined with others involved with occupational safety and health to push for reform of the Occupational Safety and Health Act, which has not been revised since its original enactment in 1970. One of the most important proposals for reform is to extend coverage under the law to public employees. Approximately 323,000 nurses work in national, state, or local governmental hospital settings, and they, as well as other public employees, are often exposed to bloodborne pathogens (as well as other risk factors) and are entitled to the same protection as their colleagues in the private sector. Other proposals for reform include requiring employers with at least 11 employees to organize health and safety committees, composed of employees and employers, to discuss and resolve employer health and safety issues.[34] The fate of the OSHA reform remained up in the air as health care reform dominated the legislative agenda.

Immunizations. One of President Clinton's domestic priorities was to improve the immunization status of the nation's children. By the early 1990s, approximately 40 percent of American children between the ages of one and four years were behind in their immunizations, with higher rates for certain minority groups. To remedy this situation, Congress enacted a new childhood immunization entitlement program to assist states in bringing more children up to date with their vaccines. The program was to augment existing funds for immunizations that had been in existence for many years. The new law was enacted in 1993, as part of the fiscal 1994 budget reconciliation bill (P.L. 103-66). It requires states to provide free vaccines to all children under age 19 who lack health insurance, are not covered by Medicaid, or are Na-

tive American. It also would assist children with health insurance who are unvaccinated, and get their immunizations at community or migrant health centers. The bill authorized an additional $1.4 billion for immunizations over five years, above ongoing categorical funding for immunizations. By the mid-1990s, annual appropriations for immunizations (combining ongoing programs and the new entitlements) totaled between $800 and $900 million.

Under the new law, HHS negotiates a discounted price for the vaccines from the manufacturers, sets up a government vaccine warehouse, and then arranges with states to administer them to eligible children. States are responsible for the administrative costs of the program, and neither states nor providers are allowed to charge the family for the costs of the vaccines, although they can charge a limited fee for administration of the vaccine. Implementation of the immunization program was delayed because of concerns that the law provided discounted and subsidized vaccinations for children who had health insurance or whose families could ostensibly afford to obtain vaccines without federal assistance. The conflicts depict how even a basic preventive program, such as childhood immunizations, can fall prey to political conflicts over eligibility, financing, and the allocating of responsibility for health care between public and private sectors.

In addition, there were concerns among child health professionals that even if the costs of the vaccines were covered, barriers to access (such as lack of available providers, cultural and language differences, poor understanding among families as to the importance of vaccines, and inconvenient clinic hours) would still make it difficult for many children to obtain necessary immunizations. Nurses have historically taken a leading role in advancing immunization programs at federal, state, and community levels and are often the ones to conduct community needs assessments and develop and implement outreach programs to ensure that as many children as possible are prevented against infectious diseases.

Women's Health. Since the early 1990s, women's health issues have catapulted to the top of the legislative agenda, prompted, in part, by the growing number of female lawmakers, staff, and interest groups that focus on women's health issues. Activities in behalf of women's health have taken several different forms. First, the Office of Research on Women's Health at NIH was formed in 1990 and mandated under federal law in 1994. Its purpose is to establish women's health priorities, implement research, report on the status of women's mortality and morbidity, advise other NIH programs, and interact with women's organizations and members of the scientific community regarding women's health issues.

Second, the Women's Health Initiative at NIH was launched in 1991, at the suggestion of Bernadine Healy, MD, who was the director of NIH at the time (and the first woman to assume that role). This initiative was to feature a $500 million study of middle-aged women, focusing on prevention of the most common causes of death and disability for women and spanning 10 NIH institutes, the Office of Research on Women's Health, and the Office of Disease Prevention.[35]

Third, in response to a report that women— especially of childbearing age—were excluded from clinical research trials, several federal agencies revised their policies. For example, in March 1993, the FDA changed its guidelines to allow more women of childbearing age in the early phase of drug trials. The 1993 NIH reauthorization bill called for increases in the numbers of women and minorities in clinical studies sponsored or regulated by NIH. The law followed a 1990 General Accounting Office study that criticized NIH for not requiring participation of women and other minorities in its funded research, and thereby overlooking differences in effects for those populations. The bill also specified that the cost of including women and minorities in research studies was not an acceptable reason for their exclusion. The guidelines for implementing the 1993 law were issued in 1994. Also in 1994, the Institute of Medicine issued a report on women and health research that made recommendations similar to those of the other government panels just described.[36]

Within the Veterans Administration, there also are efforts underway to focus attention on the special needs of women veterans. This is largely in response to the growing proportion of women within the armed forces, currently at about 12 percent.[37]

ANA and other nursing groups have been in the vanguard of the legislative and regulatory efforts on behalf of women, not only because of the large percentage of nurses who are women but also because of the concerns that nurses have in caring for women patients, regardless of the setting or condition. To that end, ANA has been a member of the steering committee for the Campaign for Women's Health, which is a broad-based coalition of over 70 organizations, working to ensure that women's issues are addressed in health care reform.

Another salient women's health issue of the 1990s was breast cancer prevention and treatment, which received a huge increase in research funding under the 1993 NIH law, largely owing to the effectiveness of the relatively new breast cancer lobby. Other important women's health issues are coverage for mammography under Medicare, reproductive health, and hormone replacement therapy. The growing support for these types of issues reflects the importance they will undoubtedly hold in years to come. Nurses interested in obtaining more information on any of these women's health policies can contact the NIH Office of Research on Women's Health at 301-496-4000, the ANA in Washington, D.C., or other women's and nursing organizations specializing in women's health.

NURSING EDUCATION, PRACTICE, AND RESEARCH

To understand the dynamics of current legislation for nursing, it is useful to establish a historical perspective. Except for the Bolton Act during World War II, it was not until Congress enacted the Health Amendments Act of 1956 that members of the health professions received any substantial government funding. This act, now a section of the Public Health Service Law, provided dollars (called traineeships) to nurses to prepare for clinical, teaching, administrative, and other aspects of public health work. The traineeship program set the stage for years of subsequent federal funding for nursing. The government agencies that focus solely on nursing and those resources designated for the use of nurses are the Division of Nursing and the National Institute for Nursing Research (NINR). Each deserves to be presented separately.

The Division of Nursing

The Division of Nursing is a subdivision of the PHS. In turn, the PHS has been a component of HHS, since it was created in 1953 (originally named the Department of Health, Education and Welfare). The PHS is an exceedingly important federal agency as far as health is concerned. Established in 1798 as a hospital service for sick and disabled seamen, the PHS has steadily expanded its scope and activities over the years and is now the federal agency charged with overall responsibility for promotion and protection of the nation's health.

The Division of Nursing is exclusively concerned with nursing education and practice. It is within the Division of Nursing that the PHS focuses on the nation's nursing situation. However, nursing's roots go far back into the history of the PHS. In 1933, the first public health nursing unit was created within the PHS, primarily to implement the health provisions of the Social Security Act and to conduct the first national census of nurses in public health work. In 1941, PHS established a unit on nursing education to administer federal programs, among them the United States Cadet Nurse corps, which produced nurses during the emergency caused by World War II. In 1946, the Division of Nursing was established within the Office of the Surgeon General. Formally, the Division of Nursing was known as the Division of Nurse Education. During 1949, PHS was reorganized to better coordinate its activities. The Division of Nursing in the Surgeon General's Office was abolished and its functions were taken over by the Division of Nursing Resources of the Bureau of Medical Services. In 1960, a restructuring of PHS again occurred, uniting the Division of Nursing Resources and the Division of Public Health Nursing into the present-day Division of Nursing.

The division's overall purpose is to work toward the achievement of high-quality nursing care for the nation's growing population and to approach this goal through aid to nursing education, consultation, and analysis and evaluation of nursing personnel, and preparation of nurses for expanded roles in the primary care and teaching of patients. The division identifies what exists in nursing, what is needed, and how improvements can be made. The division is a catalyst for progress.

The division supports programs related to the development, financing, and use of educational resources for the improvement of nurse training; conducts and supports a national program to improve the quality of nursing practice and health care, including innovative demonstration practice models; conducts studies and evaluations of nursing personnel supply, requirements, utilization, and distribution; and provides support to develop or maintain graduate nursing education programs and to prepare RNs for expanded roles in primary health care in various health care settings. It formerly funded research projects to expand the scientific base of nursing practice and education. However, its research functions and responsibilities were transferred to the National Center for Nursing Research, now the National Institute of Nursing Research, at the National Institutes of Health when the center was established in 1986.

The division (and its predecessor units) has exerted significant influence and leadership within the nursing profession. Over the years, the division has developed many significant publications as well as significant reports of special committees, such as that on the extended role of the nurse (discussed in Chap. 5) that helped launch federal financing for NPs. Consultation services in many nursing areas are available through the division. For example, schools wishing to expand enrollment of professional nursing students, or those interested in developing or expanding nursing practice arrangements in noninstitutional settings to demonstrate methods to improve access to primary health care in medically underserved communities may receive help from the division. The division also conducts data collection on a continuing basis to determine the current and projected supply and distribution requirements for nurses within the United States and each state. The National Sample Survey of Registered Nurses, initiated in 1975, is the profession's major source of comprehensive personal and professional data on RNs, whether or not they are employed in nursing.

DHHS has ten regional offices throughout the United States, each headed by a Regional Health Administrator. PHS has always recognized the importance of nursing in the total scheme of providing health services, and there is scarcely a PHS program that does not have a nurse involved in some way. At one time, there was a regional nursing program director in each region, but in the cutback of the 1970s that position was abolished. Further information may be obtained by writing the Division of Nursing, Bureau of Health Professions, Public Health Service, Health Resources and Services Administration, U.S. Department of Health and Human Services, 5600 Fishers Lane, Rockville, Maryland 20857. A complete list of publications and reports is available from the Division of Nursing.

The division will only be as successful and prominent as funding allows. With the advent of Medicare and Medicaid, and the expansion of facilities, health personnel became an urgent issue to Washington. At that same time, nurses were becoming more vocal, their organizations stronger, and their politics more sophisticated.

Nurses had a self-assured and convincing presence as they appeared before legislative committees and met with their representatives. As a result, several new laws were enacted in the early 1960s that are noteworthy.

Most significant among these was the *Nurse Training Act* of 1964 (Title VIII of the Public Health Service Act). The purpose of this law was to increase the number of nurses through financial assistance to nursing schools, students, and graduates taking advanced courses, and thus to help assure more and better schools of nursing, more carefully selected students, a high standard of teaching, and better health care for the people. Signed into law by President Lyndon B. Johnson on September 4, 1964, the original law provided $287.6 million for five years.

Over the past 30 years, nurses have fought successfully to retain federal funding for nursing education and research. This has often meant overcoming substantial political obstacles, such as budget constraints, competition with other compelling health care needs and interests, lack of presidential support, and lack of understanding among members of Congress about the importance of nursing research and graduate education. However, the profession has succeeded and even triumphed in gaining federal support and recognition. Several recent events are most noteworthy in this regard. For more details on federal funding for nursing education, see Chap. 19 in the 5th and 6th editions of *Dimensions of Professional Nursing*.

In 1985, federal funding for nursing education was reauthorized for three years, by the renamed Nurse Education Act (NEA). President Reagan signed the new law (P.L. 99-92) primarily because it represented lower funding levels compared with previous bills. Although the authorization level of $54 million was considerably lower than funding levels in the 1970s, the bill was still a political success for nursing, given the tightly constrained budgetary environment.

Federal funding for nursing education was reauthorized in 1988 and 1992. In 1994, President Clinton proposed the consolidation of over 25 categorical health professions programs, including nursing, into five categorical grants. Nursing organizations generally opposed such a move, arguing that it would force nursing to compete with other programs and would lower the funding levels for nursing and other health professions grants. The consolidation proposal failed, but it is possible that it will reemerge in the future as a way of addressing the health care needs of the public, rather than the separate education programs of each profession.

In the meantime, federal funding for nursing education followed the precedents of previous years and has gradually increased since the late 1980s. By 1995, a total of $63 million was appropriated, with the majority of funds supporting graduate programs for nurse practitioners and nurse-midwives, and advanced (mostly graduate) nurse traineeships. Other categories included special projects, education for disadvantaged and minority health professionals, CRNAs, and student loan repayments. Given budgetary constraints, which limit the extent to which funding can be increased for discretionary programs such as nursing education, these funding levels are indicative of nursing's political success. As primary care assumes greater importance under health care reform, it is unclear if federal funding for nursing education will continue under its present guise or be subsumed under other federal initiatives. In any event, it remains one of the most important federal laws affecting the profession.

Support for other health professions education (medicine, osteopathy, dentistry, veterinary medicine, optometry, podiatry, and pharmacy), known by the acronym MODVOPP, had been provided by the *Health Professions Education Assistance Act of 1963* and its successors. Nursing organizations have often been allied with groups representing the other professions as together they strive to maintain funding for the health professions.

Until lately, nursing's political strategy had been to concentrate on a select package of legislation that was exclusive to our needs. If those bills failed, the loss was tragic. Today finds sources of funding for nursing and the health professions included in a variety of places. Networking external to the field, incremental building from smaller funding sources, and education of the profession's leadership to search out new and more nontraditional sources may offer long-term protection.

The National Institute of Nursing Research

1985 was a landmark year for nurses because it marked the establishment of the National Center for Nursing Research (NCNR) at NIH. Nurses claimed the victory on November 20, when the Senate voted 89 to 7 to override President Reagan's veto of the NIH reauthorization bill. The House had already supported the bill in its 380 to 32 vote to override the veto the previous week. The bill culminated several years of negotiations among various interest groups, legislative chambers, and branches of government. It also was a compromise between House members advocating a National Institute of Nursing and senators who opposed any type of new national nursing research entity.

Within a short time, the center was up and running[38] under the dynamic leadership of a distinguished nurse scientist, Ada Sue Hinshaw, RN, PhD, FAAN. In a short time, the center was conducting collaborative intramural research (within NIH) on topics such as the frail elderly, extramural grants to schools of nursing, a research program in bioethics and clinical practice, and research initiatives for low-birth-weight infants and patients with HIV infections (see Chap. 14).

In June 1993, the NCNR was upgraded to the National Institute of Nursing Research, following two years of lobbying and advocacy on behalf of nurses in Washington and across the country. Although the change in status from center to institute did not involve a change in budget, it did reflect an increase in status and visibility for nursing research.

Generally, federal funding for nursing research seems to have fared better than funding for nursing education. By 1991, funding for nursing research had increased to $40 million (from $10 million in 1985). It reached close to $53 million in 1995. Despite these increases, many approved NINR applications go unfunded. Of the 452 NINR project grant applications reviewed in 1993, only 51 were awarded funding, for a success rate of 11.3 percent, compared with an overall NIH success rate of 24.5 percent for that year. (This success rate equals the applications funded, as a proportion of the total number reviewed.) The highest success rate for NINR applications was 19.2 percent in 1991, compared with an overall NIH success rate of 24 percent for that year. As the number of qualified applications increases, unless there is a commensurate increase in funding, the success rate will inevitably fall. Nursing organizations and leaders have continually endorsed increased funding levels, with the hope that more of the high-caliber research grants turned away could be implemented in the future.

It is interesting to note that even President Bush, a fiscally conservative Republican, supported funding increases for nursing research, implying that its significance was "catching on," and the findings of nursing studies were being disseminated in the "right circles." Nonetheless, given the overall NIH funding level of over $6 billion for five years, and the competition within NIH for these dollars, it is clear that nurses need to continue lobbying for funds to support nursing education and research and to muster all their political savvy in the process.

HEALTH CARE REFORM

Starting in the 1980s, policy makers discussed various proposals to provide health coverage for the uninsured. The major obstacles to all of these proposals were that the burden of cost would fall on different groups, depending on the policy scheme, and that invariably the plans involved increased costs and spending. In addition, each plan targeted a different group, and unless Congress accepted some form of national health insurance, there was no way to provide coverage for everyone.

Underlying all of these proposals are unanswered questions about health care as a right or privilege. If one assumes that access to affordable health care is a right, then which level of government is responsible for it? Although health care is not explicitly stated in the Constitution as a right, the federal government does devote many resources to providing health care. On the other hand, many health programs are under state jurisdiction, and perhaps health care, like education, should be left to states' discretion. Finally, the issue of equity needs to be addressed. Are all individuals entitled to the same level and quality of health care, regardless of their ability to pay for their care? Or can we accept a two-tiered level of care, wherein those who can afford to pay more are entitled to the better quality and quantity of services their money can buy? Although the answers to these questions seem elusive, they raise important issues for nurses to consider as they become increasingly involved with the health care system.

In 1992, President Clinton was elected to office on a platform that included changes in the health care system. His first two years in office, 1993–1994, witnessed the most controversial and intense deliberations pertaining to health care in recent history. His ambitious Health Security Act, a bill of more than 1,000 pages covering all aspects of the health care delivery system, was the standard against which most subsequent proposals were measured. Many nurses were part of the committees and task forces that designed the bill, and ANA endorsed the Health Security Act shortly after it was formally introduced. However, given the partisan nature of congressional politics, the controversial nature of health care as a redistributive issue, and the narrow margins by which (liberal) Democrats led the House and Senate, it was difficult for Congress to reach consensus on any one particular plan.

Despite these conflicts, there did seem to be consensus regarding major elements of insurance industry reform, for example, that health coverage should not be dependent on employment status and that nobody should be denied health insurance, regardless of preexisting condition.[39] If nothing else, the debates over health care reform raised public and government awareness about the importance of insurance reform and increased the likelihood of insurance industry changes benefiting future and potential subscribers.

There were several main approaches to health care reform. At one end of the continuum was the bill that Representative Jim McDermott (D-Washington) and Senator Paul Wellstone (D-Minnesota) introduced. It featured state-administered single-payer plans, with uniform federal benefits and federal funding. This plan most closely resembled the national health insurance policies of Canada. It would eliminate most of the administrative maze of deductibles and copayments that exist under most private health insurance plans and would be financed by a payroll tax.

At the other end of the continuum were proposals that relied on market incentives and continued much of the present system of health insurance. One such alternative, introduced by Senator John Breaux (D-LA) and Representative Jim Cooper (D-TN), featured voluntary health plan purchasing cooperatives for individuals and small businesses. These cooperatives, or alliances, would provide insurance coverage for groups of employees, as well as for others, including the unemployed and poor. Several health reform proposals built on the current system of Medicare, Medicaid, and employer provided coverage, with variations on the extent to which individuals would be required to obtain some form of health insurance. Most of the health reform proposals retained Medicare, although there was considerable discussion in the House about creating a part C Medicare program, to replace Medicaid and provide coverage to others who lack employer or Medicare coverage.

Financing of health care reform was a major issue, with options including increases in cigarette taxes, employer-employee contributions, payroll taxes, and larger out-of-pocket payments for those covered. Other issues debated

included the feasibility and timing of universal coverage, the contents of a federal benefits package, and the balance between employer and employee costs, and between employer and government responsibilities for paying for health care. How to distribute the costs of financing health care insurance for the uninsured was a major problem, with some preferring government subsidies and others leaning more toward sharing the costs among employers, providers, and state and federal authorities. Most agreed that any final plan would have to give people some sort of flexibility in choosing physicians and other practitioners. It also would emphasize managed care plans, including HMOs, to monitor usage, costs, and quality of care. Giving states the flexibility to establish their own systems was also considered important.

In the absence of a national policy for the uninsured, states launched programs of their own. Some states have expanded Medicaid eligibility, as discussed earlier in this chapter. Innovative approaches have been approved in state legislatures across the country. Each state has taken a slightly different approach, depending on its political culture, the number of under- or uninsured, and the relative power of various interest groups. There is no one solution that will work for all states across the board.

One of the most notable state initiatives was Oregon's 1989 decision to "ration" or prioritize certain types of Medicaid services (see Chaps. 10 and 22).[40] For years, the Bush administration blocked approval of Oregon's waiver, eventually claiming that it violated the Americans with Disability Act of 1990. In March 1993, the new Clinton administration granted a Medicaid waiver to Oregon to implement its plan, under the auspices of the Oregon Health Services Commission (HSC). This waiver allowed Oregon to deviate from certain Medicaid policies. For example, it was permitted to establish a basic package of health care for people with incomes at or below the federal poverty level, based on a prioritized list of condition or treatments; restrict freedom of providers in favor of prepaid managed care delivery; and delete services normally included under Medicaid's Early and Periodic Screening, Diagnosis, and Treatment (EPSDT) Program, if the HSC determined them to be ineffective. Since 1993, implementation of the Oregon plan has been delayed because of changes in the Oregon legislature, in particular, eroding Democratic control. In addition, new problems emerged regarding the financing of the plan, with small business opposing burdens or mandates placed on employers.[41] Regardless of how the Medicaid waiver fares, Oregon will always be remembered for its ground-breaking efforts in state health care reform, and for the important ethical and political questions it raised.

Hawaii is another state that has received a lot of publicity for its health care reforms. One reason that Hawaii was able to deviate from other states is that it developed its proposal before federal legislation—known as the Employee Retirement Income Security Act (ERISA) of 1974—was enacted. (ERISA prevents states from requiring employers who self-insure to offer a minimum of health benefits.)[42] This enabled Hawaii to develop an employer mandate program, which has been augmented with a subsidized insurance plan for the uninsured, created in 1989. Hawaii also has the advantage of a relatively healthy population compared with other states, in part because its major industries—tourism, government employment, and agriculture—produce less pollution and fewer health hazards than most other "smokestack environments." Since 1993, Hawaii has also been experimenting with an ambitious Medicaid reform program to enhance quality of care while providing universal access.[43]

Finally, Florida passed legislation in 1992 and 1993 that requires the state to move toward relying on a managed competition approach, through the establishment of regional purchasing cooperatives.[44] Other states (such as California, Maryland, Minnesota, New Jersey, New Mexico, and Connecticut, to name just a few) have enacted health care reforms that resemble many of those just described, in anticipation of new federal laws. However, once enacted, implementing reform often poses unpredictable problems, such as lack of funding and new political battles. Most states found that incremental reform worked best, as opposed to dramatic shifts in the delivery and administration of health services and coverage.

Throughout all of these deliberations, it is important to keep in mind the strengths and weaknesses of health care systems in other countries and to formulate one for the United States that best serves the distinctiveness of our political culture, diverse population, and economic realities. ANA and other nursing organizations continue to be active participants in these discussions, and nurses with firsthand knowledge of patient's needs have much to offer in this realm, too.[45,46] The reader is referred to Chap. 7 for a discussion of reform that considers the issue from a broader social perspective.

ABORTION AND FAMILY POLICIES

Since the 1973 Supreme Court decision, *Roe v. Wade*, which legalized abortion, there have been many legislative and judicial battles over abortion. In the late 1970s, Congress prohibited federal funding for abortion when it routinely passed the Hyde amendments to health services appropriations bills. However, approximately 14 states have been able to circumvent the Hyde amendment by allowing state funds for publicly funded abortions.

Controversies over funding and legality of abortions intensified in the 1980s with two consecutive conservative presidents, and increases in like-minded federal court appointments. Several states enacted laws restricting access to abortions, and abortion rights activists questioned many of these new laws in courts. Often, the cases were referred as high as the Supreme Court. One of the most notable cases was the 1989 case of *Webster v. Reproductive Health Services*, in which the Supreme Court upheld provisions of a Missouri law restricting access to abortions. Although the 1989 ruling left intact the *Roe v. Wade* decision legalizing abortion, it signaled the Court's willingness to reverse its previous decisions on abortion, which deemed other restrictive state laws unconstitutional. The three provisions of the Missouri law that the Court upheld in the 1989 case were:

1. Prohibition of public employees from performing or assisting in abortions other than those necessary to save a pregnant woman's life.
2. Prohibition of the use of public buildings or facilities for performing abortions.
3. Requirements that physicians perform tests on fetal viability if they believe a woman to be at least 20 weeks pregnant.

It is important to note that the *Webster* decision refers only to Missouri. Furthermore, it does not refer to abortions performed in offices or clinics where, in Missouri as in other states, most abortions are performed.[47] Despite these exceptions, the 1989 Supreme Court decision changed the scope and nature of abortion politics considerably. It seems to have set the stage for "ferocious battles" in state legislatures, and "exacerbated tensions within both political parties."

There have been other cases testing how far the Court will let states go in restricting access to abortion. Major issues have included the use of federal funds (usually meaning Medicaid) for abortions, how much information health providers must give women as part of informed consent of abortion, weighing fetal "potential" life against the well-being of the mother, and the right to require parental consent or notification when minors seek abortions. Specifically, in 1990, the Supreme Court ruled on cases from Ohio and Minnesota as to whether the Constitution allows minors to obtain abortions without first informing one or both parents, and upheld the constitutionality of parent notification.

In the aftermath of *Webster*, several proposals to restrict abortions at the state level emerged. However, over time, relatively few changes in state abortion policy were enacted. One could conclude from the outcomes of these events

that in reality, the Court did not leave a lot of room to make major changes in abortion policy. In addition, public opinion on abortion seemed to support this notion. Shortly after the Court's decision, polls indicated that the public overwhelmingly opposed severely restricting a woman's right to obtain an abortion.[48]

President Bush consistently vetoed any legislation, even major appropriations bills, that contained permissive federal abortion policies. Despite Bush's opposition, many members of Congress supported the Freedom of Choice Act (FOCA), first introduced in 1990, which would codify the *Roe v. Wade* decision. (The United States has been unique among countries in lacking legislation pertaining to abortion.) Hearings were held on the bill, and it was given serious consideration. However, the divisiveness and controversy surrounding abortion, even under a more liberal president, impeded enactment.

The one area that Congress was able to reach consensus on was the right to obtain access to abortion clinics. The bill, enacted in 1994 with strong bipartisan support, makes it a federal offense to physically obstruct women's access to a clinic, or to use force, threats, or other tactics intended to intimidate women seeking abortion.[49] The legislation was introduced in response to the rise in violent incidents at abortion clinics, and killings of physicians who performed abortions. It also provides protection to abortion clinic employees, places of worship, and pregnancy counseling centers operated by groups that are against abortion.

On another front, a 1988 ruling, known as the "gag rule," banned health care practitioners from providing abortion counseling in federally funded (Title X) clinics. In the following years, many legislators introduced legislation to overturn the gag rule, but they always were defeated. In the meantime, the ruling was declared constitutional by the Supreme Court, in May 1991, but its implementation was delayed, owing to political protests and squabbles over its implications. In 1992, HHS announced that only physicians were allowed to counsel women regarding abortion as a health care option under Title X. Nurses were outraged, and argued that this infringed on their rights to practice their profession and to assist women make informed choices. The uproar over the gag rule continued until early 1993, when as one of President Clinton's first actions, he reversed it, relaxing the restrictions placed on all practitioners in Title X clinics.

The controversies over the gag rule, the Freedom of Choice Act, and even the clinic access bill reflect how abortion remains one of the most controversial issues on the domestic political agenda. Its divisiveness extended to health care reform debates, because of differences over whether abortion should be included in a standard benefits package and receive federal subsidies under a revamped health care system.

In addition to abortion, there are several other family-related issues that Congress and interest groups such as nursing have been discussing. Two that received considerable attention during the late 1980s and early 1990s are family leave and child care. The first bill that President Clinton signed into law was the Family and Medical Leave Act of 1993. It went into effect on August 5 of that year. In previous years, Congress came close to enacting legislation on family and medical leave that would require employers to give unpaid time off to parents of newborn or sick children or dependents. Women's rights groups and organized labor supported such legislation. However, business groups (and President Bush) opposed any type of parental leave bill that made benefits mandatory.

The 1993 law allows employees to take up to 12 weeks a year of unpaid leave for the birth or care of a child born to an employee; placement of a child for adoption or foster care with the employee; care for an employee's immediate family member with a serious health condition; or a serious health condition that makes the employee unable to perform at work. It applies to all private sector businesses with 50 or more employees, within 75 miles of a given workplace. Employees may take leave intermittently or at one time. Upon returning from leave, the employer must give the employee the same position, or an equivalent one in terms of benefits, responsibilities, and pay. This legislation was very important for signaling the federal government's support for the millions of families that shoulder responsibilities for caring for family members, while also maintaining full-time jobs.[50]

As for child care, Congress enacted a landmark bill as part of the 1990 budget reconciliation act. It featured a new Child Care and Development Block Grant to assist states in improving the quality and availability of child care facilities, and it expanded the earned income tax credit. Both the block grant and the tax credit target low-income working families with children. President Clinton expanded the earned income tax credit under his 1993 reconciliation bill, and demonstrated his commitment to young children with large increases in Head Start funding, enacted in 1994.

FEDERAL POLICIES FOR PROTECTING CIVIL, PATIENT, PRACTITIONER, AND LABOR RELATIONS RIGHTS

Beginning in the 1960s, a number of laws were passed to prohibit discrimination based on sex as well as race, color, religion, and national origin. Many of these are particularly meaningful to women and are cited in Chap. 17. Some of the most important are the following:

The *Civil Rights Act of 1964*, called by some the most far-reaching social legislation since Reconstruction, intended to create a rule of law under which the United States could deal with its race problems peaceably through an orderly, legal process in federal courts. Title VII of the Civil Rights Act (the Equal Employment Opportunity Law) has affected the job status of nurses because it includes a section forbidding discrimination against women in job hiring and job promotion among private employers of more than 25 persons. Executive Order No. 11246 as amended extended the law to include federal contractors and subcontractors. Hospitals and colleges are subject to this order because of their acceptance of federal grants of various kinds.

One year later, the *1965 Voting Rights Act*, with direct bearing on the Civil Rights Act, was passed, requiring that the procedure for registering persons to vote within a given county must be the same for everyone. Intended to ensure the right to vote promised in the Fifteenth Amendment, this law attempted to eliminate the practice of disqualifying potential voters on the basis of discriminatory literacy tests. This legislation represented an alteration in federal-state power, for the states had the authority for nearly two centuries to set, for the most part, the standards for voting eligibility within their own borders.

The *Educational Amendments* of 1972 had three provisions of economic importance to women: (1) equal treatment of men and women in federally funded educational programs (especially admissions to programs); (2) minimum wage and overtime pay benefits to employees of nursery schools, private kindergartens, and other preschool enterprises; (3) extension of the federal Equal Pay Act of 1963 to executives, administrators, and professional employees. The same pay was guaranteed to men and women doing substantially equal work, requiring substantially equal skill, effort, and responsibility under similar working conditions in the same establishment. (Comparable worth issues were discussed in Chap. 17.)

The *Age in Employment Discrimination Act Amendments* of 1975 was intended to eliminate "unreasonable discrimination on the basis of age." Among other things, it banned certain kinds of mandatory retirement. The *Fair Labor Standards Act Amendments* of 1974 (originally 1938) increased the minimum wage and extended coverage to 7 million workers, including state, county, and municipal employees.

Among other civil rights that have been given new protection are the rights of patients, children, the mentally ill, prisoners, the elderly, and the handicapped (see Chap. 22). Actions to protect these rights have come through a variety of legal means at state and national levels. Protection has increasingly been specified through regulations of various laws such as the amendments and subsequent regulations of the Social Security Act.

One of the most frequently cited provisions is Section 504 of the *Rehabilitation Act* of 1973. It reads, "no otherwise qualified handicapped individual in the United States shall, solely by reason of his handicap, be excluded from the participation in, be denied the benefit of, or be subjected to discrimination under any program or activity receiving federal financial assistance." The definition of *handicapped* includes drug addicts and alcoholics, as well as those having overt physical impairment such as blindness, deafness, or paralysis of some kind. (A 1984 expansion of the definition relates to deformed newborns, as discussed in Chap. 22.) Because most health facilities and health professional education programs have some federal support, this law applies both to admission to a nursing school, for instance, and to employment in a hospital.

A major issue now is whether, and under what circumstances, AIDS and HIV-infected people come under this law. Some state and local jurisdictions have ruled that AIDS-related illness does come under their laws as a protected handicap. Those that do not consider communicable diseases as "protected" rule differently.

In recent years, there have been two types of renewed civil rights activities. First, the Americans with Disabilities Act was enacted in 1990 with the intent of barring firms from denying jobs to individuals solely on the basis of disability, as long as reasonable accommodations can be made. The legislation is aimed at protecting the approximately 43 million disabled Americans including people infected with HIV. Discrimination is prohibited in areas such as public accommodations, transportation, and private employment.

Second, the Civil Rights Act of 1991 (P.L. 102-66), signed by President Bush, was a response to Supreme Court rulings in 1989 that were blows to civil rights enforcement. Specifically, in cases where employees experience job discrimination, the new rulings shifted the burden of proof from the employer to the employee. An earlier version of the civil rights bill came one vote short of a veto override in 1990. President Bush was motivated to reach a compromise in 1991, following two events that made him less than popular in civil rights circles: the Clarence Thomas–Anita Hill hearings and the strong support in October primaries for a Louisiana Republican and former Ku Klux Klansman, David Duke. The Civil Rights Act of 1991 restored many employees' rights and left the most controversial issues open to court interpretation, thereby clearing the path toward enactment. But it did not go as far as some civil rights advocates, including ANA, would have liked. However, compromises were needed to enact the bill.

The 1991 law left to the judicial system the determination of whether an employer has set up requirements, such as educational or physical tests, that have an adverse impact on women or minorities. The law also imposed a cap on the amount of punitive damages that women, religious minorities, and the disabled can claim, and called for a commission to study the "glass ceiling" effect, referring to the lack of women and minorities in top corporate positions. Many groups, including ANA, are committed to fighting to reverse the caps, as part of their civil rights agenda.[51,52]

The right to privacy also affects nurses. Among the most important federal laws in this area are the *Freedom of Information Act* (FOIA) of 1966 and the *Privacy Act* of 1974. The purpose of the FOIA is to give the public access to files maintained by the executive branch of government. Recognizing that there were valid reasons for withholding certain records, the law exempted broad categories of records from compulsory public inspection, including medical records. To further clarify the situation, the FOI Act of 1974 was passed to amend the 1966 law. It had been necessary to set some time and expense limits for federal agen-

cies because, in their frequent reluctance to give up information, they tended to use bureaucratic red tape to delay transmission of the requested records and imposed high fees to photocopy them. The next question that arose was whether a person shouldn't have the right to see all information about himself or herself in government files. The result was enactment of the Privacy Act. Its purpose was to provide certain safeguards for an individual against invasion of personal privacy by requesting the federal government, with some exceptions, to:

1. Permit an individual to determine what records pertaining to him are collected, maintained, used, or disseminated by such agencies.
2. Permit an individual to prevent records pertaining to him and obtained by such agencies for a particular purpose from being used or made available for another purpose without his consent.
3. Permit an individual to gain access to information pertaining to him in federal agency records, to have a copy made of all or any portion thereof, and to correct or amend such records.
4. Collect, maintain, use, or disseminate any record of identifiable personal information in a manner that assures that such action is for a necessary and lawful purpose, that the information is current and accurate for its intended use, and that adequate safeguards are provided to prevent misuse of such information.
5. Permit exemptions from the requirements with respect to records provided in the act only in cases in which there is an important public policy need for such exemption as has been determined by specific statutory authority.
6. Be subject to civil suit for any damages that occur as a result of willful or intentional action that violates any individual's rights under the act.

Another step in providing access to one's own records was enactment of the *Family Educa-*

tional Rights and Privacy Act of 1974, also known as the *Buckley Amendment*. The basic intent of this law was to provide students, their parents, and their guardians with easier access to and control over the information contained in academic records. Educational records are defined broadly and include files, documents, and other materials containing information about the student and maintained by a school. Students must be allowed to inspect these records within 45 days of their request. They need not be allowed access to confidential letters of reference preceding January 1975, records about students made by teachers and administrators for their own use and not shown to others, certain campus police records, certain parental financial records, and certain psychiatric treatment records (if not available to anyone else). Students may challenge the content, secure the correction of inaccurate information, and insert a written explanation regarding the content of their records. The law also specifies who has access to the records (teachers, educational administrators, organizations such as testing services, and state and other officials to whom certain information must be reported according to the law). Otherwise the records cannot be released without the student's consent. The law applies to nursing education programs as well as others.

The rights of research subjects have also been incorporated in diverse federal laws, especially in the last decade. P.L. 94-348, the *National Research Act* of 1974, set controls on research, including the establishment of a committee to identify requirements for informed consent for children, prisoners, the mentally disabled, and those not covered by the federal regulations, and required an institutional committee to review a research project to protect the patient's rights. The 1974 Privacy Act required a clear, informed consent for those participating in research. The 1971 *Food and Drug Act* also gave some protection in regulating the use of experimental drugs, including notification to the patient that a drug is experimental. The *Drug Regulation Reform Act* of 1978 took further steps to protect the patient receiving research drugs. Other drug and narcotics laws also affect nursing (see Chap. 21).

There are many federal laws and regulations pertaining to pharmaceutical testing and administration. The main provision of the *Drug Amendments of 1962* (to the Food, Drug, and Cosmetic Act of 1938) provides that manufacturers of drugs who seek Food and Drug Administration (FDA) approval must prove through extensive preliminary clinical testing that the drug is safe to use and that it will have the intended therapeutic effect. Before undergoing clinical testing, an Investigational New Drug (IND) Application must be submitted to the FDA, followed by three phases of clinical trials, which can take many years and require substantial funding to complete. Only 20 percent of all IND applications progress to the point of being eligible to apply for a New Drug Application with the FDA.[53]

The *Comprehensive Drug Abuse Prevention and Control Act* of 1970 (Controlled Substance Act) replaced virtually all other federal laws dealing with narcotics, depressants, stimulants, and hallucinogens. It controls the handling of drugs by providers, including hospitals. The *Drug Regulation Reform Act* of 1978 took further steps in protecting the patient; at the same time, the FDA set requirements about sharing product information on drugs with consumers.

In 1993, the federal Drug Enforcement Administration (DEA) published final rules regarding the definition and registration of midlevel practitioners (a term that includes advanced practice nurses, and which most nurses prefer not to use because of its derogatory implications). The final rules allow advanced practice nurses to obtain a DEA number, which is required to prescribe controlled substances. However, only nurses (and other practitioners) who practice in states whose attorneys general have determined that they can prescribe controlled substances may apply for the DEA number.[54] Thus the importance of clarifying and advancing the prescribing privileges of nurses at the state level becomes even more important, given this new DEA provision.

Rulings by the Federal Trade Commission also have affected the rights of practicing nurses. The FTC, established pursuant to federal law in 1914, has extensive power. It can represent itself in court, enforce its own orders, and conduct its own litigation in civil courts, and it seems to have relative freedom from the executive branch of government. Its forays into the health field, with rulings on professional advertising, licensure, and other aspects of health care delivery may indicate a direction for other administrative agencies.[55]

One of the most important FTC cases for nursing was in 1982, when attached to the FTC reauthorization bill was an amendment exempting state-licensed professionals from its jurisdiction. A major supporter was AMA; an opponent, ANA. The underlying issue was whether, for instance, if professionals were exempted from fair trade practices, physicians could legally restrain the practice of competitors, such as nurse-midwives.[56] That time the FTC won, but the problem continues to resurface in various forms as more nurses engage in independent practice, obtain legislative rights to do so, and pose threats to the medical profession.

In 1990, Congress enacted the *Nutrition Labeling and Education Act*. This bill requires food companies to identify precisely the fat, sodium, and caloric, as well as other nutritional components of their products. Many nurses were staunch advocates of the law. By 1994, the strict labeling format required by the law went into effect, requiring labels to include a realistic serving size and a full description of the food's nutritional contents.

Another FDA-related bill, the Safe Medical Devices Act of 1990, mandated that health care facilities report to the FDA and manufacturer (depending on the case) all incidents that could suggest that a medical device caused or contributed to the death, serious injury, or serious illness of a patient. Facilities that fall under the jurisdiction of this act include hospitals, ambulatory surgical facilities, nursing homes, and outpatient treatment facilities, other than physician offices. The law was in response to the prolifera-

tion of medical devices and the need to protect patients and providers in the course of their use. This law has strong implications for nursing, because nurses are typically the ones who monitor and are responsible for patient well-being, and complete incidence reports, whether or not they relate to medical devices. The regulations for the law were finalized in early 1992, and nurses working in facilities that are under the law should be knowledgeable about them and how they might affect nursing practice.[57]

Also within the broad category of rights are those laws addressing labor relations. The first was the National Labor Relations Act (NLRA), one of several pieces of legislation enacted to pull the country out of the Great Depression. The logic was that labor unions could prevent employers from lowering wages, resulting in higher incomes and more spending. Initially, to allow the growth of unions, the power of employers had to be curtailed. For instance, they could no longer legally fire employees who tried to unionize. The National Labor Relations Board (NLRB), created by law, was empowered to investigate and initiate administrative proceedings against those employers who violated the law. (If these administrative actions did not curtail the illegal acts, court action followed. Only employer violations were listed.)

In 1947, the NLRA was substantially amended, and the amended law, entitled the *Labor Management Relations Act* (or *Taft-Hartley Act*), listed prohibitions for unions. Section 14(b), for instance, contained the so-called right-to-work clause, which authorizes states to enact more stringent union security provisions than those contained in the federal laws. More than twenty states have enacted such laws. Usually they prohibit union security clauses in contracts that make membership or nonmembership in a labor union a requirement for obtaining or retaining employment. Such laws prohibit the closed shop, union shop, and sometimes (right-to-work states) the agency shop in which employees who do not join a union must pay a fixed sum monthly as a condition of employment to help defray expenses.

In 1959, a third major modification was made. One of the purposes of the law, the *Labor-Management Reporting and Disclosure Act* or *Landrum-Griffin Act*, was to curb documented abuses such as corrupt financial and election procedures. For this reason, it is sometimes called the union members' Bill of Rights. The result is a series of rights and responsibilities of members of a union or a professional organization, such as ANA, that engages in collective bargaining. Required are reporting and disclosure of certain financial transactions and administrative practices and the use of democratic election procedures. That is, every member in good standing must be able to nominate candidates and run for election and must be allowed to vote and support candidates; there must be secret ballot elections; union funds must not be used to assist the candidacy of an individual seeking union office; candidates must have access to the membership list; records of the election must be preserved for one year; and elections must be conducted according to bylaws procedures.

Highly significant for nurses is the 1974 repeal of the Tyding amendments to the Taft-Hartley Act (P.L. 93-360), the *Nonprofit Health Care Amendments*. This law made nonprofit health care facilities that had, through considerable lobbying, been excluded in the 1947 law, subject to national labor laws. These employees were now free to join or not join a union without employer retribution, a right previously denied to them unless they worked in a state that had its own law allowing them to unionize. It also created special notification procedures that must precede any strike action. Included in the definition of *health care facility* were hospitals, HMOs, health clinics, nursing homes, ECFs, or "other institutions, devoted to the care of sick, infirm, or aged persons." Employers of all kinds must abide by the various civil rights and other protective laws noted earlier. The *Civil Service Reform Act* of 1978 also had an influence in the labor relations activities of nursing because its definition of *supervisor* allowed nurse supervisors to be included in collective bargaining units

(the employee status of licensed nurses was visited by the U.S. Supreme Court in May 1994. See Chap. 30.) It also wrote into law collective bargaining, previously sanctioned only by executive order. In 1988, the NLRB issued rules regarding appropriate bargaining units for the health care industry and determined that RNs constitute a separate bargaining unit and have a strong desire for separate representation. "The Board found LPNs to be appropriately included with technical employees." ANA has been an active participant in NLRB rulemaking.[58]

Another right that should be reported is the revision of the *Copyright Law*, amended in 1976 to supersede the 1909 law. The categories of work covered include writings, works of art, music, and pantomimes. The owner is given the exclusive right to reproduce the copyrighted work. The new law has some significance in this time of photocopying from journals and books; there are certain limits and need for permission to copy anything beyond certain minimums. Generally, if in doubt, it is best to seek the publisher's permission. Libraries can provide the appropriate information. Some books and journals specify their copying permission requirements.

REFERENCES

1. Katz JL: Conference oks bill creating independent agency. *Congressional Quarterly Weekly Report* 2054, July 23, 1990.
2. Social security programs in the United States, 1993. *Social Security Bulletin* 56:3–82, Winter 1993.
3. Ibid.
4. Ross JL, Upp MM: Treatment of women in the U.S. social security system, 1970–1988. *Social Security Bulletin* 56:56–67, Fall 1993.
5. US Congress, House Committee on Ways and Means: *Overview of Entitlement Programs: 1993 Green Book.* WMCP: 103–18. Washington, DC: Government Printing Office, 1993, p 69.
6. Health insurance provision helps disabled. *Nation's Health* 20:4, January 1990.
7. Marmor TR: *The Politics of Medicare.* New York: Aldine, 1970.

8. For a synopsis of Medicare legislative developments since its enactment, see Gale BJ, Steffi BM: The long-term dilemma: What nurses need to know about Medicare. *Nurs Health Care* 13:34–41, January 1992.

9. Iglehart J: The American health care system, Medicare. *N Engl J Med* 327:1467–1472, November 1992.

10. Kent V, Hanley B: Home health care. *Nurs Health Care* 11:234–40, May 1990.

11. Milone-Nuzzo PF: Third-party reimbursement for home care of clients with diabetes. *Diabetes Educ* 19:513–516, November–December 1993.

12. Randall DA: The role of the Medicare fiscal intermediary and the regional home health intermediary part 1. *J Nurs Adm* 22:47–53, June 1992.

13. Grimaldi P: Medigap insurance policies standardized. *Nurs Mgt* 23:20, 22, 24, November 1992.

14. Denega D: National practitioner data bank impacts nursing practice. *Am Nurs* 25:10, July–August 1993.

15. Culbertson RA: National practitioner data bank has implications for nursing. *Nurs Outlook* 9:102–103, May–June 1991.

16. IOM completes report on Medicare and quality care. *Capital Update* 8:6, Mar 30, 1990.

17. Shaffer F: DRGs: History and overview. *Nurs Health Care* 4:388, September 1983.

18. Hamilton J: Nursing and DRGs: Proactive responses to prospective reimbursements. *Nurs Health Care* 5:155–159, March 1984.

19. Joel L: DRGs and RIMs: Implications for nursing. *Nurs Outlook* 32:42–49, January–February 1984.

20. Physician Payment Review Commission. *Annual Report to Congress, 1993*. Washington, DC: The Commission, 1993, p 30.

21. Griffith H: Physician payment reform: Implications for nurses. *Nurs Econ* 7:231–233, July–August 1989.

22. Morrow MM: Medicare physician payment reform: Implications for nurse practitioners. *J Am Acad of Nurse Pract* 4:38–43, January, March 1992.

23. Burke SP: Reflections on the 101st Congress. *Nurs Econ* 8:15–16, January 1990.

24. Congress approves reconciliation legislation. *Capital Update* 7:1, Dec 8, 1989.

25. Keepnews D: HCFA clarifies Medicare payment for advanced nursing services. *Am Nurs* 25:18, September 1993.

26. Physician Payment Review Commission: *Annual Report to Congress, 1994*. Washington, DC: The Commission, 1994, pp 283–284.

27. For an update on the status of nurse practitioner reimbursement and scope of practice by state, see annual updates in the journal *Nurse Practitioner*, typically in the first issue of every year.

28. Sofaer S: Community health planning in the United States: A post mortem. *Community Health* 10:1–12, February 1988.

29. Most states continue planning program. *Nation's Health* 19:24, October 1989.

30. NIH Reauthorization Bill Provisions, 1993. *Congressional Quarterly Almanac, 1993*. Washington, DC: Congressional Quarterly, Inc, 1994, pp 363–369.

31. Joel L: Seizing an exceptional moment: The effectiveness initiative. *Am Nurs* 22:6, April 1990.

32. OSHA releases final standards on AIDS and Hep B exposures. *Capital Update* 9:1–2, Dec 6, 1991.

33. OSHA creates office of occupational health nursing. *Am Nurs* 25:46, July 8, 1993.

34. Government health workers to be protected under OSHA reform. *Nation's Health* 23:5, March 1994.

35. DeVries C: Publications explore women's health issues. *Am Nurs* 25:14, January 1993.

36. Institute of Medicine: *Women and Health Research: Ethical and Legal Issues of Including Women in Clinical Studies*. Washington, DC: National Academy Press, 1994.

37. Women, vets, building bills advanced by House panel. *Congressional Quarterly Weekly Report* 1313, May 21, 1994.

38. Hinshaw AC: The National Center for Nursing Research: Challenges and initiatives. *Nurs Outlook* 36:54–56, March–April 1988.

39. *Nursing's Agenda for Health Care Reform*. Washington, DC: American Nurses Publishing, 1991.

40. Capuzzi C, Garland M: The Oregon plan: Increasing access to health care. *Nurs Outlook* 38:260–263, 286, November–December 1990.

41. Fox DM, Leichter HM: The ups and downs of Oregon's rationing plan. *Health Affairs* 12:66–70, Summer 1993.

42. Gostin L, Widiss A: What's wrong with the ERISA Vacuum? *JAMA* 269:2527–2532, May 19, 1993.

43. Neubauer D: A pioneer in health system reform. *Health Affairs* 12:31–40, Summer 1993.

44. Brown L: Commissions, clubs, and consensus: Florida reorganizes for health reform. *Health Affairs* 12:7–26, Summer 1993.

45. Ward D: National health insurance: Where do nurses fit in? *Nurs Outlook* 38:206–207, September–October 1990.

46. Mundinger M: Health care reform: Will nursing respond. *Nurs Health Care* 15:28–33, January 1994.

47. Cohen S: Health care policy and abortion: A comparison. *Nurs Outlook* 38:21, January 1990.

48. Shribman D: Despite expectations of big changes high court ruling on abortion has had little impact so far. *Wall Street J* A14, Mar 9, 1990.

49. Clinic access bill clears House. *Congressional Quarterly Weekly Report*, May 14, 1994.

50. White JD: Learning to live with the family and medical leave act. *Caring* 13:10–1, 72–74, March 1994.

51. House passes civil rights measure. *Capital Update* 9:5–6, Nov 15, 1991.

52. Compromise civil rights bill passed. *Congressional Quarterly Almanac, 1991*. Washington, DC: Congressional Quarterly, Inc, 1992, pp 251–261.

53. Allen A: The high-stakes drug drawing. *J Post Anesth Nurs* 9:52–54, February 1994.

54. Final rule published on DEA numbers for mid-level practitioners. *Am Nurs* 25:22, July–August 1993.

55. Avellone J, Moore F: The Federal Trade Commission enters a new arena: Health services. *N Engl J Med* 291:478–483, August 1978.

56. Kelly L: FTC: Dragon or dragon-slayer. *Nurs Outlook* 30:490–492, November–December 1982.

57. ANA responds to FDA's Safe Medical Device Act of 1990, proposed tentative final rule. *Capital Update* 10:4–5, Feb 28, 1992.

58. National labor relations board. *Capital Update* 6:5, Nov 25, 1988.

59. Clegg R: Copyright law and the nursing professor. *Nurs Educ* 16:28–31, November–December 1991.

Licensure and Health Personnel Credentialing

ESPITE A VARIETY of patchwork reforms, the health care system remains the target of serious criticism. A major focus has been the undeniable fragmentation of services, accelerating costs, and poor utilization and maldistribution of health manpower. Therefore, credentialing of health manpower, as one of the factors that probably contributes to these problems, has been given special attention by legislative, governmental, and consumer groups. This pointed scrutiny has subsequently aroused new, or at least renewed, interest on the part of the health occupations and professions.

Licensing of individuals is the most authoritative mechanism of credentialing, because it is a function of the police power of the state. Its primary purpose is to protect the public; therefore, the state, through its licensure laws, sets standards and qualifications for the licensed practitioner and holds the power to punish those who violate the law. At the same time, licensure, as it stands currently, has definite advantages for the licensee: status, protection of title (RN, LPN, MD), and certain economic gains. Other methods of credentialing for individuals or institutions have also evolved. Whether official, quasiofficial, or voluntary most purport to provide a certain assurance of quality or safety to the public as well as benefits for the credentialed. And therein lies the dilemma. The dangers inherent in credentialing and the potential for conflict of interest were eloquently expressed almost 25 years ago and are still relevant today:

It is true that any professional society or group, no matter how socially oriented, will tend to develop barriers to protect itself .... Among the contemporary protective mechanisms for the health professions are accreditation, certification, licensure, and registration. All four of these mechanisms medicine has employed with excellent results, if not always for the benefit of society, at least for the benefit of most members of the profession. And now many of the numerous other health professions wish to adopt, if they have not already done so, the same steps which medicine had fashioned to meet the needs of society *and its own protection* (emphasis mine)[1]

This phenomenon has not escaped the notice of the consumer or the government. Because the health professions, as a whole, did not seem to show rapid progress in remedying the more questionable aspects of credentialing, particularly licensure, a series of blue-ribbon panels, high-level committees, and prestigious task forces at state and national levels were formed in the 1970s.

There is clear evidence that the recommendations made in the reports (1977) were a strong impetus to changes in the various forms of health manpower credentialing. These are reported in detail in the 5th edition of this book.

The 1971 PHS report also gave definitions for the major credentialing processes that have, since then, been used almost universally:

Accreditation: The process by which an agency or organization evaluates and recognizes an institution or program of study as meeting certain predetermined criteria or standards. [See also Chaps. 12 and 26.]

Licensure: The process by which an agency of government grants permission to persons to engage in a given profession or occupation by certifying that those licensed have attained the minimal degree of competency necessary to ensure that the public health, safety, and welfare will be reasonably well protected.

Certification or registration: The process by which a nongovernmental agency or association grants recognition to an individual who has met certain predetermined qualifications specified by that agency or association. Such qualifications may include (1) graduation from an accredited or approved program; (2) acceptable performance on a qualifying examination or series of examinations; and/or (3) completion of a given amount of work experience.[2]

Another acceptable definition of *registration* given in the working papers of the nurse credentialing study referred to in Chap. 5 and later in this chapter is: the process by which individuals are assessed and given status on a registry attesting to the individual's ability and current competency. Its purpose is to keep a continuous record of the past and current achievements of an individual.

INDIVIDUAL LICENSURE: PROBLEMS AND RECOMMENDATIONS

Among the problems addressed was licensure. As noted earlier, licensure is a police power of the state; that is, the state legislative process determines what group is licensed and with what limits. It is the responsibility of a specific part of the state government to see that that law is carried out, including punishment for its violation. Although licensure laws differ somewhat in format from state to state, the elements contained in each are similar. For instance, in the health professions laws, there are sections on definition of the profession that delineates the scope of practice; requirements for licensure, such as education; exemptions from licensure; grounds for revocation of a license; creation of a licensing board, including member qualifications and responsibilities; and penalties for practicing without a license.

Licensure laws are either mandatory (compulsory) or permissive (voluntary). If mandatory, the law forbids anyone to practice that profession or occupation without a license on pain of fine or imprisonment. If permissive, the law allows anyone to practice as long as she or he does not claim to hold the title of the practitioner (such as registered nurse).

Licensing of the health occupations was advocated in the early nineteenth century, but it was not until the early 1900s that a significant number of such licensing laws were enacted. They were generally initiated by the associations of practitioners that were interested in raising standards and establishing codes for ethical behavior. Because voluntary compliance was not always forthcoming, the associations sought enactment of regulatory legislation. To some critics, this movement is also seen as a means of giving members of an occupation or profession as much status, control, and compensation as the community is willing to give. It is true that as the health occupations proliferate, each group begins to organize and seek licensure. Because many of these occupations are subgroups of the major health professions, or are highly specialized, licensure creates problems in further fragmentation and increased cost in health care—according to the critics.

In all of the proposals for changes in health manpower credentialing, criticism of individual licensure is implicit or explicit. Particularly since 1970, the evils have been cited, but there was little recognition of actions taken to remedy the faults. Evolving changes (often slow in evolving) were dismissed as too little and too late. Some of the key criticisms of individual licensing are:

1. Most licensure laws for the health professions do not mandate continuing education or other requirements to prevent educational obsolescence. Therefore, the minimal standards of safety, theoretically guaranteed by granting the initial license, may no longer be met by some (perhaps many) practitioners.

2. Specific requirements for courses, roles, and so on are rigidly specified in statutes instead of relying on the administrative rule-making process. This makes timely responses to a changing environment difficult and slow. The result is that minimal standards and educational innovations in the health professions lag behind the practice realities.

3. Definitions of the area of practice are generally not specific, so that allocation of tasks is often determined by legal decisions or interpretations by lay people. On the other hand, some limitations of practice—ones that are not congruent with changing health care needs—are delineated.

4. Licensing boards are dominated by members of the particular profession and may not have representation by competent lay members or allied health professions. This has been negatively viewed as a means by which the profession controls entry into the field. There is the possibility of shutting out other health workers climbing the occupational ladder, and also limiting the number of practitioners for economic reasons. Moreover, the members of a one-profession board may lack overall knowledge of total expertise in the health care field, so that the scope of functions which could be delegated to other workers is not clearly determined. This creates the possibility that others capable of performing a particular activity may be prevented from doing so by another profession's licensing law. On the other hand, the inclusion of members of potentially competing health professions on licensing boards may result in the promotion of additional barriers to competition rather than growth and expansion of the profession being regulated.

5. There are always some licensed practitioners who are unsafe, and even if they lose their license in their own state, boards in other states are not notified, and the individual simply crosses a state line and continues to practice. [Physicians were particularly pinpointed, and in 1990 the government established a National Practitioner Data Bank (NPDB) to track serious disciplinary actions taken by medical boards and societies and hospitals, as well as settled malpractice cases. State boards and others are mandated to use these data before permitting a physician to practice. This also applies to dentists.]

The lack of geographic mobility that licensing causes for some health professionals is a concern. Nursing, with its state board examinations, now called the National Council Licensure Examination (NCLEX), that are used in every state, allows for licensure by endorsement in most states. That is, assuming that other criteria for licensure are met, a nurse need not take another examination when relocating to another state. Even then, nursing does not completely escape the mobility criticism, because, in the last few years, various state boards of nursing have adopted rather idiosyncratic criteria, particularly for advanced practice nurses.

Nevertheless, it seems that almost all of the established or fledgling health occupations, more than 250 at last count, consider licensing as a primary means of credentialing. The licensure problems of one health occupation obviously are not necessarily the same as those of all the others. Yet, because the majority of all kinds of health workers function in institutional settings, the various weaknesses of all health occupations' licensing laws, the inconsistencies and varying standards of those seeking licensure, and the sheer numbers involved appear to be the bases for whatever enthusiasm exists for alternatives to licensure, such as institutional licensure.

Given the many criticisms of licensure, it was not surprising that major recommendations have been made related to this form of credentialing. These include institutional licensure.

Institutional Licensure

Institutional licensure is a process by which a state government regulates health institutions;

it has existed for some 40 years. Usually, requirements for establishing and operating a health facility address administration, accounting requirements, equipment specifications, building construction and space planning, structural integrity, sanitation, and fire safety. In some cases, there are also minimal standards for occupancy including square footage per bed and minimal nursing staff requirements. The issue in the "new" institutional licensure dispute is whether personnel credentialing or licensing should be part of the institution's responsibility under the general aegis of the state licensing authority. There are various interpretations of just what institutional licensing means and how it could or should be implemented. The *Hershey model* had become synonymous with institutional licensure to many people.

Nathan Hershey, then professor of health law at the University of Pittsburgh, had criticized individual licensure for years. In a number of papers, he advocated that institutionally based health workers be regulated by the employing institution within bounds established by state institutional licensing bodies:

> Because the provision of services is becoming more and more institution-based, individual licensing of practitioners might be legitimately replaced by investing health services institutions and agencies with the responsibility for regulating the provision of services, within bounds established by the state institutional licensing bodies.
>
> The state licensing agency could establish, with the advice of experts in the health care field, job descriptions for various hospital positions, and establish qualifications in terms of education and experience for individuals who would hold these posts. Administrators certainly recognize the fact that although a professional nurse is licensed, her license does not automatically indicate which positions within the hospital she is qualified to fill. Individuals, because of their personal attainments, are selected to fill specific posts. Educational qualifications, based on both formal and inservice programs, along with prior job experience, determine if and how personnel should be employed.[3]

Hershey further suggested the development of a job description classification similar to that used in civil service. Personnel categories could be stated in terms of levels and grades, along with descriptive job titles. Under such a system, the individual's education and work experience would be taken into consideration by the employing institution for the individual's placement in a grade; basic qualifications for the position, expressed in terms of education and experience, would be set by the state's hospital licensing agency.

Thus, a professional nurse returning to work after ten or fifteen years, Hershey indicated, might be placed in a nurse aide or practical nurse (PN) position, moving on to a higher grade when she "regained her skills and became familiar with professional and technological advances through inservice programs." Hershey was, then and later, rather evasive about the role of the physician in this new credentialing picture, implying that the current practice of hospital staff review was really a pioneer effort along the same lines and might as well continue to function. However, he did list as sites all institutions and agencies providing health services, such as hospitals, nursing homes, physicians' offices, clinics, and the all-inclusive "et cetera."

There are many criticisms of institutional personnel credentialing. One concern was whether all agencies would be willing to initiate the expensive and extensive educational, evaluative, and supervisory programs necessary to fulfill the basic tenets of institutional licensure. With increasing pressure to control costs, extensive staff education programs seemed even less likely. This raised the specter of a return to the corrupted apprentice system of early hospital nursing in the United States. Probably a hospital's own personnel would be used as teacher-preceptors. Who then would do their job? How would they be compensated? How long would "students" be expected to function in their current positions with the current salary while they "practice" the new role? And with what kind of supervision? What kind of testing program for each level? Testing by whom? With what kinds of standards? Such sliding positions might well cut manpower costs, but might they not also indenture workers instead of freeing them with new mobility?

Problems of criteria for standards were obvious. If fifty states cannot agree on criteria for individual licensure, why would institutional licensure be any different? Considering the more than 6,000 profit and nonprofit hospitals with bed capacities ranging from the tens to the thousands, in rural and urban areas, with administrators and other key personnel prepared in widely varied ways, and the even larger number of extended care facilities, clinics, and home care agencies that are equally dissimilar, a state of confusion, diversity, and parochialism becomes an overwhelming probability. Instead of facilitating interstate mobility, institutional licensure would more likely limit even interinstitutional mobility. A worker could qualify for position X in institution A, with absolutely no guarantee that this would be acceptable to institution B. Moreover, the disadvantages to those health professions that have fought to attain, maintain, and raise standards might be disastrous to patient safety.

Whether or not, as was argued, many of these practices exist already—de facto institutional licensure, as one proponent asserted—it hardly seems progressive to legalize what is already considered an unsatisfactory situation. And let there be no mistake: under this proposed system, the institution would determine the specific tasks and functions of each job and indicate the skill and proficiency levels required, regardless of the employee's licensure, certification, or education. Control would be almost complete, because guidelines to be developed by the state institutional licensing agency were intended to be general.

But then, would not the state guidelines protect the consumer, if not the employee? Presumably, the state licensing agency would be empowered to review the institution's utilization and supervision of health personnel to determine whether employees are performing functions for which they are qualified. How feasible would such an evaluation be? No one believes that an army of experts knowledgeable in all the subcategories of health care could be recruited, employed, and dispersed to check the hundreds of thousands employed in the multiple subcategories of workers in the thousands of caregiving facilities in any state. Therefore, one more paper tiger would be created—inspection by paper work. To determine the effectiveness of similar surveillance schemes, look at the nursing home scandals and the admitted deficiencies of various municipal, state, and proprietary hospitals. In all of these situations, the institution reviewed was given an official blessing; in truth, the conditions varied from unsafe to life-threatening. Generally, approval was given on the basis of the written self-report, with or without a visit by harassed, overworked surveyors. (What's more, when surveyors did recommend closings of the institutions, they were frequently overruled or ignored, if it was politically expedient.) Would institutional licensure suddenly, miraculously avoid these pitfalls? Nursing led protests in opposition to the institutional licensure concept, and the issue seems to have died.

Does this eliminate the threat of institutional licensure? Not really, for it seems now that the concept is reappearing, if it ever disappeared, with or without its label.[4] In some states, overt attempts to legislate institutional licensure (which had been kept in committee or killed primarily through the efforts of organized nursing) keep emerging. It is conceivable that with the trend toward multi-institutional ownership, especially by for-profit groups, and the concomitant trend for physicians to become employees, corporate-wide credentialing may be sought by the corporate giants. It is speculative whether professional groups would have the political clout to prevent it.

Certification

Certification has also been under scrutiny. As a follow-up to the 1971 DHEW Report on Licensure and related health personnel credentialing, a project to determine the feasibility of a national certification system, aimed particularly at allied health personnel, was explored—with federal funding. The results seemed to be positive, and DHEW concluded that this concept, a voluntary national certification system, should be developed further.

By 1978, a Certification Council, later called the National Commission for Health Certifying Agencies (NCHCA), had been organized. Its general purpose was to certify the certifiers—an overall group that would include the organizations that certified allied health professionals but also set certain uniform standards and guidelines. At the same time, certification of nurses was also undergoing reorganization and expansion, as was certification for PAs. Nurse-midwives and nurse anesthetists had been certified for some time, but in the period following the credentialing reports, their system also underwent change. In general, certification was and is attracting considerable attention as a substitute for, or an adjunct to, licensure; in the latter case, it is a means of identifying specialists within a field. For instance, many of the health occupations described in Chap. 8 are only certified, but physicians with all-encompassing licensure increasingly use certification to differentiate specialists, and, as discussed later, this is the trend for nursing.

Still, certification is not a clearly understood credentialing mechanism. Two points are essential for comprehension: (1) certification is voluntary on the part of the individual, and (2) the organization or agency that certifies is nongovernmental and is usually comprised of experts or peers in that particular field. This "private credentialing" differs fundamentally from "public credentialing" (licensure) in that the latter can legally prohibit unlicensed practice. Those who lack private credentials "still possess a legal right to practice, although they may be disadvantaged in the marketplace because independent decision-makers such as consumers, hospitals, and public or private financing plans value their services less highly."[5] Havighurst and King describe private credentialing as serving solely informational purposes, a sort of "seal of approval" from the professional association or nongovernmen-tal board that grants it.[6] It gives the consumer an opportunity to make more informed decisions, in that certification indicates that the certified person has voluntarily met certain standards that similar caregivers have not. Because the public needs to know that the certifying group and its standards have some legitimacy, there is a second-tier credentialing organization, like the NCHCA noted above, that can be either voluntary or governmental. Accreditation of educational programs, as done by NLN, or of health care facilities, as done by the Joint Commission on Accreditation of Healthcare Organizations (JCAHO), are other examples of private credentialing.

There are hybrids of "private credentialing" mandated in statutes. For example, there are statutory requirements for testing professionals using professionally developed examinations to assure competence instead of licensing the individual. The government places the individual's name on a registry. Persons who are not listed on the registry cannot be hired and the institution can be penalized for not checking the registry prior to employing the individual. For example, physician assistants are often listed on Board of Medicine registry and/or cannot practice without the professional certification as required by state law.

Criticisms of certification are remarkably like those of licensure. One is that individuals as well qualified as those who are certified are denied certification and are thus disadvantaged in the marketplace. The denial may be due to the lack of a certain educational background or failure to pass an examination. The latter is a common certification mechanism. This was indeed challenged in a legal suit, and the certifying board settled out of court. The issue is often the validity of the examination and whether it discriminates against minorities, for instance—a matter that has also arisen in licensure. Examinations for both types of credentialing are now undergoing close scrutiny, with continual involvement of test experts. Nevertheless, some persons question whether *any* examination can really identify the competent practitioner.

Second, there is the question of grandfathering, also a licensure problem. Usually those who practiced a specialty before certification existed are "grandfathered in," that is, permitted to hold certification without fulfilling the usual requirements. Thus, the information given the public—that these persons fulfill certain criteria—is not accurate. Here the answer may lie in requirements to demonstrate ongoing competency for recertification—provided that that measure is valid. More certifying groups now have a recertification mechanism.

Finally, there is the concern that certification is done by the professional organization that also accredits the educational program from which the candidate must graduate in order to qualify for certification. Clearly, that mechanism provides complete control by the occupation and can also shut out potential candidates. This problem was resolved, to a large extent, by the FTC rulings that such arrangements were illegal restraint of trade.[7] Professions then gradually separated these functions into independent entities. Two examples are the nurse-midwives and nurse anesthetists, whose organizations are described in Chap. 27.

Despite these criticisms, certification is generally advocated as a way to assist the consumer in making choices.

Sunset Laws and Other Public Actions

Besides considering alternatives, improving the licensure process has become a state mandate. This is particularly true because, beginning with the Reagan administration, credentialing issues were no longer a priority on the federal level. Although the speed of the action taken has varied from state to state, steps taken almost universally at one level or another include adding consumers and sometimes other functionally related health professionals to each board, giving more attention to disciplinary procedures, and gradually developing proficiency and equivalency examinations. In a number of states, boards have been consolidated, sometimes under committees of lay people (or at least a majority of consumers), who make the decisions about licensing, with the individual boards acting in an advisory capacity. Other states have been restructured to form multidisciplinary boards, investigative and administrative functions have been consolidated, and/or other ministerial activities have been added to the duties of the professional boards. One reason given is improved efficiency, but some nurses fear that this is an indirect approach to institutional licensure because these reorganizations tend to attenuate nursing's control over its practice.

For some professions, improving the licensure laws to protect the public was a new experience. A motivating factor was the enactment of "sunset laws" which require the periodic reexamination of licensing agencies to determine whether particular boards or activities should be established. By 1984, two-thirds of the states had already enacted such laws. These laws were a result of a lobbying campaign by Common Cause, a consumer group, to bring about legislative and executive branch oversight of regulating boards and agencies of all kinds. Common Cause identified ten principles to be followed, including a time schedule. An important component was that an evaluation was to allow for public input, as well as that of the boards and occupations involved. Consolidation and "responsible pruning" were encouraged. Although the review would be done by appropriate legislative and executive committees, safeguards were to be built in to prevent arbitrary termination of boards and agencies.[8] These principles are generally adhered to, but states do vary in their management of sunset reviews. If a sunset law is in effect, the data and justification for existence are a joint staff-board responsibility, although the professional organizations are also usually helpful.

Nursing was no more ready for sunset review than other disciplines, but nurses learned, sometimes the hard way.

By 1985, most nursing boards had undergone sunset reviews, and the new or amended laws usually reflected changes in practice and society.

These changes, and some instituted earlier, also reflected the impact of the DHEW reports. Most practice acts have broadened the scope of practice, added consumers to their boards, and sometimes required evidence of current competence through various means, including continuing education. State boards have given increased attention to removing and/or rehabilitating incompetent nurses. Meanwhile, educators are working seriously on equivalency and proficiency examinations and other methods of providing flexibility and upward mobility for nursing candidates. Nurses in the field have continued to improve techniques of peer evaluation, implement standards of practice, and encourage voluntary continuing education.

NURSING ACTIONS IN CREDENTIALING

Nursing was in the thick of all these credentialing activities. Since the beginning of organized nursing, finding ways to assure the public of high-quality nursing was given a high priority by nursing leaders (see Chap. 5). Licensing for individuals and accreditation for institutions seemed to be the first solution, but as noted earlier, each has its weaknesses. Moreover the ANA had for some years been inclined to think that perhaps all voluntary credentialing, including accreditation, which was done by NLN, should be under ANA.

A major study of credentialing sponsored by ANA made some daring proposals in 1979, including suggesting the establishment of a national nursing credentialing center, run by a federation of organizations with "legitimate interests" in nursing and credentialing, "as the means of achieving a unified, coordinated, comprehensive credentialing system for nursing."[9] A follow-up task force affirmed the study's recommendations, particularly about establishing a credentialing center with a coalition of other organizations. This recommendation was not accepted by nursing, except "in principle." Then, with the increase of nurse specialists and the confusion in licensing laws described later, the

question of the best way to credential specialists became urgent. It was decided by ANA that certification rather than recognition of specialists by licensing was the best choice. The ANA Social Policy Statement says:

> Certification of specialists in nursing practice is a judgment made by the profession, upon review of an array of evidence examined by a selected panel of nurses who are themselves specialists and who represent the area of specialization . . . . the public needs clear evidence that a nurse who claims to be a specialist does indeed have expertise of a particular kind. The profession of nursing has a social obligation to the public to satisfy that need, which it does by means of certification of specialists and by accreditation of the graduate programs that educate specialists in nursing practice.[10]

Unfortunately one major problem in the certification of nursing specialists is that both ANA and certain specialty organizations each certify, so that both nurse and consumer must decide which is more reliable.

At the time, ANA was already certifying advanced clinical practitioners, but so were almost all the existing specialty organizations. When in a 1982 meeting none of the organizations was willing to be part of a multi-organization credentialing center, each fearing a loss of power, ANA created its own center. By 1985, the House of Delegates endorsed the retention of the Center for Credentialing Services as an administrative unit within ANA, and in 1991, the American Nurses Credentialing Center (ANCC) became a separately incorporated subsidiary of ANA. Interest in development of a coherent system for credentialing remained an ANA priority, but with the improvement of cooperative relations between ANA and NLN, no overt action was taken by ANA to wrest the accreditation of nursing education programs from NLN. (ANA does accredit CE programs.) Although there were House of Delegates resolutions about the need for ANA to become involved in accreditation of nursing services, that seemed to be more rhetoric than action.

In 1986, the ANA published the first of a monograph series on credentialing in nursing, which along with the credentialing study gives as comprehensive and provocative information about nurse credentialing as any publication. In this first monograph, Dr. Margretta Styles, who had chaired the original Credentialing Study, made some in-depth comparisons between credentialing of nurses in the United States and in the rest of the world.[11] She had been commissioned by the ICN, which also had many concerns about nurse credentialing, to help them develop a position on credentialing and regulation in nursing. The position paper she developed, which was accepted by the ICN Council of National Representatives in 1985, included 12 principles of regulation equally applicable to American nursing and to other countries. These principles provide a fundamental orientation for the regulation of professionals that has application beyond nursing:

- Regulation should be directed toward an explicit purpose.
- Regulation should be designed to achieve the stated purpose.
- Regulatory standards should be based upon clear definitions of professional scope and accountability.
- Regulatory mechanisms and standards should promote the fullest development of the profession commensurate with its potential social contribution.
- Regulatory systems should recognize and incorporate the legitimate roles and responsibilities of interested parties—the public, the profession and its members, government, employers, other professions—in various aspects of standard setting and administration.
- The design of the regulatory system should acknowledge and appropriately balance interdependent interests.
- Regulatory systems should provide and be limited to those controls and restrictions necessary to achieve their objectives.
- Standards and processes of regulation should be sufficiently broad and flexible to achieve their objective and at the same

time permit freedom for innovation, growth, and change.
- Regulatory systems should operate in the most efficient manner, ensuring coherence and coordination among their parts.
- Regulatory systems should promote universal standards of performance and foster professional identity and mobility to the fullest extent compatible with local needs and circumstances.
- Regulatory processes should provide honest and just treatment for those parties regulated.
- In their standards and processes regulatory systems should recognize the equality and interdependence of professions offering essential services.[12]

Basically these principles warn against overregulation, propose a flexibility that will allow practice to respond sensitively to the changing times, recognize the temptation for regulation to be self-serving and protect the fiefdoms among professionals, urge consumer input, universal standards, and the broadest practice role commensurate with the ability of the provider and social need.

In viewing United States patterns of regulation, Styles commented on our peculiarities; the mix of public and private, mandatory and voluntary mechanisms; the decentralization of controls to the state and local level, but with some federal controls still held; and the American multilevel system of higher education from diploma and certificate to doctoral degrees. She also noted that the generic term "auxiliary" used by the International Labor Organization (ILO) to designate nonprofessionals in any occupation would currently apply to our LPNs, who are of course licensed. At the other end of the clinical spectrum, "titles incorporate the terms practitioner, clinician, specialist, a variety of specialty fields, and in most instances, the noun 'nurse' as recommended by ICN."[13] Second licenses and certification as means of regulation are considered duplicative and uneven in definition; national certification is recommended. In 1989, Styles presented an extremely comprehensive study on nursing specialties, including a survey of characteristics of specialties in nursing summarized in a voluminous appendix with information on each specialty. The "composite indices of the maturity of the special interest areas (SIAs)" were identified as:

1. The practitioner is recognized as a nurse specialist, but perhaps not certified.
2. The baccalaureate in nursing is a prerequisite for further study.
3. There is support, with directed resources toward research and knowledge building.
4. A rigorous program of certification is available.
5. The interests and concerns are represented by an organized body.
6. The SIA has refereed journals publishing SIA research.
7. The SIA recognizes ANA as the official organization of nursing-at-large, but maintains a communication link with other specialty nursing organizations.
8. The SIA is identifiable as nursing through its definitions of practice and practitioners, its educational programs and knowledge base, and its relationships with nursing-at-large.[14]

She found the specialties at various stages of "maturity," according to these indices. As is seen later, clear identification of SIAs is particularly important in credentialing, since there is no clear, consistent differentiation across states. Styles believes that to empower nurse specialists, specialty credentials must be strengthened through the creation of a National Board of Nurse Specialties to review and approve specialties and their certification programs. As a corollary process, marketing may have financial as well as professional implications, as once certification is fully recognized, the person holding board certification may be reimbursed for services at a higher rate than a nurse without these credentials.[15] In 1991, the American Board of Nursing Specialties (ABNS) was established. Its objectives include setting standards for the for-

mal recognition of professional nursing specialty certification programs, establishing policies and procedures for the review and approval of certification programs, and recognizing specialty nursing certification that meets ABNS standards. Thirteen certification boards compose the membership of ABNS, collectively representing over 120,000 certified nurses, more than 65 percent of the total number of registered nurses currently certified in the United States.

Legal advisers see no problem in credentialing bodies accomplishing their goals of self-regulation and advancement of the profession as long as certain basic legal principles are followed. They expect minimal interference from court and administrative enforcement agencies.[16] Understanding the balance between internal and external regulations is important for nurses, as nurses will probably be credentialed in this manner for the foreseeable future. Before considering the next sections on nursing's licensure law, Exhibit 20-1 may be helpful in clarifying some of the differences between internal and external regulation.[17]

LICENSURE: THE LEGAL BASIS OF NURSING PRACTICE

Enactment of nurse licensure laws was one of the primary purposes of ANA at its inception. The first permissive nursing practice law in this country was enacted in North Carolina on March 3, 1903. Weak though it was compared with present-day laws, it represented a great achievement for nursing leaders, who had been working toward this goal for a decade. Within a month, New Jersey passed a state nursing practice act, followed closely by New York and Virginia. In 1904, Maryland was the only state to pass such an act, but in each succeeding year from 1905 until 1917, state legislation was enacted to govern the practice of nursing. By 1917, 45 states and the District of Columbia had nursing practice acts; by 1923 the last of the 48 states in existence adopted such an act. In 1952, all

Exhibit 20-1	Characteristics of Regulation of the Profession

Internal Regulation (within the profession)

The purpose is to ensure the advancement of nursing while serving the public interest.

- Regulation is dependent upon self-discipline, peer surveillance, and evaluation.
- Compliance is voluntary.
- Penalties for non-compliance are (a) professional censure, (b) withdrawal of credentials such as certification and accreditation, and (c) disciplinary actions such as recommendation for investigation by board of nursing.
- Standards and criterion measures are developed and revised by changing groups of selected and elected nurses from within the profession.
- The expertise and critique of a large number of nurses provide broad input for development and review of self-regulatory measures.

External Regulation (outside the profession)

The purpose is to protect the public.[1]

- Regulation is dependent upon surveillance, complaints, reports of others, investigation, and court action.
- Compliance is mandatory.
- Penalties for non-compliance are (a) dismissal from employment, (b) loss of license, and (c) court judgments such as imprisonment.
- The professional's standards and recommended nominees for appointment to boards of nursing and other agencies may or may not be used in establishing rules and regulations and in board appointments. Board of nursing appointments tend to be political. The board selects or formulates standards and adopts them.
- Statutes tend to define qualifications at a general, minimal level.

[1]There may be other purposes, such as profit or control over nurses.

Source: Hildegard Peplau, Credentialing in Nursing: Contemporary Developments and Trends. "Internal vs. External Regulation" (Kansas City, MO: American Nurses' Association 1986), p 4.

states and territories had such laws. Hawaii's first nursing practice act was passed in 1917 and Alaska's in 1941.

In every instance, the original state law was permissive. The first mandatory licensure statute was enacted in New York in 1938, but it was not put into effect until 1947. One of the real dangers of permissive licensing was the use of graduates of schools with poor curricula and inadequate clinical experience. These workers could legally use the title "nurse," although they were potentially dangerous practitioners. Such programs also tend to defraud unsuspecting students who do not know that they will not be eligible for licensure, because a school must maintain minimum standards set by the state board before graduates may sit for licensing examinations. Theoretically, any person with or without schooling can practice as a nurse if someone is willing to hire him or her. With permissive licensure, the kind of nurse most likely to be hired is one who has graduated from a legitimate program but has not been able to pass the licensing exam.

As of 1990, all states had mandatory licensure laws for professional nurses and for practical nurses. However, some states are permissive in their interpretation of mandatory. States that have such global exemption clauses in licensure laws stating that almost anyone can be a "nurse," provided that there is some kind of "supervision," are sometimes seen as permissive states regardless of a mandatory clause.

Objections to making licensure laws mandatory come from many sources. Some feel that mandatory laws are used to keep out individuals who might be capable but lack the formal education and other requirements for licensure. It is true that some laws are rigid in these requirements, but more and more states are beginning to consider the use of equivalency and proficiency examinations and other means of demonstrating knowledge and skills.

Another concern is that those already practicing in the field will be abruptly removed and deprived of their livelihood. This is, however, untrue because mandatory laws are forced, for political and constitutional reasons, to include a grandfather clause. A grandfather or waiver clause is a standard feature when a licensure law is enacted or a current law is repealed and a new law enacted. The grandfather clause allows persons to continue to practice the profession or occupation when new qualifications are enacted into law. Although the concept goes back to post-Civil War days, it is also related to the Fifth and Fourteenth amendments of the Constitution. The U.S. Supreme Court has repeatedly ruled that the license to practice a profession or occupation is a property right and that the Fourteenth Amendment extends the due process requirement to state laws. All nurses currently licensed and in compliance with state law were protected by the grandfather clause when a new law was passed or new requirements were made, although most probably never realized it. For instance, when the Wyoming Nursing Practice Act was repealed in 1983, the new law had a grandfather clause, and all nurses holding a valid license continued to be licensed. When the grandfather clause is enacted in relation to mandatory licensure, those who can produce evidence, that they practiced as, say, a PN, if applying for LPN status, must be granted a license. However, grandfathering does not guarantee employment. Thus, some employers chose not to employ "waivered" PNs, just as they had not employed them as unlicensed practitioners. Because of these problems, and often because of their need and desire to be safe, competent practitioners, many took courses to fill the gaps in their knowledge and chose to take the state board examinations later. One interesting exception was attempted with the Wyoming law: a "limited grandfather clause" for previously approved nurse practitioners, giving them two years to meet the new NP qualifications. The legislature disagreed because NPs were being treated differently from other RNs. The Mississippi Supreme Court made a similar decision.[18]

CONTENT OF NURSING PRACTICE ACTS

Unfortunately, many nurses know no more about the law that regulates their practice than that it requires them to take state board examinations in order to become licensed. More details about the procedure for obtaining a license will be given later; however, it is vital that nurses understand the components of their licensure law and how these affect their practice. (Nurse-midwives and nurse anesthetists may be included within a nursing practice act, a medical practice act, separately, or totally ignored legislatively. If mentioned, certification is usually a prerequisite for legal practice.)

Because each state law differs to a degree in its content, it is important to have available a copy of the law of the state in which you practice and the regulations that spell out how the law is carried out. These may be obtained from the state board or agency in the state government that has copies of laws for distribution. The language in all laws often seems stilted because they are written in legal terms. However, a little effort or discussion with someone familiar with the law will soon enable you to become almost as familiar with legal jargon as with nursing jargon. This is particularly important, for many states anticipate some change in their nursing practice act in the near future or have recently passed amendments related to sunset review. Changes made or contemplated are generally in relation to the definition and scope of nursing practice, the composition of the nursing board, and actions to ensure competency.

Most nursing practice acts have basically the same major components, although not necessarily in the same order: legislative mandate (why have this law?), definition of nursing, requirements for licensure, exemption from licensure, grounds for revocation, suspension or conditioning of the license, provision for endorsement for persons licensed in other states, creation of a board of nurse examiners, responsibilities of the board, and penalties for practicing in violation of the act or without a license. All states do not, unfortunately, have the same requirements in these categories. Some follow the ANA guidelines, some the model act of the National Council of State Boards of Nursing (NCSBN); others enact what is politically feasible or necessary in their particular state.

The ANA guidelines and the NCSBN Model Act will be referred to frequently. The question is often raised as to why two influential groups involved in nurse licensure should have separate recommendations for legislation. This is difficult to answer; however, they do function from different mandates. Once, certain activities relating to licensure were in a committee within ANA, but in 1978 the group decided to rename and reorganize itself outside the ANA. Despite angry protests from many ANA delegates about this action, a liaison committee between the two organizations was established. Even after many amicable meetings, an agreement on guidelines for revising the nurse practice act could never be reached. Why? Each group has its own constituents: NCSBN with its representatives from all the state boards of nursing works from the perspective of elected or appointed state officials, with an overriding responsibility to ensure that licensure protects the consumer, while ANA with its diverse group of nurses is committed to setting standards for nursing. The ANA document *Suggested State Legislation* is intended as a policy guide for "nurses, state nurses' associations, state boards of nursing and state officials who are considering changes to their state nursing practice act or overall health regulatory legislation."[19] Since ANA's beginning, their state components have suggested changes in nurse licensure as a part of their normal responsibilities. Therefore, now some important ANA members consider NCSBN's actions on formulating definitions of nursing an encroachment on the prerogatives of ANA and the state associations. It is not the business of state boards or NCSBN, they say, because boards implement nursing practice acts *after* they are enacted.

Nevertheless, NCSBN has been publishing model acts since 1982 "to serve as a guide to states in considering revisions to their Nursing Practice Acts."[20] There are useful elements in each document, but one radical change in the ANA *Suggested State Legislation* is that although now both organizations call for only one broad statement defining nursing (and one board), ANA refers to professional nursing practice and technical nursing practice; the NCSBN *Model Act* refers only to registered nursing and practical nursing. ANA is oriented to a philosophy that expects their definitions to become reality in the future, and NCSBN is dealing with current reality. The other major difference is that ANA specifies a separate act for prescriptive authority and another for "disciplinary diversion," which means that nurses with addictions or mental health problems are treated differently from others with problems in professional discipline. NCSBN does not mention either. Other major differences will be pointed out in the following sections. Though neither document has any legal clout, and states tend to use what suits their needs, those involved in nurse legislation generally study both documents. This would be a worthwhile exercise for interested nurses as well, providing provocative and stimulating food for discussion on how we see nursing.

Recent intensive discussion within the nursing community about the issue of second licensure for advanced practice nurses provided the opportunity for ANA and NCSBN to recognize the need to work together on these complex, evolving credentialing questions. So, as of the summer of 1994, ANA and NCSBN intend to develop a joint document on legislative language for a model nursing practice act that addresses the entire continuum of professional nursing practice.

Definition and Scope of Practice

The definition of *nursing* in the licensure law determines both legal responsibilities and the scope of practice of nurses. Inevitably, the definition of nursing in all nursing practice acts is stated in terms that are quite broad. This is generally frustrating to nurses who turn to the definition to determine if they are practicing legally, because it does not spell out specific procedures or activities. Often such activities are not even spelled out in the regulations of the laws. However, a broad definition is usually preferable because of the problems of including specific activities in a law. Changes in health care and nursing practice often move more rapidly than a law can be changed, and the amending process can be long and complex. If particular activities were named, the nurse would be limited to just those listed. Not only would the list be overwhelmingly long, but it is conceivable that any new technique easily and, perhaps necessarily, performed by a nurse would require an amendment to the law. An occasional state law does specify certain procedures, but always includes the phrase "not limited to."

A practicing nurse soon finds that the nursing functions taught in an educational program may differ from those expected by an employer. The differences may be small and caused by variations in the settings of nursing care. Nursing in a medical center may require knowing more sophisticated techniques or assuming more comprehensive responsibilities in nursing care. Sometimes, whether in a large or small agency, there are procedures performed that the nurse has not learned. If the nurse has not practiced for some time, this is even more likely to happen. In other cases, the responsibilities expected in the nursing role are not in nursing care but in clerical and administrative tasks. Although this may not be desirable, it is not illegal. What concerns nurses is whether the patient-oriented care expected in the employment situation is legal or in the domain of another health profession. Many of the activities in health care overlap. A common example might be the administration of drugs, which could be done by the physician, RN, LPN, and various technicians in other hospital departments if related to a diagnostic procedure or treatment. Yet dispensing a drug from the hospital pharmacy. still done by some nursing supervisors at night when no

pharmacist is on duty, is in most states a violation of the pharmacy licensing law.

Obviously, one of the greatest concerns for nurses is the possible violation of the Medical Practice Act. Nurses have gradually been performing more and more of the technical procedures that once belonged exclusively to medicine, but often these are delegated willingly by physicians. Whether nurses are always properly prepared to understand and perform them well is seldom questioned. However, as some nurses have assumed more comprehensive overall responsibilities in the care, cure, and coordination of patient care, questions have been raised by both nurses and physicians. Some are resistant to such changes; others are supportive but concerned about the legality of such acts. There are few data on nurses being disciplined for practicing medicine without a license.

In the now classic DHEW report *Extending the Scope of Nursing Practice*, there is a statement that the identical act or procedure "may be the practice of medicine when carried out by a physician and the practice of nursing when carried out by the nurse" (see Chap. 5).

> **There is an ever-widening area of independent nursing practice entailing nursing judgment, procedures, and techniques. This is due to natural evolution, commencing with the nurse's assumption of certain activities carried out under medical direction, and the subsequent relaxation or removal of that direction.**
>
> **Concomitant with increasingly complex nursing practice is the continual realignment of the functions of the professional nurse and physician. The boundaries of responsibility for nurses are not shifting more rapidly simply because of increased demands for health services. The functions of nurses are changing primarily because nurses have demonstrated their competence to perform a greater variety of functions and have been willing to discontinue performing less important functions that were once performed only by nurses.**[21]

The same report stated that there are no legal barriers to extending the scope of practice because the statutory laws governing nursing practice (the licensing laws) are broad enough to permit such extension, provided that the nurse has the proper skills and necessary knowledge of the underlying science. It did acknowledge that at times common law, essentially judge-made law, has made interpretations of nursing practice not specifically defined by statute, through legal decisions and stated that the profession must then look at these decisions to determine the need to change the statutory law. After reviewing some of the problems concerned with specific acts in changing nursing practice, the report concluded that as nursing changes, both nursing and the law must evaluate these changes and make the necessary adaptations to meet society's changing needs.[22] That is exactly what happened.

Until 1974 the nursing practice acts of most states had as their definition of nursing one similar to a model suggested by ANA in 1955:

> **The practice of professional nursing means the performance for compensation of any act in the observation, care, and counsel of the ill, injured, or infirm, or in the maintenance of health or prevention of illness of others, or in the supervision and teaching of other personnel, or the administration of medications and treatments as prescribed by a licensed physician or dentist; requiring substantial specialized judgment and skill and based on knowledge and application of the principles of biological, physical, and social science. (The foregoing shall not be deemed to include acts of diagnosis or prescription of therapeutic or corrective measures.)[23]**

The definition distinguished between independent acts that the nurse might perform, but also identified certain dependent acts and prohibited diagnosis and treatment (not preceded by the word *medical*). In the 1970s, with expanded functions being assumed by nurses, state nurses' associations (SNAs) increasingly became concerned about the adequacy of this definition. Therefore, the first states to change their laws concentrated on broadening the definition to encompass these roles.

Professional nursing literature had been distinguishing between the independent acts that a nurse must undertake and the dependent acts that must be carried out under the supervision or "orders" of the physician, such as administra-

tion of medications and treatments. The problem in the 1955 definition, in terms of the needs of the 1970s, was that although the first sentence did not *prohibit* the nurse from carrying out medical acts or making diagnoses, the last sentence effectively prohibited a broad interpretation by the courts.

As nurses in their expanded role seemed to be moving into the gray areas between medicine and nursing, it was evident that, if a state had a licensure law with a dependent clause, nurses might be seen as practicing medicine. The 1971 and 1973 credentialing reports suggested extending delegation of authority in all fields, but nursing was concerned that such delegation might mean including nurses specifically in the exception clause of medical practice acts, thus permitting the practice, but placing control totally in the hands of physicians. Perhaps as a compromise or in the hope that medicine and nursing could work together as they should in providing new health care options to the public, ANA counsel at the time suggested that a new clause be added to the ANA model definition:

> **A professional nurse may also perform such additional acts, under emergency or other special conditions, which may include special training, as are recognized by the medical and nursing professions as proper to be performed by a professional nurse under such conditions, even though such acts might otherwise be considered diagnosis and prescription.[24]**

Later, after various states had amended their laws with this phrase or changed it altogether, with varying success, an ANA ad hoc committee revised the definition entirely in 1976. This model law, recommending one nursing practice law with provisions for licensing practitioners of nursing, used the terms *registered nurse* and *practical/vocational nurse.* This definition differentiated between the independence of the RN's functions and the dependence of the LPN/LVN. It also placed the responsibility for what the RN can legally do in the hands of the nursing profession, always considered a hallmark of professionalism.

The 1980 definition spoke of professional services for the RN and technical services for the PN (vocational), probably as a manifestation of the professional-technical differentiation presented in the 1965 ANA position paper and reaffirmed by the House of Delegates in 1978. Direct accountability to the public is also a part of the definition; again, differentiation between the two types of nurses is made. In the commentary section, it was noted that the definition should recognize "the singular element that distinguishes the nurse from other nursing personnel—the breadth and depth of educational preparation that justify entrusting overall responsibility for nursing services to the judgment of the registered nurse." (The ANA is in the process of revising its publication, *Nursing: A Social Policy Statement*, which also addresses some of these issues, due to be completed by early 1995.)

In its introduction to the 1990 Suggested State Legislation, ANA stated:

> ANA is committed to state laws that provide for the licensure of persons practicing nursing. This commitment requires an understanding of the principles relating to the legal regulation of nursing practice:
>
> 1. The primary purpose of a licensing law for the regulation of the practice of nursing is to protect the public health and welfare by establishing legal qualifications for the practice of nursing. Such legal standards are recognized as the minimum standards determined as adequate to provide safe and effective nursing practice.
> 2. All persons practicing or offering to practice nursing should be licensed. Protection of the public is accomplished only if all who practice or offer to practice nursing are licensed. The public should not be expected to differentiate between competent and incompetent practitioners.
> 3. Since nursing has one scope of practice, there should be one nursing practice act which licenses all nurses. The public, as well as nurses, may be confused when there is more than one law regulating the practice of nursing.
> 4. The enactment of one nursing practice act necessitates only one licensing board for nursing in a state. The board of nursing should be composed of nurses whose practice is regulated by the licensure

law and by a representative or representatives of the public.
> 5. Candidates for licensure should complete an educational program approved by the board and pass the licensing examination before a license to practice is granted.
> 6. It is the function of the professional association to establish the scope and desirable qualifications required for specialized areas of practice, and to certify individuals as competent to engage in specific areas of nursing practice. This allows the field of nursing to expand commensurate with research findings and demands from the practice environment.[25]

The NCSBN said that their Model Act revisions were based on data identifying the need for such revision.

Exhibit 20-2 shows the difference between the ways ANA and NCSBN conceive of what might be the most important aspect of a nursing practice act, the definition of nursing. There are clearly many similarities, although the language is different. AD nurses or students may find the ANA definition confusing (or insulting) in relation to "technical nursing practice." However, the intent was to use this description for what is now the LPN position. Current AD nurses holding an RN license would be grandfathered into the "professional component." NCSBN does not address that possibility, staying with the current status of licensure laws (except for North Dakota).

Another interesting difference is the content of the legislative intent or purpose section. Both refer to the need for regulation to protect the public, but again wording (and perhaps intent) varies. NCSBN says:

> The legislature finds that the practice of nursing by competent persons is necessary for the protection of the public health, safety, and welfare and further finds that the *two levels of practice within the profession of nursing* should be regulated and controlled, in the public interest. (Emphasis by the authors.)

ANA says:

> The legislature further declares it to be the policy of this state to regulate nursing practice and those engaged in *professional nursing practice and technical*

nursing practice, as well as all who assist in the practice of nursing **through a state agency with the power to enforce the provisions of this act . . . . It is the intent of the legislature to provide clear legal authority for functions and procedures that have common acceptance and usage and to recognize the overlapping functions between individuals licensed to practice nursing and other licensed health care providers in the delivery of health care services. (*Emphasis mine.*)**

These are really quite daring statements, and it will be interesting to see how the recent commitment between ANA and NCSBN to develop joint statements on legislative language will alter existing documents.

Just how varied the state licensure laws were in 1983 was revealed by an ANA analysis of fifty-one nursing practice acts.[26] Definitions of nursing were looked at in light of the nursing process, that is, assessment, diagnosis, planning, intervention, and evaluation. ANA found that even when the concepts of the process were identifiable in the various laws, the language varied considerably. Terms such as *diagnosis of human responses, nursing diagnosis, problem* or *need identification, nursing analysis*, and *diagnosis of disease* were all used. Since 1983, all but two states have revised their Nursing Practice Acts.[27] Being that the state nurses association is the major (and often only) state lobby for nursing, the ANA "suggested state legislation" may have promoted more consistency (no subsequent analysis has been done).

A major concern in the 1970s was how states legislated for advanced nursing practice, which is related to both definition and regulations. This was reported in 1983 in considerable detail, including the practice of nurse-midwives and nurse anesthetists.[28] By 1994 a comprehensive yearly state-by-state legislative review of advanced practice nurses reported continuing serious barriers to advanced nursing practice in many states.[29] The barriers were in the areas of scope of practice, prescriptive authority, and reimbursement. These barriers remain in spite of the documented value of advanced practice nursing, and the absence of any quality-of-care problems.[30]

In an early approach to the expanding role of nurses, joint statements of practice (or function) were issued by state professional organizations concerning a specific function performed by the nurse. Such statements are usually jointly agreed upon by the nurses' association, medical association, and hospital association, and occasionally other professional groups. They are not intended to tell nurses how to practice nursing, but set criteria that attorneys believe would make it possible for them to defend a nurse if legal defense were necessary in relation to emerging, questioned areas of nursing practice.

When joint agreement is reached after a meeting of representatives and attorneys of the concerned associations, the statement is published and distributed by each group and often by the state medical licensing board and nursing licensing board. The statement usually includes specific criteria for performance of the acts concerned and always includes the need for appropriate education and training. Frequently there is a preliminary statement advocating the formation, in each health care institution, of a committee of medicine, nursing, and administration to state responsibilities of doctors and nurses and to set criteria for determining the role and responsibility of each, considering newer developments in health care and education.

Because such organizations do not have legal status in relation to changing the law (although they can initiate such changes), these statements, in a way, only formalize the custom and usage doctrine. The chances of prosecution of the nurse by the medical licensure board are slight, for usually the board has been involved in issuing the statement. However, these statements do not have the effect of law unless the groups are given the legal authority to make them. Theoretically, a case could still be made against the nurse, particularly if a civil malpractice suit is involved. To remedy this situation, some states have taken action to legalize the statements. A number of states have developed and used joint statements without legal sanction.

In the past, state legislatures have chosen three general means of dealing with advanced

Exhibit
20-2   Comparison of ANA and NCSBN Suggested Definitions of Nursing in Licensure Law

ANA

The "practice of nursing" means the performance of services for compensation in the provision of diagnosis and treatment of human responses to health or illness; "professional nursing practice" encompasses the full scope of nursing practice and includes all its specialties and consists of application of nursing theory to the development, implementation, and evaluation of plans of nursing care for individuals, families, and communities. Professional nursing practice requires substantial knowledge of nursing theory and related scientific, behavioral, and humanistic disciplines. Professional nursing practice includes, but is not limited to:

(1) assessment, diagnosis, planning, intervention, and evaluation of human responses to health or illness;

(2) the provision of direct nursing care to individuals to restore optimum function or to achieve a dignified death;

(3) the procurement, coordination, and management of essential client resources;

(4) the provision of health counseling and education;

(5) the establishment of standards of practice for nursing care in all settings, including the development of nursing policies, procedures, and protocols for a specific setting;

(6) the direction of nursing practice, including delegation to those practicing technical nursing;

(7) the supervision of those who assist in the practice of nursing;

(8) collaboration with other independently licensed health care professionals in case finding and the clinical management and execution of intervention as identified to be appropriate in a plan of care; and

(9) the administration of medication and treatments as prescribed by those professionals qualified to prescribe under the provision of (*cite state statute[s]*);

"Technical nursing practice" includes the skilled application of nursing principles in the delivery of direct care to individuals and families within organized nursing services. Technical nursing practice requires

NCSBN

The "Practice of Nursing" means assisting individuals or groups to maintain or attain optimal health, implementing a strategy of care to accomplish defined goals, and evaluating responses to care and treatment. This practice includes, but is not limited to, initiating and maintaining comfort measures, promoting and supporting human functions and responses, establishing an environment conducive to well-being, providing health counseling and teaching, and collaborating on certain aspects of the health regimen. This practice is based on understanding the human condition across the lifespan and understanding the relationship of the individual within the environment.

"Registered Nursing" means the practice of the full scope of nursing which includes but is not limited to:

(a) Assessing the health status of individuals and groups;

(b) Establishing a nursing diagnosis;

(c) Establishing goals to meet identified health care needs;

(d) Planning a strategy of care;

(e) Prescribing nursing intervention to implement the strategy of care;

(f) Implementing the strategy of care;

(g) Delegating nursing interventions that may be performed by others and that do not conflict with this act;

(h) Maintaining safe and effective nursing care rendered directly or indirectly;

(i) Evaluating responses to interventions;

(j) Teaching the theory and practice of nursing;

(k) Managing and supervising the practice of nursing;

(l) Collaborating with other health professionals in the management of health care; and

(m) Practicing advanced clinical nursing in accordance with knowledge skills acquired through graduate nursing education.

Licensed Practical Nursing means practice of a directed scope of nursing practice which includes, but is not limited to:

(a) Contributing to the assessment of the health status of individuals and groups;

the study of nursing within the context of the applied sciences. Technical nursing practice includes, but is not limited to:

(1) participation in the development, evaluation, and modification of a plan of care;

(2) the provision of direct care to individuals to restore optimum function or to achieve a dignified death;

(3) patient teaching;

(4) the supervision of those who assist in the practice of nursing;

(5) the administration of medications and treatments as prescribed by those professionals qualified to prescribe under the provisions of (*cite state statute[s]*).

(b) Participating in the development and modification of the strategy of care;

(c) Implementing the appropriate aspects of the strategy of care as defined by the Board;

(d) Maintaining safe and effective nursing care rendered directly or indirectly;

(e) Participating in the evaluation of responses to interventions, and;

(f) Delegating nursing interventions that may be performed by others and that do not conflict with this Act.

The Licensed Practical Nurse functions at the direction of the Registered Nurse, licensed physician, or licensed dentist in the performance of activities delegated by that health care professional.

Source: American Nurses Association. *Suggested State Legislation: Nursing Practice Act, Nursing Disciplinary Division Act, Prescriptive Authority Act.* Kansas City, MO: The Association, 1990. Reprinted with permission.

Source: National Council of State Boards of Nursing: *Model Nursing Practice Act.* Chicago: The Council, 1988. Reprinted with permission.

nursing practice in the legal definition of the licensure law. The first could be called the use of nonamended statutes. These states either have made no changes from the 1955 ANA model and allow for a liberal interpretation of the definition by the state board or have made minor changes. In some, the word *medical* has been inserted to describe prohibited acts. Thus, certain acts of diagnosis and treatment would presumably be identified as nursing. Other states have retained portions of the traditional definition but omitted or substituted certain other phrases. Although all these states maintain that their acts allow expanded practice, interpretation is the key, so a change in attitude or political-medical pressures could bring a rapid about-face.

The second trend, and by far the largest, is the use of administrative statutes. These permit nurses to perform expanded duties, as authorized by the professional licensing boards: nursing alone, nursing and medicine, or medicine alone. Regulations are an integral part of that mechanism. The first to use such statutes was Idaho (1971); New Hampshire enacted a slightly different version shortly thereafter.

Various reasons (with positive and negative connotations) are given for this approach: regulations can spell out specific criteria and protect the public from incompetents and promote the use of NPs by increasing competence and awareness; nursing can limit the role to nurses and exclude others; physicians can extend some control over nurse expansion; nurses and physicians can respond rapidly to changing needs and patterns of practice, because regulations do not go through the legislative process; state professional boards, familiar with both fields as well as the idiosyncrasies of regulation formulation, can act rapidly and effectively. All have some legitimacy. Some states found that at first, cooperation between the two boards went well, regulations were formulated rapidly, and nurse practitioners were able to practice freely at a time when they were badly needed. Then, physicians decided to pull back, and legal obstacles were put in the way of such practice particularly when the law required *joint* agreement. In some states, regulations could not be agreed upon, even by nurses alone, or there was considerable internal group pressure, and legal practice stayed in limbo. Others had no major problems. Two ANA concerns have been, first, that recognition of specialized practice is the function of the professional organization (through certification) and not the law, and second, that the additional acts clauses frequently require at least some medical approval for NP practice. This not only means that another profession can determine the scope of nursing's practice, but it does little to advance the concept of nurses and physicians as equal, collaborating professionals. Another problem is that the specificity of the language regarding the practices that can be performed is restrictive and potentially harmful to the expansion or evaluation of these practice areas.

Whether or not the additional acts clause is part of the law, the majority of state boards have now been granted the right to develop administrative rules and regulations for the NP, and most have developed such rules. One method of authorizing advanced practice is certification by an organization approved by the state board. (In a sense, this makes voluntary certification a mandatory legal process.) Second is separate licensure, using a term such as *advanced nurse practitioner*. With the exception of nurse-midwives and nurse anesthetists, this identification and the specific requirements are part of the general nursing practice act.

The last category of nursing definitions is termed *authorization*, chosen by the fewest number of states. These states have developed a new definition of nursing that is intended to cover expanded or advanced practice as well as what might be considered ordinary practice at this time. The first of these states was New York (1972), which pioneered the use of the phrase "diagnosing and treating human responses to actual or potential health problems." A number of other states copied this terminology almost verbatim.

While the New York law was thought to be quite daring at the time, it is now considered rather conservative, because it has no provision for independent acts of treatment. As happens in many cases, this limitation is due in part to the compromises necessary to get the law passed. Although some say that everything NPs do is nursing because they are nurses, this argument is not always accepted legally. If a practice is challenged, its legitimacy may depend on the ruling of a state attorney general or a court. For some states, challenge is not a major issue, and their nurses have done well with the authorization approach.

However, nurses in other states that adopted the New York model (including New York) have had serious problems in achieving acceptance of the overall definitions as adequate to authorize NP practice, because it included no educational training requirements or delineation of practice. Organized medicine in those states has generally insisted that medical diagnosing and treating are off limits. This has caused a schism between NPs, who are willing to accept a more limiting law in order to be able to practice without constant fear of being deemed to be illegally practicing medicine, and the SNA, which usually holds that the general definition protects them. Sometimes everyone settles for regulations anyhow or a requirement for national certification.

A breakthrough may have occurred when the Missouri Supreme Court ruled in 1983 that that particular general definition did indeed allow advanced nurse practice.[31] This landmark case, *Sermchief v. Gonzales*, was the outcome of a threat by the Missouri Board of Registration for the Healing Arts, which licenses physicians and osteopaths, to initiate proceedings against nurses in a family planning clinic. (Physicians in the area had lodged a complaint.) The nurses, working under standing orders and protocols signed by the clinic physicians, performed a variety of diagnostic and treatment functions, including breast and pelvic examinations; pregnancy testing; Pap smears; gonorrhea cultures and blood serology; the administration of all kinds of contraceptive measures, including oral contraceptives and intrauterine devices; as well as the usual teaching and counseling. The trial court judgment was that the nurses were practicing medicine without a license, but the Missouri Supreme Court judge ruled that the acts of the nurses were "precisely the types of acts the legislature had contemplated when it granted nurses the right to make assessments and nursing diagnoses." The 1975 Missouri law is similar to the ANA guidelines of the time but uses the phrase "including, but not limited to." The nursing board had not promulgated any rules and regulations regarding advanced practice, so the case stood on the interpretation of the definition alone. Although the judgment is limited to Missouri, it is considered a victory for NP practice, with the focus on how clearly a general definition can legally determine whether a nurse is practicing nursing in performing what was once considered the exclusive function of medicine. On the other hand, there is a question as to whether the case was a good example, since Missouri had been open to nurse practitioner practice for some time, which is not true of other states.

It is clear that advanced nurse practice is still in legal flux. Short of a state supreme court ruling, the legality of certain practices can change in that very state with attorney general appointments, the attitude of a judge, or simply the political climate. Health care facility lawyers can only advise on how they interpret the practice act (and they may be influenced by physicians' attitudes or advice). A strong statement for or against advanced practice made by a voluntary professional association (medicine or nursing, for instance) is quite common but has no legal authority; it *can* help mold public opinion.

The doctrines of common practice or custom and usage may also be invoked. This means basically that the act is performed in that particular community or at that current time and is accepted as being within the responsibility of the nurse by the individuals' employer and/or physicians in the area. It usually assumes appropriate training for that function. Although this has been considered acceptable in some courts, it has been denied in others. Practically speaking, statutes cannot be changed informally by mass violation, although they may be changed through the legislative process eventually, be-cause of evidence that a nurse has been taught to perform such a function and is capable of carrying it out safely.

By 1992, the varied, inconsistent approaches to regulating advanced practice nursing resulted in NCSBN issuing a draft position paper on the regulation of advanced nursing practice in order to provide guidance to member boards. The draft statement proposed a second license for the advanced practice nurse, and it generated considerable activity within the nursing community. The primary rationale for recommending a second license was the inconsistency in requirements for certification, level of education and practice, and titling. There was also recognition of the increasing overlap between medical practice and advanced practice nurses, and the need for increasing autonomy in practice.

ANA convened an Ad Hoc Committee on Credentialing in Advanced Practice to address the overall issue of regulation of advanced practice. NCSBN was invited and participated on this committee, as did representatives of the American Association of Nurse Anesthetists, the American College of Nurse-Midwives, and representatives of the advanced practice specialties. The Ad Hoc Committee initially developed a definition of the "advanced practice registered nurse" (APRN) that was subsequently modified and adopted by the ANA Congress on Nursing Practice. The definition is:

> **Advanced practice registered nurses are professional nurses who have successfully completed a graduate program in nursing or a related area that provides specialized knowledge and skills.**[32]

During 1992, the Ad Hoc Committee held hearings on the issue of second license, and the 1993 ANA House of Delegates passed a report requesting the ANA Board of Directors to provide for a state-by-state analysis outlining the steps to be taken to standardize the regulation of advanced nursing practice.[33] During the ensuing year, ANA and NCSBN developed a cordial working relationship. However, in August 1993, NCSBN's Delegate Assembly did adopt the position paper on the "Regulation of Advanced Nursing Practice" calling for the regulation of advanced practice nurses by licensure,[34] although prior to that meeting, ANA transmitted a letter to the NCSBN Board of Directors opposing the establishment of a second license and requested instead a focus on health care reform and its implications for regulation of all nurses.

It is important to note that ANA recognizes that nurses in advanced practice should be regulated. However, ANA promotes a rule-making approach rather than a statutory one. It advocates regulation of advanced practice through authorization of the Board of Nursing as the sole authority to regulate nurses in advanced practice and the promulgation of the definition of advanced practice and other requirements in the rules.[35] The 1994 ANA House of Delegates adopted another report on the regulation of nurses in advanced practice that called for continued strategies to standardize the authorization of advanced nursing practice based on the most professionally empowering approach.[36]

It is not always easy for nurses of any kind to determine immediately which or how many of these alternatives are operative in the state where they practice. Except for those practices that may be limited to a particular hospital or agency, the State Board of Nursing can usually provide information as to whether a certain activity is permitted or specifically prohibited. When this information is not available, it is essential to remember that whatever nurses do, they must be competent in their performance, which implies education, training, and current competence.

Creation of a Board of Nursing

The name of the state administrative agency varies from state to state, as does the number of members. Traditionally, this board has been made up entirely of nurses, who may or may not be designated as to area of practice and education. In most states, members are appointed by the governor from a list of names submitted by the SNA and others. Because of some public outcry against control by professionals, gradually the addition of nonnurses, either public members or other health professionals, has been legally required. Although some nurses have considered this a danger to the profession, it can be to the advantage of nursing to have the input and support of the public and others on the health team, for these public members can be educated to understand and appreciate the problems of the profession. The danger exists when political pressure seeks to force the creation of a board with a majority of nonnurses, so that nursing practice and education can be totally controlled by others. Most states had consumers or other professionals as members by 1977. The ANA supports consumer participation as does the NCSBN; the latter also includes LPNs. There is also increasing interest in having nursing specialties and advanced practice nurses on boards. Board size ranges from five to nineteen appointed members, who make policy. Staff employed by the board carry out the day-to-day activities.

Responsibilities of the Board of Nursing

The major responsibility of a board is to see that the nursing practice act is carried out. This involves establishing rules and regulations to implement the broad terms in the law itself and setting minimum standards of practice. Usual responsibilities include approval of programs of nursing and development of criteria for approval (minimum standards) such as facilities, curriculum, faculty, and so on; evaluating the personal and educational qualifications of applicants for licensure; determining by examination applicants' competence to practice nursing; issuing licenses to qualified applicants; and disciplining those who violate the law or are found to be unfit to practice nursing, sometimes holding hearings. (Investigations and hearings are sometimes done by another arm of the state government.)

Other responsibilities include developing standards for continuing competency of licensed practitioners and issuing a limited license (for someone who cannot practice the full scope of nursing, perhaps owing to a handicap). Boards have also developed prescriptive authority regulations.

Nursing boards may hold educational programs, collect certain data, and cooperate in various ways with other nursing boards or the boards of other disciplines. If they operate under an overall board, certain administrative responsibilities will be carried out on a central level.

The power of the board should not be underestimated. For instance, it was simply by changing their regulations that the North Dakota Board changed requirements for RN and LPN licensure.

Requirements for Licensure as a Nurse

Licensure is based on fulfilling certain requirements. The following points are usually included.

1. The applicant must have completed an educational program in a state-approved school of nursing and received a diploma or degree from that program; usually the school must send the student's transcript. There is some legislative pressure that the applicant not be required to have completed the program, particularly if the uncompleted courses are in a nonnursing area such as liberal arts. This is not looked on favorably by either ANA or NCSBN.
2. The applicant must pass an examination given by the board. This examination is currently the NCLEX-RN, developed under the aegis of the NCSBN and given in every state. The examination is now offered using a computerized adaptive testing approach known as CAT.
3. Some states require evidence of good physical and mental health, but this is not recommended by either ANA or NCSBN. Actual practice varies a great deal from state to state. Handicapped students have been admitted, graduated, and taken state boards in some states; in others, this is denied. Court cases often result.[37]

4. Most states maintain a statement that the applicant must be of good moral character, as determined by the licensing board, but this too is impractical. The model act suggests terminology that refers to acts that are grounds for board disciplinary action if the nurse is licensed.
5. A fee must be paid for admission to the examination. This varies considerably among states.
6. A temporary license may be issued to a graduate of an approved program pending the results of the first licensure exam.
7. Demonstrating competence in English is a relatively new recommendation.

It has been declared unconstitutional to make requirements of age, citizenship, and residence.

Provisions for Endorsement of Persons Licensed in Other States

Nurses have more mobility than any other licensed health professionals because of the use of a national standardized examination, with the exception of nurses in advanced practice. However, usually the individual must still fulfill the other requirements in the state in which he or she seeks licensure and must submit proof that the license has not been revoked. The nurse's nursing school record is usually evaluated to determine whether the program is generally equivalent to this state's program requirements of the same time period. If it is not, the nurse may be required to take the courses lacking and the examination.

If all requirements are satisfactorily fulfilled, the nurse is granted a license without retaking the state board examination. A fee is also required for this process of endorsement. Endorsement is not the same as reciprocity; the latter means acceptance of a licensee by one state only if the other state does likewise.

Renewal of Licensure

Until the early 1970s, nursing licenses were renewed simply by sending in the renewal fee when notified, usually every two years. For nurses licensed in more than one state, as long as the license was not revoked in any state, the process was the same. Theoretically the individual might be denied relicensure for certain physical or mental handicaps or drug abuse, but there was no organized way to check on this. Usually the form asked for information about employment and the highest degree (and still does), but no attempt was made to determine if the nurse was competent. At about that time (also the time of the credentialing reports), there was increased concern about the current competency of practicing health professionals, and an estimate was made that perhaps 5 percent of all health professionals were not competent for some reason. Moreover, there was some question as to whether the professions made any real effort either to rehabilitate these people or to revoke their licenses. The credentialing reports emphasized the need for CE as a requirement for relicensure. One outcome was the enactment of a mandatory CE clause in a number of licensure laws; that is, a practitioner's license would not be renewed unless she or he showed evidence of CE. A number of health disciplines have such legislation. By 1977, a number of states had made mandatory CE a requirement for relicensure (or a legal practice requirement) for about 20 health occupations. (This information is much more difficult to find now that the federal government doesn't keep complete records.) Not all such requirements are well enforced. Some states do have permissive legislation for possible later implementation. In addition, some national associations and state medical societies require continuing education for renewal of certification.

Actually, any state could use regulations to require CE without changing the law because all practice acts give the licensing boards the authority to determine standards of competence, and these are usually delineated in the regulations. Nevertheless, in the 1970s, a number of SNAs introduced legislation either requiring CE or specifically directing the state board to study or plan such a requirement. Re-

alistically, this action may have been attributable as much to the fear of externally introduced legislation that might remove control of the measure from nursing as to the conviction that this was a necessary amendment. Some of these states recognize only CE offerings approved by their boards or given by an agency, group, or institution that has been given a provider (or approval) number. This may create problems for those licensed in more than one state or living in a state other than where licensed. In the latter situation, some states permit the nurse to maintain the license on an inactive status, which can be reactivated when evidence of continuing education is shown.

Forms of CE accepted by states include various formal academic studies in institutions of higher learning converted to CEU credit; college extension courses and studies; grand rounds in the health care setting; home study programs; inservice education; institutes; lectures; seminars; workshops; audiovisual learning systems, including educational television, audiovisual cassettes, tapes, and records with self-study packets; challenge examinations for a course or program; self-learning systems such as community service, controlled independent study, delivery of a paper, preparation and participation in a panel; preparation and publication of articles, monographs, books, and so on; and special research. The required number of hours of continuing education, or CEUs, varies considerably among states.

No law requires formal education directed toward advanced degrees. In fact, although additional formal education is acceptable, the emphasis is on continuous, *updated competence in practice.* The fears and anger of many nurses have been misdirected because they assumed that advanced degrees would be required. Obviously, there are innumerable ways in which an individual can maintain competence and increase knowledge and skills. How to measure achievement for the large number of nurses concerned is the real problem.

Objections to mandatory CE focus on the difficulty of assessing true learning; the question of whether learning can be forced (attendance does not mean retention or change in behavior); the danger of breeding mediocrity; the lack of research on the effectiveness of CE in relation to performance; limitation of resources, particularly in rural areas; the cost to nurses; the cost to government; the usual rigidity of governmental regulations; the problems in record keeping; and the lack of accreditation or evaluation procedures for many CE programs.

The entire issue is far from resolved. The trend toward mandatory CE slowed considerably in the early 1980s for all occupations, although the call for continued competence did not. It is possible that another trend, peer evaluation, and other kinds of performance evaluation may provide a more effective answer to continued competence.

Exemptions from Licensure

This may also be called an *exception clause.* Generally exempted from RN licensure are basic students in a nursing program; anyone furnishing nursing assistance in an emergency; anyone licensed in another state and caring for a patient temporarily in the state involved; anyone employed by the U.S. government as a nurse (Veterans Administration, public health, or armed services); any legally qualified nurse recruited by the Red Cross during a disaster; anyone caring for the sick if care is performed in connection with the practice of religious tenets of any church; and anyone giving incidental care in a family (home) situation; and any RN or LPN from another state engaged in consultation as long as no direct care is given.

In all these cases, the person cannot claim to be an RN of the state concerned. Over strong nursing protests, some states have also incorporated in the exemptions nursing services of attendants in state institutions, if supervised by nurses or doctors, as well as other kinds of nursing assistants under various circumstances. This, of course, weakens the mandatory aspect of the law.

An interesting development is that the NCSBN model act suggests for this clause statements that permit the establishment of an independent practice and fee-for-service reimbursement.

Grounds for Revocation of Licensure

The board has the right to revoke or suspend any nurse's license or otherwise discipline the licensee. The reasons most commonly found in practice acts for revoking a license are acts that might directly endanger the public, such as practicing while one's ability is impaired by alcohol, drugs, or physical or mental disability; being addicted to or dependent on alcohol or other habit-forming drugs or a habitual user of certain drugs; and practicing with incompetence or negligence or beyond the scope of practice. Other reasons are obtaining a license fraudulently, being convicted of a felony or crime involving moral turpitude (or accepting a plea of *nolo contendere*); practicing while the license is suspended or revoked; aiding and abetting a nonlicensed person to perform activities requiring a license; and committing unprofessional conduct or immoral acts as defined by the board. The refusal to provide service to a person because of race, color, creed, or national origin may also have been added in some states.

The most common reasons that nurses lose their licenses are the same as those that apply to physicians—drug use, abuse, or theft.

Nurses' drug use and abuse may be on the increase, since this is also a trend in society, but certainly it has gotten considerably more attention in recent years, with many articles in nursing and lay publications and other media. At one time, given sufficient evidence, boards suspended or revoked nurses' licenses readily for drug abuse. Nurses impaired by drug abuse are likely to be the target of disciplinary action. Criteria for reinstatement are based on a written statement from a physician that the nurse is cured and can function in the workplace or is under treatment and can function in the workplace or that board evaluation shows that the nurse is able to function.[38] A number of boards have had the legal freedom to take no action but to provide information or recommend rehabilitative programs for the nurse to get treatment. Almost none did so.[39] Eventually state nurses associations recognized this as a professional responsibility and made such arrangements, along with counseling and support (see Chap. 10). Alcohol abuse or intemperance interfering with safe practice may also be part of what is considered substance abuse. It is probably for this reason that the ANA suggested a separate law (Nursing Disciplinary Diversion Act) that mandated that the board of nursing seek ways to rehabilitate impaired nurses and to "establish a voluntary alternative to traditional disciplinary actions."[40] Only nurses who request such diversion and supervision by a committee are permitted to participate in the program. The NCSBN does not include such a provision.

As is true in obtaining or renewing licenses, a nurse could also lose his or her license because of physical or mental impairment. Legal blindness is the most common physical condition involved, but there are many exceptions, especially since the Rehabilitation Act described in Chap. 19.

With the exception of substance abuse, it is rare that specific conditions for revocation or suspension of license are detailed in legislation or even regulations. Rather, disciplinary action may be authorized by the ubiquitous "unprofessional behavior" clause. This issue gained attention with the landmark 1977 Tuma case in Idaho. Jolene Tuma, an instructor in an associate degree program, went with a student to the bedside of a terminally ill woman to start chemotherapy after obtaining the patient's informed consent. When the patient asked Ms. Tuma about alternate treatments for cancer, she was told about several. Her son, upset because his mother stopped the chemotherapy, told the physician, who brought charges against Ms. Tuma. Subsequently, she was not only fired, but her license was suspended for 6 months by the Idaho board of nursing for unprofessional conduct, because her actions "disrupted the physi-

cian-patient relationship."[41] The case aroused a national nursing furor.[42] Ms. Tuma took her case through the courts, and on April 17, 1979, the Idaho Supreme Court handed down a decision that Ms. Tuma could not be found guilty of unprofessional conduct because the Idaho Nurse Practice Act neither defined unprofessional conduct nor set guidelines for providing warnings. The judge also questioned the ability of the hearing officer, who lacked the "personal knowledge and experience" of nursing to determine if Ms. Tuma's behavior was unprofessional.[43] Unfortunately, the court did not address itself to Ms. Tuma's actions, which leaves the nurse's right to inform the patient in some question—at least in Idaho.

While a number of states already had regulations defining unprofessional conduct, this court ruling spurred on those that did not. Depending on how licensure laws are structured, the regulations may apply to all licensed health professions (New York) or may be written into each separate law.

The courts have also played a major role in shaping interpretation. They have been opposed to trivializing the term and have held to the criteria of conduct that intellectually or morally creates jeopardy through practice. An example exists where the District Court in Nebraska reversed the Board of Nursing's denial of license finding that the plaintiff may be difficult to get along with and resistive to directions, but not unprofessional.[44] Criteria used by the state of Utah are especially clear and provide a good example:[45]

- Failing to utilize appropriate judgment in administering safe nursing practice based upon the level of nursing for which the individual is licensed.
- Failing to exercise technical competence in carrying out nursing care.
- Failing to follow policies or procedures defined in the practice situation to safeguard patient care.
- Failing to safeguard the patient's dignity and right to privacy.

- Violating the confidentiality of information or knowledge concerning the patient.
- Verbally or physically abusing patients.
- Performing any nursing techniques or procedures without proper education and preparation.
- Performing procedures beyond the authorized scope of the level of nursing and/or health care for which the individual is licensed.
- Intentional manipulation or misuse of drug supplies, narcotics, or patients' records.
- Falsifying patients' records or intentionally charting incorrectly.
- Appropriating medications, supplies or personal items of the patient or agency.
- Violating state or federal laws relative to drugs.
- Falsifying records submitted to a government agency.
- Intentionally committing any act that adversely affects the physical or psychosocial welfare of the patient.
- Delegating nursing care, functions, tasks and/or responsibilities to others contrary to the laws governing nursing and/or to the detriment of patient safety.
- Failing to exercise appropriate supervision over persons who are authorized to practice only under the supervision of the licensed professional.
- Leaving a nursing assignment without properly notifying appropriate personnel.
- Failing to report, through the proper channels, facts known to the individual regarding the incompetent, unethical, or illegal practice of any licensed health care professional.

The absence of very specific language in statutes and/or regulations is purposeful to avoid foreclosure on unanticipated types of behavior. This problem is sometimes resolved by using the phrase "not limited to," but if the legislature has a particular concern, this may be written into the law. Some states have also adopted the ANA standards of practice as criteria for incompetence.

A particular problem in both statutory and regulating language relates to such terms as *moral, ethical,* and *moral turpitude,* since these can be interpreted in various ways. The model act uses phrases such as "has engaged in any act inconsistent with standards of nursing practice as defined by Board Rules and Regulations" and "a crime in any jurisdiction that relates adversely to the practice of nursing or to the ability to practice nursing."

Another issue is what a nurse should do about reporting incompetence or unprofessional conduct on the part of physicians or other health professionals. Because the nurses' code of ethics requires that she or he safeguard the patient, incompetent or unprofessional practitioners should be reported. Most surveys indicate that a large percentage of nurses would take some sort of action, usually speaking with the doctor, head nurse, or supervisor, if the patient was endangered by medical action. Few would report the physician to a peer review or licensing board. In part, this is because they fear a lawsuit. All but a few states have laws giving immunity from civil action to any person who reports to a peer review board if there is no malice,[46] but this does not preclude being sued, even though legally the accused must be cleared. (Malice is very difficult to prove.) In New York, a statute was enacted in 1977 requiring physicians to report other physicians' misconduct on penalty of being cited for unprofessional conduct themselves; nurses and others are also encouraged to report such misconduct. (Some have interpreted the law as *requiring* such reporting by all licensed professionals.) Other states have similar statutes[47] including states requiring nurses to report nurses.[48] There is another problem: some nurses who have reported a physician have either been dismissed from their jobs or harassed, a problem difficult to combat. A supportive working environment can make a difference.[49]

Although the law seems to protect the public, data show that relatively few nurses have had licenses revoked or suspended. In part, the reason is believed to be the reluctance of other nurses to report and consequently testify to these acts by their colleagues before either the nursing board or a court of law.[50] Nursing associations and state boards are now emphasizing the responsibility of professional nurses to report incompetent practice. The model act makes nonreporting a disciplinary offense.

When a report is filed with the state board, charging a nurse with violation of any of the grounds of disciplinary action, he or she is entitled to certain procedural safeguards (due process). After investigation, the nurse must receive notice of the charges and be given time to prepare a defense. A hearing is set and subpoenas are issued (by the board, attorney general, or a hearing officer). The accused has the right to appear personally or be represented by counsel, who may cross-examine witnesses. If the license is revoked or suspended, it may be reissued at the discretion of the board. (Sometimes the individual is only censured or reprimanded.)

The effect of the National Practitioners Data Bank (NPDB) is not clear. Nursing boards are not yet required to report adverse licensure actions. However, all malpractice payments must be reported to the NPDB by insurance companies and others, and state boards get copies. The boards expect queries because all health care facilities are required to check with the NPDB concerning any health practitioner who has applied for clinical privileges, including nurses. Are clinical privileges synonymous with employment as a staff nurse, and so would all applicants for nursing positions have to be cleared through the NPDB?

Penalties for Practicing Without a License

Penalties for practicing without a license are included only in the mandatory laws. Penalties vary from a minimum fine to a large fine and/or imprisonment. Usually legal action is taken. Penalties are being strengthened to deter illegal practice.

Other Components

It has become increasingly popular to add a "good Samaritan" clause to medical and nursing laws, although it is not always a part of the licensure law. This clause protects the professional from liability for damages for alleged injuries or death after rendering first aid or emergency treatment in an emergency situation away from proper medical equipment unless there is proven gross negligence. Although such laws exist in all fifty states, there is some feeling that they are really counterproductive.

Another occasional addition has been the requirement that equivalency and proficiency exams be used to determine the qualifications of those wishing to enter RN schools.

Separate licensing laws for PNs have a similar format. It is a good idea for a nurse who is expected to supervise PNs to also become familiar with laws concerning them.

HOW TO OBTAIN A LICENSE

Almost all new graduates of a nursing program apply for RN licensure, because it is otherwise impossible to practice. Although there is nothing to prohibit you from postponing licensure, it is generally more difficult psychologically and because of lack of clinical practice to take the state board examination (NCLEX) much later.

As a rule, your school makes available all the data and even the application forms necessary for beginning the licensure procedure. Should you wish to become licensed in another state, because of planned relocation, request an application from that nursing board. Correct titles and addresses of the nursing boards of all states are found in the directory issue of the *American Journal of Nursing*. The board advises you of the proper procedure, the cost, and the data needed. For this initial licensing, you must take the state board examination in the state where licensure is sought.

As of April 1994 NCLEX has changed its administration of the licensing examination from a paper-and-pencil, twice-a-year method to year-round using computerized adaptive testing (CAT). This change in testing methodology has resulted in a slightly altered candidate registration process. Applications for the examination are made to the board of nursing in the jurisdiction you want to be licensed. You will also need to register to take the NCLEX either with Educational Testing Service (ETS) or with the board of nursing, depending on the individual state procedures. Once the licensure application has been reviewed and eligibility approved by the board of nursing, you will receive an Authorization to Test (ATT) from the ETS Data Center. A bulletin, *Scheduling and Taking Your NCLEX*, will also be forwarded that describes the examination, procedures for making an appointment, a list of available test center locations and telephone numbers, and a toll-free number to call for information on any newly opened centers. The NCLEX is administered at more than 200 Sylvan Technology Centers, with at least one located in each state and territory. The individual candidate schedules his or her own date and time for the examination. For more information on specific candidate application procedures and requirements, contact your board of nursing.[51]

The RN Field Tests and the Beta Test found that candidates perform comparably on CAT and paper-and-pencil nursing examinations, and that demographic groups were neither advantaged nor disadvantaged.[52] The CAT has been determined to be psychometrically sound. The NCSBN has produced a video, *NCLEX using CAT: A Candidate's Viewpoint*, that walks the candidate through the test experience. It is designed to answer basic questions commonly asked by candidates, and shows the test site. The video is available for $50 from the National Council, Dept. 77-3953, Chicago, IL 60678-3953.

The CAT provides for each candidate to have a unique examination because it is assembled interactively as the individual is tested. A competence estimate based on all earlier answers is calculated by the computer as the candidate answers each question. A large question bank stores all the examination questions and classifies them by test plan area and level of difficulty. The questions are then searched and the one determined to measure the candidate most precisely in the appropriate test plan area is shown on the computer screen. This process is then repeated for each question, thus forming an examination unique to the candidate's knowledge and skills.

Since that time, a number of changes have occurred including the use of a simple pass-fail score, and others are to come. However, both NCLEX (RN) and NCLEX (LPN) will continue to be based on periodic job analyses. A new RN Job Analysis has been completed, and the National Council's Examination Committee has reviewed the results. The committee's recommendations concerning the RN Test Plan were taken to the August 1994 NCSBN Delegate Assembly and approved.

The tests are the same for all nurses seeking an RN, whether graduating from a diploma, associate degree, or baccalaureate program. This has been the subject of considerable criticism, because the state goals of all three programs are different. However, proponents of a single licensing exam state that the purpose is to determine safe and effective practice at a minimal level, and that this criterion applies to all levels of nurses.

Nurses who pass the licensing examination receive a certificate bearing a registration number that remains the same as long as they are registered in that state. The certificate (or registration card) will also carry the expiration date—usually one, two, or three years hence. Failure to renew promptly may mean that you must pay a special fee to be reinstated.

It is advisable to keep your registration in effect, whether actively engaged in nursing or not. The expense is nominal, and more and more nurses who "retire" temporarily to have families return to nursing. These nurses do have the responsibility (and sometimes the legal requirement) to keep their nursing knowledge updated through CE.

To become licensed or registered by endorsement, applicants must already be registered in one state, territory, or foreign country. They must apply to the state board of nursing in the new state and present credentials, as requested, to prove that they have completed preparation equal to that required. A temporary permit is usually issued to allow the nurse to work until the new license is issued.

Nurses who wish to be reregistered after allowing their licenses to lapse should contact their state board for directions. An RN wishing to practice nursing in another country also needs to investigate its legal requirements for practice. Members of the armed forces or the Peace Corps, or those under the auspices of an organization such as the World Health Organization or a religious denomination will be advised by the sponsoring group. Registration in one state is usually sufficient.

Nurses educated in other countries are expected to meet the same qualifications for licensure as graduates of schools of nursing in the United States. The procedure for obtaining a license is the same as for graduates of schools here. However, generally nurses from other countries are now expected to take the CGFNS Qualifying Examination, which screens and examines foreign nursing school graduates while they are still in their own countries to determine their eligibility for professional practice in the United States (see next section for further details). The 1 day examination covers proficiency in both nursing practice and English comprehension; both exams are given in English. If the applicant passes, she or he is given a CGFNS certificate, which is presented to the U.S. embassy or consulate when applying for a visa and to the state board in the state where the nurse wishes to practice. The nurse still must take the state board examination and otherwise fulfill the licensing requirements for that state. (Because of the nursing shortage, some states were considering dropping the CGFNS requirement preceding NCLEX, although it would still be necessary in order to receive a temporary permit to practice. However, California's experience with this pointed out the problem—the vast majority who had not taken or passed CGFNS failed NCLEX, even after several repetitions.) Specific information about requirements for licensure must be obtained directly from the board of nursing in the state in which the foreign nurse wishes to be licensed.

On November 17, 1993, Congress approved the North American Free Trade Agreement (NAFTA). This trade pact, between the United States, Canada, and Mexico, removes most trade barriers among the three nations. This creates the world's largest free-trade zone. ANA, working with the Office of the U.S. Trade Representative and a coalition of licensed professionals, worked hard to ensure state primacy and autonomy in matters related to licensing and credentialing under NAFTA by obtaining language in the Statement of Administrative Actions clarifying that NAFTA does not permit Mexican or Canadian professionals to practice a licensed profession in the United States without meeting all applicable state licensing criteria.[53]

The Commission on Graduates of Foreign Nursing Schools (CGFNS)

In the late 1960s the United States experienced an increase in nurses migrating to the United States to practice nursing. Immigration officials were having difficulty identifying which of the nurses educated abroad, and applying for nursing occupational visas, would actually be eligible for licensure as registered nurses in the United States. At that time, only about 15 to 20 percent of the nurses educated out of the United States were passing the U.S. registered nurse licensing exam. This led the Division of Nursing at the then-Department of Health, Education and Welfare (HEW) to contract for two studies regarding RN licensure of foreign-educated nurses in the United States. The findings of these landmark studies on foreign nurse immigration were presented at a 1975 HEW conference attended by representatives from governmental and private organizations, including the U.S. Department of Labor, the Immigration and Naturalization Service, the ANA, and the NLN, among others.

The outgrowth of the conference was that in 1977, ANA and NLN agreed to cosponsor the establishment of an independent nonprofit organization for the purpose of developing an equitable system through which nurses educated outside the United States could gauge their chances of becoming licensed as registered nurses in the United States. Such an organization would have as its mission to establish an orderly process for assessing the individual knowledge and level of preparation of each nurse applicant. These efforts would also help serve to protect the public health, by assuring that nurses educated outside the United States meet standards that are comparable those of registered nurses educated in the United States. The organization created and chartered with this mission was the Commission on Graduates of Foreign Nursing Schools, or CGFNS.

Today, the commission provides a variety of services, including the CGFNS Certification Program and the Credentials Evaluation Service (CES), for nurses educated outside the United States who wish to practice nursing in the United States. To support these services, CGFNS conducts studies and surveys, and is an active participant in policy discussions concerning international nursing education, licensure, and practice.

The CGFNS Certification Program is a two-part screening and testing program for first-level general nurses educated outside the United States who wish to practice as registered nurses in the United States. It includes a credentials review, followed by a qualifying exam of nursing knowledge and English language proficiency. By meeting the credentials criteria and passing the two-part examination, nurses educated outside the United States earn a CGFNS certificate that can help them in four ways. First, nurses wishing to obtain a nonimmigration (temporary) occupational preference visa (H1-A) from the U.S. Immigration and Naturalization Service must have a CGFNS certificate or hold a full and un-

restricted license to practice as a registered nurse in the state where they plan to work, and have an offer of employment from a U.S. health care organization. Second, nurses educated abroad who wish to live in the United States permanently under an Immigrant (permanent) Occupational Preference Visa need a labor certificate from the U.S. Department of Labor, which will be issued only if a nurse holds a CGFNS certificate or a full, unrestricted license to practice as a registered nurse in the state where they will be employed. Third, approximately 80 percent of U.S. state boards of nursing require nurses who were educated outside the United States to hold a CGFNS certificate before they can take the U.S. registered nurse licensing exam, called the NCLEX-RN. Finally, nurses who pass the qualifying examination portion of the CGFNS Certification Program can be reasonably assured of success on the NCLEX-RN. This is because the CGFNS qualifying exam is modeled after the NCLEX-RN. Since the Certification Program was begun, first-time RN licensure pass scores of foreign-educated nurses holding a CGFNS certificate have shown a marked improvement, up from 15 to 20 percent prior to the program in the 1970s to 70 to 75 percent today.

To be eligible to take the CGFNS qualifying exam, a nurse must be educated and licensed (or registered) as a "first-level general nurse" as defined historically by the International Council of Nurses. A first-level general nurse is called a "registered" or "professional" nurse in most countries. CGFNS evaluates a nurse's credentials based on extensive, centralized information about nursing education around the world. Foreign-educated nurses who are found to be first-level general nurses move to the second step of the Certification Program, taking the CGFNS qualifying exam at one of the 30 to 50 sites throughout the world, frequently in their home country. Nurses who fail the qualifying exam can reapply to take the exam as many times as necessary. To help applicants prepare for the qualifying exam, CGFNS publishes study materials, including an Official Study Guide and Practice English Test Audio Tapes.

While the CGFNS Certification Program is designed to assist only first-level general nurses wishing to practice as registered nurses in the United States, the CGFNS Credentials Evaluation Service (CES) is useful to anyone with a background in nursing, regardless of where the individual was educated or licensed (or registered). This includes professional nurses, enrolled, vocational or practiced nurses, as well as nurse assistants.

The Credentials Evaluation Service is an evaluation and reporting service that uses documents received principally from source agencies to evaluate an applicant's nursing education and registration credentials earned outside the United States. The service then presents the nurse's credentials in terms of U.S. comparability. The service does not include an evaluation of knowledge through examination. The Credentials Evaluation Service is advisory in nature, unlike the credentials review portion of the CGFNS Certification Program, which evaluates an applicant for eligibility for an exam, i.e., the CGFNS Qualifying Exam. The CGFNS Credentials Evaluation Service may be required by a regulatory agency, such as a U.S. state board of nursing prior to licensure, by a governmental agency prior to immigration, by a school to assist in the admission or placement of a student working toward higher education, or by an employer in evaluating a candidate's preparation for a particular job opportunity.

CGFNS receives direction from a Board of Trustees and nine standing committees, comprised of professional nurses, educators, health care administrators, and researchers. An executive director and staff assume administrative responsibilities. CGFNS is located at 3600 Market Street, Suite 400, Philadelphia, PA 19104-2651.

ISSUES, DEVELOPMENTS, PREDICTIONS

It seems that almost every month brings information about changes in nurse practice acts or challenges as to what they permit. The scope of practice issue will not go away for quite a while.

With the accelerated change in the delivery of health care, and national and state health care reform efforts, the boundaries of advanced practice nursing are being rapidly expanded. Advanced Practice Nurses (APN) are rethinking approaches to regulation because the assumption that recognition of nurses in advanced practice would lead to reimbursement, consistency in practice, and expansion of the scope of nursing practice was dispelled.[54] Recommendations have been offered to solve the quagmire of confusion related to the regulation of nurses in advanced practice so that they can truly enhance the nation's health care delivery system.[55] State statutes and rules have been reviewed by ANA to determine how they have been used to benefit (or deter) the expansion of nursing practice. Some states are now amending nursing practice acts using the least restrictive approaches.

Nursing has made strides in the area of prescriptive authority; however, consistency remains a problem. Carson, ANA practice counsel, labels the situation a "crazy quilt of overregulation."[56] In 1983, eighteen states had formally given prescriptive authority to certain categories of nurses. By 1994, ANA identified forty-five states including the District of Columbia that had taken some action related to recognition of some form of prescriptive authority in advanced practice. The prescriptive authority may be through statutes, regulations, opinions, dependent legislation, or regulation or delegation of authority from another practice act.[57]

Even in states without legislative authority to prescribe, nurses in advanced practice manage to actively prescribe for their patients. They use one or more of the following strategies: request a physician to write the prescription, call in the prescription under the physician's name, cosign a physician's prescription pad, or follow a jointly developed protocol.[58]

Still another change that is evolving is legal approval for third party reimbursement. In 1989, 19 states had already given approval; in seven, there was direct reimbursement from insurance companies without legislative mandate;

and NPs were working diligently to get reimbursement in over fifteen other states.[59] By 1994, thirty-four states allowed APNs to receive third party reimbursement, but in ten of these states, it was very limited. Forty-nine states offered advanced practice nurses Medicaid reimbursement of which thirty-nine offered the rate at 80 to 100 percent of a physician's rate of reimbursement.[60] More detail on reimbursement and prescriptive authority can be found in Chaps. 15 and 19.

Although the focus is on NPs, all these activities include nurse-midwives, nurse anesthetists and, perhaps later other kinds of nurse specialists. Certification for specialties will certainly grow, probably with an overview organization certifying the certifying groups. As noted earlier in this chapter, the ABNS has already been established to assume this function. The growth of the many certifying groups, sometimes overlapping in functions, is quite astounding.

At the other end of the educational scale is the growing concern about the competency of nurses' aides and the increased use of unlicensed assistive personnel (UAP). New positions are growing for aides in hospitals, LTC facilities, and home care; 433,000 *new* jobs are predicted for the year 2000. As the least expensive and least prepared nursing person, the aide is still expected to detect behavioral changes that may signal a serious health problem—and isn't trained to do so. Although the need for national training standards has been agreed to, just who will implement them is still undecided. Some states, such as New Jersey, now regulate homemaker-home health aides. How can nurses who are ultimately responsible for nurses' aides ascertain that they are safe and competent?[61] Will the state board have a role? The NCSBN has developed standards for the regulation of nurses' aides to be included in a new Model Nursing Practice Act and the administrative rules. Approval of educational programs and the maintenance of registries of nurses' aides who have successfully completed training and competency evaluation are recommended.

Equal concern can be directed at the growing responsibilities of LPNs. Many state boards are put under tremendous pressure by employers to approve procedures for LPNs that are not in their curricula, such as venipuncture. Some boards approve and demand that PN programs include these procedures in their curriculum. Schools say there is already enough to cover in one year.[62] The impact is uncertain. Will patients be endangered? What of the responsibility of nurses who supervise LPNs? Might these new demands escalate the move toward AD education for LPNs?

On a less happy note, nurse disciplinary problems are likely to increase. In part, this is due to institutional staff cutbacks, with the extra stress of caring for sicker patients with fewer people. Stress has been seen to cause substance abuse, and nurses are not exceptions. It may be that there will be more state board programs to help addicted nurses to recover and return to work. This seems to work.[63] A research project to evaluate the efficacy of the different approaches used by state boards has been developed. Still another concern is nurse involvement in right-to-die issues, where their own moral and ethical philosophy is to let patients discontinue treatment if they wish and helping them to do so. The reality is that nurses can, at the least, lose their licenses in such circumstances, depending on the attitudes of the members of the state board involved.

Nursing state boards have some challenging years ahead. The 1993 Health Security Act offered by President Clinton contains a provision for federal preemption of state practice acts or licensing laws as a means of controlling costs and removing barriers to practice for nurses in advanced practice. The NCSBN believed that the provisions were imprecise and called for licensing boards to pursue crafting a more precise provision with predictable results.[64] Regardless of the outcome of health care reform efforts, it is clear that there will be an increasing push for more uniform licensing standards, and removal of statutory barriers to practice. The licensure examinations are expected to continue to change. Next on the agenda is Computerized Simulation Testing (CST), augmented by interactive video, which will allow candidates to demonstrate competence in clinical judgment and decision making.[65] (The National Board of Medical Examiners has already developed such a computer-based test.) Another activity for NCSBN is a study to determine potential item bias. NCLEX has been criticized as not taking into consideration cultural, gender, and other factors. With the large immigrant population, some of whom may go into nursing, such aspects must be considered. Other issues about licensure will include concerns about developing a mechanism to ensure competence, including that of returning nurses; the great diversity of definitions of nursing and scope of practice; what to do about temporary licenses for foreign nurses during the nursing shortage; and developing better means of verifying licensure across state lines.

Finally, the credentialing issues in health care in general are not expected to improve greatly because they are so disorganized now. More health occupations will continue to seek licensure or other legal status. All these groups will have problems similar to those of nursing with definition, scope, discipline, and testing methods. And what of the uncredentialed health worker? How best can we guarantee at least safe care for the public?

Resolution of the problems posed here could help to resolve some of the other problems of health care delivery. And if someone must take the lead in initiating cooperative action, it may well be nursing.

REFERENCES

1. *Study of Accreditation of Selected Health Education Programs*. Part I: Staff working papers: Accreditation of health educational programs. Washington, DC: National Committee on Accrediting, 1972: A-6.
2. US Department of Health, Education, and Welfare: *Report on Licensure and Related Health Personnel Credentialing*. DHEW Publ. (HSM) 72–11; 1971.
3. Hershey N: Alternative to mandatory licensure of health professionals. *Hosp Prog* 50:73, March 1969.
4. Kelly L: Oh no, not again: An old ghost rises. *Nurs Outlook* 38:121, May–June 1990.
5. Havighurst C, King N: Private credentialing of health care personnel: An antitrust perspective. Part One. *Am J Law Med* 9:131–201, Summer 1983.
6. Ibid.
7. Havighurst C, King N: Private credentialing of health care personnel: An antitrust perspective, Part Two. *Am J Law Med* 9:263–334, Fall 1983.
8. Grobe S: Sunset Laws. *Am J Nurs* 81:1355–1359, July 1981.
9. *The Study of Credentialing in Nursing: A New Approach*, vol. 1. The report of the committee. Staff Working Papers, vol 2. Milwaukee, WI: The American Nurses Association, 1979.
10. American Nurses Association: *Nursing: A Social Policy Statement*. Kansas City, MO: The Association, 1980.
11. Styles M: *Credentialing in Nursing; Contemporary Developments and Trends. USA Within a World View*. Kansas City, MO: American Nurses' Association, 1986.
12. Affara F, Styles M: *Nursing Regulation Guidebook: From Principle to Power*. Geneva: International Council of Nurses, 1993.
13. Styles, 1986, op cit, pp 24–25.
14. Styles M: *On Specialization in Nursing: Toward a New Empowerment*. Kansas City, MO: American Nurses' Foundation, 1989, pp 28–29.
15. Ibid, pp 64–66.
16. Malson L: *Credentialing in Nursing: Contemporary Developments and Trends: Legal Implications of Voluntary Credentialing*. Kansas City, MO: American Nurses' Association, 1989.
17. Peplau H: *Credentialing in Nursing: Contemporary Developments and Trends: International vs. External Regulation*. Kansas City, MO: American Nurses' Association, 1986, p 4.
18. Bouchaird J, Montueffel C: Constitutional issues related to grandfather clauses. *Issues* 8:5–6, January 1987.
19. *Suggested State Legislation: Nursing Practice Act, Nursing Disciplinary Diversion Act, Prescriptive Authority Act*. Kansas City, MO: American Nurses' Association, 1990, p 1.
20. *Model Nursing Practice Act*. Chicago: National Council of State Boards of Nursing, Inc, 1988.

21. Department of Health, Education, and Welfare: *Extending the Scope of Nursing Practice*. Washington, DC: The Department, 1971, p 12.
22. Ibid, pp 13–14.
23. American Nurses' Association: *Suggestions for Major Provisions to Be Included in a Nursing Practice Act*. Unpublished. New York: The Association, 1955.
24. Kelly L: Nursing practice acts. *Am J Nurs* 74:1314–1315, July 1974.
25. *Suggested State Legislation*, op cit, p 5.
26. Snyder M, LaBar C: *Nursing: Legal Authority for Practice*. Kansas City, MO: American Nurses Association, 1984.
27. American Nurses Association: *SNA Survey Results*. Kansas City: The Association, 1992, pp 75–76.
28. LaBar C: *The Regulation of Advanced Nursing Practice as Provided for in Nursing Practice Acts and Administrative Rules*. Kansas City, MO: American Nurses' Association, 1983.
29. Pearson L: Annual update of how each state stands on legislative issues affecting advanced nursing practice. *Nurs Pract* 19, January 1994.
30. Safriet B: Health care dollars and regulatory sense: The role of advanced practice nursing. *Yale J Regulation* 9:119, February 1992.
31. Wolff M: Court upholds expanded practice roles for nurses. *Law Med Health Care* 12:26–29, February 1984.
32. American Nurses Association: *1994 House of Delegates, San Antonio, Texas, Summary of Proceedings*. Washington, DC: The Association, 1994, p 6.
33. American Nurses Association: *1993 House of Delegates, Washington, DC, June 1993, Summary of Proceedings*. Washington, DC: The Association, 1993.
34. National Council of State Boards of Nursing, Inc: *Position Paper on the Regulation of Advanced Nursing Practice*. Chicago, IL: The Council, 1993.
35. American Nurses' Association: 1994 House of Delegates, loc cit.
36. Ibid, p 4.
37. Champagne M et al: State board criteria for licensure and disciplinary procedures regarding impaired nurses. *Nurs Outlook* 35:54–57, March–April 1987.
38. Swenson I et al: State boards and impaired nurses. *Nurs Outlook* 37:94–96, March–April 1989.
39. Champagne, loc cit.
40. Suggested State Legislation, op cit, pp 29–30.
41. Professional misconduct? Letters. *Nurs Outlook* 25:546, September 1977.
42. Follow-up letters in December 1977, pp 738–743, January 1978, pp 8–9; February 1978, p 78; March 1978, pp 142–143.
43. Jolene Tuma wins: Court rules practice act did not define unprofessional conduct. *Nurs Outlook* 27:376, June 1979.
44. Fiesta J: Why nurses lose their licenses, part 1. *Nurs Mgmt* 24:12, 14, October 1993.
45. Heinecke V: Department of Commerce, Division of Occupational and Professional Licensing, 810 P.2d 459 (Utah App 1991).
46. Swenson I et al: Interpretations of state board criteria and disciplinary procedures regarding impaired nurses. *Nurs Outlook* 35:108–110, May–June 1987.
47. Fama A: Reporting incompetent physicians: A comparison of requirements in three states. *Law Med Health Care* 11:111–117, June 1983.
48. Swenson (May–June 1987), loc cit.
49. Cerrato P: What to do when you suspect incompetence. *RN* 13:36–41, October 1988.
50. Price D, Murphy P: How—and when—to blow the whistle on unsafe practices. *Nurs Life* 3:51–54, January–February 1983.
51. National Council of State Boards of Nursing, Inc. (NCSBN): What Candidates Can Expect with NCLEX Administered by Computerized Adaptive Testing (CAT). *Issues* 14, 1993.
52. Ibid.
53. North American Free Trade Agreement (NAFTA): *Capital Update* December 3, 1993.
54. ANA: *1994 House of Delegates*, loc cit.
55. Safriet, loc cit.
56. Carson W: *Prescriptive Authority Information Packet*. Washington, DC: ANA, 1993.
57. Ibid.
58. Pearson L: 1991–92 Update: How each state stands on legislative issues affecting advanced nursing practice. *Nurs Pract* 17:14–23, January 1992.
59. How each state stands on legislative issues affecting advanced nursing practice. *Nurs Pract* 15:11–18, January 1990.
60. Pearson (January 1994), loc cit.
61. Reinhard S: Jurisdictional control: The regulation of nurses' aides. *Nurs Health Care* 9:373–375, September 1988.

62. LPNs widen their role; disagreement grows. *Am J Nurs* 90:16, 17, February 1990.

63. Penny J: Spotlight on support for impaired nurses. *Am J Nurs* 86:688–691, June 1986.

64. NCSBN: Federal preemption of state licensing. *Issues* 14:1–4, December 1993.

65. Computerized clinical simulation testing project (CST): Project overview and update. *Issues* 11:4–5, January 1990.

Nursing Practice and the Law

UNITED STATES CITIZENS who enter schools of nursing of any type take with them all of the citizen's legal rights and responsibilities. As nursing students, however, they gradually take on duties and responsibilities that may involve them in litigation, directly or indirectly, trivial or serious, that would not concern them as citizens only. Upon graduation and licensure they may be held liable for actions that apply only to RNs, as well as for other acts of a more general nature. With nursing experience and knowledge, responsibilities will increase still further, because a court of law takes these facts into consideration.

There are numerous ways in which nurses become involved with the law in their practice. The impact of statutory law has been previously discussed. In this chapter, other legal aspects will be considered, primarily within the common law of torts, that is, an intentional or unintentional civil wrong. This is the kind of law that relates to the daily practice of most nurses. When cases are used to illustrate a legal principle, it is important to remember that even a landmark decision may be overturned.

> The law . . . is not rigidly fixed, but a composite of court decisions, state and federal statutes, regulations and procedures. There are no final answers. Law is dynamic—it lives, grows and changes. . . . No book, . . . lawyer or teacher can tell you with complete assurance what is right or wrong or what the final outcome of any case will be.[1]

While this chapter includes a variety of legal topics, the emphasis is on malpractice in the clinical setting.

LITIGATION TRENDS IN HEALTH CARE

Part of the doctrine of common law is that anyone can sue anyone if she or he can get a lawyer to take the case or is able to handle it personally (as is common in a small claims court). This does not necessarily mean that there is just cause or that the person suing (plaintiff) has a good chance of winning; in fact, the defendant might be protected by law from being found liable, as when someone, in good faith, reports child abuse.

Most people are reasonably decent in their dealings with others, and unless a person sustains a serious injury, they will not institute legal proceedings. Sometimes this is because legal services are expensive, perhaps more so than paying the medical bills, and the offended person is realistic enough to know this. Often the person inflicting the injury is also realistic and prefers to settle the matter out of court, knowing that it will be less costly in the long run; or insurance may pay for the damage inflicted. One or both parties may settle their difficulties out of court because one or the other or both wants to avoid publicity and does not want to have a court record of any kind.

Once people seemed particularly reluctant to "make trouble" for nurses, doctors, or health agencies such as certain nonprofit or voluntary hospitals, either out of respect for the services offered and/or because they presumably had so little money that it seemed unfair or pointless. The latter was probably always an inaccurate generality, but today patients and families who feel aggrieved are considerably more likely to sue any or all concerned, sometimes for enormous sums. Health care is big business. The number of claims and the severity of awards began to increase in the 1930s, declined during World War II, and then rose again, with the 1980s and 1990s seeing multi-million-dollar awards. Malpractice suits against hospitals, especially, have increased.

A variety of reasons have been cited: the "litigant spirit" of the general public, what seems to be a "sue if possible; I'm entitled" attitude; changing medical technology that brought new risks, with a potential for exceptional severity of injury; sometimes high, unrealistic public expectations; the increase in specialization that has resulted in a deterioration of the physician-patient relationship; and patient resentment of depersonalized care and sometimes rude treatment in hospitals.

At the height of the malpractice crisis, a specially appointed interdisciplinary committee reported that the *prime factor in malpractice was malpractice*. However, because there are so many more medical injuries than medical claims, a major factor might be interpersonal problems between the provider and patient and frustration with the way specific complaints were handled or not handled. This was reaffirmed in 1994. However, there is also some evidence that people are being socialized into thinking that if something goes wrong, they should sue. One factor is seen to be the influence of the ubiquitous advertisements of attorneys on radio and television, promising legal help for a multitude of injuries and accidents. An AMA report also identifies other health professionals or workers as encouraging patients or families to sue because they feel that there was malpractice.

Most suits are settled out of court. The dramatic multi-million-dollar suits seldom result in awards anywhere near the original figure; sometimes they are not won at all. The largest awards have the largest elements of compensation for pain and suffering, almost exclusively occurring after some negligently caused catastrophic injury, such as severe brain damage or paralysis, which obviously has an enormous effect on the victim's life. The frequent suits and large awards were part of the reason for the mid-1970s' and 1980s' malpractice crisis, when many physicians could not get malpractice insurance, and neither hospitals nor physicians felt that they could afford it if they could get it. In 1990, malpractice fees were being reduced; state laws limiting awards and increased caution by physicians were cited as reasons. By 1992, a study of medical malpractice cases indicated that unjustified payments were rare.

The vast majority of malpractice cases are against physicians or hospitals. One policy research center reported in 1994 that such suits had increased medical costs by about $20 million in 1993 for one Indiana hospital, where, actually, owing to the state's legal reform legislation, the legal climate was deemed "favorable." Don't nurses get sued? Absolutely. As noted later, a good percentage of hospital and physician suits include nurses and may be based on the nurse's negligence. Because of the various legal doctrines also explained later, the aggrieved patient has the option of suing multiple defendants. The *deep pocket* theory of naming those who can pay has become traditional tort law strategy, as has the *fishnet theory* of suing every defendant available. Thus the likelihood of recovery from one or more defendants is greater, and a favorite defense of admitting negligence but blaming an absent party, the so-called empty chair defense, is defeated. Because presumably either or both the physician or the hospital has more money than the nurse, either may have to pay the award or at least more of the award, even if it is the nurse who is clearly at fault. Particularly in the case of the hospital whose liability and responsibility may be only secondary (vicarious liability), it may recover damages from the employee primarily responsible for the loss.

The possibilities of pretrial arbitration and no-fault insurance have been considered. Some states use an arbitration procedure that makes preliminary recommendations on the viability of a suit. The attraction of no-fault insurance is the increasing public tendency to believe that if someone is hurt, someone must pay, whether or not negligence is clearly evident. How costly this would be remains to be seen; no-fault auto insurance has been much more costly than ever contemplated. To get to the root of the problem—quality of care—government and health providers are looking at the impact of quality assurance techniques. It has also been noted that physicians, through self-owned insurance companies, are more stringently controlling the practice of their peers. Actually the majority of malpractice suits are decided in favor of the physician. Still, with all the discussions of health care reform in 1994, tort reform was also on the agenda, and it is doubtful if the issue will die, regardless of the outcome of health care reform.

BASIC LEGAL CONCEPTS AND TERMS

As in any profession, law has its own terminology. Short definitions and illustrations of key words and phrases used in tort law follow.

Abandonment—failing to continue to give services to a patient without notice; refusal to treat after accepting the patient. (Example: a nurse leaves the unit at the end of a shift without reporting off or determining that there is another RN to cover his or her assigned patients.)

Borrowed servant—an employee temporarily under the control of someone other than the employer (a hospital OR scrub nurse placed under the direction of a surgeon).

Breach of duty—under the law of torts, not behaving in a reasonable manner; in the legal sense, causing injury to someone. (Example: careless administration of drugs.)

Captain of the ship doctrine—similar to the borrowed servant concept that physicians are responsible for all those presumably under their supervision. Courts have ruled both for and against this doctrine, but the trend is to hold the individual responsible for that individual's own acts. (Example: incorrect sponge count done by nurses.) However, this does not preclude the hospital's being sued under the doctrine of *respondeat superior*.[2]

Charitable immunity—originating in English common law, holds that a hospital will not be held liable for negligence to a patient receiving care on a charitable basis. In 1969, the Massachusetts Supreme Court abolished prospectively the immunity of charitable institutions. In other states it varies, but the trend is toward recognizing the liability of charitable institutions. However, some states put a limit on how much money can be recovered from a hospital, and the plaintiff can collect the difference in the award from the negligent nurse. For government hospitals, the old *doctrine of sovereign immunity* granted them freedom from liability ("the government can't be sued" concept). However, the Federal Tort Claims Act (1946) partially waived sovereign immunity of the federal government, and a U.S. Supreme Court ruling in 1950 made the government liable for harm inflicted by its employees. Immunity of state and municipal hospitals varies, but the trend is toward liability. Immunity does not include the individual's liability. (Example: a clamp had been left in a patient's abdomen during surgery in a state hospital. Although this occurred before the state lifted the doctrine of sovereign immunity, both physicians and OR nurses were held liable for gross negligence.)[3]

Damages or monetary damages—redress sought by plaintiff for injury or loss. Nominal damages (usually $1) are token damages when the plaintiff has proved his case but actual injury or loss could not be proven or is minor. *Compensatory damages* are the actual damages, with amounts awarded for proven loss. These include *general damages* (pain, suffering, loss of limb) and special *damages* which must be proved (wage loss, medical expenses). *Punitive* or *exemplary damages* may be awarded when the defendant has acted with "wanton, reckless disregard," or has acted maliciously. Because awards may be large for "pain and suffering," this is an object of tort reform.

Defendant—person accused in a court trial.

Employee—someone who works for a person, institution, or company for pay.

Employer—one who selects, pays, can dismiss the employee, and controls his or her conduct during working hours.

Expert witness—someone with special training, knowledge, skill, or experience who is permitted to offer an opinion in court. The expert witness gives "expert testimony."

Foreseeability—holds the individual liable for all consequences of any negligent act that could or should have been foreseen under the circumstances. (Example: a suicidal patient is left unattended by an open window and jumps.)[4]

Indemnification—if the employer is blameless in a negligence case but must pay the plaintiff under *respondeat superior*, the employer may recover the amount of damages paid from the employee in a separate action. *Subrogation* means that the employer can sue the employee for the amount of damages paid because of the employee's negligence. This may also occur if the award is more than that covered by either the employer's or the nurse's insurance. It is not yet common, but does happen.[5]

Liability—being held legally responsible for negligent acts. The *rule or doctrine of personal liability* means that everyone is responsible for his or her own acts, even though someone else may also be held legally liable under another rule of law. *Vicarious liability*—liability imposed without personal fault or without a causal relationship between the actions of the one held liable and the injury (usually a case of *respondeat superior*), not a situation where individuals work as colleagues as in the case of nurse-midwife and physician.[6] *Corporate liability* relates to the legal duty of a health care institution to provide appropriate facilities (staff and equipment) to carry out the purpose of the institution and to follow established standards of conduct.[7]

Locality rule or community rule—first enunciated in 1880 in *Small v. Howard*, in which a small-town doctor unsuccessfully performed complex surgery and was held not liable. The rationale was that a physician in a small or rural community lacks the opportunity to keep abreast of professional advances. Gradually, courts took into account such facts as accessibility of medical facilities and experience. Beginning in the 1950s, various state supreme courts abandoned the locality rule on the basis that modern communications, including availability of professional journals, TV, and rapid transportation, made the rule outdated. The proper standard considered is whether the practitioner is exercising the care and skill of the average qualified practitioner, taking into account advances in the profession, as well as national standards.[8]

Long tail—the lag between the time when an injury occurs and the claim is settled. Insurance companies say that because of this lag, it is difficult to determine reasonable premiums for a malpractice insurance risk.

Malpractice—"any *professional* misconduct, unreasonable lack of skill or fidelity in professional or judiciary duties, evil practice or invalid conduct"; also, as related to physicians, "bad, wrong, or injudicious treatment resulting in injury, unnecessary suffering, or death to the patient, and proceeding from carelessness, ignorance, lack of professional skill, disregard of established rules or principles, neglect, malicious or criminal intent."[9] (Note that malpractice refers only to professionals.)

Negligence—failing to conduct oneself in a prescribed manner, with due care, thereby doing harm to another, or doing something that a reasonably prudent person would not do in like circumstances.

Criminal negligence and gross negligence are sometimes used interchangeably and refer to the commission or omission of an act, lawfully or unlawfully, in which such a degree of negligence exists as may cause a serious wrong to another. Almost any act of negligence resulting in the death of a patient would be considered criminal negligence.

Comparative negligence—takes into consideration the degree of negligence of both the defendant and the plaintiff. This allows the possibility of the plaintiff having some redress, which often is not possible if there has been contributory negligence.

Contributory negligence—a rather misleading expression used when the plaintiff has contributed to his own injury through personal negligence. This he may do accidentally or deliberately. Some authorities assert that a plaintiff who is guilty of contributory negligence cannot collect damages; others state that he may collect under certain conditions. As in most legal matters, decisions vary widely. Because contributory negligence must be proved by the defendant, as much written evidence as possible is needed. (Example: a patient died of burns when he smoked in the hospital bed, although the nurse had taken away his cigarettes and told him not to smoke.)[10]

Corporate negligence—the health care facility or an entity is negligent. This is a concept based on the landmark decision *Darling v. Charleston Community Memorial Hospital*, discussed later. It is based on two responsibilities: monitoring and supervising all professional personnel and investigating physician's credentials before granting staff privileges.

Outrageous conduct doctrine or tort of emotional distress—allows the plaintiff to base his case on intentional or negligent emotional distress caused by the defendant. This is quite hard to prove as described in two separate cases in which the women had mis-carriages and the nurses involved made extremely insensitive statements about disposal of the fetus. The courts did not find the behavior bizarre, outrageous, or intended to cause emotional distress, but rather unprofessional and insensitive and did not award damages.[11]

Plaintiff—party bringing a civil suit, seeking damages or other legal relief.

Proximate cause—the immediate or direct cause of an injury in a malpractice case. The plaintiff must prove that the defendant's malpractice caused, precipitated, or aggravated his condition. (Example: A nurse gives an unruly patient an injection of a tranquilizer. Shortly thereafter he goes into cardiac arrest and later dies. Because the medical examiner concluded that death was due to "sickle cell crisis," whether or not the injection was improper did not matter: the patient died of an underlying condition and the actions of the nurse were not the "proximate cause" of his death.)[12]

Reasonably prudent man theory—standard that requires an individual to perform a task as any reasonably prudent man of ordinary prudence with comparable education, skills, and training under similar circumstances would perform that same function. It is often described as requiring a person of ordinary sense to use ordinary care and skill. This concept is the key to determination of the standard of care.

Res gestae—all of the related events in a particular legal situation, which may then be admitted into evidence.

Res ipsa loquitor—"The thing speaks for itself," a legal doctrine that gets around the need for expert testimony or the need for the plaintiff to prove the defendant's liability because the situation (harm) is self-evident to even a lay person. The defendant must prove, instead, that he is not responsible for the harm done. Before the rule of *res ipsa loquitor* can be applied, three conditions must be present: the injury would not ordinarily occur unless there were negligence; whatever caused the injury at the time was under the exclusive control of the defendant; the injured person had not contributed to the negligence or voluntarily assumed the risk.[13] A common example involving nurses occurs when sponges have been left inside an abdomen after surgery, and the nurse had made an inaccurate sponge count.

Respondeat superior—"Let the master answer." The employer is responsible for what employees do within the scope of their employment.[14] This is a part of the vicarious liability doctrine. Independent contractors such as private duty nurses may or may not be included.

Standard of care—simply defined as the skill and learning commonly possessed by members of the profession. How the standard of care is determined is discussed in detail later.

Stare decisis—"Let the decision stand." The legal principle that previous decisions made by the court should be applied to new cases. Also called *precedent*. The decisions cited are usually made at the appellate level, including the state supreme court or the U.S. Supreme Court, highest appellate court in the land.

Statute of limitations—legal limit on the time a person has to file a suit in a civil matter. The statutory period usually begins when an injury occurs, but, in some cases, as with a sponge left in the abdomen, it starts when the injured person discovers the injury (*discovery*). In the case of an injury done to a minor, the statute will usually not "start to run" until the child has reached age eighteen. The statute of limitations that relates to malpractice actions has not been applied to nurses in all states; instead, the longer periods for statutes of limitations for negligence are applied to them (thus not considering them as professionals). However, along with other new legislation related to the NP and PA, several states have revised their statutes of limitations to include

nurses.[15] Court decisions about the inclusion of nurses in malpractice statutes of limitations have varied, with a previous but changing tendency to hold them liable for negligence, not malpractice, because they were seen as performing under specific directions. The shorter time is intended to ensure a professional a "fair chance to defend on merit and not find his defenses eroded by lapse of time." This apparently was not seen as necessary for anything less than "professional negligence." Though the length of time involved varies from state to state, it is about two years for malpractice, and four years or more for negligence by "others."

Tort—civil wrong against an individual. In order to have a cause of action based on malpractice or negligence, four elements must be present:

1. There was a duty owed to the plaintiff by the defendant to use due care (reasonable care under the circumstances).
2. The duty was breached (the defendant was negligent).
3. The plaintiff was injured or damaged in some way.
4. The plaintiff's injury was caused by the defendant's negligence (proximate cause).

No matter how negligent the health provider was, if there was no injury, there is no case. The plaintiff must also establish that a health practitioner-patient relationship existed and that the practitioner violated the standard of care.

APPLICATION OF LEGAL PRINCIPLES

With the added responsibilities nurses have assumed over the years, they are much more likely now to be involved in negligence actions by their patients. Not only must nurses follow doctors' orders, but they must use their own professional judgment in assessing a patient, reporting signs and symptoms, and taking appropriate action, sometimes very quickly. Yet most are not "in charge" of the patients' care and treatment. In addition, nurses supervise other nursing personnel, not all well trained, and agency nurses. This work is not done in a vacuum, for patients are sicker and staff often reduced. Yet even in the greatest turmoil, a nurse is required by licensure law to give, at a minimum, *safe* and effective care. It is useful to begin by understanding how the legal principles mentioned translate into real cases involving nurses. All nursing law textbooks include case examples, as do almost all nursing journals, when there are articles or columns on law.

Some are classic cases that are repeatedly cited in nursing law; others are more recent. At times, when two similar cases are judged in quite different ways, both are given. The findings may change with the changing role of the nurse and a court's concept of what a nurse is and does. For instance, one attorney who had handled nurse liability cases for many years reflects that 40 years ago a nurse client was not held responsible when she gave a wrong medication that had been ordered by the physician. She should have known it was wrong; yet she blindly administered it anyhow. But she was "just following doctors' orders." Then, in the 1980s he defended a nurse who followed routine orders for a tetanus injection without checking for patient allergy. She was judged liable because she didn't use her nursing judgment.[16]

Assuming that you are at little risk because you don't work in the ICU, the emergency room, or some other high-pressure unit is a mistake. In reviewing cases in which nurses were found liable, the sad news is that most of the incidents are everyday situations in which nurses not only did not use nursing judgment but sometimes didn't even use common sense. Quite often they neglected basic principles that they learned in their first year of nursing, such as how to give medications, or were careless about communication. Not only are RNs found liable, but also students. The following hypothetical case (although based on fact) provides

a useful illustration as well as several other legal principles.

A first-year student nurse was assigned by the instructor to care for a thin, very ill patient who required an intramuscular injection. The student had only practiced the procedure in the school laboratory. She injected the medication in the patient's sciatic nerve and caused severe damage. The patient sued the doctor, hospital, head nurse, faculty members, and school of nursing. This was a case of *res ipsa loquitor*. The student was clearly negligent because she should have known the correct procedure and should have taken special precautions with an emaciated patient. The student is held to the standards of care (*standards of reasonableness*) of an RN if she is performing RN functions. If the student is not capable of functioning safely unsupervised, she should not be carrying out those functions. The doctor may or may not be held liable, depending on the court's notion about the *captain of the ship* doctrine. However, this would have nothing to do with the drug and injection itself, assuming that it was an appropriate order. The hospital will probably be held liable under *respondeat superior*, because students, even if not employed, are usually treated legally as employees. In addition, because the head nurse is responsible for all patients on the unit and presumably should have been involved in the student's assignment, or should have assigned an RN to such an ill patient, she too would be liable, because she did not make an appropriate assignment ("appropriate delegation of duties").

The instructor might be found liable, not on the basis of *respondeat superior*—just as the head nurse or supervisor would not be liable if the student had been an RN, because these nurses are not employers in the legal sense—but on the basis of inadequate supervision. If a supervisor or other nurse assigns a task to someone not competent to perform that task and a patient is injured because of that individual's incompetent performance, the supervising nurse can be held personally liable because it is part of her or his responsibility to know the competence and scope of practice of those being supervised.[17] Although theoretically this nurse could rely on the subordinate's licensure, certification, or registration, if any, as an indication of competence, if there is reason to believe that that individual would nevertheless perform carelessly or incompetently and the nurse still assigns that person to the task, the nurse is held accountable (as is the employer under the doctrine of *respondeat superior*). The school might be found liable in the case of the student, if the court believed the director had not used good judgment in employing or assigning the faculty member carrying out those teaching responsibilities.

In another situation, the outcome would be different. A student gave an electric heating pad, per the doctor's order, to a patient who was alert and mentally competent and demonstrated to the nurse her ability to adjust the temperature and her knowledge of the potential hazards. The patient fell asleep on the pad, set at a high temperature, and burned her abdomen. In this case, there would seem to be sufficient evidence of *contributory negligence* on the part of the patient, with the student having good reason to assume that the patient was capable of managing the heating pad. Therefore, even if the patient sued, her case would be weak. If the court used the doctrine of *comparative negligence*, some liability might be assigned to the student, if for instance she or he did not check on the patient in a reasonable time. If the heating pad were faulty, the hospital would probably be liable, not the nurse.

Another case involving a student reinforces the principle of individual and teacher responsibility. In *Central Anesthesia Associates v. Worthy* (1985), Bonnie Castro, a senior student nurse anesthetist, was accused of administering anesthesia improperly, causing the patient to have a cardiac arrest and brain damage; the patient was still in a coma at the time of the case. Castro was under the supervision of a PA employed by the professional corporation that had the nurse anesthetist program. The Supreme Court of Georgia held Castro, the PA, and the three an-esthesiologist teachers liable. It rejected her argument that she should be held to the student standard; she was held to the standards of a CNA. The teachers were not on the scene and had not delegated supervision properly. The PA either did not supervise adequately or was himself not capable. This case has implications for nursing students and their staff nurse preceptors when faculty are absent.

Another case of *res ipsa loquitor*, reported in 1987, resulted in an award of over $2 million.[18] A four-day-old infant suffered trauma to her head as a result of being dropped or mishandled by the nursing staff. The hospital and staff denied responsibility, although the baby had been under exclusive control of hospital staff throughout its stay. Even when the parents visited, staff was present. It appears that whoever caused the injury chose to cover up the incident. The hospital paid under the *respondeat superior* doctrine, since all the staff were employees.

The captain-of-the-ship doctrine was negated in a case that cost the hospital $5 million. (Nelson v. Trinity Medical Center, 1988.) The physician of a woman in active labor ordered assessment of fetal heart tones, an IV, and analgesia. Standing orders in that labor unit called for continuous fetal heart monitoring, but the nurse, without checking, assumed the monitors were all in use and did not place one on the patient until an hour later. It indicated fetal distress, and despite an immediate cesarean, the infant had severe brain damage. According to the expert who testified, the damage was caused by placenta abruptio, which could have been diagnosed by earlier fetal monitoring. The defendant hospital tried to invoke the captain-of-the-ship doctrine to cover the nurse's negligence. The court ruled that even though the doctor was in charge of the case, he had no direct control over what the nurse did (as opposed to an OR situation) and that the nurse was performing a routine act.[19]

A particularly useful example from many points of view is the landmark decision of *Darling v. Charleston Community Memorial Hospital* (211 N.E. 2nd 53, Ill., 1965). A minor broke his leg playing football and was taken to Charleston

Community Memorial Hospital, a JCAH-accredited hospital. There a cast was put on the leg in the emergency room, and he was sent to a regular nursing unit. The nurses noted that the toes became cold and blue, charted this, and called the physician, who did not come. Over a period of days, they continued to note and chart deterioration of the condition of the exposed toes and continually notified the physician, who came once but did not remedy the situation. The mother then took the boy to another hospital, where an orthopedist was forced to amputate the leg because of advanced gangrene. The family sued the first doctor, the hospital, and the nurses involved. The physician settled out of court; he admitted he had set few legs and had not looked at a book on orthopedics in forty years. The hospital's defense was that the care provided was in accordance with standard practice of like hospitals, that it had no control over the physician, and that it was not liable for the nurses' conduct because they were acting under the orders of a physician. However, the appellate court, upholding the decision of the lower court, said that the hospital could be found liable either for breach of its own duty or for breach of duty of its nurses. The new hospital standards of care set by that ruling were in reference to the hospital bylaws, regulations based on state statutes governing hospital licensure and criteria for (now JCAHO) accreditation. The court reasoned that these constituted a commitment that the hospital did not fulfill. In addition, the court held that the hospital had failed in its duties to review the work of the physician or to require consultation when the patient's condition clearly indicated the necessity for such action. This is corporate negligence.

For nurses, the crucial point was the newly defined duty to inform hospital administration of any deviation in proper medical care that poses a threat to the well-being of the patients. (The hospital was also expected to have a sufficient number of trained nurses capable of recognizing unattended problems in a patient's condition and reporting them.) Specifically, the court said:

> **...the jury could reasonably have concluded that the nurses did not test for circulation in the leg as frequently as necessary, that skilled nurses would have promptly recognized the conditions that signalled a dangerous impairment of circulation in the plaintiff's leg, and would have known that the condition would become irreversible in a matter of hours. At that point, it became the nurses' duty to inform the attending physician, and if he failed to act, to advise the hospital authorities so that appropriate action might be taken (211 N.E. 2d at 258).[20]**

Because Darling-type situations are not rare, it is essential for nurses to know their legal responsibilities (and rights) in such cases, so that they can act accordingly. That this kind of notification problem may still exist after almost 30 years is shown by another $2 million award. Nurses in a VA hospital were found liable because they failed to recognize the emergency condition of a postoperative patient and failed to take prompt steps to notify attending physicians. When the physicians were slow to respond, the nurse made no effort to call another physician or anyone else because she said she thought no one else was capable of handling the situation (which was not so). This case also points out the importance of a patient's chart, which the judge called "a mess"—sketchy and unreliable with important data missing. The court stated that the lack of charting contributed to the decision against the nurses. Actually, because physicians and nurses working in a VA hospital cannot be sued separately, under the Federal Tort Claims Act, the United States was the defendant.[21]

LITIGATION INVOLVING NURSES

In the last twelve years, the number of legal suits involving nurses have increased significantly. It is difficult to say whether this is because there is actually more negligence, whether the public's litigious spirit now extends to nurses, or whether people simply are more aware of nurses' increased responsibilities and nurses are now seen as professionals responsible for their own actions. It may be that all of these factors are involved.

In late 1988, the ANA reported that each year an estimated 1,900 nurses are named in liability and malpractice lawsuits. Half of those claims against nurses resulted in payment. The ANA followed this study by establishing a National Nurses Claims Data Base in order to have some reliable data about nurses in malpractice suits, in part because questions were being raised by insurance carriers about the cost of defending nurses. Preliminary information made available in 1990 came primarily from two major insurance carriers involved with nursing liability insurance. The results showed some similarity to a study of litigation against nurses between 1967 and 1977.[22] Sites of the alleged negligence were again, hospitals first, by a large margin, and then clinics (13.5 percent). The areas most involved were obstetrics, patient room, emergency room, and operating room. The chief reasons for the claims were improper treatment, birth related; improper treatment, miscellaneous; and patient falls.

In 1994,[23] the current statistics on a national level taken from data reported in the National Practitioner Data Bank from 1990 to 1993 indicated that as of 1990, about five nurses in 10,000 are sued in a given year. The malpractice claims ranged from patient falls (the greatest number of claims) to failure to impart vital information about a patient's changing condition. More cases are involving physical procedures, and courts are using policy and procedure documents increasingly.[24] Insurance reports for one state, which are rather typical of others, listed patient falls, burns, medication errors, failure to assess adequately, failure to remove foreign objects, mistaken identity of patients, failure to clarify the physician's instructions, "bad baby" cases, and failure to restrain, as some of the most recurring cases.[25] Again, many of these are the same as those reported in the Campuzzi study mentioned earlier.

Some insurance companies have expressed concern about potential malpractice claims of advanced practice nurses, and APNs do have higher premiums than other nurses. In a survey of state boards (with a rather small sample of 45 complaints, it was found that nurse practitioners had the largest percent of complaints related to practice, such as failure to assess or intervene, misdiagnosis, and documentation errors. Almost 40 percent of all complaints about APNs were dismissed; 24 percent resulted in some kind of state board discipline. Clinical nurse specialists had the fewest complaints of any kind. It is important to note here that not all complaints to state boards are related to malpractice suits and it is possible to win a suit or have it dismissed without the information necessarily getting to the state board. Also, some of the state board cases related to drug abuse (of which the highest percentage were nurse anesthetists).[26]

MAJOR CAUSES OF LITIGATION

The kinds of incidents reported as most prevalent in causing litigation still continue to be problems. Sometimes they are caused by lack of knowledge, as when a nurse simply does not know the most current use or dangers of a drug or treatment or how to respond to a complication. Sometimes it's simply a matter of carelessness—doing something in a hurry or neglecting to do something routine because the nurse is busy. Often problems result from poor nursing judgment, as when a nurse in the emergency room sends away a patient without consulting with or calling a physician, or does not question a doctor's order or behavior despite having doubts that the action is correct. The amount of responsibility now put on nurses to judge the actions of the physician and (within their scope of practice or knowledge) to stop and/or report his action is increasing. For instance in one case, both nurse and physician knew that a baby was in footling breech position and the nurse observed symptoms of fetal distress, but the physician decided to perform a vaginal delivery anyhow. The nurse expressed her concerns to the physician (who ignored them), but she did not contact her supervisor or anyone else. The baby suffered brain damage. In the suit that followed, the courts ruled that the physician made an error, but that the nurse should have notified a supervisor immediately. The hospital was held responsible and the family was awarded damages.[27]

Other examples reinforce the fact that nurses are being held responsible for their own actions. In *Story v. St. Mary Parish Service District* (1987), a new staff nurse who had not yet taken her boards was held responsible for the death of a man because she failed to recognize an impending myocardial infarction. The man complained of pain and symptoms that typically signal such a condition. The nurse neither consulted with the charge nurse concerning his complaints nor attempted to contact any medical person. The plaintiff's attorney shored up his case by citing the Louisiana nursing practice act which states that "the practice of a registered nurse includes such activities as assessing human responses to actual or potential health problems...." Even though the nurse was not yet an RN, the law required that, until she was, she work only where direct RN supervision is available.

Being busy was not accepted as an excuse by a Texas judge, who ruled for the plaintiff. A nurse ignored a patient lying on a table when he started to vomit because she was busy having his father sign papers. He fell off the table, got hurt, and sued.[28]

Physician-Nurse Communication Problems

Do you have a responsibility to take action when a doctor writes an order that you think is incorrect or unclear? When he does not respond to a patient's worsening condition? When he does not come to see a patient even if you think it's urgent? When he does not follow accepted precautions in giving a treatment? What if he becomes angry and abusive? Even if he was right? According to court decisions in the last few years, the answer to all these questions is that it *is* the nurse's responsibility to take action. Medications seem to be a major problem. When

an order is incomplete or written illegibly and the nurse does not question it, the results can be tragic.

A classic case, *Norton v. Argonaut Insurance Co.*, 114 S. 2nd 249 (La. 1962), is cited in almost every nursing law text in detail. A nursing supervisor thought she would help out in a pediatrics unit when it was short-staffed, even though she was not familiar with current pediatric nursing practice. An order for a medication for an infant did not state the appropriate route of administration and, after asking nearby physicians whether the dose was appropriate (not the route), the nurse gave it by injection. By this route, the amount given was a massive overdose and the child died. The nurse was not aware that the drug came in an oral solution and had not called the physician who wrote the order. Both were found liable. (This case also demonstrates the dangers of not having updated knowledge.)

A nurse who follows a physician's orders is just as liable as the physician if the patient is injured because, for instance, a medication was the wrong dose, given by the wrong route, or was actually the wrong drug. If the order is illegible or incomplete, it is necessary to clarify that order with the physician who wrote it. If you doubt its appropriateness, check with a reference source or the pharmacist, and always with the physician who wrote the order.[29]

You have a right to question the physician when in doubt about any aspect of an order, and the nursing service administration should support any nurse who does so. In fact, there should be a written policy on the nurse's rights and responsibility in such matters, so that there is no confusion on anyone's part and no danger of retribution to a justifiably questioning nurse faced with an irate physician. What if the physician refuses to change the order? You should not simply refuse to carry out an order, for you may not have the most recent medical information and could injure the patient by *not* following the order. You should report your concern promptly to your administrative supervisor. The supervisor or other nurse administrator is often expected to act as an intermediary if there is a problem. However, a good collegial relationship and mutual courtesy can prevent or ease a doctor-nurse confrontation, and should be cultivated by both.

Verbal or telephone orders are another part of this problem.[30] Although they are considered legal, the dangers are evident. In case of patient injury, either the doctor, or the nurse, or both will be held responsible. There frequently are or should be hospital, sometimes legal, policies to serve as guides. Nurses should be very familiar with these, for adherence to such policies may protect them from liability. If telephone orders are acceptable, precautions should be taken that they are clearly understood (and questioned if necessary), with the doctor required to confirm the orders in writing as soon as possible. Some hospital policies require a repetition of the order; it is not unheard of to have two nurses listen together to a telephone order with the second nurse cosigning the order. In any case, most hospitals require the nurse to record the date and time of the communication. In states where PAs' orders have been declared legal (as an extension of the physician), the same precautions must be taken, with the physician again confirming the order as quickly as possible.

An incident that repeatedly shows up in litigation is the failure of a physician to see a patient either on the unit or in the emergency room. Often the nurse is held liable for not following through. More and more often, it is suggested that a system (or a policy) be set up specifying whom the nurse then contacts. If you neglect to call a doctor when the patient needs help or simply because you are not aware of the seriousness of the patient's condition, simply charting is not enough. This was clearly demonstrated in the *Darling* case. In another frequently cited case, *Goff v. Doctor's General Hospital of San Jose*, 333 P. 2nd 29, (CA 1958), the nurse did not call the physician when a pregnant woman continued to bleed excessively, "because he wouldn't come." The patient died, and the hospital was held vicariously liable because of the nurse's negligence.

Another failure in communication occurs when a nurse does not report a situation because she or he doesn't fully investigate or fully assess it. A 22-year-old suffered multiple fractures as a result of a motorcycle accident. The report of blood gases revealed that the patient was hypoxemic, but the nurse did not report it, nor did she report that the patient had vomited after being given medication ordered by the surgeon. After shift change, other nurses found the patient with unequal pupils, but it took several hours for the patient to be put on oxygen. He suffered severe brain damage. A settlement of $1.2 million was reached.[31] Still other judgments against the nurse have been given when a doctor has not followed through on appropriate technical procedures, such as the timely removal of an endotracheal tube. If you know that a particular procedure is being done incorrectly or a wrong medication is ordered (because it's within the scope of your knowledge) and do nothing about it, you can be held liable as well as the physician. A nurse may also refuse to administer a drug or treatment because it is against hospital policy.[32] However, it is important to have support from nursing management, if discussion with the physician ends with an impasse. If the supervisor refuses to help, it will be necessary to go up the chain of command.[33]

A woman sued a hospital because she maintained that the nurses had failed to notify a physician about her lab and x-ray reports. She had an exceptionally high blood count after a cesarean section, and an x-ray showed intestinal dilation. Nevertheless she was discharged. She developed gangrene, and her ileum and ascending colon had to be removed. The nurse testified that she had informed the physician. The jury found both liable and awarded the woman $2 million, 80 percent against the physician. The jury found that either the nurse had not notified the physician or that she had failed to seek direction from a superior when the doctor discharged the patient, which was clearly less-than-acceptable medical care.[34]

These examples reinforce the need for nurses to recognize their accountability to the patient, even if it means disagreeing with physicians and reporting them if the patient appears to be endangered. Some hospitals that appreciate how difficult the nurses' situation can be in such a potential confrontation have set policies that clarify everyone's responsibilities. Nurses need to take precautions anyhow.

There are a number of actions you can take. Don't hesitate to call a physician; be persistent in tracing down the attending or substitute physician; stay on the phone until you get the information you need (use nursing judgment).[35] Be especially careful about telephone orders. Make sure you're both talking about the same patient. Make certain you understand what the doctor is saying even if it requires repetition. Repeat the order. Document the order, noting physician's name, time, date, and name of the third party if there was a witness.[36]

Legal Problems in Record Keeping

It is almost impossible to overemphasize the importance of records in legal action, especially nurses' notes. They hold the only evidence that orders were carried out and what the results were; they are the only notes written with both the time and date in chronological order; they offer the most detailed information on the patient. Nurses' notes, like the rest of the chart, can be subpoenaed. No matter how skillfully you practice your profession, if your actions and observations are not documented accurately and completely, the jury can only judge by what is recorded. If you are subpoenaed, comprehensive notes will not only give weight to your testimony but will help you remember what happened. A case may not come up for years, and unless there was a severe problem at the time, it is difficult to remember exact details about one patient. General, broad phrases such as "resting comfortably," "good night," "feeling better," are totally inadequate. How could a jury interpret them? How could even another professional who did know that patient interpret them? While today's tendency is to limit the amount of charting, skimpy nurses' notes can

lose a case for a nurse or hospital. One judge noted that insufficient notes indicated substandard care.[37]

The correct way to chart, with legal aspects in mind, is probably charting as you were taught and following good nursing practice: write what you see, hear, smell, feel; don't make flip or derogatory remarks; use acceptable hospital or agency abbreviations. Be as accurate as possible, but if a mistake is made, recopy or cross out with the original attached and still legible, but marked "error." Do not use correction fluid. Never alter a record in any other way; this has been shown to influence a jury negatively. Every good malpractice attorney calls on experts to examine charts for alterations, erasures, and additions. You may make minor corrections on a "correction sheet" after reading the chart at a deposition, but nothing that changes the facts substantially. Computer records have changed correction procedures, since corrections can be made immediately. (Such "charting" does allow for more accurate, timely, and legible charting, but the issue of confidentiality discussed in Chap. 22 does present a problem.) All too often, a nurse makes a change or an omission in the chart to protect a physician or the hospital. This can lead to criminal charges, as in the case of the OR nurse who did not record the illegal participation of an equipment salesman in surgery and who was cited for falsification of records.[38]

Some of the most serious problems arising from poor charting concern lack of data, such as omission of a temperature reading or other vital signs, lack of observations about a patient's condition, or no record of oxygen liter flow in a newborn infant; these and others have resulted in liability judgments against nurses and hospitals, although in each it was contended that the "right" thing had been done. However, although it is often inaccurate, the statement "if it wasn't charted, it wasn't done" has evolved into a legal standard.[39] Because of this, new attention is being given to the "shortcuts" in charting such as a flowchart. The flowchart should be consistent with the nurses' notes. You cannot simply check off what the nurses on the previous shift checked off. If you were sued, such discrepancies would damage your credibility. Moreover, you should not depend too heavily on flowcharts; it is still important to record the patient's *response* to care in your notes.

Suggestions have been made for what should *not* be charted, in order to stay out of legal trouble.

1. Avoid using labels to describe your patient's behavior, such as "noncompliant" or "combative." Describe what happened instead.
2. Don't refer to staffing problems.
3. Refrain from mentioning that an incident report has been filed.
4. Don't try to explain a mistake or use words like "accidentally" or "somehow," which opposing attorneys look for. Just record what was done.
5. Avoid airing your "dirty laundry"—disputes with, or criticism of, your colleagues, both nurses and physicians.
6. Never chart that you've "informed" a colleague of a certain event if you really only mentioned it. Informing means to clearly state why she is being notified.
7. Never refer to another patient by name. Use "roommate," initials, or bed number.[40]

None of this means that you should withhold pertinent information, since this is no different from altering information. It is important to record accurately oral conversations with physicians, family, and others. If there is a later dispute about who said what, if the patient is injured, a clear description of the conversation recorded at the time it was held will generally be considered accurate by the court.

Information in the patient's record that is particularly important from a legal point of view includes names and signatures of the patient, nurses, and doctors; notations of the patient's condition on admission, with progress notes on changes for the better or worse while in the hospital; accounts of injuries sustained accidentally while in the hospital, if any; a de-

scription of the patient's attitude toward the treatment and personnel; medications and other treatments given (what, when, how); vital signs; visits of doctors, consultants, and specialists; receiving the patient's permission for therapy and all special procedures such as surgery. Gaps in documentation can be as dangerous as errors. Another potentially dangerous practice occurs when a nurse must chart what an aide says he or she did or what occurred when the nurse has not personally seen it (as is usual). Some lawyers advise adding a statement that clarifies the facts to protect yourself.

Checking doctors' orders and following through might seem to be an ordinary act, but when neglected, it can have dire consequences. Nurses failed to pick up and transcribe a surgeon's postoperative order to remove rectal packing four hours after insertion. Two days later, noting that it had not been done, he removed it himself, but it was too late. The patient had become septic and later died. When surgeon and hospital were sued, the hospital paid the bulk of the settlement because of nursing negligence.[41]

Other Common Acts of Negligence

Among the acts of negligence a nurse is most likely to commit in the practice of nursing are the following (not in order of importance):

1. *Failure to respond or to ask someone else to respond promptly to a patient's call light or signal* if, because of such failure, a patient attempts to take care of his own needs and is injured. This might happen when he attempts to get out of bed to go to the bathroom or reaches for a bedpan in the bedside stand. Sometimes the bedpan or urinal is not even at hand. After prostate surgery, a 79-year-old man rang to go to the bathroom. The nurse said an orderly would help him. Despite the flashing call light, no one came. The patient got out of bed, fell, and injured himself. The court faulted the nurse; she had not left a

urinal, and she did not see to it that he got help. It was deemed her responsibility, even though the orderly didn't come.[42]

2. *Failure to use adequate precautions to protect the patient against injury.* As a nurse, you know that drugs, or hot liquids, or potentially harmful implements, such as scissors, must be kept out of the reach of a young child or a delirious or confused patient. You know the necessity of staying with—or having someone else stay with—a patient on a stretcher or narrow treatment table to keep him from falling, or with a helpless or irresponsible person at any time. (Remember, falls are most frequently the cause of malpractice suits against nurses.)

Even if there is a staff shortage, nurses have a responsibility to use good judgment. A man was admitted with a serious case of pneumonia; he was confused, uncoordinated, and weak. He was placed in a room with a balcony. The wife stayed with him, but when she left, he was seen on the balcony calling to workers below to bring a ladder. The nurses restrained him and called the wife to sit with him. She asked them to call her mother, who lived only five minutes away, to come until she could get there and asked that someone sit with him until her mother arrived. The nurses said that they were short-staffed and couldn't. By the time the mother got there, the patient was on the ground below. In part because an aide had been sent to supper and other staff were performing routine duties that could have waited, the court ruled in favor of the plaintiff.[43]

The injuries that occur to patients are often the result of the nurse breaking a basic rule of nursing care. As a student you learn what to do to avoid harming the patient. You learn that every medicine must be given accurately to the right patient, whether it is five grains of aspirin or an injection of a highly potent drug; that a sponge count is a very important step in certain surgical operations and must

never be neglected; that sterility of equipment is essential for safety in caring for a venous catheter,[44] or doing sterile dressings as well as for use during surgery; that particular care must be exercised when performing treatments involving delicate tissues; that strict precautions must be observed to prevent infections and cross-infections, such as diarrhea in the nursery for newborn babies; that injections and other procedures must be done with care; and that restraints, siderails, and other protective measures should be used with appropriate nursing judgment.

Carelessness in giving an injection can cause serious injury. A patient who had received several injections contracted an infection, eventually requiring plastic surgery. In the resulting trial, a nurse expert witness testified that the cause was improper sterile technique (*Tripp v. Humana Inc.* (1985).[45]

Medication errors are a particularly serious problem. Studies have shown that drugs were the major cause of iatrogenic illness and injury to patients in hospitals, 20 percent of which caused a serious disability. Medication-related incidents comprise 40 percent of all reported errors. The major errors are wrong dose, wrong drug, omission of a dose, wrong rate of administration, wrong route, and wrong time.[46] Nurses who are imprudent and take unsafe shortcuts or otherwise fail to adhere to what they know is competent nursing practice are being negligent. If harm to a patient or coworker can be traced to a nurse, and it often can, she or he may be held liable. Negligence tends to involve carelessness as much as lack of knowledge.[47] As an example, in *Baines v. St. Francis Hospital and School of Nursing*, a patient sued because of injuries sustained after an injection of Dramamine subcutaneously. Expert witness testimony established that nurses should know that it must be given intramuscularly if ordered by hypodermic, even if the physician's order was not specific.[48]

Recommendations from the American Society of Hospital Pharmacists (ASHP) to help nurses stop medication mishaps follow:

- *Review* the medications of all patients, assessing drug interactions. If you have questions, get the information from pharmacists or other resources. If you're not satisfied, don't administer the medication until you've checked with the physician ordering it.
- *Verify* all new drug orders before you carry them out by checking the original order, the medication itself, and the patient's ID.
- *Inspect* the medication, checking expiration date and general appearance. If it doesn't look right, check with the pharmacist.
- *Confirm* calculations for drug dosage, flow rate, and anything else that requires a mathematical formula with another nurse or the pharmacist.
- *Administer* medications at the scheduled time. Don't remove identifying information until just before administration. Chart immediately.
- *Follow up* after administering a drug like an analgesic or antihypertensive to be sure it has had its intended effect.
- *Check* with the pharmacy if the patient's medication hasn't arrived. Don't substitute or borrow from another patient's medication. Return all unfinished or discontinued drugs to the pharmacy.
- *Question* unusual orders, particularly for large dosages.
- *Counsel* patients and their caregivers about the prescribed medications, making sure they understand the purpose, how taken, and side effects to watch for.
- *Listen* to patients who question or object to the use of a particular drug. If concerns remain after you explain the medication's purpose, double-check the order and the dispensed medication with the doctor and pharmacy before giving it.

ASHP calls nurses "the final point of the checks and balances triad" that starts with the physician and pharmacist.[49]

Still further carelessness and haste is demonstrated in *Breit v. St. Luke's Memorial Hospital* (1987). A patient had had a laminectomy; by the next day he had full use of his extremities and could walk. When the patient complained of pain, the nurse took as unwise shortcut: she gave him the injection when he was in an upright position. Soon he lost all sensory and motor function and became an invalid. Two expert nurse witnesses testified that the morphine should not have been given in that way, because it could cause hypotension and the pooling of blood in the legs could precipitate a stroke. The nurse admitted that she knew this. She was found liable.[50]

3. *Inadequate or dated nursing knowledge.* Since having current knowledge is a professional responsibility, there seems to be little excuse for this kind of negligence. However, on occasion, even the most competent nurse has a problem. If an entirely new type of treatment or piece of equipment is introduced on your unit, it is your responsibility, as well as that of the head nurse or supervisor, to get the appropriate information on it. Further problems can come from "floating" and short staffing. In these cases, you may be placed in a specialty area with which you are not familiar, with or without a more experienced nurse. There is no clear answer to this dilemma, since some courts have ruled that shifting staff is the employer's privilege and refusal can be considered insubordina-

tion. The supervisor, of course, is also responsible for any damage done because he or she is supposed to delegate safely. The float nurse must be especially careful and report any change in a patient's condition. (See also Chap. 30.)

4. *Abandoning a patient. Abandonment* simply means leaving a patient when your duty is to be with him. One example would be leaving a child or incompetent adult without the protection you would have offered. The results can be fatal. In one case, a circulating nurse went, at a doctor's demand, to assist in another operating room, while the OR technician was removing the surgical drapes at the end of a patient's surgery. No one else was in that OR, and when the patient went into cardiac arrest, the technician could not handle the situation alone. The patient became permanently paralyzed and semicomatose. Although the physician and anesthesiologist were also held liable, the court focused on the duty of the circulating nurse, as spelled out in the hospital procedure book. The jury concluded that the nurse was negligent for leaving the unconscious patient's side.

5. *Failure to teach a patient.* Nurses sometimes neglect to teach a patient in preparation for discharge, either because of the time it takes or because the physician objects. Nurses are responsible for providing appropriate teaching to the patient and/or caregiver. An increasing number of suits are being filed because such teaching was not done or not done thoroughly or understandably. In one case, where a child had Bryant's traction applied, one of the complaints was that the nursing staff did not provide proper discharge instructions.[51] Written instructions are often considered necessary to help the patient and family remember the information.

6. *Failure to make sure that faulty equipment is removed* from use, that crowded corridors or hallways adjacent to the nursing unit are cleared, that slippery or unclean floors are taken care of, and that fire hazards are eliminated. This is an area of negligence that, in most instances, would implicate others just as much as, or more than, the professional nurse. For example, the hospital administration would certainly share responsibility for fire hazards and dangerously crowded corridors, and the housekeeping and maintenance departments would not be blameless either. This does not lessen your responsibility for reporting unsafe conditions and following up on them, or in checking equipment you use. Report persistent hazards in writing and keep a copy for personal protection.

SPECIALTY NURSING

As nurses assume more responsibility in nursing, particularly in specialty areas, they often seek help in determining their legal status. Frequently their concern has to do with the scope of practice: are they performing within legal bounds? Negligence, whether in a highly specialized unit, an emergency, or a self-care unit, is still a question of what the reasonably prudent nurse would do. Therefore, although a nurse might look for a specific answer to a specific question, the legal dangers lie in the same set of instances described earlier, simply transposed to another setting.

Nevertheless, there are some areas such as OR, psychiatric, and obstetric units, which have been mentioned, that merit some special attention. Nurses in emergency rooms have particular problems in these days of overcrowding and lack of beds for emergency patients. Policies and procedures for admitting or transferring patients should be in place, but this is not always so. Using nursing judgment is particularly important when hospitals or doctors order the arriving patient to be sent on to another hospital without seeing the patient. The revised (1990) Emergency Medical Treatment and Active Labor Act of 1986 protects patients requiring emergency care, and they should never be told that they cannot be examined or treated unless they pay, or have health insurance.[52] Cushing reports at least two cases where the nurse was found liable for the death of a patient who was not admitted. One involved a 4-month-old infant seriously ill with diarrhea. The court stated that the nurse should have recognized the "unmistakable emergency," and the hospital was held liable for the actions of its agent. In another, the nurse met the ambulance in the courtyard and directed the driver to take the 83-year-old patient with congestive heart failure to another hospital. The court ruled that the patient should at least have been admitted until stabilized.[53] A vast number of other cases are the result of poor physician-nurse communication.

With the increased interest in home health care, more attention is being given to the nurse's liability in providing such care. Among the concerns are the use of equipment (knowing how to operate it, monitor it, and provide associated care, such as suctioning) and teaching the family to use it properly and to be alert for specific problems. Still another concern is knowing how to get action if the patient has an emergency and must be seen by a physician promptly. What can be even more serious is having the family threaten to sue *you* because of something the home health aide has done, like letting the patient fall out of bed. In this case, it is particularly important that aides have proper training, that the duties performed are within the scope of that training, and that they are properly supervised.[54]

Office nurses also have special problems. The most frequent cause for liability is the patient who falls, often from an examining table, and is injured. Equally important is what information the nurse gives to a patient over the phone and how she gives it. The nurse and physician should agree on the type of information that is appropriate.[55]

STANDARD OF CARE

The standard of care basically determines nurses' liability for negligent acts. If this stand-ard is based on what the "reasonably prudent" nurse would do, who makes that judgment? In litigation, it is the judge or jury, based on testimony that could include the following:

1. *Expert witness.* Did the nurse do what was necessary? A nurse with special or appropriate knowledge testifies on what would be expected of a nurse in the defendant's position in like circumstances. The expert witness would have the credentials to validate his or her expertise, but because the opposing side would also produce an equally prestigious expert witness to say what was useful to them, the credibility of that witness on testifying is critical.[56]

2. *Professional literature.* Was the nurse's practice current? The *most current* nursing literature would be examined and perhaps quoted to validate (or invalidate) that the nurse's practice in the situation was totally up-to-date.

3. *Hospital or agency policies.* Were hospital policies, especially nursing policies (in-house law), followed? Example: If side rails were or were not used, was the nurse's action according to hospital policy? On the other hand, if a nurse followed an outdated policy or followed policy without using nursing judgment (according to the expert witness), it could be held against her or him.

4. *Manuals or procedure books.* Did the nurse follow accurately the usual procedure? Example: If the nurse gave an injection that was alleged to have injured the patient, was it given correctly according to the procedure manual?

5. *Drug enclosures or drug reference books.* Did the nurse check for the latest information? Example: If the patient suffered from a drug reaction that the nurse did not perceive, was the information about the potential reaction in a drug reference book, such as the *PDR (Physicians' Desk Reference)*, or a drug insert?

6. *The profession's standards.* Did the nurse behave according to the published ANA or a specialty group's standards?[57]
7. *Licensure.* Did the nurse fulfill her responsibilities according to the legal definition of nursing in the licensure law or the law's rules and regulations? Example: Did she teach a diabetic patient about foot care?

If the judge or jury is satisfied that the standards were met satisfactorily, even if the patient has been injured, the injury that occurred would not be considered the result of the nurse's negligence. Different judgments in different jurisdictions must be expected. Nevertheless, a nurse who knows the profession's standards and practices accordingly is in a much firmer position legally than one who does not.

OTHER TORTS AND CRIMES

The average nurse probably will not get involved in criminal offenses, although in the last several years, a number of nurses have been accused of murder.[58] Nurses, like anyone else, may steal, murder, or break other laws. Crimes most often committed are criminal assault and battery (striking or otherwise physically mistreating or threatening a patient); murder (sometimes in relation to right-to-die principles); and drug offenses. If found guilty of a felony, the nurse will probably also lose her or his license.

Sometimes nurses will be involved in litigation as *accessories*; that is, they are connected with the commission of a crime but did not actually do it themselves, although present and promoting the crime or near enough to assist if necessary.

An *abettor* encourages the commission of a crime but is absent when it is actually committed. The term *accomplice* is similar in meaning to both *accessory* and *abettor*, although a distinction may be made in some jurisdictions. A nurse (or anyone else for that matter) found guilty of any of these crimes may be held equally guilty with the person who commits the crime. However, whether the nurse is a perpetrator, a victim, or simply has to deal with people who are, it is useful to know the definition and scope of the most common criminal offenses. These can be found in most nursing law texts. Several will be discussed here. Not discussed but worth noting are some torts and crimes in which nurses occasionally are involved in their professional lives: *forgery*—fraudulently making or altering a written document or item, such as a will, chart, or check; *kidnapping*—stealing and carrying off a human being; *rape*—illegal or forcible sexual intercourse; and *bribery*—an offer of a reward for doing wrong or for influencing conduct.

Assault and Battery

In general, every time one person touches another in an angry, rude, or insolent manner and every blow or push that is delivered with an intent to injure, or to put the person in fear of injury, constitutes an assault and a battery in the context of criminal law. Legal action can result from any of these acts unless they can be justified or excused.

Also, every attempt to use force and violence with an intent to injure, or put one in fear of injury, constitutes an *assault*, such as striking at a person with or without a weapon; holding up a fist in a threatening attitude near enough to be able to strike; or advancing with a hand uplifted in a threatening manner with intent to strike or put one in fear of being struck, even if the person is stopped before he gets near enough to carry the intention into effect.

A *battery*, as distinguished from an assault, is the actual striking or touching of the body of a man or woman in a violent, angry, rude, or insolent manner. But every laying on of hands is not a battery. The person's intention must be considered. If someone slaps a person on the back in fun or as an act of friendship, for example, it does not constitute a battery, for there is no intent to injure or put the person in fear of injury. To constitute a battery, intent to injure or put one in fear of injury must be accompanied by "unlawful violence." However, the slightest degree of force may constitute violence in the eyes of the law.

As in so many legal matters, the terms used to describe the acts are much less important than the acts themselves as far as the nonlegal public is concerned. In legal proceedings, however, terminology has a significant bearing on the outcome of a case. For example, should a nurse be either the plaintiff or defendant in a case of assault or battery, or both, the terms used might influence considerably the conduct of the case and the settlement made. In day-to-day practice, however, the nurse need only be aware of the acts related to nursing that might conceivably be considered as assault or battery, or both, and therefore subject to legal action. Assault and battery in the context of civil law is discussed in Chap. 22.

Defamation, Slander, Libel

As is true of so many legal terms, there is some overlapping of meaning and interpretation of the terms *defamation, slander*, and *libel*.[59] In general, however, it is correct to consider *defamation* as the most inclusive because it covers any communication that is seriously detrimental to another person's reputation. If the communication is oral, it is technically called *slander*; if written or shown in pictures, effigies, or signs (without just cause or excuse), it is called *libel*. All three are considered wrongful acts (torts) under the law, and a person convicted of one or more of these in criminal or civil court is ordered to make amends, usually by paying the defamed person a compensatory fee.

In both slander and libel, a third person must be involved. For example, one person can make all kinds of derogatory statements directly to another without getting in trouble with the law *unless* overheard by a third person. Then the remarks become slanderous. Moreover, the third person must be able to understand what has been said. If it is spoken in an unfamiliar language, for example, it is not slanderous under the law. Likewise a person can write anything

she or he wishes to another, and the communication will not be considered libelous unless it is read and understood by a third person. A malicious and false statement made by one person to another about a third person also comprises slander.

Statements of a strong and uncomplimentary nature are not necessarily slanderous or libelous. They must be false, damaging to the offended person's reputation, and tending to subject him to public contempt and ridicule. The best and often the only defense allowed for the person accused of slander or libel—under the law—is proof that she or he told the truth in whatever type of communication used.

It is evident that there are many "if's" "and's" and "but's," associated with defamation, slander, and libel. Wise nurses avoid becoming embroiled in such litigations by being extremely careful in what they say or write about anyone. They also proceed with caution when they are the victims of slander and libel, knowing that litigation is expensive and time-consuming and, in many instances, hardly worth the trouble. On the other hand, they should not be overly meek in accepting unfair and untrue statements about them that are likely to adversely affect their reputations and future in nursing, as well as the good name of nursing in the community. There have been documented cases in which nurses were slandered by a physician, for instance, and collected damages.

Homicide and Suicide

Homicide means killing a person by any means whatsoever. It is not necessarily a crime. If it is unquestionably an accident, it is called *excusable homicide*. If it is done in self-defense or in discharging a legal duty, such as taking a prisoner, putting a condemned person to death, or preserving the peace, it is termed *justifiable homicide*. The accused must be able to prove justification, however.

Criminal homicide is either murder or manslaughter. *Murder* means the unlawful killing of one person by another of sound mind and with malice aforethought. It may be by direct violence, such as shooting or strangling, or by indirect violence, such as slow poisoning. Murder is usually divided into two degrees: *first degree* when it is premeditated and carried out deliberately; and *second degree* when it is not planned beforehand but is nonetheless performed with an intent to kill. In both, there must be a design to effect death.

Suicide is considered criminal if the person is sane and of an age of discretion at the time of his action. An unsuccessful attempt to commit suicide is a misdemeanor under the law. If there is doubt as to whether a person has committed suicide, a court of law usually presumes that he has not, although this judgment may be reversed by evidence to the contrary. A person who encourages another to commit suicide is guilty of murder if the suicide is effected. Statutes vary from state to state.

As a professional person, it is not unusual for a nurse to become implicated in cases of murder and suicide, usually associated with patients. Following are a few suggestions for keeping as free of legal involvement as possible:

1. Any indication on the part of any patient or employee that she or he has suicidal tendencies should be taken seriously and reported to the appropriate person.
2. Generally, a patient with known suicidal inclinations should not be left alone unless completely protected from self-harm by restraints or confinement.
3. Items that a depressed person might use for suicidal purposes should be kept out of reach.
4. Observations should be accurately reported on the patient's chart.
5. Help should be sought for individuals or their families immediately upon becoming aware of suicidal tendencies.
6. Cooperation with the police and hospital authorities guarding a patient who is accused of homicide is important.
7. Unethical discussions of a homicide case involving a patient or employee should be avoided.
8. Complete and accurate records of all facts that might have a bearing on the legal aspects of the case should be kept.

GOOD SAMARITAN LAWS

The enactment of good samaritan laws in many states exempts doctors and nurses (and sometimes others) from civil liability when they give emergency care in "good faith" with "due care" or without "gross negligence." The first state to pass such a law was California in 1959; in 1963, California enacted such legislation specifically for nurses. By 1979, all states and the District of Columbia had good samaritan laws, not all including nurses in the coverage. No court has yet interpreted these statutes, and prior to their enactment, no case held a doctor or nurse liable for negligence in care at the site of an emergency. The law is intended to encourage assistance without fear of legal liability. As far as the law is concerned, there is no obligation or duty to render aid or assistance in an emergency. Only by statutory law can the rendering of such assistance be made obligatory.

RNs engaged in occupational health nursing are likely to be called upon to give first-aid treatment to patients with wounds and other injuries as part of their job responsibility. Such emergency treatment in a health care setting is not covered under the good samaritan laws. These nurses, just like nurses in an emergency room, should take every precaution to make sure they are operating within the bounds of legally authorized practice for nurses in their position.

Because of the lack of clarity of terms and the many differences in the law from state to state, many health professionals are still reluctant to give emergency assistance.[60] One lawyer gives this advice: don't give aid unless you know what you're doing; stick to the basics of first aid; offer to help, but make it clear that you won't interfere if the victim or family prefers to wait for other help; don't draw any medical or diagnostic conclusions; don't leave a victim you've begun to assist until you can turn his care over to an equally competent person; whether you do or do not volunteer your services, be absolutely certain to call or have someone else call for a physician or emergency medical service immediately.[61]

DRUG CONTROL

In 1914, the United States adopted an anti-narcotic law—the *Harrison Narcotic Act*, to be administered by a bureau of narcotics within the Department of the Treasury. It was amended frequently to meet the demands of changing times. For example, in 1956, a strong *Narcotic Control Act* was passed, and in 1961 a new law gave federal authorities broader control of drug preparations containing small amounts of narcotics. This came about largely because teenagers were reported to have become addicted by taking preparations such as cough medicines containing a small percentage of narcotics, which they could obtain without a prescription. As noted in Chap. 19, the *Comprehensive Drug Abuse and Control Act* of 1970 (*Controlled Substance Act*) replaced virtually all earlier federal laws dealing with narcotics, stimulants, depressants, and hallucinogens. Sections in the law prohibit nurses from prescribing controlled substances, but they may administer drugs at the direction of legalized practitioners (who are registered). All registrants must follow strict controls and procedures against theft and diversion of controlled substances.[62] New state laws are based on the federal law, although there are variations.

Some other drugs subject to federal or state control, or both, are poisons, caustics, corrosives, methyl or wood alcohol, drugs for sexually transmitted disease treatment, and amphetamines. Marijuana has been subject to changing legal patterns. In many states, its use but not its sale has been decriminalized. Barbiturates, principally used therapeutically as sedatives, but also a part of the illegal drug scene, have been state regulated through the so-called lullaby laws—aimed originally at the legitimate user, not the addict. New drugs are also being given closer scrutiny because of misuse and consequent dangerous effects.

Knowledge of the laws controlling the use of drugs will help you to understand the reasons for the policies and procedures established by an institution or agency for the mutual welfare of the employer, employee, and patient. It also helps you to keep free of legal involvements and to intelligently direct and advise others whom you may supervise or who may look to you for guidance in such matters. Nurses should all be alert to changes in drug laws on either the state or national level.

LIABILITY (MALPRACTICE) INSURANCE

Almost all lawyers in the health field now agree that nurses should carry their own malpractice or professional liability insurance, whether or not their employer's insurance includes them. The employer's insurance is intended primarily to protect the employer; the nurse is protected only to the extent needed for that primary purpose. It is quite conceivable that the employer might settle out of court, without consulting the nurse, to the nurse's disadvantage. The nurse has no control and no choice of lawyer.[63] There are a number of other limitations. The nurse is not covered for anything beyond the job in the place of employment during the hours of employment. If the nurse alone is sued and the hospital is not, the hospital has no obligation to provide legal protection (and may choose not to). Moreover, if the nurse carries no personal liability insurance, there is the possibility of subrogation. Should there be criminal charges, the employer or insurance carrier may choose to deny legal assistance, or the kind offered could be inadequate. A nurse must remember that no matter how trivial, how unfounded a charge might be, a legal defense is necessary and often costly, aside from the possibility of being found liable and having to pay damages.[64]

Professional liability insurance should be bought with some care so that adequate coverage is provided. The most important distinction to be made in selecting insurance is whether it is on an "occurrence based" or a "claims made" basis. If the insurance policy is allowed to lapse, an incident that occurred at the time of coverage will be covered in an occurrence based policy, but not on a claims made policy. The latter may be less expensive but will require almost continuous coverage, which might be a problem for a nurse planning to take time out for child rearing or for one close to retirement. Benefits usually include paying any sum awarded as damages, including medical costs, paying the cost of attorneys, and paying the bond required if appealing an adverse decision. Some policies also pay damages for injury arising out of acts of the insured as a member of an accreditation board or committee of a hospital or professional society, or when a nurse gives advice or care to a neighbor or friend, personal liability (such as slander, assault, libel), and personal injury and medical payments (not related to the individual's professional practice).

Here are some questions you should ask:

1. What does this insurance cover and at what cost?
2. What will the insurance company do if I'm sued?
3. How are the terms defined?
4. How long is a policy in effect?
5. What are the exclusions?
6. What happens if I'm involved in an incident?[65]

Generally speaking, an ANA or state association policy is the best buy. Until a few years ago, nurse-midwives and nurse practitioners had no difficulty buying malpractice insurance. Then, in 1985, in response to the general malpractice crisis, the American College of Nurse-Midwives (ACNM) was notified by its insurer that its members would no longer be covered. Actually there were no data to justify this action, even

though it would effectively put nurse-midwives out of business. Finally, after intense efforts, a consortium of insurance companies and ACNM began to provide the insurance. It was noted by insurance journals that the claims experience was very favorable. In like fashion, this kind of action was threatened against NPs, who also have had few claims against them. In response, ANA made arrangements with a new insurance carrier that covers all nurses, including NPs and nurses in private practice (the only one that does). Premiums depend on the position of the nurse. Only nurse anesthetists and nurse-midwives are not covered.

IN COURT: THE DUE PROCESS OF LAW

Yes, you can be sued. What happens if you become involved in litigation? What steps should you take to try to make sure that the case will be handled to the best advantage throughout? The answers to these questions will depend upon (1) whether you are accused of committing the tort or crime; (2) whether you are an accessory, through actual participation or observance; (3) whether you are the person against whom the act was committed; or (4) whether you appear as an expert witness.

Assuming that this is a civil case, five distinct steps are taken:

> **(1) the filing of a document called a complaint by a person called the *plaintiff* who contends that his legal rights have been infringed by the conduct of one or more other persons called *defendants*; (2) the written response of the defendants accused of having violated the legal rights of the plaintiff, termed an *answer*; (3) pretrial activities of both parties designed to elicit all the facts of the situation, termed *discovery*;[66] (4) the *trial* of the case, in which all the relevant facts are presented to the judge or jury for decisions; and (5) *appeal* from a decision by a party who contends that the decision was wrongly made.[67]**

The majority of persons who are asked to appear as witnesses during a hearing accept voluntarily. Others refuse and must be subpoenaed. A *subpoena* is a writ or order in the name of the court, referee, or other person authorized by law to issue the same, which requires the attendance of a witness at a trial or hearing under a penalty for failure. Cases involving the care of patients often necessitate producing hospital records, x-rays, and photographs as evidence. A subpoena requiring a witness to bring this type of evidence with him contains a clause to that effect and is termed a *subpoena duces tecum*.

The plaintiff, defendant, and witnesses may be asked to make a *deposition*, an oral interrogation answering various questions about the issue concerned. It is given under oath and taken in writing before a judicial officer or attorney.[68,69] You may be asked the same questions as a witness. A witness has certain rights, including the right to refuse to testify as to privileged communication (extended to the nurse in only a few states) and the protection against self-incrimination afforded by the Fifth Amendment to the Constitution. The judge and jury usually do not expect a person on trial or serving as a witness to remember all of the details of a situation. Witnesses in malpractice suits are permitted to refer to the patient's record, which, of course, they should have reviewed with the attorney before the trial.

Only under serious circumstances is someone accused (and convicted) of *perjury*, which means making a false statement under oath or one that she or he neither knows nor believes to be true.

There are certain guidelines on testifying that are the same whether serving as an expert or other witness or if the nurse is the defendant:

1.   Be prepared; review the deposition, the chart, technical and clinical knowledge of the disease or condition; discuss with the lawyer potential questions; educate the lawyer as to what points should be made. Trials are adversary procedures that are intended to probe, question, and explore all aspects of the issue.
2.   Dress appropriately; enunciate clearly.
3.   Behave appropriately: keep calm, be courteous, even if insulted; don't be sarcastic or angry; take your time (a cross-examiner attorney may try to put you in a poor light).
4.   Give adequate and appropriate information: if you can't remember, notes or the data source, such as the chart, can be checked. Answer fully, but don't volunteer additional information not asked for.
5.   Don't use technical terminology, or, if use is necessary, translate it into lay terms.
6.   Don't feel incompetent; don't get on the defensive; be decisive.
7.   Don't be obviously partisan (unless you're the defendant).
8.   Keep all materials; the decision may be appealed.

In the expert witness role,[70] the same precepts hold, but in addition the nurse should present her or his credentials, degrees, research, honors, whatever else is pertinent, without modesty; the opposing expert witness will certainly do so.

Expert witnesses are paid for preparation time, pretrial conferences, consultations, and testifying. Nurses are beginning to act officially in this capacity more frequently, and several state nurses' associations accept applications for those interested in placement on an expert witness panel, screen applicants in a given field for a specific case, submit a choice of names to attorneys requesting such information, and have developed guidelines and CE for nurse expert witnesses.

Should you be sued, here are some tips for defending yourself:

*   Cut all communication with the claimant; simply tell whoever contacts you that your insurer will be in touch. (Then find out why they haven't been already.)
*   Educate the insurer; claims adjusters may know little about nursing.
*   Keep tabs on the claim. Don't be afraid to ask questions.
*   Be sure that your claim is supervised adequately. You have a right to ask that it be handled by an experienced and attentive professional.

- Seek input on settlement decisions. You might not have the right, but you can ask your insurer to check with you before making an offer.
- Remember that the defense attorney is *your* attorney. If you really think his or her qualifications are inadequate, ask for a change.
- Dictate all memories of the patient to the attorney. Do it as soon as possible, but not until an attorney has been assigned to your case, or your information may not be considered "privileged."
- Retrieve medical records. You have access if you still work at the same place and can get access before the attorney does.
- Review the records.
- Compile a list of experts; the case may hinge on getting the best. (Although in some courts, physicians have been allowed as expert witnesses on a nursing case, ordinarily it should be the nurse/s who are most knowledgeable about the type of situation involved.)
- Have a reference list available on the topics related to nursing care of the patient involved so that you have backup for your actions.
- Speak up in court; you must project self-confidence.[71]

Other attorneys also point out that you shouldn't talk to anyone about the case at your hospital except the risk manager, or with anyone involved in any way with the plaintiff, or to reporters. Certainly don't hide any information from your attorney, and never, never alter the patient's record.

RISK MANAGEMENT

No matter how strong the defense, everyone agrees that prevention is better than any suit. Therefore, hospitals have now adopted risk-management programs in which nurses are very much involved, as part of the team and also sometimes in one of the risk-management positions, including patient representative or advocate. Risk management must be a team effort involving everyone.

Risk management initiatives are now required by JCAHO and more and more by state legislation. The purpose is not only to protect the interest of the hospital and its personnel but also to improve the quality of patient care. Risk management means taking steps to control the possibility that a patient will complain and minimizing any risks *before* complaints are filed. Nurses are often involved in risk management, which includes focusing on the review and improvement of employee guidelines, personnel policies, incident reports, physician-nurse relationships, safety policies, patient records, research guidelines, and anything else that might be a factor in legal suits.[72]

Nevertheless, patient injuries do occur. In case of patient injury, most hospitals and health agencies require completion of an "incident report." The purpose is to document the incident accurately for remedial and correctional use by the hospital or agency, for insurance information, and sometimes for legal reasons. The wording should be chosen to avoid the implication of blame and should be totally objective and complete: what happened to the patient; what was done; what his condition is. The incident report may or may not be discoverable, depending on the state's law. It is considered a business record, not part of the patient's chart, but some courts rule that it is not privileged information. The incident *must* be just as accurately recorded in the patient's chart. This kind of omission casts doubt on the nurse's honesty if litigation occurs. However, the fact that an incident report was filed should not be charted.

Appropriate behavior by nurses and other personnel is often a key factor as to whether or not the patient or family sues after an incident, regardless of injury. Maintaining a good rapport and giving honest explanations as needed is very important.

All of this involves nurses. For individual nurses who have specific concerns about the legal aspects of their practice, it may be possible to get some information from the employing agency's legal counsel or state licensing board. Keeping abreast of legal trends is always necessary. Observing some basic principles will also help to avert problems:

1. Know your licensure law.
2. Don't do what you don't know how to do. (Learn how, if necessary.)
3. Keep your practice updated; CE is essential.
4. Use self-assessment, peer evaluation, audits, and supervisor's evaluations as guidelines for improving practice and follow up on criticisms and knowledge and skill gaps.
5. Don't be careless.
6. Practice interdependently; communicate with others.
7. Record accurately, objectively, and completely; don't erase.
8. Delegate safely and legally; know the preparation and abilities of those you supervise.
9. Help develop appropriate policies and procedures (in-house law).
10. Carry liability insurance.

The ANA also points out that nurses have a stake in tort reform, since many of the suggested changes do not consider nurses and the changes in their status and responsibilities.[73] It is clear that nurses' involvement with legal issues extends beyond the workplace, and also involves the nurse as a citizen.

REFERENCES

1. Hemelt M, Mackert ME: *Dynamics of Law in Nursing and Health Care*. Reston, VA: Reston Publishing, 1978, p 3.
2. Feutz-Harter S: *Nursing and the Law*, 4th ed. Eau Claire, WI: Professional Education Systems, 1991, pp 142–143.
3. Calfee B: *Nurses in the Courtroom*, Cleveland: ARC Publishing, 1993, pp 197–198.
4. Ibid, pp 214–216.
5. Aiken T, Catalano J: *Legal Ethical and Political Issues in Nursing*. Philadelphia: Davis, 1994, pp 166–167.
6. Jenkins S: The myth of vicarious liability. *J Nurse-Midwifery* 39:98–106, March 1994.
7. Fiesta J: The evolving doctrine of corporate liability. *Nurs Mgt* 25:17–18, March 1994.
8. Mehlman M: Assuring the quality of medical care: The impact of outcome measurement and practice standards. *Law Med Health Care* 18:4, Winter 1990.
9. Creighton H: *Law Every Nurse Should Know*, 5th ed. Philadelphia: Saunders, 1986, p 141.
10. Feutz-Harter, op cit, pp 20–21.
11. Calfee, op cit, pp 128–129.
12. Ibid, pp 210–211.
13. Northrop C, Kelly M: *Legal Issues in Nursing*. St Louis: Mosby, 1987, pp 49–50.
14. Aiken and Catalano, op cit, pp 192–93.
15. Cournoyer C: *The Nurse Manager and the Law*. Rockville, MD: Aspen, 1989, pp 148–149.
16. Horsley J: Why it's harder to defend nurses now. *RN* 9:56–59, November 1986.
17. Feutz-Harter, op cit, pp 18–19.
18. Northrop C: Current case law involving nurses: Lessons for practitioners, managers and educators. *Nurs Outlook* 37:296, November–December 1989.
19. Cushing M: Law and orders. *Am J Nurs* 90:29–32, May 1990.
20. Murchison I, Nichols T: *Legal Foundations of Nursing Practice*. New York: Macmillan, 1970, pp 139–143.
21. Northrop (1989), op cit.
22. Campazzi B: Nurses, nursing and malpractice litigation: 1967–1977. *Nurs Adm Q* 5:1–18, Fall 1980.
23. Lupia I: Who gets sued and why: Malpractice trends and issues update. *NJ Nurse* 24:14–15, July–August 1994.
24. Moniz D: The legal danger of written protocols and standards of practice. *Nurse Pract* 17:58–60, September 1992.
25. Lupia, op cit, p 14.
26. Advanced practice discipline survey results. *Issues* 14:1, 4–5, 10, 2, 1993.
27. Calfee, op cit, pp 40–41.
28. Tammelleo D: The high cost of not paying attention. *RN* 10:61–62, March 1987.
29. Legal questions: dose dilemma. *Nurs 94* 24:23, June 1994.

30. Carson W: What you should know about physician verbal orders. *Am Nurs* 26:30–31, March 1994.

31. Fiesta J: Failure to assess. *Nurs Mgt* 24:16–17, September 1993.

32. Following hospital policy: A legal risk? *Nurs 94* 24:26, May 1994.

33. Doctor's IV order: Edging toward liability. *Nurs 94* 24:30, April 1994.

34. Cushing M: Million-dollar errors. *Am J Nurs* 87:435–436, 420, April 1987.

35. Katz B: Reporting and review of patient care: The nurse's responsibility. *Law Med Health Care* 11:76–79, April 1983.

36. Tammelleo D: When a phone call is your liability lifeline. *RN* 12:69–70, February 1989.

37. Calfee, op cit, pp 83–84.

38. Greenlaw J: What to do if your supervisor orders a "cover-up." *RN* 45:81–82, October 1982.

39. Fiesta J: Charting—one national standard, one form. *Nurs Mgt* 24:22–24, June 1993.

40. Calfee B: Seven things you should never chart. *Nurs 94* 24:43, March 1994.

41. Cushing (1990), op cit, p 29.

42. Tammelleo, op cit, p 61.

43. Cushing M: Short staffing on trial. *Am J Nurs* 88:161–162, February 1988.

44. Carroll P, Maher V: Legal issues in the management of central venous catheters. *AD Clin Care* 5:11, July–August 1990.

45. Rhodes AM: Judging nursing practice. *MCN* 14:123, March–April 1987.

46. Smith L: Those medication error dilemmas! *AD Clin Care* 5:50–51, September–October 1990.

47. Cushing M: Drug errors can be bitter pills. *Am J Nurs* 86:895, 899, August 1986.

48. Feutz-Harter, op cit, p 89.

49. Lippman H: Rx: Error-free meds. *RN* 56:65–66, June 1993.

50. Cushing C: Two caveats: Listen and use your knowledge of science. *Am J Nurs* 89:1434, November 1989.

51. Fiesta J: Premature discharge. *Nurs Mgt* 25:17–20, April 1994.

52. Tammelleo A: How the law protects emergency patients. *RN* 55:67–68, October 1992.

53. Cushing M: In case of emergency. *Am J Nurs* 88:1175–1177, September 1988.

54. Sullivan G: Home care: More autonomy, more legal risks. *RN* 57:63–69, May 1994.

55. Fiesta J: Liability issues for the office nurse. *Nurs Mgt* 23:17–18, January 1992.

56. Rhodes AM: The expert witness. *MCN* 14:49, January–February 1989.

57. Fiesta J: Legal aspects—standards of care, part II. *Nurs Mgt* 24:16–17, August 1993.

58. Yorker B: Nurses accused of murder. *Am J Nurs* 88:7–13, October 1988.

59. Klein C: Defamation: Libel and slander. *Nurse Pract* 11:49–50, January 1986.

60. Northrop C: How good samaritan laws do and don't protect you. *Nurs 90* 20:50–51, February 1990.

61. Horsley J: You can't escape the good samaritan role—or its risks. *RN* 44:87–92, May 1981.

62. Creighton, op cit, pp 237–238.

63. Think twice about relying on employer liability coverage. *Am Nurse* 25:35, 40, March 1993.

64. Brooke P: Shopping for liability insurance. *Am J Nurs* 89:171–172, February 1989.

65. Northrop C: 6 questions about malpractice insurance. *Nurs 87* 17:97–98, August 1987.

66. Rhodes AM: Nursing and the discovery process. *MCN* 13:53, January–February 1988.

67. Cushing M: How a suit starts. *Am J Nurs* 85:655–656, June 1985.

68. Chenowith S: Tips on giving pre-trial testimony. *RN* 8:67–68, February 1985.

69. Rhodes AM: Defining depositions. *MCN* 13:89, March–April 1988.

70. Guido G: Be an expert witness for critical care nursing. *AACN Crit Issues* 5:66–70, February 1994.

71. Quinley K: Twelve tips for defending yourself in a malpractice suit. *Am J Nurs* 90:37–38, 40, January 1990.

72. Harrison B, Cole D: Managing risk to minimize liability. *Caring* 13:26–30, May 1994.

73. Nurses have a stake in tort reform. *Am Nurse* 24:29, March 1992.

Health Care and the Rights of People

THE CIVIL RIGHTS MOVEMENT of the late 1950s and early 1960s had a profound effect on American society. Not only were there major and obvious changes in public policy, but it seems American citizens learned to *think* differently. We learned to think and speak much more in terms of individual *rights*.

The consumer movement (described in Chap. 6) was an outgrowth of the civil rights movement. It further led us all to think in terms of our *rights* as purchasers or users of goods and services. Especially as health care has come to be perceived as an essential public good upon which all members of the community have legitimate claims, it seems natural that Americans increasingly speak about health care in the language of "rights."

Until recently, people felt helpless in their patient role—and small wonder. Stripped of their individuality as well as their belongings, they are thrust into an alien environment where they feel that they have little control over what happens to them. They are surrounded by unidentified faces and unidentifiable equipment. Their privacy is invaded. Their dignity is lost. They hesitate to complain or criticize for fear of reprisals from the staff. They may be reluctant to press for answers to their questions because, too often, the idea that the doctor or nurse is too busy is conveyed. Underlying all is fear for their health, and even their lives.

Now, an increasing number of consumers are no longer willing to put up with this state of affairs, will no longer accept the traditional role

of "good" patient: the one who does as he's told and asks no awkward questions. The frequent denial of their fundamental rights—among them, to courtesy, privacy, and, most of all, information—has brought about the ultimate form of patient rebellion—malpractice suits. More than twenty years ago, a national Commission on Medical Malpractice declared that "to ignore these and other rights of the patient is both to betray simple humanity and to invite dissatisfaction that may lead to malpractice suits."[1] The 1982 President's Commission for the Study of Ethical Problems in Medicine and Biomedical and Behavioral Research (hereafter called the President's Commission) made equally strong statements and recommendations.

PATIENT RIGHTS

Most of the rights about which patients are concerned are theirs legally as well as morally and have been so established by common law. They are also stated in the codes of ethics of both physicians and nurses (although, to be honest, much is stated by implication and thus open to considerable personal interpretation). Moreover, they closely reiterate the four basic consumer rights President John F. Kennedy enunciated in his consumer message to Congress in 1962:

1. The right to safety
2. The right to be informed

3. The right to choose
4. The right to be heard

Since the well-publicized American Hospital Association's (AHA) "A Patient's Bill of Rights" was presented in 1972 (Exhibit 22-1), a spate of such "rights" statements has followed: for the disabled, the mentally ill, the retarded, the old, the young, the pregnant, the handicapped, and the dying. By the end of the 1970s, many state legislatures had made these statements the basis of new statutory law.

The vagueness of the AHA statement and the inability to force compliance without legal intervention have made it a butt for some bitter humor. George Annas, an attorney in the health field, quotes a commentator who likened the document to a fox telling the chickens what their rights are. Nevertheless, commenting on the required posting in hospitals of the Minnesota bill, Annas noted that the "trend toward publishing rights is important because it not only reminds people that they have rights, it also encourages them to assert them and to make further demands."[2] It might also remind the staff, for there is some evidence that they, too, are often unaware of the patient's rights, even legal rights.

In 1974, new Medicare regulations for skilled nursing facilities included a section on patient's rights. Just how disgraceful the violation of rights of this captive group was might be judged when reviewing the rights: the right to send and receive mail; the right to have spouses share rooms if both are patients, or allow privacy for visits; the right to have restraints used only if authorized by the physician and only for a limited time; the right to use one's own clothes and possessions, as space permits; and the right to require both written permission by the patient, and accounting, for management of his or her funds. And, as in other laws, patients had to be told what their rights were.

Since that time the continuing scandals involving violation of patients' and residents' rights in so many long-term care (LTC) facilities have resulted in legislation in various guises, usually requirements under Medicare and Medicaid. For the LTC facilities not certified, there is still some control by state regulation. The regulations on rights are enacted and enforced erratically, sometimes depending on the political climate. However, now nursing home residents have the right to talk directly to state surveyors, who ensure that the facilities meet the standards set by the Health Care Financing Administration (HCFA), which include rights statements. Nursing homes also may have a volunteer ombudsman and teaching nursing homes have students and faculty who observe what goes on. Such facilities are not usually problem sites. Some states have also given legal attention to the rights of residents in continuing care communities, including such aspects as complete disclosure of costs and other financial data, posting of the last state examination report, freedom to form a resident's organization, and other mechanisms to avoid fraud and deception.

Many rights advocates have little enthusiasm for most of these declarations, particularly the AHA statement, as they tend to hedge about some or many of the rights, ethical or legal. This is probably because few if any evolved out of some massive "goodness of heart" by the institutions or by government. The AHA bill, for instance, came about because of pressures from consumer advocates in health centers affiliated with larger general hospitals, where their clientele, mostly black and Hispanic, were mistreated even when treated. They were subjected to long waiting times, never seeing the same physician twice, little or no explanation of the patient's diagnosis or treatment, loss of confidentiality of records, no real effort to get *informed* consent, multiple student access without consent, involvement in research without consent, and overall loss of dignity. This history is clearly reflected in the AHA statement. Therefore, because the neighborhood health centers' bills of patients' rights were keyed to the basic agenda of the Office of Economic Opportunity (OEO), that is, raising the personal expectations of the people of those communities, the stage

Exhibit 22-1	A Patient's Bill of Rights

Introduction

Effective health care requires collaboration between patients and physicians and other health care professionals. Open and honest communication, respect for personal and professional values, and sensitivity to differences are integral to optimal patient care. As the setting for the provision of health services, hospitals must provide a foundation for understanding and respecting the rights and responsibilities of patients, their families, physicians, and other caregivers. Hospitals must ensure a health care ethic that respects the role of patients in decision making about treatment choices and other aspects of their care. Hospitals must be sensitive to cultural, racial, linguistic, religious, age, gender, and other differences as well as the needs of persons with disabilities.

The American Hospital Association presents *A Patient's Bill of Rights* with the expectation that it will contribute to more effective patient care and be supported by the hospital on behalf of the institution, its medical staff, employees, and patients. The American Hospital Association encourages health care institutions to tailor this bill of rights to their patient community by translating and/or simplifying the language of this bill of rights as may be necessary to ensure that patients and their families understand their rights and responsibilities.

Bill of Rights*

1. The patient has the right to considerate and respectful care.
2. The patient has the right to and is encouraged to obtain from physicians and other direct caregivers relevant, current, and understandable information concerning diagnosis, treatment, and prognosis.

   Except in emergencies when the patient lacks decision-making capacity and the need for treatment is urgent, the patient is entitled to the opportunity to discuss and request information related to the specific procedures and/or treatments, the risks involved, the possible length of recuperation, and the medically reasonable alternatives and their accompanying risks and benefits.

   Patients have the right to know the identity of physicians, nurses, and others involved in their care, as well as when those involved are students, residents, or other trainees. The patient also has the right to know the immediate and long-term financial implications of treatment choices, insofar as they are known.
3. The patient has the right to make decisions about the plan of care prior to and during the course of treatment and to refuse a recommended treatment or plan of care to the extent permitted by law and hospital policy and to be informed of the medical consequences of this action. In case of such refusal, the patient is entitled to other appropriate care and services that the hospital provides or transfer to another hospital. The hospital should notify patients of any policy that might affect patient choice within the institution.
4. The patient has the right to have an advance directive (such as a living will, health care proxy, or durable power of attorney for health care) concerning treatment or designating a surrogate decision maker with the expectation that the hospital will honor the intent of that directive to the extent permitted by law and hospital policy.

   Health care institutions must advise patients of their rights under state law and hospital policy to make informed medical choices, ask if the patient has an advance directive, and include that information in patient records. The patient has the right to timely information about hospital policy that may limit its ability to implement fully a legally valid advance directive.
5. The patient has the right to every consideration of his privacy. Case discussion, consultation, examination, and treatment should be conducted so as to protect each patient's privacy.

*These rights can be exercised on the patient's behalf by a designated surrogate or proxy decision maker if the patient lacks decision-making capacity, is legally incompetent, or is a minor.

6. The patient has the right to expect that all communications and records pertaining to his/her care should be treated as confidential by the hospital, except in cases such as suspected abuse and public health hazards when reporting is permitted or required by law. The patient has the right to expect that the hospital will emphasize the confidentiality of this information when it releases it to any other parties entitled to review information in these records.

7. The patient has the right to review the records pertaining to his/her medical care and to have the information explained or interpreted as necessary, except when restricted by law.

8. The patient has the right to expect that, within its capacity and policies, a hospital will make reasonable response to the request of a patient for appropriate and medically indicated care and services. The hospital must provide evaluation, service, and/or referral as indicated by the urgency of the case. When medically appropriate and legally permissible, or when a patient has so requested, a patient may be transferred to another facility. The institution to which the patient is to be transferred must first have accepted the patient for transfer. The patient must also have the benefit of complete information and explanation concerning the need for, risks, benefits, and alternatives to such a transfer.

9. The patient has the right to ask and be informed of the existence of business relationships among the hospital, educational institutions, other health care providers, or payers that may influence the patient's treatment and care.

10. The patient has the right to consent to or decline to participate in proposed research studies or human experimentation affecting his care and treatment or requiring direct patient involvement, and to have those studies fully explained prior to consent. A patient who declines to participate in research or experimentation is entitled to the most effective care that the hospital can otherwise provide.

11. The patient has the right to expect reasonable continuity of care when appropriate and to be informed by physicians and other caregivers of available and realistic patient care options when hospital care is no longer appropriate.

12. The patient has the right to be informed of hospital policies and practices that relate to patient care, treatment, and responsibilities. The patient has the right to be informed of available resources for resolving disputes, grievances, and conflicts, such as ethics committees, patient representatives, or other mechanisms available in the institution. The patient has the right to be informed of the hospital's charges for services and available payment methods.

The collaborative nature of health care requires that patients, or their families/surrogates, participate in their care. The effectiveness of care and patient satisfaction with the course of treatment depend, in part, on the patient fulfilling certain responsibilities. Patients are responsible for providing information about past illnesses, hospitalizations, medications, and other matters related to health status. To participate effectively in decision making, patients must be encouraged to take responsibility for requesting additional information or clarification about their health status or treatment when they do not fully understand information and instructions. Patients are also responsible for ensuring that the health care institution has a copy of their written advance directive if they have one. Patients are responsible for informing their physicians and other caregivers if they anticipate problems in following prescribed treatment.

Patients should also be aware of the hospital's obligation to be reasonably efficient and equitable in providing care to other patients and the community. The hospital's rules and regulations are designed to help the hospital meet this obligation. Patients and their families are responsible for making reasonable accommodations to the needs of the hospital, other patients, medical staff, and hospital employees. Patients are responsible for providing necessary information for insurance claims and for working with the hospital to make payment arrangements, when necessary.

A person's health depends on much more than health care services. Patients are responsible for recognizing the impact of their lifestyle on their personal health.

was set for a consumer assault on hospitals. The various arms of government followed, sometimes for political purposes.

Some statements are better than others, but Annas's Model Patient Bill of Rights aimed at all facilities is indeed a model, covering many of the loopholes in the various institutions' statements. Recognizing that most people are in health care facilities because they have a debilitating health problem and therefore are probably not as aggressive about assuring their rights as they might otherwise be, the final statement in the model recognizes the right of all patients to have 24-hour-a-day access to a patients' rights advocate to assert or protect the rights set out in this document.[3]

It would seem that consumer action has some ongoing effect on patient rights. Annas says that the patients' rights movement is as slow as a glacier, equally relentless in changing the landscape, but ultimately healthy.[4] In addition to the organizations built around specific populations and diseases (children; AIDS), there is one national patient rights organization, the Peoples' Medical Society. These groups generally provide excellent information. A list with addresses is found in Annas's *The Rights of Patients*, as well as many other useful resources.

INFORMED CONSENT

For years, when patients have been admitted to hospitals, they signed a frequently unread universal consent form that almost literally gave the physician, his associates, and the hospital carte blanche in determining the patient's care. There was some rationale for this because civil suits for battery (unlawful touching) could theoretically be filed as a result of giving routine care such as baths. Patients undergoing surgery or some complex, dangerous treatment were asked to sign a separate form, usually stating something to the effect that permission was granted to the physician and/or his colleagues to perform the operation or treatment. Just how much the patient knew about the hows and whys of the surgery, the dangers and the alternatives, depended on the patient's assertiveness in asking questions and demanding answers and the physician's willingness to provide information. Nurses were taught *never* to answer those questions, but to suggest, "Ask your doctor." Health professionals, and especially physicians, took the attitude, "We know best and will decide for you."

Many patients probably still enter treatment and undergo a variety of tests and even surgery without a clear understanding of the nature of the condition they have and what can be done about it. Although they may very well be receiving care that is medically acceptable, they have no real part in deciding what that care should be. Most physicians have believed that anything more than a superficial explanation is unnecessary, for the patient should "trust" the doctor. Kalisch has elaborated this point, calling it *Aesculapian authority*.[5] Yet the patient has always had the right to make decisions about his own body. A case was heard as early as 1905 on surgery without consent, and the classic legal decision is that of Judge Cardoza (*Schloendorff vs. The Society of New York Hospital*, 211 NY.125, 129-130, 105 NE 92, 93-1914): "Every human being of adult years and sound mind has a right to determine what shall be done with his own body."

A noted hospital law book later stated:

> **It is an established principle of law that every human being of adult years and sound mind has the right to determine what shall be done with his own body. He may choose whether to be treated or not and to what extent, no matter how necessary the medical care, nor how imminent the danger to his life or health if he fails to submit to treatment.[6]**

In nonlegal terms, informed consent simply means that a doctor cannot "touch or treat a patient until the doctor has given the patient some basic information about what the doctor proposes to do, and the patient has agreed to the proposed treatment or procedure."[7] In what is still considered the most important study of informed consent, the President's Commission concludes that "ethically valid consent is a process of shared decision-making based upon mutual respect and participation, not a ritual to be equated with reciting the contents of a form that details the risks of particular treatments."[8]

The patient's need for and right to this kind of knowledge is highlighted by the increasing number of malpractice suits that involve an element of informed consent. (Some lawyers are advocating the use of the term *authorization for treatment*, implying patient control). For many years, in such suits, courts have tended to rule that the physician must provide only as much information as is general practice among his colleagues in the area, as determined by their expert testimony. Later decisions, however, are changing this attitude, most of them hinging on informed consent. The landmark decisions have involved situations in which the surgery was done effectively but patients sued because of complications or results about which they had not been warned. In one such case, a patient who had numerous complications after surgery for a duodenal ulcer had been informed of the risks of the anesthesia but not the surgery. He received a verdict against both hospital and surgeon.[9] In another case, when a child never regained consciousness after administration of anesthesia by a nurse anesthetist, the jury was instructed that there had been no informed consent, because the family had been told of the potential dangers of the surgery, but not of the anesthesia.[10]

In these and other cases, judges disallowed the right of the medical profession to determine how much the patient should be told; rather, they said, the patient should be told enough, in understandable lay language, to make a decision. The relative importance of the risk or facts to be disclosed by the physician "is to be determined by applying the standards of a reasonable man, not a reasonable medical practitioner."[11]

There continue to be similar judgments and some legislation supporting the same concept. The trend now is for the courts to view the doctor-patient relationship as a partnership in decision making. They are expected to pay increased attention to the "physician's fiduciary duty to disclose fully to his patients the condition of their bodies" even where this is caused by the physician's own negligence.[12]

Principles of Informed Consent

Consent is defined as a free, rational act that presupposes knowledge of the thing to which consent is given by a person who is legally capable of consent. *Informed consent* is not expected to include minutiae but to delineate the essential nature of the procedure and the consequences. The disclosure is to be "reasonable," without details that might unnecessarily frighten the patient. The patient may, of course, waive the right to such explanation, or any teaching.[13] Consent is *not* needed for emergency care if there is an immediate threat to life and health, if experts agree that it is an emergency, if the patient is unable to consent and a legally authorized person cannot be reached, and when the patient submits voluntarily.

The essential elements of an informed consent include (1) an explanation of the condition; (2) a fair explanation of the procedures to be used and the consequences; (3) a description of alternative treatments or procedures; (4) a description of the benefits to be expected; (5) an offer to answer the patient's inquiries; and (6) freedom from coercion or unfair persuasions and inducements.[14]

The last has special significance, because the legal concept of informed consent really became viable with the Nuremberg Code, originating from the trials of Nazi physicians who were convicted of experimenting on prisoners without their consent. The principles were then formalized in the Declaration of Helsinki, adopted by the Eighteenth World Medical Assembly in 1964, and revised in 1975.

Informed consent is *a process, not a form*. A consent form is a piece of physical evidence that the process took place. That is, one can have true informed consent without producing a form and a form without true informed consent. The relationship between consent and the piece of paper is exactly the relationship between a nursing assessment and the record of that assessment in the patient chart. One must not confuse a complex, interactive process with its documentation. However important it may be to maintain good records, good records are not a substitute for good care and may even camouflage bad care.

Trends in Informed Consent

The principle is that each person of sound mind and adult years has the right to consent to or refuse any or all medical treatment. However, like all principles, this one is not absolute. For example, in circumstances that vary among states, courts may grant requests to override a patient's refusal if that refusal threatens the patient's life. The trend seems to be that these circumstances are being narrowed and that, increasingly, the patient's right to refuse is being upheld, even when the medical interventions at issue would almost surely save the patient's life.

For example, a Jehovah's Witness refuses a blood transfusion, even though it might mean his life, because taking such transfusions is against his religious beliefs. The rulings have varied,[15] although tending to be in favor of allowing him to make his own decision; in fact, the Witnesses and AMA in 1979 agreed upon a consent form requesting that no blood or blood derivative be administered and releasing medical personnel and the hospital for responsibility for untoward results because of that refusal. (This particular problem has been lessened to some extent as better blood substitutes have become available.) However, in 1990 a Jehovah's Witness sued a major medical center and five physicians because he was given blood after a serious automobile accident. Although he was unconscious and it was an emergency situation, he claimed his rights were violated. If a minor child of a Witness needs the blood and the parent refuses, a court order requested by the hospital usually permits the transfusion.[16] This is based on a 1944 legal precedent when the Supreme Court ruled that parents had a right to be martyrs, if they wished, but had no right to make martyrs of their children. On the other hand, if the child is deemed a "mature minor," able to make an intelligent decision, regardless of chronological age, the child has been allowed to refuse the treatment.

In another type of case, a seventy-nine-year-old diabetic refused to consent to a leg amputation. Her daughter petitioned to be her legal guardian so that she (the daughter) could sign the consent. The judge ruled that the woman was old but not senile, and had a right to make her own decision. In a slightly different situation, an alcoholic derelict was found unconscious on the street and taken to a hospital. When he became conscious, he refused to have his legs amputated for severe frostbite. The court order sought by the hospital was denied because, although the man was alcoholic, he was competent at the time of making his decision. (As it happened, he lost only a few toes from his frostbite.) In still another case, a young man on permanent kidney dialysis decided he did not want to live that way and refused continued treatment. He was allowed to do so and died within a short time. Other cases can also be cited. The right of a competent patient to refuse treatment seems more firmly established than ever.

Is Informed Consent Practical?

Some physicians do not believe that it is feasible to obtain an informed consent because of such factors as lack of interest or education and high anxiety level, in which case a patient might refuse a "necessary" treatment or operation. The physician may invoke "therapeutic privilege," in which disclosure is not required because it might be detrimental to the patient.[17]

Although reasonable people would allow for *some* place for such "therapeutic privilege," the circumstances in which withholding information can be justified are *very* rare—on the order of once or twice in a career. Most times, when physicians plead that full disclosure (and, hence, truly informed consent) would be too distressing, it is evidence of an "old-fashioned" (i.e., pre–civil rights era) notion that patients' rights are relatively less important than physicians' responsibility to do good.

Most often, failures of informed consent seem to be a communicating function of physicians who simply are "not good at" talking or not inclined to take time to talk with patients or family members. As is true of nurses, those physicians who enjoy or otherwise derive rewards from genuine personal interaction at an intimate level are those who will be the most effective teachers, counselors, and advocates for their patients.

Although the President's Commission avoided recommending *legal* alternatives, the members came out in unequivocal support of "shared decision-making" and full disclosure to patients except in unusual circumstances. Their surveys (like others before) indicated that people *do* want full information even when they

trust their doctor completely and will probably go along with his recommendations. They may not always remember the details later, but with a full explanation, given in lay terms, and with enough time for questions and answers, they can understand. However, many patients are still reluctant to ask for fear of appearing stupid or "bothering the doctor."

The written consent form that is generally accepted as the legal affirmation that the patient has agreed to a particular test or treatment has undergone a number of changes in the last few years. The patient rights movement has motivated hospitals, especially, to review and revise their consent forms. The catchall admissions consent has already been ruled as legally inadequate for anything other than avoiding battery complaints, because it does not designate the nature of the treatment to be given.[18] What has emerged are forms that contain all the required elements for the informed consent process, usually individualized by the physician for each patient. Often they are available in the foreign languages most prevalent in the area. One of the key points is having a form that avoids unnecessary technical terms or compound-complex sentences. Communications specialists who have developed and tested such forms conclude, "A comprehensible consent form is not, of course, a guarantee that physician and patient have communicated to either's satisfaction. It is, however, at least an indication of good faith and a reflection of the physician's sincere attempt not only to enable the patient to understand, but also to educate the patient."[19] A question sometimes arises as to whether a patient can waive his right to sue even if there is malpractice. In one hospital where a patient signed such a waiver as part of the consent form, the court ruled that it was null and void, that is, not allowable as a condition of treatment.[20]

Although many people think of informed consent only in terms of hospitalization, there are already some court cases that indicate that the concept embraces the continuum of health care, such as a clinic or doctor's office. In one court case, the physician was held to have breached his duty by failing to inform the patient of the risks of *not* consenting to a diagnostic procedure, in this case a Pap smear. The patient died of advanced cervical cancer.[21]

The Nurse's Role in Informed Consent

What is the nurse's role in informed consent? To provide or add information before or after the doctor's explanation has been given? To refer the patient to the doctor? To avoid any participation? The advice given varies. Some suggest that getting involved in informed consent is simply not a nurse's business and is best left to the doctor; others consider it a professional responsibility.[22]

It is generally agreed that nurses do not have the primary responsibility for getting informed consent. However, the President's Commission noted that "nurses as a practical matter, typically have a central role in the process of providing patients with information,"[23] and that NPs, including nurse-midwives, have *full* responsibility for informing patients about their conditions, tests, and treatment, and obtaining consent. The American Nurses Association has stated that the nurse has a responsibility to facilitate informed decision making. There was also at least one serious court case in which a patient sued because the physician *and* nurses withheld information about his condition. Both were held liable.[24] Nevertheless, the question asked by most nurses is how much can be told, especially if the physician chooses not to reveal further information. The Tuma case[25] did not resolve the nurse's right to supply the missing information, and the nurse may be taking a personal risk. Greenlaw suggests that patients' questions may range over a variety of topics, including what you are doing to the patient and your qualifications (if so, answer honestly) to interpretation of what the doctor said (explain in lay terms) to "What's wrong with me?" (don't answer directly) or "Is my doctor any good?" (tell the patient that he has a right to ask his doctor for his qualifications and experience or to get a second opinion).[26] A variety of other opinions are offered, but a point that is always made is that the patient's lack of information should always be discussed with the doctor and, if there is no response, with administrative superiors. There is nothing wrong with questioning the patient to see what he or she really understands and clarifying points, provided you know what you are talking about. If you decide to give further information, it should be totally accurate and carefully recorded, and the fact that it was given should be shared with the physician and others. Nurses have found ways to make the patient aware of knowledge gaps so that they ask the right questions, but it's unfortunate that most are still employed in situations in which it could be detrimental to them to be the patient's advocate. Of course, if the patient is coaxed or coerced into signing without such an explanation, the consent is invalid. Moreover, if the patient withdraws consent, even verbally, the nurse is responsible for reporting this and ensuring that the patient is not treated. This is a legal responsibility not only to the patient but also to the hospital, which can be held liable.

Hospitals are beginning to use a clerk to witness the consent form, after the physician provides an explanation, on the theory that only the signature is being witnessed, not the accuracy or depth of the explanation. Other hospitals ask the physician to bring another physician, presumably to validate the explanation. Where nurses still witness the form, it should be clear *what* they are witnessing—the signature or the explanation.[27] Hospital policy can clarify this.

It has been suggested that the nurse's role in informed consent is threefold: to perform a patient assessment to evaluate the patient's readiness to understand and respond intelligently to the consent form; to determine the best approach to obtain informed consent (time, environment, presence of a supportive person); patient and staff follow-up (reaffirmation that the patient understood), supporting the patient's decision, reinforcement of information, apprising staff and physician of the patient's understanding.[28]

The nurse's specific responsibility is to explain nursing care, including the whys and hows.

An interesting idea to contemplate is whether you should tell patients about the risks of the *nursing* procedures you do, even though this is not a legal requirement. (Nor does it prevent you from doing so.) The answer seems to be— maybe, but carefully.[29]

THE RIGHT TO DIE

Because improved technology has succeeded in artificially maintaining both respiratory and cardiac functions when a person can no longer do so, the definition of *clinical death* as the irrevocable cessation of heartbeat and breathing is no longer sufficient. (Physicians have had the sole authority and responsibility to pronounce a patient dead, even though a nurse may quite accurately do so. The law has caught up with reality in New Jersey, where nurses can now pronounce death.)

In common law, there had been a strongly entrenched cardiac definition of death until, in 1977, in Massachusetts, the Supreme Judicial Court officially recognized the use of "brain death" criteria. In 1970, Kansas was the first state to adopt a brain death statute, thus offering two alternative definitions of death to be used at the discretion of the attending physician. Since then, all the states have passed similar legislation. Various types of criteria have been adopted by state legislatures, but all are based on cessation of brain functioning. Black notes an important aspect of brain death:

> Patients with brain death are not merely perpetually unresponsive: they are patients whose brain destruction, including loss of respiratory and cardiovascular control, means that life of all kinds is soon to be lost as well.[30]

Translated into statutory language, the concept is typically expressed as follows:

> An individual who has sustained either (1) irreversible cessation of circulatory and respiratory functions, or (2) irreversible cessation of all functions of the entire brain, including the brain stem, is dead. A determination of death must be made in accordance with accepted medical standards.[31]

Use of the term "brain death" has [u]nfortunate. It has perpetuated the mistak[en no]tion that there are two *kinds* of death, b[rain] death and real death. The more accurate ter[m,] and the one less likely to confuse both professionals and the general public is "death as determined by neurological criteria." Such semantic precision is important. Twenty-five years after the concept was developed, otherwise careful nurses and physicians still betray their confusion by such inappropriate behavior as labeling as "brain dead" patients who are comatose or by hesitating to remove life support from patients who are certifiably dead.

The determination of death by neurological criteria is a common diagnosis only in specialized units, particularly trauma centers. In such settings, staff members are clear that "dead is dead." They recognize that the diagnosis, though painstaking and time-consuming, is rarely difficult. They speak to family members in terms of "death" as they continue to test for signs of brainstem responsiveness. Finally, when they are convinced that death has occurred, they turn off the ventilator rather than asking family permission to do so. Thus "brain death" illustrates a general truth: There is nothing so practical as a clear concept and nothing so mischievous as a confused concept.

The popular label of "right to die" has been applied to a long series of famous court cases in which patients and, more often, their surrogates have fought to have life-sustaining treatment discontinued. The label is misleading because, strictly speaking, there is no "right to die." The rights to which these patients and their families have actually appealed are either (1) the right to freedom from undue state interference, often called the right to privacy, and (2) the right to self-determination. The first of these rights involves an appeal to constitutional guarantees. The second is based in our long tradition of common law.

Most of the "right to die" cases have been heard exclusively in state courts because they have not entailed legal questions appropriate to federal judicial review. Hence, it is not surpris-

...ates have evolved different
...iew of selected "landmark"
5...ate the point.

...ewicz case, the high court in Mas-
...upheld a decision not to give a se-
...tarded 67-year-old more chemother-
...at would be unpleasant for the sake of a
short extended life span. (He died a month later of pneumonia.) That court ruled that such decisions on behalf of incompetent patients should be made only with explicit permission of the courts. A very different procedure was established by the New Jersey Supreme Court in the Quinlan case. In this case, a 22-year-old woman received severe and irreversible brain damage that reduced her to a persistent vegetative state (PVS). Her father petitioned the court to be made her guardian with the intention of having all extraordinary medical procedures sustaining her life removed. The court ruled that the father could be the guardian and have the life support systems discontinued with the concurrence of her family, the attending physicians, who might be chosen by the father, and the hospital ethics committee. (After disconnection of the respirator, Karen Quinlan continued to live another ten years, sustained by fluids and other maintenance measures, in a nursing home.)[32] In a long series of subsequent cases the New Jersey Supreme Court has held to its initial stance that such decisions belong in the traditional control of family and primary caregivers. However, courts in some other jurisdictions have continued to insist on a role for judicial review.

One might suppose that nonemergency cases involving competent patients would be clearer. In such cases, there can be no question about whether the elements of informed consent have been satisfied. When someone wants to discontinue kidney dialysis today because the quality of life is unacceptable, there is relatively little objection. That may be because the patient is ambulatory and may simply choose not to come back for treatment. Yet when a competent 77-year-old California man with multiple serious ailments, but not at the point of dying, wanted the right to have his respirator turned off be-

cause *he* found the quality of life unbearable, neither the hospital, nor the doctors, nor the court would allow him to do so, and no other hospital or doctor would accept him. (He had signed a living will and other documents.) His arms were restrained to prevent any action on his part; the hospital said he continued to "live a useful life." His medical and hospital expenses were by then almost $500,000.[33] William Bartling died the day before the state appeals court heard his case. Six weeks later the court ruled that he did have the constitutional right to refuse medical treatment, including the respirator. The family sued the hospital.

Also in California, a 26-year-old woman almost totally paralyzed from cerebral palsy found the quality of her life intolerable and had herself admitted to a hospital and asked the staff to keep her comfortable and pain-free, but to let her starve herself to death. They refused, and a court supported that decision. She was described by psychiatrists as "mentally stable," not clinically depressed. She finally signed herself out to a nursing home in Mexico, but found that she would have been force-fed there also and consented to eat. Later that year Elizabeth Bouvia returned to California and again appeared in court because doctors in the facility in which she was now a patient cut down her medication for pain. Again the court supported her.[34] Ironically (or, perhaps, understandably from a psychosocial point of view), the patient ceased her efforts as soon as her right to do so had been affirmed by the court. In New Jersey, a lower court agreed to removal of a nasogastric tube on an eighty-four-year-old incompetent (but not brain-dead) woman, Ms. Conroy, at the request of her nephew. The case was appealed, but the patient died before a final appellate decision was reached.

In the Conroy decision, the New Jersey Supreme Court ruled that termination of any medical treatment, including artificial feeding, on incompetent patients is lawful as long as certain procedures are followed. (Ms. Conroy had indicated, but not in writing, that she would not have wanted to live under those conditions.)

The decision came too late for Ms. Conroy, who died with the feeding tube in place. This case was considered different because the person was in a nursing home, but Annas maintains that the distinction should not have been made. Another problem with the final decision was that, although the court articulated the right of competent adults to refuse treatment, it failed to provide any way to require proxies to exercise the right on behalf of incompetent patients.[35]

This was demonstrated again in the similar Hilda Peters case in New Jersey, this time in part because the ombudsman mandated by the Quinlan decision forbade the removal of her feeding tubes even though the man with whom she lived had her medical power of attorney and there was verbal (not written) evidence that she, too, would not have wanted to survive in this condition. (The ombudsman said that he didn't want to rule in this way because he believed Peters would not want to live, but that he had a legal obligation to do so because a 1985 ruling by the Supreme Court said that a feeding tube could be removed only if the patient were expected to die within a year. (Expected by whom?) However, in 1987, the New Jersey Supreme Court made three rulings, for Peters and two others, that was expected to influence other states. The court said, first of all, that these life-or-death decisions should be made not by a court, but personally or through a surrogate. The rulings also provided immunity from civil and criminal liability for those making such decisions "in good faith."

It is interesting to note that the New Jersey court decided that the care setting *did* matter. Because Ms. Conroy was in a nursing home, rather than in a hospital, the court modified its principle of leaving such decisions entirely in local hands. Citing a history of rights abuses in nursing homes and noting that nursing homes are less open to multidisciplinary scrutiny by highly trained professionals, the court insisted on review by the independent state Office of the Ombudsman before any withholding or withdrawing of life-sustaining treatment. This outside review applies only to elderly persons institutionalized in nursing homes and psychiatric hospitals and is justified wholly in terms of their perceived special vulnerability.

In the years since the Conroy decision, nursing homes have increasingly come under scrutiny. In most states, regulatory oversight has been extended and, in some ways, improved. The efforts of professional organizations and the further development of geriatric specialization in medicine, nursing, and social work are having a general, if unevenly distributed, effect. Even ethics committees are becoming more common in nursing homes.[36]

These cases are presented in some detail to show some of the legal and ethical factors that can affect decisions that would seem to be relatively clear-cut, although very painful to the family or other surrogate. Especially during the 1980s, many similar situations were reported, with court decisions varying in each state according to the way the judges interpreted the law or how they were influenced by their own moral or religious beliefs. Most often these cases arose when physicians or an institution refused to allow treatment to be discontinued.

Such legal processes can take a long time. The Paul Brophy case in Massachusetts is an example.[37] It took 2 years and the refusal of the U.S. Supreme Court to review the case (which would have taken even longer) before, after many contrary rules, his wife, a nurse, could have him transferred to a hospital that was willing to do what he would have wished and removed his feeding tube. He died 8 days later, kept comfortable but not fed, and cared for by his wife.

People like Mrs. Brophy and the parents of Karen Ann Quinlan, though motivated by the plight of their own family member, have ended by doing a service to the entire community. These cases are called "landmark" because the decisions had implications far beyond the persons whose names they bear.

The idea of having a loved one die of thirst or starvation, as the pro-life group describes it (although there is little evidence that a PVS patient has such sensations),[38] is naturally repugnant to families, and the pressures on them are great. Some advocates with a religious affiliation are strongly opposed to removal, although others are not.[39] Physicians and nurses are likewise divided in their feelings. Nurses have occasionally criticized families contemplating removal of life support (especially artificial feeding) and in some cases have reported them to authorities or alerted right-to-life organizations. The nurse who had cared for Ms. Conroy testified in the case, in detail, as to Ms. Conroy's condition; she thought that the tube should not have been removed. Others have stated the opposite point of view. In all such cases, the nurses are the ones in intimate contact with the patient; if the decision is to let the patient die, it is their responsibility to keep the patient as comfortable as possible.

In 1986, the AMA Council of Ethical and Judicial Affairs issued a statement on "Withholding or Withdrawing Life Prolonging Medical Treatment," declaring that "life-prolonging medical treatment and artificially or technologically supplied respiration, including nutrition and hydration, may be withheld from a patient in an irreversible coma even when death is not imminent."[40] In January 1988, the ANA Committee on Ethics issued guidelines on the subject, saying, in essence, that there are few instances under which it is morally permissible for nurses to withhold or withdraw food and/or fluid from persons in their care.[41] This position is now outdated. In 1992, the ANA Board of Directors adopted a new "Position Statement on Forgoing Artificial Nutrition and Hydration." This new stance is in essential agreement with that of the AMA and the Hastings Center's "Guidelines on the Termination of Life-Sustaining Treatment." Its central assertion is "Like all other intervention, artificially provided hydration and nutrition may or may not be justified."[42] Thus the ANA has distinguished tube feeding from assisting dependent people with feeding by mouth, an ancient and continuing form of care that is always obligatory.

It was inevitable that, given the controversy on these issues and the fact that there may be several hundred thousand PVS patients, a case would eventually reach the U.S. Supreme Court, probably as a privacy (Fourth Amendment) issue. The first right-to-die case to go before the court was that of Nancy Cruzan, a 32-year-old woman who was injured in an auto accident in 1983 and was eventually determined to be in a persistent vegetative state. In 1988, her case was the first in Missouri to raise the question of whether feeding tubes can be equated with other life-sustaining medical treatments and whether patients in Nancy's condition have any rights regarding their care. The parents, stating that this would have been Nancy's wish, wanted to have the implanted gastrointestinal tube removed. A probate judge ruled that they could, but was overruled by the Missouri Supreme Court, which relied on a Missouri statute requiring "clear and convincing" evidence of a patient's prior wish that life support be removed.

The United States Supreme Court's decision in *Cruzan* is complex. The court upheld the general concept, implied or asserted in so many cases from *Quinlan* onward, that there is a constitutional right to refuse life-sustaining treatment. Moreover, the court ruled that artificially delivered nutrition and hydration is not legally distinct from other kinds of medical intervention and thus may be withheld or withdrawn in the same way as other treatment. Finally, the court upheld the right of the Missouri legislature to insist on "clear and convincing" evidence of prior wishes. While clearly not requiring other states to adopt such a strict standard, the court ruled that Missouri's statute does not violate the United States Constitution. (Only New York and Missouri have laws insisting on "clear and convincing" evidence, a test difficult to meet by any means short of a "living will.") Eventually, the family came up with enough "clear and convincing" evidence to satisfy the Missouri legal system, and Nancy was allowed to die.

Advance Directives

"Advance Directives" is the generic name embracing both instruction directives (living wills) and proxy directives (appointment of someone to act when the directive maker is incapacitated). Living wills are written documents or statements by competent persons setting forth how they wish to be cared for at the end of their lives. The beginning statement of a living will generally says that the maker is "emotionally and mentally competent" and that he or she directs the physician and other health care providers, family, friends, and any surrogate appointed by him or her to carry out the stated wishes if the maker is unable to do so. The intent is to withhold life-sustaining treatment if there is no reasonable expectation of recovery from a seriously incapacitating or fatal condition. The directive also has space for specific directions about treatments the individual may refuse, such as "electrical or mechanical resuscitation of my heart when it has stopped beating"; "nasogastric tube feedings when I am paralyzed or unable to take nourishment by mouth"; "mechanical respiration if I am no longer able to sustain my own breathing." If such a list is already present in the document, the person is directed to cross out all that do not reflect his or her wishes and/or to add others. Two witnesses sign the document; sometimes it must be notarized. Of course, the living will can be withdrawn at any time by the maker, but otherwise it stands as a clear indication of his or her wishes.

In 1977, California enacted a Natural Death Act, the first "legal" state living will. The next year, Arkansas, Idaho, Nevada, New Mexico, North Carolina, Oregon, and Texas followed with similar statutes. By 1990, at the time of the Supreme Court decision in the Cruzan case, forty-one states and the District of Columbia had enacted such laws and others were being debated. All granted civil and criminal immunity for those carrying out living will requests. All states now have such laws.

In 1984 California enacted a law entitled the Durable Power of Attorney for Health Care, which was the first of its kind. This law allowed terminally ill patients to designate another individual to make life-or-death decisions in the event that the patient was unable to do so. The agreement conveys the authority to consent, refuse, or withdraw consent "to any care, treatment, service, or procedure to maintain, diagnose, or treat a mental or physical condition." Like living wills, durable power of attorney provisions are now recognized throughout the United States. They are also known as "proxy directives," and the person who has been designated may variously be known as the "proxy" or the "health care representative" or the "person with durable power of attorney for health care." Some forms include designation of an alternate surrogate, "should my surrogate be unwilling or unable to act in my behalf." The document must also be witnessed. Sometimes both components, will and proxy, are combined in one document.

Although probably a generic living will, that is, not the official state document, would be seen as a clear indication of a person's intent, legally the forms specific to the particular state in which the individual lives should be used. These can be obtained from the state or from the organization, Choice in Dying, 200 Varick Street, New York, NY 10014-4810; phone 1-800-989-WILL.

Federal law now requires all health care institutions receiving Medicare or Medicaid reimbursement to maintain policies and procedures regarding advance directives. The Patient Self-Determination Act of 1989 (PSDA) applies to hospitals, nursing homes, hospices, and home health agencies. It further requires that each newly enrolled patient be asked whether he or she has an advance directive. If the answer is "yes," a copy is to be placed in the patient record. If the answer is "no," the patient must be offered information about the right to execute such a document. The PSDA also requires institutions to provide education on advance directives both to staff and to the community.

The American Nurses Association has adopted a position paper on the nurse's role regarding advance directives.[43] The ANA insists that nurses should assume a major role in facilitating informed decision making by patients, including, but not limited to, advance directives.

The position paper recommends that the legally mandated questions about advance directives be made a part of the nursing admission assessment. In fact, this recommendation has not been implemented in most hospitals. Where it has been, nurses are obliged to learn about advance directives and about the applicable state law regarding advance directives. On the whole, nurses who are thus aware and knowledgeable feel empowered in their role as patient advocates.[44] For example, the laws of many states require that a physician who will not or cannot in good conscience honor an advance directive must withdraw from the case. Nurses who know this feature of the law can and often have broken a decisional stalemate by simply reminding the physician or the proxy of this legal requirement.

Of Principles and Practice

In what is probably the most comprehensive part of their 1983 report, *Deciding to Forgo Life-Sustaining Treatment*, the President's Commission supported the patient's right to refuse treatment[45] and the right of the family of an incapacitated patient to make that decision with the physician. (The data presented are unusually detailed.) The next year, a group of experienced physicians from various disciplines and institutions came to the conclusion that in relation to these issues, "the patient's role in decision-making is paramount, and a decrease in aggressive treatment when such treatment would only prolong a difficult and uncomfortable process of dying" is acceptable.[46] In summary, several important points were made. In dealing with a competent patient, the treatment should "reflect an understanding between patient and physician and should be reassessed from time to time." Patients who are determined to be brain-dead require no treatment. With patients in a persistent vegetative state, "it is morally justifiable to withhold antibiotics and artificial nutrition and hydration, as well as other forms of life-sustaining treatment, allowing the patient to die. (This requires family

agreement and an attempt to ascertain what would have been the patient's wishes.)" Severely demented and irreversibly demented patients need only care to make them comfortable. It is ethically appropriate not to treat intercurrent illness. Again, the patient's previous desires and the family's wishes must be considered. With elderly patients who have permanent mild impairment of competence, the "pleasantly senile," emergency resuscitation and intensive care should be provided "sparingly."

Professionally Assisted Suicide

Meanwhile, on both the ethical and the legal fronts, the current big "right to die" issue is physician-assisted suicide, sometimes called professionally assisted suicide. This subject has been under discussion for some time and is usually brought into open debate after highly publicized physician-assisted suicides like the Debbie case or the suicide device used by Dr. Jack Kevorkian and a woman who requested help in dying, which is also mentioned in Chap. 10. A poll after the latter incident in 1990 found that 53 percent of those polled thought that a doctor should be able to assist a patient who wants to die. More recent polls suggest that this figure is rising. The AHA has estimated that 70 percent of the 6,000 deaths that occur in the United States each day are somehow timed or negotiated by patients, families, and doctors, who decide not to do all they can do and to let a dying patient die.[47] It apparently seems to many citizens that, at least in some circumstances, *helping* to die is a small and legitimate extension of *allowing* to die. Many doctors admit that the known elderly suicide rate is twice that of younger groups, and many other deaths may well come from the mixed array of very powerful drugs the elderly have at hand. The issue is further accelerated with the AIDS epidemic bringing what is almost certain death under painful circumstances. In addition, more cases of family members or friends assisting in suicide are being reported. (These may simply have been unreported before.) Sometimes these people are charged with murder; those charged are often acquitted or lightly sentenced.

One fear of doctor-assisted suicide is the possible abuse of such power. Some people think the possibility would cause patients to fear doctors. Yet, actions are being taken to legalize euthanasia.[48] When a panel of distinguished physicians was brought together to consider the issue, 10 of the 12 members agreed that "if a hopelessly ill patient believes his or her condition is intolerable, it should be permissible for a physician to provide the patient with the medical means and the medical knowledge to commit suicide."[49] In the Netherlands, euthanasia has gained a degree of social acceptance. Beginning in 1984 it was no longer prosecuted in certain approved circumstances,[50] and in 1993, the Dutch Parliament approved a law that sanctioned euthanasia under strict conditions. Although public and medical sentiment were on the side of this law, about 11 percent of doctors said that they would not practice euthanasia. Other countries have organizations that will assist a person to commit suicide, and the international Hemlock Society, which advocates that people have a right to "die well," is gaining members.

Despite many articles in the professional and lay press, and several unsuccessful attempts to pass enabling legislation, professionally assisted suicide generally remains unapproved in both law and professional policy. However, fanned into periodic flames by such proponents as Dr. Kevorkian (who was not convicted after publicly assisting a number of people), best-selling books, petitions to get the matter on state ballots, debates at professional meetings, and court cases, the issue will persist. For instance, although Michigan passed a law forbidding physician-assisted suicide, it and similar laws in other states have been declared unconstitutional by various federal courts. In 1994, Oregon was the first state to legalize physician-assisted suicide—with limits.

Certainly physicians are beginning to face the many issues surrounding euthanasia.[51] Nurses

need to do the same. Some health professionals think that prescribing or injecting a fatal dose of a carefully chosen drug could be, under the right circumstances, a natural and legitimate extension of their duty to suffering patients.[52] Many remain uneasy about taking such actions, or are opposed to any easing of the conventional prohibitions often for religious reasons.[53] A number of nurses are known to have disconnected life support on comatose patients; it has probably happened more often than is known. Legally they have been charged with everything from murder to practicing medicine without a license. However individual nurses feel about these difficult ethical problems, they are on the firing line; they deal with the patients and families as well as physicians. They simply cannot ignore these matters.

THE RIGHTS OF THE HELPLESS

Children, the mentally ill, the mentally retarded, and certain patients in nursing homes are often seen as relatively helpless, because they have been termed legally incompetent to make decisions about their health care for many years. Often the rights overlap, as when a child or elderly person is mentally retarded (as in the Saikewicz case). Some of the rights of the elderly are being protected by a legalized bill of rights.

The Mentally Disabled

For mental patients, state laws and some high court decisions have served the same purpose. Both have focused on mental patients' rights in the areas of voluntary and involuntary admissions; kind and length of restraints, including seclusion; informed consent to treatment, especially sterilization and psychosurgery; the rights of citizenship (voting); right of privacy, especially in relation to records; rights in research; and especially, the right to treatment. Although rulings have varied, the trend is toward the protection of rights. The landmark decision of

Wyatt v. Stickney (325 Federal Supplement, Alabama, 1972) clearly defined the purposes of commitment to a public hospital and the constitutional right to adequate treatment.[54]

Later, an Oklahoma court's decision in *Rogers v. Okin* that gives a voluntary mental patient the right to refuse psychiatric medication created a furor. The appeals court modified the ruling, holding that voluntary patients could be forced to choose between leaving the hospital or accepting the prescribed treatment. (Or physicians could modify the treatment.) Later, a Massachusetts court ruled that an *incompetent* person could refuse medication if he was able to express a "sensible" opinion, unless there was a proven danger to the public. For certain extraordinary medical treatments, the courts would have the ultimate authority to decide whether treatment is given. However, a number of states have enacted legislation protecting the right of the mentally ill to refuse medication.[55]

In some situations, a structured internal review system in which patients could appeal treatment decisions has seemed to work. On the other hand, follow-up on patients who refused treatment showed a deterioration in their functioning when they were released to the community.[56] In large and small cities, the evening television news shows disquieting pictures of apparently undermedicated, mentally ill persons whose lives are endangered by harsh environments they are not equipped to negotiate safely.

In issues of informed consent, other rulings have determined that if the mentally incompetent cannot understand the benefits or dangers of treatment, the family must be fully informed and allowed to make the decision.[57] According to a Supreme Court decision in 1990, prison officials are permitted to treat mentally ill prisoners with psychotropic drugs against their will without first getting permission in a judicial hearing. The prisoner who objects is entitled to a hearing and other protections first.

Some legal decisions relate to sterilization of the retarded, which came to a head when it was found that retarded adolescent black girls were being sterilized with neither the girls nor their mothers apparently having a clear notion of what that meant. Restraints were increasingly put on sterilization until, in 1979, DHEW tightened the regulations for federal participation in funding of sterilization procedures. Regulations included requirements of written and oral explanations of the operation, advice about alternative forms of birth control to be given in understandable language, and a waiting period. In addition, no federal funding was allowed for sterilization of those under 21, mentally incompetent, or institutionalized in correctional facilities or mental hospitals. However, this does not mean that a parent cannot have a mentally disabled child sterilized; it means that more precautions are being taken by the courts and the government to ensure that the child's rights are not violated. There is general concern for the rights of young people in the mental health system, but parents maintain considerable control. In 1979, the Supreme Court upheld the constitutionality of state laws that allow parents to commit their minor children to state mental institutions; several states have such laws.

Children and Adolescents

The rights of young people and children in health care relate primarily to consent for treatment or research and protection against abuse.[58] It is a general rule that a parent or guardian must give consent for the medical or surgical treatment of a minor except in an emergency when it is imperative to give immediate care to save the minor's life. Legally, however, anyone who is capable of understanding what he or she is doing may give consent, because age is not always an exact criterion of maturity or intelligence. Many minors are perfectly capable of deciding for themselves whether to accept or reject recommended therapy and, in cases involving simple procedures, the courts have refused to invoke the rule requiring the consent of a parent or guardian. If the minor is married or has been otherwise emancipated from his or her parents, there is likely to be little question legally. In addition, states cite different ages and situations in which parental permission is needed for medical treatment. The almost universal exception is allowing minors to consent to treatment for sexually transmitted diseases, drug abuse, and pregnancy-related care. Although it has been understood that health professionals have no legal obligation to report to parents that the minor has sought such treatment, a few states are beginning to add statutes that say that the minor does not need parental permission, but that parents must be notified. In 1983, the Reagan administration issued a rule that would require parents to be notified whenever children under eighteen received any contraceptives from federally funded family planning clinics. After a number of court challenges, this was overruled as infringing on a woman's right to privacy.

In 1972, the Supreme Court ruled that state statutes prohibiting the prescription of contraceptives to unmarried persons were unconstitutional because they interfere with the right of privacy of those desiring them. However, it did not rule on a minor's right to privacy in seeking or buying contraceptives. This was left to the states, and a number still set age limitations from 14 to 21. In many, however, doctors and other health professionals may provide birth control information and prescribe contraceptives to patients of any age without parental consent. Changes in federal and state laws also required welfare agencies to offer family planning services and supplies to sexually active minors. In general, there had been a national trend toward granting minors the right to contraceptive advice and devices, but the political power of conservative groups who oppose this trend is being felt, and state legislatures frequently attempt to put limits on young people in these areas.[59]

An even more dramatic change has occurred in relation to abortion. In 1976 the Supreme Court held that states may not constitutionally require the consent of a girl's parents for an abortion during the first 12 weeks of pregnancy. In addition, parents cannot either prevent or force an abortion on the daughter who, in the eyes of the court, is now "a competent minor mature enough to have become pregnant."

Since that time the reproductive rights of teenagers have been gradually eroded by state legislation and federal edicts influenced by conservatives and right-to-life groups. More than half the states have laws requiring teenagers to notify one or both parents, even if divorced, and/or to get permission from them before an abortion.

The Justices of the Supreme Court ruled five to four, in June 1990, that states had a right to make such a requirement of unmarried women under 18 as long as there was an alternative of judicial bypass (speaking to a judge instead) if the law requires notice to both parents. The five conservative justices did not allow for the fact that one or both parents might be abusive, alcoholic, or drug-addicted or even that the pregnancy might be due to incest. Undoubtedly, prochoice forces will continue to work to overturn these restrictive state laws. Should the young woman decide against an abortion and elect to bear the child, she can receive care related to her pregnancy without parental consent in almost every state. An unwed mature minor may also consent to treatment of her child. Meanwhile, state laws on parental consent and notification are still a hodgepodge, differing from state to state.

Groups such as the American Academy of Pediatrics (AAP), the Society for Adolescent Medicine, and the National Association of Children's Hospitals and Related Institutions have taken stands on protecting the rights of minors in health care. For example, the AAP Committee on Youth has presented a model act for consent of minors for health services, recommended for enactment in all states. The Pediatric Bill of Rights may also be a forerunner to legal action, as was the AHA Patient's Bill of Rights. (Unless such a statement is incorporated into law, the effect is that of a professional guideline to encourage protection of rights, with no enforcement powers.) The Pediatric Bill of Rights deals with the rights of young people in the areas of counseling and treatment for birth control, abortion, pregnancy, drug or alcohol dependency, sexually transmitted diseases, confidentiality, and information about her or his condition, as well as protection if a parent refuses consent for needed treatment. A psychologist suggested an extension to the Pediatric Bill of Rights, believing that "children will be as competent as society allows them to be."[60] Actually, cases in which mature minors are being permitted to make life-and-death decisions are increasing. An example is the case of a 13-year-old who chose not to have a bone marrow transplant because of religious beliefs and potential danger to her donor sister. In 1994, another young person refused further chemotherapy for his cancer and decided to try to live a reasonably normal life until he died, which he did.

The question of whether parents may make a decision for a child if the child's well-being is their prime consideration, as in giving Laetrile to a leukemic child, has not been decided with any consistency. (For that matter, neither has the legality of Laetrile.) Two very divergent cases can be cited in relation to these issues.

In 1986, two-year-old Robin Twitchell died of a bowel obstruction because his parents, who were Christian Scientists, did not seek medical help. They believed prayer would take care of the situation. In 1990, a jury found them guilty of manslaughter and they were sentenced to probation and community service; they also had to pledge to seek medical care for their other children. In another case, a New York court overruled a mother who refused surgery for a 15-year-old who had a massive tumor on his face. Because the surgery held some danger, she was afraid. There are also similar cases.[61] The legal principles involved are *parental autonomy*, a constitutionally protected right; *parens patriae*, the state's right and duty to protect the child; the *best interest doctrine*, which requires the court to determine what is best for the child; and the *substituted judgment doctrine*, in which the court determines what choice an incompetent individual would make if he or she were competent. (The last could be applied properly

only to a once-competent person and, thus, not to young children or to severely retarded persons of any age.)

Another unresolved issue is whether the grossly deformed neonate should be allowed to die. Few judges will rule to let it die, but often the decision is quietly made by parents and health personnel. These situations are especially difficult for a nurse who cares for the infant. Ethical and moral considerations weigh strongly.

The so-called Baby Doe case began with a child born in Indiana with Down's syndrome and a correctable esophageal fistula. The parents refused surgery, and their decision was upheld by the courts. The child was deprived of artificial nutritional life support and died. Although similar action had been taken in other cases, this one came to the attention of President Reagan. It resulted in a DHHS regulation that threatened hospitals that neglected such children with loss of funds under Section 504 of the Rehabilitation Act of 1973 (which protects the handicapped). Large signs had to be posted alerting people to a "hot line" number to call to report such incidents. After a series of legal challenges, this regulation was ruled unconstitutional—"arbitrary and capricious," among other things. Eventually, an alternative suggestion by the American Academy of Pediatrics was agreed on: establishment of infants bioethics committees (IBC) with diverse membership whose responsibility, in part, would be to advise about decisions to withhold or withdraw life-sustaining measures.[62] This was encouraged in the "Baby Doe" law, the federal Child Abuse Amendment of 1984, which labeled withdrawal or withholding of medically indicated nutrition "child abuse." However, a regulation basically left the decision as to whether such nutrition might be "virtually futile" up to the physician.[63]

In 1983, a child known as Baby Jane Doe was born in New York with multiple serious congenital conditions, one of which required immediate surgery. The family was told that even if she lived, she would be in a vegetative state, so after consultation with a physician and religious adviser, they opted for conservative treatment. A right-to-life attorney from Vermont learned of the case and managed to be appointed guardian by a like-minded judge, but this was overruled by an appeals court. Other right-to-life groups attempted to intervene; so did the federal government, which demanded the child's medical records to see if Section 504 was being violated. After considerable time, effort, and money had been spent, the government finally gave up. The child survived on conservative treatment and went home, where she required constant care for some time because of her paralysis and lack of mental development. Years later, she was reported as slightly retarded but generally all right.

Many questions are raised by these cases, and all are concerns of nursing. Creighton discusses a number of similar cases, as well as a Yale study in which some malformed infants were allowed to die with parental and physician consent. She notes how a nurse can influence a family to accept their deformed baby by emphasizing the normal.[64] Such cases will certainly continue, and the issue is not easily resolved; it is not just the rights of the infant that must be considered, but also those of the family and society.

Follow-up on the "Baby Doe" law indicates that many who are concerned about these infants agree that the federal regulations are an ethically inadequate response to the complex needs of the handicapped child, the family, the health care professions, and society as a whole.[65] An ethics committee, if functioning well, can be helpful to the physician and family in making decisions, but the decisions lean toward preserving life.[66] It has also been reported that discriminatory denial of medical treatment has not dramatically changed since the Child Abuse Amendment of 1984, although others claim that overtreatment is more likely to be the result. One author feels that the fact that treatable infants and children do not receive therapy because state legislation allows parents and religious healers to avoid their obligation to treat is a completely neglected problem that

has not been covered by the Child Abuse Act.[67] Several cases have been tried since then. One major tragedy caused by this law is not easily resolved—that some infants will have their lives prolonged and suffer "a fate worse than death" because the physicians are afraid of the legal consequences of letting them die.[68] On balance, the situation is similar to the so-called right to die situation for elderly adults. Though often cited as a reason for indecision and questionable treatment, "the law" rarely requires life-sustaining treatment contrary to the wishes of loving and sensible parents.

A newer right-to-die situation involving a minor came to the Maine courts in 1990. Chad Swan, persistently vegetative and being tube fed after an accident, developed several serious medical complications. With the concurrence of his physician, his family filed for a court order permitting the termination of the feeding. The court ruled that there was clear evidence, based on Chad's statements reported by his family, that he would not want to be maintained in a vegetative state, but the state attorney general appealed because Chad was only 17 years old. The Maine Supreme Court then expanded a previous right-to-die decision to include minors capable of making a serious decision to forgo treatment.

Well before this development, however, many specialized adolescent units in hospitals had developed the practice of routinely obtaining "assent" from older minors before doing invasive procedures. Although not a legal substitute for parental consent, assent of teenaged patients is defended by its proponents as respectful toward the young patients and nurturing of their developing responsibility.

RIGHTS OF PATIENTS IN RESEARCH

The use of new, experimental drugs and treatments in hospitals, nursing homes, and other institutions that have a captive population—for example, prisons or homes for the mentally retarded—has been extensive. Nurses are often involved in giving the treatment or drugs. As noted earlier, DHHS regulations now require specific informed consent for any human research carried out under DHHS auspices, with strong emphasis on the need for a clear explanation of the experiment, possible dangers, and the subject's complete freedom to refuse or withdraw at any time.

In addition, the National Research Act of 1974 established a commission to, among other things, "identify the requirements for informed consent procedures for children, prisoners, and the mentally disabled and determine the need for a mechanism to assure that human subjects not covered by HEW regulations are protected."

An interesting trend is toward including very young children in making decisions about research in which they are asked to participate. In the past, as a rule, parents were asked whether they consented to their child's participation in research—medical, educational, psychological, or other. There has always been some concern as to whether children should be subjected to such research if it was not at least potentially beneficial to them (such as the use of a new drug for a leukemic child). The child was seldom given the opportunity to decide whether or not to participate. New knowledge of the potential harm that could be done to the child, however innocuous the experiment, and appreciation of the child as a human being with individual rights have now resulted in recommendations that even a very young child be given a simple explanation of the proposed research and allowed to participate or not, or even to withdraw later, without any form of coercion.[69] Given that choice, some children have decided not to participate. Overall, the support for using healthy children in research or being volunteered for procedures not beneficial to themselves is eroding. In 1983, DHHS published rules requiring children's consent to participate in research.

Nurses were in the forefront of the move to protect subjects, with a statement in the ANA Code of Ethics, "The nurse participates in research activities when assured that the rights of individual subjects are protected," as well as an extensive ANA document on research guidelines (see Chap. 10). When a nurse is participating in research, at whatever level, ensuring that the rights of patients are honored is both an ethical and a legal responsibility. Nurses should know the patients' rights: self-determination to choose to participate; to have full information; to terminate participation without penalty; privacy and dignity; conservation of personal resources; freedom from arbitrary hurt and intrinsic risk of injury; as well as the special rights of minor and incompetent persons previously discussed. For instance, nurses have been ordered to begin an experimental drug knowing that the patient has not given an informed consent. The nurse is then obligated to see that the patient does have the appropriate explanation. This is one more case in which institutional policy that sets an administrative protocol for the nurse in such a situation is helpful.

If the nurse is the investigator, she or he must observe all the usual requirements, such as informed consent and confidentiality.[70,71] An interesting debate concerns the problems related to written informed consent and whether it could not as well be oral.[72,73] Still another concern is how consent can be obtained from mentally incompetent subjects.[74]

Any institution that applies for research funding from DHHS is required to have in place an Institutional Review Board (IRB). Some multidisciplinary panels are charged with protecting human subjects from both unduly dangerous procedures and from abuses of their rights. These IRBs vary widely in the rigor of their processes, despite being tightly regulated. Some IRBs subject proposals for research to very careful scrutiny; others are much less effective.[75]

There is no requirement that there be nurses on these boards, even if the boards are in hospitals or other health care agencies. Nurses can bring a useful perspective and should probably propose themselves for membership where not already invited.

Unfortunately, these boards may be less protective of patients' rights than they should be, especially in the area of informed consent. There is usually no follow-up to determine whether the plans to preserve subjects' rights that are presented in the proposals are really carried through. There is also criticism about lack of consistency in proposal approval. However, the IRB is generally seen as a safeguard to patients.[76]

PATIENT RECORDS: CONFIDENTIALITY AND AVAILABILITY

There is some evidence that, in situations other than the legally required ones, confidentiality of patients' records is frequently violated. From birth certificates to death certificates, the health and medical records of most Americans are part of a system that allows access by insurance companies, student researchers, and governmental agencies, to name a few. The information is often shared illegally with others, such as employers.

One physician, after completing a survey of the number of health professionals and hospital personnel who had access to the chart of one of his patients, called the principle of confidentiality "old, worn-out and useless; it is a decrepit concept." Seventy-five people had a legitimate access to that medical record.[77] Annas also says that it is not realistic for hospital patients to think that medical information about them will be kept confidential, even when staff follow all the basic rules about not discussing patients except in clinical situations. In part, of course, confidentiality is even less likely since the advent of computerized recordkeeping, which has grown tremendously in the last decade. Even in the 1970s, a position paper on confidentiality adopted by the American Medical Records Association said:

> The tremendous growth of computerized health data, the development of huge data banks, and the advancements in record linkage pose an enormous threat to the privacy of medical information. The public is generally unaware of this threat or of the serious consequences of a loss of confidentiality in the health care

system. Adequate measures to control medical privacy in the light of electronic information processing can and must be established....

By 1994, the organization's concern was even greater, and the AMRA suggested that reproductions of health records provided to authorized outside users should be accompanied by a statement prohibiting use for other than the stated purpose.[78]

Nevertheless, maintaining patient confidentiality is a part of both nursing and medical ethical codes, and practitioners have a responsibility to safeguard patients' privacy as much as possible. That includes the privacy of patient records. Many states have enacted laws to protect medical records, and the federal Freedom of Information Act (FOIA) denies access to an individual's medical record without that person's consent. In addition, the Fair Health Information Act of 1994 addresses the need for federal law to protect confidential material. Still some feel that the law would not be able to protect the confidentiality of records because of computerization.[79] There are also practical problems: if certain data are needed, as in following through on occupational health hazards, can exceptions be made for research that would be beneficial to the well-being of people? The problem does not lie in the aggregate figures but occurs when individual records must be scrutinized. The Supreme Court, recognizing the right of privacy, which protects certain personal information from public disclosure, has applied a test that balances the individual's constitutional right against the state's interest in maintaining open records. Most states have followed suit.[80]

Physicians and health administrators have historically been hostile toward the concept of sharing the record with the patient. Some attorneys serving health care facilities tend to share that feeling, often because they fear that patients may detect errors or personal comments that will result in a legal suit. (Actually, patient access has been mandated in Massachusetts since 1946 without a single reported adverse incident.) Whether or not any person involved in health care still feels that way is immaterial. Almost without exception, the patient's medical record is available to him or her upon request—and sometimes without request.

It is interesting to review the literature over the last twenty years to see the changes in attitudes and legislation. There were always physicians and others who saw sharing the record with the patient as not only fair, but sensible. Rather than worry that a patient would be too frightened or too stupid to understand, these practitioners had a philosophy of openness. More than twenty years ago, a health care center associated with the University of Vermont stated in its "Principles of Practice":

> **The best care of the patient is assured when the patient is part of the team and he shares his medical records with the providers of care. This is best effected by assuring that the record is complete, well organized, and available to the patient so that he can review the record for reliability, the subjective data and clarity of plans for treatment and education.[81]**

Choice in the matter of sharing the record is ending. Whereas it is legally recognized that the patient's record is the property of the hospital or physician (in his office), the information that the record contains is not similarly protected. Both states and the federal government have legislated access—either direct patient access, with or without a right to copy, or indirect access (physician, attorney, or provision of a summary only). The majority of states allow patients direct access to their records. In the others, individuals have a probable legal right to access without going to court.[82] States may differentiate between doctors' and hospital records and have other idiosyncratic qualifications. Of course, one certain way in which the patient can get access is through a malpractice suit in which the record is subpoenaed, a costly process for both provider and consumer.

The Privacy Protection Study Commission, created by the 1974 Privacy Act, also included recommendations on patient access. One federal step in this direction was the same FOIA and Privacy Act that prevented unauthorized access. Included are any records under the control of any agency of the federal government that contain an individual's name or any other identifying information. Medical records are specifically cited and include those of patients in the Veterans Administration and other federal hospitals. It also gave VA patients access to their own medical records, with some restrictions.

Does the nurse have any legal responsibility to be an intermediary? The answer is more complex than just yes or no. A nurse generally would not hand a patient the chart at request, for that would be inappropriate. Most states, as well as health care agencies that permit access to records, have a protocol to be followed. This usually involves providing both privacy and an opportunity for the physician and/or another person to explain the content. Nurses should know the specific procedure in their agencies so that they can tell patients who to ask. However, the advice of one prominent health care attorney is that patients should simply demand to see their records.[83]

Privacy

Nurses and others who work with patients must be especially careful to avoid invading the patient's right to privacy. There are a number of special concerns. For instance, consent to treatment does not cover the use of a picture without specific permission, nor does it mean that the patient can be subjected to repeated examinations not necessary to therapy without express consent. Undue exposure during examination should also be avoided.[84]

Exceptions to respect for the patient's privacy are related to legal reporting obligations. The nurse may be obligated to testify about otherwise confidential information in criminal cases. All states have laws requiring hospitals, doctors, nurses, and sometimes other health workers to report on certain kinds of situations, because the patient may be unwilling or unable to do so. The nurse often has responsibility in these matters because, although it may be the physician's legal obligation, the nurse may be the only one actually aware of the situation. Even if such reporting is not explicitly required by a law, regulations of various state agencies may require such a report. Common reporting requirements are for communicable diseases, diseases in newborn babies, gunshot wounds, and criminal acts, including rape.

Every state requires that suspected child abuse or neglect be reported to the child protective agency. Although other kinds of reporting are relatively objective, there are problems in reporting abused children because of the varying definitions of *child* and the question of whether there was abuse or an accident, with the consequent fear of parents suing. Usually, however, the person reporting is protected if the report is made in good faith, i.e., without malice and honestly.[85] It is not necessary that one be sure that abuse has taken place; the obligation is to report *suspected* abuse. The responsibility to "prove" abuse belongs with the child protective agency. In some states, there are penalties for *not* reporting. Spouse abuse and elder abuse are also reportable in most states. Procedures vary greatly, but in elder abuse, in each state, the nurse is included as a reporter. In most states, the abuses covered are physical abuse, fiduciary abuse, neglect, and abandonment.[86]

As the AIDS epidemic grew, new reporting problems arose. By 1987 all states had added AIDS to the list of reportable diseases. Many, but by no means all, require reporting of AIDS carriers, that is, the reporting of positive test results for the human immuno-deficiency virus (HIV). Physicians have been willing to make these reports because of the virulence of the disease and the need to maintain the best possible epidemiological records. However, the problem arises of whether to notify the family, especially a wife or lover, of a person with AIDS. Many patients object to notification and therefore will not come for testing, creating a situation that may be even more serious. The laws are not clear on notification, although in cases related to other infectious diseases judges

have ruled that the physician had a duty to inform the third party. Theoretically the third party could sue the physician if infected and not warned. As a rule, this kind of reporting is a public health department's responsibility, but it hasn't yet been determined whether, for instance, a home health nurse with information on AIDS-related conditions has a duty to tell the family.[87] What Northrop described as a breach of duty is the action of a nurse, formerly in an AIDS clinic, who passed on an AIDS-infected person's confidential record to the physician in charge of pre-employment physicals when the individual applied for a job in the hospital. Northrop said that the nurse could have been sued for breach of confidentiality and violation of privacy, although in this instance she was not named in the suit. The hospital paid.[88]

Ethical and legal practice prohibits the professional person from divulging any confidential information to anyone else, unless possibly to another physician or nurse who serves as a consultant. Neither does the ethical person engage in gossip based on this information, trivial and harmless though it may seem at the time. Moreover, the professional nurse has an obligation to set a good example for others in nonprofessional groups who may be less aware of their responsibilities in this respect.

Confidential information obtained through professional relationships is not the same as *privileged communication*, which is a legal concept providing that a physician and patient, attorney and client, and priest and penitent have a special privilege. Should any court action arise in which the person (or persons) involved is called to testify, the law (in many states) will not require that such information be divulged. Not all states acknowledge that nurses can be recipients of privileged communication, but there are specific cases in which the nurse-patient privilege has been accepted, especially in the case of advanced practice nurses.[89] Another issue is that psychiatric nurses, like other psychotherapists, have a responsibility to warn potential victims about their homicidal clients (the "Tarasoff principle," named after a case in which a psychiatrist did not do so). The same may be true of NPs in the case of warnings to the sexual partners of AIDS patients.[90]

As a rule, intentional torts, such as assault and battery, are not covered by malpractice insurance.

ASSAULT AND BATTERY

Assault and battery, although often discussed with emphasis on the criminal interpretation, also has a patients' rights aspect that is related to everyday nursing practice, especially when dealing with certain types of patients. Grounds for civil action might include the following:

1. Forcing a patient to submit to a treatment for which he has not given his consent either expressly in writing, orally, or by implication. Whether or not a consent was signed, a patient should not be forced, for resistance implies a withdrawal of consent.
2. Forcefully handling an unconscious patient.
3. Lifting a protesting patient from his bed to a wheelchair or stretcher.
4. Threatening to strike or actually striking an unruly child or adult, except in self-defense.
5. Forcing a patient out of bed to walk postoperatively.
6. In some states, performing alcohol, blood, urine, or health tests for presumed drunken driving without consent. There are some "implied consent" statutes in motor vehicle codes that provide that a person, for the privilege of being allowed to drive, gives an implied consent to furnishing a sample of blood, urine, or breath for chemical analysis when charged with driving while intoxicated. However, if the person objects and is forced, it might still be considered battery. This may also be true in relation to taking blood samples from unwilling individuals in potential criminal cases. Several states, acknowledging this, have enacted legislation to insulate hospital employees and health professionals from liability.

FALSE IMPRISONMENT

As the term implies, *false imprisonment* means "restraining a person's liberty without the sanction of the law, or imprisonment of a person who is later found to be innocent of the crime for which he was imprisoned." The term also applies to many procedures that actually or conceivably are performed in hospital and nursing situations *if they are performed without the consent of the patient or his legal representative*.[91] In most instances, the nurse or other employee would not be held liable if it can be proved that what was done was necessary to protect others.

Among the most common nursing situations that might be considered false imprisonment are the following:

1. Restraining a patient by physical force or using appliances without written consent, especially in procedures where the use of restraints is not usually necessary. This is, or may be, a delicate situation because if you do not use a restraint, such as siderails, to protect a patient, you may be accused of negligence, and if you use them without consent, you may be accused of false imprisonment. This is a typical example of the need for prudent and reasonable action that a court of law would uphold.
2. Restraining a mentally ill patient who is dangerous neither to himself nor to others. For example, patients who wander about the hospital division making a nuisance of themselves usually cannot legally be locked in a room unless they show signs of violence.
3. Using arm, leg, or body restraints to keep a patient quiet while administering an intravenous infusion may be considered

false imprisonment. If this risk is involved—that is, if the patient objects to the treatment and refuses to consent to it—the physician should be called. Should the doctor order restraints for the patient, make sure that the order is given in writing before allowing anyone to proceed with the treatment. It is much better to assign someone to stay with the patient throughout a procedure than to use restraint without authorization.

4. Detaining an unwilling patient in the hospital. If a patient insists on going home, or a parent or guardian insists on taking a minor or other dependent person out of the hospital before his condition warrants it, hospital authorities cannot legally require him to remain. (An exception can be made, in some states, for a "hospital hold" in the case of a child thought to be in imminent danger of abuse or neglect.) If a patient insists on leaving, the doctor should write an order permitting the hospital to allow the patient to go home "against advice," and the hospital's representative should see that the patient or guardian signs an official form absolving the hospital, medical staff, and nursing staff of all responsibility should the patient's early departure be detrimental to his health and welfare. If the patient refuses to sign, a record should be made on the chart of exactly what occurred and an incident report probably should be filed. Take the patient to the hospital entrance in the usual manner.

5. Detaining for an unreasonable period of time a patient who is medically ready to be discharged. The delay may be due to the patient's inability to pay his bill or to an inordinate wait, at his expense, for the delivery of an orthopedic appliance or other service. In such instances, the nurse or nursing department may or may not be directly involved, but it is always wise to know the possibility of legal developments and to exercise sound judgment in

order to be completely fair to the patient and avoid trouble.[91,92]

LEGAL ISSUES RELATED TO REPRODUCTION

Laws permitting abortion have varied greatly from state to state over the years. In early 1973, the Supreme Court ruled that no state can interfere with a woman's right to obtain an abortion during the first trimester (twelve weeks) of pregnancy. During the second trimester, the state may interfere only to the extent of imposing regulations to safeguard the health of women seeking abortions. During the last trimester of pregnancy, a state may prohibit abortions except when the mother's life is at stake (*Doe v. Bolton* and *Roe v. Wade*). Legislation relating to abortion is discussed in Chap. 19; other aspects are covered in Chap. 6.

Theoretically, all hospitals are required to perform abortions within these guidelines, and it is legal to assist with such a procedure. However, because of religious and moral reasons, some institutions are exempted from complying with the law, and individual doctors and nurses have refused to participate in abortions. Individual professionals or other health workers may make that choice, and there is legal support for them (conscience clause). This does not preclude the right of the hospital to dismiss a nurse for refusing to carry out an assigned responsibility or to transfer her to another unit. There have been some suits by nurses objecting to transfer, but rulings have varied.

More than twenty years after the *Roe v. Wade* decision, opinions were still strong on abortion issues and now appear even more so; generally the same arguments are heard.[93]

Immediately after *Roe v. Wade*, with a liberal Supreme Court, the rulings were almost consistently directed at freedom of choice, in opposition to restrictions on abortion being put by the states and later by the conservative Reagan administration. The rulings changed dramatically with appointments of conservative judges by

President Reagan, until there was a five-to-four conservative majority with the only woman Justice, Sandra O'Connor, considered the sometime swing vote. (However, she tended to be conservative on abortion issues.)

The following list shows the tilt of the court and the diversity of cases, generally brought by states. It is important to remember that the U.S. Supreme Court rules only on issues related to the Constitution. In these cases, the Court rules that the state or other petitioner does or does not have a constitutional right to behave in a particular way.

1973 The Court struck down restrictions on places where abortions could be performed, allowing for abortion clinics.

1976 The Court said that states could not give husbands veto power over their wives' decision to abort their pregnancies. It also said that parents of minor unwed girls cannot be given an absolute veto over abortions.

1977 The Court ruled that states have no constitutional obligation to pay for "nontherapeutic" abortions (referring to Medicaid patients).

1979 The Court said states may seek to protect a fetus that has reached viability, but the determination of viability is up to doctors.

1979 The Court implied that the states may be able to require a pregnant unmarried minor to obtain parental consent to an abortion as long as the state provides an alternative procedure, such as a judge's permission.

1980 The Court said that neither federal nor state government was constitutionally obligated to pay for even medically necessary abortions of women on welfare.

1981 The Court ruled that states may require doctors consulted by "immature" or dependent minors to try to notify their parents before an abortion.

1983 The Court heard three abortion-related cases, ruling that states and communities cannot require that all abortions for women more than three months pregnant be performed in a hospital. Also struck down were regulations requiring a 24-hour waiting period between consent and procedure.

1986 The Court said that states could not require doctors to tell women seeking abortions about potential risks and available benefits for prenatal care and childbirth.

1987 The Court split four to four, invalidating an Illinois law restricting access to abortion for some teenagers.

1989 In *Webster v. Reproductive Health Services*, considered a turning point,[94] the Court provided the states with new authority to limit a woman's right to abortion by upholding a Missouri law that banned abortions in tax-supported facilities except to save the mother's life, even if no public funds are spent; banned any public employee (doctors, nurses, others) from performing or assisting with abortions except to save a woman's life; and required testing of *any* fetus thought to be at least 20 weeks old for viability.

1990 The Court ruled constitutional the Ohio and Minnesota laws requiring parental notification by unmarried teenagers.

1992 In *Planned Parenthood v. Casey*, the Court upheld most of the restrictions passed by the Pennsylvania legislature and in doing so, established a new legal standard: restrictions are constitutional so long as they do not impose "undue burdens" on a woman's right to choose.[95]

The aim of many of these cases was to force the overturn of *Roe v. Wade*. That did not quite happen, but some state legislatures passed increasingly restrictive laws (even forbidding abortion in case of incest and rape), in part to try to force the Supreme Court to hear the cases. Governors vetoed some of these, but the very fact that they had gotten through two Houses was appalling to many men and women alike. Some young women have already sought back-alley abortionists with the expected dire results. Both pro-choice and pro-life forces concentrated their efforts on legislators and candidates to bring about state laws that supported their particular point of view. The end is not in sight.

How does this affect nurses? Nurses support both sides of this issue, as was clear by the anger or joy expressed by nurses when ANA took a pro-choice stand. But regardless of their personal feelings they will care for women and young girls regardless of their choices. Ethically, nurses must give all patients good care, but who gets what care and why, as in the Webster case, may affect nurses professionally as well as personally. As citizens, nurses must stay abreast of such important issues. For instance, many pro-life groups also object to sex education and contraceptive use, yet an astounding number of teenagers get pregnant every year. What should the role of the nurse be in this aspect? It is educational to see how other countries handle these issues.[96] It is also important to see how some of these issues interrelate. For instance, groups opposed to abortion are now becoming involved in right-to-die issues, taking a "life-is-sacred" stand.

There have already been court rulings that bar women from jobs (usually higher-paying) that might endanger the fetus of a pregnant woman, even if the woman isn't pregnant and doesn't plan to have children. In another case, a dying woman was forced to have a caesarean to "save" her fetus. Both died, and later the action was ruled illegal. In still another case, a woman in a coma was denied an abortion, but later, in a similar case, one was permitted—even though a right-to-life lawyer who didn't even know the woman tried to become her guardian to prevent it. And what of the Baby Doe-saved children? Who will be responsible for them? Will the family be forced to care for and pay for a severely deformed child? What of all the issues related to the fetus? Will new technology that has been successful in intrauterine surgery save some of these babies? Cure them? How will new techniques of birth control including the abortion pill, RU 486 and the use of other new drugs, or

changed use of drugs already approved for other conditions that are found to act as abortifacients, change the family planning scene?

There are a number of other reproduction-related rights that are also important, such as sterilization, artificial insemination of various kinds, and surrogate parenthood. *Sterilization* means "termination of the ability to produce offspring." Both laws and regulations have been in the process of change. If the life of a woman may be jeopardized if she becomes pregnant, a therapeutic sterilization may be performed with consent of the patient and sometimes her husband, although the latter rule is being challenged. If there is no medical necessity, the operation is termed *sterilization of convenience* or *contraceptive sterilization*. In some states, this is illegal; in other, arguable. Only a few states regulate nontherapeutic sterilization. Here too, consents are often required from the individual and spouse, and there may be a mandatory waiting period. The consequences of the operation must be made clear to all concerned, and often a special consent form is required. Some physicians have been advised not to perform sterilizations if the law is not clear. There seems to be little legal concern about male sterilization, *vasectomy*, which is being done with increasing frequency. The legal consequences of unsuccessful sterilization, both male and female, have resulted in suits. Called *wrongful birth*, these suits usually seek to recover the costs of raising an unplanned or unwanted child, normal or abnormal—but usually the latter. Judgments have varied, but are more likely to favor the plaintiff if the child is abnormal. (The same term may be used if an abnormal child is the result of incorrect information negligently given to the parents by a professional,[97] and the child may sue.)

Eugenic sterilization is the attempt to eliminate specific hereditary defects by sterilizing individuals who could pass on such defects to their offspring. Once, approximately half the states authorized eugenic sterilization of the mentally deficient, mentally ill, and others, but since the case mentioned earlier, only a few do so; in fact, judges have refused to grant permission in the absence of a law. There have also been suits after sterilization.[98] Legality where no law exists is questionable; civil or criminal liability for assault and battery may be imposed on anyone sterilizing another without following legal procedure or specific legal guidelines.

Laws on *family planning*, in general, also vary greatly. Some laws appear to be absolute prohibitions against information about contraceptive materials, but courts usually allow some freedom. It is important, however, that the information be complete and accurate.[99] Nurses are particularly involved, for they do much of this counseling, either as specialists or as part of their general nursing role. Moreover, new contraceptive drugs such as Norplant[100] and the use of RU486 require continual updating. Because there are still some state limitations and, as noted earlier, the federal government is becoming more involved, it is important for the nurse to keep up to date in this area.

Artificial insemination, the injection of seminal fluid by instrument into a female to induce pregnancy, has evolved into an acceptable medical procedure used by childless couples. (Consent by the husband and wife is generally required.) Homologous artificial insemination (AIH) uses the semen of the husband and appears to present no legal dangers for doctors or nurses. Heterologous artificial insemination (AID) uses the semen of someone other than the husband and does raise the question of the child's legitimacy. On occasion, the question of adultery also arises in the courts if the husband's consent has not been obtained. Few states have enacted statutes to deal with the AID situation. When a woman, for a fee, is artificially inseminated with a man's sperm and bears a child, who is then turned over to the man and his wife, this is termed *surrogate motherhood*. It has already created some legal problems, such as when the woman decided not to give up the child and again when neither wanted a baby born with a birth defect.[101]

One case in which the surrogate refused to give up the baby became a news sensation and stimulated some legislatures to introduce bills that, more often than not, would make illegal surrogate motherhood for profit. In the Baby M case, the New Jersey Supreme Court eventually awarded custody of the child to the natural father and his wife who had contracted for the baby, but the natural mother was given visiting rights somewhat like those in a divorce case. Not everyone thought that was best for the baby, but other decisions appear to be going in that direction also. Equitable laws seem to be slow in coming, although badly needed.[102] Annas also contends that laws are needed in relation to "full surrogacy" in which new scientific methods (in vitro fertilization and embryo transfer) are used to implant an embryo into a woman not genetically related, making her an "incubator."[103] This point is reinforced by a 1990 case where a woman carrying an embryo-transfer baby not genetically hers went to court to keep the baby. In fact, among the most controversial legal concerns related to reproduction are the issues of *in vitro fertilization* and *surrogate embryo transfer*, each of which is intended to enhance the fertility of infertile couples. Just one of the issues is related to patenting the process. Annas suggests that such commercial patenting should be rejected unless the patent holder can assure quality control and reproductive privacy.[104] Other questions are being raised, such as: will the government put restrictions on such techniques as embryo freezing? (There has already been a case in which frozen embryos were awarded to a woman in a divorce settlement, somewhat like a child!) There are also cases of lesbian couples, one of whom has borne a child by artificial insemination, fighting for custody of the child in court when they separate. Still another issue seen as ethical, but possibly becoming legal, is whether lesbians or "geriatric" women have the right to have children.[105]

One relatively new legal aspect of human reproduction concerns the field of *genetics*, with which nurses, physicians, and lay genetic counselors must be concerned. Some of the issues have to do with human genetic disease, genetic screening, *in vitro* fertilization (IVF), and genetic data banks. In addition, legislation, such as the National Sickle Cell Anemia, Cooley's Anemia, Tay-Sachs, and Genetic Diseases Act, has encouraged or forced states to expand genetic screening to cover other disorders. Neonatal screening, for instance, will probably be expanded considerably and offers new opportunities and responsibilities for nurses. But with what is still a relatively new science, many legal questions will be evolving.

Confidentially is of major importance. If a genetic disease is discovered, health professionals probably should not contact other relatives, even if it would benefit those relatives, without the screenee's consent. However, one can easily think of a clinical example in which the Tarasoff principle would seem to require that a relative be told. Imagine, for instance, a patient newly diagnosed as a carrier of a serious congenital disorder, whose estranged sibling is now four months pregnant. If the specific inheritance pattern indicates that there is a *high* likelihood of the fetus being affected, and if efforts fail to persuade the patient to disclose, it is arguable that the duty to warn outweighs the duty to maintain confidentiality. One emerging problem is *wrongful life*, which occurs when a deformed baby is born, although abortion was an option, because the physician or other counselor neglected to tell parents of the risk.[106] Informed consent that enables the patient to make such serious decisions as having an abortion, sterilization, or artificial insemination is also vital.

TRANSPLANTS AND ARTIFICIAL PARTS

Since Dr. Christian Barnard performed the first human heart transplant in 1967, the question of tissue and organ transplants has become a point of controversy. Tissue may be obtained from living persons or a dead body. In recent years, improvement in immunosuppressive therapy has lessened the need for close tissue matches in most cases, thus permitting most transplants to shift from living donors to cadaver donors. As that shift occurred, the need to clarify "brain death" became more apparent. Thus the rising need for cadaver organs accelerated the process of legal acknowledgment discussed above, the development of medical standards for determination of death by neurological criteria, and the growth of a nationwide network of tissue- and organ-sharing agencies.

While cadaver organs are donated by newly bereaved families from hospitals everywhere, the largest numbers come from regional trauma centers. Not only do such centers tend to concentrate those patients who are prime candidates for donation, but it is in such centers where the staffs develop the familiarity with and expertise in recognizing potential donors and asking the next-of-kin for permission to harvest organs. Such hospitals are also apt to approach the determination of death by neurological criteria with relatively greater efficiency and more nearly according to established standards.

Many potential opportunities for harvesting organs are missed because physicians and nurses are reluctant to broach the subject of organ donation or even to acknowledge in a timely and forthright fashion that their patient is or may soon be "brain dead." A reluctance to be "the bearer of bad news" or a belief that grieving family members are best served by indirect communication and "maintenance of hope" is almost surely the major factor in avoidance of timely determination of death and hence of requests for donation.

"Timing is everything." This often repeated statement is especially applicable here. Highly vascularized organs are lost if the blood supply is interrupted for any significant period. Meanwhile, the ethically correct and psychosocially sensitive behavior is not to ask for organ donation until *after* the next of kin has been told that death has apparently occurred. ("Apparently" because of the standards requiring repeat examinations and/or confirmatory tests.) Nurses and physicians with the most extensive experience in securing family consent for organ donation insist that the ethically correct and psychosocially sensitive timing is also the timing that assures the highest yield of donation from newly bereaved family members.

Common law once prevented the decedent from donating his own body or individual organs if the next of kin objected and statutes prohibited mutilation of bodies. However, all 50 states have adopted, in one form or another, the *Uniform Anatomical Gift Act*, approved in 1968 by the National Conference of Commissioners on Uniform State Laws. The basic purposes are to permit an individual to control the disposition of his own body after death, to encourage such donations, to eliminate unnecessary and complicated formalities regarding the donation of human tissues and organs, to provide the necessary safeguards to protect the varied interests involved, and to define clearly the rights of the next of kin, the physician, the health institution, and the public (as represented by the medical examiner) in relation to the dead body. As a practical matter, however, organs are ordinarily not harvested without the explicit permission of the next of kin, regardless of the decedent's prior wishes. Of course, such permission is very likely if the newly dead family member had previously expressed a desire to donate.

Since 1987, hospitals have been required to ask the next of kin of all potential donors whether or not they wished to donate. This "required request" law has resulted in widespread changes in hospital policies and stimulated some staff education. Most importantly, it resulted in designation of a person or set of persons who could be called when a prospective donor is identified. Such designated requesters are often both more knowledgeable about donation and more psychologically skilled than the primary physicians and nurses.

An ideal hospital procedure for securing organ donation might include such features as these:

- The attending physician tells the family the patient has died (usually brain-death).
- The physician, nurse, chaplain, or organ-procurement coordinator makes the request for donation.
- The donor's spouse (or other family in a specific legal order) may consent.

- Find out what you can about the family before you make the request.
- Explain to the family that they can donate as few or as many organs as they like.
- If the family is opposed, support their decision, thank them, and leave them a number to call in case they change their minds.
- If the family is uncertain, give them time alone to discuss it.
- If the family agrees, have the appropriate donation card ready.
- Answer the family's questions honestly.

For a quarter of a century, various attempts to get people to donate organs have been generally disappointing. The need for organs continues to far exceed the supply. While most people express positive attitudes toward organ donation, few take specific steps to make it more likely that their own organs will be harvested. Chief among those steps would be repeated, open conversations within families about organ donations and other aspects of end-of-life care. The problem for those who seek quick solutions to the persistent shortage of organs is that the discomfort of professionals and the public is not readily addressed by legislative initiatives and institutional rule making.

As in so many other situations, ethics and law are closely related here. Because of the scarcity of organs, the criteria are not so limited as they once were, and new scientific findings have opened new frontiers of transplantation. However, ethical concerns, made into law, have had an impact, good and bad, on transplantation. For instance, PL 98-507 (1984) prevents the sale of human organs, and court cases have forbidden the transplantation of the organs of anencephalic newborns or fetal tissue transplants.[107] With the Clinton administration, there is more willingness to allow fetal tissue transplants and research, but there are still objections by certain groups. These issues must be resolved, and so must development of a better system of matching the available organs with those who need them. Another concern is how long transplants will be paid for by government funds. And finally whether an individual such as Barney Clark, who received the first artificial heart, would have the right to disconnect the equipment if the quality of life was found to be untenable.

POSITIVE RIGHTS: ANOTHER MATTER ALTOGETHER

Much of what has been discussed in this chapter falls under the heading of "negative rights." As we have seen, these include the right to chart one's own course, the right not to be intruded upon, the right to be protected—in short, freedom *from*. "Positive rights," on the other hand, are those rights that assure the freedom *to*. They are rights that support an individual's claims on the community, which define what each person may justifiably demand as his or her rightful share of the common stock of goods and services. For example, when George is admitted to the Veterans Administration Hospital, he is exercising a positive right; only honorably discharged veterans are eligible. However, when George signs the general consent that the admitting clerk hands him, he is exercising a negative right, namely, the right to control who may touch him or obtain his medical record.

As Americans have gradually come to see health care as a public good, "patients' rights" increasingly have come to refer to *access to health care*, as well as to protection from intrusion. In our culture, with its constitutional heritage of negative rights, we are only now developing a firm consensus about whether there really *is* such a thing as a general, universal right *to* health care. These positive rights and their enormous implications for our system of health care services are discussed in other chapters.

RIGHTS AND RESPONSIBILITIES OF STUDENTS

When students of nursing begin their course of study, they in effect, if not in writing, enter into a contract with the school that does not expire until they graduate. It is understood that both the students and the school will assume certain responsibilities, many of which have legal implications,. Most legal cases related to education have involved institutions of higher education (junior and senior colleges, or universities) or general education.

Most legislation and judicial decision affecting education, however, probably can be applied to nursing education as well. Every approved school of professional nursing must meet the criteria for approval set by the state board of nursing, a legally appointed body found in every state, sometimes under a different name. The state-approved school must conduct an educational program that will prepare its graduates to take state board examinations and become licensed to practice as RNs. No matter where the students receive education and experience, the nursing school is still responsible for the content of the course of study. The board's minimum standards require the school to provide a faculty competent to teach students to practice nursing skillfully and safely. Students are expected to be under the supervision of a faculty member who is also an RN, and the school and teacher are responsible, with the student, for the student's errors. As discussed in Chap. 21, most legal experts hold that when students give patient care, they are, for legal purposes, considered employees of the hospital or agency. They are liable for their own negligence if injury results, and the institution and faculty will also be liable for the harm suffered. Carrying malpractice insurance is a wise precaution, and many schools recommend or require its purchase by all students. Many state student nurses associations offer low-cost insurance with membership.

Whether it is wise educationally and practically for nursing students to perform nursing functions as regular, paid employees is debatable, because then they can legally function in only those capacities not restricted to licensed nursing personnel. State laws governing the practice of nursing vary widely and are subject to misinterpretation by the employing agency. Most laws classify students working part time as employees. In this capacity, students performing tasks requiring more judgment and skills than the position for which they are employed are subject not only to civil suits but also to criminal charges for practicing without a license.

Traditionally, the relationship of institutions of higher education to a student under twenty-one years of age had been that of *in loco parentis*, which means that the school stands "in the place of the parent" and has the right to exercise similar authority over the student's physical, intellectual, and moral training. Since the early 1960s, courts have overturned this concept, and it is no longer considered to have much legal validity. However, the student's enrollment in a particular college, generally is an implied contract, which requires that the student live up to the reasonable academic and moral standards of the college, with the school also having certain responsibilities. For instance, if the student lives in a dormitory connected with the school, it must meet safety and sanitation standards established by local regulations. However, the school rarely assumes responsibility for the student's loss of personal property.

Undesirable student conduct may result in some discipline, including suspension or expulsion, and there has been considerable disagreement on the school's power in such circumstances. Generally, it is expected that the school's rules of conduct are made public and that the student has the right to a public hearing and due process. Legal rulings may be different when applied to private or public universities. Private universities have greater power in many ways, particularly if they do not accept federal monies directly, which then exempts them from certain federal laws such as the Rehabilitation Act of 1973.[108]

Constitutional rights are most frequently cited by students in complaints: the First Amendment (freedom of speech, religion, association, expression); the Fourth Amendment (freedom from illegal search and seizure); and the Fifth and Fourteenth amendments (due process of law). The courts recognize the student first as a citizen, so that they will consider possible infringements of these rights. Most commonly, First Amendment rights involve dress codes and personal appearance. Although schools do not possess absolute authority over students in this sense, some lower court rulings have approved the establishment of dress codes necessary for cleanliness, safety, and health. Beginning with *Dixon v. Alabama State Board of Education* in 1961, random, unannounced searches that schools had carried out previously were no longer allowed without student permission or a search warrant; otherwise, evidence found is inadmissible in court. If material uncovered is proscribed by *written* institutional policy, it may be used in institutional proceedings.

Due process has been a major issue of legal contention, especially since the landmark case of *Dixon v. Alabama State Board of Education* (1961), where several black students were expelled during civil rights activities. They sued, and the court held that they had a right to a notice and disciplinary hearings.[109] In essence, this term means that the purpose of the rule or law must be examined for fairness and reasonableness. Is the student and faculty understanding of the rule the same? Did the student have the opportunity to know about the rule and its implications? What is the relationship between the rule and the objectives of the school? A decade ago, few schools had a grievance procedure, and this situation was believed by students to be a serious violation of rights. In 1975, the National Student Nurses' Association (NSNA) developed grievance procedure guidelines as part of a bill of rights for students. This was revised in 1991, and may be purchased from NSNA. Besides suggesting the makeup of the committee[110] (equal representation of students and faculty on the committee), and general procedures, such issues as allowing sufficient time, access to information and appropriate records, presentation of evidence, and use of witnesses were included.

The usual steps in any grievance process are also followed for academic grievances, with the formal process consisting of a written complaint and suggested remedy by the student grievant, followed by a written reply, a choice between a private or public hearing, permission for the student to have counsel present, a student's right to remain silent,[111] a hearing with presentation of evidence on both sides, a decision by the committee within a specific time, right of appeal, and sometimes arbitration. With students, the right to continue with classes during the total process is considered necessary, although in nursing, if the situation relates to a clinical problem and the safety of patients is considered at risk, further clinical experience may be put on hold until the matter is settled. In any case, a full and complete record of the hearing should be made. Due process is considered crucial for students who are expelled or suspended for disciplinary reasons or who feel that they are discriminated against in their extracurricular activities because of race, religion, sex, or sexual preference.

There seem to be an increasing number of grievances filed or legal complaints made because of academic concerns, especially grades. The courts have been reluctant to enter this area of academic freedom. There has yet to be a definitive ruling on curriculum and degree requirements. The attitude is demonstrated by a highly significant statement made by one court (45 Federal Rules Decisions, 133[1968], 136):

> **Education is the living and growing source of our progressive civilization, of our open repository of increasing knowledge, culture and our salutory democratic traditions. As such, education deserves the highest respect and the fullest protection of the courts in the performance of its lawful missions ....Only when erroneous and unwise actions in the field of education deprive students of federally protected rights or privileges does a federal court have power to intervene in the educational process ....[112]**

This statement has a number of counterparts in other jurisdictions. A major case involved a female fourth-year medical student who, after receiving many documented warnings, was dismissed because of her attitude in the clinical area, her unacceptable personal hygiene, inappropriate bedside manner, and tardiness. However, she had an excellent academic record. She fought this issue to the Supreme Court (in *Board of Curators of the University of Missouri v. Horowitz*) charging violation of her constitutional rights to liberty and property. She lost, in part because her clinical evaluations had been consistently unsatisfactory and she had been given sufficient warning,[113] and the court accepted the faculty's judgment. This was considered an "academic" case, as opposed to a dismissal for disciplinary reasons. It has implications for nursing. For instance, a nursing student was dismissed in her second year of a community college program for "unsafe clinical behavior." After a grievance procedure, in which her dismissal was upheld, she sued, alleging bad faith on the part of the faculty. The court refused to overturn the decision. A similar case in a diploma school resulted in the same decision by another court.[114]

Most colleges now have grievance procedures for students who think that they have received unfair grades, and these procedures must be followed first before any lawsuit can be filed. It is generally advised that before the student wages an all-out battle, the situation should be considered practically. The student must prove that the grade is arbitrary, capricious, and manifestly unjust, which is generally very difficult. Furthermore, unless that particular grade is extremely important to a student's career, the cost and time involved are greater than even a favorable result might warrant.

Cases in which the results have been more favorable to the student are related to inadequate advisement,[115] and the school catalog as a written contract. In the latter situation, a case that went to the Supreme Court (*Russell v. Salve Regina*) related to an obese woman who was admitted to a nursing program and did well. However, because she did not lose weight as agreed to in a "side contract," she was asked to withdraw before her senior year. She transferred to another college, eventually graduated and attained licensure. Then she sued with a variety of allegations, including contract violation. After a number of appeals, she was awarded $25,000 on her contract claim (a year's salary) and $5,153 for additional costs in obtaining her baccalaureate. The court also commented negatively on how the faculty had treated her about her obesity. This case had a number of other interesting points of law.[116] Earlier, also in relation to a contract issue, a landmark case was heard by the Supreme Court, which ruled that an all-women's nursing school could not refuse to admit a male student.[117]

Because those schools receiving federal money directly are subject to federal laws, the Americans with Disabilities Act of 1990, the Civil Rights Restoration Act of 1987, and Section 504 of the Rehabilitation Act of 1973 have created rights for students with disabilities. In one case, a prospective student with a severe hearing problem sued because she was not admitted to a community college nursing program. The court upheld the school's decision because the applicant's hearing disability made it unsafe for her to practice as a nurse. At another school, an applicant with Crohn's disease was refused because her disease process would probably cause her to miss too many classes. Although the court required the school to admit the student, the decision was later overturned on a procedural issue. In other disciplines, students have been dismissed because of contracting tuberculosis, AIDS, and other diseases; this may yet occur in nursing.[118]

Another type of student right involves school records. The types of student records kept by schools vary. They may consist of only the academic transcript, or may include extracurricular activities and problem situations, which are kept in an informal file. The enactment of the Buckley Amendment, described in Chap. 19, has clarified the issue of student access to records. The individual loses the right to confidentiality by waiving the right or by disclosing the information to a third person. A student's academic transcript is the most common document released, particularly to other schools and employers. Students might also be interested in a landmark decision affecting their teachers—the Supreme Court ruling in 1990 that required the disclosure of tenure committee files when bias was charged.[119]

As more student activists, most of whom are now voting citizens, request or demand certain rights as part of the academic community, more legal decisions are made. One example is the "truth in testing" laws, the first of which was passed in New York State in 1979. It required manufacturers of standardized admission tests, such as the Scholastic Aptitude Test and the Graduate Record Examination, to file test questions and correct answers with the New York Commissioner of Education after student scores are released. A federal version also allowed the students to see their answers and the correct answers after release of scores. But school rules that were once ironclad have become flexible, even without legal intervention. Students can often bring about desirable changes through participation in committees intended for this purpose. Nevertheless, it is also helpful to know one's basic legal rights as an individual and a student.

The concept of rights need not be seen as an adversary proceeding. Both the student and the school have a new accountability. In the long run, it might be more meaningful to look at certain student rights as freedoms and responsibilities. The following have been suggested:[120]

1. Freedom to learn
2. Freedom to explore ideas
3. Freedom to help choose educational goals
4. Freedom to invite and hear any person within the institution's acceptable realm
5. Freedom to express opinions publicly and privately
6. Freedom to disagree

These freedoms are based on mutual respect and commitment by faculty and students, and enhance not only the educational process, but also nursing professionalism.

REFERENCES

1. U.S. Department of Health, Education and Welfare: *Secretary's Commission on Medical Malpractice Report*, DHEW Pub. (OS) 73-88. Washington, DC: Government Printing Office, 1973. p 71.
2. Annas G: The hospital: A human rights wasteland. *Civil Liberties Rep* 9:20, Fall 1974.
3. Annas G: *The Rights of Patients: The Basic ACLU Guide to Patient Rights*, 2d ed. Carbondale, IL: Southern Illinois University Press, 1992, pp 9–12.
4. Ibid, p 1.
5. Kalisch B: Of half gods and mortals: Aesculapian authority. *Nurs Outlook* 23:22–28, January 1975.
6. Hayt E, Hayt L, Groeschel A: *Law of Hospital, Physician and Patient*, 3d ed. Berwyn, IL: Physicians' Record Company, 1972, p 478.
7. *The Rights of Patients*, op cit p 83.
8. President's Commission for the Study of Ethical Problems in Medicine and Biomedical and Behavioral Research: *Making Health Care Decisions*. Washington, DC: Government Printing Office, 1982, pp 2–3.
9. Creighton H: *Law Every Nurse Should Know*, 5th ed. Philadelphia: Saunders, 1986, pp 34–36.
10. Northrop C, Kelly M: *Legal Issue in Nursing*. St Louis: Mosby, 1987, p 86.
11. Creighton, op cit, pp 34–36.
12. LeBlang T: Disclosure of injury and illness: Responsibilities in the physician-patient relationship. *Law Med Health Care* 9:4–7, September 1981.
13. McWeeny M: The patient's right to learn or not to learn. *Nurs Admin Q* 4:83–87, Winter 1980.
14. *The Rights of Patients*, op cit, pp 86–87.
15. Ibid, p 204.
16. Ibid, p 112.
17. Ibid, pp 91–92.
18. Ibid, pp 93–94.
19. Kaufer D et al: Revising medical consent forms: An empirical model and test. *Law Med Health Care* 11:155–162, September 1983.
20. *The Rights of Patients*, op cit, p 96.
21. Creighton H: The right of informed refusal. *Nurs Mgt* 13:48, September 1982.
22. Kelly L: Neither maverick nor martyr. *Nurs Outlook* 28:644, October 1980.
23. *President's Commission for the Study of Ethical Problems in Medicine and Biomedical and Behavioral Research. Making Health Care Decisions*. Washington, DC: President's Commission, 1982, p 147.
24. Court case: What went wrong? *Nurs Life* 2:88, March–April 1982.
25. Northrop and Kelly, op cit, pp 414–416.
26. Greenlaw J: When patient's questions put you on the spot. *RN* 46:79–80, March 1983.
27. Cushing M: Informed consent; An MD responsibility? *Am J Nurs* 84:437–438, April 1984.
28. Varricchio C et al: Issues related to informed consent. *JET Nurs* 20:14–20, January–February 1993.
29. Trimberger L et al: Should you tell your patients about the risks of nursing procedures? *Nurs Life* 3:26–32, November–December 1983.
30. Black P: Brain death. *N Engl J Med* 299:398, Aug 24, 1978.
31. Bernat J et al: Defining death in theory and practice. *Hastings Cent Rep* 12:5–9, February 1982.
32. *The Rights of Patients*, op cit, pp 204–206.
33. Annas G: Prisoner in the ICU: The tragedy of William Bartling. *Hastings Cent Rep* 14:28–29, December 1984.
34. Annas G: Transferring the ethical hot potato. *Hastings Cent Rep* 17:20–21, February 1987.
35. Annas G: When procedures limit rights: From Quinlan to Conroy. *Hastings Cent Rep* 15:24–26, April 1985.
36. Price D: The ombudsman experience: Administrative protection for vulnerable patients. *Trends in Health Care, Law and Ethics* 8:49–56, Spring 1993.
37. Annas G: Do feeding tubes have more rights than patients? *Hastings Cent Rep* 16:26–27, February 1986.
38. Crawford R: The persistent vegetative state: The medical reality (getting the facts straight). *Hastings Cent Rep* 18:27–32, February 1988.
39. Meilaender G: On removing food and water: Against the stream. *Hastings Cent Rep* 14:11–13, December 1984.
40. American Medical Association, Council on Ethical and Judicial Affairs: Opinion—with-

drawing or withholding life prolonging treatment, Mar 15, 1986.

41. Fry S: New ANA guidelines on withdrawing or withholding food and fluid from patients. *Nurs Outlook* 36:122–123, 148–150, May–June 1988.

42. American Nurses Association: Position statement on forgoing artificial nutrition and hydration, Apr 2, 1992.

43. American Nurses Association: Position statement on nursing and the Patient Self-determination Act, Nov 18, 1991.

44. Price D, Murphy P: PSDA: Practical help for conscientious nurses. *J Nurs Law* 1:51–56, 1 1993.

45. Williams C: Deciding to forgo life-sustaining treatment: Recommendations on ethics. *Nurs Outlook* 31:294–295, November–December 1983.

46. Wanzer S et al: The physician's responsibility toward hopelessly ill patients. *N Engl J Med* 310:955–959, April 12, 1984.

47. Malcolm A: Giving death a hand: Pending issue. *New York Times*, June 9, 1990, p 10.

48. Angell M: Euthanasia. *N Eng J Med* 319:1348–1350, Nov 17, 1988.

49. Simons M: Dutch Parliament approves law permitting euthanasia. *New York Times*, Feb 10, 1993, p A10.

50. Orentlicher D: Physician participation in assisted suicide. *JAMA* 262:1844–1845, Oct 6, 1989.

51. Wanzer S et al: The physicians' responsibility toward hopelessly ill patients: A second look. *N Eng J Med* 320:844–849, Mar 30, 1989.

52. Brock D: Voluntary active euthanasia. *Hastings Cent Rep* 22:10–22, February 1992.

53. Kowolski S: Assisted suicide: Where do nurses draw the line? *Nurs Health Care* 14:70–76, February 1993.

54. Curran W et al: *Health Care Law: Forensic Science and Public Policy*. Boston: Little, Brown, 1991.

55. Clayton E: From Rogers to Rivers: The rights of the mentally ill to refuse medication. *Am J Law Med* 13:7–52, 1 1987.

56. Oriol M, Oriol RD: Involuntary commitment and the right to refuse medication. *J Psychosocial Nursing* 24:15–20, November 1986.

57. Trandel-Korenchuck D, Trandel-Korenchuk K: Informed consent and mental incompetency. *Nurs Admin Q* 7:76–78, Fall 1983.

58. Holder A: Disclosure and consent problems in pediatrics. *Law Med Health Care* 16:219–228, Fall–Winter 1988.

59. Isaacs S, Swartz A: *The Consumer's Legal Guide to Today's Health Care*. New York: Houghton Mifflin, 1992, pp 183–185, 244–247.

60. Medenwald N: Children's liberation—in a hospital. *MCN* 5:231–232, July–August 1980.

61. Isaacs, op cit, pp 246–247.

62. Taub S: Withholding treatment from defective newborns. *Law Med Health Care* 10:4–10, February 1982.

63. *The Rights of Patients*, op cit, pp 213–214.

64. Creighton H: Shall we choose life or let die? *Nurs Mgt* 15:16–18, August 1984.

65. Huefner D: Severely handicapped infants with life-threatening conditions: Federal intrusions into the decision not to treat. *Am J Law Med* 12:171–205, 2 1986.

66. Fleischman A: Parental responsibility and the infant bioethics committee. *Hastings Cent Rep* 20:21–22, March–April 1990.

67. Nolan K: Let's take Baby Doe to Alaska. *Hastings Cent Rep* 20:3, January–February 1991.

68. Weir R: Pediatric ethics committee: Ethical advisers or legal watchdogs? *Law Med Health Care* 13:99–109, Fall 1987.

69. Stantz ML: Defining informed consent. *MCN* 13:98, March–April 1985.

70. Institute of Medicine: *The Responsible Conduct of Research in the Health Sciences*. Washington, DC: National Academy Press, 1989.

71. Northrop and Kelly, op cit, pp 333–338.

72. Noble MA: Written informed consent: Closing the door to clinical research. *Nurs Outlook* 33:292–293, November–December 1985.

73. Oberst M: Another look at informed consent. *Nurs Outlook* 33:294–295, November–December 1983.

74. Floyd J: Research and informed consent. *J Psychosocial Nurs* 26:13–17, March 1988.

75. Northrop and Kelly, op cit, pp 338–340.

76. *The Rights of Patients*, op cit, pp 148–156.

77. Ibid, pp 178–179.

78. Computerized records' confidentiality a growing concern, attorney explains. *BNA's Health Reporter* 3:810–811, June 16, 1994.

79. Ibid.

80. Grad F: *The Public Health Law Manual*, 2d ed. Washington, DC: American Public Health Association, 1990, pp 282–283.

81. Given Health Care Center: *Principles of Practice*, unpublished, Burlington, VT: University of Vermont, 1974, p 1.

82. Philipson N, McMullen P: Medical records: Promoting patient confidentiality. *Nurs Connections* 6:48–50, Winter 1993.

83. *The Rights of Patients*, op cit, pp 171–172.

84. Ibid, pp 189–191.

85. Fiesta J: Protecting children: A public duty to report, *Nurs Mgt* 23:14–17, July 1992.

86. Thobaben M, Anderson L: Reporting elder abuse: It's the law. *Am J Nurs* 85:371–374, April 1985.

87. Brent N: Confidentiality and HIV status: A duty to inform third parties? *Home Healthcare Nurse* 8:27–29, April 1990.

88. Northrop C: Rights versus regulation: Confidentiality in the age of AIDS. *Nurs Outlook* 36:208, July–August 1988.

89. Silva A: Confidentiality crucial to nurse-patient relationship. *Am Nurse* 25:16, October 1993.

90. Henry P: Nurse practitioners and the duty to warn. *Nurse Pract Forum* 1:4–5, June 1990.

91. *The Rights of Patients*, op cit, pp 70–71.

92. Aiken T, Catalano J: *Legal, Ethical, and Political Issues in Nursing*. Philadelphia: Davis, 1994, pp 151–152.

93. McIntyre R: Abortions and the search for public policy. *Trends Health Care, Law Ethics* 8:7–16, 3, 1993.

94. Rhodes AM: Webster versus Reproductive Health Services. *MCN* 14:423, November–December 1987.

95. Benshoff J: Planned Parenthood v. Casey. *Trends Health Care, Law Ethics* 8:21–31, March 1993.

96. Cohen S: Health care policy and abortion: A comparison. *Nurs Outlook* 38:20–25, January–February 1990.

97. Isaacs, op cit, pp 179, 233–235.

98. Creighton, *Law Every Nurse Should Know*, op cit, p 212.

99. Isaacs, op cit, pp 171–178.

100. Moseley C, Beard M: Norplant: Nursing's responsibility in procreative rights. *Nurs Health Care* 15:294–297, June 1994.

101. Creighton H: The nurse and the surrogate mother. *Nurs Mgt* 16:40–43, June 1985.

102. Andrews L: The aftermath of Baby M: Proposed state laws on surrogate motherhood. *Hastings Cent Rep* 17:31–40, October–November 1987.

103. Annas G. Death without dignity for commercial surrogacy: The case of Baby M. *Hastings Cent Rep* 18:21–24, April–May 1988.

104. Annas G: Surrogate embryo transfer: The perils of patenting. *Hastings Cent Rep* 14:25–26, June 1984.

105. Curtin L: Lesbian, single and geriatric women: To breed or not to breed. *Nurs Mgt* 25:11–16, March 1994.

106. Nolan K, Swenson S: New tools, new dilemmas: Genetic frontiers. *Hastings Cent Rep* 18:40–42, October–November 1988.

107. Robertson J: Rights, symbolism, and public policy in fetal tissue transplants. *Hastings Cent Rep* 18:5–12, December 1988.

108. Weiler K, Helms L: Responsibilities of nursing education: The lessons of Russell v Salve Regina. *J Prof Nurs* 9:131–138, May–June 1993.

109. Lessner M: Avoiding student-faculty litigation. *Nurse Educ* 5:29–32, November–December 1990.

110. National Student Nurses' Association: *The Bill of Rights and Responsibilities for Students of Nursing*. New York: The Association, 1991.

111. Lessner, op cit, p 32.

112. Pollok C et al: Faculties have rights, too. *Am J Nurs* 77:636, April 1977.

113. Parrott T: Dismissed for clinical deficiencies. *Nurs Educ* 18:14–17, November–December 1993.

114. Ibid, p 17.

115. Liability issues related to advising and counseling on health issues. *Nurse Educ* 17:3–4, January–February 1992.

116. Weiler and Helms, op cit.

117. Greenlaw J: Mississippi University for Women v Hogan: The Supreme Court rules on female-only nursing school. *Law Med Health Care* 10:267–269, December 1982.

118. Helms L, Weiler K: Disability discrimination in nursing education: An evaluation of legislation and litigation. *J Prof Nurs* 9:358–366, November–December 1993.

119. Blum D: Supreme Court rejects privacy claim for tenure files, says university must disclose information in bias case. *Chron Higher Ed* 33:A1, A17–20, Jan 17, 1990.

120. *The Bill of Rights and Responsibilities for Students of Nursing*, op cit.

Part III

Professional Components and Career Development

Organizations
and
Publications

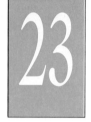

Organizational Procedures and Issues

THE MORE COMPLEX and highly organized society becomes, the harder it is for a single individual to exert any significant influence or power. There are exceptions to this rule, of course. There will be always be pioneers and crusaders—individuals who through sheer force of personality, conviction, and determination succeed in making an impact. But by and large, the concerted effort of a group of people working in an organized manner is necessary today to accomplish a given purpose, to effect a change in the status quo.

This is as true in nursing as in any other field on both student and graduate levels. One student alone, for instance, can do little to change what may seem to be the out-of-date or autocratic practices of the nursing school administration, but working through the student association in the school or through a unit of the National Student Nurses' Association (NSNA), she or he may very well bring about improvements. Similarly, one nurse, no matter how dedicated or determined, would never have been able to make it easier and less expensive for older citizens to get needed hospital and medical care. Yet the strong voice of the ANA, speaking out in favor of health insurance coverage for the aging under the Social Security system, was one of the factors that brought about Medicare. ANA took this stand because the majority of its members indicated that this was what *they* wanted. So, working through the professional organization, the individual *was* heard, *did* have influence, *did* help to bring about change.

There are many persons who are inclined to do nothing more than grumble to themselves and others about what they don't like or what they would like to see accomplished. But so long as they do no more than complain and unless they join with their colleagues to act in an organized, effective way, they will probably continue to be powerless and dissatisfied. That doesn't mean that a person should simply become a "joiner"—someone who seems to become a member of almost any organization. Such a process only scatters the person's interests and energies in many directions and provides no focus. But there are many organizations concerned with health and nursing that a nursing student or RN will want to either join, support, or at least be familiar with. By joining some of them, individuals will be able to work with colleagues in advancing their own nursing interests or those of nursing as a whole; in others, they will find the companionship of those with the same, perhaps more specific, concerns; and in still others, they will be able to keep abreast of the forces that are influencing nursing and health care today.

The nature and purpose of these nursing and health organizations will be discussed in the following chapters. Of concern in this chapter is the nurse's role—or anyone's role, for that matter—as an organization member. Presumably, people join an organization because its concerns and goals are the same as their own. Joining is not enough. An association's success depends on intelligent, industrious, and conscientious leadership; a willing, enthusiastic, and well-informed membership; adequate financial support; and sound business organization and administration. It is the responsibility of each member to help make all of these things realities.

MEMBERSHIP RESPONSIBILITIES

Members of any organization should feel responsible for learning as much as possible about it—its history, purposes, the number and composition of its membership, and its principal activities. They should study the constitution and bylaws, the code of ethics if there is one, and subscribe to its official publication. They should learn the names of the organization's principal current officers and preferably their background. When attending meetings, they should listen carefully to the discussion, and become familiar with the most important issues under consideration and the conditions and facts that influence the decisions to be taken. This will take time, but spending just a few hours can prepare new members for rewarding participation in the organization's work.

As soon as a person is ready to take a more active part in the meetings, he or she can enter into discussions, ask relevant questions, help clarify issues by presenting a fresh and knowledgeable point of view, accept appointments to committees, and volunteer to help as time and ability dictate. Restraint, diplomacy, and a sense of good timing should guide new members as they find their place in any group.

Individuals who hold or want to hold office should have a copy of authoritative rules of order for organizing and conducting an organization's business and should become familiar enough with the publication so that they can readily find the information needed. Whoever presides over formal business meetings in any other capacity must know how to do so efficiently, without referring to the book of rules, except for an answer to unusually difficult questions. The rules of order used by a particular association are usually named in its bylaws.

Most members do not need to be as familiar as an officer with the minute details of parliamentary procedure, but should know how to address the presiding officer; formulate, present, and vote on a motion; and be familiar with other basic procedures that facilitate the progress of the meeting. This knowledge will enhance their ability to express views and contribute to the discussion without embarrassment or lack of confidence. On the other hand, it would be naive not to recognize that parliamentary procedure can be used as a manipulative tool to bring about certain action or lack of action. For instance, if an item is not placed on the agenda by the presider, other officers, or members, it is not likely to be discussed and certainly not acted on. If the item is placed in an unfavorable position—at the end of a long session when people are less alert, at a point when a certain voting constituency is present for a short time (some bylaws allow any member present to vote), or at a point when certain information is not yet available, or after a controversial, emotional, related item—the action taken might be quite different than it would be if the topic were discussed at another time. There are also those who misuse the intricacies of parliamentary procedure by complex motions to amend, substitute, or amend the amendment of a motion repeatedly so that the members may be totally confused about the real issue in the motion to be voted on. Those speaking to a motion may also be deliberately or inadvertently obscure, incorrect, or inappropriate in their statements, which, if the usual procedure in speaking from the floor is observed, may make the point difficult to correct and clarify. (And then there are always those who like to be heard whether or not what they say is pertinent.) Therefore, the average member should be alert to these machinations and learn how to combat them. If a motion seems to have been railroaded through, it is particularly useful to know how that action can be reversed before the final adjournment. Because any organization has its political aspects, those who are interested in seeing that a certain action is taken seldom take a chance on this simply occurring during a business meeting. An effort is made to sell individuals or sub-groups within the organization on the idea before formal action is taken—that is, lobbying. The formal action can be orchestrated: who makes the motion, who speaks to it, what supporting information must be introduced, is it best referred to a task force or committee, and, most important of all, are the votes there? A politically astute member tries to estimate at what point the issue is more likely to be voted in the desired direction, delaying the vote by some form of postponement if necessary.

WHO DOES THE WORK?

Even the most careful plans and the finest constitution and bylaws do not ensure a healthy, productive, organization. The plans and directions must be put into action. Who does this? Every officer, every committee member, every member at large shares the responsibility for knowing what that person as an individual can do for the good of the entire membership and for doing it—unless health or some other serious problem is a deterrent.

An incapacitated officer or committee chair should resign promptly and give the organization the opportunity of deciding whether or not to choose another. Members who accept an appointment to a committee and later find themselves unable to assist with its work should withdraw, leaving the chairman or other authorized person free to appoint another, more productive member.

Members in today's organizations can be categorized as owners, potential owners, the unambitious, or dissidents. The owners of an organization know the system and how to work it; are adept at organizational politics; are the leaders or the supporters of leaders; make decisions and dispense rewards. The owners are satisfied members, highly involved, and make up about 10 percent of an organization's membership. Potential owners comprise about 50 percent of the membership and are usually too busy to participate in leadership although they might like to have some kind of organizational power. Potential owners pay dues and may be an untapped bounty for an organization as they have opinions and views that are not sought out but might be important for the organization to have. Dissidents are those who are generally very involved in organizations but are dissatisfied—dissatisfied with leadership, policy, programs, or positions. The dissident often enjoys the role of the contrarian, seeking recognition through opposition. Dissidents comprise about 10 percent of an organization's membership. The fourth category of member is the unambitious. Approximately 30 percent of an organization's members are satisfied with the organization's work but have little involvement in the organization. They would rather "pay than do," shun power and enjoy watching from afar.[1]

President, Chairperson, Moderator

Although the elected or appointed head of an association does a great deal of work behind the scenes during a term of office, the membership thinks of this person most frequently as the one who presides at meetings. This is one of the most important responsibilities for which a leader needs particular skills, talents, and personality assets.

The individual should be in complete control of emotions; avoid distracting mannerisms; speak clearly; be discreet, impartial, and courteous; have considerable stamina; and be businesslike. However, a good sense of humor is a decided asset. A good leader should be able to sense the atmosphere of a meeting and prevent it from becoming explosive or detrimental to progress. It is even important to be sensitive to the physical comport of the assembly and to do what is possible to improve ventilation, lighting, seating arrangements, or whatever else is indicated to keep everyone alert and interested. The presiding officer should be prompt for every meeting, ready to function at the appointed time, and, as soon as a quorum is present, call the meeting to order. This encourages habitual latecomers to be on time and helps to assure prompt adjournment.

The president must have a thorough knowledge of the history of the organization, what it has done in the past, and what it plans to do in the future. Rarely should a question find this person completely unprepared; if the president doesn't know the answer, he or she should know who does or where it can be found. Sometimes the questions are referred to someone else even if the chair knows the answer. This might happen when a question is asked about the organization's finances, and the president asks the treasurer to answer. Any officer must know when it is appropriate to withhold information as well as when to disclose it. It is important always to be in control of the situation and to keep the audience informed about the discussion before the group to avoid the confusion that results when members do not understand the issue.

Generally, the presiding officer should not express a personal opinion on an issue. This is because of the need to maintain a neutral attitude and because one of the chief duties of a leader is to encourage others to participate. It is a good policy to subtly encourage the less assertive member to speak up and discourage the individuals who always want to express their views at length. In doing this, the presiding head must be eminently fair and unbiased, allowing all the right to air their views.

The chair (whoever is presiding) must be thoroughly familiar with the agenda of every meeting over which she or he presides and know how to complete it expeditiously and in accordance with the rules of procedure adopted by the organization. This is learned through studying the rules, observing other presiding officers in action, and experience. Every meeting will bring confidence and learning from successes and failures.

A president may have exhibited considerable ability to lead discussions but may not have had extensive practice in handling motions, one of the major responsibilities of a presiding officer. Sometimes this is a simple procedure, but it can

become involved. The chair who understands the intricacies guides the action deftly and gains the respect of the group; the one who gets confused about what step takes precedence over another, for example, may create a chaotic situation that will leave the members dissatisfied and possibly highly critical. Some organizations use a parliamentarian to avoid problems.

It is vital to be acquainted with as many members of the organization as possible and to become familiar with their interests and abilities. This will help in making appointments to committees and selecting members for other assignments. If the organization is widespread, visits to several different areas or constituent associations each year, giving necessary help, often stimulate the members in their work. On social occasions the president should mingle with members; this will establish rapport with the various groups and will tend to promote interest and enthusiasm.

The president must keep in touch with the work and progress of other officers and the committees in the organization and cooperate amicably and constructively with them. Democratic principles must be observed, allowing each person to use the initiative and authority necessary to discharge assigned duties and responsibilities without interference while, at the same time, demanding first-rate performance. If the organization has a paid chief staff officer or director and a headquarters staff, the officers must observe the same principles, carrying the appropriate responsibilities but never usurping prerogatives that are rightfully those of the staff.

The head of any organization needs leadership qualities in large measure. Although every individual elected to such an office probably will not possess all of them, there will be many opportunities to develop them.

Vice President

Although, theoretically, a vice president—particularly a first vice president—is as capable as the president, because she or he must be prepared to function in the president's absence or in an emergency, the qualifications tend to be less exacting. Many persons with outstanding leadership ability are unwilling to accept the relatively inactive post of the vice presidency. This happens in organizations of all sizes and types, from a local volunteer group to the federal government.

To make the office more challenging, some associations declare in their bylaws that the vice presidents shall also be heads of committees or assume other responsibilities. Among the most common are chairperson of the program, policy development, or bylaws committees. Vice presidents may also represent the organization in meetings, interorganizational committees, or task forces. This gives the vice president an opportunity to make a specific contribution to the organization and also gives visibility. Sometimes large organizations have more than one vice president, all with specific responsibilities.

One trend that seems to be occurring is to include a president-elect on the board, preparing that person for assumption of the presidential office with minimal orientation. There are some disadvantages: a double-term commitment on the part of that individual and probable inability to prevent that person from succeeding to the presidency if she or he proves to be ineffectual at the board level.

Secretary

The secretary often takes the minutes and may deal with correspondence. If the organization is large enough to have a professional staff, the actual taking of detailed minutes and handling of correspondence are done by staff, but both are checked, and sometimes signed by the secretary, president, or other appropriate person. Nevertheless, the functions of the secretary are spelled out in the bylaws and may be the responsibility of an elected person or duly authorized staff.

In a smaller organization, the secretary who thinks and writes clearly, is well informed about

the association's business, and has the necessary knowledge and skill to write appropriate minutes is invaluable. The secretary must be able to keep alert throughout meetings that can be both tedious and frustrating, and maintain an outward attitude of equanimity, neutrality, and cooperation regardless of inner conflicts. She or he must be objective and impartial in all reports in spite of the fact that at times it is necessary to "interpret the interpretations" of others when transcribing the notes taken at a meeting. It is important to be methodical, reliable, and prompt in getting out all reports and memoranda. The corresponding secretary needs to be a master of the courteous and appropriate phrase, because these responsibilities have important public relations connotations. Neatness and promptness in correspondence are highly desirable.

Treasurer

It is not unusual for the treasurer of an organization to be selected more carefully than the president, and almost as much is expected. The principal qualifications should be honesty, accuracy, and conscientiousness in keeping records, and knowledge of bookkeeping procedures, budgeting, and financial reporting. Business experience is a decided asset. The membership, even when it knows better, often judges the treasurer's ability by the balance on hand in the treasury.

The treasurer of any organization is often chair of its committee on finance. This post requires the usual skills necessary to conduct a committee meeting plus additional ability to discuss facts and figures intelligently, often before board members who may not be well versed in financial matters but are vitally interested in the organization's purse strings. The president's work is also made easier by a competent treasurer because so many of the organization's activities depend on its financial status. Even if the details of the financial management of the organization are carried out by skilled employees, the board has fiduciary responsibility for the association. Budgets cannot be properly developed or adhered to and intelligent financial decisions cannot be made, nor a myriad of state and federal reports filed, if accurate information is not available. Therefore, board members and especially the treasurer must have at least a basic understanding of financial management.

Committees

An organization's bylaws usually call for standing committees, with the number depending more on the scope of the activities than on the volume.

The quantity and quality of work done by each special group greatly influence the status and progress of the organization, although sometimes so indirectly that the general membership is unaware of their extent. For example, the nominating committee is responsible for finding persons who are willing and eligible to fill elected offices and who have the qualifications for them. This requires diligence and excellent salesmanship, especially if the prospective candidate is initially reluctant to serve. In large or widely scattered organizations, many members don't know the candidates personally. They must depend on the nominating committee to select the best available people; they then base their voting decisions on whatever information about them is released through official channels.

Members of the nominating committee, therefore, must always seek the best person or persons regardless of friendships, school ties, personal obligations, or any such influencing factor. And it follows logically that the persons responsible for appointing or electing members of this committee must consider integrity to be one of their most important personal qualifications. Their influence on the future of the organization is considerable: a ballot can be set up in such a way that a certain individual or someone representing a particular constituency is sure to win that election. This is especially true with a mail ballot, where a strong write-in vote

is almost impossible to achieve unless it is highly organized.

The work of other committees often is equally important. Some aspects may be obvious; others may need definition and delineation of responsibilities.

PARLIAMENTARY PROCEDURES

The purpose of the business meetings of any organization is to transact business efficiently while recognizing the rights of individual members and giving minority and opposing groups ample opportunity to air their views, yet assuring that the wishes of the majority prevail. To achieve this purpose, a methodical order of conducting the meetings is essential.

When early American congresses first organized, they borrowed from the British Parliament many practices, which they adapted for their own use. Further changes were made from time to time until a distinctive American system evolved. The terms *parliamentary procedure* and (incorrectly) *parliamentary law* are used, however, in referring to both the American and British systems, which still have a good deal in common.

The procedures that have been used for many years by the United States Senate and House of Representatives developed from four sources:

1. The Constitution of the United States.
2. Jefferson's *Manual of Parliamentary Procedure*, which he prepared while he was vice president and presided over the Senate.
3. Rules that have been adopted by the House since its beginning and that may be changed with each Congress; these rules are sometimes called the *legislative manual*.
4. Decisions rendered by the presiding officer and the chairman of the Committee of the Whole House.

The transactions of less imposing bodies than the United States Congress are governed similarly. Each usually has a constitution and by-laws citing the officers and their duties in general, the order of business, voting regulations, and other matters related to the conduct of business meetings. The presiding officer makes decisions consistent with his or her authority, often with the advice of a parliamentarian employed by the organization. Each major meeting of the membership or house of delegates may produce changes in rules or the formulation of new ones needed to expedite its own activities, and each organization adopts a manual of parliamentary procedure to guide the business transactions.

The most popular guide for formal business procedure is *Robert's Rules of Order, Revised*. This reference work, written by General Henry M. Robert of the United States Army and published originally in 1876, is based upon the rules and practices of Congress. It is generally considered the most authoritative book of its kind, and some organizations attempt to follow it to the letter. Others use it only as a final authority to settle a controversial point. Still others select simpler but equally reliable rules of order to guide their transactions, such as *Sturgis' Standard Code of Parliamentary Procedure* by Alice F. Sturgis, and *Parliamentary Law* by F. M. Gregg.

As stated in *Robert's Rules of Order, Revised*:

> **Parliamentary procedure, properly used, provides the means whereby the affairs of an organization or club can be controlled by the general will within the whole membership. The "general will" in this sense does not always imply even near unanimity or "consensus" but rather the right of the deliberate majority to decide. Complementary to this is the right of the minority—at least a strong minority—to require the majority to be deliberate—that is—to act according to its considered judgment after a full and fair "working through" of the issues involved.[2]**

Although *Robert's Rules of Order* and other such publications include duties of officers and committees and other information, the discussion here will be concerned with the conduct of a business meeting because duties of officers and other details are defined in an organization's constitution and bylaws, which supersede any other rules.

Some of the principles and techniques of parliamentary procedure can perhaps be best presented by following an imaginary annual meeting of the NSNA from beginning to end. This organization, described in the next chapter, is the membership organization for nursing students. When the NSNA bylaws do not specify a procedure, *Robert's Rules of Order, Revised* is used as a guide.

Most formal meetings have an order of business. A classic example follows.

1. Call to order.
2. Minutes of previous meetings.
3. Reports of officers, boards, and standing committees.
    Executive reports.
    Executive announcements.
    Order and procedure of reports.
       President.
       Vice president.
       Secretary.
       Treasurer.
       Board of directors.
    Standing committees.
4. Reports of special committees.
5. Announcements.
6. Unfinished business.
7. New business.
8. Adjournment.

In this meeting, these steps will be considered one at a time and others, which are often included in the order of business, will be added.

Although the following discussion implies that the NSNA's business is completed in one session, it usually takes several sessions to finish it. This is usual at convention meetings and may be required in the bylaws by certain wording, such as the need for the nominating committee to report the ticket at a certain time.

An order of business must be flexible enough to be realistic. For example, if there is good reason for having the reports of special committees given ahead of the standing committees, the president is privileged to make that change simply by announcing it from the chair. The president is also privileged to make announcements or have others make them and to invite the headquarters staff members and guests to address the assembly whenever it appears appropriate and helpful. A major reordering of the agenda by the presiding officer or another member may require approval of the total group.

Call to Order

The president calls the meeting to order by rapping a gavel for attention if necessary and saying, "Will the meeting please come to order?" or words to that effect. The secretary then presents the agenda for the meeting and the parliamentarian explains the basic rules of parliamentary procedure that will be followed.

To make sure that a quorum (as defined in the NSNA bylaws) is present, the president asks the secretary to call a roll of delegates. If a quorum is present, the president so states; if not, he or she may declare a recess or fill in the time with matters of a nonbusiness nature until enough members arrive. (To simplify the use of pronouns, it will be assumed for this discussion that the president is female.)

Minutes of the Preceding Meeting

Although the NSNA's secretary keeps accurate and complete files on all business transacted at every meeting of the association, it is highly improbable that minutes of the association's last meeting will be read, because these would be long, detailed, and time-consuming. So, in lieu of reading the minutes, most large membership organizations distribute mimeographed copies of the previous meeting's minutes or make them available upon request.

However, in meetings of smaller groups within the NSNA, such as the executive board or one of the committees, the second step in the order of business could be the reading of the minutes of the preceding meeting. This is done by the secretary at the request of the chairman or silently by the members. It is also possible that minutes will have been distributed and read before the meeting. When this is finished, the chair asks the members if they wish to make any additions or corrections. A member wishing to make a change rises and after being recognized makes a statement that might be something like this: "Madame Chairman, my name is Helen Gibson [or simply "Helen Gibson"], Kentucky. The secretary reported that the president of the New Jersey association moved that the executive board investigate the feasibility of promoting a national student nurse week. The motion was actually made by the president of the New York State association."

Small groups in which members know each other may not need to identify themselves. Nonetheless, it is correct parliamentary procedure. The chairman and the recording secretary *must* know who is speaking and other members *like* to know.

The president says "Thank you" to the member and asks the secretary to change the record, unless the correction is contradicted by someone. When all requests for additions or corrections have been made, the president states, "The minutes will be (or are) accepted as corrected." If no changes are indicated, she says, "The minutes will be (or are) accepted as read."

Report of the President

The president usually presents her own report but has the privilege of asking the secretary or someone else to read it. If presenting it personally, she will ask the first vice president to take the chair until the report is completed. This is because correct parliamentary procedure requires that a meeting must always have a presiding officer and the president cannot preside and present a report at the same time.

Although the president's report may contain some facts and figures, it is not usually a business report. Rather it is of a general nature and greatly influenced by the president's personality. Included will be an account of the progress made by the association during the past year, the satisfactions and perhaps the disappointments; some of the things done while president, such as visiting state nurses' associations and speaking at meetings; plans and ambitions for the future with implied and possibly formulated recommendations based on needs as she sees them; and expressions of appreciation to others for their support and assistance.

No formal acceptance procedure of the president's report is indicated. If reports are not captured electronically, a copy is given to the secretary for the record and the president resumes the chair.

Report of the Secretary

The secretary's report includes information about his or her personal activities in the office, stressing the broad scope of official duties. When the report has been completed, the president accepts it as presented without asking for a vote by the delegates.

Report of the Treasurer

The treasurer's report is a statement showing the income and expenses of the association during the past year and its financial status at the end of the fiscal year. When the treasurer has finished presenting the report, the president says, "The treasurer's report is accepted as presented," and may add, "And it is filed for audit."

Any questions about the treasurer's report should be asked at this time. The president may reply or may ask the treasurer to do so. General discussion is permitted at the president's discretion.

Report of the Committee on Nominations

Much of the work of the nominating committee—deciding upon appropriate candidates for office, securing their permission to be nominated, and compiling their biographies—is done prior to the annual meeting. At the meeting the chairperson (sometimes simply called chair) of the nominating committee, when called upon by the president, reads the slate of officers to the assembly. When finished, she or he says, "Madame President, I move the adoption of this slate of officers." The president then asks the house if there are other nominations. If there are none, a delegate will move that the nominations be closed. This motion will be seconded and voted promptly.

A *nomination from the floor* can be made by any delegate by addressing the chair, naming the proposed candidate, and giving briefly the proposed nominee's qualifications for the post. A special form supplied by the nominating committee, containing detailed information about the candidate, is submitted to the nominating committee if the nomination is seconded. Nominations from the floor are closed by house vote.

Following the meeting, the nominating committee reviews the information about candidates who were nominated from the floor and may post their names and offices for which they are candidates near the voting place where balloting is done. It is also possible that a convention paper or other form of written communication will be distributed to members with election information and the nominees' names and qualifications. It may or may not be possible to have the new names printed on the ballot in time for the election. If not, the names may be written in by the delegates wishing to vote for them.

Voting is done at a time and place designated by the executive board. Delegates must present credentials before they are allowed to vote. When voting is completed—usually within a few hours—the tellers who were appointed by the president at the first meeting count the ballots and prepare a report to be given at the NSNA's closing business session. A plurality vote (more votes than any other candidate for the same office) is required for election by the NSNA. If a majority vote were required, a candidate would need at least one more than half the votes cast to be elected.

Reports of Other Committees

As the NSNA president calls for reports of the association's other committees, the chairperson of each goes to the platform—if invited by the president—or to a microphone or other place where she or he can be seen and heard easily by the entire assembly, addresses the chair, and presents the report. If any action is to be taken (usually recommendations), the committee chair or someone else says, "Madame President, I move the acceptance of this report" or "adoption of the recommendation." A delegate may second the motion, and the motion is handled like any other. If no action is required on any sections of the report, the preceding step may be omitted and the president will thank the reporting person. At times, reports are presented in a book of reports and are not read if the business of the committee does not appear controversial or call for action. They can still be discussed, however, if members desire.

Unfinished Business

At this point the president makes sure that any items of business left incomplete because of time limitations, absent persons, and so on, are satisfactorily completed.

New Business

New business is often the most interesting and exciting part of the agenda. If the issues are controversial, debate may be heated and lengthy. Even if they're not, the topics discussed indicate the course the association will take during the months ahead.

Resolutions

Resolutions may be one of the most important parts of a major meeting, because they are indications of the organization's position on key issues. Resolutions are submitted by individual members, groups, or committees within the organization to a resolutions committee and/or the board of directors. A resolutions committee may, usually with the permission of the originators, combine similar resolutions or change some aspect of a resolution.

The board has the privilege of supporting or not supporting the resolution, and in some organizations it can withhold it from the voting body. Some organizations hold preliminary hearings to expedite action and/or agreement without the formality of strict parliamentary procedure. This often clarifies misunderstandings and saves time during the business meeting. Generally, a member whose resolution has been rejected for presentation has the right to introduce it from the floor.

Resolutions, except courtesy resolutions, are often meant to be acted upon by the organization after the meeting. For instance, a resolution may call for a letter to the President of the United States requesting better federal funding of nursing education, or it could direct long-term activities of the organization. Although the wording is often formal, with one or more *whereas* clauses giving the reasons for the resolution preceding the resolution, there's no reason why the wording can't be clear and concise, so that the message is understood by all. Reviewing the past resolutions of an organization gives an excellent picture of its philosophy and goals and is one means of judging its quality. Therefore, although resolutions frequently come toward the end of a meeting, they should be given thought before voting.

Adjournment

After the amenities have been observed, such as the passing of other resolutions expressing appreciation for services and courtesies, and perhaps introduction of the new officers, the meeting is adjourned by motion and vote.

MANAGING MOTIONS

The work of a business session goes much better if officers and members know and practice the proper methods of handling motions according to parliamentary procedure. A motion is a proposal or suggestion intended to initiate action, effect progress, or allow the assembly to express itself as holding certain views. It is through these motions—made, seconded, discussed, and approved by a majority of the delegates—that the association is enabled to transact its business, make decisions, and move forward.

Uncomplicated motions may be passed very quickly by *silent assent*, such as accepting the secretary's report as read; or by *viva voce*, which means responding "aye" or "no" ("yea" or "nay") in response to a request from the presiding officer; *viva voce* may also be used in voting on involved issues. However, if the vote is, or is likely to be, close, the chair will ask for a *show of hands* or a *standing vote*, because they permit an actual count. Some organizations now use electronic systems to give an instant count, which saves time and arguments about accuracy. A *written vote*, or *ballot*, may be indicated and is usually required for elections.

To Make a Motion

A member who wishes to make a motion always:

1. Stands and goes to microphone when indicated.
2. Waits, if necessary, until the speaker ahead has stopped talking. In general, it is advisable to remain seated until the previous speaker has finished, but if several members have motions to present, it's better to "get in line."
3. Waits for the chair's signal to go ahead. This may be done with a nod of the head or verbally.
4. Addresses the presiding officer as Madame (or Mister) Chairman, Chairperson, President, or Speaker.
5. Identifies oneself by name and state or other designation as indicated. Sometimes stating the name of the office held, the

committee, or some other affiliation is appropriate.
6. States the motion clearly and succinctly. When time permits, it is a good idea to write out a motion before rising to make it. This helps the individual say what is intended and also to repeat it verbatim, if requested. Frequently, a written motion is given to the secretary to be sure it will be recorded accurately in the minutes.

Most motions require seconding before action. The chair will call for a second, if indicated, particularly when there is likely to be discussion of the motion. The member who does the seconding rises, addresses the chair, and after identification, says, "I second the motion." If no one seconds a motion calling for seconding, the motion is automatically lost and the president so states. No mention of it is made in the official records.

Discussion

Assuming that a motion is seconded, the chair next says, "It has been moved and seconded that…Is there any discussion?" If there is none, she asks for a vote by one of the methods previously mentioned. A member wishing to ask a question or make a comment follows the usual procedure for recognition.

Sometimes discussion is prolonged, heated, and confused, involving proposed amendments to the original motion and perhaps even amendments to the amendment, known as *subsidiary amendments*. The presiding officer must be fair and skillful to permit all persons to express their views and yet not seriously impede the progress of the meeting. The action must then be guided back to the original motion, disposing of the last-mentioned items first.

Discussion of a motion may be terminated if a member calls for "the question." This means that the member feels that the matter has been discussed sufficiently for the members to vote intelligently on it. Because to terminate the discussion without the approval of the assembly would infringe on the privilege of unlimited debate, the chair then asks, "Are you ready for the question?" If a sufficient number, as predetermined by the association's rules of order, vote in the affirmative, the motion is put to a vote. Otherwise, debate must be reopened or some other method must be used to handle the motion before the house.

Decision

The ultimate disposition of a motion depends on the majority decision of the delegates. If more than half of them vote "yes," it is passed; if the majority vote "no," the motion is, of course, defeated. Sometimes a motion is passed "as amended," that is, not in its original form, but with one or more changes in it, or additions to it, as proposed from the floor during the discussion. Some organizations require a two-thirds vote for passage of a motion or of motions in certain areas. These requirements are spelled out in the association's bylaws.

When there is obvious conflict or confusion about a particular motion, especially when it may have become complicated or unclear as a result of several proposed amendments, a motion to *refer it to a committee* may be made. This motion in itself may be debated. If it is passed, then the original motion goes to an appropriate committee for further study and possible presentation at some later date.

It is also possible to vote to *table* a motion; this means that it is set aside temporarily, permitting the chair to move on with the agenda, but will be taken up again later in the same session or meeting. A vote to *postpone* action on the motion until some other time may also be taken. Decisions to table or postpone action on a motion are most likely to be made when the matter at hand is a complicated or hotly debated issue. Any of these actions gives the members more time to clarify their thinking about it. It also permits more time to marshal arguments pro and con and, finally, permits the president, possibly aided by the parliamentarian, to study the motion so that at some later date it may be

reviewed clearly for the delegates. Sometimes a tabled motion never comes for action again, because everyone agrees that it's better not acted on (or it's forgotten).

Occasionally, members pass a motion that they later regret, either because the decision was made hastily, with incomplete information, or in a state of confusion. To bring that same motion before the assembly again, an individual voting on the prevailing side may move to reconsider. Anyone can second. The motion to reconsider takes precedence over other motions, and therefore is acted on at once, regardless of what else is being discussed. It is debatable, and if passed, the entire issue of the previously passed motion is open for discussion, with the opportunity to clarify or to introduce needed information. It is then handled in the usual manner.

The responsible member and, especially, the officer of any organization will not want to depend on this necessarily brief presentation of parliamentary procedure as the sole guide to informed action. If a meeting is not run efficiently and fairly, members become rapidly disenchanted with the entire organization. Meetings may be the only way in which members participate in the decision-making process of the organization, and if they see it as disorganized or a setup, many will withdraw completely. The knowledge and skill of both officers and members are required to ensure that meetings are conducted as they should be, so that the voice of the members prevails.

MEMBER-STAFF RELATIONSHIPS

As nursing organizations grow larger, many acquire professional staff, supported by clerical and sometimes technical assistants. Not too long ago, an executive secretary was a retired member of a nursing association, untutored in association management, who learned on the job. Today, the professional executive is seen as essential, for she or he deals with complex issues, policies, structure, and human and financial resources, and, frequently, thousands of volunteers.

Although the professional staff of nursing associations may consist of nurses, members of the same organization, with voting and office-holding rights, the *job* role is different. The members make policy through the volunteer board and officers; the staff carries out policy. Because volunteers are transient—a board of directors inevitably changes after each election—it is often only the staff who have continuity. Yet, should their opinions as to a certain action be in direct opposition to the board's or committee's, unless they can sell their point of view, it is the staff's responsibility to do what the volunteers decide. Staff may try very hard, directly or indirectly, to influence the key members of the organization.

Many members don't have a clear concept of the careful balance needed between board and staff lines of authority and responsibility. Just as volunteers should expect to devote an adequate amount of time to the association and bring to it the same amount of intellectual commitment and judgment used in their professional pursuits, staff members are expected to provide not just services but leadership, and must create confidence in their judgment and in the program. Staff are expected to synthesize and analyze issues and prepare materials and options for decision making so that volunteers' time is not wasted and they can react to specifics, not generalities. Staff and volunteers should regard each other as valuable colleagues with whom bad news as well as good news is shared. Staff must learn to identify the special abilities of volunteers so that they are put to use.

It is also important that staff identify their roles, responsibilities, and activities, so that expectations are real. Volunteers should not get involved in what is not their responsibility. An executive director (ED) manages the office and personnel. When volunteers attempt to interfere in personnel matters, problems inevitably result. If the ED is incompetent, she or he should be terminated by the board.

The ED is an employee of the board, the only employee of the board. Often a search committee reviews and selects candidates to recommend to the board. Criteria for selection should be carefully thought through to meet the needs of that organization. A study done by the Foundation of the American Society of Association Executives noted that the qualities considered most important for a successful association executive for the twenty-first century are sevenfold. First, the association executive must have a desire to serve others manifested through a commitment to board, staff, members, and external publics. A vision of the future and ability to succeed through change, to forge partnerships, and to manage information and technology are also key ingredients for success. Dealing with diversity and maintaining a personal and professional life balance are qualities the association executive must carry into the next century as well.[3] The most significant point to remember in staff-volunteer relationships is that it is a partnership; both are supposed to be working toward the same goals, and when there are unusual tensions between the two, it is often the result of misunderstanding or disagreement on how these goals are to be achieved. As in any other professional and human relationship, good communication is essential.

Issues and Concerns

Probably because of the proliferation of professional associations, there are many more concerns about them. At one time, organizations were run by volunteers in their spare time, typing notices with two fingers or with the help of somebody's sister; now they are a form of big business, including powerful unions and well-funded professional organizations. All seek economic and other advantages for their members, as well as the power necessary to succeed. Politicians do not want a strong, organized group against them, and there is no doubt that organizational lobbying gets action, especially if associations cooperate with each other. Still, there is also concern that the power of such organizations is not good for the public, and trade associations and professional organizations have been found subject to the Sherman Act and the Federal Trade Commission Act, which relate to price fixing and restraint of trade. In nursing, this has raised questions about certification and accreditation by the professional organizations. In addition, the tax-exempt status of many associations is under scrutiny and challenge.

Because of this growth and power, or potential power, the concerns of voluntary organizations have become more and more similar to those of their for-profit counterparts. Recently, for instance, attention has been given to ethical dilemmas of staff and management, whereas previously this was considered more of a theoretical topic relating to a profession or business in general. An important factor is good management, since a voluntary organization, like any business, must be solvent. Few, if any, can expect an automatic increase in members or can retain members without considerable effort. Today's members expect an association to be sensitive to their needs and to be instantly responsive in meeting those needs. Members expect quality products and services. Such products or services might take the form of liability insurance, professional and technical publications, and videos or computerized information systems.

Most members look to organizations for two basic things—information and networks. Prospective members should query association members about the quality and speed of service, information and networks provided, and how often the association assesses member needs. The answers to these questions will determine the value of joining and the viability of an organization. The organization that survives into the twenty-first century will be fast, friendly, flexible, and focused.[4]

Most critical is the issue the president of one professional organization called the *internal crisis of identity and mission*.[5] The key question asked about this professional organization for university professors is also pertinent to nursing's professional organization: recognizing that the heterogeneity of the professionals generates threatening tensions and divisions within the organization, is there a sufficient residue of *common* concern to justify the creation of one body to bring together all who call themselves professional nurses?

One problem in nursing is that so many nurses do not understand what the functions of a professional association are and therefore have inappropriate expectations. Sociologist Robert Merton in his classic article has delineated the functions in three categories: functions for individual practitioners, for the profession, and for society. For individuals, the association (1) gives social and moral support to help them perform their roles, especially in terms of economic and general welfare (salary, conditions of work, opportunities for advancement), CE, and working toward legally enforced standards of competence; and (2) develops social and moral ties among its members so that each becomes his brother's keeper. For the profession, the organization must set rigorous standards and help enforce them (quality of those recruited, of education, practice, and research). The profession must always press for higher standards. For society, the organization helps furnish the social bonds through which society coheres, providing unity in action.

> **The association mediates between the practitioner and profession on the one hand, and on the other, their social environment, of which the most important parts are allied occupations and professions, the universities, the local community, and the government.[6]**

The membership of most organizations is and probably always will be made up of people with varying degrees of commitment. No association can please them all. Yet, it is widely agreed that unless there is one voice for a profession, no one will listen. Adequate numbers of participating members are crucial. Nevertheless, although ANA is the largest nursing organization in the United States, the lack of internal agreement on issues is often evident and the multitude of other nursing organizations that have evolved have kept it from reaching its full potential.

In the following chapters, it will be seen how the increasing numbers of organizations that nurses can and do join overlap, compete, and frequently disagree. Add to that the trade unions that some nurses are choosing to represent them, and it is small wonder that the public asks, "Which is nursing's real association? Who speaks for nursing?"

REFERENCES

1. Perlo D: Our members, in *Working Papers of Consensus Management Group*. New York: The Group, 1991.

2. Robert H: *Robert's Rules of Order, Revised*. New York: Morrow, 1985.

3. Bethel S: Beyond management to leadership, in *Designing the 21st Century Association*. Washington, DC: The Foundation of the American Society of Association Executives, 1993.

4. Kanter R: *When Giants Learn to Dance*. New York: Simon and Schuster, 1989.

5. Steiner P: The current crisis of the association. *AAUP Bull* 64:135–141, September 1978.

6. Merton R: The functions of the professional association. *Am J Nurs* 58:50–54, January 1958.

CHAPTER 24

National Student Nurses' Association

THE NATIONAL STUDENT NURSES' ASSOCIATION, INC. (NSNA), established in 1953, is the national organization for nursing students in the United States and its territories, possessions, and dependencies. NSNA's mission is to:

- Organize, represent, and mentor students preparing for initial licensure as registered nurses, as well as those nurses enrolled in baccalaureate completion programs.
- Promote development of the skills that students will need as responsible and accountable members of the nursing profession.
- Advocate for high-quality health care.[1]

The functions of the organization, as listed in the bylaws, are as follows:

1. To have direct input into standards of nursing education and influence the educational process.
2. To influence health care, nursing education, and practice through legislative activities, as appropriate.
3. To promote and encourage participation in community affairs and activities toward improved health care and the resolution of related social issues.
4. To represent nursing students to the consumer, to institutions, and to other organizations.
5. To promote and encourage students' participation in interdisciplinary activities.
6. To promote and encourage recruitment efforts, participation in student activities,

and educational opportunities regardless of a person's race, color, creed, sex, age, lifestyle, national origin, or economic status.

7. To promote and encourage collaborative relationships with ANA, NLN, and the International Council of Nurses, as well as the other nursing and related health organizations.[2]

The NSNA is autonomous, student financed, and student run. It is the voice of all nursing students speaking out on issues of concern to nursing students and nursing.

MEMBERSHIP

Students are eligible for active membership in NSNA if they are enrolled in state-approved programs leading to licensure as an RN or are RNs enrolled in programs leading to a baccalaureate degree in nursing. Students are eligible for associate membership if they are prenursing students enrolled in college or university programs designed to prepare them for programs leading to a degree in nursing. Associate members have all of the privileges of membership except the right to hold office as president and vice president at state and national levels.

Application for membership is made directly to NSNA. Dues paid to NSNA are a combination of national and state association dues; the latter vary from state to state. The dues structure is decided by a vote of the membership.

NSNA also has two categories of membership not open to students. Sustaining membership is open at the national level to any individual or organization interested in furthering the development and growth of NSNA. Sustaining members receive literature and other information from the NSNA office. Dues vary for sustaining members, which may include NSNA alumni, other individuals, local organizations, and national organizations. Honorary membership is conferred by a two-thirds vote of the House of Delegates upon recommendation by the board of directors on persons who have rendered distinguished service or valuable assistance to NSNA. This is the highest honor NSNA can bestow upon an individual.

History

Just when or where the idea of a national association of nursing students originated will probably never be known. But for many years and in increasing numbers, students had been attending the national conventions of ANA and NLN, eager to learn of the activities of these two associations that would soon be affecting them as graduate nurses. Special sessions were arranged at these conventions so that students could meet together and discuss mutual problems. At the same time, some student nurses' organizations had been formed on the state level, giving students an awareness of both the strength and the values of group association and action. It was inevitable, of course, that sooner or later, the idea of a national association would arise. Once it did, nursing students throughout the United States began to work enthusiastically in that direction.

In June 1952, approximately 1,000 students attending a national nursing convention in Atlantic City, New Jersey, voted to start preparations for the formal organization in 1953 of a national student nurses' association under the sponsorship of the Coordinating Council of the ANA and NLN. In the intervening year, a committee of nursing students and representatives of ANA and NLN worked on organization plans, and in June 1953 the National Student Nurses' Association was officially launched. Bylaws were adopted and NSNA's officers were elected.

In its first few years, NSNA had little money, a small membership, no real headquarters of its own, and no headquarters staff. Its main assets at the time were the persistence, determination, and dedication of its members, plus financial and moral support from ANA and NLN. A year after NSNA's founding, these two organizations appointed (and paid) a coordinator to help NSNA function; many of the association's activities were transacted through correspondence. Each organization also provided a staff consultant to NSNA and helped finance the association's necessary expenses and publications. Among the latter were the bylaws and a newspaper. The next step was a headquarters office. Today NSNA rents its own office at 555 West 57th Street, New York, New York 10019.

Even in its early years, NSNA was able to help finance itself. And year after year, NSNA's share of the costs increased. Membership grew, and annual dues, which had originally been fifteen cents per year, were raised to fifty cents in 1957. Finally, in 1958, only five years after its inception, NSNA became financially independent. The original coordinator appointed in 1954, Frances Tompkins, became the executive secretary (the title was later changed to *executive director*) and headed a staff of two. In 1959, NSNA became legally incorporated as the National Student Nurses' Association, Inc., a nonprofit association. Today the association pays for headquarters offices, a staff, and all the other expenses incidental to running the business of a large association. It holds and finances its own annual convention. And, at the same time, it has initiated and financed several important projects in the interests not only of its members but of the nursing profession as a whole.

General Plan of Organization

The policies and programs of NSNA are determined by its House of Delegates, whose membership consists of elected representatives from the school and state associations. The delegates at each annual convention elect NSNA's three officers; six nonofficer directors, one of whom will become editor of *Imprint*, the official journal of NSNA; and a four-member nominating committee. Officers serve for one year or until their respective successors are elected.

Two consultants are appointed, one each by the ANA and NLN, in consultation with the NSNA board of directors. They serve for a two-year period or until their respective successors are appointed. According to the bylaws, these consultants are charged with providing an interchange of information between their boards and NSNA. All consultants are expected to serve only as resource persons, consulting with officers, members, and staff and attending the meetings of the association. Consultants and advisers serve several major purposes:

- To assist elected and appointed officers to identify issues, problems, and alternatives as they carry out their legal, fiduciary, and organizational responsibilities.
- To provide students in leadership positions with information about professional issues and positions taken by the appointing organization.
- To strengthen organizational ties between the student association and the appointing organization by serving as a liaison with these organizations.
- To provide continuity to the organization where the student leadership is short-term, and changes composition from year to year.
- To act as a professional role model and mentor.[3]

The board of directors manages the affairs of the association between the annual meetings of the membership, and an executive committee, consisting of the president, vice president, and secretary/treasurer, transacts emergency business between board meetings. There are two standing committees, the nominating and elections committee; the board has the authority to

establish other committees as needed. State and constituent organizations may or may not function in a similar manner; their bylaws must be in conformity with NSNA's bylaws.

In 1976, the NSNA House of Delegates mandated a change in the structure of the association, giving school chapters the eligibility for constituency status and delegate representation. Under this system, school chapters must verify that their bylaws are in conformity with NSNA's bylaws and must have fifteen members. If a school has fewer than fifteen students enrolled, membership by 100 percent of the students entitles the school to constituency status. Delegate representation is based upon the number of students in the school who are members. State associations that have two recognized school chapters and their own bylaws in conformity are recognized as NSNA constituents and are entitled to one voting delegate.

Projects, Activities, Services

NSNA has a wide variety of activities, services, and projects to carry out its purpose and functions. Even in its early years, the association sought participation in ANA and NLN committees and sent representatives to ICN.

Early projects were the Minority Group Recruitment Project (which has developed into Breakthrough to Nursing) and the Taiwan Project. The latter project, carried out in cooperation with the American Bureau for Medical Aid to China, grew out of NSNA members' interest in nursing students in other countries, coupled with a desire to assist whenever possible. After a firsthand report about the inadequate, overcrowded living conditions for nursing students at the National Defense Medical Center, Taiwan, delegates to the 1961 NSNA convention voted to raise $25,000 to build and equip a new dormitory for this group. By 1965, through vigorous fund-raising drives carried out at all levels of NSNA, the larger sum of $37,000 had been accumulated. The completed fifty-student residence, named the NSNA Dormitory, was officially dedicated in March 1966, with American government officials cutting the traditional ribbon at the ceremony and representing both NSNA and the United States government.

Today, NSNA collaborates with several nursing and other health organizations. In 1990, the organization was made an affiliate member of the National Federation of Specialty Nursing Organizations (NFSNO). NSNA is also a leading participant in the student assembly of the ICN, and the NSNA president served as its chairperson during the 1977 ICN in Tokyo. NSNA served as host for the 1981 student assembly. Through a special program funded by the Helene Fuld Health Trust, in 1993 NSNA sent a delegation of 52 nursing students to the 20th ICN Quadrennial Congress in Madrid, Spain. The 1993/94 NSNA president led the delegation and served as chair of the student assembly.

NSNA members are involved in community health activities such as hypertension screening, health fairs, child abuse, teenage pregnancy, and education on death and dying. Some of these activities are carried out in cooperation with other student health groups. In addition to health- and nursing-related issues, social, women's, and human rights issues are supported by NSNA.

Community health activities receive major emphasis by NSNA, and projects planned and implemented by NSNA members cover a wide variety of community health needs, such as heart attack risk reduction education programs, aid to homeless families, disaster relief efforts, and health fairs for all age groups.

Breakthrough to Nursing

NSNA has always been involved in recruiting qualified men and women into nursing. In 1965, however, NSNA launched a nationwide project directed toward the recruitment of blacks, Native Americans, Hispanic, and other minority group members into the nursing profession. Known as the National Recruitment Project, this long-term effort grew out of an increasing awareness on the part of nursing students of their collective responsibility for supporting the civil rights movement, for recruiting for nursing, for alerting young men and women in minority groups to the opportunities in a nursing career, and in recognition of the value of such nurses in improving the care of their own ethnic groups.[4]

The national project was proposed at the 1965 NSNA convention by the 1964–1965 NSNA Nursing Recruitment Committee, whose recommendations were based on results of pilot projects conducted in Colorado, Minnesota, and Washington, D.C. The delegates voted to undertake the project on a national scale.

By early 1967 the project was well underway in many different areas of the country, with the state associations tackling the problem in various ways. In collaboration with other appropriate community groups—the Urban League, those associated with Head Start or other antipoverty programs, and civil rights groups—nursing students throughout the United States worked diligently not only to interest minority group members in nursing but also to help them financially, morally, and educationally to undertake such a career.

In 1971, NSNA set the Breakthrough to Nursing Project, as it is now called, as a priority and sought funds to strengthen and expand the existing program. Later that year, NSNA was awarded a contract for $100,000 by the Division of Nursing, DHEW. In 1974, a three-year grant expanded Breakthrough to forty funded target areas. The grant ended in June 1977, but students are still involved in Breakthrough to Nursing on a nonfunded basis.

The objectives of the project were (1) to develop and implement a publicity campaign to inform and interest potential nursing candidates in a nursing career; (2) to coordinate nursing student recruitment efforts with community organizations and schools of nursing in support of the program to reach more minority students; (3) to participate in recruitment program activities such as conferences, workshops, and career days focused on increasing the number of minority students recruited into nursing; (4) to work with public school counselors, teachers, school nurses, and other secondary school personnel to assist with the identification, motivation, and encouragement of disadvantaged and/or minority group students interested in a career in nursing; and (5) to inform the public and the nursing community of the goals of the project.

In order to carry out these objectives, the involvement and support of nursing student volunteers, faculty, and heads of schools of nursing were essential. Student volunteers in Breakthrough areas carried out such activities as career fairs, education of school counselors, working with schools and community groups to provide tutorial and counseling services, development and distribution of brochures, help with the application and registration procedures in colleges, and provision of information about financial resources.

To raise the level of awareness of the need for minority nurses, a publicity campaign was developed using various media. Breakthrough to Nursing guidelines and materials are available for distribution nationally. Although there are still problems such as racial polarization and retention of students after recruitment, there is no doubt that the project has had an impact on nursing, on NSNA members, and on the community. Over the years, the Breakthrough to Nursing Project has evolved to reflect the needs of contemporary society. For example, in addition to those groups already cited, the Breakthrough to Nursing Project also focuses on nontraditional students (returning students) and encourages all qualified people to enter the profession.

Legislation

One of the most impressive NSNA developments in recent years is the active and knowledgeable participation of NSNA members in legislation. Excellent resources on legislative activities and political education on a national level and assistance and support in legislation provided by NSNA to constituent associations resulted in legislative committees in most states. During the various crises of federal funding for health, students have testified before congressional committees and supported the passage of the Nurse Education Act by their active participation in the political process. They have also urged passage of social and health care reform legislation. Students are also encouraged to work with state nurses' associations (SNAs), state political action committees (PACs), and other groups on health legislation on the local and state levels, and to educate members in such areas as state nurse practice acts and political activism.

Interdisciplinary Activities

NSNA has shown a forward-looking interest in the health and social problems of society, often combined with like interest in interdisciplinary cooperation. With the American Medical Student Association (AMSA), Student American Pharmaceutical Association (SAPhA), and American Student Dental Association (ASDA), individual nursing students have participated in Head Start, Appalachian and Indian health, migrant health, and Job Corps projects. Recently reinstated as the Coalition of Health Care Professional Students, students from various health-related disciplines meet routinely to discuss mutual interests and concerns.

One major interdisciplinary activity in which NSNA participated was Concern for Dying's Interdisciplinary Collaboration on Death and Dying. This student program recruited representatives from the AMSA, the Law Student Division of the American Bar Association, and students from social work and theology schools. The Collaboration, begun in 1977, introduced students to a variety of professional perspectives on death and dying and created a dialogue among future professionals. Concern for Dying, now known as Choice in Dying, continues to provide NSNA members with information on nursing's role in death and dying issues.

Other Professional Activities

Almost since the inception of NSNA, members have been invited to participate in the committees of ANA and NLN. Such participation has increased as NSNA has sought to take an active part in the debates, discussions, and decisions concerning nursing. Usually the resolutions of NSNA support the goals of the ANA and NLN, and, at times, they move ahead of the others in their acceptance of change. The support of both organizations is often asked on issues that require the support of nurse executives, educators, or others. Some of the issues involved have been in relation to curriculum change, clinical experience opportunities, education for practice, career mobility, and accreditation.

Scholarship Funds

The Foundation of the National Student Nurses' Association administers its own scholarship program. The Foundation was established in 1969 as the Frances Tompkins Educational Opportunity Fund to enable individuals and organizations to contribute funds to educate nursing students and others to study and understand the scope of present and future community health needs with a view to developing innovative programs. The fund is incorporated and has obtained federal tax exemption. Scholarship monies are obtained from various organizations, and contributors have included both commercial enterprises and professional organizations. Individual contributions are accepted for the Mary Ann Tuft Scholarship Fund. Scholarship applications become available in the fall of each year.

Also under the aegis of NSNA is the Laura D. Smith Scholarship Fund. Each year the NSNA has awarded a $600 scholarship for graduate study. The nurse must have been a member of NSNA while in nursing school. This scholarship was established in 1962 in honor of Laura D. Smith, former senior editor of the *American Journal of Nursing* and NSNA adviser, who died in 1961. Application for the scholarship should be made to its administrator, Nurses' Educational Funds, AJN Company, 555 West 57th Street, New York, N.Y. 10019.

Publications and Resources

Imprint, the official NSNA magazine, came into existence in 1968, and a subscription is given to members.[5] Subscriptions are also available to other interested groups, schools, and individuals. *Imprint*, published five times during the academic year, is the only publication of its kind specifically for students. It is the only nursing magazine written by and for nursing students, and students are encouraged to contribute articles and letters. Students may also take advantage of the annual Springhouse Nursing/NSNA Essay Contest, which offers cash awards.

Other publications include the *NSNA News*, a newsletter that keeps organization leaders at state and school levels informed of pertinent issues and activities; *The Dean's Notes*, a newsletter for deans and directors of schools of nursing; the *Business Book*, which serves as an annual report and is printed for the annual convention; *Getting the Pieces to Fit*, a yearly handbook for state and school chapters; and informational, supportive materials on students' rights, guidelines for faculty evaluation, and guidelines for clinical evaluation. Most states and some schools also publish newsletters.

At the 10th anniversary of its founding, NSNA had accomplished a great deal.[6] Before its 30th, it had become an involved group whose activities demonstrated committed professionalism.[7] Gone were the talent shows and uniform nights of the early days. "Students learned to conduct meetings and to use parliamentary procedure, they showed concern about their education and their future practice, and they showed concern for others."[8] They were involved in many of the same issues as ANA and NLN and often seemed to show more foresight. With their 40th anniversary NSNA had reason to celebrate their history and their future.[9]

Education was of prime interest, and among the issues discussed in their meetings were curriculum planning, accreditation, entry into practice, and student rights. In 1976, the NSNA House of Delegates recognized the need for baccalaureate education in nursing and encouraged the increased availability of baccalaureate programs in nursing and increased enrollment of registered nurses in baccalaureate programs. NSNA urges the gradual movement of all programs preparing for practice as RNs to the baccalaureate level. NSNA also recognizes the contributions of associate, baccalaureate, diploma, generic master's, and doctoral programs that prepare students for RN licensure. As early as 1969, NSNA delegates also encouraged the development and demonstration of nursing education programs that would recognize an individual's previously acquired knowledge and skill. For the next decade, convention resolutions called for pathways for career mobility for AD and diploma nurses.

As in other fields, nursing students have also fought for their own rights, and NSNA has maintained a commitment to student rights. In 1970, a guideline for a student bill of rights was distributed to all constituents, a mandate of the 1969 delegates. In 1975, a comprehensive bill of rights, responsibilities and grievance procedures was accepted and published. The statement was adopted in schools throughout the country. The document was revised by the 1991 House of Delegates and is available from NSNA.

In the area of practice, students have taken positive stands on the concept of mandatory licensure, maldistribution of nurses, national standards for practice, substitution of unlicensed personnel for nurses, and use of student nurses as a substitute for nurses. They have supported economic security and the ANA position that in the event of a non-RN strike, students would not substitute for striking workers unless patients were endangered. They also supported ANA acting as the collective bargaining agent for nursing (as opposed to trade unions).

Finally, NSNA members have been involved in issues affecting the public's health—for instance, by participating in projects to educate children and young people about the dangers of drugs. NSNA has taken numerous positions on contemporary issues such as women's health and social issues, pregnancy, infant and child health, sexually transmitted diseases, AIDS-HIV prevention and education, smoking and health, drug and alcohol abuse, infection control, and promotion of a positive image of nursing. NSNA offers the opportunity for nursing students to be heard, becomes a forum for debates on health and social issues as well as nursing issues, provides opportunities for interdisciplinary contacts, and is a testing ground for leadership skills. Participation and involvement can be a meaningful and valuable part of the nursing student's education.[10] Many involved NSNA members go on to leadership positions in nursing organizations and continue their lifelong commitment to advancing the profession of nursing.

REFERENCES

1. *Getting the Pieces to Fit.* New York: National Student Nurses' Association, 1994.
2. National Student Nurses' Association: *Bylaws.* New York: The Association, 1994.
3. National Student Nurses' Association: *Guidelines for Planning for School Advisors and State Consultants.* New York: The Association, 1992.
4. Johnson N: Recruitment of minority groups—A priority for NSNA. *Nurs Outlook* 14:29–30, April 1966.
5. Byrne M: Imprint, the NSNA Journal, 1968–1973: A profession's messages to its students in turbulent times. *Imprint* 37:97–105, April–May 1990.
6. *NSNA's Ten Tall Years.* New York: National Student Nurses' Association, 1963.
7. NSNA today. *Am J Nurs* 77:624–626, April 1977.
8. *NSNA '77: A Retrospective.* New York: National Student Nurses' Association, 1977.
9. NSNA's 40th Anniversary Issue. *Imprint,* 39, April–May 1992.
10. Fitzpatrick ML: NSNA: Path to professional identity. *Imprint* 34:63–66, April–May 1987.

American Nurses Association

THE AMERICAN NURSES ASSOCIATION (ANA), a federation of state associations, is nursing's professional organization, with membership in its state constituent associations open only to registered professional nurses. Through their state membership, nurses decide upon the functions, activities, and goals of their profession. ANA serves as spokesperson and agent for nurses and nursing, acting in accordance with the expressed wishes of its membership. ANA membership is voluntary and in 1994 totaled more than 200,000 nurses.

The ANA was established in 1897 by a group of nurses who, even then, recognized the need for a membership association within which nurses could work together in concerted action. Its original name was the Nurses' Associated Alumnae of the United States and Canada, but in order to incorporate under the laws of the state of New York, it was necessary to drop the reference to another country in the organization's title. This was done in 1901; however, the name remained Nurses' Associated Alumnae of the United States until 1911, when it became the American Nurses Association. The Canadian nurses formed their own membership association.

History shows that ANA's primary concern has always been individual nurses and the public they serve. Thus, in its early years ANA worked diligently for improved and uniform standards of nursing education, for registration and licensure of all nurses educated according to these standards, and for improvement of the welfare of nurses. The need for such actions and the difficulties involved become apparent if one remembers that in the early 1900s many hospitals opened schools for economic reasons only, with no real interest in the education or employment of the nurses, and the public had no guarantee that any nurse gave safe care. ANA's efforts served to protect the public from unsafe nursing care provided by those who might call themselves nurses but who had little or no preparation. In recent years, ANA has continued to give major attention to setting standards of practice and education, although the National League for Nursing (NLN) has retained the accreditation functions for nursing education programs. The ANA subsidiary, the American Nursing Credentialing Center, does accredit continuing education providers.

PURPOSES AND FUNCTIONS

Throughout its existence, ANA's functions and activities have been adapted or expanded in accordance with the changing needs of the profession and the public. As a changed or changing major function becomes crystallized, it is incorporated in the bylaws by vote of the ANA House of Delegates. Thus the purposes of ANA, as stated in the current bylaws, are to:

1. Work for the improvement of health standards and the availability of health care services for all people.

2. Foster high standards of nursing.
3. Stimulate and promote the professional development of nurses and advance their economic and general welfare.

These purposes are unrestricted by considerations of nationality, race, creed, lifestyle, color, age, religion, disability, gender, health status, or sexual orientation.

ANA's current functions, also as outlined in the bylaws, are to:

- Establish standards of nursing practice, nursing education, and nursing services.
- Establish a code of ethical conduct for nurses.
- Ensure a system of credentialing in nursing.
- Initiate and influence legislation, governmental programs, national health policy, and international health policy.
- Support systematic study, evaluation, and research in nursing.
- Serve as the central agency for the collection, analysis, and dissemination of information relevant to nursing.
- Promote and protect the economic and general welfare of nurses.
- Provide leadership in national and international nursing.
- Provide for the professional development of nurses.
- Conduct an affirmative action program.
- Ensure a collective bargaining program for nurses.
- Provide services to constituent members.
- Maintain communication with members through official publications.
- Assume an active role as consumer advocate.
- Represent and speak for the nursing profession with allied health groups, national and international organizations, governmental bodies, and the public.
- Protect and promote the advancement of human rights related to health care and nursing.[1]

MEMBERSHIP AND DUES

ANA is made up of state and territorial associations (SNAs). While the bylaws say constituent member, the "vernacular" still is the SNA. The SNA consists of district or regional associations (DNA), the number varying with geography, population distribution, and other factors. There are presently fifty-three SNAs, one in each of the fifty states plus the District of Columbia, the Virgin Islands, and Guam.

From the inception of ANA, individual nurses could become members, usually by joining their district association. They then automatically became members of the SNA and ANA. This began to change in the 1970s, when a number of SNAs began experimental programs (some sanctioned by ANA) allowing members to join at any level without having to join all three—or pay dues for all three. Certain states, especially those with many collective bargaining units, felt that this would attract more members to the SNAs, and perhaps to ANA, since, of course, dues would be less and since a number of nurses were not interested in national professional issues or vice versa. It was also expected that the SNA with an increased membership would have more power in state legislative and political affairs. Some of these states did gain a larger membership; few nurses chose only ANA as the level at which to join. Finally, at the 1982 House of Delegates, after a heated debate, the bylaws were changed and a new organizational entity was born—the federation. No longer could an individual become a member of ANA. Now ANA is composed only of state or territorial associations. Qualifications are delineated in the bylaws:

A constituent member is an association that—
a. **is composed of individual members and may include organizational members/affiliates.**
b. **has articles of incorporation and bylaws that govern its individual members and regulate its affairs.**
c. **has stated purposes and functions congruent with those of ANA.**
d. **provides that each of its individual members has been granted a license to practice as a registered**

nurse in at least one state, territory, or possession of the United States and does not have a license under suspension or revocation in any state, or has completed a nursing education program qualifying the individual to take the state-recognized examination for registered nurse licensure as a first-time writer.

e. may, in accord with its policies and procedures, include in its membership the impaired nurse, in recovery, who has surrendered a license to practice.

f. provides that each of its organizational members or affiliates—

1) has a mission and purpose harmonious with the constituent member.

2) has a governing body composed of a majority of registered nurses. This shall not preclude the participation of organizations of associate nurses. The rights and privileges of the organizational members or affiliates shall be determined by and limited to participation in the constituent member.

g. serves a geographic area such as a state, territory, or possession of the United States or any combination thereof where there is no other recognized constituent member.

h. maintains a membership that meets the qualifications in these bylaws, unrestricted by consideration of age, color, creed, disability, lifestyle, nationality, race, religion, sexual orientation, or health status.

i. is not delinquent in paying dues to ANA.

Responsibilities

The bylaws of each constituent member shall—

1) provide for the obligation of the constituent member to pay dues to ANA in accordance with policies adopted by the ANA House of Delegates.

2) provide for individual members of the constituent to elect delegates and alternates to the ANA House of Delegates according to provisions of these bylaws.

3) protect individual members' right to participate in the constituent member.

4) specify the obligations of individual members.

5) provide for disciplinary action and an appeal procedure for individual members pursuant to common parliamentary and statutory law.

6) provide for the recognition of disciplinary action taken by any constituent member against its individual member.

7) provide for official recognition of constituent associations of the constituent member.

8) provide that additional dues shall not be required from nor refunded to individual members transferring from another constituent member if the individual member has made full payment of dues.

Each constituent member shall—

1) apprise individual members of the constituent of their right to—

a) receive a membership card and *The American Nurse.*

b) be candidate for ANA elective and appointive positions in accordance with these bylaws.

c) participate in the election of constituent member delegates to the ANA House of Delegates in accordance with these bylaws.

d) attend the meetings of the ANA House of Delegates, the convention, and other unrestricted ANA activities.

e) attend the congress of the International Council of Nurses.

f) affiliate with ANA councils in accordance with provisions of these bylaws.

2) require that individual members of the constituent member abide by the *Code for Nurses.*[2]

Dues are set by policy adopted by the House of Delegates, and are based on the annual dues revenue of the SNA. To this would be added SNA dues and DNA dues.

GENERAL PLAN OF ORGANIZATION

From time to time, ANA's organizational structure undergoes some minor or major changes to enable the association to function more efficiently in the light of changing circumstances or needs. The major changes made in 1989 by the House of Delegates are included in the following description of how ANA is organized and how it functions.

House of Delegates, Officers, Board

The business of the association is carried on by its House of Delegates and board of directors. The House of Delegates, made up of a designated number of membership representatives elected by the SNAs, is the highest authority in the association. It meets every year to transact the association's business and to establish policies and programs; once in two years, it meets at the ANA convention. Until 1985, it had met biennially at conventions. It also elects ANA's board of directors and officers, the majority of the members of its nominating committee, and some members of its congresses (to be described later). Thus, control of the association remains always in the hands of its membership.

Throughout the years, ANA's House of Delegates has made many important decisions related to nursing and nurses. At many successive conventions, for instance, it went on record as supporting the principle underlying the legislation that eventually brought Medicare into being. As early as 1946, it made several decisions designed to discourage discriminatory policies in regard to nationality, race, religion, or color within the nursing profession. In 1964 it voted to revise the bylaws so that ANA's responsibility for nursing education and nursing services might be more explicitly stated. In 1966 it adopted a national salary goal with a differential for nurses with a baccalaureate degree. In 1968 the Congress on Practice was created, reemphasizing ANA's concern with practice. In 1970, even with the news that ANA was in a financial crisis because of mismanagement of funds and a consequent cutback of programs, the delegates resolved to recruit more of the disadvantaged into nursing, to help reduce the many threats to the environment, to become more deeply involved in health planning, and to develop closer working relationships with consumers of health care.

In 1972, some of the priorities set were directed toward defining requirements for high-quality nursing services, clarifying the scope of nursing practice, providing for continuing peer review, recognizing excellence and continued competence among practitioners of nursing, expanding and improving all aspects of education, and assisting SNAs with their economic security activities. Also adopted was an affirmative action program, which called for appointment of an ombudsman to the ANA staff.

In 1974, convention action gave major emphasis to national health insurance, nurses' participation in Professional Standards Review Organizations (PRSOs), implementation of standards for nursing practice, certification for excellence in practice, reaffirmation of support of individual licensure (as opposed to institutional licensure), support of CE programs and a mandate to the ANA board of directors to establish a system of accreditation of CE programs and to study the possibility of accrediting other nursing education programs, efforts to effect direct fee-for-service reimbursement for NPs, the role of the ANA in collective bargaining, and a series of activities related to foreign nurses to eradicate their exploitation and assist in their becoming qualified to practice.

In 1976, the bicentennial convention year, the House passed resolutions on nurse advocacy for the elderly, responsibilities of nurses in nursing homes, alternatives to hospitalization for the mentally disabled and retarded, and involvement of nurses in health planning. The 1978 and 1980 Houses set as priorities for the next biennium: improving the quality of care provided to the public; advancing the profession so that the health care needs of people are met; enlarging the influence of the nursing profession in the determination and execution of public policy, and strengthening ANA so that it may better serve the needs and interests of the profession. Also approved were major resolutions on national health insurance, quality assurance, human rights, career mobility, and identifying, titling, and developing competency statements for two categories of nursing practice.

In 1982 and 1984, the House adopted the following statement of association priorities for the biennium: "To promote and protect the economic worth, the education and the practice of nurses." Specific goals were related to better communication with the public, standard setting for nursing, influencing health policy, and strengthening ANA's role in credentialing. The action taken in the House and the actions taken by the association throughout the year focused on these efforts. For instance, proposals accepted by the House in 1984 were related to smoking and other hazards of the workplace; the role of nurses within the prospective payment system, in home care, and in long-term care; implementing the goal of entry into practice at the baccalaureate level; supporting ERA; action to improve the economic status of women and children; nurse accountability and ethics; and protection of collective bargaining rights.

In 1986, the ANA adopted a long-range strategic and business plan for the organization. The plan set forth eight long-range goals:

1. Expand the scientific and research base for nursing practice.
2. Clarify and strengthen the educational system for nursing.
3. Develop a coordinated system for credentialing in nursing.
4. Restructure the organizational arrangements for delivery of nursing services.
5. Develop comprehensive payment systems for nursing.
6. Achieve effective control of the environment in which nursing is practiced and services are offered.
7. Enhance the organizational strength of ANA.
8. Maintain and strengthen nursing's role in client advocacy.

Between 1987 and 1990, priority was given to goals 2, 6, and 8 and to the maintenance of the organization. The 1988 House of Delegates mandated that ANA establish its headquarters in Washington, D.C. ANA relocated to Washington, D.C., in March 1992.

In 1989, the ANA House adopted the recommendations of the Commission on Organizational Assessment and Renewal (COAR), which was the result of a broad study undertaken to address all aspects of function, structure, membership base, and interorganizational relationships of ANA.

In 1990, the House of Delegates concentrated on social issues, such as drug abuse, human rights, the right to health care, and homeless-ness. These are all illustrations of the wide scope of House of Delegates' decisions and ANA activities and the directions in which the efforts of the organization are moving.

In 1992, the ANA focused a great deal of attention on health care reform. The ANA and the National League for Nursing articulated *Nursing's Agenda for Health Care Reform* that calls for a health care system that assures access, quality, and services at an affordable cost. *Nursing's Agenda for Health Care Reform* is supported by over seventy nursing and nonnursing organizations.[3]

In 1994, the ANA House of Delegates continued to discuss health policy and the impact of the nation's changing policy on employment of registered nurses. The delegates reaffirmed commitment to universal coverage, ensuring that third-party payers directly reimburse advanced practice nurses; essential benefit packages that include health promotion, restoration of health, disease prevention, and long-term care. The delegates opposed taxation of individual health benefits or health care providers.

The 1994 ANA House of Delegates also deliberated ANA policy direction for the nineties and acknowledged that the organization must be focused and responsive to the rapidly changing environment. The house adopted a vision statement.

VISION STATEMENT
To have the health care system be restructured in such a way that the fundamental principles of "Nursing's Agenda for Health Care Reform" and the protection of nursing practice are accomplished and that nurses are *essential* providers *in all* practice settings. Throughout development of innovative programs and services, ANA and the nursing profession will be strong and unified, meeting evolving needs of all nurses in all settings with an emphasis on collective bargaining and workplace advocacy.[4]

In the intervals between the House of Delegates' meetings, the board of directors transacts the general business of the association. This is a fifteen-member body, consisting of ten directors and the association's officers: a president, two vice presidents, secretary, and treasurer. Terms of office are staggered to prevent a complete turnover at any one time and to provide for continuity of programs and action.

Serving to implement ANA policies and programs is the headquarters staff, made up of RNs, economists, attorneys, lobbyists, statisticians, writers, and other professionals, as well as a support staff. They carry out the day-by-day activities of the association in accordance with the policies adopted by the House of Delegates and ANA's general functions. ANA headquarters is 600 Maryland Ave., S.W., Suite 100, Washington, D.C. 20024-2571.

Standing Committees

Like other large organizations, ANA has its standing committees, those that are written into the bylaws and that continue from year to year to assist with specific, continuing programs and functions of the association. There are three such committees of the House of Delegates: bylaws, nominating, and reference. These standing committees differ from what are called *special committees*, which are appointed on an ad hoc basis to accomplish special purposes. Special committees may be board committees or House of Delegates committees.

Except for the nominating committee and committees of the congresses and councils, committee members are appointed by the board. The standing committees are accountable to the house and submit reports to the board. The board also appoints its own committees to carry out its work.

Other Organization Entities

There are a number of other organizational entities. A *congress* is an organized, deliberative body that focuses on long-range policy development essential to the mission of the association. There is a *Congress on Nursing Economics* and a *Congress of Nursing Practice*, which came into effect after the 1990 convention. Congresses are accountable to the Board of Directors and report to the ANA House of Delegates.

According to the bylaws, the major responsibilities of the *Congress on Nursing Economics* are to:

- Develop long-range policy essential to the mission of the association.
- Establish a plan of operation for carrying out its responsibilities.
- Develop and adopt standards.
- Develop and evaluate programs.
- Address and respond to concerns related to equal opportunity and human rights, ethics, and to nursing education, research, and services.
- Recommend policies and positions to the Board of Directors and the ANA House of Delegates.
- Evaluate trends, developments, and issues.[5]

Major responsibilities of the *Congress of Nursing Practice* are to:

- Develop long-range policy essential to the mission of the association.
- Establish a plan of operation for carrying out its responsibilities.
- Develop and adopt standards.
- Develop and evaluate programs.
- Address and respond to concerns related to equal opportunity and human rights, ethics, and to nursing education, research, and services.
- Recommend policies and positions to the Board of directors and the ANA House of Delegates.
- Evaluate trends, developments, and issues.
- Formulate revisions of the *Code for Nurses* and recommend them to the ANA House of Delegates, and interpret the *Code for Nurses.*[6]

In 1990, the House of Delegates established an *Institute of Constituent Members on Nursing Practice*, which reports directly to the Congress of Nursing Practice. It consists of one representative from each SNA.

The *Institute of Constituent Member Collective Bargaining Programs* was put into place in 1990. It consists of one elected representative from each SNA with a collective bargaining program and is autonomous in respect to the development of operational standards, positions, policies, practices, and all other matters related to SNA collective bargaining programs. More details about the institutes can be found in the ANA bylaws.

The *Commission on Economic and Professional Security* is an organized, deliberative body to which the Congress on Nursing Economics assigns specific responsibilities related to the economic and professional security of individual nurses or groups of nurses. Its major responsibilities are to:

- Evaluate trends, developments, and issues related to the economic and professional security of individual nurses or groups of nurses.
- Develop standards, positions, and policies for recommendation to the Congress on Nursing Economics.[7]

Councils have a clinical or functional focus and are established by the board. They provide the one mechanism through which the individual SNA member can participate or join directly in ANA activities. Their primary purpose relates to providing a forum for discussion; continuing education; consultation; and proposing standards and certification offerings.

The *Constituent Assembly* is made up of the president and chief administrative officer of each SNA or their designees. The purpose is to discuss nursing affairs of concern to ANA, SNAs, and the profession. *The Nursing Organization Liaison Forum* (NOLF) is made up of duly authorized representatives of ANA and other nursing organizations, who meet for the purpose of discussing issues of concern to the profession and promoting concerted action on them.

The American Academy of Nursing (AAN)

A significant action taken by the 1966 House of Delegates was the creation of an Academy of Nursing to provide for recognition of profes-

sional achievement and excellence. Because of the financial problems of ANA in the late sixties, the Academy was not established until early 1973. At that time, thirty-six nationally prominent nurses were selected as charter fellows of the Academy by the ANA board of directors. Included were practitioners, researchers, academicians, and administrators from thirty-four states.

The vision of the American Academy of Nursing is to transform health care so as to optimize the well-being of the American people and the world in general.

The mission of the Academy is to:

- Provide visionary leadership to the nursing profession.
- Potentiate the contributions of nursing leaders.
- Advance the development and synthesis of knowledge.
- Shape the formulation of effective health care policies and practices.

The AAN goals are to:

- Anticipate national and international trends in health care and address resulting issues of health care knowledge and policy.
- Inform public and professional constituencies of the state of health care knowledge and policy issues.
- Elect and sustain a distinguished, diverse, and active membership.
- Augment the senior-level leadership skills of distinguished nurses, and encourage the deployment of these nurse leaders in a wide array of policy forums.
- Communicate effectively the accomplishments and values of the AAN to ensure public and private funding for articulated priorities.
- Develop an effective and efficient organizational structure to achieve aforementioned goals.

The Academy was constituted as a self-governing affiliate of ANA to insulate its work from the inevitable politics of membership associations. The Academy has its own dues structure, bylaws, and elected officials. Using AAN as the vehicle, the leadership corps for the profession provides thinking on the critical issues confronting nursing. Their ability to create, speak, and disseminate intellectual products must be unencumbered by political pressure. The AAN has responded well to the challenge of shaping the future. The Magnet Hospital Study of 1983 set the stage for the current Magnet Hospital Recognition Program instituted by ANCC to pay tribute to departments of nursing service that are exemplary. The Teaching Nursing Home Program contributed significantly to the nursing home reforms of 1987.[8] The AAN Clinical Scholars Program accorded advanced practice nursing intellectual respect, and moved practice toward the level of distinction it currently enjoys. The faculty practice initiative of the 1980s gave credibility to service-education unification efforts that have since become the standard to bring the best of nursing to both students and patients. The AAN has accomplished its work through demonstration projects, annual meetings, smaller interest groups that are a mechanism for continuing problem solving and discussion around issues, dissemination of ideas through *Nursing Outlook* (the Academy's official journal), and the wide reach of its influential members.

Nurses who wish to become Fellows must be sponsored by two current Fellows in good standing. The Academy's Fellow Selection Committee reviews the applications according to established procedures and determines those applicants who meet the criteria for fellowship.

Criteria for selection of Fellows are as follows:

1. **Member in good standing in ANA (of an SNA).**
2. **Evidence of outstanding contributions to nursing, such as:**
   a. **Pioneering efforts that contribute information useful in surmounting barriers to effective nursing practice or facilitating excellence in nursing practice.**
   b. **Successful implementation of creative approaches to curriculum development, defini-**

tion of specialized areas for practice, or development of specialized training programs.
   c. **Research or demonstration projects that contribute to improvement in nursing and health service delivery.**
   d. **Creative development, utilization, or evaluation of specific concepts or principles in nursing education, nursing practice, nursing management, or health services.**
   e. **Authorship of books, papers, or other communication media that have had significant implications for nursing practice, health policy, or health planning** (*published by date of application only*).
   f. **Successful development of health policy or health planning.**
   g. **Leadership in nursing organizations at the local, state, or national level.**
3. **Evidence of potential to continue contributions to nursing and to the academy, such as the following:**
   a. **Efforts, projects, or other activities that relate to contemporary problems.**
   b. **Efforts, projects, or other activities that reflect broad perspective on nursing including social, cultural and political considerations.**
   c. **An expressed willingness to actively participate in and support academy activities.**

Members designated as Fellows of the American Academy of Nursing are entitled to use the initials FAAN following their names.

MAJOR ANA PROGRAMS AND SERVICES

The programs and services of ANA represent the total results of the efforts of members and staff, elected officers, committees, forums, congresses, institutes, commissions, and councils. These include meeting with members of other groups and disciplines; planning or attending institutes, workshops, conventions, or committee meetings; developing and writing brochures, manuals, position papers, standards, or testimony to be presented to Congress; and implementing ongoing programs, planning new ones, or trying to solve the problem of how to serve the members best within the limitations of the budget. Every issue of the *American Journal of*

Nursing and of *The American Nurse* carries reports of these many and varied activities. Presented here are brief descriptions of some (but not all) of the major ANA programs and services.

Nursing Practice

ANA works continually and in many ways to improve the quality of nursing care available to the public. In its role as the professional association for RNs, it defines and interprets principles and standards of nursing practice and education. These publications are available from ANA.

ANA's concern for quality nursing care is clearly demonstrated by the development of the practice standards, with their implications for peer review, and the consequent action of ANA and many state associations to assist nurses to implement the standards. The *Standards of Clinical Nursing Practice* (see Chap. 9) and standards in areas of nursing specialty are general enough to encompass the variety of practitioners. They are intended as models to measure the quality of nursing performance, another assurance to the public that quality care will be delivered. As the need for standards in highly specialized areas of practice was identified, various ANA divisions, now councils, cooperated with specialty organizations to formulate standards. The many excellent publications are part of the overall plan to assist SNAs and individuals in the utilization of the standards of practice. Many workshops, seminars, and other programs were also held to provide nurses with new knowledge to facilitate implementation and thereby improve nursing care. Major papers and/or proceedings of these conferences were made available. ANA's concern for quality nursing care is also manifested through its Center for Ethics and Human Rights and *Code for Nurses*. One of the center's purposes is to develop and disseminate information on ethical and human rights issues facing the profession of nursing. The center provides consultation and resources in addressing practice dilemmas and controversies. For example, the center helps nurses and SNAs with application of the *Code for Nurses* and prepares documents such as the Position Statements on the Nurse's Role in End-of-Life Decisions.

Certification

The ANA established a certification program in 1973 to recognize professional achievement and excellence in practice, both to help practitioners maintain motivation for superior performance and to provide another means to establish and maintain standards of professional practice to the end that all citizens will have quality nursing care.

The impetus for establishment of the certification program is found in the adoption by the 1958 House of Delegates of Goal Two: "To establish ways within the ANA to provide formal recognition of personal achievement and superior performance in nursing."[9] In 1968, interim certification boards began to work with the Congress for Nursing Practice to establish criteria for certification. Action slowed during the period of financial crisis, but by 1973 ANA was completing arrangements for its certification program. Included was an arrangement with the Educational Testing Service (ETS) of Princeton, New Jersey, to provide technical support in the development of systems for certification, including appropriate examinations. (ANA-appointed groups provided the content for these tests, and ETS the test development expertise.) By 1974, criteria had been fully delineated for geriatric nursing, psychiatric and mental health nursing, pediatric nurse practitioners, and community health nursing. Any licensed RN who could demonstrate current knowledge and excellence in practice regardless of the basic program from which the nurse graduated was eligible to take the examination.

The first examinations were taken by approximately 300 pediatric and geriatric nurses in May 1973, but more than 5,000 applications had been received, attesting to the significance members attached to the program. Until then, nurses had rarely been recognized or rewarded for excellent patient care; monetary rewards, prestige, and promotion had been via the administrative route or through educational achievement.

ANA became one organizational entity among several who certified nurses. ANA's program was predated by successful certification offerings from the American Association of Nurse Anesthetists and the American College of Nurse Midwives. Other specialty societies also expressed the intent to begin to certify in their areas of practice.

In 1976, the ANA announced that it would certify at two levels: (1) certification for competence in specialized areas of practice with distinctive eligibility requirements, and (2) certification for excellence in practice, with diplomate status in a proposed American College of Nursing Practice for certified nurses who met additional criteria. The proposal was given a hostile reception, primarily because the diplomate status called for a master's degree, and many of those certified for excellence had no degree at all. In other words, the model provided for three levels of practice distinction: competence, excellence, and diplomate. In rethinking the program, two levels of certification were identified: competence in specialized areas of practice (generalist), and acknowledged achievement as a specialist. The former will require a bachelor's degree by 1995, and the latter calls for the master's degree. Each is based on the assessment of knowledge, demonstration of current practice ability, and endorsement of colleagues.

During its 1989 review of ANA's organizational structure and functions, the Commission on Organizational Assessment and Renewal (COAR) recommended that the ANA Board of Directors establish a separately incorporated center through which ANA would serve its credentialing programs. At the House of Delegates meeting in June 1989 it was voted to adopt the recommendations of COAR and establish a separately incorporated center for credentialing. As a result in 1991 the ANA certification program became a separately incorporated entity called the American Nurses Credentialing Center (ANCC). The ANCC philosophy of credentialing is based upon, and is consistent with, the adopted ethical codes of ANA and its policies, standards, and positions on nursing practice, education, and service.

ANCC offers certification, accreditation, and recognition programs that reflect a commitment to professionalism in nursing. Certification by ANCC provides tangible recognition of professional achievement. The ANCC Accreditation program administers a national system for the evaluation and recognition of continuing education in nursing. The Magnet Recognition Program recognizes excellence in nursing services. Together these programs contribute to ANCC's position of national leadership.

The Board of Directors is the governing body of ANCC and is responsible for the supervision, control, and direction of ANCC. All board members are appointed by ANA and six ANCC members are sitting members of the ANA Board of Directors. The ANCC Commission on Certification is responsible for implementing the certification program. Among its functions, the commission sets certification program policy, establishes boards on certification; serves as the final appellate body for certification candidate appeals; receives, reviews, and comments on proposals from the ANA Congress on Nursing Practice for new certification programs; and provides a mechanism for the systematic evaluation of the certification program. There are nine boards on certification composed of representatives of each of the Test Development Committees (TDCs) within their specialty fields. Each TDC is responsible for one certification examination and is composed of certified nurses who are content experts in their specialty field. TDC members typically represent a variety of practice settings and educational backgrounds.

In 1994, certification examinations were being offered at the generalist level, and at the advanced practice level to nurse practitioners and clinical specialists. Examinations were offered in twenty-four practice areas: Community Health

Nurse, General Nursing Practice, Gerontological Nurse, Medical-Surgical Nurse, Nursing Administration, Pediatric Nurse, Perinatal Nurse, Psychiatric and Mental Health Nurse, School Nurse, College Health Nurse, Continuing Education/Staff Development Nurse, Home Health Nurse, Adult Nurse Practitioner, Family Nurse Practitioner, Gerontological Nurse Practitioner, Pediatric Nurse Practitioner, School Nurse Practitioner, Clinical Specialist in Adult Psychiatric and Mental Health Nursing, Clinical Specialist in Child and Adolescent Psychiatric Mental Health Nursing, Clinical Specialist in Gerontological Nursing, Clinical Specialist in Medical-Surgical Nursing, Nursing Administration Basic and Advanced, Clinical Specialist in Community Health Nursing. Testing technology is forever evolving and ANCC is keeping pace with all technological advances. As evidence of this the first Nursing Informatics examination will be offered in October 1995. ANCC will also offer the Acute Care Nurse Practitioner certification examination for the first time in early 1995. In October 1994 over 100,000 nurses were certified by ANCC.

The eligibility criteria for each certification vary according to the specialty area. Specified documents are examined and evaluated to determine eligibility. These documents include evidence of continuing education, educational transcripts, and nurse colleague endorsement forms. Some of the specialty areas require both past and present practice while all require current licensure as a registered nurse in the United States or its territories. Once certified, the certification is valid for five years and may be renewed by submitting a stipulated amount of continuing education or by taking an examination. Specific information on eligibility criteria for each specialty area and the cost of the exam may be obtained by contacting ANCC.

The accreditation program, which is also administered by ANCC, was established in 1974 by ANA as a voluntary system for accreditation of continuing education in nursing. The essential purpose of this system is to provide professional nursing judgment on the quality of the continuing education offered. Accreditation is a peer review system based on designated standards and criteria for continuing education in nursing. The ANCC Commission on Accreditation, utilizing the ANA's *Standards for Continuing Education in Nursing*, is responsible for developing and administering the operational policies, procedures, and criteria that govern the accreditation and approval processes. The commission defines accreditation as a voluntary process for appraising and granting recognition to an organization or institution that meets established standards based on predetermined criteria. The two categories of accreditation available in the ANCC system are (1) accreditation as an approver of continuing education in nursing and (2) accreditation as a provider of continuing education in nursing.

The Magnet Recognition Program was introduced by ANCC in 1994 and is built upon the 1983 Magnet Hospital Study conducted by the American Academy of Nursing (AAN). The baseline for its development is the ANA *Standards for Organized Nursing Services and Responsibilities of Nurse Administrators Across All Settings* (1991). The program is a joint endeavor of ANA and ANCC. The goal of the Magnet Recognition Program is to identify excellence in nursing services and to recognize institutions that act as a "magnet" by creating a work environment that recognizes and rewards professional nursing. Related outcomes could result in a nursing department's ability to recruit and retain high-caliber professional staff as well as the ability to provide a consistent quality of patient care.

In a major effort to promote professionalization through standardization of criteria for national nursing certification programs, ANCC and other nursing leaders worked together to create The American Board of Nursing Specialties (ABNS). The main function of ABNS is to develop and maintain standards and criteria for the review and approval of national specialty certification boards and their certification programs. Eight of the ANA boards on certification have been recognized by ABNS as meeting national standards for certifying organizations. This recognition by ABNS strengthens the certification process and promotes the quality of specialty practice. More information on certification is found in Chap. 20.

Nursing Education

The important ANA function of setting standards and policies for nursing education has been demonstrated in many ways. The 1965 Position Paper was the beginning of a series of specific actions toward implementing the position that education for entry into professional nursing practice should be at the baccalaureate level (see Chap. 12). ANA has made a number of other important educational statements in the last few years; these are available from ANA.

The topic of CE has also been given considerable attention by ANA, gaining impetus in 1971 with the establishment of the Council on Continuing Education and the awarding of a grant for a project entitled "Identification of Need for Continuing Education for Nurses by the National Professional Organization." See Chaps. 12 and 13 for discussion of issues in CE, as well as information on CE units and accreditation.

ANA endorsed the concept of CE for all nurses as one of the means by which they can maintain competence. ANA believes that maintaining competence is primarily the responsibility of the practitioner. Because of a practical and philosophical reluctance to transfer this responsibility to government, the association, by a vote of its 1972 House of Delegates, opposed mandatory CE as a condition for renewal of a license to practice. This was reversed by the ANA house in 1974, and particular emphasis was put on SNA control rather than government control. The house directed ANA to provide support to those states that choose to establish CE as one prerequisite for relicensure, as well as to those states that choose to encourage CE through a voluntary program. By 1979, most SNAs had some sort of CE approved programs. However, as NP programs continued to proliferate on a CE basis, some type of accreditation of these educational programs was also adjudged essential. Extensive planning was done, with the result that since 1975, the association has provided a mechanism for voluntary national accreditation of continuing education in nursing (now carried out by the American Nurses Credentialing Center).

Legislation and Legal Activities

ANA's legislative program is an important one that often affects, directly and indirectly, the welfare of both nurses and the public (see Chaps. 18 and 19). The association's legislative endeavors are concentrated on matters affecting nurses, nursing, and health, but in today's society these matters represent an extremely broad area of activity, ranging from child care to gun control.

ANA's legislative program comprises three main endeavors: (1) to help SNAs promote effective nursing practice acts in their states in order to protect the public and the nursing profession from unqualified practitioners; (2) to offer consultation on other legislative and regulatory measures that affect nurses; and (3) to speak for nursing in relation to federal legislation for health, education, labor, and welfare, and for social programs such as civil rights.

The first ANA Committee on Legislation was established in 1923, with the responsibility of watching federal legislation affecting nursing and representing ANA in such matters. The ANA board also determined at that time to confine the association legislatively to matters of health, nurses, and nursing. ANA now has a board-appointed legislative committee that recommends legislative priorities to the board on a yearly basis. Legislative decisions are based on ANA policy statements, house resolutions, and, of course, the ANA goals and priorities.

The major responsibility for coordinating legislative information and action lies with the ANA governmental affairs arm. It was not until late 1951 that ANA opened an office in Washington, with one staff person to act as full-time lobbyist, and even then direction for the legislative program emanated from ANA headquarters (then in New York). From that time on, the Washington staff has expanded considerably, and their responsibilities have increased and broadened to include lobbying (through its registered lobbyists); development of relationships with congressional members and their staffs and committee staffs; contacts with key figures in the executive branch of government; maintaining relations with other national organizations; preparing most of the statements and information presented to congressional committees; drafting letters to government officials; presenting testimony; acting as backup for members presenting testimony; and representing ANA in many capacities.

Over the years, ANA has represented nursing in the capital on many major issues: funds for nursing education, pension reform, national health insurance, quality of care in nursing homes, collective bargaining rights, pay equity, health hazards, civil rights, Federal Trade Commission authority and regulations, problems of nurses in the federal service, tax revision, higher education, problems of health manpower, direct reimbursement to nurses, and health care reform. In addition, ANA lobbies for or against legislation that may affect nursing directly and immediately, such as funding for nursing education, collective bargaining, and reimbursement for nurses. For instance, ANA has always monitored the status of the Nursing Education Act (NEA), which has funded so much of nursing education and research.

Major newspapers and journals have commented on nursing's clout. It is important to note that as invaluable as the ANA Washington staff is, with its behind-the-scenes and visible lobbying activities, there would be no success without the active backup of nurses, as well as consumers, labor, and other health groups. Participation in the legislative process, as described in Chap. 18, is essential for nurses if the profession is to have any impact in influencing health policy.

ANA has often cooperated and coordinated with other health disciplines but has also faced areas of disagreement (such as early opposition of AMA and other groups to funding for nurse education). Such philosophical differences still occur, but there has been increasing cooperation with both health and other groups to achieve mutual legislative goals.

Communication about legislative matters is particularly important to help members keep abreast of key legislative issues. Beginning in 1955, *Capital Commentary*, first called *Legislation News*, was sent to state associations, schools of nursing, state boards of nursing, state boards of health, chief nurses in federal services, and selected individuals. The demand and the need became so great that news of a legislative and regulatory nature is now incorporated in *The American Nurse*. A monthly newsletter, *Capital Update*, is sent to individuals and groups, including SNAs.

Special communications are sent out from ANA headquarters when membership support is needed for legislative programs. Periodically, discussion guides and manuals have been developed for the use of SNAs, and the government relations staff frequently participates in state and national conventions and other meetings. For many nurses, the real excitement has occurred on the state level, particularly in the last few years, when issues of health care, health education, and especially new nurse practice acts have been the focus of legislative attention. ANA is noted for its grassroots network, the Congressional District and Senatorial Coordinators (CDC/SC). Designated SNA members have established personal relationships with each member of Congress and use that position of influence to educate about nursing issues.

In addition to specific legislative action, ANA becomes involved in various legal matters that affect the welfare of nurses. In some cases, ANA acts as a friend of the court, providing information about the issues involved. Since 1973, ANA has filed charges of discrimination in various district offices of the Equal Employment Opportunity Commission (EEOC), some of which it won and some of which are still unsettled.

ANA has also presented oral arguments and briefs on various matters before the National Labor Relations Board and the United States Supreme Court. (SNAs advocate for nurses before state legislatures and state and federal courts.) The number of such services that ANA offers expands yearly.

American Nurses Association Political Action Committee

Important components of nursing lobbying efforts are the nursing political action groups. Most professional organizations have such groups, which are independent of the organization but related to it. This is because a tax-exempt, incorporated professional organization such as ANA (or AMA) is under definite legal constraints as far as partisan political action is concerned. In 1971, a small group of nurses in New York formed the Nurses for Political Action (NPA) to serve as a political arm for ANA by providing financial support for candidates and engaging in other political activities, as well as providing political education to nurses. In 1973, ANA directed an ad hoc committee to explore the possibility of a political action committee (PAC). For various reasons, a new organization evolved: Nurses' Coalition for Action in Politics (N-CAP), which was officially organized in 1974 with a $50,000 ANA grant, as a voluntary, unincorporated, nonpartisan political action group. This is now called the American Nurses Association Political Action Committee (ANA-PAC). ANA does not give money to ANA-PAC to give to candidates but does provide funds for ANA-PAC administrative support. ANA-PAC has a single purpose: to promote the improvement of the health care of the people through political action. Its two major functions are education and support. Education is directed toward encouraging nurses and others to take a more active part in governmental affairs, educating them on the political process and political issues relevant to health care, and assisting them in organizing themselves for effective political action. For this purpose, ANA-PAC has sponsored workshops and prepared educational materials. It has also encouraged and assisted PACs on the state level. Many states now have active PACs that primarily give attention to state issues but are also able to coordinate collective action on national legislation.

Support is offered to political candidates (regardless of political affiliation) whose acts demonstrate dedication to constructive health care legislation. This support may be in the form of endorsement or include monetary contributions. Endorsements are made in consultation with state PACs whenever possible. State political action coalitions endorse state candidates. The fact that nurses, or at least SNA members, are perhaps more politically active than other citizens was shown by one survey: 91 percent are registered to vote, 75 percent have written a letter to an officeholder expressing an opinion, 58 percent have attended a political meeting or rally, and about 58 percent have contributed money to a candidate.

To support these activities, ANA-PAC accepts donations from nurses and others. It is headquartered at 600 Maryland Ave., S.W., Suite 100 West, Washington, D.C. 20024-2571.

Economic and General Welfare

The ways in which ANA has worked to promote the welfare of its membership have varied with the times. When it was first incorporated, it gave as one of its purposes "To distribute relief among such nurses as may become ill, disabled, or destitute." Today, thanks to an economic security program established in 1946 and steadily expanded and strengthened since that time, it works actively to ensure that nurses have a voice in determining their employment conditions, that nursing salaries are appropriate to nursing responsibilities, and that employment conditions are of the kind to enable nurses to give high-quality care.

ANA's economic security program promotes the concept that nurses have a right to form a group to choose a representative to negotiate for them with their employer, and to have the mutually agreed-upon provisions put in writing. It endorses the constructive use of collective bargaining techniques in nurses' negotiations with their employers. Although ANA does not serve as bargaining agent for groups of nurses, many SNAs do so. ANA helps to develop the principles and techniques for such employer-employee negotiations and advises and assists the SNAs with their economic security activities as much as possible. In addition, a major role of the ANA on the national level is to develop policy positions, as shown in the bylaws. Because of its status as a collective bargaining organization, ANA must follow the requirements of the Labor-Management Reporting Act of 1959 (Landrum-Griffin Law), which affects voting rights and elections of officers.

Overall, ANA is concerned not only with improving salaries, fringe benefits, and working conditions but has also expanded its activities to improve the quality of nursing care, to assure the public of the individual and collective accountability of qualified professional nurses, and to increase accessibility of health care services for the public. This is accomplished by nurses achieving the right to make decisions affecting themselves, their practice, and the quality of care. Although this approach to collective bargaining might be considered new to individuals who think of economic security only in terms of salaries, fringe benefits, and working conditions, job action by nurses has often been in protest of inadequate patient care, which has not been improved by the employer.

The ANA economic and general welfare program is often misunderstood by members, nonmembers, and others. Seeing that the economic security of its members is maintained is one of the classic roles of a professional association, and, especially in recent years, economic security has been seen as extending beyond purely monetary matters and conditions of employment to involvement of nurses in the decision-making aspects of nursing care. An example might be that, through an agreed-upon process, perhaps including a formal committee structure,

nurses' objections to inadequate staffing or illegal or inappropriate job assignments would be instrumental in bringing about changes that would provide improved care.

In the last few years, the nurse's right to adequate monetary compensation has been recognized almost universally, although in many places, salaries and benefits are still abysmal, and there is still a struggle involved for improvement, with or without SNA representation as a bargaining agent. There is still significant employer resistance to allowing nurses a voice in policy-making, both because of the possible financial impact and because of fear of loss of control, as well as on the basis of general philosophic disagreement.

Over the years, the ANA House has made many major decisions in relation to economic security issues. In 1968, ANA's 18-year-old no-strike policy was rescinded, and in 1970 the 20-year-old neutrality policy (that nurses maintain a neutral position in labor-management disputes between their employers and nonnurse employees) was also rescinded.

The 1974 passage of a NLRA amendment to include employees of nonprofit health care institutions created a flurry of activity. In 1975, as the result of a legal brief presented by ANA, NLRA ruled that a separate collective bargaining unit of RNs is appropriate under the normal local unit determination criteria, and by early 1980, the professional organization was the largest collective bargaining representative for RNs. Also in 1975, the ANA board of directors established the Shirley Titus Award in recognition of individual nurses' contributions to the association's economic and general welfare program. Finally, the formation of the Commission of Economic and General Welfare in 1976 was a further indication of increased ANA membership interest and commitment to economic and general welfare issues.

In the years following the 1974 NLRA amendments, ANA and SNAs were frequently involved in legal actions regarding various aspects of collective bargaining that are unique to nursing: whether nurses could be in separate units, the status of head nurses and supervisors as management, and whether the fact that supervisors and directors of nursing may sit on the board of directors of a SNA means that the collective bargaining agent (the SNA) is controlled by management. Decisions favoring unions have been less frequent in the last few years, as unions have lost ground. Such cases are not settled with one ruling, and frequently further action is taken through appeal mechanisms or legislation. One major victory was a 1990 decision by the U.S. Court of Appeals for the Seventh Circuit to allow nurses to organize in separate (all-RN) bargaining units. (The decision was ultimately upheld by the U.S. Supreme Court.) The NLRB had made such a ruling, but a suit by AHA had enjoined the NLRB from implementing it. In a more negative decision of May 1994, the U.S. Supreme Court ruled that a licensed practical nurse who directed lesser prepared personnel in a nursing home was considered a supervisor and therefore exempt from any legal employee protections. This could potentially challenge the right for nurses to organize and bargain collectively and to join in any concerted activity about patient care or employment conditions, whether or not they are represented by a union. In other words, the majority of the justices said that the direction of assistive workers was a responsibility the nurse assumed as an agent of the employer, rather than as an agent of the patient, since the consumer looked to the employer to guarantee service and safety. The decision holds implications far beyond nursing and may have to be addressed through legislation. In a minority opinion, one justice noted that every professional's work involves to some degree directing the work of others.[10] More discussion on labor and collective bargaining is included in Chaps. 19 and 30.

Because ANA recognizes that other employee groups also have the right to organize, guidelines have been developed in the event of a job action (strike) that involves an organized group of nonnurses. Nurses were urged to continue to perform their distinctive nursing duties; press for action in the interest of safe patient care to reduce the patient census; refuse to assume duties normally discharged by other personnel unless a clear and present danger to patients exists; and coordinate their activities and efforts through their local unit organizations and SNAs, using established channels for intercommunications with management and the other employee groups.

Unions, which have been successful in organizing nonprofessional health workers and a number of professionals, have been giving priority to organizing nurses. There is serious concern that large unions with strong economic backing and single-purpose goals to increase monetary and working benefits, may prove competitive, for nurses frequently do not see the professional organization as a strong or even appropriate bargaining agent. Because past experience has shown that unions have taken little action to negotiate contracts involving nurses in decisions that could improve patient care, and because many nurses are not even aware that such participation is possible, one of the most worthwhile purposes of collective bargaining could be lost. Currently, ANA finds itself competing with several powerful unions. Nevertheless, in 1993, SNAs represented over 150,000 RNs in 27 states.

It should be noted that concern for the economic security of nurses is not limited to the American scene. In 1973, an unprecedented committee meeting was held jointly by the World Health Organization and the International Labor Organization to discuss urgent and radical measures to alleviate international problems of shortage, maldistribution, and poor utilization of nurses. A major objective of the meeting of health care experts from nineteen nations was to set viable recommendations covering factors influencing conditions of life and work in the nursing profession. Among the proposals presented were the right of collective bargaining, a forty-hour basic week, payment for overtime, two consecutive days of rest, and four weeks' compulsory paid leave per year. The meeting, initiated by the International

Council of Nurses (ICN) of which ANA is a member, may have had positive effects on nursing around the world.

But the issues are not easily resolved. At ICN meetings, economic issues are discussed extensively, and in meetings of the Council of National Representatives, the subject of social and economic welfare affecting nurses is a top priority. Reports indicate that unions in many countries are attempting to represent nursing and control the profession.

Although the economic benefits gained through collective bargaining are obvious, the test of nurses' commitment to patient care will come as they acquire the right to become joint decision makers about conditions to improve patient care.

Human Rights Activities

ANA works toward integrating qualified members of all racial and ethnic groups into the nursing profession and tries to achieve sound human rights practices. From the time of its founding, ANA as a national organization has never had any discriminatory policies for membership in the association. Until 1964, however, a few of its constituent associations denied membership to black nurses. In these instances, ANA made provision for black nurses to bypass district and state associations and become members of ANA directly. At that point (1950), the National Association for Colored Graduate Nurses (NACGN) voluntarily went out of existence on the basis that there was no longer a need for such a specialized membership association. At the same time, strong pressure from ANA and the other state associations was exerted until now all state and district associations have discontinued such discriminatory practices, and minority group nurses are appointed and elected to committees and offices at district, state, and national levels. ANA has also strongly supported every major civil rights bill affecting health, education, public accommodations, nursing, and equal employment opportunities. In 1956, long before most health and professional associations had taken a

positive stance on civil rights, ANA's board of directors adopted a statement supporting the principle that health and education should not be supported by tax funds if there are any discriminatory practices. Testimony along these lines was presented at federal hearings.

Even so, there was some feeling that a greater effort was necessary, and in 1972 the House of Delegates passed the Affirmative Action Resolution, calling for a task force to develop and implement a program to correct inequities. The program was defined as "a positive ongoing effort which is results-oriented and specifically designed to transcend neutrality." It was aimed at not only nondiscriminatory programming but action to correct past deficiencies at all levels and in all segments of an organization. An ombudsman was also provided for and appointed.

The program went into action in 1973, and a task force of minority and nonminority members met with ANA units to identify problems and make plans. A minority position statement was developed, recommending methodology for change on such issues as recruitment and retention of minority students, lack of data on career patterns of minority group RNs, and the need to include information in nursing education about the health needs of minority groups. In the years that followed, several regional conferences were held on quality care for ethnic minority clients, and the papers were published. A bibliography, *Minority Groups in Nursing*, was also published by the Task Force in 1973, and an updated bibliography was published in 1976 after the establishment of the Commission on Human Rights. Both were a compilation of the literature on ethnic people of color, men, and people with different lifestyles who are in nursing, as well as other pertinent topics relating to minorities and the provision of health care to minorities.

In 1974, ANA was awarded a 6-year grant by the Center for Minority Group Mental Health Programs of the National Institutes of Mental Health to establish and administer the Registered Nurse Fellowship Program for Ethnic/Racial Minorities. The program continues today and supports a number of minority nurses in doctoral study in psychiatric mental health nursing or a related behavioral or social science. Over half of the fellows have earned doctorates. Most are teaching or doing research on the health needs of minorities.

ANA's human rights activities, which had been under the aegis of a commission, are now the focus of a newly created staff structure, the Center for Ethics and Human Rights.

ANA has taken positive legal action on minority rights and women's rights (salary and pension discrepancies). With the support of most members, ANA also made a major statement on reproductive health and took action in the Cruzan case to uphold patients' rights (see Chap. 22).

Since 1974, ANA has taken a position in support of the Equal Rights Amendment (ERA) and participates in various women's rights programs and activities. There is no doubt that activities related to human rights will continue. It is important that the valuable services of all nurses be fully utilized and the nursing needs of the American pluralistic society met.

The American Nurses' Foundation

The American Nurses' Foundation (ANF) was created by ANA to meet the need for an independent, permanent, nonprofit organization devoted to nursing research. It was an outgrowth of the ANA's expanding research activities, particularly the 5-year *Studies of Nursing Function*, which was undertaken by ANA after the 1950 convention, both because of a mandate by membership nationally and as an assumption of the profession's responsibility to determine its own functions.

Initial financing of this project was provided by the SNAs, but by the third year the ANA board of directors decided to finance the program from the association's budget. Between 1950 and 1955, twenty-seven studies were funded. *Nurses Invest in Patient Care*, a preliminary report, was prepared and published by ANA in 1956. *20,000 Nurses Tell Their Story*, by Everett C. Hughes, Helen MacGill Hughes, and

Irwin Deutscher, was published in 1958; it was a synthesis of the findings of the studies.

So that such research could be continued and expanded, the ANA board recommended that the 1954 House of Delegates "authorize the incoming board of directors to secure information and to develop a foundation or trust for receiving tax-free funds for desirable charitable, scientific, literary or educational projects in line with the aims and purposes of the American Nurses Association." After 6 months of committee study, the establishment of the American Nurses' Foundation was approved by the new board. It was incorporated in 1955, and its tax-exempt status was approved in 1956. The foundation was organized exclusively for charitable, scientific, literary, and educational purposes.

Between 1955 and 1973, the major objectives of ANF were to provide financial support for research and to disseminate and promote dissemination of research findings through publications, conferences, and other communications media.

In 1979, the ANF board established major new objectives focusing on analysis of health policy issues of priority to nursing, support for the career development of nurses, and assistance to the educational and research activities of ANA.

ANF has continued its Nursing Research Grants Program, funded through the contributions of corporations, nursing organizations, and individuals. In 1983, the ANF Distinguished Scholar Program was established. The purpose of the program was to permit nurse health policy analysts and scholars to analyze selected policy issues related to economics, delivery of nursing services, nursing practice, and nursing education as identified by the nursing profession. In 1980, in collaboration with the American Nurses Association Council of Nurse Researchers, ANF also established a Distinguished Contribution to Nursing Science award to recognize nurse researchers who have made significant contributions to the nursing profession. The Professional Practice for Nurse Administrators in Long-Term Care Facilities Project (NA/LTC) was co-sponsored by ANF and the Foundation of the American College of Health Care Administrators, Inc. (FACHCA), and was supported by a grant from the W. K. Kellogg Foundation. The primary goal of this 3-year project (completed in April 1984 and then re-funded) was the continued professional development of nurse administrators and directors of nursing in long-term care. A health education project involving Missouri elementary schools was another early ANF project.

The American Nurses' Foundation solicits, receives, and/or administers funds for a variety of projects such as the W. K. Kellogg Foundation award of 1.3 million dollars for the community-based Health Care Project. ANF also receives and administers funds for ANA and AAN. Grants have been received from various sources for work on HIV prevention, managed care, immunization, managing genetic information, and nursing informatics.

Obviously, funding is of vital concern to ANF. In 1959, in order to establish a strong base upon which to operate, the foundation launched a nationwide drive for funds, enlisting support from the nursing community, the business community, and the general public. In 1992, ANF concluded a successful "Nursing on the Move" campaign, raising $1.5 million toward the relocation of headquarters to Washington, D.C. In 1993, ANF received a two-million-dollar bequest from the estate of Julia Ondo Hardy, RN, the largest bequest in the history of nursing in the United States.

ANF is governed by its bylaws and directed by a nine-member board of trustees; six of the trustees are RNs. A finance committee and a research advisory committee report to the board of trustees. The finance committee monitors budget preparation, the investment portfolio, and fund-raising activities. The research advisory committee establishes guidelines for administering the small grant program and recommends recipients to the board for final approval. The executive director of ANA is the executive director of ANF. There is also a professional headquarters staff involved in fund-raising and managing grant-funded projects.

Requests for information about completed ANF research projects or applications for grants (which should include an outline of the research question and the proposed design) may be sent to ANF headquarters at 600 Maryland Ave., S.W., Suite 100 West, Washington, D.C. 20024-2571.

Communication and Information Services

ANA is a veritable goldmine of information. The association publishes *The American Nurse* monthly which reports recent activities and happenings important to the nursing community. Many of the staff units, as already described, have specific newsletters that are published on a regular basis; such as *Capital Update, Center for Ethics and Human Rights Communique, Legal Developments*, and *E&GW Update*, to name a few. ANA is also a clearinghouse for information on the state-specific statutory requirements for nursing, language in collective bargaining contracts, the prevailing demographics of practicing nurses, as some examples. *Facts about Nursing* is also published periodically, a statistical summary of information about nurses, nursing, and related health services and groups.

American Nurses Publishing (an arm of ANA and ANF) publishes standards of practice, the Code for Nurses, major reports, monographs, papers presented at meetings, and certain publications of the AAN and ANCC. The association also publishes position statements, guidelines for practice, bulletins, manuals, and brochures for specialized groups within the organization and sends out news releases and announcements concerning activities of interest to the public. Available from American Nurses Publishing upon request is its periodically revised *Catalogue*. ANA also conducts an ongoing educational and informational service to interpret ANA's activities, programs, and goals to nurses, allied groups, government, special agencies, and the public, and monitors news and public opinion trends affecting the profession. ANA has created "ANA Net," which enables the electronic exchange of information between ANA and the SNAs.

ANA Participation with Other Groups

In the conduct of business, the ANA staff, officials, and members meet with some 300 organizations and groups. Much of this participation is in the form of official liaisons and coalitions. There are also many occasions for cosponsorship of conferences, educational programs, and projects. The association is very much aware that where policy or programs that impact on other groups are evolving, representatives of these constituencies must be included in the developmental process. It is this sensitivity that prompted the creation of the Nursing Organization Liaison Forum (NOLF). Over 75 nursing organizations come together as the members of NOLF, and under the sponsorship of ANA, to share common concerns and to respond to the implications that ANA policy and programs hold for their constituents. The existence of NOLF has eliminated much of the fragmentation that once existed in the ranks of organized nursing, and established the leadership role of ANA.

The other formal liaison that warrants mentioning is the Tri-council, composed of ANA, NLN, the American Organization of Nurse Executives (AONE), and the American Association of Colleges of Nursing (AACN). The origins of the Tri-council are in the ANA/NLN Joint Coordinating Committee which dates back to 1952. The 1952 reorganization of nursing associations resulted in a strengthened and expanded ANA, the establishment of the NLN, and the need for a coordinating mechanism. Over time, AONE and AACN were added. The Tri-council strategizes around the most basic issues, and consolidates their governmental affairs and public relations resources to position nursing strongly.

Other Activities and Services

Among other ANA benefits for nurses is insurance of various kinds, available at favorable group rates at national and state levels. Many educational programs, seminars, workshops, clinical conferences, scientific sessions, and so on are available at all levels at reduced rates for members. They are geared to current issues and new developments in health and nursing.

Nurses are also increasingly interested in international nursing. ANA was one of the three charter members of the ICN and is an active participant in the work of this international nursing organization. Essentially, ICN is a federation of national associations of professional nurses (one from each country), and ANA is the member association for the United States (see Chap. 28).

ANA established an International Nursing Center in 1992 through the ANF. The Center sponsors an international talent bank comprised of nurses with expertise in international work and foreign language capability. The Center was awarded a grant by the World AIDS Foundation in 1993 to train nurses in Sri Lanka and India in HIV/AIDS prevention and care.

AMERICAN JOURNAL OF NURSING COMPANY

The American Journal of Nursing Company, a nonprofit corporation, is the oldest nursing journal company in the United States, and is owned by the American Nurses Association. AJN Company has a broad range of products and services that it offers to the nursing and health care community, including publication of three major journals and the International Nursing Index. Corporate offices are located at 555 East 57th Street, New York, New York 10019.

The American Journal of Nursing

Oldest of the nursing periodicals now in existence and first started by and for nurses, the *American Journal of Nursing* (*AJN*) first appeared in October 1900 and has been published monthly ever since. *The Trained Nurse and Hospital Review* (later *Nursing World*) antedated the *Journal* by twelve years but was not nursing owned and nursing run. It ceased publication in

1960. *AJN* is the refereed professional journal of ANA.

AJN, intended for all nurses, cuts across all fields and levels of nursing practice, administration, and education, with special emphasis on the clinical practice of nursing. As fast as new nursing care principles or techniques evolve, they are reported in the *Journal* in clinical news reports or in articles written by nurse experts.

New ideas about nursing in general—its scope, its definition, and its problems—are found in the pages of *AJN*. And, not least important, *AJN*, as the official journal of nursing's professional organization, ANA, carries up-to-date information about ANA's programs and activities. *AJN* news ranges from local (legislative efforts of individual states, for instance) to international (reports of ICN congresses and interim activities). In addition, drug and equipment supplements, columns on ethical dilemmas, legal decisions, pain interventions, computers, books, and films are other examples of the diversity of important information available to readers. *AJN* also publishes a programmed instruction monthly for which CEUs are granted on request. In addition, *AJN* sponsors major clinical conferences several times a year.

MCN, The American Journal of Maternal/Child Nursing

MCN, The American Journal of Maternal/Child Nursing, first appeared in January 1976 and quickly acquired interested subscribers. It is a bimonthly publication established to help the practicing nurse so that care given to individuals and families during the childbearing and childrearing phases of the life cycle can be of high quality. *MCN* is a refereed journal whose review panel is made up of practicing nurses and nurse researchers who are active in the field of maternal-child nursing.

MCN primarily focuses on clinical practice, with particular emphasis on nursing intervention. The topics range from preconception through adolescence. Many issues have a spe-

cial section that highlights such areas as human sexuality, mother-child relationships, or the school-age child. Occasionally, an entire issue of the journal is devoted to one subject, such as nutrition or the family. Every issue carries a column on research authored by a noted nurse researcher and one that focuses on a particular drug. Equally important, space is devoted to the discussion of other issues about which practicing nurses must be knowledgeable. Each issue carries book reviews and notices of major meetings in the field of maternal/child care. *MCN* also sponsors a major convention focused on maternal/child issues and nursing care.

Nursing Research

Still another publication of the American Journal of Nursing Company is *Nursing Research*, a bimonthly journal established in 1952 for the purposes of stimulating and reporting research and specific studies in nursing. The idea for a magazine such as *Nursing Research* came initially from the Association of Collegiate Schools of Nursing, an organization that was merged into NLN in 1952. *Nursing Research* has an editorial advisory committee and nurse editors who are qualified nurse researchers. *Nursing Research* carries reports of research projects, articles on research methods, and news about research activities.

Other American Journal of Nursing Company Services

In addition to the magazines, the AJN Company publishes the quarterly *International Nursing Index* and the annual *AJN Guide: A Review of Nursing Career Opportunities*. It also provides a variety of other services related to the publications and communications fields.

Educational Services Division The Educational Services Division was established in 1970. Since then, its activities have expanded through the company's production of multimedia and print materials and the acquisition of distribu-

\

tion rights to audiovisual materials produced by others.

Today, the Educational Services Division distributes a wide range of multimedia programs for generic and inservice nursing education. These programs are listed for purchase or rental in a catalog that is available on request.

The AJN Company through its educational services division was awarded a grant from the Division on Nursing to develop and put into operation an electronic information system that would bring expert opinion and professional updating to rural nurses. This initiative signifies the inauguration of a new service line in electronic interactive information systems.

Publication Awards To recognize excellence in the official publications of all ANA constituent members, the AJN Company makes awards every two years to state publications for excellence in a number of categories. To achieve fairness in making the awards, the association publications are grouped according to the size of association membership. Outstanding editors and professional nurses serve as judges in the various categories, and awards are presented at an event held in conjunction with each ANA biennial convention.

During the ANA convention, the Educational Services Division conducts a Media Festival, awarding plaques to producers of films, videotapes, and slide tape programs judged to be outstanding. These are screened throughout the convention week, providing educators and other interested persons with the opportunity to view them for possible later use.

The AJN Company also gives "Book of the Year" awards to publications in a variety of categories.

Sophia F. Palmer Memorial Library For many years, the AJN Company has maintained a library at its headquarters. Intended originally for the use of the magazines' editors and the staffs of ANA and NLN, the library's facilities have for some years been available to a limited number of nurses and graduate students. They must make an appointment to use the library, however; there is no mail or loan service, and no material may be taken out of the library.

In 1953 the library was named the Sophia F. Palmer Memorial Library in honor of *AJN*'s first editor. Under the administration of a professional librarian, the library contains a wealth of nursing literature, including textbooks, periodicals, numerous bulletins, reports, and official publications of all kinds, as well as rare and old material about nursing not available elsewhere.

International Nursing Index One of the AJN Company's most significant services to the profession is the *International Nursing Index (INI)*, which it publishes in cooperation with the National Library of Medicine. This quarterly publication, whose first issue appeared in the spring of 1966, provides a categorized listing of the articles published in nursing journals throughout the world, many of them in languages other than English, plus articles relevant to nursing that appear in journals indexed in *Index Medicus*. The first three issues of *INI* each year are paperbound and noncumulated; the fourth issue is a cloth-bound cumulation of the three previous issues plus new material to the end of the year.

Representing a comprehensive and continuing index of the world literature pertaining to nursing, *INI* is important to nursing and nurses. Copies are found in many nursing and health profession libraries.

THE INDIVIDUAL NURSE AND ANA

A classic article by sociologist Robert Merton cites the functions of any professional organization as including social and moral support for the individual practitioner to help him perform his role as a professional, to set rigorous standards for the profession and help enforce them, to advance and disseminate research and professional knowledge, to help furnish the social bonds through which society coheres, and to speak for the profession. In carrying out some of these functions, the association is seen as a "kind of organizational gadfly, stinging the profession into new and more demanding formulations of purpose."[11] Not all members agree with their organization's goals, and the difficult task of achieving a flexible consensus of values and policies must be accomplished with full two-way communication between the constituencies and the organizational top. However, the key to the success of any organization is the participation of its members. This review of the ANA and its activities is at best an overview. As the needs of members and the demands of society require, changes occur, rapidly, inevitably, and, it is hoped, appropriately—but not always easily. The best way for a nurse to keep up with and share in the changes taking place is through active membership. ANA speaks for nurses; nonmembers have no part in that voice and have no right to complain if it is not representing them. The strength in the organization and in nursing lies in thinking, communicating nurses committed to the goal of improving nursing care for the public and working together in an organized fashion to achieve this goal.

REFERENCES

1. American Nurses Association: *Bylaws*. Washington, DC: American Nurses Publishing, 1993, pp 1–2.
2. Ibid, pp 3–4.
3. American Nurses Association: *Nursing's Agenda for Health Care Reform*, Kansas City, MO: The Association, 1992.
4. American Nurses Association: *Summary of 1994 House Action*. Washington, DC: The Association, 1994, pp 1–33.
5. *Bylaws*, 1993, op cit, p 18.
6. Ibid, pp 18–19.
7. Ibid, p 20.
8. Mezey M et al: The teaching nursing home program. *Nurs Outlook* 32:146–150, May–June 1984.
9. American Nurses Association: *Summary of 1958 House Action*. Kansas City, MO: The Association, 1958.
10. Joel L: The ultimate gag rule. *Am J Nurs* 94:7, August 1994.
11. Merton R: The functions of the professional association. *Am J Nurs* 58:50–54, January 1958.

National League for Nursing

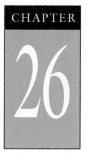

THE MAIN PURPOSE of the National League for Nursing (usually referred to as NLN or the League) is best expressed in this phrase from its certificate of incorporation: "that the nursing needs of the people will be met." ANA is concerned with the same goal, but these two major nursing organizations approach this objective in different ways. ANA, as the membership organization for registered nurses, works primarily through nurses and within the profession. NLN, whose membership includes not only nurses but other members of the health team, interested lay people, and agencies concerned with nursing education and service, works within the community and in association with individuals and groups outside of, but interested in, nursing. In pursuit of the same general end of better nursing care, each organization has its own programs, responsibilities, and functions.

HISTORY

It is easier, perhaps, to understand the distinction between NLN and ANA if the events that led up to the establishment of the NLN in 1952 are reviewed. In many ways, NLN is older than the date suggests, because it grew out of several preexisting nursing organizations and absorbed many of the functions they had carried (see Chaps. 3 and 4).

In the mid-1940s the nursing profession decided to take a long, hard look at its entire organizational structure. At this time there were six national nursing organizations and a host of jointly sponsored committees, activities, and services. This somewhat cumbersome arrangement resulted not only in an overlapping expenditure of time, effort, and resources, but also in confusion in the minds of both nurses and the public as to the purpose and functions of each organization.

Starting in 1944, nurses, under the leadership of the Committee on Structure of National Nursing Organizations, began to study the way in which their profession was organized. The culmination of this long and painstaking self-examination came in 1952. At that time, nurses voted in favor of having two major organizations: a strengthened and reorganized ANA, which would continue to serve as the membership association for RNs, and a new organization, the National League for Nursing, through which nurses and others interested in nursing, along with institutions (both educational and service), could work together to strengthen nursing education and nursing services.

The six organizations prior to the 1952 decision were ANA, the National League of Nursing Education (NLNE), the National Organization for Public Health Nursing (NOPHN), the Association of Collegiate Schools of Nursing (ACSN), the National Association of Colored Graduate Nurses (NACGN), and the American Association of Industrial Nurses (AAIN). NACGN voluntarily went out of existence in 1951, because ANA required all its constituents to admit to membership RNs without discrimination on the basis of color. AAIN decided to continue as a separate organization. The newly created NLN, however, inherited the major functions of the other three organizations—excluding, of course, ANA.

NLNE was the first nursing organization in the United States. Established in 1893 under formidable title of the American Society of Superintendents of Training Schools for Nurses of the United States and Canada (it became NLNE in 1912), its purpose was to standardize and improve the education of nurses. Originally for nurses only, it broadened its membership policies in 1943 to admit lay members.

NOPHN was established in 1912. As its title implies, it was an organization concerned not only with public health nurses but also with the development of public health nursing services. It provided for both agency and individual membership—the latter, except in NOPHN's very early years, open to nonnurses as well as nurses.

The prime objective of ACSN, started in 1933 when baccalaureate degree education for nurses was just beginning to make headway, was to develop nursing education on a professional and collegiate basis. Membership was open principally to accredited programs offering college degrees in nursing.

PURPOSES AND FUNCTIONS

In 1993, NLN revised its mission statement as follows:

> **The National League for Nursing advances the promotion of health and the provision of quality health care within a changing health care environment by promoting and monitoring effective nursing education and practice through collaborative efforts of nursing leaders, representatives of relevant agencies, and the general public.**

To carry out its stated mission, the National League for Nursing, with its diverse constituencies, set forth the following goals for the 1993–1995 biennium:

I. Participate in implementing a national health plan on behalf of the nursing community that assures affordable quality care to all Americans.

II. Promote quality nursing education as critical to quality health care.

III. Promulgate creative approaches to the resolution of health care problems.

IV. Enhance a consumer partnership to advance the mission and attain the goals of the organization.

V. Ensure the financial solvency of the organization through sound management of resources and creation of additional revenue-generating activities.

NATIONAL LEAGUE FOR HEALTH CARE

Over the course of several years, the National League for Nursing, through its Long Range Planning Committee, investigated how to best approach an organizational restructuring. It became apparent that a more flexible structure was needed to accommodate the growth and diversity of activities of the League. A proposal for restructuring was fashioned along those lines in the spring of 1987.

The formation of the National League for Health Care (NLHC, Inc.) as a holding organization was recommended to provide a structure that could easily adapt as new ventures and possibilities presented themselves. The NLN Board endorsed this recommendation during the 1989 biennium, when it voted to establish NLHC, Inc.

The Community Health Accreditation Program (CHAP) was established on April 7, 1988, as the first subsidiary of NLHC. NLN underwrote this program and worked hard to have CHAP gain deemed status in 1992. The Health Care Financing Administration (HCFA) designated CHAP as an organization to accredit home care agencies, in order for them to be reimbursed by Medicare.[1,2]

Because of some confusion about the legal status of NLHC and its executive during the

1993–1995 biennium, alternative reorganizational models for NLHC and NLN were brought to the membership in 1994, but no membership action was taken at that time.

NATIONAL LEAGUE FOR NURSING

Board of Governors, Officers, Committees

The 1989 organizational restructuring process resulted in a streamlined version of the NLN governing body. Previously known as the board of directors, the new NLN Board of Governors consists of three elected officers (president, president elect, and treasurer), the membership council chairs, three governors at large, and the chief executive officer of NLN, who serves as secretary. This configuration amounts to 18 members. Under the previous structure, the board of directors consisted of 30 officials. (In the 1993–1995 biennium, the elected president of NLN served as executive president of both NLN and NLHC.)

The officers of the League and three members of the committee for nominations are elected by the membership every two years. Governors-at-large are elected to a four-year term, not to exceed a maximum of two consecutive terms. Membership council chairs are elected by their respective groups every two years.

Balloting is done by mail, with both individuals and agency members entitled to vote. All of these offices and elected positions are open to both nurse and nonnurse NLN members. In the 1979–1981 biennium, the first nonnurse president served.

Business sessions of the individual councils are held at annual meetings and the full organization membership meets at a biennial convention. Decisions are made by the individual and agency members present. Each individual membership means one vote, and each member agency has five or ten votes, depending on their membership category.

The NLN has two types of committees, standing and special, which may be elected or ap-

pointed. The composition and methods of election or appointment and the term of office of committees are spelled out in the bylaws. The Committee on Nominations is currently the only elected committee of the overall organization. In the appointed category are three standing committees: the Committee on Constitutions and Bylaws, the Committee on Finance, and the Committee on Accreditation. Also considered standing committees are the executive committees of each membership council. Members of these committees are elected by their membership every 2 years.

From time to time the League appoints other special committees to deal with matters of general, and often continuing, concern to the organization as a whole. The Committee for Long Range Planning, responsible for the League's organizational restructuring proposal, was a special committee. Additional recent examples of these committees include: Convention Program Advisory Committee, Committee on Long Term Care, Public Policy Committee, and Committee on Resolutions. The Public Policy Committee studies current, significant issues related to the nation's health care delivery, with particular emphasis on nursing; identifies those issues on which the committee believes NLN should take a stand; and prepares position statements on them for presentation to the board. The Committee on Long Term Care explores and responds to issues in long-term care, advises the board on policies and programs relative to long-term care, and promotes collaborative action related to long-term care among the councils of the League.

COMMUNITY HEALTH ACCREDITATION PROGRAM (CHAP)

The Community Health Accreditation Program (CHAP) is the only independent evaluating body for home care and community health care organizations driven solely by considerations of management, quality, and client outcomes. In 1987, CHAP became a fully independent subsidiary of the National League for Nursing. CHAP's purpose is to employ accreditation to elevate the quality of home care in this country and to counter public fears about a quality crisis in this increasingly crucial health care arena. Its goal is to see home care organizations not only prosper but also gain strength in the overall health care industry. CHAP is committed to ensuring that this nation's home care and community health providers adhere to the highest standards of excellence and that those standards are maintained through specific guidance for self-improvement.

CHAP accreditation offers organizations both professional assistance and consumer recognition. CHAP is committed to providing management consultation, along with a broad network of professional resources, and clear guidance on how to move forward and build on organizational strengths as a component piece to the accreditation process. CHAP accreditation certifies to the public that CHAP-accredited organizations have voluntarily met the highest standards for home care and community health care in the nation. Agencies seeking CHAP accreditation perform an extensive self-study, which is submitted to CHAP offices for preliminary analysis of specific areas. A site visit is then performed by visitors selected to assure a range of expertise, including both management and service delivery areas, and come from an agency similar to that of the applicant organization. Site-visit findings along with the agency's self-report are then studied by a peer-member board of review. There is a process of appeal if the board's decision is not acceptable to the agency. Organizations are accredited for a three-year cycle, during which additional site visits occur, focusing on specific standards.

NLN Membership

As in the past, there remain two major classes of membership within NLN, individual and agency. Individual membership is open to anyone interested in fostering the development and improvement of nursing service, education, and health care. Individual members are eligible to vote in the League's national affairs, constituent (state) league activities, and specialty council elections. Agency membership is for organizations or groups providing various nursing services and for the various schools conducting educational programs in nursing. In 1989, agency membership expanded into two subdivisions, category 1 and category 2. Category 1 membership entitles an agency to ten votes, category 2, five votes. Membership dues and available services vary within each category.

Until 1967, NLN, like ANA, was structured on a local-state-national basis. At that time, however, it was decided that the "constituent units" (formerly state leagues) of NLN need not necessarily follow state lines. A constituent league may now take in only part of a state (a large metropolitan center, for instance), a whole state, parts of several different states, or several different states as a whole. The emphasis is on organization according to interests and needs in given regions or areas rather than in given states. (This change reflects the emphasis now given in many other fields to regional organization or planning). Forty-eight constituent leagues for nursing implement national goals and objectives through statewide programming. Many have local units to stimulate community interest in cooperative planning for nursing and health care services and present programs at the local level.

Individual members join NLN and the constituent league in the area in which they reside or work. As was the case with agency membership, individual membership also underwent restructuring in 1989. Whereas previously an individual might belong to the national organization and not to a constituent league, or vice versa, now individual membership includes three avenues for influence and activity: at the national level, within a more local constituent league, and also within a council focused on a more particular concern. Individual members may also belong to any number of these membership councils.

General Plan of Organization

Both individual and agency members are concerned with the "further development and improvement of nursing services, education and the achievement of comprehensive health care." The groups approach the task through membership opportunities in various NLN councils.

Individual members are expected to work through their constituent leagues and their chosen specialty councils. Under the revised (1989) bylaws, agencies and individuals are eligible for voting membership in all councils. In addition, agencies can elect to join more than one council, as category 1 or category 2 members. This new structure provides opportunities for agency and individual members to jointly pursue interests common to both groups.

Membership Councils

Through eleven councils, agency and individual members may influence the policies of the NLN, receive information, attend programs, participate on committees, present ideas, and vote.

The four educational councils are:

1. Council of Associate Degree Programs (CADP). The general purpose of the Council of Associate Degree Programs is the continuous development and improvement of education for nursing. The primary purpose of the council is the development and improvement of associate degree programs in nursing to allow them to make their appropriate contributions to a changing society. Associate degree nursing programs are the fastest-growing program type in the nation today, and likewise, the Council of Associate Degree Programs in one of the League's busiest. Just one example of the crucial work this council is engaged in speaks to the vitality and creativity of its members. In October 1994, this council held the First National Videoconference Faculty Meeting, a W. K. Kellogg–funded event, linking faculty from every state in a national discussion.

2. Council of Baccalaureate and Higher Degree Programs (CBHDP). The general purpose of the Council of Baccalaureate and Higher Degree Programs is to provide leadership in matters related to high-quality nursing education and to represent and speak for educational programs leading to baccalaureate and higher degrees. The primary purpose of the council is to support the development and improvement of baccalaureate and higher degree educational programs in nursing. Changes in accreditation criteria, focusing on outcome measures and public accountability, make up a vital part of this council's agenda. In the context of national health care reform, this council's membership is focusing on the two issues of nurse practitioners and community-based nursing education.

3. Council of Diploma Programs (CDP). The primary purposes of the Council of Diploma Programs is the development and improvement of diploma programs in nursing and the exercise of leadership in all activities that stimulate sound planning for and advancement of diploma education in nursing. Its general purpose, as for all other educational councils, is the continuous development and improvement of education for nursing. In accordance with its mandate the CDP is conducting a survey on how diploma programs might promote concern for quality in home care to its graduates.

4. Council of Practical Nursing Programs (CPNP). The general purpose of the Council of Practical Nursing Programs is to provide leadership in matters related to high-quality nursing education and to represent and speak for educational programs leading to a certificate or diploma in practical nursing. The primary purpose of the council is the development and improvement of educational programs in

practical nursing. The issue of assuring quality care in long-term care is of particular importance to this council, especially as it relates to the role of unlicensed assistive personnel.

The practice and multidisciplinary councils listed next provide opportunities for participants to play key roles in shaping nursing practice and its relationship to nursing education.

1. Council of Community Health Services (CCHS). The purpose of the Council of Community Health Services is to provide leadership in matters related to nursing and the delivery of quality health care by community health agencies and to assist community health agencies in the development and improvement of their programs. One of the most diverse councils of the League, the Council of Community Health Services encompasses professionals from community health departments, family planning agencies, occupational health, home health agencies, managed care programs, and hospices.

2. Council for Nurse Executives (CNE). The purpose of the Council for Nurse Executives is to provide opportunities among members who currently hold executive or associate executive responsibilities in their employment settings. Their unique mandate is to develop programs for leadership development and executive preparation, develop important policy positions on national health issues, encourage the development of quality programs of graduate education, and identify and promote the singular needs of council members.

3. Council for Nursing Informatics (CNI). The purpose of the Council for Nursing Informatics is to create a multidisciplinary network for assessing needs, providing information, and presenting programs on the impact of the information age and computer technology upon nursing education, administration, clinical practice, and

research. This "user friendly" council views technology as the bridge between nursing education and practice. One of the fastest-growing councils, its members are committed to using technology to facilitate one's professional role, whether it lies in education, clinical settings, or research.

4. Council for Nursing Centers (CNC). The purpose of the Council for Nursing Centers is to promote the development of nursing centers as sources of affordable quality health care and to provide a network for nurses who offer nursing services directly to consumers. A nursing center is defined as an organization that provides nursing services and may include other health services and is owned, operated, or controlled by nurses. The members of this productive council are actively managing nursing centers and are part of a nationwide network for nurses who directly serve the public. A Metropolitan Life-funded grant is tapping their considerable expertise to develop the criteria for exemplary models of nurse-managed delivery systems. Council members plan to use these criteria to promote the concept of nursing centers and their significance for health care delivery.

5. Council for Nursing Practice (CNP). The purpose of the Council for Nursing Practice is to continually develop and improve nursing practice. With one of the broadest agendas, this council's activities appeal to a wide range of direct care providers. Members are currently planning programs that address key nursing practice issues like delegation, priority setting, empowerment, and ethical concerns. In addition, this council is addressing the very significant issues related to the restructuring and reengineering occurring within acute care institutions.

6. Council for the Society for Research in Nursing Education (CSRNE). The purpose of the Council for the Society for Re-

search in Nursing Education is to improve education in the practice and academic settings through the development, dissemination, and use of research and theory in nursing education. Its members are unique in their expertise, interest, and specific focus on research in nursing education. They further their goals of grounding nursing education with sound research by publishing an annual research review, a monograph series, and a monthly column in *Nursing and Health Care*. In addition, they seek funding for research projects in nursing education.

The Council of Constituent Leagues for Nursing (CCLN) completes the membership council roster. All individual members of constituent leagues become members of CCLN through the new membership structure.

7. Council of Constituent Leagues (CCLN). The CCLN serves as a national forum where constituent leagues may exchange ideas, discuss action taken and problems encountered, and make recommendations. It provides guidance and direction to its membership and constituent leagues. Leadership opportunities are found at the state and local levels, through involvement in one of the 48 Constituent Leagues. Constituent League members have organized extremely effective campaigns against the AMA's Registered Care Technologist concept and those directed at the negative public image of nursing.

Each council works within its own readily identifiable field of interest, but there are certain activities in which all engage. All are expected to facilitate collaboration among councils and non-NLN groups, assure consumer involvement in council activities, and develop goals that are not only relevant to individual council activity but are also congruent with those of the NLN. Workshops and programs are held regionally and nationally. The four education councils also

have accreditation as part of their programs. Council committees vary according to each council's needs, but according to NLN bylaws, each must have an executive committee of six members, including a chair and vice chair. At least one member of the executive committee guides and administers the affairs of the council under the direction of the board of governors. The executive committee also determines what meetings, other than the mandated annual meeting, are held.

SERVICES AND PROGRAMS

More or less permanent components within the League are a variety of services and programs carried out through its organized staff divisions.

Division of Accreditation

The NLN accrediting service has been a stimulant to the improvement of nursing education since its inception in 1949 under the name of the National Nursing Accrediting Service. Related to nursing education, it is a service that reviews and evaluates nursing education programs of various types such as those preparing PNs; diploma, associate degree, and baccalaureate degree programs for RNs; and programs leading to a master's degree in nursing. Those meeting NLN criteria within each category are granted NLN accreditation.

To operate legally, each school of nursing must have the approval of the state government, as represented by its board of nursing. But standards vary from state to state, despite efforts to standardize them as much as possible; in some, the requirements for school approval are minimal. Criteria for NLN accreditation, however, are nationally determined; they represent the combined thinking of experts in the various kinds of programs. League accreditation, therefore, symbolizes a nursing education program of high quality in all respects—admission and achievement standards, curriculum, faculty preparation, library, laboratory and other facilities, and the like. NLN accreditation is voluntary. The school requests this service and pays for the evaluation. There is no guarantee that the end result will be accreditation.

NLN accreditation is peer evaluation. The visitors who come to the program to amplify, verify, and clarify the data and to make a recommendation relative to a school's accreditation program are faculty and/or faculty administrators of like programs, who have been selected and especially trained by NLN to review programs.

Often NLN visits are made cooperatively with regional or specialty accrediting associations or state board visits. NLN visitors may be able to point out weaknesses in the report, which can be corrected, and also give supplementary information to the board of review, which meets in New York several times a year to review the materials for accreditation that have been sent from the schools and the visitors' reports.

Recommendations for improvements are sent to the school, with or without the granting of accreditation. If a program is accredited, interim reports of the status of the program are sent to NLN at specified intervals before another major accreditation visit. If the program is not accredited, there is an appeal procedure, and, of course, the opportunity to correct the deficiencies and reapply for accreditation. In recent years, there has been greater flexibility in the acceptance of ways to meet accreditation standards, so that programs of greatly varying educational approaches are being accredited. The common denominator is quality. Increasingly, NLN accreditation is sought and worked toward, because of the significance of this accreditation to the prospective student, the faculty member, and the community. In addition, only NLN-accredited schools are eligible for the nursing education funds made available through the Nurse Training Act of 1964 and later amendments. NLN is officially recognized by the national voluntary accrediting bodies and the U.S. Department of Education as the accrediting agency for master's, baccalaureate, associate degree, diploma, and PN programs.[3]

Each year, a list of NLN-accredited programs of nursing is published in the NLN journal. There are also pamphlets issued listing all state-approved and accredited nursing programs. By 1994, more than 1,550 educational programs held NLN accreditation; over 75 percent of the total basic RN programs were accredited by the League.

NLN Consultation Network

NLN's newly expanded consultation network offers a wide range of consultation services through a cadre of experts in the fields of nursing education, practice, research, testing and evaluation, and communication/video. Traditionally, nursing schools have utilized NLN consultation services for help with their educational programs; thus, a school failing to meet accreditation standards may be helped to achieve them, or one just starting or seeking to improve its program can be helped by consultation expertise. Recent developments in the health care arena, like spiraling costs and personnel shortages, have increased the demand for assistance from individuals, hospitals, and community health services. Consequently, NLN consultants are involved in crisis management for nurse executives and fiscal and organizational management concerns. Additional types of consultation available through network affiliates include the design and use of evaluation techniques, establishment of new community health services, and assistance with research proposals.

Consultation fees are determined by the type of consultation needed. Expertise may be provided through a review of mailed materials, a scheduled meeting at NLN headquarters, a telephone consultation, or an on-site visit.

Division of Assessment and Evaluation

NLN conducts one of the largest professional testing services in the country. Test batteries have been developed by NLN using experts in tests and educational measurements and in nursing. The tests available through NLN fall into several categories: guidance and placement of students for schools of professional and practical nursing, achievement of professional and practical nursing students while in nursing school, the preimmigration screening examination and nursing tests prepared for the Commission of Graduates of Foreign Nursing Schools, tests designed for nurse practice settings, and certification tests for nursing specialties. All objective tests are machine-scored under the direction of the NLN Test Service. There are separate sets of tests for practical nursing and for professional nursing. Also included are achievement tests for baccalaureate students. In addition, tests have been developed for schools to use in making advanced placement relative to educational mobility.

Depending on the nature and purpose of the tests, they may be given at central locations within a state or the nation, or at individual schools. They are all returned to NLN headquarters for scoring, and the scores are then released to the schools of nursing. Preadmission test results are available directly to the examinees. The League does not make the decision as to whether an individual's score means that she or he is qualified for admission to a school or has a satisfactory achievement in the subjects tested. This judgment is left to the individual schools, although NLN provides national standards as a guide.

The League's testing services are offered on a voluntary basis; no school or state is required to use them. The tests undergo continual evaluation and revision to maintain their validity and ensure appropriateness of content. League policy stipulates that tests must be current, and they are updated annually or every two or three years, depending on the content area and level of usage.

Division of Communications

As NLN works to achieve its objective of improving nursing education and service, it maintains a constant flow of information to both its membership and the general public. Therefore,

it distributes a wide variety of informative materials.

Some of this information is promotional, explaining the nature and purpose of the League, at the same time providing the public with a glimpse of the League's newest products. Other publications are statistical or highly factual, such as school directories and lists of accredited schools of nursing. The bulk of NLN publications are references and texts, written by leading nursing and health care authorities on topics such as administration and management, career guidance, community health care, curriculum, ethics, public policy, research, theory, and long-term care. In addition, videotapes are available on a wide range of subject matters pertinent to the health care arena, with a growing segment developed for the general public.

Each year NLN issues a publications catalog that is available on request from its headquarters office and is also sent to all members. The official journal, *Nursing and Health Care*, is published ten times a year. A subscription to this journal is included with NLN membership. Periodic bulletins help members keep informed of current federal and state legislation, important health care issues, and League positions on major issues.

Division of Research

Since 1953, NLN's Division of Research has maintained and updated a data bank on the entire universe of nursing education and supply. NLN Research conducts the annual Survey of Nursing Education Programs, the biennial Nurse Faculty Census, and the biennial Newly Licensed Nurse Study. NLN surveys consistently yield an outstanding response rate of up to 90 percent, making NLN data highly reliable. NLN disseminates the results of these surveys in a number of comprehensive publications and in addition provides customized data searches.

NLN Research is fully equipped to conduct large-scale surveys and to perform detailed qualitative and quantitative analyses. With a highly skilled, experienced staff, NLN Research is uniquely qualified to collect and analyze data. NLN possesses sophisticated computing capabilities and state-of-the-art software capable of handling and manipulating large quantities of data. NLN's mainframe system is accessible through an ethernet local area network. This network infrastructure gives staff access to statistical, database, spreadsheet programs, documents, and datasets. NLN produces publications using desktop publishing and scores tests using multi-thousand-item-per-hour scanners. In addition, NLN is evaluating intelligent character-recognition devices for more sophisticated data and image collection.

NLN is currently planning to become the Internet source for a wide range of information and raw research data of importance to many constituents. The league will soon acquire Primary Rate ISDN communication capabilities, which will expand and better manage the organization's telecommunications channels and provide new opportunities in worldwide multimedia interactivity and video teleconferencing.

NLN, as need and resources permit, surveys or studies other selected aspects of nursing education or nursing service programs. In addition, it carries on both short-term and long-term research projects. Some of these projects are financed by the League itself; some are financed through grants from other agencies. (NLN, unlike ANA, enjoys tax-exempt status, and funds granted to it are not considered taxable income.)

Interorganizational Relationships

NLN works closely with ANA, AACN, and AONE (especially as part of the Tri-Council). However, throughout its entire program NLN also maintains active liaison with many other national agencies, both governmental and voluntary. Among them are NSNA, APHA, the National Federation of Licensed Practical Nurses, the National Association for Practical Nurse Education and Service, the American Association of Community Colleges, the National Council of State Boards of Nursing, the American Council on Education, the National Heath Council, and the National Council on Patient Information and Education, as well as several consumer groups and health care coalitions.

Other Services and Activities

Because of its tax-exempt status as an educational and charitable organization, the League (and its constituent leagues) is prohibited from participating in any political campaign on behalf of or in opposition to any particular candidate, and no substantial part of its activities may consist of influencing legislation. However, this prohibition does not extend to dealing with administrative agencies or the executive branch of the government. The League is also permitted to inform members fully of proposed legislation, engage in nonpartisan analysis or study and disseminate results, and give factual testimony and information. Preferably these presentations are made on request of the legislators. Within this framework, NLN has been involved in legislation affecting nursing and has been helpful in its implementation.

In 1973, the NLN chose the National Library of Medicine in Bethesda, Maryland, home of the world's largest collection of health sciences literature, as the official repository of NLN's historical documents and records. These include the history of NLN, old photographs of American nurses, correspondence by Florence Nightingale and other nursing leaders, and the history of NOPHN. League officials also plan to join in a campaign to identify and acquire other nursing memorabilia for the library.

The impact of NLN on nursing does not lie only in the services and activities of the organization and its component groups. It is equally important to look at some of the major pronouncements made by NLN in taking stands on nursing issues. Among these is a 1965 resolution on nursing education that recommended community planning to "implement the orderly movement of nursing education into institutions of higher learning in such a way that the flow of nurses into the community will not be interrupted." A 1970 statement on open curriculum urged changes in programs to aid mobility in nursing without lowering standards, and in 1976 a new and stronger version was approved by the board of directors. A 1971 statement (revised 1976) about degree programs with no major in nursing was intended, in part, to help RNs who were seeking degrees to make informed choices. In 1972 *Nursing Education in the Seventies* spelled out the needed characteristics of an effective system of nursing education and the actions needed to attain these characteristics. A 1966 statement encouraged continuity of nursing care, and in 1973, the statement on *Quality Review of Health Care Services* urged intra- and interprofessional review of care standards; the updated 1979 version urged greater participation of nurses in Professional Standards Review Organizations (PSROs). Other position papers are national health insurance, nursing's responsibility to minorities and disadvantaged groups, and NLN's role in continuing education in nursing.

A controversial NLN statement was made in 1979, "Preparation for Beginning Practice in Nursing," in which support for all four types of nursing education programs was reiterated, "for the present." Because the League accredits all four types of programs, this position was not surprising to some, although the 1965 NLN resolution that was never rescinded seemed to present a contradictory view. A report of the NLN Task Force on Competencies of Graduates of Nursing Programs, also released in 1979, identified differences in the knowledge base and in minimal expectations of the new graduate of the four types of nursing programs studied (PN, AD, diploma, and baccalaureate), as well as differences in the practice role in terms of structured and unstructured settings, focus of care, and accountability.

The NLN membership has reaffirmed its commitment to the community and to an agenda that positions nursing in the center of the health care delivery system. Membership has chosen to ratify resolutions that support NLN development of a national health care system and strengthen nurses' involvement in national health care issues. Care for the indigent and homeless, community and long-term care, involvement in AIDs-related care, and utilization of resources for improvement of the image of nursing are current areas of focus. Progress in this last area has been greatly enhanced with the development of the League's "Nurses of America" program. This project, funded by the Pew Charitable Trust and administered by NLN, was a national, multimedia effort designed to inform the public about the role of contemporary nursing.

The NLN headquarters is located at 350 Hudson Street, New York, N.Y. 10014.

REFERENCES

1. Davis C: Deemed status for CHAP: A new standard for health care. *Nurs Health Care* 13:294–295, June 1992.
2. Mitchell M: Nursing's legacy of leadership. *Nurs Health Care* 13:296–302, June 1992.
3. Millard R: The accrediting community: Its members and their interrelationships. *Nurs Health Care* 5:451–454, October 1984.

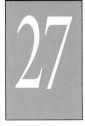

Other Nursing and Related Organizations in the United States

W ITHIN THE LAST 10 years, an increasing number of specialty organizations for nurses has been added to those already well established. Although all nurses can find a place for themselves within ANA, some, particularly those in clinical or occupational specialties, have elected to join one of the other nursing organizations instead of, or in addition to, ANA. The aegis of these organizations varies. Some are totally independent; others are part of another organization. Some restrict membership to nurses; others include medical-technical personnel.

It would be impossible to describe all the organizations in nursing today. This chapter lists primarily those that are part of the Nursing Organization Liaison Forum (NOLF) or the National Federation for Specialty Nursing Organizations (NFSO). Information was provided by each organization; some are omitted because they neglected to do so. A directory of organizations appears annually in the *American Journal of Nursing*.

Although there have always been other organizations, ANA has generally been accepted as *the* professional organization that speaks for nursing. The first of the specialty organizations that still exists was the American Association of Nurse Anesthetists (1931). In the 1940s and 1950s, the American Association of Industrial Nurses (AAIN), now the American Association of Occupational Health Nurses (AAOHN), the Association of Operating Room Nurses (AORN), and the American College of Nurse-Midwives (ACNM) followed, but beginning in 1968, literally dozens of others were organized. They were either splinter groups that broke off from ANA and formed their own association or others that evolved as the profession became more specialized.

Special-interest groups seem to have several things in common, such as providing a forum of peers for sharing experiences and problems related to a particular specialty or interest, continuing education, and standard setting and leadership development. Some certify for specialty practice but in time establish a separate corporate entity for certification. The separation of standard setting or the peer group from the certifier is necessary for credibility. Most of these special-interest groups indicate that they intend to remain autonomous organizations.

COALITIONS

National Federation for Specialty Nursing Organizations

The proliferation of nursing organizations, although meeting the special needs of some nurses, has also caused some confusion among nurses, other health workers, and the public. Do these organizations speak for nursing in addition to ANA? In place of ANA? Members of these nursing organizations were also concerned. A perceived or real lack of unity can frustrate the achievement of desired goals. Therefore, in November 1972, ANA hosted a meeting of ten specialty groups and NSNA to "explore how the organizations can work toward more coordination in areas of common interest." It was found that concerns were similar and that such a meeting was generally considered long overdue.[1]

In its second meeting, hosted by the American Association of Critical Care Nurses (AACN) and held at the Western White House in San Clemente, California, in January 1973, federal nurses and representatives from the National Commission on Nursing and Nursing Education were also invited, and the group was asked to consider forming a National Nurses Congress. Although this suggestion was rejected, the participants accepted the importance of the specialty, at the same time recognizing the unique role of ANA.

At the third meeting of presidents and executive directors of the specialty nursing organizations, ANA, and NSNA, held in June 1973, this group adopted a name—The Federation of Specialty Nursing Organizations and American Nurses Association. They identified a specialty nursing organization as a "national organization of registered nurses governed by an elected body with bylaws defining purpose and functions for improvement of health care; and a body of knowledge and skill in a defined area of clinical practice." Those attending expressed mutual support and agreed on some of the issues of the times.

Meetings of the group were held on a semi-annual basis in the following years, with the member organizations alternating as hosts, responsible for arranging and conducting the meeting and writing the minutes. The nursing press and auditors were permitted to attend meetings. The focus of the meetings was usually on current issues, but often related to CE accreditation procedures and certification, about which ANA and the other organizations seldom agreed. However, the federation did support ANA on certain issues and various legislative proposals. Resolutions on issues raised by other members were also supported from time to time.

In 1981, the title of the organization was changed to National Federation for Specialty Nursing Organizations (NFSNO), which more clearly defined the membership.

The mission of the National Federation for Specialty Nursing Organizations is to promote specialty nursing practice and its contributions to the health of the nation through the collaborative and educational efforts of member organizations and provide a forum for networking and addressing areas of mutual concern.

The goals of the federation are to:

- Facilitate collaboration and action in areas of mutual interest related to specialty nursing practice.
- Influence public policy issues pertinent to specialty nursing.
- Improve the exchange of information on specialty nursing issues and positions to member organizations and relevant external groups.
- Increase organizational viability and financial stability.

Eligibility for membership is limited to those nursing organizations that meet the following general criteria:

- Are national in scope.
- Are composed of a majority of registered nurses.
- Are governed by an elected body with bylaws defining purpose and functions.
- Have been in existence for two or more years.
- Have a mission compatible with that of NFSNO.
- Are an independent organization, or if a subunit of a multidisciplinary organization, shall show evidence of a separate structure for nursing groups.

There are two classifications for membership: regular members and affiliates. To be a regular member an organization must both meet the general criteria and:

1. Have, as part of its purpose, a focus on issues related to direct provision of care to a clearly defined patient/client population with one or more specific health needs.
2. Have a body of knowledge and skills in a defined area of clinical practice, supported by documentation, which might include a core curriculum, nursing publications and research, standards of care/practice, or other documents.

Affiliate members meet the general criteria but do not meet the specific criteria for regular membership. They also are allowed to enter into debate at federation meetings but are not permitted to make motions and vote.

NFSNO is governed by an Executive Board that is elected by the regular member organizations. The federation meets annually in July to discuss issues and share information of interest to its member organizations. A quarterly newsletter, *Focus on the Federation*, keeps members informed of NFSNO activities between annual meetings. NFSNO also conducts the Nurse in Washington Internship (NIWI) programs to enhance the ability of registered nurses to influence the legislative and regulatory processes.

The federation's membership continues to grow. As of 1994, NFSNO consisted of 34 regular and 5 affiliate members. ANA participates as an auditor since all the NFSNO members belong to NOLF. Furthermore, ANA's direct care and specialty agenda is addressed through its councils.

The mailing address for NFSNO is Box 56, East Holly Avenue, Pitman, NJ 08071.

National Alliance of Nurse Practitioners

In 1986, in response to the need for a united voice among nurse practitioner (NP) groups, the National Alliance of Nurse Practitioners (NANP) was formed. The alliance evolved out of several earlier meetings of NP leaders, including an attempt in 1984 to center NP issues within the ANA Council of Primary Health Care NPs. However, the consensus among NPs was to build a national organization that would encompass the ANA Council as well as other NP groups. For those interested, the NANP has a fact sheet summarizing its history.

The purpose of the alliance is to address the health care of the nation by promoting the visibility, viability, and unity of NPs. The organization is committed to achieving cost-effectiveness in health care, improving organization and delivery of health care services, and supporting education of health professionals. Its focus is on legislative and political action, public relations and marketing of NPs, and communication among its members and with other health professions, other nurses, and the public. All national, state, regional, or local NP organizations qualify for membership based on the four NANP categories:

1. National organization.
2. Freestanding organization with greater than 500 members.
3. Freestanding organization with less than 500 members.
4. State organization with a national parent body.

Currently, NANP represents 30,000 NPs through its organizational members, which comprise its governing body:

American Academy of Nurse Practitioners

American College Health Association (Nurse/NP Sections)

ANA, Council of Nurses in Advanced Practice

National Association of NPs in Reproductive Health

National Association of Pediatric Nurse Associates and Practitioners

National Conference of Gerontological NPs

For more information on the NANP, contact any member of the governing body, or send inquiries directly to the NANP, 325 Pennsylvania Ave., SE, Washington, DC 20003.

Nursing Organization Liaison Forum

ANA also made an effort to bring together the various nursing organizations. A change in the 1982 bylaws provided for the formation of a Nursing Organization Liaison Forum (NOLF) to promote unified action of allied nursing organizations under the auspices of ANA.[2] In December 1983, ANA invited 45 nursing organizations to Kansas City to explore the possibilities of coming together in such a forum. The meeting was cordial, but the results were somewhat noncommittal. There was a question of whether NOLF and NFSNO would be duplicative efforts. Over time, NOLF has grown and flourished, uniting 73 nursing organizations. Its members are regularly updated on the work of ANA, their opinions sought, and they frequently speak for both ANA and their specialty organization to the media, the Congress, and in a variety of instances. NOLF organizations have voluntarily shared their resources with ANA to help fund the AMA-RCT battle in the late 1980s and again in the 1990s to promote nursing's agenda for health care reform.

Tri-Council for Nursing

The Tri-Council traces its roots to the ANA-NLN Coordinating Council, established with the ANA reorganization in the 1950s. In time, the American Association of Colleges of Nursing (AACN) and the American Organization of Nurse Executives (AONE) were added to this coalition. The Tri-Council agenda addresses broad-based issues such as public image, the nursing shortage of the 1980s, recruitment to the field, and legislative and regulatory concerns. Despite the addition of AONE as a fourth member in 1986, the name of Tri-Council was retained. The presidents and executive directors of the Tri-Council organizations meet regularly and frequently engage in joint lobbying on the federal level.

Such collaborative activities among nursing organizations show a new maturity in nursing that not only recognizes the importance of joining together on major health issues but also fosters positive cooperative action. This action will enable nurses to be a stronger force in the planning and delivery of health care services. As Margretta Styles, then ANA president, noted at a meeting of NFSNO, "For a profession to be successfully self-regulating, to speak a common language, and to develop and disseminate its science and skill, it is necessary that the education, credentialing, organizational, and practice components of the field develop in substantial synchrony."

The nursing organizations noted in this chapter are not all clinical specialty groups; some exist to serve other needs of nurses, educationally, socially, or spiritually. It is evident that still more nursing organizations will evolve as nurses assume new and diverse roles. Those discussed here appear to be most firmly established and active at this time. All are national organizations and a few are or aspire to an international constituency. The exceptions are the four regional associations—NEON, MAIN, SCCEN, and WIN—presented later in the chapter.

MEMBERSHIP ORGANIZATIONS

Alpha Tau Delta

The Alpha Tau Delta (ATD) Nursing Fraternity, Incorporated, is a national fraternity for professional nurses founded on February 15, 1921, at the University of California, Berkeley. Chapters are established only in schools of nursing where baccalaureate or higher degree programs are fully accredited by NLN. ATD has many active collegiate and alumnae chapters. Membership is based upon scholarship, personality, and character and has no restriction as to race, color, creed, or sex. Members must be enrolled in a baccalaureate or higher degree program. Because ATD is a professional fraternity, its membership is limited to those in the nursing profession, and it organizes its group life to promote professional competence and achievement within the field of nursing.

The purposes of ATD are to further higher professional and educational standards, to develop character and leadership, to encourage excellence of individual performance, and to organize and maintain an interfraternity spirit of cooperation. Besides the chapter scholarships, financial aid is given annually through the Miriam Fay Furlong National Grant Awards and the PRN Alumni Awards. Other awards are the National Chapter Members of the Year, and award keys and merit awards to individuals for outstanding accomplishments.

The governing body of ATD is its biennial national convention. It is composed of elected delegates from each college and alumnae chapter, and the national council officers.

The national paper, *Cap'tions of Alpha Tau Delta*, is published in the spring and fall of each year. ATD is a member of the Professional Fraternity Association, and through this organization is represented in the Interfraternity Research and Advisory Council. National headquarters for ATD is located at 5207 Mesada Street, Alta Loma, CA 91701.

American Academy of Ambulatory Care Nursing

The American Academy of Ambulatory Care Nursing (AAACN) was formally chartered in 1978. Its purpose is to promote high standards of ambulatory care nursing administration and practice through education, exchange of information, and scientific investigation. In 1993, AAACN revised its standards for nursing administration and practice in the ambulatory care setting. It offers the bimonthly newsletter, *Viewpoint*, as a benefit of membership. It also sponsors an annual convention. Membership is about 1,400. For more information contact AAACN, Box 56, East Holly Avenue, Pitman, NJ 08071.

American Association of Colleges of Nursing

The American Association of Colleges of Nursing (AACN) was established in 1969 to answer the need for a national organization dedicated exclusively to furthering nursing education in America's universities and 4-year colleges.

For approximately 2 years prior to that date, a group of deans of NLN-accredited graduate programs in nursing had been meeting informally to discuss the kind of organization needed to focus on nursing higher education and to provide a forum for deans and directors to meet and take rapid and concerted action on significant issues. In May 1969, 44 deans of nursing gathered in Detroit and voted to establish an independent Conference of Deans of College and University Schools of Nursing, composed of the deans and directors of NLN-accredited baccalaureate and graduate programs in the United States.

The first general meeting of the newly organized group was held in Chicago in October 1969. In February 1972 the name of the organization was changed to the American Association of Colleges of Nursing. AACN meets twice yearly.

AACN's mission is to advance the quality of baccalaureate and graduate nursing education, promote nursing research, and develop academic leaders. AACN works in the public interest to prepare clinicians, research scientists, educators, administrators, consultants, and policymakers for leadership and health promotion through nursing, the nation's largest health profession.

Membership in the association is institutional, represented by the dean or other highest administrative officer of a baccalaureate or graduate program leading to a degree in nursing. From an original 80-member institutions in 1969, AACN today represents more than 460 schools of nursing at public and private universities and senior colleges nationwide.

In 1986, AACN directed the national panel that defined the knowledge, practice skills, values, and other essential components in the education of America's professional-level nurses. AACN publishes and disseminates the *Essentials* document to schools of nursing and policymakers throughout the nation and reviews and revises these teaching components to remain current with changing conditions in nursing and health care.

Through its government relations and other advocacy programs, and as a member of the Tri-Council for Nursing, AACN works to advance public policy on nursing education and research. AACN has been a vigorous leader in securing federal support for nursing education and research; influencing legislative and regulatory policy affecting nursing education, practice, and health care delivery; and in obtaining continuing financial assistance for nursing students.

AACN also operates the Institutional Data System, a central data source publishing current reports on enrollment, graduations, and other trends in baccalaureate and graduate nursing education. Other AACN publications provide policymakers with critical information and guidance on key issues facing the profession. An example is AACN's 1989 report, *The Economic Investment in Nursing Education: Student, Clinical and Institutional Perspectives*, funded by a 2-year grant from the Pew Charitable Trusts. This groundbreaking study provided educators, federal legislators, and health care agencies with data not previously available on the financial costs to students of a nursing education and on the benefits and costs of such education to hospitals and other clinical service agencies that serve as training facilities.

Published in 1994 in cooperation with AACN, Peterson's *Guide to Nursing Programs* is the only comprehensive guide to accredited baccalaureate and graduate nursing education programs nationwide. In addition, AACN conferences provide deans and other education administrators enhanced skills in areas such as student recruitment and retention, legal issues, and master's and doctoral program development. Begun in 1989, a new AACN executive development series prepares new and aspiring deans in the skills necessary to carry out successfully the responsibilities of the deanship.

AACN publications include *Syllabus*, the bimonthly AACN newsletter; the bimonthly *Journal of Professional Nursing*; and a variety of books and reference directories for nursing

educators, administrators, researchers, and students. AACN is located at One Dupont Circle, Suite 530, Washington, DC 20036.

American Association of Critical-Care Nurses

The American Association of Critical-Care Nurses (AACN) was founded in 1969 as the American Association of Cardiovascular Nurses. The association was reincorporated in California in 1972 under its present name, which more accurately reflects the professional practice of its members. The present membership totals over 78,000, with over 275 chapters located throughout the United States and in other countries. The association's growth has directly paralleled the increasing importance of nursing specialties that deal with human responses to life-threatening health problems. The major function of AACN is to provide education directed at advancing the art and science of critical-care nursing and promoting environments that facilitate comprehensive professional nursing practice for people experiencing critical illness or injury. The AACN vision is one of a health care system driven by the needs of patients in which critical care nurses make their optimal contribution.

The association prepares critical care nurses for continuing challenges and demands of the profession by offering a series of programs throughout the year. The largest and most widely attended program is the National Teaching Institute and Critical Care Exposition held annually in May.

Membership benefits currently include subscriptions to the two AACN publications: *Critical Care Nurse* and the *American Journal of Critical Care*. Other official AACN publications include *AACN Clinical Issues*, a quarterly peer-reviewed hardbound journal available by subscription, *AACN Nursing Scan in Critical Care* and *Technology for Critical Care Nurses*. AACN encourages professional accountability and has established its *Standards for Nursing Care of the Critically Ill, Outcome Standards for Nursing*

Care of the Critically Ill, and *Education Standards for Critical Care Nursing* to define and frame nursing care of the critically ill and injured.

Through its affiliate, the AACN Certification Corporation, CCRN certification in adult, pediatric, and neonatal critical care nursing is offered to nurses who meet the eligibility requirements. Certification examinations are offered by computer-based testing at hundreds of sites, and certification is valid for a 3-year period, after which time recertification is available through continuing education or retesting. Currently over 50,000 nurses hold the CCRN certification credential. An agreement was finalized in 1994 between the AACN Certification Corporation and the American Nurses Credentialing Center jointly to develop and offer a certification for NPs in acute care.

Other membership benefits include reduced registration fees at AACN programs, professional liability and other group insurance programs, and professional discounts on AACN publications. Membership and program information is available from AACN, 101 Columbia, Aliso Viejo, CA 92656. Certification information is available from the Certification Corporation at the same address.

American Association for the History of Nursing

The American Association for the History of Nursing (AAHN), formerly the International History of Nursing Society, was incorporated in October 1982. Its purpose is to educate the public regarding the history and heritage of the nursing profession by stimulating interest and national and international collaboration in promoting the history of nursing; supporting research in the history of nursing; promoting the development of centers for the preservation and use of materials of historical importance to nursing; serving as a resource for information related to nursing history; and producing and distributing to the public educational materials regarding the history and heritage of the nurs-

ing profession. Membership is open to individuals interested in the purpose and work of the association. The AAHN's *Bulletin* is published quarterly. AAHN sponsors two awards that recognize exemplary historical research and writing: the Lavinia A. Dock Award for established historians of nursing and the Teresa E. Christy Award for work conducted in a student status. The address for AAHN is P.O. Box 90803, Washington, DC 20090-0803.

American Association of Neuroscience Nurses

The American Association of Neuroscience Nurses (AANN) was founded in 1968 as the American Association of Neurosurgical Nurses. Its purpose is to foster the health, education, and welfare of the general public through promoting education, research, and high standards of care of the patient with neurologic dysfunction and to promote the growth of nursing as a profession.

Criteria for membership include:

1. Active involvement or primary interest in neurosurgical nursing
2. A license to practice as an RN in the United States or Canada

AANN currently has a membership of over 3,000, and all members are also members of the World Federation of Neuroscience Nurses.

Major publications of AANN include the *Journal of Neuroscience Nursing* (six issues a year); "Synapse," the membership newsletter, also published bimonthly; and the *Core Curriculum for Neuroscience Nursing,* third edition. Other materials include a research directory, which lists nurses involved in neuroscience research; a speaker's bureau; and *Neuroscience Nursing Practice: Process and Outcome Criteria for Selected Diagnoses* (published with ANA). CE programs are offered nationally and through a series of regional chapters (over sixty) throughout the country.

Certification is provided through the American Board of Neurosurgical Nursing, which offers examinations twice a year. Information may be obtained from AANN. The association holds its annual meeting each spring and another meeting in the fall. AANN is headquartered at Suite 204, 218 No. Jefferson, Chicago, IL 60606.

American Association of Nurse Anesthetists

Organized in 1931, the American Association of Nurse Anesthetists (AANA) is the professional organization for nurses who have specialized in anesthesia. Certified Registered Nurse Anesthetists (CRNAs) and student nurse anesthetists are eligible for AANA membership. AANA represents 96 percent of the nation's CRNAs and its members automatically become members of their state associations. There are approximately 26,500 members nationwide.

To become a CRNA, a registered nurse must be a graduate of an accredited program of nurse anesthesia and have passed the national certification examination administered by the AANA's Council on Certification of Nurse Anesthetists. In 1952, the AANA developed an accreditation program for schools for nurse anesthetists, currently administered by the AANA's Council on Accreditation of Nurse Anesthesia Educational Programs. A third credentialing council, the AANA's Council on Recertification of Nurse Anesthetists, oversees the recertification process.

Ongoing activities of the AANA include developing standards that ensure high-quality anesthesia care to safeguard patients; offering a continuous quality and risk management program for anesthesia departments, group practices, and individual practitioners; facilitating the nurse anesthesia education process and research; taking a leadership role in efforts to ease the CRNA shortage; seeking private and public sector funding sources for educational advancement and research; providing educational opportunities and professional recognition; and monitoring, assessing, and working with legislative and regulatory bodies regarding governmental initiatives.

AANA also promotes a professional and equitable work environment by addressing legal and ethical issues facing CRNAs; facilitates effective cooperation between nurse anesthetists and other health care groups; works with state nurse anesthetist associations on projects of mutual interest; disseminates information about nurse anesthesia by publishing a scientific journal, a newsletter, and miscellaneous monographs; and conducts an annual membership survey regarding the practice of anesthesia by CRNAs.

The association holds an annual convention. Sessions are open to AANA members as well as others in the health care field.

The *AANA Journal*, the official publication of the American Association of Nurse Anesthetists, is published bimonthly, and the *AANA NewsBulletin* is published monthly for members only. The headquarters building is at 222 South Prospect Avenue, Park Ridge, IL 60068-4001, along with an office maintained in Washington, DC.

The American Association of Nurse Attorneys

The idea of organizing nurses who were attorneys was proposed in 1977, when it became apparent that no national association addressed the needs and interests of this growing group of professionals. Meetings were held in areas where nurse attorneys were clustered. The American Association of Nurse Attorneys (TAANA) was incorporated in 1982.

The aims and purposes of the association are to assist the professional development of nurse attorneys and to educate the public on matters of nursing, health care, and law. Specific goals are to educate the membership on relevant issues; to facilitate information sharing among nurse attorneys and with related professional groups; to establish an employment network; to provide mutual support among nurse attorneys; to develop the nurse attorney profession; to become well-known experts, consultants, and authors in nursing and law; to educate nurses about legal aspects of the profession; and to offer educational seminars and workshops for nurse attorneys.

An annual meeting whose educational component addresses issues of national concern to nurse attorneys occurs every fall in different areas of the country. Educational and social gatherings are held at regular intervals in approximately twenty-five metropolitan areas. *Inside TAANA*, the official newsletter of TAANA is published four times a year.

Current membership is over 600. Membership is open to any nurse attorney, nurse in law school, or attorney in nursing school. Information regarding TAANA or its activities may be obtained from the national office at 720 Light Street, Baltimore, MD 21230.

American Association of Occupational Health Nurses

The American Association of Occupational Health Nurses (AAOHN) was organized in 1942 as the American Association of Industrial Nurses, and in 1977 changed its name to reflect the broadened scope of practice and its settings.

The professional association for registered nurses who provide on-the-job health care for the nation's workers, AAOHN has about 12,500 members. Its mission is to advance the profession of occupational health nurses by promoting professional excellence in achieving workers' health and safety through education and research; establishing professional standards of practice and code of ethics; influencing legislative and regulatory issues that have an impact on health and safety; and fostering internal and external communications in order to facilitate AAOHN's goals and objectives.

AAOHN has developed a comprehensive professional affairs program covering academic education, continuing education, professional practice, research, and association leadership training. Specific projects include assisting constituent associations with program planning, offering continuing education opportunities, and publishing resource documents.

The association maintains a strong governmental affairs program, which publishes the *Governmental Affairs Program Guide for Constituent Associations*. It represents occupational health nurses in public policy discussions that affect their day-to-day practice. It also studies and attempts to influence legislative actions. AAOHN believes that increased professional competency is the method for the occupational health nurse to achieve economic opportunity and security. Its goal is to promote the occupational health nurse as a professional worker.

AAOHN's annual meeting is held in conjunction with that of the American College of Occupational and Environmental Medicine, with the combined meeting called the American Occupational Health Conference. Symposia and workshops are also held on other occasions. In addition to its official monthly magazine, *AAOHN Journal*, AAOHN provides a comprehensive communications program, including a monthly newsletter, *AAOHN News*. The organization's headquarters is located at 50 Lenox Pointe, Atlanta, GA 30324.

The American Association of Office Nurses

The American Association of Office Nurses (AAON) was founded and incorporated in 1988. It has a membership of approximately 4,000, with local chapters in most states.

AAON views the office practitioner as one of the physician's most important professional assistants and allies, helping to facilitate the delivery of quality care to patients and to manage the daily operation of the office. It is committed to the continuing education and long-term welfare of all professional personnel working in the physician's office, ambulatory nursing, and clinic settings. Because AAON believes that comprehensive, quality care is dependent on the medical office team, it offers various levels of membership and invites registered nurses, nurse educators, nurse practitioners, licensed practical nurses, nursing assistants, and office managers to avail themselves of educational opportunities.

The mission of AAON is to enhance the delivery of effective patient care by providing continuing education specific to the field of office nursing, patient education, leadership, and office management. It is dedicated to promoting the professionalism of the office nurse and recognition of this specialized field of nursing among its peers. AAON also provides a networking forum for office professionals to share ideas and knowledge to help in delivering comprehensive, safe, and effective patient care.

AAON offers a bimonthly journal, *Office Nurse,* and a bimonthly newsletter, *Nurses Exchange Office News (NEON),* as benefits of membership. It also sponsors an annual convention each fall and regional meetings each spring that highlight office nursing care, nursing assessment, patient education, interpersonal communications, organizational management, and leadership classes. In addition to the annual and regional meetings, CE programs include local seminars and monthly meetings, and home study programs offered in *Office Nurse.* Standards of office nursing practice are being developed and will be available by 1995. Headquarters is located at 109 Kinderkamack Road, Montvale, NJ 07645.

American Association of Spinal Cord Injury Nurses

The American Association of Spinal Cord Injury Nurses (AASCIN) is a national specialty nursing organization formed in 1983 to promote excellence in meeting the health care needs of individuals with spinal cord injury. Its goals include the advancement and improvement of nursing care of spinal cord injured individuals, promotion of education and research, and dissemination of information. There are about 1,500 members.

AASCIN publishes a quarterly journal, *SCI Nursing,* as well as *SCI Nursing: Educational Guidelines for Professional Nursing Practice,* *Standards of Spinal Cord Injury Nursing Practice,* and *SCI Patient/Family Education Manual for Nurses.* AASCIN also sponsors a research program, prepares position papers on key issues on spinal cord injury, and convenes an annual education conference. Additional information is available from offices at 75-20 Astoria Boulevard, Jackson Heights, NY 11370-1177.

American College of Nurse-Midwives

The philosophy of the American College of Nurse-Midwives (ACNM) is based on the beliefs that every childbearing family has a right to a safe, satisfying experience with respect for human dignity and worth; for variety in cultural forms; and for the parents' right to self-determination. ACNM defines a certified nurse-midwife (CNM) as an individual educated in the two disciplines of nursing and midwifery, who possesses evidence of certification according to the requirements of the organization.

The mission of the ACNM is to develop and support the profession of nurse-midwifery in order to promote the health and well-being of women and infants within their families and communities. In pursuit of its goals, and working frequently in cooperation with other groups, ACNM identifies areas of appropriate nurse-midwifery practice; studies the activities of the nurse-midwife; establishes qualifications for those activities; approves educational programs in nurse-midwifery; sponsors research and develops literature in this field; and serves as a channel for communication and interpretation about nurse-midwifery on regional, national, and international levels.

The American College of Nurse-Midwifery was established in 1955; it merged in 1969 with the American Association of Nurse-Midwives, founded in 1929, to become the American College of Nurse-Midwives. Membership is limited to ACNM-certified nurse-midwives, although they do not have to live in the United States.

Accreditation is done by the ACNM's Division of Accreditation, which functions autonomously. Certification activities have been handled by the ACNM Division of Competency Assessment. In 1990, the ACNM membership voted to separately incorporate the Division of Competency Assessment as the ACNM Certification Council, Inc., effective September 1991. This sister organization provides certification for professional nurse-midwives for entry into practice.

ACNM and its 4,800 members conduct or take part in conferences, institutes, and workshops concerned with the practice of nurse-midwifery and with the improvement of services in the maternal and child health fields. A national meeting is held annually. The official newsletter is the bimonthly *Quickening*, and the official publication, *The Journal of Nurse-Midwifery*. ACNM is located at 818 Connecticut Avenue, NW, Suite 900, Washington, DC 20006.

American Holistic Nurses' Association

The American Holistic Nurses' Association (AHNA) was organized in 1980 by a group of nurses and others dedicated to the principles and practice of holistic nursing. Its purposes are to promote the education of nurses in the concepts and practice of the health of the whole person and to serve as an advocate of wellness. AHNA strives to support the education of nurses, allied health practitioners, and the general public on health-related issues; to examine, anticipate, and influence new directions and dimensions of the practice and delivery of health care; and to improve the quality of patient care through research on holistic concepts and practice in nursing.

Local, area, regional, and national educational programs, workshops, seminars, and conferences are presented. *Beginnings*, the official newsletter of AHNA, is published ten times each year. *The Journal of Holistic Nursing* is published annually.

Membership is open to nurses and others interested in holistically oriented health care practices. AHNA can be contacted at 4101 Lake Boone Trail, Suite 201, Raleigh, NC 27607.

American Nephrology Nurses' Association

The American Nephrology Nurses' Association (ANNA) is the professional organization for registered nurses practicing in nephrology, transplantation, and related therapies. It was founded in 1969 as the American Association of Nephrology Nurses and Technicians. In 1984, it was reorganized and retitled. The purpose is primarily educational with numerous national, regional, and local programs, seminars, and conferences given. Other major activities include a registry for continuing education credit, and provision of standards of nursing practice in the hemodialysis and transplantation areas. The objectives of ANNA are to develop and update standards for the practice of nephrology nursing, provide the mechanisms to promote individual growth, and promote research, development, and demonstration of advances in nephrology nursing.

There are more than 9,000 members of the national organization. ANNA provides membership services through an organizational structure that includes a national board of directors, 4 membership regions, and more than 66 local chapters. Any RN interested in the care of patients with renal disease is eligible for full membership. Dietitians, social workers, LPNs, and technicians may participate as associate members. Major publications are *ANNA Update, Standards of Clinical Practice*, a journal entitled *ANNA Journal, Core Curriculum for Nephrology Nursing, Nephrology Nursing—A Guide to Professional Development*, and a number of clinical monographs and other publications on topics such as scope of practice, core curriculum, careers, and nephrology nursing research. ANNA headquarters is located at East Holly Avenue, Box 56, Pitman, NJ 08071-0056.

American Organization of Nurse Executives

The American Organization of Nurse Executives (AONE) is a corporate subsidiary of the American Hospital Association (AHA). It has been so since 1988 when the boards of each group approved a restructuring proposal to enhance the role of nursing at the AHA. As the national organization representing nurse executives and managers, AONE provides direction and leadership for the advancement of nursing practice and patient care in organized health care systems, for the achievement of excellence in nurse executive practice, and for shaping policy affecting health care delivery from the perspective of the nurse manager.

AONE includes two types of members: nurse executives and nurse managers. The executives are represented through AONE, and the managers are represented through the Council of Nurse Manager Affiliates. AONE conducts its business operations through an elected governing board and board committees. National initiatives are reinforced through chapters at the state and regional level.

The council is charged by the AONE to facilitate the professional development and promote the leadership role of nurse managers. It is geared to meet the special needs of head nurses and nurse supervisors. The council conducts its business through an elected governing board, committee structure, and representation on the AONE board of directors.

AONE publishes a monthly newsletter, *The Nurse Executive*, as well as other monographs and publications. In 1989, it collaborated with the ANA in issuing six monographs on strategies for the nursing shortage. AONE and the Council of Nurse Managers each sponsor annual meetings, educational conferences, and teleconferences, which address issues central to nursing management, administration, and leadership.

As part of the AHA, AONE participates directly in policy development through involvement on AHA committees, and the AHA board of trustees. Additionally, AONE holds ex-officio membership on AHA regional policy boards, observer status in the AHA House of Delegates, and appointment to the AHA Committee of Commissioners to the Joint Commission on Accreditation of Health Care Organizations (JCAHO).

AONE is part of the Tri-Council for Nursing. It also has extensive liaison relationships with other major nursing and health care organizations. Headquarters is at 840 North Lake Shore Drive, 10E, Chicago, IL 60611.

The American Public Health Association Public Health Nursing Section

The American Public Health Association (APHA), established in 1872, is the largest organization of its kind in the world, with a membership of some 32,000, in addition to the approximately 25,000 members of its affiliates. As a professional organization, it represents over 75 disciplines in public health concerned about shaping national and local public health policies; as a communications network, it circulates new knowledge through the internationally respected *American Journal of Public Health* and a publishing house operation of major proportions. *Nation's Health* is the official monthly newspaper of the association.

Of the twenty-four specialized sections that comprise APHA, the Public Health Nursing Section is one of the largest, with almost 2,200 members and one of the oldest, having been established in 1923. Highly active and influential, the Public Health Nursing Section provides a voice for nursing interests within the APHA structure, and nationally through that structure. Section members participate on APHA's program development board, action board, task forces and committees, and with other sections of the association. Through cooperative relationships with other nursing groups, such as ANA (where the section participates as a member of NOLF), the Association of Community Health Nursing Educators, Association of State and Territorial Directors of Nursing, and NLN, it strives for improvement of nursing and education services within the broad perspective of public health. This section has been instrumental in establishing the Quad Council (ANA, ACNE, ASTDN, and APHA) to promote a strong, coordinated voice for public health nursing.

Over the six decades of its existence, the Public Health Nursing Section has studied numerous aspects and issues of public health nursing, including the definition and roles of public health nursing, relationships between hospitals and public health agencies, planning services to certain high-risk populations, salaries, educational and professional qualifications, quality assurance, staffing issues, research priorities, and the role of public health nursing in health care reform.

In its investigation of these issues, the Public Health Nursing Section has continuously been in the organizational forefront of the APHA structure. Over the years, numerous nurses have been elected members of APHA's governing council, including the executive board. Nurses Marion Sheahan, Margaret Dolan, and Iris Shannon served as president of the APHA in 1960, 1973, and 1988, respectively, and several nurses have held the office of vice president. In addition, Marion Sheahan, Margaret Arnstein, and Doris Roberts have won the Sedgwick Memorial Medal, one of APHA's highest citations; the Albert Lasker and Martha May Eliot Awards have been won by nurses several times; and the prestigious Bronfman Prize was given to Ruth B. Freeman in 1971.

The APHA annual meeting provides an excellent forum for the Public Health Nurses' scientific and business exchanges and social events, but meetings of the various section councils and committees are also held throughout the year. The Ruth B. Freeman and the creative achievement awards are given by the section at each annual meeting to recognize nurses who have made outstanding contributions to public health nursing. A fascinating and detailed *History of the Public Health Nursing Section, 1922–1972*, by Ella E. McNeil, is now out of print, but on file in the APHA archives. In 1977, the Margaret B. Dolan Lectureship Fund was established by the Public Health Nursing Section. At the 1978 APHA Convention, the first Dolan lecture was presented as the keynote address. The lectures have continued as an annual keynote convention event.

The first century of public health nursing came to a close at the 1993 annual APHA meeting, following a year focusing on the history, accomplishments, and future role of public health nursing. Archives of the PHN Section of APHA are located at Mugar Library, Boston University. APHA headquarters is at 1015 15th Street, NW, Washington, DC 20005.

American Radiological Nurses Association

The American Radiological Nurses Association (ARNA) was founded in 1981. The purposes of ARNA are to promote health and wellness by defining the functions, qualifications, and educational criteria of radiology nurses; to promote the practice; to assess, recommend, and evaluate radiological nursing standards; to facilitate efficient networking among radiological nurses and allied health care professionals; and to promote scientific research in the professional publications to radiological nursing.

ARNA is governed by an elected board of directors and various standing committees that constitute the association's executive committee. The association publishes a quarterly journal, *ARNA Images*, and an annual membership directory. ARNA holds an annual business meeting and educational program in conjunction with the RSNA and an educational program with SCVIR. Association headquarters is at 2021 Spring Road, Suite 600, Oak Brook, IL 60521.

American Society for Parenteral and Enteral Nutrition

Founded in 1975, the American Society for Parenteral and Enteral Nutrition (ASPEN) is the nation's only multidisciplinary group of health professionals chiefly concerned about the nutritional support of patients. ASPEN's staff manages the daily operations of the society for a membership of 7,200 individuals comprised of physicians, dietitians, pharmacists, and nurses. Student membership and membership for individuals not included in one of the above disciplines is available under an affiliate status category. They receive all benefits of membership except voting rights and holding a position on committees or the board of directors.

ASPEN is committed to promoting quality patient care, education, and research in the field of nutrition and metabolic support in all health care settings. Its specific objectives are to promote communication among professional disciplines in the field; promote proper applications of clinical and research experience in the practice of nutritionally sound medicine; and encourage professional competence in the field.

ASPEN publishes two bimonthly journals, the *Journal of Parenteral and Enteral Nutrition (JPEN)*, and *Nutrition in Clinical Practice (NCP)*. *JPEN* contains original research, reviews, and editorials, whereas *NCP* provides reliable, practical, "hands on" information for health professionals concerned about nutrition. In addition, the society publishes bibliographies, textbooks on core curriculum, course syllabi, standards of practice, and guidelines for proper administration of parenteral and enteral nutrition (PEN).

The society holds an annual educational convention entitled Clinical Congress, which attracts over 3,500 attendees. It gives six research awards at this event. In 1993, the ASPEN Rhodes Research Foundation was established to promote further and fund new research in the field of parenteral and enteral nutrition.

ASPEN produces certification exams for both nurses and dietitians that are administered and scored by Professional Testing Corporation twice a year. In addition, its board of directors has approved preparation of a certification program in PEN for physicians, with the target exam date planned for September 1995. The exam will be carefully designed and administered under the auspices of ASPEN's National Board of Nutrition Support Certification (NBNSC). Although the NBNSC is legally a part of the society, it functions as an independent credentialing agency. ASPEN is located at 8630 Fenton Street, Suite 412, Silver Spring, MD 20910-3805.

American Society of Ophthalmic Registered Nurses

Organized in 1976, the American Association of Ophthalmic Registered Nurses, Inc. (ASORN), is open to all professional RNs engaged in ophthalmic nursing. ASORN's purpose is to unite professional ophthalmic RNs in order to promote excellence in ophthalmic nursing for the better and safer care of the patient with an eye disorder or injury. Specific objectives are to study, discuss, and exchange knowledge, experience, and ideas related to ophthalmic nursing in order to provide CE to its members; to hold regular meetings to advance the purpose of the society; and to cooperate with other professional associations, hospitals, universities, industries, technical societies, research organizations, and governmental agencies in matters affecting the purposes of the society.

A national meeting is held annually in conjunction with the American Academy of Ophthalmology meeting. *Insight*, the official journal, is published quarterly. Local chapters, which are independent of the national organization, meet at regular intervals in ten regional areas.

Current membership is about 1,800. The address of ASORN is P.O. Box 193030, San Francisco, CA 94119.

American Society of Plastic and Reconstructive Surgical Nurses

The American Society of Plastic and Reconstructive Surgical Nurses (ASPRSN) is a national voluntary nursing specialty organization committed to the enhancement of quality nursing care delivered to the patient undergoing plastic and reconstructive surgery. The organization supports and encourages the collaborative relationship between nurses engaged in the areas of clinical practice, education, administration, and research. The purpose of ASPRSN is to promote high standards of plastic and reconstructive surgical nursing practice through education, exchange of information, and scientific inquiry. The organization cooperates fully with other professional nursing associations, medical associations, hospitals, universities, industries, technical societies, research organizations, and governmental agencies in matters affecting the purpose of ASPRSN.

An annual convention is held each fall. Membership includes about 1,500 nurses. Local and regional chapters provide supplementary seminars throughout the year. ASPRSN publishes the *Journal of Plastic and Reconstructive Surgical Nursing*. ASPRSN's *Core Curriculum* is available from the national office, which is located at East Holly Avenue, Box 56, Pitman, NJ 08071.

American Society of Post Anesthesia Nurses

The American Society of Post Anesthesia Nurses (ASPAN) is the national association representing nurses practicing in all phases of postanesthesia care. The purposes for which ASPAN was organized are educational, scientific, and charitable. Founded in 1980, ASPAN has over 10,000 members representing 41 state and regional associations.

The association provides members with a bimonthly newsletter, the *Breathline*, and a scientific journal, the *Journal of Post Anesthesia Nursing*. Other reference publications offered include the *Standards of Nursing Practice*, the *Review Text, Redi-Ref*, and numerous videotapes on post anesthesia nursing. An annual conference is held in April. ASPAN also offers a certification exam twice a year to all members meeting the criteria. As of July 1994, over 3,400 nurses were certified. An ambulatory postanesthesia certification was initiated in November 1994.

The first week in February is recognized as National Post Anesthesia Nurses Week and is celebrated throughout the country. The national office is located at ASPAN, 11512 Allecingie Parkway, Richmond, VA 23235.

American Urological Association, Allied

Organized in 1972, the American Urological Association, Allied (AUAA) is an organization dedicated to advancing the cause of professionalism and better patient care in the field of urology. The care of the urologic patient requires a high degree of education, skill, and dedication. Education is the key to achieving these objectives; thus, AUAA was organized to supplement and extend the urology curriculum provided by nursing schools.

The purposes of AUAA are to serve as a vehicle for the distribution of all available information in the field of urology; to point the way to advanced nursing technique and new equipment; and to help those who wish to become urology specialists

The AUAA board of directors plans educational meetings on national, regional, and local levels. An annual conference is held in conjunction with that of the American Urological Association, the professional association for urologic surgeons.

AUAA provides certification and recertification for members and nonmembers, through the American Board of Urologic Allied Health Professionals. Certification is based on assessment of knowledge, demonstration of current clinical practice, and endorsement by colleagues. A newsletter, *Urogram*, is published six times a year. *Urologic Nursing*, the official journal of the AUAA, is published quarterly by Mosby-Yearbook, Inc. Active membership is open to persons in the health care professions who are engaged in care of the urologic patient. Current membership is over 2,400. AUAA is divided into eight geographic sections with a total of forty-four chapters. The administrative offices are located at 11512 Allecingie Parkway, Richmond, VA 23235.

Association of Child and Adolescent Psychiatric Nurses

The purposes of the Association of Child and Adolescent Psychiatric Nurses (ACAPN) are to recognize the uniqueness of and promote communication among child psychiatric nurses, and to promote the mental health of infants, children, adolescents, and their families through advocacy, practice, education, and research. ACAPN's specific goals involve advocating for policy, legislation, and funding to meet the mental health needs of youth and their families; promoting and maintaining standards for the delivery of mental health care to youth; promoting advanced practice in child and adolescent psychiatric nursing; promoting educational programs that prepare nurses sensitive to the mental health needs of youth and their families; and encouraging the development of nursing research and theory specific to the mental health of youth and their families. ACAPN is an organizational member of the Coalition of Psychiatric Nursing Organizations (COPNO), and participates with its other member organizations as well as ANA and nursing, mental health, and consumer groups to support cost-effective, accessible mental health care. As a COPNO organization, ACAPN collaborates in developing psychiatric nursing practice statements and standards.

ACAPN membership is comprised of nurses and student nurses with an interest in and commitment to child and adolescent psychiatric nursing and the mental health of children, adolescents, and their families. Each member belongs to a local chapter and a region, and has representation in decision making through individual, chapter, regional, and national activities. Membership opportunities for organizations and an associate status are currently under consideration.

An annual national conference addresses trends and issues in the mental health care of youth, and provides education and professional development for child and adolescent psychiatric nurses regarding innovations in clinical practice, advocacy, and research. All members receive the *Journal of Child and Adolescent Psychiatric and Mental Health Nursing*, the organization's official journal, published quarterly, and the quarterly *ACAPN Newsletter*. Another publication is a membership directory.

In 1993, ACAPN established the Robert O. Gilbert Foundation, a memorial educational and research fund that recognizes and supports the work of child and adolescent psychiatric nurses in research and educational endeavors related to the mental health of youth and their families. ACAPN and the foundation are located at 1211 Locust Street, Philadelphia, PA 19107.

Association of Nurses in AIDS Care

The Association of Nurses in AIDS Care (ANAC) is a nonprofit professional nursing organization committed to fostering the individual and collective professional development of nurses involved in the delivery of health care to persons infected or affected by the Human Immunodeficiency Virus (HIV), and to promoting the health, welfare, and rights of all infected persons. Founded in 1987, ANAC has grown to a membership of 2,600 nurses, 33 local chapters, and 3 international affiliates.

ANAC active members include registered nurses, and associate members, licensed practical or vocational nurses, and student nurses. Services to members include publishing the *Journal of the Association of Nurses in AIDS Care* six times a year and a quarterly organization newsletter, the Annual National Conference, local meetings, conferences, support groups, and publication of other educational materials. ANAC's *Core Curriculum for HIV/AIDS Nursing* will be published in 1995. Two ANAC Fellowship Awards are awarded annually to nurses pursuing graduate education in the field of HIV/AIDS.

The organization has 11 active committees including a Government Relations Committee addressing health care policy issues, an Education Committee producing educational programs and materials, and a Clinical Issues Committee to address new research and clinical information of interest and importance to the members. ANAC's address is 704 Stony Hill Road, Suite 106, Yardley, PA 19067.

Association of Operating Room Nurses

The Association of Operating Room Nurses (AORN) is a voluntary organization of professional registered nurses with national and international members and a universal interest in the care of the surgical patient. Founded in 1954, AORN has over 49,000 members and more than 380 chapters throughout the world.

AORN's mission states that it is the professional organization of perioperative nurses that unites its members by providing education, representation, and standards for quality patient care. AORN believes that the OR nurse must be responsible for patients undergoing surgery. Its philosophy recognizes its responsibility to health care and the OR by setting standards of practice, contributing to essential nursing education, and providing opportunity for continuous learning through a broad program of educational activities.

AORN sponsors activities to meet the educational needs of its members. Continuing education offerings are sponsored throughout the United States and in foreign countries. These include the national AORN Congress, the biennial World Conference, National Seminars, week-long courses, and self-directed study materials. An extensive list of publications is available including the *AORN Standards and Recommended Practices in Perioperative Nursing*, which is widely recognized in the field, and the *AORN Journal*, which is published monthly.

A registered professional nurse who currently manages, teaches, or practices perioperative nursing either full or part time is eligible for active membership. A registered professional nurse enrolled in formal nursing education or engaged in perioperative research may retain active status. Associate membership is available to registered professional nurses who are engaged in an allied field of nursing. AORN headquarters is at 2170 S. Parker Rd., Suite 300, Denver, CO 80231.

Association of Pediatric Oncology Nurses

The Association of Pediatric Oncology Nurses (APON) is an organization of RNs who are either interested in or engaged in pediatrics, on-cology, and/or pediatric oncology nursing. The group was formally begun in 1976, as a result of increasing demands for education and support for nurses who care for and about children with cancer and their families. The overall objective of APON is to promote an optimal level of nursing care for pediatric oncology patients and their families. This is achieved through an annual national educational conference, the quarterly *Journal of Pediatric Oncology Nursing*, and many other publications. In addition, APON promotes implementation of standards of pediatric oncology nursing practice and encourages research in nursing care of children with cancer.

Membership is open to all RNs in the United States, Canada, and foreign countries, and is currently over 1,900. Members receive a newsletter, chapter directory, an official journal, and other publications.

The most frequently expressed benefit of APON membership is the opportunity to network with nurses with common goals, interests, and values, as there is an ongoing improvement in the quality of life and life expectations for children with cancer. APON is located at 11512 Allecingie Parkway, Richmond, VA 23235.

Association of Rehabilitation Nurses

The Association of Rehabilitation Nurses (ARN) is the membership organization for professional nurses who work with individuals with physical disabilities or chronic illness. Formed in 1974, ARN has over 10,000 members who practice in a variety of settings. There are 88 local chapters throughout the country and 10 special-interest groups. ARN's mission is to promote and advance professional rehabilitation nursing practice through education, advocacy, and research to enhance the quality of life for those affected by disability. Rehabilitation nurses work in general hospitals, rehabilitation and long-term care facilities, insurance companies, home health care operations, educational institutions, and private consulting firms.

ARN offers a certification program through its Rehabilitation Nursing Certification Board (RNCB). Over 10,000 rehabilitation nurses have met the qualifications to be Certified Rehabilitation Registered Nurses (CRRNs). The CRRN program is a member of the American Board of Nursing Specialties.

Over the years, ARN has focused much of its energies on education programming for rehabilitation nurses. In 1975, it established an education and research foundation, the Rehabilitation Nursing Foundation (RNF), and prepared a comprehensive educational plan in 1993. ARN and RNF have developed many educational and communications resources including annual educational conferences; regional seminars; a rehabilitation nursing management seminar; an intermediate level seminar that concentrates on current rehabilitation concepts and skills applicable to various rehabilitation nursing practice roles and settings; a basic rehabilitation nursing course; standards and scope of practice; and a core curriculum.

The organization publishes ten times a year the *ARN News*, a newsletter, *Rehabilitation Nursing*, a bimonthly journal, and the quarterly journal, *Rehabilitation Nursing Research*. The Rehabilitation Nursing Foundation continues to develop educational resources and has strengthened its role as the research and development resource for rehabilitation nursing.

The organization funds annual grants for rehabilitation nursing research and will offer a novice researcher grant beginning in 1995. It conducts its own research project on rehabilitation nursing diagnoses. A biennial research symposium has been instituted. External activities include working with other organizations and participating in national health care improvement efforts. ARN provides testimony to government bodies, such as the National Center for Nursing Research, the National Center for Medical Rehabilitation Research, and the National Institute for Disability and Rehabilitation Research, to share rehabilitation nursing's perspective where appropriate. The national office is located at 5700 Old Orchard Road, First Floor, Skokie, IL 60077.

Association of State and Territorial Directors of Nursing

The Association of State and Territorial Directors of Nursing (ASTDN) was established in 1935 as the public health nursing leadership affiliate of the Association of State and Territorial Health Officials. Its primary purposes were to encourage state and local health authorities to improve the quality and extend the volume and scope of their public health nursing services; to encourage the development of nursing leadership for all public health nursing within the respective states; to participate in joint efforts with federal and national nursing groups in the promotion of a unified approach to existing public health nursing problems; and to promote the establishment of sound educational facilities for the preparation of additional public health nurses. Public health nursing directors for the official state or territorial health department comprise the membership. If the position is vacant, a liaison member may be appointed by the State Health Officer.

ASTDN members hold an annual meeting and continuing education session for members and guests, which include nurses in leadership positions within the federal government and current presidents of the affiliating organizations of the Quad Council (the Association of Community Health Nursing Educators, the Public Health Nursing Section of the American Public Health Association, the Community Health Nursing Council of the American Nurses' Association, and ASTDN). Additionally, the executive committee meets in conjunction with the fall meeting of APHA. Membership services include these meetings, a quarterly newsletter, assorted committee assignments, and networking opportunities with colleagues across the country.

Research activities have focused on public health nursing staffing and career ladders, leadership positions with state health departments, utilization of nurse practitioners in local health departments, and other similar work. The association has an active research committee, with research disseminated at the annual meeting. Legislative activities concern funding for nursing education and public health's structure, function, and financing under health care reform.

For mailing purposes, the address of ASTDN's president can be obtained through the office of the Association of State and Territorial Health Officials, 415 Second Street, NE, Suite 200, Washington, DC 10002.

The Association for Women's Health, Obstetric and Neonatal Nurses

The Association for Women's Health, Obstetric and Neonatal Nurses (AWHONN) was originally established in 1969 within the American College of Obstetricians and Gynecologists as the Nurses' Association of the American College of Obstetricians and Gynecologists (NAACOG). In 1993, the organization became an independent, nonprofit association as AWHONN. Its purpose is to promote excellence in nursing practice with women and newborns. AWHONN's nearly 28,000 members represent a rich diversity of skills and experience, and demonstrate why the association is considered the voice for women's health, obstetric and neonatal nursing.

AWHONN is divided into nine geographic districts in the United States, its territories, and Canada, plus one district to include armed forces members wherever stationed. Districts further divide into sections, which subdivide into chapters. Members interact at these grassroots levels to coordinate workshops, educational outreach, and other programs that improve career skills, help provide better service to the community, and set a course for future professional success.

The organization concentrates on nursing education, research, and practice. Through video and audio tapes, computer-assisted instruction, video satellite seminars, and a fetal heart monitoring program offered nationwide, it offers many continuing education opportunities. It also encourages individual member research projects through grants presented annually. Additionally, the Department of Research coordinates national research utilization projects. In everyday practice, AWHONN has consistently been known for its standards, guidelines, and position statements that specifically address women's health, obstetric and neonatal nursing practice issues. In the present era of health care reform, it contributes as a resource to legislators and participates in many nursing coalitions.

AWHONN's monthly newsletter, the *AWHONN Voice*, informs members about the association's activities and reports on new developments that affect perinatal and women's health nursing. The *Journal of Obstetric, Gynecologic and Neonatal Nursing (JOGNN)* reflects the latest in practice and research in these nursing specialties. For information on membership, contact AWHONN's Member Services, 700 14th St., Suite 600, Washington, DC 20005-2019.

Chi Eta Phi Sorority

Chi Eta Phi Sorority, Inc., is an international sorority of registered and student nurses. Founded in 1932, its purposes are to encourage the pursuit of CE among members of the nursing profession; to have a continuous recruitment program for nursing and the health professions; to stimulate a close and friendly relationship among the members; and to constantly identify a corps of nursing leaders within the membership who will function as agents of social change on national, regional, and local levels.

Its national projects include those designed to stimulate interest in nursing; facilitate recruitment and educational preparation for nursing and the health professions; increase retention of students in nursing programs; and provide scholarship funding for educational advancement. Service programs involve health screening, health education, and tutorial programs.

There are seventy chapters throughout the United States, St. Thomas, U.S. Virgin Islands, and Africa. The national headquarters is located at 3029 13th Street, NW, Washington, DC 20009.

Consolidated Association of Nurses in Substance Abuse

The Consolidated Association of Nurses in Substance Abuse (CANSA) International was founded in 1979, becoming the first nursing organization to certify chemical dependency nurses in 1986. CANSA International's goals and objectives are to establish and promote standards for the practice of nursing in the field of chemical dependency; to develop criteria for the protection and rehabilitation of the chemically dependent nurse; to provide health professionals and the community at large with quality educational programs on chemical dependency; to promote public health and safety through the development of standards of practice, rehabilitation programs, educational programs, and certification of nurses in the field of chemical dependency; to foster the growth of the profession of chemical dependency nursing through networking and unifying with other nurses working within the specialty; and to increase unity within the field of chemical dependency by networking with other professionals, paraprofessionals, and professional organizations that address themselves to chemical dependency issues.

CANSA International offers active membership to RNs, LVNs or LPNs, and LPTs. Student membership is open to those registered in a program of RN, LVN, LPN, or LPT studies, although not yet licensed; corporate membership is available to institutions and treatment providers. Any individual who holds an interest in the field of chemical dependency may apply for associate membership. Benefits include a subscription to the *Behavioral Health Management* magazine, and *The Dove Newsletter*, along with discounts for CANSA activities.

CANSA International offers two certifications: Chemical Dependency Nurse Specialist (CDNS) and Certified Chemical Dependency Nurse (CCDN). CDNS certification is available to RNs only, with at least two years or 4,000 hours experience in chemical dependency within the last five years. Eligible RNs, LVNs, LPNs, and LPTs may apply for CCDN certification. Every applicant must test to be certified; recertification is required every two years. CANSA International certifications are valid throughout the United States and in Canada. For more information write to CANSA International, 303 W. Katella Ave., Suite 202, Orange, CA 92667.

Dermatology Nurses Association

The Dermatology Nurses Association (DNA) was established in 1982. Its mission is to provide quality education, to foster high standards of nursing, and to promote wellness.

An annual convention and business meeting are held each December in conjunction with the annual meeting of the American Academy of Dermatology. Since 1986, 25 local DNA chapters have been formed in several states. Membership numbers over 2,000 and is open to nurses, medical assistants, and technicians involved in dermatology.

DNA publishes *Dermatology Nursing* as its official journal, as well as a bimonthly newsletter, *Focus*. Headquarters is located at East Holly Avenue, Box 56, Pitman, NJ 08071.

Emergency Nurses' Association

The Emergency Nurses' Association (ENA) was incorporated in December 1970, and since that time has grown to an active membership in excess of 23,000. It was founded to represent nurses faced with all the problems of providing emergency care so that these nurses could pool their knowledge and seek solutions to these problems, set standards, and develop improved methods for practicing efficient emergency care. Eligible for membership are RNs engaged in emergency care who have special skills or knowledge related to emergency nursing. Any other health professional may join the association as an affiliate member.

The major objective of ENA is to provide optimum emergency care to patients in emergency departments. Members are urged to promote a positive attitude toward education on all levels within the emergency department by continuing study through the ENA organization, to support formal programs of instruction for emergency techniques and for postgraduate courses on the professional level, and to participate in community planning of total emergency care.

In 1993, CEN certification became available in Canada for the first time. That same year, the organization offered a certification examination for flight nurses, and 403 candidates became the world's first certified Flight Registered Nurses (CFRN). Over 21,000 nurses in the United States and Canada hold either the CEN or CFRN credential.

Since 1975, ENA has published the *Journal of Emergency Nursing*, which provides articles on all aspects of emergency nursing. The association also publishes an emergency nursing core curriculum, a trauma nursing core course, a pediatric emergency guide, and several new resource materials to assist members.

During the annual ENA Scientific Assembly, business and clinical programs are presented. The ENA national office is located at 230 E. Ohio, Suite 600, Chicago, IL 60611.

Home Healthcare Nurses Association

Founded in 1993, the Home Healthcare Nurses Association (HHNA) is a nursing organization of more than 3,000 individual members involved in home health care practice, education, administration, or research. Its goals are to develop the specialty of home health care nursing, foster excellence in practice, influence public policy as it affects home health care nursing practice; and enhance communication among members and other publics with the outcome of quality health care services for home health care clients.

Membership is comprised of registered nurses engaged in any aspect of home health care. At present, no provision exists for institutional, student, associate, or nonnurse membership. Membership dues include a subscription to *Home Healthcare Nurse* and the bimonthly *HHNA News*.

HHNA is the first and only organization specifically targeted toward nurses in home health care. It is an organization of, for, and by the nurses caring for clients and their families in the home. Headquarters is located at 437 Twin Bay Drive, Pensacola, FL 32534-1350.

Hospice Nurses Association

The Hospice Nurses Association (HNA) was established in 1986 for the purpose of exchanging information, experiences, and ideas among hospice nurses, and promoting understanding of the specialty of hospice nursing within the wider health community and general public.

Its mission is to foster excellence in hospice nursing by promoting the highest professional standards; studying, researching, and exchanging information, experiences, and ideas leading to improved nursing care for terminally ill patients and their families; encouraging nurses to specialize in the practice of hospice nursing; fostering the professional development of nurses; responding to the changing needs of HNA members and the population they represent; and promoting the recognition of hospice care as an essential component of the health care system.

Although primarily a professional membership association for practicing hospice RNs, HNA offers categories for associate members and students. Benefits include access to regional groups organized locally and supported and managed from the national office. Also, members receive the quarterly *Fanfare*, which features topical issues, news of association activities, clinical articles, and other information relevant to hospice nursing.

HNA has a certification program that grants successful candidates the title of Certified Registered Nurse in Hospice (CRNH). The organization funds research on hospice nursing, including a spiritual care perspectives study to determine the attitudes and practices of hospice nurses in this area.

Address inquiries to 5512 Northumberland Street, Pittsburgh, PA 15217-1131.

International Association of Forensic Nurses

The International Association of Forensic Nurses (IAFN) is the only international professional organization of registered nurses formed exclusively to develop, promote, and disseminate information about the science of forensic nursing.

The forensic nurses provide services to individual clients and consultation services to nursing, medical, and law-related agencies. They give expert court testimony in areas dealing with trauma and/or questioned death investigative processes, adequacy of services delivery, and specialized diagnoses of specific conditions as related to nursing.

Several groups of nurses in various specialties are eligible to join IAFN ranging from sexual assault nurse examiners to nurses in clinical or community-based nursing practice involving victims of injuries. Categories are regular members, associate members (for non-RNs), and students and retired members.

IAFN issues a quarterly *Journal of Forensic Nursing*, an annual directory of membership, free copies of protocols and guidelines for identifying crime victims and evidence collection, and several other materials. The organization sponsors an annual Scientific Assembly, which features papers and research of renowned scientists.

For further information, contact IAFN at 6900 Grove Road, Thoroughfare, NJ 08086.

International Society of Psychiatric Consultation Liaison Nurses

The International Society of Psychiatric Consultation Liaison Nurses (ISPCLN), formerly a Special Interest Group of the American Nurses' Association Council on Psychiatric and Mental Health Nursing, was inaugurated at the 8th National PCLN Conference in March 1994. It aims to provide critical leadership in uniting diversity and linking intricate strategies to respond to health care needs in a rapidly changing environment; to be the future of nursing in mind-body interaction and systems consultation; to be the leader in promoting the integration of social, cultural, psychological, and biological issues within the psychiatric nursing community; to be the professional home for PCLNs where we can get support and encouragement and creatively share our ideas with one another; and promote psychiatric consultation liaison nursing as a subspecialty of psychiatric–mental health nursing.

Membership in ISPCLN is open to nurses practicing in or having an interest in psychiatric consultation liaison nursing. The categories include charter member, founding member, and executive member for individuals who wish to provide additional financial support for ISPCLN.

ISPCLN members enjoy networking opportunities with others in the specialty; an annual conference; a bimonthly newsletter; free listing in the membership directory; participation on committees such as Core Curriculum, Bylaws, and Research; a peer consultation program; team building; and access to publications that are state-of-the-art tools prepared for the novice to expert practicing in the field. ISPCLN headquarters is located at 437 Twin Bay Drive, Pensacola, FL 32534.

Intravenous Nurses' Society

The Intravenous Nurses' Society (INS), formerly the National Intravenous Therapy Association, is a nonprofit professional nursing association established in 1973, which represents nurses involved in the practice of intravenous (IV) therapies both in hospitals and at alternative clinical practice settings. The INS mission is to enhance the practice of intravenous nursing through education, standards, and research to achieve the highest level of patient care.

INS has developed its Intravenous Nursing Standards of Practice, which relate to all the major areas of the IV nursing specialty (e.g., blood and blood component therapy, total parenteral nutrition, and oncology). The INS Certification Corporation was established in 1983 and annually provides a national certification exam to credential the practicing IV nurse.

Membership is offered on an active or an associate basis. Membership currently numbers about 6,000. INS publishes a professional journal, the *Journal of Intravenous Nursing*, and a newsletter, *INS Newsline*, both of which are bimonthly. An annual 4-day meeting and three 2-day Advanced Study programs provide, on an annual basis, continuing education and professional networking opportunities.

INS has more than 50 chapters nationwide that hold bimonthly meetings and annual seminars. The Society's headquarters is located at Two Brighton Street, Belmont, MA 02178.

National Association for Health Care Recruitment

The National Association for Health Care Recruitment (NAHCR), formerly the National Association of Nurse Recruiters, was founded in 1975. It seeks to promote and exchange principles of professional health care recruitment. The association maintains appropriate but separate relationships with voluntary and government hospitals, leading community health care organizations, educational institutions, nursing organizations, and advertising media. NAHCR serves its members by strengthening the recruitment and management skills needed to be effective in the profession and gives health care recruiters an opportunity to meet with their peers to exchange ideas and discuss mutual concerns. An annual conference featuring speakers, exhibits, workshops, and a new recruiter orientation is held. Problem solving is the emphasis of free, informal discussions held frequently in each of NAHCR's nine regions. There are 28 NAHCR regional chapters.

NAHCR also holds fall, spring, and regional one-day workshops.

Recruitment Directions, NAHCR's newsletter, is published ten times per year. This publication reports on industry trends, events, and association happenings. An annual recruitment survey provides up-to-date data of importance to health care recruiters. A membership directory and resource guide is published annually. A recruitment and retention manual is also available.

Membership, currently numbering over 1,500, is open to those working in a hospital or health care agency who are actively involved in nurse and allied health recruitment. Nonvoting associate membership is available to individuals interested in supporting NAHCR activities. Subscriptions are available to *Recruitment Directions*. Institutional membership is open to organizations interested in promoting and supporting the association's development. The NAHCR address is P.O. Box 5769, Akron, OH 44372.

National Association of Hispanic Nurses

The National Association of Hispanic Nurses (NAHN) was formed in June 1976 in Atlantic City, New Jersey, under the name National Association of Spanish Speaking/Spanish Surnamed Nurses. Evolving from an ad hoc committee of the Spanish Speaking/Spanish Surnamed caucus formed at the 1974 ANA convention, it brought together for the first time Hispanic nurses from all Hispanic subgroups—Mexican-American, Puerto Rican, Cuban, and Latin American—to provide a forum for exchange of information and experiences about health care services to the Hispanic community. Its name was changed in 1979.

The objectives of NAHN include providing a forum in which Hispanic nurses can analyze, research, and evaluate the health care needs of the Hispanic community; disseminating research findings and policy perspectives dealing with Hispanic health care needs to local, state, and federal agencies to influence policymaking and the allocation of resources; identifying Hispanic nurses throughout the nation to ascertain the size of this group of health care professionals available to provide culturally sensitive nursing care to Hispanic consumers; identifying barriers to the delivery of health services for Hispanic consumers and recommending appropriate solutions to local, state, and federal agencies; identifying barriers to quality education for Hispanic nursing students and recommending appropriate solutions to local, state, and federal agencies; assessing the safety and quality of health care delivery services for the Hispanic community; working for the recruitment and retention of Hispanic students in nursing educational programs, so as to increase the number of bilingual and bicultural nurses who can provide culturally sensitive nursing care to Hispanic consumers; and providing an opportunity for Hispanic nurses from all over the United States and Puerto Rico to share information dealing with their professional concerns, experiences, and research.

Membership is open to any Hispanic nurse in the United States, the Commonwealth of Puerto Rico, or other jurisdiction of the United States. Non-Hispanic nurses and nursing students interested and concerned about the health delivery needs of the Hispanic community as well as the professional needs of Hispanic nurses are welcome to become members.

The NAHN publishes a newsletter, *The Hispanic Nurse* and a *Directory of Hispanic Nurses in the United States*. The organization holds biennial national conferences (even years) and national conventions (odd years). NAHN's mailing address is 1501 Sixteenth St., NW, Washington, DC 20036.

National Association of Nurse Practitioners in Reproductive Health

The National Association of Nurse Practitioners in Reproductive Health (NANPRH), established in 1980, is the only national organization exclusively representing nurse practitioners in obstetrics, gynecology, family planning, reproductive endocrinology, and infertility.

NANPRH members can be found in state and federally funded family planning and maternal child health programs, sexually transmitted disease clinics, health maintenance organizations, the armed forces, private practices, and a variety of other settings. The association's purpose is to assure quality reproductive health services that guarantee reproductive freedom and to protect and promote the delivery of these services by NPs.

The association's objectives include advocating the NP role, educating the public about the value and cost-effectiveness of NPs in reproductive health, functioning as a clearinghouse for information and consultation on current issues, accrediting women's heath nurse practitioner programs, and monitoring state and national legislation. The association also has standards of practice for women's health nurse practitioners, as well as for colposcopy and clinical training.

There are nearly 2,000 members, comprising five membership categories: active membership for registered nurses who have completed a NP program or are certified (or eligible for certification); associate membership for nurses and other clinicians who support the purpose of NANPRH; student membership; corporate membership; and supporting membership, for executives, employers, physicians, and other individuals who uphold the purpose of NANPRH.

Membership benefits include a newsletter published three times a year, and continuing education programs. The NANPRH is headquartered at 2401 Pennsylvania Avenue, NW, Suite 350, Washington, DC 20037.

National Association of Orthopaedic Nurses

The National Association of Orthopaedic Nurses (NAON) is organized to promote, in cooperation with all members of the health team, the highest standards of nursing practice and research and to maintain effective communication between orthopaedic nurses and other interested persons and groups.

NAON's 7,000 members comprise five geographical regions, 130 chapters, and four divisions: clinical practice, education, communication, and management. The association also offers certification exams for orthopaedic nurses, the *Orthopaedic Nursing* journal, a newsletter, a bibliography on orthopaedics, a core curriculum, patient education videos, and other monographs and videos.

In addition to awards for excellence in orthopaedic nursing practice, writing, and research, NAON also offers its active members competitive scholarships for continuing education. The address for NAON is Box 56, East Holly Avenue, Pitman, NJ 08071.

National Association of Pediatric Nurse Associates and Practitioners

The National Association of Pediatric Nurse Associates and Practitioners (NAPNAP) was established in 1973 to provide continuing education relevant to the needs of pediatric nurse practitioners; provide standards for PNP education and practice; develop and maintain a certification process to ensure the public of competent PNPs; and support legislation designed to improve the quality of infant, child, and adolescent health.

NAPNAP has over 4,200 members, organized in 40 local chapters across the country. It sponsors an annual convention, the *Journal of Pediatric Health Care*, a bimonthly newsletter, and opportunities for continuing education. It also has published brochures on the role of PNPs and their scope of practice. NAPNAP has had an active role in influencing legislation relevant to PNP practice, especially in the areas of child abuse, child care and safety, and reimbursement of PNPs.

The association is located at 1101 Kings Highway North, Suite 206, Cherry Hill, NJ 08034.

National Association of School Nurses

The National Association of School Nurses (NASN) was formed in 1969 as a department of the National Education Association (NEA). In 1977, the name was changed to its current one. In 1979, the NASN incorporated and became an affiliate of the NEA, a status that still exists. The mission of NASN is to advance the practice of school nursing and provide leadership in the delivery of quality health programs to the school community.

To become an active member, a registered professional nurse must meet the requirements for school nursing in the member's state, and fulfill other qualifications or requirements set forth in the bylaws. Other membership categories are associate, student, retired, corporate, and institutional. Currently there are almost 8,000 members.

Besides initiating a variety of projects aimed at educating school nurses, NASN sponsors a newsletter, the *Journal of School Nursing*, an annual conference, and two regional conferences. It has developed several publications including *School Nursing Practice: Roles and Standards*, and *Guidelines for School Nursing Documentation: Standards, Issues, and Models*. NASN also offers a certification examination for school nurses.

NASN sponsors "School Nurse Day" the fourth Wednesday in January each year and monitors federal legislation that pertains to school health, testifying on important health issues. NASN is located at 16e Route One, P.O. Box 1300, Scarborough, ME 04070-1300.

National Black Nurses' Association

The National Black Nurses' Association (NBNA) was formed at the end of 1971 as an outgrowth of the Black Nurses' Caucus held during the 1970 ANA convention.[3] These nurses believed that black Americans and other minority groups "are by design or neglect excluded from the means to achieve access to the health mainstream of America" and that black nurses have the "understanding, knowledge, interest, concern, and experience to make a significant difference in the health care status of the Black Community."

Membership is open to all RNs, LPNs, and nursing students, regardless of race, creed, color, national origin, age, or sex. The first national conference was held in 1972, and annual conferences have continued to be held. Further information may be obtained from the National Black Nurses' Association, Inc., 1511 K Street, NW, No 415, Washington, DC 20005.

National Council of State Boards of Nursing

The National Council of State Boards of Nursing (NCSBN) was created in 1978 by boards of nursing throughout the United States and its territories, who are its members. It is an organization through which the boards act and counsel together on matters of common interest and concern affecting the public health, safety, and welfare, including the development of licensing examinations in nursing. To accomplish its mission of promoting public policy related to the safe and effective practice of nursing, NCSBN provides services and guidance to its members in performing functions that regulate entry to nursing practice, continuing safe practice, and nursing education programs.

Under the direction of its member boards, NCSBN develops the National Council Licensure Examinations for Registered Nurses (NCLEX-RN) and Practical Nurses (NCLEX-PN). The exams are used by each member board to test the entry-level competence of candidates for nursing licensure. To assure that the content is relevant to current nursing practice, the organization conducts job analysis studies and monitors trends in nursing practice and education.

The NCLEX is administered using computerized testing at more than 200 Sylvan Technology Centers nationwide, with at least one testing location in each state or territory. Appointments to test are available year-round, with testing available 15 hours a day, six days a week, and on Sundays to meet peak demands.

NCSBN provides support for boards of nursing through collecting and analyzing information pertaining to the licensure and discipline of nurses (including a disciplinary data bank), developing model nursing legislation and administrative rules, and sponsoring educational programs.

The organization publishes a quarterly newsletter, *Issues*, and offers a series of videotapes on the NCLEX as well as numerous other resource materials. Its members consist of 61 boards of nursing. A delegate assembly meets annually to determine policies and provide future direction. National headquarters is located at 676 North St. Clair St., Suite 500, Chicago, IL 60611-2921.

National Gerontological Nursing Association

Established in 1984, the National Gerontological Nursing Association (NGNA) aims to provide a forum in which gerontological nursing issues are identified and explored; develop and support educational programs for nurses, health providers, and the general public; and educate and inform the general public on health issues, particularly those affecting the elders.

NGNA's mission also supports innovative approaches in gerontological health care, disseminating information and research related to gerontological nursing, and enhancing the professionalism of gerontological nurses.

Among membership benefits are a subscription to *Geriatric Nursing*, which has a special NGNA section; continuing education programs; networking at local chapters; and *New Horizons*, the official bimonthly newsletter.

Membership is open to registered nurses, nursing students, nursing assistants, and non-nurses in the associate member category. There are about 1,700 members. NGNA headquarters is located at 7250 Parkway Drive, Suite 510, Hanover, MD 21076.

National Nurses Society on Addictions

The National Nurses Society on Addictions (NNSA), formerly a component of the National

Council on Alcoholism, is an association of nurses interested in chemical dependency problems. The purposes are to extend knowledge, to disseminate information and to promote quality nursing care for the addicted patients and their families, and to become involved with public policy and social issues concerning addiction. This organization serves as a forum for nurses who wish to share their knowledge and experience and to continue their education.

Membership is available to all currently licensed nurses in any of the fifty states, the District of Columbia, Puerto Rico, territories of the United States, and other countries of North America. Candidate membership may be given to student nurses in their senior year.

NNSA meets annually, and the National Forum proceedings, other than the business meetings, are open to nonmembers. NNSA participates in conferences, panel discussions, and teaching sessions. The society is governed by an elected board.

Since 1989, NNSA has been conducting certifying exams, which its Addictions Nursing Certification Board administers. The society also worked with ANA to develop and publish a scope of practice, standards of nursing practice, and diagnosis-related criteria sets. NNSA publishes the *NNSA Newsletter* quarterly for distribution to its members. The society can be reached at 4101 Lake Boone Trail, Suite 201, Raleigh, NC 27607.

National Nursing Staff Development Organization

Established in 1989, the National Nursing Staff Development Organization (NNSDO) exists to foster the art and science of nursing staff development; promote the image and professional status of nursing staff development educators; encourage and support nursing research and its application of findings in practice; and provide a platform for nurses engaged in staff development practice to discuss issues related to the continuing evolution of the field of nursing staff development. NNSDO also provides a forum

for members to further define staff development practice. In addition, it offers staff development services for members through disseminating information, meetings, conferences, consultation, mentoring, and other formats. Members include individual nurses engaged in any aspect of nursing staff development.

The organization holds an annual convention, publishes a bimonthly newsletter, *TrendLines*, and offers a discount on subscriptions to the *Journal of Nursing Staff Development*. It conducts workshops on various topics relating to staff development.

NNSDO collaborates in developing the certification examination for continuing education and staff development through the American Nurses Credentialing Center. It offers certification preparation courses under contract with its affiliates (local groups of nursing staff development educators). The organization recently initiated a research fund to stimulate projects. Headquarters is located at 437 Twin Bay Drive, Pensacola, FL 32534-1350.

North American Nursing Diagnosis Association

The North American Nursing Diagnosis Association (NANDA) was formally organized in 1982 for the purpose of developing, refining, disseminating, and promoting nursing diagnostic terminology as well as taxonomic structure for use by professional nurses. NANDA was begun by a small group of nurses at St. Louis University concerned about the unavailability of specific patient data that could be computerized and used for providing patient care in a team approach. In 1973, they organized the first invitational conference of the National Conference Group for the Classification of Nursing Diagnoses to identify, develop, and classify nursing diagnoses. At the fifth conference (1982), formal bylaws were adopted and the name North American Nursing Diagnosis Association adopted to recognize the significant contribution made by Canadian nurses.

NANDA has assumed responsibility for developing and maintaining a nursing diagnosis classification system or taxonomy for professional nursing. The NANDA database is included in the Metathesaurus of the Unified Medical Language System of the National Library of Medicine, and in the International Classification of Nursing Practice developed by the International Council of Nurses. NANDA classification, titled *NANDA Nursing Diagnoses: Definitions and Classification*, has been translated into numerous foreign languages. It is updated and published every two years. The organization has a process for review and inclusion of new nursing diagnoses into the taxonomy, and encourages interested individuals and groups to submit new diagnoses.

Membership is organized into seven geographic districts of the United States and Canada, which may consist of smaller regional or local groups. Affiliate membership is available for regional groups along with individual and institutional membership. Membership numbers about 900, including many international members. Registered professional nurses are eligible to be members as well as students and those with associate status.

The national organization holds a biennial conference while regional and smaller groups may hold more frequent meetings. NANDA has liaisons with many similar nursing diagnosis groups internationally, which are developing nursing language systems.

The organization publishes a quarterly journal, *Nursing Diagnosis*. Its address is NANDA, 1211 Locust Street, Philadelphia, PA 19107.

Nurses Christian Fellowship

Established in 1948, Nurses Christian Fellowship (NCF) is both a professional organization and a ministry by and for Christian nurses and nursing students. It is a division of InterVarsity Christian Fellowship and aims to bring the good news of Jesus Christ to nursing education and practice. NCF is concerned for the nurse as whole person and advocate of quality nursing care. The goals are to (1) develop a network of nurses who listen to God and pray with expectation; (2) equip nurses with a biblical world view that prepares them to represent Jesus Christ in nursing education and practice; (3) proclaim the gospel of Jesus Christ so that others will hear the good news of Christ's relevancy to people and issues in nursing; (4) demonstrate Christ's righteousness and justice through teaching biblical ethical standards and advocating health care for the poor and underserved; (5) develop leadership qualities and skills in Christian nurses who will communicate the gospel of Jesus Christ in nursing locally, nationally, and internationally.

NCF provides a local, regional, national, and international network for Christian nursing. Local groups meet for prayer, Bible study, mutual encouragement, and outreach. NCF staff and volunteers provide mentoring, vision for ministry, and help to establish campus and areawide groups. Area, national, and international continuing education programs and conferences provide spiritual and professional growth opportunities. Topics include Christian growth, spiritual care, suffering, death, healing, stress and conflict management, ethics, and values.

Written materials include guidelines for starting groups, textbooks on spiritual care and Christian ethics, Bible study guides, and the quarterly *Journal of Christian Nursing*. Some workshops are available on videotape. Members receive regular newsletters and prayer updates. Specific resources are available for students, faculty, and graduate students, including the student newsletter, *Campus Vitals*, and listings of theses and dissertations that include the spiritual dimension from a Christian perspective.

Membership is open to nurses and nursing students who affirm NCF's vision and faith and are committed to involvement in some aspect of the ministry, both financially and practically. For more information contact Nurses Christian Fellowship, P.O. Box 7895, Madison, WI 53707-7895.

Oncology Nursing Society

The Oncology Nursing Society (ONS) was founded in 1975. The purposes of the society include promoting the highest professional standards of oncology nursing; studying, researching, and exchanging information, experiences, and ideas leading to improved oncology nursing; encouraging nurses to specialize in oncology nursing; and fostering the professional development of oncology nurses, individually and collectively. Registered nurses practicing in or interested in oncology are eligible to apply for membership. Today, ONS is the largest professional membership oncology association in the world.

A primary goal of ONS is to provide a network of peer support and exchange for oncology nurses on both the national and local levels. Currently, there are more than 179 local chapters and over 25,000 members. In 1988, ONS established Special Interest Groups, a formal structure to facilitate national networking of ONS members in an identified subspecialty or interest area.

Members receive a subscription to the society's official journal, the *Oncology Nursing Forum*, and to the newsletter, the *ONS News*. They also can receive a reduced rate on a variety of publications developed by ONS and benefit from a reduced registration fee at the ONS Congress and Fall Institute.

In 1981, the Oncology Nursing Foundation, an affiliate organization of ONS, was established to provide research grants, research fellowships, scholarships, cancer public education projects, and career development awards to oncology nurses.

A second affiliate organization, the Oncology Nursing Certification Corporation, was established in 1984 to develop, administer, and evaluate a program for the certification of oncology nurses. For additional information, contact ONS, 501 Holiday Drive, Pittsburgh, PA 15220.

The Philippine Nurses Association of America

The Philippine Nurses Association of America (PNAA) was formed in response to a growing need to address the issues and concerns of Filipino nurses in the United States. Since its inception in 1979, PNAA has organized 26 chapters in the nation.

The organization's purpose is to uphold the image and foster the welfare of Filipino nurses as a professional group. It promotes activities to further this goal; networks with other groups to develop and implement programs relevant to nursing practice and research; influences legislation and public policies directly affecting nursing; participates in community activities; and collaborates with organizations and agencies to enhance the adjustment of Filipino nurses in the United States.

Categories of membership include active, associate, international associate, honorary, and member-at-large. PNAA publishes *The Philippine American Nurse* twice a year and holds an annual convention and midyear conference.

PNAA aims to develop a database to identify the health status of Filipino–Asian Americans, assist in restructuring alternative models of health care programs that are culturally competent, and identify learning behaviors of Filipino American nursing students to verify areas of failure and success. Headquarters' address for 1994–1996 is PNAA, 7728 Hillandale Avenue, San Diego, CA 92120.

Respiratory Nursing Society

The Respiratory Nursing Society (RNS) is the professional association for nurses who care for clients with pulmonary dysfunction and who are interested in promoting pulmonary health. RNS was created in 1990 to promote coordinated, comprehensive high-level nursing care for these clients by fostering respiratory nurses' personal and professional development. To accomplish this, the organization provides educational opportunities that help nurses enhance their knowledge and skills; has created standards of care in collaboration with the American Nurses' Association; promotes and disseminates research; and serves as a formal network for communications in the field of respiratory nursing.

The purpose of RNS is twofold: to promote

the specialty practice of respiratory nursing through professional development of its members and to promote safe and effective respiratory health care for society through activities related to health promotion, disease prevention, and care through all phases of illness and across all age spans and cultures.

RNS publishes a quarterly newsletter, *Perspectives in Respiratory Nursing*, which provides information on clinical practice issues, current research, and a calendar of events. The quarterly *RNS Bulletin* provides up-to-date information on organizational and member news. An annual educational conference offers programs covering basic pulmonary assessment, strategies for intervention, concepts in managed care, advanced techniques and skills, and new product information. The national RNS office is located at 5700 Old Orchard Road, First Floor, Skokie, IL 60077.

Society for Vascular Nursing

Founded in 1982, the Society for Vascular Nursing (SVN) is an international association dedicated to promoting excellence in the compassionate and comprehensive management of persons with vascular disease. The society aims to assume the leadership role in defining the vascular component of fundamental nursing education; establish and implement research-based standards of practice for vascular nursing; collaborate with other professions to address the unique needs of the vascular patient; and enhance public awareness of vascular disease.

SVN offers active membership to licensed nurses as well as associate membership to non-nurse health professionals, and corporate membership to related industry. Benefits include subscriptions to the quarterly *Journal of Vascular Nursing* and the bimonthly newsletter, *SVN...prn*. SVN features an annual national symposium each spring. A Vascular Nursing Fellowship Grant program provides funding for approved research projects by SVN members. A task force is currently exploring a specialty certification program.

SVN also sponsors a nationwide health education and screening campaign for peripheral arterial disease, "A Step Ahead," and assists in the coordination of screening programs across the country and in Canada. Currently there are approximately 900 members. Headquarters is located at 309 Winter Street, Norwood, MA 02062-1333.

Society of Gastroenterology Nurses and Associates

Formed in 1974, the Society of Gastroenterology Nurses and Associates (SGNA) works to advance the science and practice of gastroenterology and endoscopy nursing through education, research, advocacy, and collaboration. SGNA has a current roster of 6,700 individual members who practice in a variety of roles, providing care for patients with digestive diseases. Included in the membership are registered nurses, licensed practical nurses, medical technologists, x-ray technicians, and physicians' assistants.

SGNA issues a bimonthly journal, a monthly newsletter, and several resource materials. It offers certification through the Certifying Board of Gastroenterology Nurses and Associates. Headquarters is located at 1070 Sibley Tower, Rochester, NY 14604.

Society of Pediatric Nurses

Established in 1990, the Society of Pediatric Nurses (SPN) aims to improve the nursing care of children and their families, and to further the development of pediatric nursing as a subspecialty within the nursing profession. Members include staff nurses, school and outpatient nurses, clinical nurse specialists, practitioners, administrators, educators, and researchers.

The society offers a SPN newsletter, membership directory, educational scholarships, and a small grants research program. Chapters are located throughout the nation, with 2,000 members to date.

SPN holds an annual meeting each spring. An awards program recognizes outstanding contributions to pediatric nursing. Send inquiries to SPN, 7250 Parkway Drive, Suite 510, Hanover, MD 21076.

REGIONAL NURSING ASSOCIATIONS

Midwest Alliance in Nursing

The Midwest Alliance in Nursing (MAIN) is a thirteen-state nonprofit association of nursing service and nursing education agencies whose common purpose is to enhance the health of persons in the Midwest region. MAIN works with its member agencies and others to advance education in nursing, improve nursing practice, and promote nursing research.

MAIN was organized in 1979 as a unique mechanism to serve the public good, following a two-year regionwide feasibility study supported by a grant from the Division of Nursing, DHHS, and by subsequent five-year funding by the W. K. Kellogg Foundation. The thirteen states in the MAIN region are Illinois, Indiana, Iowa, Kansas, Michigan, Minnesota, Missouri, Nebraska, North Dakota, Ohio, Oklahoma, South Dakota, and Wisconsin.

The primary mission of MAIN is to facilitate regional investigation, planning, communication, and collaboration toward obtaining shared goals and resolving issues and problems arising from health care delivery. The ultimate goal is maximum utilization of nursing resources to achieve cost-effective health care in communities in the region.

To fulfill this mission, the organization attempts to foster productive relationships and better communication between personnel in nursing education, nursing service institutions, and liaison agencies and organizations. MAIN's special status as a regional association with four kinds of member agencies—hospitals, nursing education institutions, community health agencies, and long-term care and rehabilitation facilities—provides a broad base for sharing nursing talents and resources.

MAIN agency membership includes agencies giving direct nursing care or teaching persons to give such care. Identified as liaison agencies are those groups not eligible for membership but wishing to establish formal liaison with MAIN, such as nursing, hospital, or other health professional organizations.

MAIN has received funding for several projects and studies that have a direct impact on nursing. Specifically, the Division of Nursing, DHHS, funded three projects: (1) Geriatric Education for Nurses in Long Term Care, (2) Impact of DRGs on Nursing: Report of the Midwest Alliance, and (3) Continuing Education for Consensus on Entry Skills. The W. K. Kellogg Foundation funded a MAIN study entitled "Associate Degree Nursing: Facilitating Competency Development."

Publications include fact sheets on important nursing matters, including comparisons of the Midwest with other areas of the country; the *MAIN Journal*, published three times a year; *Mainlines*, the organization's quarterly newsletter; proceedings of conferences; and reports of studies. A list of MAIN's publications can be obtained from the MAIN headquarters, BR108, 1226 West Michigan, Indianapolis, IN 46202-5180.

North East Organization for Nursing

The North East Organization for Nursing (NEON) was formed in the mid-1980s through the combined resources of the Mid-Atlantic Regional Nursing Association and the New England Organization for Nursing. The merger brought together nurse leaders from the New England and Middle Atlantic states.

NEON's primary purpose is to promote cooperative planning and collaboration between and among nursing service and nursing education agencies, toward the ultimate goal of improving the quality of health services available to people in the northeast.

Agency membership with voting privileges by a designated official agency representative is available to educational institutions with a major in nursing, and to health care agencies offering nursing services and nursing departments administered by a registered nurse. Liaison membership (nonvoting) is open to individuals and related health care groups.

NEON holds an annual meeting that features lectures and panel discussions on timely issues and provides an opportunity to network. As the organization's research arm, the Eastern Nursing Research Society presents a conference each spring. Further information can be obtained by contacting NEON Office, Department of Nursing, University of New Hampshire, Durham, NH 03824.

Southern Council on Collegiate Education for Nursing

The Southern Council on Collegiate Education for Nursing (SCCEN), in affiliation with the Southern Regional Education Board (SREB), engages in cooperative planning and activities to strengthen nursing education in colleges and universities in the South. The Southern Regional Education Board, the nation's first interstate compact for higher education, appointed a Committee on Graduate Education and Research in Nursing in 1948 to establish graduate programs in nursing. In 1963, the Council on Collegiate Education for Nursing was formed as the major mechanism for working toward strengthening and expanding nursing education programs at all levels. Two successive 5-year grants (1962–1972) from the W. K. Kellogg Foundation of Battle Creek, Michigan, supported a variety of activities addressing statewide planning, new instructional techniques, curriculum theory and development, and inservice programs for faculty and administrators. In 1972, SREB and the Council, with funding from the Division of Nursing, DHHS, developed plans for conducting regional activities on a more permanent basis.

The Council on Collegiate Education for Nursing became a membership organization, maintaining an affiliation with the Southern Regional Education Board, in 1975. (*Southern* was added to the council's name in 1980.) Regionally accredited colleges and universities that provide nursing education programs leading to the associate degree, baccalaureate, and higher degrees are eligible for membership. Each member institution pays an annual fee that is established by the council. The current membership is 200 institutions.

SCCEN functions as a forum where the chief administrator of college-based nursing programs can obtain information, discuss developments at national, state, and local levels, and conduct regional planning. This group generates ideas for and implements nursing-related projects administered by the Southern Regional Education Board. Projects address relevant issues and concerns of nursing education in the 15 SREB-member states (Alabama, Arkansas, Florida, Georgia, Kentucky, Louisiana, Maryland, Mississippi, North Carolina, Oklahoma, South Carolina, Tennessee, Texas, Virginia, West Virginia). Notable among the projects are: Regional Action to Improve Curriculum in Nursing Education (1972–75), Increasing Opportunities for Disadvantaged in Nursing Education (1972–75); Regional Action to Implement Curricular Change in Nursing Education (1976–82); Nursing Research Development in the South (1977–80); Faculty Development for Associate Degree Nursing Education (1982–85); Continuing Nursing Education in Computer Technology (1985–1990); Faculty Preparation for Teaching Gerontological Nursing (1989–92); and Faculty Development for Graduate Nurse Educators (1992–1995).

SCCEN is housed at SREB headquarters at 592 Tenth Street, NW, Atlanta, GA 30318-5790.

Western Institute of Nursing

The Western Institute of Nursing (WIN), a nonprofit organization, was established in 1986 and represents nurses in the 13 western-state region (Alaska, Arizona, California, Colorado, Hawaii, Idaho, Montana, Nevada, New Mexico, Oregon, Utah, Washington, Wyoming). The institute expands on the 29-year heritage of the Western Council on Higher Education for Nursing (WCHEN) to provide leadership and representation for nursing in the West by joining practice and education in a full and active partnership. Over the years, WIN has developed into the western region's comprehensive, knowledgeable, and action-oriented organization involved with regional and national issues, concerns, and trends in nursing.

Recognizing the complex needs within the region, WIN has a proven track record of helping nurses address common interests as well as special problems. WIN has acquired the capacity and expertise to improve health care and advance the profession. Through the assistance of WIN, the efforts of individual and agency members are leveraged, creating diverse benefits for nurses. The mission of WIN is to influence positively the quality of health care for people in the West through monitoring relevant issues and trends and through designing, implementing, and evaluating regional action-oriented nursing strategies in nursing education, nursing practice, and nursing research.

Constituent memberships are open to all registered nurses, students, nursing education programs offering associate degree, baccalaureate, and higher degrees, and nursing service agencies in the 13 western states. Associate memberships are open to registered nurses outside the West, nonnurses and organizations that support the mission and goals of WIN. An elected board of governors manages the affairs of the institute. The board includes representation from educational programs, health care agencies, and individual members.

Membership in the institute's Western Society for Research in Nursing (WSRN) is open to constituent, individual, student, and agency members and associate members. WSRN supports research efforts, providing a network for researchers and sponsoring an annual research conference.

WIN holds an annual assembly that provides a forum and networking for discussion of relevant issues, trends, and activities related to the mission and goals of the institute and a business session for organizational matters. Through the annual Communicating Nursing Research Conference, nursing research is presented and discussed. Papers are selected for the quality of the research and the impact of the research on the discipline of nursing. Proceedings of the combined WIN/Assembly/Nursing Research Conference are published annually.

In 1992, WIN celebrated its 35th anniversary and the 25th anniversary of its research conference series. Subsequently, two publications were produced, *The Cumulative Index of Communicating Nursing Research Conference Proceedings: Volumes 1 to 25*, and *The Anniversary Book: A History of Nursing in the West: 1956–1992*.

To recognize outstanding leadership and the promotion of excellence, WIN has established an awards program. Each year, the Carol A. Lindeman Award for a New Researcher is given. WIN has conducted workshops to increase understanding of ethnic groups, and on the scope of the problem of substance abuse with a focus on prevention and treatment models. Proceedings are available.

The institute launched a project designed to enhance the knowledge and skills of registered nurses involved in the care of the elderly in the thirteen western states. "A Western Project to Improve Training in Geriatric Nursing," funded by the Division of Nursing, DHHS offered the opportunity for nurses in the West to participate in a continuing education program, "Essentials of Quality Nursing Care for the Elderly." A training manual based on these programs is available. The address for WIN is P.O. Drawer P, Boulder, CO 80301-9752.

NURSING-RELATED ORGANIZATIONS

There are a variety of organizations that allow for the participation of nurses through some form of exclusive or general membership. They are too varied to begin to list. The American Heart Association, the American Cancer Society, and the Catholic Hospital Association are just three examples.

In addition, there are those organizations that can either trace their roots to nursing or service a constituency closely involved with the registered nurse. The practical nurse organizations and the American Red Cross are of that nature and are presented here.

American Red Cross

The American Red Cross was founded in 1881 by Clara Barton, a volunteer who cared for soldiers during the Civil War. She became committed to ensuring that the U.S. government ratified the Geneva Convention and established an organization in the United States that would alleviate human suffering. The American Red Cross is a humanitarian organization, led by volunteers, that provides relief to victims of disasters and helps people prevent, prepare for, and respond to emergencies. It does this through services consistent with the 1905 Congressional Charter and the fundamental principles of the international Red Cross movement. The 50-member all-volunteer board of governors directs the American Red Cross and establishes the policies under which chapters and blood regions across the country operate. The Red Cross is a nongovernmental agency and relies primarily on the generosity of the American people for support.

The Division of Nursing was formally reestablished in the American Red Cross in July 1992. Its function is to provide support for nurse involvement throughout the organization. Nurses are recognized through nurse enrollment within the American Red Cross, after providing a minimum number of hours of service.

Ever since it was founded, Nursing and Health Services has been one of the important units in many Red Cross societies. In the United States, a Division of Nursing Services was established in the American Red Cross in 1909, with Jane A. Delano as its first director. The maintenance of a reserve of qualified professional nurses who could be mobilized quickly in emergencies such as disaster or war was the initial purpose of the Red Cross Nursing and Health Services.

Red Cross Nursing and Health Services today are designed to extend community re-
sources in helping to meet the health needs of people at home and in the community. Policies and standards for all Red Cross services are determined at the national level. At the local level, the chapter Nursing and Health Services committees are responsible for planning and implementing the nursing services. Not all chapters have identical services because community needs, resources, and interests vary. However, standardized educational courses are available throughout the nation. Although the services may vary, Nursing and Health Services maintains a reserve of volunteer nurses who become enrolled as Red Cross nurses for the following activities:

Disaster relief, education, and preparedness. The Red Cross responds to more than 60,000 hurricanes, floods, earthquakes, tornadoes, fires, hazardous material spills, and transportation accidents each year. Trained Red Cross paid and volunteer staff members are ready to respond when a disaster threatens or strikes. Nurses are prepared through a series of training courses to adapt their nursing skills to meet needs brought about by disasters. Basic training is offered for emergency mass care, emergency assistance, and long-term recovery. Through advanced training and experience on disaster operations, nurses can be prepared to serve at the supervisory and director levels on national disasters.

Emergency communications and assistance to members of the Armed Forces and their families. The Red Cross provides emergency communications, financial assistance, and counseling to members of the Armed Forces, their families, and veterans during both peacetime and conflict, on U.S. military installations within the United States and around the world.

Biomedical services: Blood and tissue services. Red Cross volunteers help collect blood donations that amount to almost half of the nation's blood supply. Red Cross develops tests and implements training programs in areas such as the operations of blood testing laboratories and selection of donors. Red Cross tissue services collect, process, and distribute human tissue products.

Health and safety services. The Red Cross is a recognized provider of first aid, CPR, swimming and water safety, lifeguarding, and other health and safety programs. An average of 10 million people are trained each year. The Red Cross teaches people how to prevent HIV infection and works to increase understanding of the realities facing those who are living with HIV infection and AIDS.

International services. As a major part of the international Red Cross movement, the American Red Cross supports humanitarian relief around the world in areas affected by natural disasters and war, and educates the public in international humanitarian law and the fundamental principles of the Red Cross. International tracing and location services are offered by every chapter of the American Red Cross to help locate, reunite, and exchange messages between people separated from their loved ones because of war, civil disturbance, or natural disaster.

National Association for Practical Nurse Education and Service

The National Association for Practical Nurse Education and Service (NAPNES) is the oldest organization for practical nurses (PNs) in the United States. It was founded in 1941 by a group of nurse educators for the purpose of improving and extending the education of the PN to meet the critical need for more nursing personnel. Founded as the Association of Practical Nurse Schools, the name was changed to the National Association for Practical Nurse Education in 1942; *and Service* was added to the title in 1959.

Within a few years, after professionally planned curricula had been set up and duties of the PN defined, NAPNES expanded its activities to include a broad program of service to schools of practical nursing and the licensed practical/vocational nurse (LP/VN). At one time this included accreditation of PN programs.

NAPNES serves as one of the spokesmen of the LPN on federal and state levels on such matters as licensing, laws governing LP/VN practice, educational opportunities for the LP/VN, and matters of general welfare. NAPNES headquarters is at 1400 Spring Street, Suite 310, Silver Spring, MD 20910.

National Federation of Licensed Practical Nurses

The membership of the National Federation of Licensed Practical Nurses (NFLPN), a federation of state associations organized in 1949, is made up entirely of LPNs and LVNs. In states with a PN association affiliated with the federation, members enroll through the state association. In other states, individual LPN and VNs may join NFLPN as members at large. Each member participates in formulating policies and programs through election of a House of Delegates, which meets during the annual convention. Students may attend meetings with voice but no vote.

Some of the major purposes of the NFLPN are to preserve and foster the ideal of comprehensive care for the ill and the aged; to bring together all LPNs or persons with equivalent titles; to secure recognition and effective utilization of the skills of LPNs; to promote the welfare and interests of LPNs; to improve standards of practice in practical nursing; to speak for LPNs and interpret their aims and objectives to other groups and the public; to cooperate with the other groups concerned with better patient care; to serve as a clearinghouse for information on practical nursing; and to continue improvement in the education of LPNs. A code of ethics for LPNs that stresses many of the same points as the ANA code has been developed by the NFLPN as a "motivation for establishing and elevating professional standards."

To help carry out its objectives, NFLPN maintains a government relations consultant in Washington, D.C., and other consultants on labor relations. In 1962, NFLPN established the National Licensed Practical Nurses' Educational Foundation "for scientific, educational, and charitable purposes."

Seminars, workshops, and conferences are financed by the federation, as well as leadership training conferences for persons engaged in PN association activities at the national, state, or local level.

Both ANA and NLN work with NFLPN in matters of mutual concern, principally through liaison committees. NFLPN supports NLN as the recognized agency for accreditation. NFLPN also supports NLN efforts in the development and improvement of PN programs. Members of NFLPN staff or appointed representatives serve on committees with other health personnel and organizations.

Publications on practical nursing, such as the *Statement on Standards of Practice*, are available from NFLPN headquarters at 1418 Aversboro Road, Garner, NC 27529.

REFERENCES

1. Nursing organizations meet at ANA Headquarters to plan greater coordination of activities. *Am J Nurs* 73:7, January 1973.
2. American Nurses Association: *Bylaws*. Washington, DC: American Nurses Publishing, 1993, p 26.
3. Smith G: From invisibility to blackness: The story of the National Black Nurses' Association. *Nurs Outlook* 23:225–229, October 1975.

CHAPTER 28

Major International Organizations

THE ORGANIZATIONS DISCUSSED in the preceding chapters have all been national ones, although some have international affiliations. Included in this chapter are the major international organizations related to nursing and health.

INTERNATIONAL COUNCIL OF NURSES

Nursing claims the distinction of having the oldest international association of professional women, the International Council of Nurses (ICN).[1] Antedating by many years the international hospital and medical associations, ICN is the largest international organization primarily made up of professional women in the world. (There are, of course, men in ICN member organizations.)

The originator and prime mover of ICN was a distinguished and energetic English nurse, Ethel Gordon Manson (Mrs. Bedford Fenwick), who first proposed the idea of an international nursing organization in July 1899.[2] Among the American nurses present in London at that time, attending a meeting of the International Council of Women, was one whose name figures prominently in the nursing history of our own country, Lavinia Dock. She was quick to support Mrs. Fenwick's idea and, shortly thereafter, a committee of nurses from nine different countries began laying the groundwork and drawing up a constitution for the proposed new organization. When ICN was officially established in 1900, Mrs. Fenwick became its first president. Miss Dock became its first secretary, a position she held for the next twenty-two years. Annie Goodrich became the first ICN president from the United States.

The essential idea for which the ICN stands is, in Miss Dock's words,

> ...self government of nurses in their associations, with the aim of raising ever higher the standards of education and professional ethics, public usefulness, and civic spirit of their members. The International Council of Nurses does not stand for a narrow professionalism, but for that full development of the human being and citizen in every nurse, which shall best enable her to bring her professional knowledge and skill to the manysided service that modern society demands of her.[3]

Today ICN is sometimes referred to as the "United Nations of Nurses," an appropriate enough title. Although nonpolitical, and certainly less affluent than the UN, ICN does bring together persons from many countries who have a common interest in nursing and a common purpose, the development of nursing throughout the world.

Membership

From the beginning, ICN was intended to be a federation of national nursing organizations. The association was a little ahead of its time, however, because in 1900 very few countries had organized nursing associations. Until 1904, therefore, ICN had individual members. (These included male nurses, although the first time men were specifically mentioned as attending an ICN Congress was in 1912 in Cologne, where greetings were given from the president of the association of male nurses in Berlin.) In 1904 three countries reported that their national nursing organizations were "ready and eager to affiliate with the International Council of Nurses," and thus Great Britain, the United States, and Germany became the three charter members of ICN.[4]

ICN today is a federation of national nurses' associations. The requirements for membership have been, essentially, that the national association be an autonomous, self-directing, and self-governing body, nonpolitical, nonsectarian, with no form of racial discrimination, whose voting membership is composed exclusively of nurses and is broadly representative of the nurses in that country. Its objectives must be in harmony with ICN's stated objective: to provide a medium through which national nurses' associations may share their common interests, working together to develop the contribution of nursing to the promotion of the health of people and the care of the sick. A majority vote by the ICN's governing body determines the admission of national associations into membership.

At the 1973 meeting of ICN, a constitutional change was made to broaden the criteria for membership to include nurses who constitute a section or chapter of a national organization composed of other health workers as well as nurses. The ICN definition of *nurse* (the basis for national membership eligibility) was also broadened. In 1989, this definition (for membership purposes only) was "A nurse is a person who has completed a programme of basic nursing education and is qualified and authorized in his/her country to practice nursing."

A reiteration of the principle of nondiscrimination was also reinforced at this meeting through a resolution requiring the South African Nursing Association (SANA) to take action to enable nonwhite nurses to serve on SANA's

board of directors or face the possibility of expulsion from ICN. (This discrimination apparently exists because of certain clauses in that country's nursing practice act, which must therefore be changed.) Later that year, SANA withdrew from ICN because of its inability to comply with the mandate.

Each country may be represented in ICN by only one national nursing organization. For the United States, the ICN member is ANA, which allocates a small percentage of membership dues to the support of ICN. Thus, even though individual nurses are not ICN members, those who are SNA members can consider themselves part of this great international fellowship.

Organization

The governing body of ICN, according to a new constitution adopted in 1965, and revised in 1993, is the Council of National Representatives (CNR), consisting of the presidents of the member associations. This group meets at least every two years to establish ICN policies. It also has the responsibility of electing the members of the board of directors.

ICN's board of directors consists of its four officers (president and three vice presidents), plus eleven additional members, all elected by the Council of National Representatives. Nearly half of the board is elected by geographic area. The board, which meets at least once a year, carries on the general business of ICN, reporting to the council. The ICN president and vice presidents constitute its executive and planning and finance committee, responsible for general administration of ICN affairs and advice in relation to investments.

Finally, the ICN constitution calls for one standing committee on professional services (PSC). This committee studies and makes recommendations in relation to the four broad areas with which ICN is concerned—nursing education, nursing practice, nursing research, and the social and economic welfare of nurses. The membership committee of the board investigates the eligibility of national associations

---

ICN Member Associations as of 1994

Argentina	Guatemala	Pakistan
Aruba	Guyana	Panama
Austria	Haiti	Paraguay
Bahamas	Honduras	Peru
Bahrain	Hong Kong	Philippines
Bangladesh	Hungary	Poland
Barbados	Iceland	Portugal
Belgium	India	St. Lucia
Bermuda	Ireland	Salvador
Bolivia	Israel	São Tomé and Principe
Botswana	Italy	Seychelles
Brazil	Jamaica	Sierra Leone
British Virgin Islands	Japan	Singapore
Brunei	Jordan	Slovenia
Burkina Faso	Kenya	Solomon Islands
Canada	Korea	Spain
Chile	Kuwait	Sri Lanka
Colombia	Latvia	Sudan
Cook Islands	Lebanon	Swaziland
Costa Rica	Lesotho	Sweden
Croatia	Liberia	Switzerland
Cuba	Lithuania	Taiwan
Cyprus	Luxembourg	Tanzania
Czech Republic	Malawi	Thailand
Denmark	Malaysia	Togo
Dominican Republic	Malta	Tonga
Ecuador	Mauritius	Trinidad and Tobago
Egypt	Mexico	Turkey
Estonia	Monaco	Uganda
Ethiopia	Morocco	UK
Fiji	Mozambique	USA
Finland	Myanmar	Uruguay
France	Nepal	Venezuela
Gambia	Netherlands	Western Samoa
Germany	Netherlands Antilles	Zaïre
Ghana	New Zealand	Zambia
Greece	Nicaragua	Zimbabwe
Grenada	Norway	

---

applying for membership and makes appropriate recommendations to the Council of National Representatives. Continued eligibility is now handled administratively.

Carrying out ICN's day-to-day activities is its headquarters staff—a group of professional nurses, including ICN's executive director. These nurses represent ICN's executive staff, but in their relationships with and services to the member associations, they serve in an advisory and consultative capacity. Staff members are selected from various member countries. In 1981, an American nurse became the executive director. Usually all executive staff speak more than one language and have special qualifications in one or more of ICN's areas of activity and service.

ICN headquarters is located at 3 Place Jean Marteau, 1201, Geneva, Switzerland. For many years, its headquarters had been in London. The move to Geneva, however, locates ICN close to the many other international bodies in that city.

ICN Congresses

Once every four years, the ICN holds what is always referred to as its Quadrennial Congress: a meeting of the members of the national nurses' associations in membership with ICN. Nursing students are usually eligible to attend ICN congresses, too, if they are sponsored and their applications are processed by their national nurses' association. Students meet as a Student Assembly during the congresses, where they discuss issues of concern across national borders, such as students' rights.

ICN met less regularly in its early years, and the two world wars also caused the canceling of meetings during these periods. The first meeting, which was to have been held in the United States in 1915, was disrupted by World War I. Instead, the business of ICN was carried on during the ANA convention in San Francisco that year, attended by American nurses and a few intrepid English nurses who braved the submarine-infested Atlantic Ocean. The seventeenth congress was held in the United States in 1981; the 1985 congress was in Israel; the 1989 congress was in Korea; the 1993 congress was in Spain; a 1997 quadrennium is planned for Vancouver, Canada. ICN congresses are usually reported in *AJN* and other nursing journals, including *International Nursing Review*.

During the last several congresses, discussions and resolutions ranged from those focusing specifically on nursing issues to general social concerns. Included, for instance, were career ladders, socioeconomic welfare, educational and practice standards, research, autonomy, nurse's role in safeguarding human rights, nurse's role in the care of detainees and prisoners, and nurse participation in national health policy planning and decision making. Related to general health care were such topics as primary care, excision and circumcision of females, increased violence against patients and health personnel, the uncontrolled proliferation of ancillary nursing personnel, environment quality, care for the elderly, and affirmation of the World Health Organization's "Health for all by the year 2000" theme (HFA/2000). On an even broader scale were the concerns about refugees and displaced persons, nuclear war, poverty, and the status of women.

Functions and Activities

In the foreword to its 1981 constitution, ICN points out that the primary purpose of nurses the world over is "to provide and develop a service for the public," and that ICN, as a federation of national nursing associations, provides for sharing of knowledge so that "nursing practice throughout the world is strengthened and improved." In pursuit of this objective, ICN promotes the organization of national nurses' associations and advises them in developing and improving health service for the public, the practice of nursing, and the social and economic welfare of nurses; provides a means of communication, understanding, and cooperation among nurses throughout the world; establishes and maintains liaison and cooperation with other international organizations; and serves as a representative and spokesman for nurses at an international level.

From the very beginning, ICN has been concerned with three main areas—nursing education, nursing service, and nurses' social and economic welfare. Nursing research was added later. Two of its first objectives were to provide for the registration of trained nurses in order to protect the public from practice by unqualified practitioners and to promote a standardized and upgraded system of nursing education. Important statements on basic beliefs about and principles of nursing education, practice, and service and social and economic welfare were agreed upon in 1969. The nursing education statement indicates that nursing education should be conducted in institutions where education is the primary concern and that supervised experience related to theory should be gained in preventive and curative facilities. The nursing practice statement stresses health care and security as a basic human right, and the economic welfare statement calls for joint consultation in determining conditions of employment and the right of nurses to participate in their national organization.

Those who have attended any of the congresses will testify to the fact that they fully live up to the pomp and ceremony of their name. Held in various countries, upon invitation of the national nurses' association of that country, the congresses are inspiring demonstrations of international communication and fellowship in nursing. In conjunction with each congress, the Council of National Representatives (CNR) holds its meeting, with all those in attendance at the congress free to observe open sessions of the ICN council's deliberations. The official language of the congress is English, but facilitating communication is a system of simultaneous translation into the official congress languages, English, French, and Spanish. There is also a daily convention paper in all three languages distributed during the congress.

One of the interesting traditions of the congress is that each outgoing president leaves a watchword for the next four years. The first, left by Mrs. Fenwick in 1901, was *work*. That left by an American, Dorothy Cornelius, in 1977, was *accountability*. Each watchword is engraved on a link of the silver chain of office of the ICN president and becomes a permanent part of ICN history.

At the congress, special program sessions are held, usually linked to one unifying theme. Among the most outstanding achievements of the CNR has been the acceptance of a new code of ethics in 1953, which was revised in 1973 and reaffirmed in 1989. The code makes explicit the nurse's responsibility and accountability for nursing care. Eliminated, for instance, were statements that abrogated the nurse's judgment and personal responsibility and stressed a dependency on physicians, which nurses throughout the world no longer saw as appropriate. There was also a major statement on the developing role of the nurse, which read:

> In the light of scientific and social change and the goals of social and health policy to extend health services to the total population, nursing and other health professions are faced with the need to adapt and expand their roles.
>
> In planning to meet health needs it is imperative that nurses and physicians collaborate to promote the development and optimum utilization of both professions. A variety of practices may evolve in different settings, including the creation of new categories of health workers.
>
> Although this may require nurses to delegate some of their traditional activities and undertake new responsibilities, the core of their practice and their title should remain distinctly nursing, and education programs should be available to prepare them for their expanding role in the various areas of nursing practice.[5]

Whenever possible, ICN has sought common denominators in education and practice throughout the world. One such common denominator, for instance, is the international Code of Ethics adopted by ICN and equally applicable to nurses in every country. Another example is the classic ICN publication *ICN Basic Principles of Nursing Care*, now available in twenty-four languages and useful to nurses throughout the world.[6] At the same time ICN has always recognized the autonomy of its member associations and the principle that each country will develop the systems of education and practice best suited to its individual culture and needs. On the other hand, the definition of *nurse*, approved by the PSC in 1990, is suggested as an indicator of future directions for nursing (Exhibit 28-1).

Throughout the years, ICN has collected and disseminated data on patterns of nursing education and service throughout the world and provided information and advisory and consultative services in both areas to member associations requesting such service. In recent years, ICN has given special attention to primary care as a means of achieving HFA/2000, and a number of workshops have been held in Asia, Africa, and South America.[7]

Some of ICN's activities in the educational field are financed, in whole or in part, by the

Exhibit 28-1	Definition of Nurse	.

The nurse is a person who has completed a programme of basic, generalised nursing education and is authorized by the appropriate regulatory authority to practice nursing in his/her country. Basic nursing education is a formally recognized programme of study providing a broad and sound foundation in the behavioural, life, and nursing sciences for the general practice of nursing, for a leadership role, and for post-basic education for specialty or advanced nursing practice. The nurse is prepared and authorized (1) to engage in the general scope of nursing practice, including the promotion of health, prevention of illness, and care of physically ill, mentally ill, and disabled people of all ages and in all health care and other community settings; (2) to carry out health care teaching; (3) to participate fully as a member of the health care team; (4) to supervise and train nursing and health care auxiliaries; and (5) to be involved in research.

Source: International Council of Nursing, 1990.

Florence Nightingale International Foundation (FNIF), which is associated with it. FNIF was established in 1934 as an educational trust in honor of Nightingale. FNIF trust funds have also been used by ICN to encourage and stimulate research activities in nursing. One document developed by FNIF is *Ethics in Nursing Practice—A Guide to Ethical Decision-Making* by Dr. Sara Fry, an American ethicist, published in 1994. ICN also administers several scholarships. In 1990, another foundation was created, the ICN Foundation, to raise money for educational purposes.

In recent years, ICN has been particularly active in the area of nurses' social and economic welfare, and its staff has carried on field work to assist national associations in this area. *An Underestimated Problem in Nursing: The Effect of the Economic and Social Welfare of Nurses on Patient Care* by Ada Jacox was published in 1977. The economic and general welfare of nurses is still considered a concern of top priority.

At one time, facilitating arrangements whereby nurses from one country could observe, study, or work in another was an ICN activity. As of 1969, direct participation in such arrangements was discontinued, and arrangements are now made with the individual countries. Each member association provides guidance and assistance for nurses planning to come into or go out of its particular country.

Providing liaison for nurses with other international groups is one of ICN's most significant contributions to world nursing. Among the organizations, governmental and nongovernmental, with which ICN is associated in some way are the World Health Organization, the World Federation of Mental Health, the International Labor Organization, the World Medical Association, the International Hospital Federation, the International Federation of Red Cross and Red Crescent Societies, the International Committee of the Red Cross, United Nations Educational, Scientific and Cultural Organization (UNESCO), Council of International Organizations of Medical Sciences (CIOMS), and the Union of International Associations.

Publications

Since 1929, ICN's official organ has been the *International Nursing Review*, published six times a year from ICN headquarters in Geneva. In addition to reports of ICN activities, the *Review* carries nursing articles of international interest, usually written by nurses from the ICN member countries. Occasionally it reprints articles from the official or other publications of member countries. It is published in English, but some associations translate certain articles into their own languages. Subscription requests to the *Review* should be addressed to ICN headquarters. The journals of member associations—the *American Journal of Nursing*, for instance—also carry reports of ICN activities and actions.

Every year ICN celebrates the International Nurses Day (IND) on a theme selected by the ICN board of directors by preparing a resource kit with a background paper, posters, and ideas for action and suggestions for planning and organizing IND activities. Themes on the recent past have included quality and cost-effectiveness of nursing, healthy aging, mental health, safe motherhood, school health, nursing and the environment, etc.

ICN has sponsored a variety of projects to study issues critical for the development of nursing. Most recent ventures have been the International Classification of Nursing Project,[8] the Regulation Project,[9] costing nursing services,[10] nursing and AIDS, nursing research, the use of assistive personnel,[11] mental health services, to name a few. Most of these initiatives produce publications that are available through headquarters, some free and others for a fee.

The Past and the Future

The preamble to ICN's original constitution stated, "We, nurses of all nations, sincerely believing that the best good of our Profession will be advanced by greater unity of thought, sympathy and purpose, do hereby band ourselves in a confederation of workers to further the efficient care of the sick, and to secure the honour and interests of the Nursing Profession." From the beginning, ICN and its officers were farsighted and pioneering. Included were members of every race and creed. The courageous Mrs. Fenwick stood firmly for her beliefs in women's suffrage and often spoke of the organization as a federation of women's organizations (for all its male members), with women's suffrage as one of its objectives. In 1901 she also stated a need for nursing education to be in colleges and universities and for nurses to be licensed. (Lavinia Dock missed one major ICN meeting because she was too busy lobbying for women's suffrage.)

In conservative 1900, at the ICN program meeting in London, one subject discussed was venereal disease. Nurses demanded early sex education for children and accessible treatment with no moral stigma attached. The members greeted this with a storm of applause. At other meetings they tackled such subjects as criminal assault on young girls, the role of nurses in prisons, and many other taboo topics. They reached out to effect change and for 90 years have been carrying on activities to meet their broadening objectives. It is impressive to see how an international group of nurses with such diverse membership can agree on common goals on education, practice, and economic security when often nurses within an individual country, including the United States, cannot agree.

In 1993, the Council of National Representatives approved in principle the ICN's Strategic Plan 1994–1999, Towards the 21st Century.[12] It identifies two major goals and a number of objectives and strategies related to each goal. The goals are as follows:

- To influence matters of health and social policy, professional and socioeconomic standards worldwide.
- To empower national nurses associations (NNAs) to act on behalf of nurses, nursing, and the public well-being.

Embodied in these goals are elements of strategic action that are as bold and risk taking as the history of international nursing. ICN offers the support to nurses in every country to come together as a critical mass and make their voices heard. For this, organizational structures need to be established and strengthened. High standards of education, practice, and management are the ultimate vision. For many countries, this requires slow steps toward a system of credentialing, with the necessary vigilance to protect autonomy. ICN pledges to work to make nursing prominent on the world stage and to work with nurses in their countries to achieve similar prominence in the best interest of the people they serve.

There are clear financial problems with which ICN must cope, reflecting perhaps the financial problems of each country's association, and there are disagreements about policy. However, the strategic plan is a good example of cooperative thinking and goal setting.

In Seoul, ICN celebrated its 90th anniversary and a new book, *ICN: Past and Present*, that brings the history of ICN up to date. ICN's history has indeed been illustrious; with its many member countries and close ties with WHO, it has helped to change the health care of the world.

SIGMA THETA TAU INTERNATIONAL

Sigma Theta Tau International is the international honor society of nursing, comparable to other professional honor societies. Founded in 1922,[13] Sigma Theta Tau's Greek name means "love," "courage," and "honor." Its six founders believed that those attributes were critical values for leadership in nursing, and they continue to be inherent in all the association's interactions. Research and scholarly development through Sigma Theta Tau International's programs and services respond to the ethical, moral, and humanistic values of society, while also enhancing scientific discovery to shape nursing's responses to societal needs.

In 1994, the honor society had 345 chapters in accredited colleges and universities offering baccalaureate and higher-degree programs in nursing. It had chapters in all 50 states and in Puerto Rico, Canada, Korea, Taiwan, and Australia. Sigma Theta Tau's membership of some 105,000 active members makes it the second largest individual member nursing association in the United States and the largest organization comprised of all baccalaureate and higher-degree nurses.

Sigma Theta Tau International members are chosen from among students enrolled in NLN-accredited nursing programs leading to a baccalaureate or higher degree. Criteria for selection are high scholastic achievement, exhibition of leadership qualities, and demonstrated capacity for personal and professional growth. Graduate nurses holding a baccalaureate or higher degree may also be awarded membership on the basis of having shown marked achievement in the field of nursing. The overall purposes of this prestigious society are to recognize superior achievement and the development of leadership abilities, to foster high professional standards, to encourage creative work, and to strengthen commitment to the ideals and mission of the profession.

The board of directors, composed of Sigma Theta Tau's five elected international officers, six elected directors, and the executive officer, meets four times a year.

The house of delegates includes two representatives from each chapter, in addition to the board of directors and standing committee chairs. It is the governing body of the society and meets biennially. During the academic year, chapters at colleges and universities conduct at least four meetings, which are usually educational in nature. Regional conferences are held in each of the seven geographic areas in years alternate to the international convention. In 1983, Sigma Theta Tau began to cosponsor international research conferences and is committed to a conference coordinated with the ICN Quadrennial Congress. Research programs are also presented at the Sigma Theta Tau, ANA, and NLN conventions.

Many affiliated chapters grant scholarships and research funds. A research fund, from which grants are given to nurses engaged in research, has been established at the international level. Awards are also presented in recognition of creativity and excellence in practice, research, education, leadership, professional goals, and chapter programming. Other awards recognize outstanding programs or publications by nurses and others. The Baxter Foundation Episteme Award; Mead Johnson Nutritionals Perinatal Nursing Research Award, Glaxo Inc. Research

Grant, and Audrey Hepburn/Sigma Theta Tau International Award for Contributions to the Health and Welfare of Children are also major honors.

Sigma Theta Tau International publishes *Image: Journal of Nursing Scholarship*, the most widely circulated nursing scholarly journal, and *Reflections*, a newsletter, on a quarterly basis. Various nursing-related monographs and publications are compiled and widely disseminated to members, other health care professionals, and the general public.

The society has distinguished itself in the development of two businesslike strategic plans—the "Ten-Year Plan," promulgated in 1981, and the more recent "Actions for the 1990's." Both focus on the mission of the not-for-profit organization and enumerate goals and objectives for the priority areas of knowledge development, dissemination and use, and resource development. Sigma Theta Tau's commitment to improving the health of people worldwide through increasing the scientific base of nursing practice is emphasized.

As a result of the "Ten-Year Plan," a member demographic study, philanthropic market study, and architectural analysis, Sigma Theta Tau realized that not only a society headquarters but also an entire center for nursing scholarship was desired—one that would bring together nurses throughout the world to encourage excellence, research, leadership, collegiality, professional growth, and matters of public policy vital to world health. It determined in 1987 that it should develop an International Center for Nursing Scholarship and Nursing Library. A national capital funds campaign, the first in the history of nursing, was launched to secure the $5 million required to provide for the facility. Approximately 16,000 nurses, 300 Sigma Theta Tau chapters, 100 nursing groups and associations, 60 corporations and foundations, and 100 friends of nursing invested in the center, making possible its construction and dedication in late 1989.

The society is now engaged in a $7.5 million 75th Anniversary Campaign that will provide funds for the Virginia Henderson International Nursing Library, Research Fund, and Nursing Leadership Institute and maintenance of the headquarters facility. The campaign culminates in the 1997 celebration of the association's 75th anniversary.

The International Center for Nursing Scholarship today serves as a focal point for nursing scholarship and excellence. The building is located on the Indiana University–Purdue University Indianapolis campus. It contains a state-of-the-art electronic library featuring a unique scientific database that may be directly accessed by individuals across the nation and internationally using Internet. The Virginia Henderson International Nursing Library exists to provide information systems and communications technology to enhance access to nursing information and knowledge; form electronic communication networks among nurse researchers; provide a directory for information about existing nursing and health care data sources; provide a structure and classification scheme to organize nursing research; and disseminate nursing research findings to the public. The library serves as a registry of nurse researchers and their research projects, including publication and conference history. Many of the projects are termed "fugitive" literature, which is unpublished and not easily obtained. Its *Directory of Nurse Researchers* is the printed form of the registry and is currently being developed into a knowledge registry incorporating names of variables studied, findings, and the clinical and statistical significance of the research.

Sigma Theta Tau International's headquarters and its International Center for Nursing Scholarship and Nursing Library are located at 550 West North Street, Indianapolis, IN 46202.

WORLD HEALTH ORGANIZATION

The World Health Organization (WHO), established in 1948, is one of the largest of the specialized agencies of the United Nations.[14] WHO's constitution states as one of its beliefs:

"The enjoyment of the highest attainable standard of health is one of the fundamental rights of every human being without distinction of race, religion, political belief, economic or social condition" and defines *health* as "a state of complete physical, mental, and social well-being and not merely the absence of disease or infirmity."

Membership in WHO is open to all countries, including those that do not belong to the United Nations. WHO is organized on a regional basis so that WHO and the nations within each region or zone can work together on matters of mutual concern. The six regions are Southeast Asia, the Eastern Mediterranean, Western Pacific, Africa, Europe, and the Americas. The American region is also served by the Pan American Health Organization (PAHO), whose Pan American Sanitary Bureau acts as the WHO regional organization.

An executive board directs the work of WHO, which is administered by a director-general. Among its working force, known as the *secretariat*, are members of the health professions, including nurses. (However, at WHO headquarters, physicians outnumber nurses by far.) WHO's activities are largely financed by assessments on the member countries, on the basis of a scale authorized by the World Health Assembly.

World Health Assembly

WHO's governing body is the World Health Assembly. It is made up of delegates from all member countries and meets once a year in May. The United States was the only country to include a nurse (Lucile Petry Leone) in its delegation to the first World Health Assembly but has not done so on many occasions thereafter. Twenty countries now include nurses in their delegations. The United Kingdom includes its chief nurse and several officers of the Royal College of Nursing in its delegation every year.

National and International Services

WHO's services are divided into three broad areas: (1) assisting governments, on request,

with their health problems, (2) providing a number of worldwide health services, and (3) encouraging and coordinating international research on health problems. The trained staff of technical advisers, doctors, dentists, sanitary engineers, nurses, and others who are dispatched to help and advise any nation requesting aid works with the national ministry of health, the main emphasis being on making health care accessible to all persons.

Personnel are trained to initiate problem-solving programs and, when progress toward solution is assured, to teach people in the locality or country to carry on by themselves. WHO personnel recognize the influence of a people's social and economic status on health practices and attempt to effect improvement in those areas also.

Among WHO's major programs in individual countries are aid to strengthen local health services through better administration; eradication or control of such communicable diseases as malaria, typhoid fever, tuberculosis, leprosy, AIDS, syphilis, trachoma, and yaws; provision of better care for mothers and babies; development of better sanitation facilities; and improvement of mental health. WHO also provides fellowships, usually short-term, to enable health workers to observe or study in other countries, with the goal of improving practice or services in their own country. U.S. nurses are among those eligible for these fellowships.

WHO, in cooperation with member nations, collects and disseminates epidemiological information, develops and administers international quarantine regulations, establishes a uniform system of health statistics, promotes standards of strength and purity for drugs and recommends names for pharmaceutical products, keeps countries advised of the possible dangers in the use of radioisotopes and helps train personnel in protection measures, and institutes international vaccination programs as, for example, those against poliomyelitis.

Within the last several years, WHO has emphasized primary care. At the WHO/UNICEF Alma-Ata (USSR) conference in 1978, primary health care was introduced as the key approach to achieving an acceptable level of health throughout the world. The HFA/2000 goal introduced at that meeting was adopted by the World Health Assembly in 1979, and member nations have been encouraged and assisted in various ways to work toward that goal. In 1983 a proposal was adopted to monitor and evaluate progress.

ICN, which has supported the primary care concept, was among the first to follow up on the Alma-Ata conference through a workshop that identified and recommended changes required in nursing education, practice, and legislation to prepare nurses for primary health care. In 1983, when the executive director reported to the WHO secretariat on these ICN activities and recommendations, many members from around the world noted the importance of nursing in primary health care.

In other actions WHO has also intensified its promotion of the health systems used by the majority of people. In the Third World countries, most people depend on traditional healers, who have often been quite effective in caring for people. Their integration into the general health system is considered essential at this point of development and health care delivery

Nursing within WHO

Delegates at the first World Health Assembly realized that more and better nurses were needed in every area of the world. In some countries—in 1948—there was not a single fully qualified nurse. Health care was given entirely by aides, who often had little or no training. In other countries, as in the United States, there were adequate nursing services that could have been even better if more nurses were available. Between these two extremes were countries with widely varying numbers of nurses and vastly different educational patterns for preparing them. The largest part of WHO's nursing support has naturally been directed toward the relatively less developed, underprivileged countries with the most urgent health and nursing

needs. In May 1992, the World Health Assembly passed a resolution in recognition of the central role nurses and midwives play in primary health care. In response to this action of the assembly, a Global Advisory Group (GAG) on nursing has been constituted to give nursing more prominence and advocacy in international health affairs. The nursing GAG has 8 or 9 nurse members, and 4 nonnurse participants.

WHO nurses work primarily in an advisory capacity, helping the nurses in a country with their specific problems. Sometimes, however, WHO nurses must temporarily assume operational responsibilities until one of the country's own nurses has been prepared for the job. Thus, in establishing a postgraduate nursing program in a university, the WHO nurse may have to serve as director of the program in its early stages.

The areas in which WHO is called upon to provide assistance cover practically all of nursing—nursing education, organization and administration of hospital and public health nursing services, mental health, maternal and child health, clinical nursing specialties, and community health care planning. Improved midwifery services and education are vitally needed in many countries; so are programs to upgrade the training of auxiliary nursing personnel. WHO helps in these areas by cooperating with health workforce planning. Assistance from WHO is also available to governments and their nursing divisions (if any) to plan for the development of nursing in those countries and to promote nursing legislation in the interests of both nurses and the public.

Another WHO nursing activity is the sponsorship, sometimes in cooperation with other agencies, of regional conferences and seminars that focus on the changing role of the nurse in relation to current health policies. These enable nurses with similar backgrounds and problems to exchange information and work toward solutions, under the guidance of expert nurses from WHO or other international health agencies. Many of these nurses have never before had an opportunity to meet with members of their profession from other countries, and they derive not only knowledge but encouragement and moral support from such conferences.

It is obvious that WHO's nursing activities call for highly qualified nurses, expert in at least one of the fields in which WHO offers advisory services. Language requirements depend upon the country of assignment, but it is desirable for nurses to be proficient in at least one language other than their own. The official languages of WHO are Spanish, English, French, Russian, Chinese, and Arabic. In addition to its more or less regularly employed nursing staff, WHO engages nurses for limited periods of time to carry out special projects in various countries. WHO nurses often work in collaboration with nurses from other agencies who are also helping with nursing development in a given country.[15]

In addition to its advisory services, WHO has published a variety of documents in relation to nursing, most of them basic and intended to be widely applicable in many countries. WHO also publishes *World Health*, a monthly magazine on world health intended for the lay public, and a variety of technical papers, journals, and reports.

WHO has had a part in many of the major developments in the international health field such as increase in the average life span; decrease in infant mortality; total eradication of smallpox; major reduction in poliomyelitis and malaria; and increase in medical and other health profession schools.

The WHO address is Avenue Appia, 1211 Geneva 27, Switzerland. The Pan American Health Organization address is Pan American Sanitary Bureau, WHO Regional Office for the Americas, 525 23d St. NW, Washington, DC 20037.

AGENCY FOR INTERNATIONAL DEVELOPMENT

The Agency for International Development (AID), administered by the U.S. Department of State, is one of a succession of agencies through which the United States has assisted other countries in their social and economic develop-

ment, with nursing one of the areas in which assistance has been provided. AID is a national rather than an international agency but is included in this section because of the worldwide nature of its activities.

The distinguishing feature of the health and other technical assistance programs that have been carried out by AID and its predecessor agencies is that they have been bilateral—that is, undertaken cooperatively with the government of the country being assisted, upon the request of that country and with both nations sharing in the determination of the programs to be carried out and the goals to be achieved. These bilateral health programs had their beginnings in 1942 with the establishment of the Institute of Inter-American Affairs to work cooperatively with Latin American countries in improving their health and welfare services. Since that time, U.S. technical assistance in nursing has been provided under a variety of administrative auspices (Economic Security Administration, Foreign Operations Administration, International Cooperation Administration, and others), culminating in the establishment of AID in 1961.

The overall objective of AID's health activities is to increase life expectancy, primarily through reduction in infant mortality and mortality in other high-risk groups, and to improve the quality of life through reductions in morbidity. The goal is to assist countries to become self-sufficient in providing broad access to cost-effective preventive and curative health services.

The Office of Health provides broad technical and research support for the agency's health program. Its program focuses on the development and promotion of health technologies to reduce child mortality and increase life expectancy, prevent the transmission of disease, and promote a healthier environment.

The early nursing assistance projects were highly concerned with the development and improvement of public health nursing services; this was the most pressing health need in Central and South America in the 1940s. The U.S. nurses working in these programs, however, soon discovered that public health nursing services could not be permanently strengthened without a continuing supply of well-prepared nurses, which would, of course, require improved nursing school systems and facilities. In turn, if nursing students were to have their clinical experience in a true learning environment, hospital nursing services also needed improvement.

These three areas—public health nursing, nursing education, and hospital nursing services—have been the target of most nursing assistance projects carried out under AID's auspices. Like WHO, however, AID has also provided assistance in other nursing areas, such as midwifery services, the preparation of auxiliary personnel, and the establishment of postgraduate programs to prepare nurses for teaching and administrative responsibilities, among others. AID also operates a participant training program whereby qualified individuals—nurses among them—in the assisted countries are given an opportunity to get the basic or advanced education they need in educational institutions in this country or elsewhere.

AID employs nurses on a short- or long-term basis to carry out its nursing assistance projects. Some AID nurses have been with the agency or one of its predecessors for many years, assisting with projects in various countries. Others are recruited on a more limited basis or act as consultants.

USAID currently funds very few nursing projects. The trend is for bilateral, multidisciplinary partnership projects between medical centers in the United States and medical centers in countries throughout the world. Nurses are involved on a short- or long-term basis on many of these and other grant projects funded and managed by USAID and carried out by nongovernmental organizations. Nurses are recruited on a limited basis as consultants to the agency.

SUMMARY

The purpose of this chapter was to provide an overview of international health and nursing activities. Therefore, only the largest and most significant organizations and agencies operating in this area have been included. There are many other organized groups—religious and lay, private and governmental, societies and foundations—carrying on similar or related functions. For additional information, the heading *international* in any nursing, hospital, or medical literature index will provide additional information about the activities being carried on around the world in behalf of the health and nursing needs of its people.

REFERENCES

1. Bridges DC: Events in the history of the international council of nurses. *Am J Nurs* 49:594–595, September 1949.
2. Breay M, Fenwick EB: *The History of the International Council of Nurses, 1899–1925*. Geneva: The Council, 1931. This is a detailed, fascinating, and informative account of ICN's founding and first twenty-five years, throwing considerable light on the nursing problems and personalities of this period.
3. According to ICN records, Miss Dock wrote these words as part of a foreword to the program of ICN's Second Quinquennial Meeting, held in London in 1909.
4. Roberts MM: *American Nursing: History and Interpretation*. New York: Macmillan, 1954, pp 80–81.
5. ICN: *Am J Nurs* 73:1388, 1352, August 1973.
6. Henderson V: *ICN Basic Principles of Nursing Care*. London: International Council of Nurses, 1958
7. Entire issue on primary health care. *Int Nurs Rev* 29, November–December 1982.
8. ICN: *Nursing's Next Advance: An International Classification for Nursing Practice (ICNP)*. Geneva: The Council, 1993.
9. Affara F, Styles MM: *Nursing Regulation Guidebook: From Principle to Power*. Geneva: The Council, 1993.
10. ICN: *Costing Nursing Services*. Geneva: The Council, 1993.
11. ICN: *Nursing Support Workers*. Geneva: The Council, 1993.

12. Council of Nurse Representatives: *Towards the 21st Century, ICN's Strategic Plan—1994–1999.* Geneva: ICN, 1993.

13. Widmer C: Sigma Theta Tau: Golden anniversary. *Nurs Outlook* 20:786–788, December 1972.

14. World Health Organization: *The First Ten Years of WHO.* Geneva: WHO, 1958, p 391.

15. Almost the entire issue of May–June 1988 *Int Nurs Rev* focuses on WHO and ICN relationships.

Transition into Practice

Making Choices: Job Selection

G RADUATION AT LAST! And now what? For most nurses, "what" means it's now time to get a job. For some, the job is predetermined—commitment to the armed services, the Veterans Administration, or another agency that funded their education. Another group may have decided early on exactly the kind of nursing they prefer and the place they want to do it. If all goes well and there are no problems, such as an oversupply of nurses for that specialty or geographic area, at least one major decision is made. But for all graduates, choosing that crucial first job and preparing for it are big considerations.

There are many employment opportunities for nurses today, although the place of employment preferred may not offer the exact hours, specialty, opportunities, or assistance a new graduate might want. Pockets of unemployment most often result from budgeting factors and a tightening of the economy. Although nurses may be *needed*, some employers tend to retain workers on lower salaries, although less qualified, and to eliminate patient care services. Another problem is maldistribution, with not enough nurses opting to work in ghettos or poor rural areas, although the need there is serious. Conversely, small communities may be flooded by nursing graduates of a community college who wish to stay in that area. Still, today, almost everywhere qualified nurses are in demand.

Even with social and economic factors that create problems of perceived oversupply of nurses, new nursing opportunities are constantly emerging. And certainly there is no overabundance of nurses with graduate degrees (or baccalaureate degrees, for that matter). How, then, can you decide what is the best job for you? How do you maximize the chances of getting it?

SOME BASIC CONSIDERATIONS

Personal and Occupational Assessment

It's a good idea to start thinking about career choices while you are still in your educational program. Since most schools have rotations through the various clinical specialty areas, this gives you a chance to compare as you learn. Generally, there is also access to someone who can advise you about the pros and cons of certain types of nursing—or at least there's a more experienced nurse, often a faculty member, to talk to.

More important than anything else, though, is to take a considered look at yourself—your own qualities and what you want out of life.[1] There are a variety of approaches to this sort of self-assessment that are interesting to explore in depth, but there are certain commonalities. Some questions you might ask are:

What are my personality characteristics? Do I like to do things with people or by myself? Am I patient? Do I like to do things quickly? Am I good at details, or do I like to take the broad view? Do I like a structured and quiet environment or one that is constantly changing? Am I relatively confident in what I undertake or do I look for support? Am I easily bored? Do I like to tackle problem situations or avoid them? Do I have a sense of humor? Am I emotional? Am I a risk taker? Do I care about the way I look? Do I care what others think of me?

What are my values? Do I believe in the right to life or the right to die? Do I think everyone should have access to health care? Do I have some religious orientation? Do I think that too many people today are too rigid or too loose in their beliefs and behavior? Can I accept and work with those who have very different values? How do I feel about my responsibility to myself, my employer, my patient, the doctors, my profession, society? Do I believe strongly that my way is the right way? Am I intolerant of others' beliefs?

What are my interests? In the broad field of nursing? In certain specialties? In the health field? In my private and social life? In the community? Do I like to travel?

What are my needs? Am I ambitious? Do I like to direct others? Is money important to me? Status? Do I need intellectual stimulation? Is academic success important? What about academic credentials? Am I willing to relocate? Does a city, suburb, or rural area fit my desired lifestyle? Is success in my field important? Am I willing to sacrifice personal and family time for success? Do I think that my first responsibility is to my family at this point? Is part-time work an option? Do I want plenty of time for family, friends, and leisure activities? Do I see nursing as a career or a way to earn a living as long as that is necessary? Do I really like nursing? If not, why not, and what can I do about it?

What kinds of abilities do I have? In manual skills? In communication? In intellectual/cognitive skills? In analyzing? In coordinating? In organizing? In supervising? In dealing with people? Do I have a great deal of energy and stamina? Are there certain times, situations, or climate conditions in which I have less? Am I good at comforting people? Am I able to give some of myself to others?

It's good to prioritize some of these lists, since life and a job are usually a compromise. What's most important? What would make you miserable? It might also be very helpful to share this list with others. Is this the way you are seen by them? Have you missed something? If some of your friends and peers are involved in their own decision making, get together with them and/or a trusted teacher or mentor to brainstorm about the possibilities in the field now or later in order to match your own profile most accurately with nursing opportunities. When compromises are necessary, you can decide ahead of time which ones are tenable or even perfectly acceptable at that point.

Since there will probably be economic constraints in the health care system for a long time, one way to look at the job market is in terms of future growth. For instance, you may choose a hospital for a first job in order to hone your new skills, but have you considered an investor-owned hospital or, later, a long-term care facility, home care, or an ambulatory-care outreach center? All are part of the trends in health care. You should examine those job prospects as carefully as any other. They may have components that do not fit in with your own self-assessment. But don't close doors because of preconceived notions.

Licensure

Regardless of the results of your self-study, a basic and essential step in your professional nursing career is becoming licensed, since you cannot practice in any state without an RN. Information about how to apply to take the state board examination leading to licensure and other significant information is found in Chap. 20. The procedure for becoming licensed and getting the results is now very quick since the use of computer testing.[2] State boards of nursing in most states permit nurses to practice temporarily pending results of their exam. Theoretically, then, you can be employed as a *graduate nurse* until you pass the licensure exam. However, in reality, many, perhaps most, hospitals will interview you but not employ you until you become licensed. The administration feels that the cost of orientation is too great to take a chance that the nurse will fail. If a nurse fails after employment, he or she may be dismissed or must work as some type of nursing assistant.

What if you decide not to work right away? Stay home with your family? Take a long vacation? It's probably wise to study for and take the exam anyway. Unused knowledge has a way of disappearing from the mind, and it might be much more difficult to pass the exams later, without intervening learning and practice. Moreover, in most states, you are expected to take the exam within a certain time after graduation. Should you take a nursing board review course? It depends on the confidence you have in your nursing knowledge and test-taking ability. The good courses can be very helpful, and may provide backup materials as well as lectures. However, be careful that you select a reputable company. These are profit-making operations, expensive to you, and always attract some borderline operators. Another way of preparing is to study with a group of peers, perhaps using board review workbooks or texts designed for that purpose.[3]

PROFESSIONAL BIOGRAPHIES AND RÉSUMÉS

Now that you have done your self-assessment and thought about career alternatives, it's time to write your résumé. No matter how you obtain a position in nursing, you will probably be asked to submit a résumé or summary of your qualifications for the job. This might include a personal history, education and experience, character and performance references, and professional credentials such as your license registration number.

Some universities and other educational programs still maintain a file with updated information about your career provided by you, and references that you have solicited. This has the advantage of eliminating the need to ask for repeated references from teachers who may scarcely remember you or to write again and again to a variety of places for records. However, this service is gradually fading away, and that may not be bad. As you and your career develop, a reference from your first teacher or your first staff position says little other than how you were perceived at that time. Newer references may be far more useful. Your academic record or simply evidence of your graduation may still be requested, and your school always provides that information, but today a well-prepared résumé is considered appropriate.

A résumé is a relatively short professional or business biography. In academia, a curriculum vitae (CV), which is somewhat lengthier and contains slightly different and more detailed information, is the appropriate form of professional biography. Résumés are usually shorter than CVs. However, the terms are often used interchangeably.

The résumé should be businesslike, typed neatly on one side of good-quality plain white, off-white, or light gray paper measuring $8\frac{1}{2}$ by 11 inches, with a good margin all around. No more than two pages are usually recommended. A word processor is useful in writing résumés because it allows you to tailor the résumé to a particular job opportunity without making a total revision. However, make sure that the word processor prepares a good-looking résumé. Some experts suggest that you have a professional printer duplicate your résumé on a newer photocopier that produces a sharp copy, absolutely free of dark areas or smudges. It can be reproduced on paper with texture and a subtle tint. Quick-copy shops may specialize in making a résumé look good, doing layouts, typing, printing, and copying.

There are various ways to write a résumé; however, the content areas are generally the same.[4,5] They start with name, address, and telephone number, with the name written as you would sign it, but including appropriate degrees or credentials, for example, Mary Smith RN BSN or RN MSN CCRN. Periods are not necessary in these abbreviations as long as you are consistent in their use. Some nurses prefer to put the degree before the RN. Be sure your address and telephone number are complete. Include your business address if you can accept calls there, although this is often omitted when you are seeking another job, especially if you haven't told your current employer. An answering machine may be useful so that important calls from potential employers are not missed.

Résumés are usually organized in a chronological or functional, sometimes called topical, format. In a chronological format, you list your experience in reverse chronological order. The functional format calls for separate categories such as clinical experience, teaching, education, and so on. The most common format is probably a combination in which the various areas of work experience, education, honors, publications, and other activities are listed separately, but in reverse chronological order in each section. Nowak and Grindel, cited in the bibliography, give multiple examples of résumés with a detailed discussion. Remember that a résumé is a marketing tool that should show you to advantage. Therefore, while you must never be dishonest, the way you present your talents and credentials, especially after you have accumulated some work experience, may make the difference between whether you are interviewed or ignored, especially in a competitive situation. Although format is a matter of taste and style, a sample résumé that might be used by a new graduate is shown in Exhibit 29-1.

The following points may also be helpful. Stating a professional objective is not a must, especially if you are not sure exactly what you want to do. If you choose to write one, it should match the job for which you are applying, and thus may need to be changed accordingly. For instance, someone with a master's degree in perinatal nursing may be interested in either a teaching or a clinical specialist position. Both the objective and the emphasis in the résumé must focus on the position for which the person is applying. Needless to say, if you are applying for your first or second staff nurse position in a hospital, the decision on what to write is less complex.

All relevant work experiences should be included, with the most recent listed first. The usual format is to list the agency and date, followed by a brief description of duties performed, using "action" verbs—*developed, initiated, supervised*. Some experts suggest that if you have not had impressive positions, you should attempt to bury this fact in statements that focus on your personal qualities, such as: "Leadership—Demonstrated my ability to lead others—as night nurse on a pediatric unit at X hospital, such and such address." No one really knows whether this is more effective, but again, style is a matter of personal choice.

The education section should also begin with the most recent academic credential, and should include the major and such additions as research projects, special awards, academic honors, extracurricular activities, and offices held. Information on other honors, professional memberships and activities, and community activities might also be given in separate sections.

Under federal law, you cannot be required to include personal data such as your age, marital status, place of birth, religion, sex, race, color, national origin, or handicap. If you choose to do so, decide whether this makes you a more desirable candidate. For instance, a second language or extensive travel might be a plus in certain situations. It is usually best not to list specific references on your résumé, since this omission allows you to select the most appropriate reference for a particular position. If your school does maintain a file, you can state this, giving the correct address.

It is not necessary to say "References on request"; you would hardly refuse to give them. When you give the references, include

Exhibit 29-1	RÉSUMÉ

LESLIE B. SMITH

120 Pine Street   Home Phone (213) 456-7890
Clearview, CA 91110   Message Phone (213) 482-6132

Professional Objective: Staff nursing in a community hospital

Experience:

1994–1995	University Hospital, Los Angeles, CA.
	Nursing extern. Performed basic nursing activities under supervision on medical-surgical and pediatrics units.
1991–1994	Clearview General Hospital, Clearview, CA.
	Unit clerk on medical-surgical units, evening shift. Assisted charge nurse in (list activities); trained new clerks; developed end of shift report between clerks.
1990, 1991 (Summer)	Williams General Hospital, Williams, CA.
	Nurse's Aide on medical-surgical units. Responsible for care of thirty patients under direction of RNs including (list major activities.)

Education:

1993–1995	Blank University School of Nursing
	Bachelor of Science (to be awarded May, 1995)
1991–1993	Clearview Community College
	Associate in Science (1993)

Honors:

1993–1995	Dean's List
	Member, Sigma Theta Tau, International Honor Society for Nursing
1993–1995	Honor Scholarship
1992	Outstanding Student Leader Award, Blank Community College

Professional Activities:

1993–1995	Member, National Student Nurses' Association
1994	Chair, Program Committee
March 1995	Presented paper "When Students Teach Patients."
1995	Member, Curriculum Committee, Blank University School of Nursing
1995	Debate: "Be It Resolved: Everyone Has a Right to Health Care." NSNA convention.
1994	Attended ANA convention
1993–1995	Art Club, Blank University

Community Activities:

1991–1995	Volunteer for public television telethon
1989–1995	Volunteer for March of Dimes
1988–1990	Candy-striper at Clearview General Hospital, Clearview

the full names, titles, and business addresses of about three persons who are qualified to evaluate your professional ability, scholarship, character, and personality. Most suitable are teachers and former employers. New graduates should probably include a clinical instructor from the desired clinical practice area. Ask permission to use their names as references in advance. Choose carefully. If the individual, no matter how prestigious, really doesn't know you, your talents, and your abilities, and the reference is noncommittal, it can do more harm than good. When you contact a reference, however, it is acceptable, even good sense, to offer to send a résumé to refresh that person's memory. For instance, almost everyone forgets the dates they knew you, as you are not likely to be the only student or employee they know. If the individual is reluctant, don't push; the result can be a reference that says nothing much and the potential employer may read it as negative. You might also keep in mind that employers frequently telephone the reference, either because they want a quick answer or because they want to ask questions that are not on a reference form or to explore some aspect of the written reference (particularly if it was noncommittal). Therefore, if your reference is inclined to be abrupt, unpleasant, or irritated on the phone, choose another. As a rule, don't ask for a "To whom it may concern" letter and have it recopied. Most sophisticated employers see that as an uninterested response. Suppose you didn't get along with your last employer and, even though you left with appropriate notice, you fear a poor reference. Sometimes someone else who was your positional superior can be substituted or another person such as a clinical specialist who knows your work is suitable. (A peer's opinion may be discounted.) However, administrators often know each other, and your potential employer may know that you did not name the person who would be the usual reference and may check with him or her by phone. That could result in a really negative reference. Therefore, as lists of references are often not requested until after the interview,

you could simply say then that you did not have a positive relationship. Be careful not to speak negatively of the former employer; try to be objective or neutral. Though references can be important, the impression you make in an interview can be much more important in the long run.

LOOKING OVER THE JOB MARKET

The potentials for a particular job are assessed both before and after applying for and/or being offered a nursing position. Chapter 15 should be helpful as an overview of the opportunities available in terms of both specialties and professional development (career ladder, internships), but reading the literature, talking to practitioners in the field, and, if possible, getting exposure to the actual practice sometime during your educational program will help answer some specific questions. Moreover, having written at least a basic résumé gives you a clearer picture of the kind of position suitable to your talents and interests.

Today, even if an employer is actively recruiting for nurses, an application, a formal letter of interest, and often a résumé are necessary before a position is actually offered. Although there are those who feel that going through the entire process is worthwhile for the experience alone, unless you have at least some interest, it is rather unfair to take an employer's time to review an application and go through an interview for nothing. Therefore, after self-assessment, it is useful to do at least a potential job assessment in advance. The first logical consideration is a place with which you have already had experience.

Hospitals or other agencies affiliated with schools of nursing may offer new graduates staff positions. That has several advantages for the employer and usually for the student as well. Nurses who are familiar with the personnel, procedures, and physical facilities may require a shorter orientation period, which saves time and money. In addition, the student has a track record; he or she is not an unknown entity. There are also benefits for new graduates. During these first months after graduation, you can gain valuable experience in familiar surroundings. There are opportunities to develop leadership and teaching skills and to practice clinical skills under less pressure because the people, places, and routines will not be totally strange. The potential trauma of relocating and readjusting your personal life is not combined with the tension of being both a new, untried graduate and a new employee. And it may be a wonderful place to work.

However, if the experiences offered do not help you to develop, if the milieu is one that eventually makes you resistant, resentful, indifferent, unhappy, or disinterested, the tone may be set for a lifetime of nursing jobs, not a professional career. Of course that can also happen in other places, but if you're alert, you can often get a pretty good notion of how it would be to work at the agencies in which you have had student or work experience. This evaluation can be a little more difficult if you don't know a place at all, but the opinion of someone you respect, word-of-mouth information, the institution's newsletter, brochures, and even the way someone replies to your inquiry provides indirect as well as direct information.

On a more concrete level, you can give some thought to what you are willing to accept in terms of salary, shifts, benefits, and travel time. (Don't underestimate the value of the fringe benefits, which may not be taxable.) Balancing these with other advantages and disadvantages as determined by your self-assessment is important. And realistically, if the job market is tight, your choices may be fewer than they would be in times of nursing shortage.

All of these factors must be considered seriously. You'll never have another first job in nursing, a job that could set the tone of your professional future. At best, you'll have wasted time. It's much better to move carefully and make sure that your choice is the best possible one for moving you toward your goal, whatever it may be.[6,7]

SOURCES OF INFORMATION ABOUT POSITIONS

Three principal sources of information are available to nurses who are looking for a position: (1) personal contacts and inquiries, (2) advertisements, and (3) recruiters. At one time, employment agencies were also a common source, but over the years, hospitals and other health care agencies employed recruiters themselves and did not find it cost-effective to pay employment agencies. However, at another level of job seeking—executive positions—well-known agencies of good reputation (headhunters) are used by both employers and potential employees to match the best possible person to a suitable position.

Personal Contacts and Inquiries

The nursing service director or someone on the nursing staff of a student-affiliated agency, instructors, other nurses, friends, neighbors, and family may suggest available positions in health agencies or make other job suggestions. Hospitals not affiliated with schools of nursing sometimes ask the heads of nursing schools to refer graduates to them for possible placement on their staff. Often, letters or announcements of such positions are posted on the school bulletin board or are available in a file. Your own inquiries are likely to be equally productive in turning up the right position.

Never underestimate the value of personal contacts. People seldom suggest a position unless they know something about it. That gives you the opportunity to ask questions early on, and the information can help you decide as well as prepare you better for the interview. Moreover, if your contact knows the employer and is willing (better yet, pleased) to recommend you, your chances of getting the position are immediately improved. (This kind of networking, discussed more fully in Chap. 16, will be useful throughout your career.) One business executive has said, "Eighty percent of all jobs are filled through a grapevine...a system of referrals that never see the light of day." When equally qualified people compete for the same position, the network recommendation could make the crucial difference. Asking for job-seeking help is neither pushy nor presumptuous, but you should be prepared to discuss your interests intelligently. A résumé will help too. Most people like to be asked for advice and want to be helpful, but they have to be asked. On the other hand, you need to use some common sense in deciding how much and how often you ask for help from whom.

Advertisements and Recruiters

Local newspapers and official organs of district and state nurses' associations often carry advertisements of positions for professional nurses. National nursing magazines list positions in all categories of employment, usually classified into the various geographic areas of the country. There are also regional nursing publications focused entirely on local nursing news and information, with major emphasis on nurse recruitment. National medical, public health, and hospital magazines carry advertisements for nurses, but they usually are for head nurse positions or higher, or for special personnel such as nurse anesthetists or nurse consultants. In times of shortage, employers also use billboards, radio and television announcements, and even letters.

All publications carry classified advertisements for information only, and, of course, as a source of revenue. Rarely, if ever, does the publisher assume responsibility for the information in the advertisement beyond its conformity to such legal requirements as may apply. If you accept an advertised position that does not turn out to be what was expected, you cannot hold the publication responsible. Read the advertisement very carefully. Is the hospital or health agency well known and of good reputation? Is the information clear and inclusive? Does it sound effusive and overstress the advantages and delights of joining the staff? What can be read between the lines? How much more information is needed before deciding whether the

job is suitable? Some of these questions can be resolved through correspondence or telephone contact or your network.

At some time, you may want to place an advertisement in the "Positions Wanted" column of a professional publication. In that event, obtain a copy of the magazine and read the directions for submitting a classified advertisement. They will be very explicit and should be followed to the letter; otherwise publication of the advertisement may be delayed. The editor will arrange the information to conform to the publication's style, but will not change the material sent unless asked to. Therefore, all the information needed to attract a prospective employer within the limits of professional ethics should be included clearly and concisely.

Career directories published periodically by some nursing journals or other commercial sources are free to job seekers. They have relatively extensive advertisements with much more detailed information than appears in the usual ad. The other advantage is instant comparison and geographic separation, with pre-printed, prepaid postcards that can be sent to the health agency of interest. (Most are geared to hospital recruitment.) Directories are frequently available in the exhibit section of student and other nursing conventions. Some carry reprints of articles on careers, licensure, job seeking, and other pertinent information. Some journals also do periodic surveys on job salaries and fringe benefits that can be useful when considering various geographic areas.

Recruiters are a major source of information and job opportunity. They represent hospitals and other agencies and are usually present at representative booths in the exhibit areas of conventions. Some also have suites where they have an open house. Recruiters, who may or may not be nurses, also visit nursing schools or arrange for space in a hotel for preliminary interviews. Notices may be placed in newspapers or sent to schools. There are advantages to the personalized recruiter approach because your questions can be answered directly, and you can get "a feel" for the employer's attitude, especially if nurses accompany the recruiter. However, remember that recruiters are selected for their recruiting ability.

Under ordinary circumstances, the so-called temporary nurse service is another option (see Chap. 15). These services function quite differently from agencies or registries, since they themselves employ the nurses and then, according to requests and a nurse's choices, send her or him to an institution or other agency for a specific period of time. Nurses are usually placed in short-term situations in hospitals, but some services advertise home care. The single most important factor that seems to attract nurses to temporary nurse services is control over working conditions, including the time, place, type of assignment, and so on. New graduates may find this type of employment attractive as a temporary measure, since the nonavailability of fringe benefits may not be important to them. There is also an opportunity to try out different types of nursing, but for the new nurse, the lack of individual support and supervision is a disadvantage.

PROFESSIONAL CORRESPONDENCE

New nursing graduates today have a wider variety of personal and educational backgrounds than they did a few years ago. Many have held responsible positions in other fields, and even more have worked part- or full-time before or during their educational programs.

Therefore, the suggested procedures for application and resignation presented are just that. They review generally accepted ways to handle certain inevitable professional matters in a sophisticated and businesslike way, and may serve as a refresher for those already familiar with these or other equally acceptable ways of relating and communicating in professional business relationships. For the younger, less experienced nurse, this material provides a convenient reference and guide.

The first contact with a prospective employer is usually made by letter, followed by a personal interview, telephone conversation, and, occasionally, telegrams, faxes, or mailgrams. Every business letter makes an impression on its reader, an impression that may be favorable, unfavorable, or indifferent. To achieve the best effect, the stationery on which it is written should be in good taste; the message accurate and complete, yet concise; the tone appropriate; and the form, grammar, and spelling correct.

Stationery and Format

Business letters should be neatly and legibly typed or, if necessary, handwritten in black or blue ink on unlined white stationery. Single sheets no smaller than 7 by 9 inches or larger than $8\frac{1}{2}$ by 11 inches are more suitable than folded sheets. Probably the more standard size gives a better impression. Personal stationery is generally acceptable if it is of the right size; white, light gray, or off-white; and used with unlined envelopes. It should not look like social stationery. Notebook paper should never be used for business correspondence; neither should someone else's personal stationery or the stationery of a hospital, hotel, or place of business. Good-quality typing paper is always in good taste if a suitable envelope is used with it.

If you type the letter, which is usually considered most desirable, use a fresh black typewriter ribbon and avoid erasures or carelessness in the general appearance of the letter. Use of a word processor is becoming more common and because of its flexibility has a number of advantages. There is mixed feedback on its acceptance in formal correspondence, in part because of the variability in appearance. If it looks good, use it; it can certainly save a lot of time. Always keep copies of your correspondence.

At one time, an attractive handwritten letter might have had certain advantages over a typed one. For example, it can show your ability to prepare neat and legible records and reports, and can indicate precision and careful attention to details. This was seen as especially true of a nicely handprinted letter, perhaps because so few individuals have the patience and skill to do it. However, a number of employers and recruiters look on handwritten correspondence negatively. They suggest that anyone can get a letter typed or put on a computer, and the interested applicant would see to it.

Books on English composition and secretary's handbooks include correct forms for writing business letters. Two or more variations may be given; the choice is yours.

The block form is employed most widely in business correspondence, and therefore is selected for illustration here (Exhibit 29-2). The left-hand words or margins are aligned throughout the letter, with extra space between paragraphs. Commas are used sparingly in this form, and a colon is used following the salutation. No abbreviations are used. If personal stationery on which the name and address are engraved or printed is used, this information should be omitted from the heading of the letter and only the date given.

In business correspondence, it is always advisable to address a person exactly as the name appears on her or his own letters. The full title and position should be used on the envelope as well as in the letter, no matter how long they may be. It is better to place the lengthy name of a position on the line below the addressee's name, and break up a long address, in the interest of a neat appearance. Indent continuation lines as follows:

Ms. Selma T. Henderson, RN
Director, School of Nursing and Inservice
    Education Program for Nurses
The Reddington J. Mason Memorial
    Hospital School of Nursing
1763 Avenue of the Nineteenth Century
Chesapeake-on-Hudson, Ohio 00000

People are sensitive about their names and titles; be accurate. If you do not know the name of the person to whom you are writing to inquire about a position it might be a good idea to call and get the correct name and title from the person's secretary or other staff. The telephone number is usually in the ad. (At the same time you could ask to be sent any information about the position and the institution.) Often the name of the person to whom an applicant should respond is also in the ad, but more often than not, that person is a recruiter or someone from the Human Resources Department. At times the ad may state that you may call collect. If it is not practical to make multiple phone calls, address the letter to the recruiter and say, "Dear Recruiter."

It is correct to give a title before the name in an address in the heading and on the envelope—not in the form of initials after the name—for example, "Dr. Constance E. Wright" rather than "Constance E. Wright, EdD." In a signature, however, it is preferable to reverse this order and place the degree initials after the name of the signer of the letter. Never use both the title and the initials in an address; "Dr. Constance E. Wright, EdD" is incorrect.

It is quite suitable, and even desirable, for a (licensed) nurse to use "RN" after his or her name, particularly in professional correspondence. Many nurses with doctorates sign their names with "RN, PhD," or "EdD, RN," added to clarify that they are nurses as well as holders of a doctorate. They should be addressed as Dear Dr. Whatever.

A professional or business woman usually does not use her husband's name at all in connection with her work. Probably most business or professional women without a doctorate prefer to be addressed as "Ms." in correspondence. However, a woman can use the title "Mrs." to identify herself as a person who is, or has been, married if she desires. "Mrs." goes in parentheses before her typed name under her signature. "Ms." or "Mr." are not used at this point in a letter as a rule.

Cover Letter

The information included in any business letter should be presented with great care, giving all pertinent data but avoiding unnecessary details. It is often helpful to outline, draft, and edit a business letter, just as you would a term paper. This requires you to think it through from be-

Exhibit 29-2	COVER LETTER

Applicant's address
Applicant's phone number
Date of letter

Employer's or recruiter's name and title   (Use complete title and address)
Employer's address

Salutation:

Opening paragraph: State why you are writing. Name the position or type of work for which you are applying. Mention how you learned of the opening.

Middle paragraph: Explain your interest in working for this employer and specific reason for desiring this type of work. Describe relevant work experience, pointing out any other job skills or abilities that relate to the position for which you are applying. If appropriate, state your academic preparation and how it relates to the job description. Be brief but specific; your résumé contains details. Refer the reader to your enclosed résumé.

Closing paragraph: Have an appropriate closing to pave the way for an interview and indicate dates and times of availability. A telephone number is useful. If you cannot be reached during the day, give a number for messages.

Sincerely,

Signature
Name typed

Enc. (probably your résumé)

ginning to end in order to ensure completeness and accuracy. It is also helpful to tailor it to fit a well-spaced single page, if possible, or two at the most.

Your writing style is your own, and how you word your message may be part of what you are judged on. The tone of a business letter has considerable influence on the impression it makes and the attention it receives. It is probably better to lean toward formality rather than informality. Friendliness without undue familiarity, cordiality without overenthusiasm, sincerity, frankness, and obvious respect for the person to whom the letter is addressed set the most appropriate tone for correspondence about a position in nursing. Although there are those who suggest very unusual, dramatic, or "differ-

ent" formats, the reality is that they may backfire. A sample cover letter is shown in Exhibit 29-2.

If you feel that you need more information before seriously considering a position (for instance, whether tuition reimbursement is a benefit or a particular specialty area has an opening), you can indicate your interest in a separate letter, simply asking for the information, or ask directly within the same application letter. The kind of response you get in terms of courtesy, promptness, and general tone will tell you a lot about the prospective employer.

If you decide not to apply for the position after all, or not to follow through with an interview, it is courteous to inform the person with whom you have corresponded. Specific reasons need be given (briefly) only if such a decision is made after first accepting the position. This is not only courteous, but advisable, because you may wish to join that staff at another time or may have other contacts with the nurse executive or recruiter.

Applications

Applications are not just routine red tape. Whether or not a résumé is requested or submitted, the formal application, which is developed to give the employing agency the information it wants, can be critical in determining who is finally hired. Even if the information repeats information offered in the résumé, it should be entered. It is usually acceptable to attach the résumé or a separate sheet if there is not adequate space to give complete information. It's a good idea to read through the application first so that the information is put in the correct place. Neatness is essential. Erasures, misspellings, and wrinkled forms leave a poor impression. Abbreviations, except for state names and dates, should not be used as a rule.

If the form must be completed away from home, think ahead and bring anticipated data— Social Security and registration numbers, places, dates, and names. Although occupational counselors say that it is not necessary to give all the information requested (such as arrests, health, or race, some of which are illegal to request), it is probably not wise to leave big gaps in your work history without explanation.

THE JOB INTERVIEW

An interview may be the deciding factor in getting a job. Anyone who has an appointment for a personal interview should be prepared for it physically, mentally, emotionally, and psychologically. The degree of preparation will depend on the purpose of the interview and what has preceded it. Assuming that you have written and sent a résumé to a prospective employer and an interview has been arranged, preparation might include the following:

Physical Preparation

Be rested, alert, and in good health. Dress suitably for the job, but wear something in which you feel at ease. It is important to be well groomed and as attractive as possible. First appearances are important, and given a choice, no one selects a sloppy or overdressed person in preference to someone who is neat and appropriately dressed. Have enough money with you to meet all anticipated expenses. If you are to be reimbursed by the employing agency, keep an itemized record of expenses for submission later. Get accurate directions to the interview site. Arrive at your destination well ahead of time, but do not go to your prospective employer's office earlier than 5 minutes before the designated time.

Mental Preparation

Review all information and previous communications about the position. You should have considerable background information before you go for an interview. Showing that you know about the hospital or agency is desirable and impressive. Make certain that you know the exact name or names of persons whom you expect to meet and can pronounce them properly. Decide what additional information you want to obtain during the interview. Consider how you will phrase your leading questions. Carry a small notebook or card on which you have listed the names of references and other data that you may need during the interview. If you bring an application form with you, place it in a fresh unsealed envelope. Have it ready to hand to the interviewer when she or he asks for it; if it seems indicated, offer it at the appropriate time.

Emotional and Psychological Preparation

If you have any worries or fears in connection with the interview, try to overcome them by thinking calmly and objectively about what is likely to take place. (Role playing an interview with a colleague who may have been through the experience can be helpful.) Be ready to adjust to whatever situation may develop during the interview. For example, you may expect to have an extended conversation with the nurse executive or at least someone in nursing administration, and find when you arrive that a personnel officer or recruiter who is not a nurse will interview you; this is becoming more usual. She or he may interview you in a very few minutes and in what seems to be an impersonal way. Or you may have visualized the job setting as quite different.

Accept things as you find them, reserving the privilege of making a decision after thoughtful consideration of the total job situation. If a stimulating challenge is inherent in the position, you will sense it during the interview, or you may have reason to believe that it will develop after you assume your duties. However, you cannot demand a challenge, and if one is "created" for you spontaneously by the interviewer, take the promise with the proverbial grain of salt, knowing that an employment situation rarely adjusts to the new employee.

During the Interview

Usually, the interviewer will take the initiative in starting the conference and closing it.[8] You should follow that lead courteously and attentively. Shake hands. Be prepared to give a brief overview of your experiences and interests, if asked. At some point, you will be asked if you have any questions, and you should be prepared to ask for additional information if you would like to have it. Should the interviewer appear to be about to close the conference without giving you this opportunity, say, "May I ask a question, please?"

If you did not get this information in the handouts, you may wish to ask about the nursing delivery system, educational opportunities, advancement opportunities, staff participation in decision making, nurse-physician relationships, and the placement of the nursing department in the organization. It is perfectly acceptable to ask, before the interview is over, about salary, fringe benefits, and other conditions of employment, if a contract or explanatory paper has not been given to you. In fact, it would be foolish to appear indifferent. A contract is desirable, but if that is not the accepted procedure, it is important to understand what is involved in the job. The job description should be accessible in writing, and it is best that you have a copy. Most interviewers agree that an outgoing candidate who volunteers appropriate information is likable. On the other hand, many use the technique of selective silence, which is anxiety-provoking to most people, to see what the interviewee will say or do. A good interviewer will try to make you comfortable, in part to relax you into self-revelation; most do not favor aggressive methods. Good eye contact is fine, but don't stare. Be sensitive to the interviewer's being disinterested in a certain response; maybe it's too lengthy. Don't interrupt. Don't smoke. Don't mumble. Watch your body language (and observe that of the interviewer). It can denote indifference or irritation. Be enthusiastic but don't gush.

Some questions that are likely to be asked in an average one-hour interview are:[9]

- What position interests you most? (Be specific)
- Why do you want to work here? (Know something positive)
- What are your strengths and weaknesses? (Play up your strengths, and, although you should be honest, play down your weaknesses. Give examples, perhaps of what people say about you.)
- What would you do if…? (Show your decision-making and judgmental skills.)
- What can you do for us? (Tell about your special qualities and experience.)
- Tell me about yourself. (Keep it short; don't give more information than necessary to reassure the interviewer that you are suitable for the job, physically, mentally, and in terms of preparation. Stress your reliability.)

- What did you like most and least in school, or on your last job? (Be honest, but don't list a series of gripes.)
- How would you describe your ideal job? (Take the opportunity to do so, but let the interviewer know that you know that nothing's perfect.)
- Where do you think you'll be 5 years from now? (Emphasize goals that show your interest in growing professionally.)
- Do you have any questions? (Be prepared.)

In a survey of directors of nursing service in various settings, the characteristics valued most highly in rating a nursing job applicant were: promptness to interview, completion of application prior to interview, neatness and completeness of application, well-groomed personal appearance, and questions asked. As other qualities that might be more important were bypassed, this list may show how important the external aspects of an interview can be.

When the interview is completed, thank the interviewer, shake hands, and leave promptly. A tour of the facility may be offered before or after the interview. This gives you a chance to observe working conditions, and sometimes interpersonal relationships.[10] You may or may not have been offered the position, or you may not have accepted it if it was offered. If it was offered to you, it is usually well to delay your decision for at least a day or two until you have had time to think the matter over carefully from every practical point of view. Perhaps you will want more information, in which case you may write a letter, send a telegram or fax, or make a phone call to your prospective employer. It is always courteous and sometimes acts as a reminder to send a thank-you letter.

Sometimes during the procedure of acquiring a position, you may have occasion to discuss some aspect of it over the telephone with the prospective employer. If you make the call, be brief, courteous, and to the point, with notes handy, if needed. It may be helpful to make notations on the conversation. It is sensible to listen carefully and not interrupt. If you receive a call and are unprepared for it, be courteous but cautious and, perhaps, ask for time to think over the proposal—or whatever may have been the purpose of the call.

Agreements about a position made over the phone should be confirmed promptly in writing. If it is your place do so, you might say, while speaking with the person, "I'll send you a confirming letter tomorrow." If it is the responsibility of the other party to confirm an agreement but she or he does not mention it, ask, "May I have a letter of confirmation, please?"

After any interview or conversation, it's useful to make notes about what happened for future use and reference. If any business arrangements are made by fax, mailgram, or telegram, file this information with other related correspondence.

For positions sought through a registry or employment agency, the same courteous, thorough, and businesslike procedures used when dealing directly with a prospective employer are appropriate. A brief thank-you note for help received shows consideration of the agency's efforts in your behalf.

Evaluation

What if you didn't get the job you wanted? There may simply have been someone better suited or better qualified. Still, it is helpful to review the experience in order to refine your interview skills. Were you prepared? Did you present yourself as someone sensitive to the employer's goals? Did you articulate your personal strengths and objectives? Did you look your best? Sometimes discussing what happened with another person also gives you a different perspective. And there's no reason why you cannot reapply another time.

CHANGING POSITIONS

There seems to be an unwritten rule that nurses should remain in any permanent position they accept for at least a year. Certainly, this is not too long—except in the most unusual circumstances—for you to adjust to the employment situation and find a place on the staff in which to use your ability and talents to their fullest. Furthermore, persons who change jobs frequently in any profession or occupation soon gain a reputation for this, and some employers are reluctant to hire them. However, should it be desirable or necessary to change positions, a number of points might be observed. Consider your employer and coworkers as well as yourself, and leave under amicable and constructive circumstances.

Depending on the reasons for leaving and how eager you are to make a change, some writers suggest that before you definitely accept a new position, the present employer should be informed about your desire to leave and why. It may be that, depending on the employer's concept of your value to the institution, a new, more desirable position might be offered.

It is important to give reasonable notice of your intention to resign. If there is a contract, the length of the notice will probably be stipulated. Two weeks to a month is the usual period, depending principally upon the position held and the anticipated difficulty in hiring a replacement. Don't tell everyone else before you tell your immediate superior, privately and courteously.

Try to finish any major projects you have started; arrange in good order the equipment and materials your successor will inherit; and prepare memos and helpful guides to assist the nurse who will assume your duties. Check out employment policies about benefits, including accrued vacation or sick leave.

A letter of resignation should state simply and briefly, but in a professional manner, your intention of leaving, the date on which the resignation will become effective, and the reasons for making the change. A sincere comment or two about the satisfactions experienced in the position and regrets at leaving will close the letter graciously. There should be no hint of animosity or resentment, because this will serve no constructive purpose and may boomerang (see Exhibit 29-3). Don't burn your bridges. You may

want to come back to that place at another time. At the least you may need a reference and if you appear vindictive or childish, the employer is unlikely to give you any enthusiastic reference, even if you did your job satisfactorily. In these days of litigation, nothing may be written specifically, but employers are adept at reading between the lines of a bland reference. The administrative network (via a personal phone call) may paint you as an undesirable employee, and you'll never know.

Terminal interviews are considered good administrative practice and are sometimes used for a final performance evaluation and/or a means to determine the reasons for resignation. There is some question of how open employees are about discussing their resignation (unless the reason is illness, necessary relocation, and so on), perhaps because of fear of reprisal in references or even a simple desire to avoid unpleasantness. This is a decision you must make in each situation.

What if you're fired? The most common reasons for being fired are poor job performance, chronic tardiness, excessive absenteeism, substance abuse, or inappropriate behavior.[11] Usually you are given a warning about any of these problems, and if you haven't done anything about correcting your problem (assuming that the charge is justified), you'd better take a good look at yourself. Those kinds of uncorrected problems may make your future prospects look dim.

Whether or not you're caught by surprise when you're told, try to maintain your composure. If you can't pull your thoughts together, request another interview to ask questions and find out about the termination procedure. If you are at fault, make a clean, fast break. If you are not at fault, try to clarify the situation to avoid negative references. You may choose to contest the action. This is discussed in Chap. 30. However, weigh whether it's worth it. You may need to clear your name, but it might be unpleasant or impossible to stay in that setting and work productively. If the dismissal is a layoff for economic reasons, it is a good idea to have a letter

Exhibit 29-3	SAMPLE LETTER OF RESIGNATION

240 North Street
San Diego, California 00000
Date

Ms. Ruth Green, RN, MSN
Vice President of Nursing
West Central Hospital
20 California Avenue
San Diego, California 00000

Dear Ms. Green:

I will be relocating to Phoenix, Arizona, in May and have accepted a position there at General Hospital as head nurse of the pediatric unit. Therefore, I wish to resign effective April 14, 1995.

Being at Central Hospital has been a very satisfying personal and professional experience. The atmosphere is one in which a nurse can grow, and I appreciate the support given by the staff of 4B and the head nurse, Melanie Rones. She has especially helped me to develop my managerial skills and encouraged me to take advantage of the hospital's tuition reimbursement. I expect to finish my degree in Phoenix. I am proud to have been a part of a group of practitioners and administrators who are committed to caring, competent patient care.

If there is anything I can do to help in the transition, I will be happy to do so.

Sincerely,

(Signature)
John Collins, RN

cc: Melanie Rones
    Head Nurse 4B

---

to this effect, both in terms of professional security and in order to get unemployment benefits, if necessary.

When leaving a job is not your choice, it sometimes helps to talk with a supportive person, to ventilate and analyze what happened. Choose someone you can trust, but who can help you see things as objectively as possible. Then it's time to get back to career planning. Perhaps you should look at the possibility of further education or training in a different kind of nursing. If not, be sensible about conserving your economic resources until you find another job. Try to select the next job, keeping in mind what made you unhappy in the last one, and of course, correcting those problems that got you fired. You need not volunteer to your prospective employer that you were fired, but if asked, don't lie. Just say that you were asked to leave and why. Don't criticize your previous employer and try to be as positive as possible about your last job. Your honesty and determination to do well could be a plus.

It's doubtful that you will stay in the same institution throughout your career. This is a very mobile society, and there are many job opportunities for nurses throughout the country (and world). Without closing the doors to unexpected opportunities, beginning early to think in terms of a career will make nursing more satisfying and interesting in the long run.

REFERENCES

1. Finn MA: Discovering who you are and what you want from your career. *Healthcare Trends Transition* 3:42–44, March 1992.
2. Stein A, Licht B: Questions and answers on the computerized NCLEX exam. *Imprint* 41:9–11, January 1994.
3. White A: Getting the most from group study sessions. *Imprint* 41:61, 63, February–March 1994.
4. O'Keefe N: How to open the right doors, in *Career Guide for 1994*. New York: American Journal of Nursing Company, pp 11–12.
5. Vogel D: Writing a résumé. *Imprint* 40:35–36, January 1993.
6. Filoromo T: Finding the right job. *Imprint* 37:27–35, December 1990–January 1991.
7. Huey F: Your first job: Great news or giant nightmare? *Am J Nurs* 88:452–457, April 1988.
8. Vogel D, Jackson P: The interview: Reflections from the recruiter's side of the desk. *Healthcare Trends Transition* 3:24–26, March 1992.
9. Bruce S: A blueprint for better job interviews. *Nurs 87* 17:64B–64F, June 1987.
10. Hannan J: Site seeing: Touring prospective employers. *Healthcare Trends Transition* 3:31, 34–36, March 1992.
11. Marriner A: Surviving being fired. *Nurs 86* 16:16N, 16P, January 1986.

Career Management

SOCIALIZATION AND RESOCIALIZATION

EVENTUALLY, GRADUATION *does* come, and for most nurses, the next step, with hardly a break, is that first nursing job. What can you expect?

Experts say that the transition from student to RN is a psychological, sociological, and legal phenomenon. The student has spent two to four years being socialized into nursing in the education setting; now resocialization into the work world is necessary. Socialization into a new role is not usually a conscious process, although both the individual being socialized and those doing the socializing consciously make certain efforts. These statements are accurate but trivialize the fact that the professions are set apart by their social position. Socialization should be anticipated and planned.

In reality, the educational experience for any field of work will differ from the expectations when you are being compensated for your services. For the most part, students are not integral to the systems of care, look to faculty for their cues and rewards, and are allowed to falter somewhat in their practice. Further, the socialization-resocialization phenomena (student to full-fledged professional) is often presented as a one-time occurrence. In fact, given today's rapidly changing health care system with the movement from hospitals into community practice, down-sizing of hospital nursing staffs, and new markets for health services, nurses will be con-

fronted with resocialization many times during their career life.

All of these circumstances caution that the only way to accomplish a comfortable transition time after time after time is to know yourself and conceptually to understand the dynamics of a situation. There is nothing so unexpected or mystical about role transition and socialization. All of us have been through the process at least once (but really many times) as we took on the attributes of a participating member of society.

Role is an abstract idea that can be assumed only through the presence of certain cues allowing you to infer its presence. A role is a constellation of rights and responsibilities that characterize a social position. Since the individual role occupant is embedded in a social structure, the role behaviors are derived from the expectations of both the individual and the social systems with which that individual interfaces. Socialization is the process by which an individual acquires the behaviors necessary for acceptance by these interfacing groups or systems. This is accomplished through a reciprocal process of role shaping and role taking, with the eventual assimilation of the behaviors within one's repertoire as follows:[1]

Step 1. Interaction with primary groups who mirror the expected behaviors (exposure)

Step 2. Development of an interpersonal attachment with significant others from that group (identification)

Step 3. Clarity on expectations; covert messages are made overt (empathy)

Step 4. Negotiation to resolve differences between the ideal and the real, and determine how much freedom there is to modify the role to personal preference (role shaping)

Step 5. Continuing support to allow movement to behavioral synthesis; accommodated behavior becomes assimilated (role taking)

Successful role transition is closely related to your personal desire to become part of the mainstream of nursing. The possibilities are greatly enhanced where there is a good feeling (chemistry) between you and your group of peers (staff nurses). This alerts you to the need to meet the people you will be working with on a day-to-day basis when applying for a position. The best of organizations go further, providing a preceptorship or "buddy" arrangement with someone who is senior in the staff nurse role.[2] Make sure you ask questions until you fully understand what is expected of you, and be cautious in bending the rules until you have established yourself. However, make inquiries that help predict how much personal role shaping will be possible. Some cues of an organization that allows little flexibility in role development are:

Highly precise and detailed job descriptions

Management by memo in situations where personal communication would have sufficed

Guarded interdisciplinary boundaries that hamper smooth operation

A hierarchy that is an obstacle as opposed to facilitating your work

Policies, procedures, and documentation systems that are cumbersome and even inconsistent with current practice

Absence of staff nurse autonomy in caring for patients

Verbalized discontent from staff, but no evidence of any attempt to change things

High turnover rate

Individuals will enact roles based on their own knowledge, the modeling they have observed, and the social structure within which the role is situated. There is always some liberty or flexibility in role enactment, but this can vary quite dramatically from situation to situation. One ingredient of success will be how accurately you can estimate these degrees of freedom.

Successful role transition includes identifying with the right group, interpreting their expectations accurately, negotiating to the extent that is possible while maintaining your unique identity, and merging with the group on terms that are mutually acceptable. This is the best of worlds. In less perfect situations, you have parties that refuse to tolerate any variance; individuals who are unable to "read" the expectations accurately or refuse to become fully involved. The latter situation has been labeled the "marginal man" syndrome.[3] This is the nurse who hangs on the periphery of a system, never quite becoming part of it or bothering to know the personalities involved and refusing to assimilate nursing with the other aspects of their life. This is particularly common in women who try to juggle multiple aspects of life, keeping each separate…obligations everywhere, multiple lists of things to do, each with a first-place priority, a comprehensive plan nowhere. The wiser strategy is to integrate the dimensions of your life, professional colleagues becoming personal friends, family participating in workplace and professional events, and so on (one list with one rank ordering of priorities).

For all but a few graduates, the first job is as an employee in some bureaucratic setting, the antithesis of professionalism. For instance, a bureaucracy has specialized roles and tasks; professionals have specialized competence with an intellectual component. The bureaucracy is organized into a hierarchical authority structure; professionals expect extensive autonomy in exercising their special competence. The bureaucracy's orientation is toward rational, efficient implementation of specific goals and tends toward impersonality; professionals have influence and responsibility in the use of their specialized competence and make decisions governed by internalized standards.[4] On these differences alone, and there are others, professionals in a bureaucracy find themselves in conflict.

Kramer, in an extensive longitudinal study that is still relevant after 20 years, has identified the problems of new graduates in establishing their roles in the midst of bureaucratic-professional conflict, and has termed it *reality shock*, "the specific shocklike reactions of new workers when they find themselves in a work situation for which they have spent several years preparing and for which they thought they were going to be prepared, and then suddenly find that they are not."[5] The phenomenon is seen as different from but related to both culture shock and future shock.

Thus, when the new nurse, who has been in the work setting but not of it, embarks on the first professional work experience, there is not an easy adaptation of previously learned attitudes and behaviors, but the necessity for an entirely new socialization to practice and simultaneous resolution of conflict with the bureaucracy. Kramer describes the steps as follows:

1. Skills and routine mastery: The expectations are those of the employment setting. A major value is competent, efficient delivery of procedures and techniques to clients, not necessarily including psychological support. New graduates immediately concentrate on skill and routine mastery.
2. Social integration: getting along with the group; being taught by them how to work and behave; the "backstage" reality behaviors. If individuals stay at stage one, they may not be perceived as competent peers; if they try to incorporate some of the professional concepts brought over from the educational setting and adhere to those values, the group may be alienated.
3. Moral outrage: With the incongruencies identified and labeled, new graduates feel angry and betrayed by both their teachers and their employers. They weren't told how it would be and they aren't allowed to practice as they were taught.
4. Conflict resolution: The graduates may and do change their behavior, but maintain their values, or change both values and behaviors to match the work setting; or change neither values nor behavior; or work out a relationship that allows them to keep their values, but begin to integrate them into the new setting.[6]

The individuals who make the first choice have selected what is called *behavioral capitulation*. They may be the group with potential for making change, but they simply slide into the bureaucratic mold, or more likely they withdraw from nursing practice altogether. Those who choose bureaucracy (*value capitulation*), may either become "rutters" (staying in a rut), with an "it's a job" attitude, or they may eventually reject the values of both. Others become organization men and women, who move rapidly into the administrative ranks and totally absorb the bureaucratic values. Those who will change neither values nor behavior, what might be called "going it alone," either seek to practice where professional values are accepted or try the "academic lateral arabesque" (also used by the first group), going on to advanced education with the hope of new horizons or escape. The most desirable choice, says Kramer, is *biculturalism*.

> In this approach the nurse has learned that she possesses a value orientation that is perhaps different from the dominant one in the work organization, but that she has the responsibility to listen to and seek out the ideas of others as resource material in effecting a viable integration of both value systems. She has learned that she is not just a target of influence and pressure from others, but that she is in a reciprocal relationship with others and has the right and responsibility to attempt to influence them and to direct their influence attempts on her. She has learned a basic posture of interdependence with respect to the conflicting value systems.[7]

Even though complicated by bureaucratic-professional conflict, our original paradigm for socialization is visible in biculturalism.

New graduates do indeed go through variations of the reality shock experience. That there was little change in the adjustment process for decades can be seen by reviewing journals in the interim and by the nomadic patterns of nursing that must reflect deep-seated job dissatisfaction. Turnover may be a response to boredom, lack of involvement, and apathy and trace its origin to incomplete socialization.

It is interesting that the shortage of the 1980s and subsequent workplace enrichment programs greatly enhanced the retention of nurses. Those enrichments most commonly took the form of strategies to professionalize the workplace, and presumably decrease the bureaucratic-professional conflict:

- Clinical ladders to recognize competence in direct care positions
- Peer review
- Shared governance and participatory management
- Increased practice autonomy
- Decentralization of operations
- Integrated documentation systems

The realities of the workplace, albeit generally a bureaucracy, could certainly be softened if faculty were to bring more of these insights to their students, or if students had more chances for "rehearsal." The following deserve consideration:

- A synthesis semester at the end of the educational experience that incorporates, as far as legally possible, all the ingredients of full-time employment
- Work-study programs that alternate semesters with work placements in your anticipated field
- A curriculum that progresses toward more independence and personal accountability with students and faculty moving to a collegial relationship, as opposed to superiors and subordinates[8]
- Service-education partnerships with faculty teaching students on their own panels of patients[9]

- Summer externships, and new graduate internships or residencies[10]
- Patient areas exclusively dedicated to the clinical learning needs of students
- Assignment of each student to a staff nurse
- Preceptor or "buddy" systems involving more advanced students as well as agency staff (see Chaps. 12 and 15)

Even with the most smoothly negotiated transition, reality finds most nurses as employees in large, complex bureaucracies. And the role of nursing becomes more complex as the system of caring increases in size and sophistication, and as nursing becomes more prominent. One should never lose sight of the fact that systems (large, small, simple, complex) exist to secure their goals and preserve their values. They accomplish this through responding to changing conditions, achieving solidarity among their parts, a division of labor to accomplish work, controlling the environment, maintaining order, and the efficient use of resources. Efficiency has caused a move to accomplish many things through ad hocracy, systems established for a very limited goal and then disbanded. Specialization is another rational response to a highly complex world. Subcontracting as opposed to the creation of internal departments allows greater flexibility to adjust to change. The nursing role will be forced to readjust to maintain organizational stability, so resocialization becomes a continuing process.

STRESS AND STRAIN: THE PERSISTING OCCUPATIONAL HAZARD

Stress and strain are synonymous with nursing, stress being the factors external to you and strain being those internal feelings of frustration and tension. Sometimes stress creates strain. Some individuals have the capacity to tolerate stressful conditions, putting them in perspective. In other instances strain is internally triggered and the search for external blame is fruitless. There are endless experts who can tell you how to deal with these frustrations and tensions. From Selye,[11] the father of the concept of stress, to Peplau,[12] the pioneer of psychiatric nursing, to Kobasa, who introduced the descriptor of "hardiness" to explain why some people rise above it all,[13] interpretations vary. In summary, there is little predictability about who will respond negatively to stressful situations, but group cohesiveness or interpersonal support seem to have a positive effect. This has been noticed in comparing emergency nurses (high-stress environment) to other staff nurses.[14] The only available responses are to fight (and you never win), run, let the tension take its toll on you physically, or use the opportunity to learn more about yourself and cope productively.

Stress and strain are predictable in situations that include ambiguity, incongruity, conflict, under- and overload and where the role occupants see themselves as under- or overqualified.[15] Ambiguity usually relates to a lack of structure and clarity. Incongruity stems from a poor fit between the person's abilities and their expectations or the expectations of the systems they interface with. Role conflict indicates contradictions within the role behaviors themselves. The staff nurse feels an obligation to provide quality care, but then finds it impossible to achieve satisfactory outcomes within the limits of a predetermined length of stay. Over- and underload often require a more objective opinion. Being over- or underqualified moves us into areas of competence. Some individuals may consider themselves overqualified because they never strain to see the complexities of a situation. Peer discussion of such clinical situations is helpful to verify your opinion of yourself. Feelings of being underqualified must be talked through and validated, or they result in living the life of an "imposter."[16]

The stress and strain that come with most of the service occupations are labeled codependency or burn-out in the literature. In codependency, a person controls through the assurance that he or she is needed, and works to keep things that way. "Unable to determine who owns a problem, they become angry and intolerant. The natural impulse to feel for their patients and occasionally bring home their frustrations is played out with exaggeration, and eventually rejected. Where once they felt too much, they now feel too little in defense of their ego. The result is poor judgment, insensitivity and burnout."[17] The codependent personality is particularly at high risk for burnout, which results in poor judgment, insensitivity, negativism, and the severe loss of self-esteem as one's clinical competence is questioned.[18]

There's no one prescription for coming to terms with an unmanageable personal or professional life. The problems are relative to the personality of the afflicted, and solutions must be individualized. "The ultimate goal is to establish control and identity that is driven by internal strength" rather than being captive to the volatility of the environment. Given that your best investment is in self-care, consider:[19]

- Learn to use distance therapeutically. Allow people to fail and learn from their own mistakes. Find a comfortable and private place to retreat to when you are stressed. If you can't physically distance yourself, try meditation techniques.
- Decide who owns a problem. If you don't own it, you have no obligation to fix it, especially if it requires self-sacrifice.
- Examine the quality of the peer support you give and get, and correct the situation if needed. Sometimes support systems become habits as opposed to helps.
- Invest in upgrading yourself. Expose yourself to new experiences; learn new skills. Plan your self-care as seriously as you plan your patient care.
- Consciously schedule routine tasks, and those requiring physical exertion as a break from complex and stressful activities.
- Learn to trust your instincts. Every problem does not have a rational and logical solution. Sometimes think in terms of what could be the worst consequence.
- Identify one person who would be willing to serve as your objective sounding board.

This may be one way to find out how you come across to people.

- Make contact with your feelings about situations. Feelings are neither good nor bad; they just are.
- Create options for yourself. Identify those circumstances that you need to personally control, those that are just as well controlled for you, and those that you choose to wait out.

THE WORKPLACE: RIGHTS AND HAZARDS

The prevailing theme of this chapter has been successful career management through personal control. Aspects of that control were to understand how you move toward acceptable and satisfying role enactment, and how you deal with stress and strain while protecting a personality that may be naturally vulnerable. An additional dimension of control is to know your rights and responsibilities as an employee—and to confront the hazardous conditions that will affect your work life from start to finish as a nurse. You have protections under the law, and other quasi-legal guarantees that are included in personnel policies (employee handbooks, personnel policy manuals). Even though you may have nothing in writing, an expressed contract takes shape as you discuss the terms and conditions of your employment.

A comprehensive overview of workplace rights would include issues of minimum wage, unemployment and disability, workmen's compensation, family leave, continuing health benefits after termination of employment, discrimination, job safety, pensions, unfair labor practices, and collective bargaining. The growing number of workplace concerns addressed through legislation and the courts is one circumstance that has contributed to the general decline in unionization. Unions appeared on the American scene when there were few legal workplace protections. Today's growing governmental involvement in professional practice, the workplace and health care facilities makes it important to understand the interrelationships between administrative codes or regulations, employment law, and practice acts. When is the RN acting as an agent of the employer versus as an autonomous professional? If administrative codes allow nurses professional staff privileges in a hospital, can a specific facility deny this status? The degrees of complexity are endless, but you have the right to answers to any questions.

Given the broad range of issues, and the degree to which they multiply once they are interrelated, the focus here will be on the most common questions:

Can I be fired without reason?

Is it possible to refuse an assignment?

What protections do I have against discrimination?

Do I have a right to withhold information about myself from an employer?

What are the most prevailing workplace hazards and what is the employer's responsibility?

Are there laws that guarantee fringe benefits including health insurance, pension, and family leave?

Are there any protections for whistle-blowing?

Most employment relationships are not protected by any formal contract and are for an indefinite period of time. Such an arrangement is termed *employment-at-will*, and the relationship may be terminated by either the employee or employer at any time, with cause or for no cause at all. A growing number of court decisions in such situations have recognized employee handbooks and a variety of other internal employer-generated documents as having a quasi-legal status. Thus, where an at-will dismissal violates one of these policies, the employer could be held liable. Above and beyond this presumed contractual protection, a number of states are moving forward to protect at-will employees through legislation.[20]

Simply put, no employer is justified in an arbitrary and capricious dismissal of an employee. It is important to note what circumstances will cause an episode of dismissal to be found in favor of the employee if the situation goes to grievance, arbitration, or court. The most common conditions for a successful appeal on the employee's behalf are:[21]

The charges for the termination are not proved.

The severity of the consequence is inappropriate to the charge.

The reason for dismissal is unrelated to job performance.

Proper or customary disciplinary procedures were not used.

Most dismissals come as a result of growing dissatisfaction between employee and employer, not a single episode. The situation should have produced documentation, and a series of warnings, written notices, attempts to counsel, and so on. For more detail on the proper handling of grievances, refer to ANA's *Survival Skills in the Workplace.*

Is it possible to refuse an assignment? That is not an idle question today as we deal with clinical situations that may be contrary to our personal conscience, hazardous, or require our participation in circumstances that are potentially unsafe for patients. This last situation is particularly common with reduced staffing and the substitution of less prepared personnel in order to cut costs.

Nursing administration has the right to assign you where needed (providing you don't have a written contract that says otherwise), but they also have the responsibility of *appropriately* assigning duties.[22] Some nurses' associations have now negotiated contracts to prevent inappropriate assignment or compulsory overtime. Others have developed a form that says, in essence, that in the nurse's professional judgment, the current assignment is unsafe and places the patients at risk, but that it will be carried out under protest. The form documents the assignment, number,

and condition of patients and number and type of staff. The legality of this process has not yet been tested, and there are some other concerns. If a nurse has stated that an assignment is unsafe and then takes it, she or he is vulnerable in case of a later negligence suit. And, of course, the use of the form can be abused.

When refusing an assignment, however, one of the dangers is being accused of abandoning your patients. Just what that means in any specific case is not clear, but it could result in the loss of your license. On the other hand, supervisors use the term loosely to frighten the nurse into staying on the job. You should discuss the inappropriate assignment with the supervisor, putting her or him on notice about your limitations; to identify your options (sharing or trading the assignment); and to document the situation.[23] In the end, it is your decision, and not an easy one, but almost inevitable in many institutions. It's best to think it through ahead of time.

Whether you can safely refuse an assignment in other circumstances is not clear. Employers are usually required to offer an alternate position if the refusal is on the basis of a conscience clause. However, if you refuse that assignment, you have little recourse. One situation that has been gaining attention is fair treatment for nurses who cannot work on certain days for religious reasons. As might be expected, rulings have differed, but in 1985, the U.S. Supreme Court ruled that there was no constitutional right involved; that in fact it was unconstitutional for a state to legislate an unqualified right not to work on the Sabbath. From a practical point of view, the nurse may be willing to accept alternatives, such as working other holidays or weekend days.

Whistle-blowing remains a very difficult moral choice for nurses. "Whistleblowers are employees who disclose information about an agency's violation of a law, rule or regulation; mismanagement; gross waste of funds; abuse of authority; or a substantial and specific danger to the public health or safety."[24] The range of situations for whistle-blowing is obviously broad, and in many situations the protections are few.

The whistle-blower is restricted from disclosing information that is classified. It is critical to have your facts straight. Since whistle-blowers must often proceed on good faith, every effort should be made to verify the correctness of information. Since 1981, twenty states have passed legislation to protect whistle-blowers. Most of these protections are for public employees, but ten states extend this protection to the private sector. On several occasions in the 1980s and 1990s, bills had been introduced in the Congress to preempt state laws and provide mandatory protection where no state laws apply. In 1988, a California nurse was awarded a significant cash settlement for damages incurred when she was dismissed for reporting what she considered to be an unethical termination of respiratory and nutritional support of a comatose patient. This case had a strong influence on policy development for "termination of treatment." (See also Chap. 10.)

A host of *discriminatory areas* could be involved in your workplace relations. Besides the protections for race and ethnicity, gender and age are of particular interest in nursing. The discrimination against male nurses continues, especially in obstetric practice. Commentary on several cases is included in the April 1994 *American Nurse*. The U.S. District Court in Arkansas gave the opinion that "The fact that the plaintiff is a health care professional does not eliminate the fact that he is an unelected individual who is intruding on the obstetrical patient's right to privacy. The male nurse's situation is not analogous to that of the male doctor who has been selected by the patient."[25]

There has been significant progress through federal and state laws that protect against age discrimination in the workplace. Some laws have no upper limits; others specify protection until a certain age, perhaps 65, 70, or 75. Effective in 1994, the Age Discrimination in Employment Act of 1967 covers those who work in academia, including nurse faculty (academics were excluded before 1994). The burden of proof in age discrimination is often difficult, and nurses should be vigilant, as there is a growing trend to cut back on the numbers of nurses on staff. A typical case is reported from California where the courts awarded damages to two nurses who sued on the basis of age discrimination. These nurses, 59 and 60, respectively, were 30-year employees of the same hospital. Each had been publicly recognized for the quality of her practice. When a clinical ladder was put in place, they consciously decided to remain at a lower level of the clinical nurse category. After being told that it was mandatory for them to participate in a career advancement program and qualify for a higher status, they were both dismissed on grounds of the inability to demonstrate the competencies for the new level. Both of these nurses are now successfully employed elsewhere.[26] There is fear that these will no longer be isolated cases in nursing. This becomes an especially significant issue with the "aging" of nurses described in Chaps. 11 and 13.

The Americans with Disabilities Act of 1990 extends protection in employment to individuals with HIV/AIDS, and also to people who are regarded to be infected, or in close association with persons with HIV/AIDS. The issues of the *HIV-infected nurse* and the workplace go beyond class protection and must be detailed. The ANA has assumed the leadership role for over a decade in providing policy direction to nurses and other health care professionals in dealing with HIV/AIDS. The ANA's 1994 publication *Nursing and HIV/AIDS* is a state-of-the-art resource. Nursing's continuous presence on the health care scene and commitment to comprehensive care created the need for ANA to speak out early and loudly in the course of this pandemic.

ANA opposes perpetuation of the myth that mandatory testing and mandatory disclosure of the HIV status of patients and/or nurses is a method of preventing the transmission of HIV disease, and therefore does not advocate mandatory testing or mandatory disclosure of HIV status. ANA supports the availability of voluntary anonymous or confidential HIV testing that is conducted with informed consent, and pre- and posttest counseling. ANA continues to support education regarding the transmission of HIV/AIDS,

and the use and monitoring of universal precautions to prevent HIV/AIDS transmission.[27]

In every situation, the nurse's first concern is the protection of the patient. Therefore, the following policy provides direction for the HIV-infected nurse:[28]

> Nurses who know they have a transmissible bloodborne infection should voluntarily avoid exposure-prone invasive procedures that have been epidemiologically linked to HIV or other bloodborne infection transmission. The nurse has a duty to report exposure of a patient to bloodborne infection. Support and protection of the nurse with a seropositive status has been a long-standing position of ANA. The association supports the confidentiality of all information about the HIV-infected nurse.

An additional dimension of the HIV-infected health care provider issue involves offers of employment. An employer may require a physical examination, including serology with HIV testing, once a conditional promise of employment has been made, but not before the promise of employment. If the anticipated employee tests HIV positive, the offer may not be withdrawn based on the positive status unless the results indicate that the employee is not qualified to perform the essential job functions. The results must be kept strictly confidential.[29] There can often be a narrow line of interpretation here, and the possibility of frequent abuse. Some states are expanding their civil rights acts to prohibit employers from requiring HIV testing. Again, state-specific inquiries are in order.

The converse of patient exposure to the HIV-infected provider is the risk of infection to the provider from the patient. This risk has been compounded by the significant incidence of tuberculosis in HIV-infected individuals. The cutback in public health funds to allow proper follow-up of TB patients, and the presence of HIV-infected individuals with compromised immune systems and frequent drug therapy has resulted in the development of *multidrug-resistant strains of TB (MDR-TB)*.

MDR-TB and HIV/AIDS have increased our awareness of workplace hazards. Nurses have

for the most part accepted the inherent risk that comes with their practice. However, recent years have prompted a new philosophy that places a high value on their own physical and psychological well-being.

The obligation of the employer is to provide environmental safety, work practice controls, and personal protective equipment to minimize or prevent exposure, and postexposure programs including counseling. The Center for Disease Control and Prevention has developed guidelines for the management of health care workers following occupational exposure to HIV. A program would include information, immediate evaluation, prophylactic intervention, counseling, and supportive care. The nurse who seroconverts should be guaranteed workers' compensation and continued health insurance coverage. Workmen's compensation still presents difficulty due to probable underreporting and the burden of proving occupational transmission. Some occupational groups such as firefighters and coal miners have been successful in legislation that assumes occupational transmission for certain conditions and places the burden of proof on the employer to prove that the condition is not work-related.[30] The important observations for the new employee are what policies exist for postexposure management and whether adequate precautions are in place to reduce the risk of exposure. MDR-TB prevention requires "a high index of suspicion for TB and early recognition of symptoms which may trigger the need for respiratory precautions.... All efforts boil down to containing the infectious agent from becoming airborne."[31] When this is impossible, most facilities are using "disposable particulate respirators that fit snugly around the face."[32]

For the protection of both patients and workers against transmission from one another, universal precautions should be used when dealing with blood and other body fluids including semen, vaginal secretions, cerebrospinal fluid, and synovial fluid, among others. The precautions include guidelines for handling sharps and laboratory specimens, use of gloves and gowns, hand washing, protective eyewear, disposal of linen, resuscitation procedures, and care of reusable equipment. As of 1993, the CDC had received reports of only 37 documented cases of HIV infection acquired through occupational transmission, and 13 were nurses.[33]

Ergonomic hazards, though less dramatic, are job and process design problems that are common and harmful. Examples are improper work methods and inadequate work and rest patterns or repetitive tasks that result in back injuries, carpotunnel syndrome, and stress disorders. *Toxic substances*, most particularly chemotherapeutic agents, are frequently handled by nurses, and cautions should be posted and personal protective equipment provided.

Violence has been a constant threat to nursing in the workplace. Incidents have rarely been reported because of the poor public image it would create for the health care facility. Currently caught in violent times, the incidence of workplace violence is increasing. Weapons that are easy to obtain, deinstitutionalized chronically mentally ill, substance abuse, and a generally angry underclass all contribute to an increasing danger of violence and assault. In Los Angeles, 25 percent of trauma patients were found to be carrying lethal weapons. Assaults on inpatient units account for 13 percent of incidents in hospitals.[34] A comprehensive review of the literature identified the following factors to be associated with assault in the health care workplace:[35]

- Inexperienced health care workers are at increased risk of assault.
- The largest number of injuries occur while attempting to contain patient violence.
- Short staffing and temporary staffing have been associated with increased assaults.
- Assaults seem to occur during times of high activity and high emotion on patient units.

The presence of policies that show sensitivity to these factors is necessary, as is the establishment of peer assistance and postassault assistance programs in environments where the incidence of violence is high.

Fringe benefits and pension are of growing importance to nurses. Although most employers provide fringe benefit packages, there is no federal or state requirement, with the exception of employer contributions to Social Security, workers compensation, and unemployment insurance. However, there are a number of legislative protections that the employee should be aware of. The Family Leave Bill of 1993 requires that employees be allowed a time limited period for a new baby, adoption, or to care for a disabled family member. You are assured the right to return to a position comparable with the one you left, and your health benefits must be continued for the period of the leave. In a similar fashion, you are given the right to personally pay for the continuation of your health insurance for up to 36 months after you leave a job (see also Chap. 19). Over the years, pensions have also increased in their protections for the worker. Benefit plans, including pensions, must satisfy nondiscriminatory requirements, treating men and women equitably. Pension benefits have mandatory vesting schedules, guaranteeing 100 percent nonforfeiture of accrued benefits after five years of service, or the option to phase in 100 percent vesting over three to seven years. In short, no benefits or pensions are guaranteed with the exception of Social Security, but where these fringes are provided there are increasing protections.

Ideally there should be a written employment contract that follows a more or less standard form and details conditions of employment such as salary, vacation, sick leave, holidays, social security coverage, pension, and duration of the contract. More usually, these things are shared verbally, and may be found written in personnel policies. For more detail on employment contracts refer to Chap. 22 of the sixth edition of *Dimensions*.

Collective Bargaining: The Process and the Issues

Some employment issues are resolved by collective bargaining. The process of collective bargaining, because it is set by law, is similar regardless of who the bargaining agent is, and details can be found in any book on labor relations. In the context of state nurses' associations (SNAs) as collective bargaining agents, the following is presented as a brief overview.

1. The nurses (or group of nurses) in an institution, discontented with a situation or conditions, and having exhausted the usual channels for correction or improvement, ask the SNA for assistance.

2. A meeting is held outside the premises of the institution and always on off-duty time. SNA staff and the nurses explore the problems, and the nurses are given advice about reasonable, negotiable issues and how to form a unit; for instance, they are told who can be included in a unit. Administrative nurses are excluded, but the question of supervisors is still being debated in some places.

3. Authorization cards, which authorize the SNA to act as the nurses' bargaining representative, must be signed by at least 30 percent of the group to be represented. Membership forms are also suggested because the SNA cannot provide service without funds. All collective bargaining activity must be carried out in nonwork areas where the employee is protected from employer interference. (There are a series of NLRB rules governing employee distribution and solicitation.)

4. If sufficient cards are signed, the SNA notifies the employer that an organizing campaign is in process, calling attention to the fact that the activity is protected. Copies of the notice are distributed to the nurses so that they know they are protected.

5. An informational meeting is held for all nurses and SNA staff.

6. If it is agreed that the SNA will represent the nurses, a bargaining unit is formed and officers are elected.

7. To seek voluntary recognition of the unit by the employer, a majority of the nurses must sign designation cards; this will probably be checked by a mutually accepted third party.

8. If the employer chooses not to recognize the unit, or if the designation is challenged by another union, a series of actions takes place, including an NLRB-conducted election. To petition for election, any union must have designation cards signed by 30 percent of the nurses in the proposed unit. The election is won or lost by the majority of nurses *voting*. They may vote for a particular union or specify none at all. The NLRB then certifies the winner as the exclusive bargaining agent. If the majority of nurses vote against *any* bargaining agent, the NLRB certifies this as well.

9. Assuming that the SNA wins the election, the SNA representative, at the direction of the unit, attempts to settle the problems and complaints of the nurses by negotiating with administration. There are specific rules about what is negotiable. *Mandatory* subjects include salaries, fringe benefits, and conditions of employment, and both sides must bargain in good faith about these issues. *Voluntary* subjects can be almost anything else that both sides want to discuss, except for *prohibited* or illegal subjects such as a requirement that all workers become members of a union before being employed for thirty days. It should be remembered that the nurse executive, both through position and under law, is an administrator. Even though the person might be in complete support of the nurses' demands, he or she cannot join them. Quite often the director has previously tried unsuccessfully to help them achieve their goals.

10. An agreement may or may not be reached, probably with some compromise on both sides. If there is agreement, a contract is voted on and signed outlining agreed-upon conditions and the responsibilities of each group. Contracts are rene-

gotiated at set time periods, usually of several years. If no agreement can be reached, the dispute may be referred to binding or nonbinding arbitration by an outside group, or some job action such as picketing or a strike may occur. Picketing may be merely informational, to communicate the issues to the community, or it may be intended to prevent other employees or services from entering the institution. The latter, combined with a strike, is the very last resort, to be used when all other efforts fail. If such action is decided upon, sufficient notice is given to allow for disposition of patient care. Even if strikes are successful, there is often a lingering, unpleasant feeling between participants and nonparticipants. However, as ANA members agreed as they gradually removed no-strike clauses from ANA and SNA policies, the strike is an ultimate weapon that may be necessary when the employer refuses any attempt to resolve the issues.

Once a labor contract is in place, there are times when individual nurses are in dispute with the employer. A grievance procedure is generally used to resolve the problem. A grievance may be caused by "an alleged violation of a contract provision, a change in a past practice, or an employer decision that is considered arbitrary, capricious, unreasonable, unfair, or discriminatory." Simple complaints are not considered grievances. If informed discussion does not resolve the issue, a grievance procedure is followed. The steps include (1) written notice of the grievance, with a written response within a set time; (2) if the response is not satisfactory, an appeal to the director of nursing follows; (3) the employee, SNA representative, grievance chairman, and/or delegate, director of nursing, and director of personnel meet; (4) if no resolution occurs, the final step is arbitration by a neutral third party selected by both parties involved. The technique for carrying out the process involves interpersonal, adversary, and negotiating skills.

For nurses, the collective bargaining environment has always been covered with landmines. Nurses are predominately salaried professionals. They are consequently concerned with employee-employer issues. These issues were historically settled internal to the workplace, and health care workers were of little interest to traditional trade unions in the heyday of the labor movement. With increasing government control of unions, the declining industry and manufacturing market, and the 1974 repeal of the Tyding Amendments that since 1947 exempted the nonprofit health care industry from the requirements of the National Labor Relations Act (the right to organize for collective bargaining), health care workers were targeted for organizing. See Chap. 19 for more detail on labor legislation. While unionization has declined from a one-time high of over 30 percent of American labor to a current low of less than 15 percent, over 20 percent of health care workers are represented, with a significant increase in the last decade. The largest single constituency in health care is RNs. They have traditionally avoided unionization, but when forced to seek more leverage through collective bargaining, their preferred choice for representation has been the state nurses association (the state affiliate of the ANA). The uniqueness of nurses, their chosen representative, and their practice patterns have given rise to a number of problems, some resolved and others still pending:

- Supervisory domination. In an attempt to thwart organizing activity by the state nurses association, employers have claimed that nurse-managers who hold office in a state nurses association create a situation of management intrusion into the collective bargaining activities of the association. Organizational structure, reporting relationships, and policy-making bodies have been created to insulate union activity while maintaining the program under the aegis of the professional association. The adequacy of these designs has been tested in the courts on a number of occasions.[36] This issue will continue to surface from time to time.

- The RN-only bargaining unit. In April 1991, after a 17-year struggle with the hospital industry and a unanimous U.S. Supreme Court decision, nurses were given the right to organize into bargaining units comprised solely of RNs.[37] The hospital industry found it more strategic to dilute nursing issues by folding them into units with other workers. Beyond a fair wage and benefits package, the issues most compelling to RNs have always been those of patient care. This has not been the priority for other groups of employees. The unique community of interest among RNs was no longer debatable after this decision.

- Nurses as categorical supervisors. The latest potential obstacle to RN organizing surfaces from a U.S. Supreme Court decision of May 1994, and is also discussed in Chap. 25.[38] It has been common to separate RNs as employees from their practice role as professionals wherein they are directly accountable to the patient. More is said about this relationship in Chap. 9. Within this professional role, it is common for the RN to delegate or assign select activities to a nursing assistant while continuing to be personally responsible. Justice Ruth Bader Ginsburg in her minority opinion observes that it is rare that a professional does not occasionally work through someone else. In contrast, the majority opinion (in this case, which involved licensed practical nurses) declared that the nurse was an agent of management in this relationship with subordinates. Though not directly involving RNs and the incident being in a nursing home, still there are serious implications. The RN frequently works with both nursing assistants and environmental support personnel (transport, messengers). The presence of these workers is increasing with restructuring. Legislation may be necessary to set the record straight for the 1990s.

- Human resource techniques building cooperation between labor and management. The last 20 years have been witness to a variety of strategies to encourage employee participation in workplace decisions. They have been called alternately work teams, quality circles, quality of work life committees...and in nursing, shared governance.[39] The old brand of unionism built on adversarial relationships is counterproductive for the 1990s.[40] A large number of American industries and unions have proved this point. In response, the federal government has applauded such initiatives. Meanwhile, those whose thinking is frozen in another generation challenge these collegial efforts as "company unions" and consequently illegal. This is another example of the need for updating of labor law to serve the twenty-first century.[41]

CAREER MAPPING

You have sought the best educational preparation to enter the field of nursing. You have hopefully done so with the intent of building a career. No field offers such variability or such opportunity to advance. Each decision you make can strategically build toward your long-term goal. Additionally, for the professional there is the obligation to remain current, which is no simple task given the rate at which the science of nursing is expanding. Try to dream about where you would like to go professionally, at least in broad terms. Remember the fastest route between two points is a straight line.

Experience Is No Myth

You have already reviewed the process of searching and courting employment in Chap. 29. You have also been counseled to take time for a personal assessment. Identify the route in nursing you would like to take. Given today's complex clinical environment, your competence as a generalist will be short-lived. You will take on the characteristics of a specialized practice area in very short order. Build your career cautiously, laying each brick in a predetermined pattern. It is a valid goal to seek out a position with the patient population that intrigues you most, and resolve to provide the best possible care to those patients, growing through experience and keeping current with a well-planned program of continuing education. It is just as acceptable to have a vision of a lateral move into education, and formal schooling that stretches on for many years, and perhaps many degrees. It is also acceptable to fail, to reconsider and change courses many times. The only thing that is unacceptable is to have no goals at all.

While you are considering your lateral moves and vertical climbs, pay proper respect to the fact that nursing is a practice discipline. You definitely grow in your ability to care as you minister to patients and as you invest hours and years in your art. Experience is not a myth, but one essential ingredient to bring you from novice to expert.[42]

Maintaining Competence

Process is content in the 1990s. Your educational experience is adequate only if it taught you how to think and where to go to find the information you need. Most of the content you currently hold will be outdated in five years. The most established professions have learned that lesson. Case material in law only provides the substance through which to cultivate analytic skills. The activities that constitute your role will be no more stable than your knowledge. During your career lifetime, the activities that are part of your practice will shift. Some will disappear, and others will be delegated by you to lesser prepared individuals. New role functions currently foreign to you will become part of your day-to-day repertoire. Beyond your own personal security and flexibility to move with the times, you need reliable sources of continuing education, and access to information. Besides

what your employer provides on their own behalves to assure your safety and currency, it is your personal obligation to maintain a curiosity and thirst for better ways to nurse.

The term continuing education (CE) has been interpreted many ways. Most agree that it includes any learning activity after the basic educational program. Courses of study or programs leading to an academic degree are separated out. The basic and overriding purpose of CE in nursing is the maintenance of continued competence so that the care of the patient is safe and effective. Continuing education is provided through your employing agency, or you may choose (or the employer may encourage you) to seek outside programs. The variety of continuing education programs is limitless. The secret is to be a discerning consumer and select those which are most immediately valuable to your practice. Continuing education need not be only clinically oriented. You must also remain conversant with current issues in the discipline, and with the thinking of nursing leaders. Employer funding and time off for continuing education is often a workplace benefit. The types of educational experiences that staff are approved to attend are often an indication of how administration views nursing, as a technical or professional field. From another perspective, it provides insights on the staff who will be your peers. The professions have always recognized the fact that learning for practice was lifelong. Florence Nightingale was eloquent on the subject:

> Nursing is a progressive art, in which to stand still is to go back. A woman who thinks to herself, "Now I am a full nurse, a skilled nurse, I have learnt all there is to be learnt"—take my word for it, she does not know what a nurse is, and never will know; she is gone back already. Progress can never end but with a nurse's life.

With CE programs proliferating (and getting more expensive), better give some thought to what is worth spending time and money on. One suggested plan for diagnosing your continuing education needs is to develop a model of required competencies, assessing your practice in relation to the model, and identifying the gaps between your knowledge and skills and those required. Some of this preliminary testing can be done by taking some of the tests in journals, and by carefully evaluating your own practice and getting feedback from peers and supervisors as well.

Other methods of CE learning, besides formal classes or conferences, are well worth investigating, although, of course, there is often the added value of interaction with other nurses in group activities. Many nursing journals offer monthly self-study programs.

Another aspect of maintaining competence is the ability to locate the information you need for your practice, and access those information sources. Your educational program should have prepared you to find the information you need, and impressed on you that you are responsible for the changing standard of practice. In some situations, physicians are being held liable for not conducting literature searches when appropriate; nurses may be similarly at risk (and in fact will be, as our salaries increase and our services grow in prominence).

You will find your most updated indexes of the nursing and allied health literature in computerized databases (of course, print versions do exist also). With the technical aspects of reviewing the literature computerized, searching becomes a highly exciting learning experience, and librarians, health care professionals, and students increasingly conduct computerized literature searches. Librarians use search software that requires extensive training and background; students and health professionals search using easy-to-learn, menu-driven software.

How are searches run on databases from a microcomputer? Through a *modem*, a device that communicates through phone lines, searchers are connected to mainframe computers of database vendors and producers. In some institutions, database tapes are leased and mounted locally for campus use. Other institutions purchase databases on small compact discs, called CD-ROM (Compact Disc-Read Only Mem-

ory). These laser discs are "read" by a compact disc drive connected to a microcomputer.

The indexes and databases most commonly used in nursing are the *Cumulative Index to Nursing and Allied Health Literature* (CINAHL), the *International Nursing Index* (INI), *Index Medicus*, and MEDLINE. Known as the "Red Books," CINAHL is found in most libraries serving nurses. Published by the Glendale Adventist Medical Center in Glendale, California, it provides subject/author access to the English-language nursing journal literature from 1956 to date. It also includes pertinent articles from the biomedical, education, behavioral sciences, management, and popular literature. Since 1977, many allied health journals are included. New books as well as dissertations in nursing and related fields are also indexed. Students and graduate nurses find the publications of the American Nurses' Association and the National League for Nursing extremely valuable; they are indexed by CINAHL as well as by the *International Nursing Index* (see below).

CINAHL indexing from 1983 to the present is available electronically as an online database and on CD-ROM. In these formats, abstracts from many of the journal articles are also available. The online database is updated monthly, the CD-ROM every 2 months.

As noted earlier, INI is published by the American Journal of Nursing Company in cooperation with the National Library of Medicine (NLM), a federal agency. All of the citations appearing in INI are part of MEDLINE, the massive, world-renowned biomedical database produced by NLM and updated twice a month. Some 360,000 citations from 3,500 journals are added each year to MEDLINE. A selected number of nursing journals appear in *Index Medicus*, its print counterpart.

Although an excellent source for general bio-medical information, MEDLINE is not as efficient as CINAHL for retrieving nursing literature. However, because it is federally supported, MEDLINE is extremely inexpensive and is widely available in online, locally mounted, and CD-ROM formats. An advantage for the researcher is that it contains data as far back as 1966.

NLM provides access to a number of related databases of interest to nurses. Among some 30 NLM databases are AIDSLINE, which consists of citations on acquired immunodeficiency syndrome; BIOETHICSLINE, a database containing citations covering ethics and public policy in health care and biomedical research; several cancer databases; DIRLINE, a directory of organizations; and HEALTH, a database developed in cooperation with the American Hospital Association on nonclinical aspects of health care delivery.

For nurses, the institution's library can serve as an important vehicle for keeping up with changes in health care and in a particular specialty. In addition to literature searches, the library offers valuable services for staying current. These include:

- Table-of-Contents Service: On a regular basis, the library routes the table-of-contents page from a number of just-published journals in the nurse's field of interest. After scanning the titles of the articles, the nurse checks the ones of particular interest. The library then photocopies the articles and routes them to the nurse. This invaluable service saves health care professionals hours of time and enables them to keep up with the latest trends.
- SDI-line: Known as a Selective Dissemination of Information, the SDI-line is another way to keep up with what's being published on a number of topics. The librarian prepares a profile of the clinician's main interests. This information is provided to a database vendor, and every time a particular database, e.g., MEDLINE or NURSING & ALLIED HEALTH (CINAHL), is updated, a printout is produced of citations to just-published articles on the profiled topics.
- Scanning tools: A number of publications specialize in scanning the literature in spe-

cific fields, e.g., women's health issues, nursing research. Abstracting services are also available. These publications can be purchased by the library to keep staff updated.
- End-user searching: In some situations, the nurse may want to search the literature directly. The library may offer these services directly or will be able to recommend particular vendors.
- Services to obtain literature relating to patient care: It is possible for the library to provide the nursing unit with copies of articles on specific patient diagnoses or on clinical problems.
- Borrowing or purchasing books and other materials: The library can usually borrow books from nearby libraries. Although the library may follow standard guidelines in purchasing materials (such as the widely accepted Brandon-Hill lists), the staff usually welcomes recommendations for adding books, journals, audiovisuals, software, and other materials to the collection to assist staff.

To find what services are available, the nurse's first step is to contact the librarian. To continue benefiting from these services, professionals need to maintain regular contact with the library and to prove use of the materials once they have been provided. In today's era of budget cuts, administrative decision makers need to understand that access to research findings and current information is necessary in order to maintain high-quality, cost-effective care. The nurse can provide much-needed documentation of the library's role as a vital disseminator of clinical information.

Formal Higher Education

Besides participating in CE programs, the graduate of a diploma or associate degree program may want to give serious consideration to formal education leading to a baccalaureate degree, and the nurse with a baccalaureate degree may want to think about getting a master's.

There is no question but that educational standards for all positions in nursing are growing steadily higher. If you really want to advance professionally to positions of greater scope and challenge, you will, in the very near future, need at least a baccalaureate degree. The process of obtaining this and higher degrees not only will serve you well professionally but will add considerably to the enrichment of your personal life and interests. In fact, these are the reasons given most by nurses.

Although it would be difficult to denigrate the value of any good-quality educational program, give some thought to your future goals. The joy of exploring new fields and studying whatever you wish without the pressure of time or the need to fulfill requirements for a program may be especially tempting. If these interests are in any of the liberal arts or the social or physical sciences, which may be required, or can be used as electives in many programs, a dual purpose will be accomplished in that you are also started toward a degree.

Because baccalaureate programs with a nursing major have not always been available (or affordable) to nurses in a particular geographic area, a number of programs have sprung up offering a degree in nursing or another field, giving credit for the lower-division nursing courses and offering no upper-division nursing courses. Evaluate them in relation to your career goals. These program is *not* usually acceptable for future graduate studies in nursing, and you may not be able to enroll in a graduate program without having taken upper-division nursing courses. Some nurses have found it necessary to complete a second baccalaureate program, this time with a nursing major, in order to continue into a master's program.

As noted in Chap. 12, RNs will find that they receive varying amounts of recognition or credit for their basic nursing courses, and may perhaps need to take challenge examinations. Nursing baccalaureate programs vary a great deal in this respect, but more and more nursing programs are offering some form of educational articulation, self-pacing, or other means of giving credit for previous knowledge, skill, and ability such as the external degree. There are also a large number of baccalaureate programs that only admit RN students. NLN publications listing baccalaureate, master's, and doctoral programs are helpful.

Many of the same points apply to graduate education. Consider carefully what you want from a program and prepare yourself for this more competitive admission procedure. Some nurses complete graduate programs in the various sciences or education, with or without any nursing input. Again, you must consider your specific career goals. Someone with a nursing major or at least a minor may be given preference in a position requiring a graduate degree, particularly in educational positions. Many state boards of nursing require faculty in basic nursing education programs to have a graduate degree with a major in nursing. Or if you are hired now, there is no guarantee that later, when there are more nurses with graduate nursing degrees, you may not be bypassed for promotion or may be required to take a second graduate degree in nursing in order to hold the current position. These are practical considerations presented here for information. You must still make the educational decisions you wish, but with as complete a knowledge of the pros and cons as possible.

Suppose you simply don't want any degree? Or suppose you enroll in an accredited nursing program but then, in time, drop out? That's your decision. There is no reason why you can't function at an acceptable level of competence, maintaining and improving that competence through CE, thereby making a valuable contribution to the profession and society. If, however, you withdrew because of disappointment or lack of interest in that particular program, it may well be that the program is not congruent with your philosophy. Consider a second try, taking time to determine whether a program's philosophy, objectives, approaches to teaching, and attitudes are what you want. Some of this information can be obtained from the catalog, the faculty or adviser interviews, informal contact with students or *recent* graduates (programs do change). Sometimes, if some courses may be taken without need for full matriculation, a sampling of courses will prove especially informative.

For RNs, going back to school is not easy, particularly if you have a family. One nurse who did it (and has a sense of humor) suggests:

1. Begin the course only if you're 100 percent committed.
2. Prepare yourself financially.
3. Unless you can afford days off without pay, start accumulating vacation days; you may need them for a clinical rotation.
4. If you don't type, learn; there are lots of papers to write.
5. Invest in a computer early; it saves time and effort.
6. Use your hospital library; that saves time, too.
7. Decide before beginning that you don't really need a 4.0 average to be successful; you don't need the extra stress.
8. Enlist the support of your coworkers and manager.
9. Refuse extra assignments at work.
10. Schedule something fun every week.
11. Cross off each week on a calendar.
12. Remind yourself that others completed the course and you can, too.
13. Delegate everything possible to your children.
14. Have regular study times.
15. Give yourself a mental health break by skipping a routine class occasionally.
16. Frequently visualize what you'll feel like when it's over.
17. Nourish yourself physically, spiritually, and socially, enough to feel healthy and supported.
18. When it's over, celebrate with everyone who made your dream come true.[43]

In addition:

19. Create study space for yourself that is comfortable and seclusive.

That's not bad advice for any nontraditional student!

Sources of Financial Aid

The problem of finances is undoubtedly the most common deterrent to advanced education for able professional nurses. First consider whether there are any educational benefits available from your workplace. Tuition reimbursement for most nurses working in acute care is still a reality. Seven in ten full-timers have these benefits, and 53 percent of part-timers, 10 percent more than two years ago. Although the benefit has remained intact, the $1,400 average tuition subsidy has not increased since 1991, meaning that the value has declined.[44] Next, review your financial resources realistically before embarking on this new venture. If you are going to request financial aid, you will need to estimate as accurately as possible your expected income and expenses. Major educational expenses will include tuition, books, educational fees, and perhaps travel. Related personal expenses depend on where and how you live. Economizing may mean enrolling in a community college for the liberal arts and later transferring to a local or state college. Economy should not include enrolling in a poor program. Graduating from a nonaccredited nursing program may create difficulties in advancing to the next higher degree. Not all nonaccredited programs are poor, but this risk does exist.

The major sources of income for a self-supporting graduate nurse in an advanced educational program are savings or other personal resources, part-time work, scholarships, and loans. If you plan to do part-time work while attending college, make reasonably sure that a position is available at a satisfactory salary and that it seems to be professionally suitable, including enough flexibility to make it possible to take courses. Consider also your mental and physical health under this double load. Can you manage?

There are a number of scholarships, fellowships, and loans earmarked for educational purposes for which professional nurses are often eligible if they seek them out and apply. Some sources of financial assistance are well known and used regularly; others are not used simply because people do not know about them. The financial aid officer at the institution where you plan to enroll is an excellent source of information.

In most instances educational scholarships, fellowships, and loans are defined as follows: (1) *scholarship*—a financial grant that does not involve repayment; (2) *fellowship*—a grant for graduate study not requiring repayment; (3) *loan*—a grant for educational purposes to be repaid by the recipient either with or without interest after completion of the course or education. Grants-in-aid are outright grants at both the undergraduate and graduate levels for accomplishment of a specific project. There may also be an outright grant to meet an immediate financial emergency or a grant to a student with a claim to a restricted scholarship fund. The term *traineeship* has also been used in recent years to denote federal grants with stipend and tuition costs, which need not be repaid, awarded to students in nursing programs, under the Nurse Education Act and its legislative successors.

Some funds are available to members of certain organizations or religious denominations or to students who meet other special requirements. Others are offered to any deserving person who has demonstrated such qualities as good character, leadership ability, and academic achievement. In general, scholarships, loans, and grants are available from both private and governmental sources and agencies.

The manner in which you apply for financial assistance may have considerable bearing on whether or not you get it. Correspondence, personal interviews, application forms, and references should all show the same meticulous attention that is given to an application for a new position.[45]

Financial assistance may be found at the local, state, regional, national, or international level. Where you should apply will depend upon how you plan to use the money. For example, some funds are only available for advanced study in certain clinical specialties; others are designed to prepare nurses for teaching, supervisory, or administrative positions; still others have different stipulations; and many are unrestricted as long as the applicant meets the designated personal qualifications.

The National League for Nursing, 350 Hudson Street, New York, NY 10014, sells a publication entitled *Scholarships and Loans for Nursing Education*. It contains a great deal of specific information that may help you decide where to apply first for financial assistance, thus saving valuable time in making applications.

The professional nursing journals frequently carry news items and articles about such funds, which can be found through the annual and cumulative indexes. Most college catalogs also list sources of student financial support. Given here, in more general terms, are some of the possible sources of funds. Some give relatively small amounts of money, but these sums do add up.

Local Sources. Local sources of funds include both professional and civic groups in the nursing school, community, district, and state. The alumni association of a school of nursing often has appropriations for scholarships and loans that are available to graduates of the school. The president of the association or the director of the school will have information about such sources of financial assistance. Some district and state nurses' associations and NLN constituencies have funds for advanced study and other special purposes, either as direct gifts or on a reasonable interest and repayment basis. Some state legislatures have apportioned money to prepare selected professional nurses to work on state health problems and, more rarely, to provide loans and scholarships to nursing (and other) students. The state board of nursing and the operational institutions involved will have information about such appropriations.

Other local sources of funds include chapters of national sororities, fraternities, and clubs whose memberships are not restricted to nurses but offer financial aid to anyone who meets their qualifications. These are churches that have educational funds as do church-affiliated groups; the Elks, Masons, Altrusa Club, American Legion Auxiliary, and other similar organizations; unions; corporations; and private foundations and institutes. Other good sources of information are local or state colleges or universities and the hospital associations. Your place of employment may also offer grants and loans, or pay part or all of the tuition fees.

In some instances, scholarships and loans are available to nurses in a region of the country comprising more than one state. Information about these funds is often carried in some of the previous sources mentioned.

National Sources. In a recent years, professional nurses interested in applying for a national scholarship, fellowship, or loan would, with the assistance of the advanced nursing programs in which they were enrolled, have turned to the federal government. Both general scholarships and loans, as well as some designated especially for RNs, grants, fellowships, and full-time nurse traineeships, have been of increasing and invaluable aid to the RN. Although there are never enough to meet all needs, without them a large majority of RNs could not have completed advanced education. However, beginning in 1973, the federal administration became less interested in providing any financial aid to nurses, and some loans and funds were cut back. Since 1975, funds for nurse traineeships have been progressively cut. Loans and special scholarships for service in underserved areas continue to be available, but there are predictions that federal money for all health professions will gradually dry up. Much depends on the amount of pressure put on Congress to legislate funds. Such congressional action appears to fluctuate from year to year but has been leaning in the direction of fewer and more restricted funds.

The Nurses' Educational Funds, Inc. (NEF), was established in 1954 to honor nursing pioneers. It was initiated largely through the efforts of NLN, which saw the need for centralized administration of the three separate educational allocations for nurses that existed at that time: the Isabel Hampton Robb Memorial Fund, the Isabel McIsaac Loan Fund, and the Nurses' Scholarship and Fellowship Fund. Since then, other funds have been initiated and turned over to NEF for administration. Many of the awards given are in the names of nurses who contributed greatly to the nursing profession. NEF is an independent organization that grants and administers scholarships and fellowships to RNs for post-RN study. It is governed by a board of trustees, mainly leaders in nursing education, and supported by contributions from business corporations, foundations, nurses, and persons interested in nursing.

Application forms and information about the necessary qualifications of applicants can be obtained from Nurses' Educational Funds, 555 W. 57th Street, New York, NY 10019.

Financial aid is also available from the National Student Nurses' Association (see Chap. 24), miscellaneous private foundations, and some health organizations that may give financial assistance to nurses for advanced work in that organization's major area of interest. In addition, the armed services and the Veterans Administration subsidize the advanced education of some nurses (see Chap. 15).

International Sources. The national nursing organizations may be able to supply information about scholarships, fellowships, and loans, accessible to RNs who wish to study abroad. It would be well to contact these organizations first, although the International Council of Nurses, the World Health Organization, and the U.S. Public Health Service are also possible sources of information. As more professional nurses become interested in international nursing, governmental, professional, educational, and philanthropic groups may originate new scholarships, fellowships, and loans to assist them. The competition for available funds for international study is likely to be increasingly keen, however, because many other professional and occupational groups also are becoming more eager for education and experience in other countries.

Individuals and groups who contribute scholarships, fellowships, and loans want them to be used to the best possible advantage. If they are left unused for several years, the administering authority may decide to allocate the money elsewhere (if it is legally empowered to do so), or at least will be inclined to feel it unnecessary to try to increase the amounts or promote the establishment of new funds. Effective use of scholarships could increase the supply. Occasionally nursing and other journals list sources of educational funds, with guidelines for application and other useful information. These make good up-to-date references.

Community Activities as a Professional

Active participation in community activities that allow you to share and utilize your professional background in full is very rewarding. Some activities are directly related to nursing, such as attending alumni and nurses' associations meetings and accepting appointments to committees and offices. Others include volunteer work on a regular or special basis, such as participating in student nurse recruitment programs or career days, soliciting donations for various health organizations, helping with the Red Cross blood program, assisting with inoculation sessions for children, acting as adviser to a Future Nurse Club, or volunteering time at a free clinic.

The importance of nursing input into the various community, state and national joint provider-consumer groups that study means of improving the health care delivery system is obvious. Although participation at a state or national level may not be immediately feasible for a nurse who hasn't yet achieved professional recognition, just showing interest and volunteering your services will often open doors at a local level. Nurses involved in direct patient care activities are particularly welcome, because there is the feeling that they can more specifically delineate some of the problems and suggest logical, down-to-earth solutions. Participation of this kind is essential if nurses are to have a part in making policy decisions (see Chap. 16).

Consumer activism has caused the formation of other groups concerned with health delivery, and nurses offering their expertise and understanding of health care services problems can make valuable contributions. Sometimes you need to convince these groups that you have a sincere interest in improved health care services and are willing to work cooperatively with the consumer to achieve that end. The American Nurses Association and National Consumer League have joined forces to initiate nurse-consumer partnerships at the local and state level that will ultimately result in public policy reform. This project has been funded through the Kellogg Foundation, and targets projects in Florida, Wisconsin, and Virginia. In some areas, ethnic and minority groups are especially suspicious of professional health workers outside of their own group, because unfortunate experiences have shown some of them to be more concerned with defending their own interests than the consumer's well-being, as the consumer sees it. In these groups, it is even more important to listen than to talk. Such participation can lead to development of free clinics, health fairs, health teaching classes, recruitment of minority students for nursing programs, tutoring sessions for students, liaison activities with health care institutions, programs for the aged, and legislative activities directed toward better health care. The opportunities, challenges, and satisfactions are unlimited.

Consumer health education is being stressed more and more today, and in what better area can professional nurses offer their expertise? Classes can be held under the auspices of health care institutions, public health organizations, and public and private community groups, and include teaching for wellness as well as teaching those with chronic or long-term illnesses. Nurses who like to teach and are skilled and enthusiastic can participate in programs already set up, and, equally important, can work to develop other programs and involve others on the health team.

Keeping the public informed about nursing and the changes that have occurred in recent years in both education and practice is a contribution to the community. Offers to present programs about modern nursing are often welcome in the many community, social, business, professional, and service groups that meet frequently and are interested in community service.

Activities such as these involve you in the community and are stimulating and satisfying. They also require time, effort, and often patience. But besides the satisfaction of being of service, you will gain in self-development and growth as a professional and as an individual, a dual reward that can't be bought.

WRITING FOR PUBLICATION

Nurses are leaders. Leaders have things to communicate. Communicate your ideas in writing. Nurses who have any inclination toward writing should respond to the "urge" early in their career. The first requirement is to have something to say, something to share with others. Sometimes it is to react to an issue, a concern, an event, or situation in nursing or elsewhere that affects nursing. It may be in response to an article read that could result in a letter to the editor, a reaction paper, or a follow-up article. A logical reason is that there has been little if anything in the literature on that particular topic, especially if this is in the area of clinical practice. Or a nurse may be involved in development of new techniques, use of new equipment, or an innovative approach to caring for a particular kind of patient. Sharing such information is satisfying in itself, but it is also a contribution to the profession. The most important reason for nurses to write (always assuming, of course, that what is written has substance) is the survival of the profession.

A profession must have an adequate body of literature documenting the theoretical and philosophical base of its practice and how its practitioners operate to provide the service that is the essence of professionalism. Informational voids encourage the multiple misconceptions and stereotypes of nursing that already exist and tempt others to fill the void on the basis of their own prejudices and interests.

It is true that both the quantity and quality of the nursing literature have grown in all its dimensions. In journals alone, the increase in clinical articles attests to nurses' interest in improving their clinical practice. Many journals concentrating on a clinical specialty have sprung up. Functional specialties such as administration and education or broad specialties such as school and occupational nursing also have their journals and their interest groups. New authors are emerging. Many nurses, who were traditionally not seen as writers, through a broader formal educational base or writing workshops, have discovered that they have something to say and are learning to express it in writing. Usually they do not yet have a long wait from the time of submission of an article to publication, as is true of many other disciplines, although some journals are developing backlogs.

Nevertheless, there are still a number of informational gaps in the nursing literature in the clinical area, because research and practice follow-through are just beginning to hit their stride. No doubt, a number of nonclinical topics also come to mind. Yet, in meetings, workplaces, and schools, some nurse is talking about a concept, an experiment, or a practice that excites a whole group.

So why don't nurses write? Or at least as much as other professionals do? Perhaps the first reason is that too many nurses think that writing is for the academician, who must function in a "publish or perish" environment, or for the researcher who, in somewhat obscure language, adds to the theory of nursing. The average nurse has a string of excuses, "I don't have anything to say"; "I don't have a degree"; "I don't have time"; "I don't know how." All those *don'ts* can be overcome. A person has to start somewhere, and except for the handful who have an innate talent and inclination for writing, a little self-discipline and maybe some tutoring are needed.

It may not be easy, as shown by this litany of pains—the need for discipline, finding the time, searching out and documenting sources, having one's cherished ideas (or pet phrases) criticized, finding the right editors, even being rejected. For those who want to write but feel that they don't know how, there are various practical steps. Anyone who has graduated from a nursing program should have the basic tools of writing: a firm grasp of grammar, punctuation, spelling, and word usage. If not, there is no excuse for not remedying the situation. To go a step further, for the purpose of writing, there are three indispensable tools: a good dictionary; *Roget's Thesaurus* (a dictionary of synonyms and antonyms to turn to when you know the meaning but can't think of the word); and William Strunk Jr. and E. B. White's *The Elements of Style*, third edition (New York: Macmillan Publishing Co., Inc., 1979), which is easily read and includes basic rules of composition, grammar, punctuation, and word usage. In addition, there is a new surge of "how to" articles and books that can be extremely helpful, some of which are directed specifically to nurses.

Here are some generally accepted guidelines to writing: the best writers write so that they are understood; there is little that cannot be said without the use of long words,[46] and there is absolutely no excuse for pretentious prose or jargon. This does not mean that the technical words that may be essential to a clinical article should be omitted. It does mean that a simple collection of noun, active verb, participle, clause, or whatever makes sense serves as well as, if not better than, a convoluted sentence that says nothing more. (See the bibliography for other sources on writing.)

Today, the use of nonsexist gender is also desirable, whenever possible. The most common writing weaknesses cited by a group of editors were overly formal and pedagogic writing; poor organization; absence of an introduction and summary; poor sentence structure (too long and "doesn't flow"); poor or fabricated documentation; and use of jargon.

A good way to break into writing is through a letter to the editor. These are almost always published, unless they're totally inappropriate. Editors love comments on articles, editorials, or other parts of their publication because it adds interest, sometimes controversy, or new information or simply indicates that someone was motivated enough by what was published to write. (They don't mind compliments on how good the journal is, either.) Few journals are overwhelmed by letters, as too often people "never get around to it," even if they are especially pleased or upset about what's written. If you choose this first step to publication, remember that it *is* a demonstration of your writing ability, perceptiveness, good sense, understanding of the issues, and/or knowledge about another aspect of what was published. Keep it short and to the point. It may be edited if it's too long, generally only with your approval. An emotional tirade may be published, but often makes the writer look foolish. However, a difference of opinion is perfectly appropriate, and as the original author may respond in print, it can be the start of an interesting new professional relationship. If you're really good, the editor might keep you in mind to serve as a reviewer or even request an article.

Don't dismiss the idea of publishing for the general public. Nurses are very consumer-friendly, and the lay public is in need of much of the information that we can give. Inquire about a "health piece" for your local paper, and any other publications that have a general readership. Propose writing about something that is timely and perhaps a bit controversial.

Another way to be published is to write a book review. Although someone who presents papers or has already written articles may be invited by an editor to review a book in his or her area of expertise it's not necessary to wait to be asked. It's perfectly acceptable to write to the editors of one or more journals, in care of the book review editor, and describe your qualifications and interests, perhaps including a résumé or curriculum vitae. Most editors will follow up, and you may be asked to be on the book-reviewer list. It is *not* appropriate to send a self-selected book review. The book and the reviewer may already have been selected, or the book may not be slated for review.

There may or may not be reimbursement for the review, and the decision on whether you may keep the reviewed book (which is sent to you) or must return it varies with the publisher. Although most reviewers develop their own style of reviewing, some journals have a general format and desired length. It's also useful to review the guidelines suggested by book review editors, or at least to read reviews already published in the selected journal.

For those who are ready to write an article and have selected a topic, there are certain basic guidelines as a beginning:[47]

1. Know as much as possible about your subject (review the literature). Research those areas you're not sure about (library, interviewing people involved or who have an opinion to offer).
2. Assemble all the ideas, arguments, facts, data, and illustrations you can think of.
3. Sort and classify them.
4. Develop an outline.
5. Write a first draft. Establish the what, where, when, why, how, and who for your beginning paragraphs.
6. Revise (a second look brings amazing insights).
7. Ask for peer review. Sometimes a friend who writes or who is an editor can be helpful in making suggestions. However, it is the writer's responsibility to see that the content is accurate and that the references and bibliography are properly cited.
8. Revise again; *proofread*.

Selecting the appropriate journal for submission of an article is crucial. Some editors will return an article with a suggestion that another journal might be better for that type of paper, but most do not. (Nor do most bother to critique it, in part because of the volume of mail they must deal with). One way to determine which journal is right is to check several recent issues of the journals that might be suitable, or at least the major journals listed in respected indexes. The table of contents presents a quick overview, and several issues should give a fairly clear picture of that journal's areas of interest. In addition, some publish authors' guidelines that include their mission or purpose. It may be helpful to check the masthead for the credentials of the editors and of an editorial advisory board and peer review panel, if any. Colleagues can also give information, or at least an opinion, on the quality and reputation of the journal. It's always useful to read some of the articles; this not only gives some indication of the journal's quality but also provides some information on its style (since most journals are edited by their editorial staff). If you have a major disagreement with the style or philosophy of a journal, you should probably not send a manuscript there. Whether to choose a journal with a large circulation or a specialized journal that reaches the particular audience desired is another important decision. In the last few years, there have been some helpful publications that compare the various journals in which nurses may want to publish.

However, one ethical point is overriding: a manuscript should be sent to *only one journal at a time*. If rejected, it can then go to another. Acceptance and publication by two journals (this does not refer to reprinting by permission) is considered a serious, and sometimes unforgivable, embarrassment. For one thing, the author has then presumably given the copyright to two separate owners.

At times, authors, especially if they have no track record, may choose to approach an editor first to see whether there is any interest in a particular type of article. This procedure is called a *query*. Opinion is mixed as to whether this is worthwhile, especially if you are reasonably sure that the article is suitable for that journal and that a similar one has not been published within the last few years. However, should such an article be in the editor's file for future publication, it saves the author time and money to know it.

The usual procedure is as follows:

1. Write to the editor. If you know a particular editor of that journal, address it to him or her. However, check a recent journal for accuracy. Editors do not appreciate getting letters addressed to a long gone predecessor, and it does imply that you have not even looked at a current issue. Explain what you would like to write about; send an outline of major points; give brief autobiographical information to indicate that you are qualified to write on the subject; list previous writings, if any; and state whether or not you expect remuneration other than what the journal usually pays. (Only if you feel strongly about the last; nursing journals are not noted for extravagant fees, and may pay no cash fee.)

2. Wait for the editor's reply. If your idea is appealing, a letter or telephone call will follow with instructions regarding the length and sometimes the due date, and possibly with suggestions about content, development, and style.

3. In preparing the manuscript, follow the journal's guidelines. If no details are given, it is usually appropriate to type the manuscript, double-spaced, leaving 1-inch margins at the top, bottom and right-hand side and a 1½-inch margin at the left. Include the references or bibliography and your (brief) autobiography as you would like to have it published with your article, but using that journal's style.

4. Send a cover letter and the article with as many copies as specified (often at least three) to the editor, via first class mail, together with pictures or other illustrations, protected with cardboard. Keep a copy.

5. You should receive an acknowledgement of receipt of the manuscript and, later, a letter stating whether or not your article has been accepted for publication. How long that will be depends on how the article is reviewed—by one or more editors or a peer review panel, whether it appears to be a clear-cut winner, or whether it will require additional editorial conferences or reviews. Probably three months should be allowed before inquiring about the manuscript's status. It is permissible to withdraw it if you wish. Some journals return declined manuscripts with the critiques of the reviewers and/or editors. If a revision and resubmission is requested, suggestions (or directions) for revision are made.

6. If the manuscript is accepted, the editor may or may not be able to give to you a publication date, but you can ask. Much depends on the timeliness of the article, the production plans for future journal issues, and the number of articles on hand.

7. The magazine's editorial staff will edit and prepare the article for the printer. They may send the edited copy for you to check and approve, or they may send you the galley proofs after the article is set in type. Sometimes both the edited copy and proof are sent. Read the copy promptly, request only such changes as you feel are necessary for clarity and accuracy, and return it to the editor's office right away. Delay may mean that your article will not appear in the issue it was planned for and may disrupt the magazine's production schedule.

8. One or more complimentary copies of the issue in which your article is published will be mailed to you. If you wish extra copies, you will usually find the cost per copy noted on the magazine's table of contents page. If you want reprints, write at once to the magazine's business office for information regarding the policy for ordering and the price.

9. Much the same process occurs when an unsolicited manuscript is submitted. For those scholars who wish to publish their research, a similar approach is used, but depending on where and how the research is to be published (as a research paper or a narrative article), the style may vary. Again, it is wise to check with poten-

tial publishers. If the research is a thesis or dissertation, it is helpful to look at strategies that make the research publishable.

Should you write with a colleague, a coauthor?[48] This may be a good idea, provided you know your coauthor and are sure that you can work together. It's possible that each of you has a particular expertise to bring to a topic that gives the reader a broader perspective, or that one of you writes better than the other, who is willing to do most of the literature search. (Make sure he or she knows how and what to focus on.) If several of you are involved in research, an article is frequently coauthored by two or more people. Ask these questions: Are we in reasonable distance for meeting and discussing? Can each of us meet deadlines? Are we each willing to take the time to do this? What exactly is each of us going to do? If we all write, who puts it together? Can we agree, or compromise, if there have to be content or style revisions? How do we share expenses for typing, for illustrations? Who is first author? (This becomes important in academia.) The person whose idea it was? The one who did the most work? The one who needs credit most for promotion? If you come to a parting of the ways, who has the right to publish the article? Do you have mutual respect and trust so that there is no concern about the accuracy and originality of either what is written or the activity or research it was based on? These are important questions because, if left to chance, you could end with no publication or, worse, a legal complication.

Suppose you followed all the rules (or didn't) and your manuscript is rejected? If the editor or reviewers gave you helpful suggestions, with which you agree, you can revise the article and send it to another suitable journal. (Usually you don't send it back to the first, unless the editor specifies that a revision could make it suitable for reconsideration.) You might very well be angry but, if the suggestions sound reasonable after reflection, consider revision seriously. It may be simpler than starting with a new topic. If you don't agree with the criticism, get some other advice and send the article to another journal. Neither reviewers nor editors are infallible, and some have hidden prejudices even they don't recognize. It's particularly difficult if you get two quite different sets of suggestions and the editor gives you no guidance. You'll then simply have to decide, perhaps with some help from reliable peers, which if any advice to follow. If the problem is your writing style, get some editorial help. However, the most common reason for rejection is related to content, primarily because it is found to be inaccurate, not important, undocumented, has a poor research design, or was covered recently.

One warning: some reviewers tend to be too hasty, sarcastic, or thoughtless in wording their critiques and the editor may not do anything about it. This is very discouraging and a blow to the writer's ego. Try not to get too upset or give up. Every author has had rejections, some not with kind words.[49] Just try again.

The procedure for writing a book is similar to that for a journal article, but it is often more exacting and usually much more time-consuming. There is more of everything, including satisfactions and remuneration. As there is also more expense to the publisher, usually even an experienced writer has to present a book proposal to a publisher (or to more than one).

In addition to the manuscript for the main portion or body of the book, the author is usually responsible for writing the foreword or preface, sometimes preparing the index, and reading the galley proof. You must obtain written permission to use material quoted or adapted from other sources, being sure that credits are included in the book as indicated in order to avoid any embarrassment, difficulty, or lawsuit.

The editorial staff of a book publishing company is willing to help the author in every way possible. But only in unusual instances does the staff relieve the author of the responsibility of checking data and presenting them in proper form.

It is customary for a book publisher and an author to negotiate a contract covering the main considerations in the preparation of the manuscript, responsibilities for illustrative materials, revision, and royalty rates. Because royalties, support or advances, and marketing vary among publishers, it is wise to "shop around" to find the one most suitable. Sometimes a lawyer or someone who has had considerable experience with publishers can be extremely helpful.

Not all nurses have writing skills, but many do have ideas that are worth sharing. There are two solutions—developing those skills through practice, study, and workshops, or joining forces with someone who does write well, keeping in mind the possible pitfalls of coauthorship.

The important point is that the person who has something worthwhile to say finds a way to say it and takes the time to do it. This is a professional responsibility and satisfying one.

THERE CAN NEVER BE A LAST WORD

Nursing is noble work, and you have chosen it wisely. You enter the profession in times of upheaval and paradox, but also at a point of its renaissance. This book has tried faithfully to portray the picture of a profession that is moving with the times. It is a profession that has often been the conscience of health care, speaking out on social issues with a fervor that has sometimes been self-destructive. Our past has been greatly influenced by the woman's movement and the growth of modern medicine and the health care industry. Through all of the change that has characterized human affairs, nursing has stayed positioned at the bedside, in the home, in the community…often the only human link between our patients and an intimidating experience in the health care delivery system.

There can never be a last word, because you will live every chapter of the profession as it unfolds, and hopefully contribute new, exciting episodes.

REFERENCES

1. Hardy ME, Conway ME: *Role Theory.* Norwalk, CT: Appleton and Lange, 1988, pp 73–110.
2. Andrusyszyn MA, Maltby HR: Building on strengths through preceptorships. *Nurse Educ Today* 13:277–281, August 1993.
3. Reid M: Marginal man: The identity dilemma of the academic general practitioner. *Symbolic Interaction* 5:325, February 1982.
4. Kramer M: *Reality Shock.* St Louis: Mosby, 1974, p 15.
5. Ibid, pp vii–viii, 3.
6. Ibid, pp 155–162.
7. Ibid, p 162.
8. Watson J, Bevis E: Nursing education coming of age for a new age, in Chaska N (ed): *The Nursing Profession: Turning Points.* St Louis: Mosby–Year Book, 1990, pp 100–105.
9. Smith DM: Thoughts about caring. *Image* 25:147–149, Summer 1993.
10. Miller MM: A study of the effects of a nursing internship program on job satisfaction and the development of clinical competence. The University of North Carolina at Chapel Hill, Ph.D. dissertation, 1990.
11. Selye H: *Stress without Distress.* Philadelphia: Lippincott, 1974.
12. Forchuk C: *Hildegard E. Peplau: Interpersonal Nursing Theory.* Newbury Park, CA: Sage Publications, 1993.
13. Tartasky DS: Hardiness: Conceptual and methodological issues. *Image* 25:225–229, Fall 1993.
14. Burns C, Harm NJ: Emergency nurses' perceptions of critical incidents and stress. *J Emerg Nurs* 19:431–436, October 1993.
15. Hardy, op cit, pp 159–239.
16. Arena DM, Page NE: The imposter phenomenon in the clinical nurse specialist role. *Image* 24:121–125, Summer 1992.
17. Joel LA: Maybe a pot watcher but never an ostrich. *Am J Nurs* 94:7, April 1994.
18. Chappelle LS, Sorrentino EA: Assessing co-dependency issues within a nursing environment. *Nurs Mgt* 24:40–42, May 1993.
19. Joel, loc cit.
20. Murphy E: Professional autonomy v. "at will" employee status. *Nurs Outlook* 38:248, September–October, 1990.
21. Stevens B: *The Nurse as Executive.* Rockville, MD: Aspen, 1985, pp 361–362.
22. Fiesta J: Staffing implications: A legal update. *Nurs Mgt* 25:34–35, June 1994.
23. Fear of floating. *Am J Nurs* 94:56, March 1994.
24. Flanagan L: *Survival Skills in the Workplace.*

Kansas City: American Nurses' Association, 1990.

25. Ketter J: Sex discrimination targets men in some hospitals. *Am Nurs* 26:3, 24, April 1994.

26. Horsley J: Fighting age discrimination on the job. *RN* 57:57–60, April 1994.

27. American Nurses' Association: *Nursing and HIV/AIDS.* Washington, DC: American Nurses Publishing, 1994, p 78.

28. Ibid, p 79.

29. Ibid, pp 95–96.

30. Ketter J: Nurses, HIV exposure and the burden of proof. *Am Nurs* 26:14, 21, May 1994.

31. American Nurses' Association, loc cit.

32. Carmon M: Legal challenges of tuberculosis in the workplace. *AAOHN-J* 41:96–100, February 1993.

33. American Nurses' Association, op cit, p 57.

34. American Nurses' Association: *Health and Safety in the Workplace.* Report to the 1993 ANA House of Delegates, Washington, DC.

35. Ibid.

36. Insulation from supervisory influence. *SNA Legal Developments*, Special Issue, Dec 22, 1989.

37. Supreme Court upholds NLRB's rulemaking in determining RN-only bargaining units: NLRB issues guidelines. *SNA Legal Developments*, July 26, 1991.

38. Joel LA: The ultimate gag rule. *Am J Nurs* 94:7, August 1994.

39. Labor relations considerations to alternate organizational arrangements for the governance of nursing services. *SNA Legal Developments*, May 20, 1988.

40. Flarey DL et al: Collaboration in labor relations. *J Nurs Adm* 22:15–22, September 1992.

41. McGuiness JC: Blunting America's competitive edge. *Industry Week* 63, Oct 21, 1991.

42. Benner P: *From Novice to Expert: Excellence and Power in Clinical Nursing.* Menlo Park, CA: Addison-Wesley, 1984.

43. Le Roy A: How to survive as a non-traditional nursing student. *Imprint* 35:73–74, 79–86, April–May 1988.

44. Lippman H: 1993 earnings survey: How your fringe benefits stack up. *RN* 40–45, December 1993.

45. Germain CP et al: Help yourself to a nursing scholarship. *Imprint* 41:84–85, April–May 1994.

46. Camilleri R: On elegant writing. *Image* 20:169–171, Fall 1988.

47. Dracup K: Writing for publication. *Focus Crit Care* 10:11–14, April 1983.

48. Boykoff S: Coauthorship: Collaboration without conflict. *Am J Nurs* 89:1164, September 1989.

49. Plawecki HM: Write right! *J Holistic Nurs* 12:135–137, June 1994.

Bibliography

This bibliography is organized in a way that should make it easy to find appropriate sources.

Under each part, title, or section heading, general sources related to more than one chapter in that part or section are listed first. Then appropriate specific sources are listed under each chapter heading.

With rare exceptions, such as with books that cover the entire topic, citations already appearing in each chapter reference list are not reprinted in the bibliography. It is possible that some of these references are cited in more than one chapter, as appropriate.

As a rule, works published prior to 1985 are not included. Most are 1990 or later. Exceptions are publications of historical significance. Other useful works published prior to 1975 are cited in the third (1975), fourth (1981), fifth (1985), and sixth (1991) editions of *Dimensions of Professional Nursing*.

The selection of books and journals is broad in order to include fields other than nursing, so that readers who are interested may explore some other perspectives.

Many of the sources cited have extensive bibliographies.

PART I
DEVELOPMENT OF MODERN NURSING

Birnbach N, Lewenson S: *First Words: Selected Addresses from the National League for Nursing 1894–1933.* New York: National League for Nursing, 1993.

Birnbach N, Lewenson S: *Legacy of Leadership: Presidential Addresses from the Superintendents' Society and the National League of Nursing Educa-tion, 1894–1952.* New York: National League for Nursing, 1993.

Bullough V, Bullough B: Achievement of eminent American nurses of the past: A prosopographical study. *Nurs Res* 41: 120–124, March–April 1992.

Bullough V: History, nature, and nurture. *J Prof Nurs* 9:128, May–June 1993.

Bullough V, Bullough B: *The Care of the Sick: The Emergence of Modern Nursing.* New York: Prodist, 1978.

Carnegie ME: Black nurses at the front. *Am J Nurs* 84:1250–1252, October 1984.

Carnegie ME: *The Path We Tread: Blacks in Nursing, 1854–1990.* New York: National League for Nursing, 1991.

Christy T: *Cornerstone for Nursing Education.* New York: Teachers College Press, 1969.

Dolan J, Fitzpatrick L, Herrman E: *Nursing in Society: A Historical Perspective,* 15th ed. Philadelphia: Saunders, 1983.

Donahue P: *Nursing: The Finest Art.* St Louis: Mosby, 1985.

Ehrenreich B, English D: *Witches, Midwives, and Nurses: A History of Women Healers.* Old Westbury, NY: The Feminist Press, 1973.

Fitzpatrick ML: *Historical Studies in Nursing.* New York: Teachers College Press, 1978.

Flanagan L: *One Strong Voice: The Story of the American Nurses Association.* Kansas City, MO: American Nurses Association, 1976.

Jones A: *Images of Nurses: Perspective from History, Art, and Literature.* Philadelphia: University of Pennsylvania Press, 1988.

Kalisch B, Kalisch P: *The Advance of American Nursing.* Boston: Little, Brown, 1986.

Kaufman M (ed): *Dictionary of American Nursing Biography.* New York: Greenwood Press, 1988.

Miller H: Registering the history of nursing. *Image* 24:241–245, Fall 1992.

Moore J: *A Zeal for Responsibility*. Athens, GA: University of Georgia Press, 1988.

Rosenberg C: *The Care of Strangers: The Rise of America's Hospital System*. New York: Basic Books, 1987.

The entire issue of *Imprint*, April–May 1990, is devoted to nursing in history, as is most of the October 1990 *American Journal of Nursing* and the March 1993 and February 1994 issues of *Nursing and Health Care*.

The American Journal of Nursing Company has published a compilation of the articles on nursing history published in its journals called *Pages from Nursing History*, 1984.

Other references may be found in the libraries of major university and college libraries with schools of nursing and in nursing history centers such as those at the University of Pennsylvania and at Teachers College, Columbia University in New York. Sigma Theta Tau archives contain oral histories and videos of some of nursing's leaders, as do some of the nursing history centers.

Section One
EARLY HISTORICAL INFLUENCES

Chapter 1
Care of the Sick: A Historical Overview

Bullough VL, Bullough B: Medieval nursing: *Nurs Hist Rev* 1:89–104, 1993.

Ellis H: Royal operations: A contrast to modern surgery. *AORN J* 17:101–109, May 1973.

Mish I: Nursing process–Medieval style. *Nurs Forum* 18:196–203, February 1979.

Chapter 2
The Influence of Florence Nightingale

Benson E: On the other side of the battle: Russian nurses in the Crimean War. *Image* 24:65–68, Spring 1992.

Berges F, Berges C: A Visit to Scutari. *Am J Nurs* 86:811–813, July 1986.

Bullough V et al: *Florence Nightingale and Her Era: A Collection of New Scholarship*. New York: Garland Publishing, 1990.

Bullough V: Nightingale, nursing and harassment. *Image* 22:4–7, Spring 1990.

Calabria M, Macrae J: *"Suggestions for Thought"* by *Florence Nightingale*. Philadelphia: University of Pennsylvania Press, 1994.

Hays J: Florence Nightingale and the India sanitary reforms. *Public Health Nurs* 6:152–154, September 1989.

Hegge M: In the footsteps of Florence Nightingale: Rediscovering the roots of nursing. *Imprint* 37:74–79, April–May 1990.

Henry B et al: Nightingale's perspective of nursing administration. *Nurs Health Care* 11:200–206, April 1990.

Seymer L: *Selected Writings of Florence Nightingale*. New York: Macmillan, 1954.

Slater V: The educational and philosophical influences on Florence Nightingale, an enlightened conductor. *Nurs Hist Rev* 2:137–152, 1994.

Uhl J: Nightingale—The international nurse. *J Prof Nurs* 8:5, January–February 1992.

Vicinus M, Negaard B (ed): *Ever Yours, Florence Nightingale: Selected Letters*. Cambridge, MA: Harvard University Press, 1990.

Widerquist J: Dearest friend—The correspondence of colleagues Florence Nightingale and Mary Jones. *Nurs Hist Rev* 1:25–42, 1993.

Widerquist J: The spirituality of Florence Nightingale. *Nurs Res* 41:49–55, January–February 1992.

Woodham-Smith C: *Florence Nightingale*. New York: McGraw-Hill, 1951.

See also the sections on Nightingale in the Bullough and Bullough, Dolan, and Kalisch and Kalisch books. An outstanding collection of Nightingale's writings can be found in the Adelaide Nutting Historical Nursing collection at Teachers College, Columbia University, New York. Some of her most noted works are listed below in chronological order. Some of these are found in Seymer.

The Institution of Kaiserswerth on the Rhine for the practical training of deaconesses under the direction of the Rev. Pastor Fliedner, embracing the support and care of a hospital, infant and industrial schools, and female penitentiary; 1851.

Notes on matters affecting the health, efficiency, and hospital administration of the British Army. Founded chiefly on the experience of the late war. Presented by request to the Secretary of State for War; 1858.

Subsidiary notes as to the introduction of female nursing into military hospitals in peace and in war. Presented by request to the Secretary of State for War; 1858.

A contribution to the sanitary history of the British Army during the late war with Russia; 1859.

Notes on hospitals, 1859, 3d ed. Almost completely rewritten; 1863.

Notes on nursing: What it is, and what it is not; 1859.

Observations on the evidence contained in the statistical reports submitted to the Royal Commission on the Sanitary State of the Army in India; 1863.

Suggestions on a system of nursing for hospitals in India; 1865.

Suggestions on the subject of providing, training and organizing nurses for the sick poor in workhouse infirmaries. Paper No. XVI in the government report of the committee appointed to consider the cubic space of metropolitan workhouses; 1867.

Introductory notes on lying-in institutions together with a proposal for organizing an institution for training midwives and midwifery nurses; 1871.

On trained nursing for the sick poor; 1876.

Nurses, training of, and nursing the sick, from A Dictionary of Medicine, Sir Robert Qwain, Bart, MD, ed; 1882.

Sick-nursing and health-nursing. Paper read at the Chicago Exhibition; 1893.

Health teaching in towns and villages—rural hygiene. Paper read at the Conference of Women Workers, Leeds; 1893. Published 1894.

Section Two
NURING IN THE UNITED STATES

Christy T: Portrait of a leader: M. Adelaide Nutting, *Nurs Outlook* 17:20–24, January 1969.

Christy T: Portrait of a leader: Isabel Hampton Robb. *Nurs Outlook* 17:26–29, May 1969.

Christy T: Portrait of a leader: Lavinia Lloyd Dock. *Nurs Outlook* 17:72–75, June 1969.

Christy T: Portrait of a leader: Isabel Maitland Stewart. *Nurs Outlook* 17:44–48, October 1969.

Christy T: Portrait of a leader: Lillian D. Wald. *Nurs Outlook* 18:50–54, March 1969.

Christy T: Portrait of a leader: Annie Warburton Goodrich. *Nurs Outlook* 18:46–50, August 1970.

Christy T: Equal rights for women: Voices from the past. *Am J Nurs* 71:288–293, February 1971.

Christy T: Portrait of a leader: Sophia F. Palmer. *Nurs Outlook* 23:746–751, December 1975.

Dock L: What we may expect from the law. *Am J Nurs* 50:599–600, October 1950.

Chapter 3
The Evolution of the Trained Nurse, 1873–1903

Alcott LM: *Hospital Sketches*. Boston: James Redpath, 1863.

Baer E: Nursing's divided loyalties: An historical study. *Nurs Res* 38:166–171, May–June 1989.

Christy T: Nurses in American history: The fateful decade 1890–1900. *Am J Nurs* 75:1163–1165, July 1975.

Culpepper M, Adams P: Nursing in the Civil War. *Am J Nurs* 88:981–984, July 1988.

Denker E (ed): *Healing at Home: Visiting Nurse Service of New York, 1893–1993*. New York, Visiting Nurse Service, 1994.

Doona Me: At least as well cared for . . . Linda Richards and the mentally ill. *Image* 16:51–56, Spring 1984.

Fitzpatrick ML: Lillian Wald: Prototype of an involved nurse. *Imprint* 37:92–95, April–May 1990.

Flaumenhaft E, Flaumenhaft C: American nursing's first textbooks. *Nurs Outlook* 37:185–188, July–August 1989.

Hamilton D: Faith and finance. *Image* 20:124–127, Fall 1988.

Lippman D: Early nursing textbooks. *Imprint* 37:109–112, April–May 1990.

Maker MD: *To Bind Up the Wounds*. New York: Greenwood Press, 1989.

Mosley M: Jessie Sleet Scales: First Black public health nurse. *ABNF J* 5: 45–51, March –April 1994.

Pryor E: *Clara Barton: Professional Angel*. Philadelphia: University of Pennsylvania Press, 1987.

Samson J: A nurse who gave her life so that others could live. *Imprint* 37:81–89, April–May 1990.

Chapter 4
The Emergence of the Modern Nurse, from 1904

Baas L: An analysis of the writing of Janet Geister and Mary Roberts regarding the problems of private duty nursing. *J Prof Nurs* 8:176–183, May–June 1992.

Breckinridge M: *Wide neighborhoods: The Story of the Frontier Nursing Service*. New York: Harper & Row, 1952.

Buhler-Wilderson, K: *False Dawn: The Rise and Decline of Public Health Nursing 1900–1930*. New York: Garland Publishing, 1989.

Chaney J, Falk P: A profession in caricature: Changing attitudes toward nursing in the American Medical News, 1960–1989. *Nurs Hist Rev* 1:181–202, 1993.

Chesler E: *Woman of Valor: Margaret Sanger and the Birth Control Movement in America*. New York: Simon and Schuster, 1992.

Kalisch B, Kalisch P: Nurses under fire: The World War II experience of nurses in Bataan and Corregidor. *Nurs Res* 6:409–429, November–December 1976.

Kalisch P: How Army nurses became officers: One bar on a shoulder strap is worth two regulations in a book. *Nurs Res* 25:164–177, June 1976.

Kalisch P et al: Louise Bougeois and the emergence of modern midwifery. *J Nurse-Midwifery* 26:3–17, July–August 1981.

Lagemann E: *Nursing History: New Perspectives, New Possibilities*. New York: Teachers College Press, 1983.

Moments in American history. *Nurs Res* 39:126–127, March–April 1990.

Norman E: *Women at War: The Story of Fifty Military Nurses Who Served in Vietnam*. Philadelphia: University of Pennsylvania Press, 1990.

Progress and promise 1900–1990. *Am J Nurs*, anniversary issue, October 1990.

Weinberg D, Buhler-Wilkerson K: The changing face of nursing. *Nurs Res* 41:40–42, January–February 1992.

Wuthrow S: Our mothers' stories. *Nurs Outlook* 38:218–222, September 1990.

Chapter 5

Major Studies of the Nursing Profession

In the text of Chap. 5, the publisher and date of publication are cited for older studies that were widely available. Many of these reports are now out of print. However, some libraries have photocopies, and microfilmed editions of most of them are also available. For information on the latter, address inquires to University Microfilms, 300 N. Zeeb Rd., Ann Arbor, MI 48106.

The following references are primarily commentaries about the various studies.

Aiken L: Nursing's future: Public policies, private actions. *Am J Nurs* 83:1440–1444, October 1983.

Bowman M, Walsh W Jr: Perspective on the GMENAC Report *Health Affairs* 1:55–66, Fall 1982.

Christy T et al: An appraisal of "An Abstract for Action." *Am J Nurs* 71:1574–1581, August 1971.

Credentialing in nursing: A new approach. *Am J Nurs* 79:674–683, April 1979. Also in *Nurs Outlook* 27:263–271, April 1979.

Deback V: Nursing today and tomorrow: The role of NCNIP. *Nurs Health Care* 7:130–132, March 1986.

Lipson J: Esther Lucille Brown: A Memorial. *Image* 24:313–317, Winter 1992.

Lysaught JP: *Action in Affirmation: Toward an Unambiguous Profession of Nursing*. New York: McGraw-Hill, 1981.

Matejski M: Nursing education, professionalism, and autonomy: Social constraints and the Goldmark report. *Adv Nurs Sci* 2:17–30, April 1981.

Rawnsky M: The Goldmark report: Midpoint in nursing history. *Nurs Outlook* 21:380–383, June 1973.

PART II

CONTEMPORARY PROFESSIONAL NURSING

Donabedian A: The role of outcomes in quality assessment and assurance. *Qual Rev Bull* 18:356–360, November 1992.

Estes PR, Estes CL: *The Nation's Health*. Boston: Jones and Bartlett, 1994.

Kovner A: *Health Care Delivery in the United States,* 4th ed. New York: Springer, 1990.

McCloskey J, Grace HK: *Current Issues in Nursing*. St Louis, MO: Mosby, 1994.

Section One

THE HEALTH CARE SETTING

American Nurses Association and National League for Nursing: *Nursing's Agenda for Health Care Reform*. Kansas City: The Associations, 1991.

Barer ML, Evans RG: Interpreting Canada: Models, mind-sets, and myths. *Health Affairs* 44–61, Spring 1992.

Betts VT: The best buy in health care. *Am Nurs* 93:7, November 1993.

Boston C, Vestal KW: Work transformation: Why the new health care imperative must focus both on people and progress. *Hosp Health Netw* 68:50–54, Apr 5, 1994.

Buerhaus PI: Managed competition and critical issues facing nurses. *Nurs Health Care* 15:22–26, January 1994.

Coopers and Lybrand Health Decisions Resource Group: Healthcare reform: Innovations at the state level. *Nurs Mgt* 25:30–40, April 1994.

Danzon MD: Hidden overhead costs: Is Canada's system less expensive? *Health Affairs* 21–43, Spring 1992.

Feingold E: Health care reform—more than cost

containment and universal access. *Am J Public Health* 84:727–728, May 1994.

Oregon's plan to ration health care. *Am Nurs* 93:9, May 1993.

Simmons HE et al: Comprehensive health care reform and managed competition. *N Engl J Med* 327:1525–1528, 1992.

Chapter 6

The Impact of Social and Scientific Chages

Biggar RJ: The global challenge of HIV/AIDS. *Am J Public Health* 83:1383–1384, October 1993.

Bridges W: The end of the job. *Fortune* 62–64, 68, 72, 74, September 19, 1994.

Bushy A: Women in rural environments: Considerations for holistic nurses. *Holistic Nurs Pract* 8:67–73, July 1994.

Cowley G: The rise of cyberdoc. *Newsweek* 52–53, September 26, 1994.

Ehrlich P, Ehrlich A: *The Population Explosion*. New York: Simon and Schuster, 1990.

Ernst RL, Hay JW: The U.S. economic and social costs of Alzheimer's Disease revisited. *Am J Public Health* 84:1261–1263, August 1994.

Fenton MV: Alma Ata, at last. *J Prof Nurs* 10:4–5, January–February 1994.

Flynn BC et al: Developing community leadership in healthy cities: The Indiana model. *Nurs Outlook* 40:121–126, May–June 1992.

Forrest JD, Fordyce RR: Women's contraceptive attitudes and use in 1992. *Fam Plann Perspect* 25:175–179, July–August 1993.

Gold R: *Abortion and Woman's Health: A Turning Point for America?* New York: Alan Guttmacher Institute, 1990.

Harlap S et al: *Preventing Pregnancy, Protecting Health: A New Look at Birth Control Choices in the United States*. New York: Alan Guttmacher Institute, 1991.

Holtzman D et al: Changes in HIV related information services, instruction, knowledge, and behaviors among US high school students, 1989 and 1990. *Am J Public Health* 84:388–393, March 1994.

Kark SL et al: Commentary: In search of innovative approaches to international health. *Am J Public Health* 83:1537–1543, November 1993.

Krieger N: Analyzing socioeconomic and racial/ethnic patterns in health and health care. *Am J Public Health* 83:1086–1087, August 1993.

The landscape: The changing faces of the American college campus. *Change* 25:57, September–Octobr 1993.

Lumshon K: Baby boomers grow up. *Hosp Health Netw* 67:24–34, Sept 20, 1993.

The new delivery and financing realities. *Hosp Health Netw* 68:86–88, August 5, 1994.

Pappas G: Elucidating the relationship between race, socioeconomic status, and health. *Am J Public Health* 84:892–893, June 1994.

Quinn JB: The luck of the Xers. *Newsweek* 66–67, June 1994.

Schorr T: The term is "health care." *Nurs Health Care* 14:294–295, June 1993.

Schwartz LL, Stanton MW: Social problems that escalate America's health care costs. *The Internist* 15–17, July–August 1992.

Teitelbaum RS: The smart way to plan health care takeover. *Fortune* 129:27–29, June 1994.

Terris M: Towards a new, "independent-cooperative model" of international health. *J Public Health Policy* 14:365–375, Autumn 1993.

Ugarriza DN, Fallon T: Nurses' attitudes toward homeless women: A barrier to change. *Nurs Outlook* 42:26–29, January–February 1994.

United Nations Commission on the Status of Women: *Preparations for the Fourth World Conference on Women*. New York: The Author, 1994.

United Nations Department of Public Information: *Conference to Set Women's Agenda into the Next Century*. New York: The Author, 1993.

Wood S. Ransom V: The 1990s: A decade for change in women's health care policy. *JOGNN* 23:139–143.

Many of the data on population and family planning were taken from reports of the Alan Guttmacher Institute, 360 Park Avenue South, New York, NY 10010. This institute also publishes *Family Planning Perspectives*. Also useful is *Population Reports* (Johns Hopkins University Population Information Program).

The *Chronicle of Higher Education* is a weekly newspaper that presents reports and discussions of the trends and issues in the field.

The publications of the World Health Organization (WHO) and the International Council of Nurses (ICN) are useful for their presentation of international health perspectives.

Both the *American Journal of Public Health* and *The Nation's Health*, publications of the American Public Health Association, publish numerous articles and reports on population, environmental hazards, and other aspects of public health.

Chapter 7

Health Care Delivery: Where?

Armstrong DM, Stetler CB: Strategic considerations in developing delivery. *Nurs Econ* 9:112–115, February 1991.

Arnst C, Zellner W: Hospitals attack a crippler: Paper. *Business Week* 104–107, February 1994.

Aydelotte M, Gregory M: *Nursing Practice: Innovative Models.* New York: National League for Nursing, 1989.

Barber GM et al: Public's perceived need for adult day care versus actual use. *Home Health Care Services Q* 14:53–56, February 1993.

Barger S, Rosenfeld P: Models in community health: Findings from a national study of community nursing centers. *Nurs Health Care* 14:426–431, October 1993.

Bovbjerg R et al: U.S. Health care coverage and costs: Historical development and choices for the 1990s. *J Law Med Ethics* 21:141–162, Summer 1993.

Bruce P: Off-site preadmission unit supports hospital ambulatory surgical unit, *J Post Anesth Nurs* 8:262–269, August 1993.

Cerne F: The fading stand alone hospital. *Hosp Health Netw* 68:28–32, June 1994.

Clearly A: A better place to be: Integrated capitated care gives frail elderly a choice over nursing homes. *Hosp Health Netw* 68:58–60, June 1994.

Davis JE: Ambulatory surgery . . . how far can we go? *Med Clin North Am* 77:365–375, March 1993.

Ernst D: Total quality management in the hospital setting. *J Nurs Care Qual* 3:1–81, January 1994.

Fielo SB, Crowe RL: A nursing center in Brooklyn. *Nurs Health Care* 13:488–493, November 1992.

Gray AP: Can nursing centers provide health care? *Nurs Health Care* 14:414–417, October 1993.

Guild SD et at: Development of an innovative nursing care delivery system. *J Nurs Adm* 24:23–29, March 1994.

Hackman B: Early discharge: There's no place like home. *Nurs Times* 89:28–30, September 1993.

Inglehart JK: The American health care system—Managed care. *N Engl J Med* 327:742–747, Septembr 1992.

Kinzer D: The decline and fall of deregulation. *N Engl J Med* 318:112–116, January 1988.

Knauth DG: Community nursing centers: Removing impediments to success. *Nurs Econ* 12:140–142, May–June 1994.

Lumsdon K: It's a jungle out there: One hospital adapts to future risks with a new care delivery model. *Hosp Health Netw* 68:68–72, May 1994.

Magiling J et al: Circles of care: Home care and community support for rural older adults. *Adv Nurs Sci* 16:22–33, March 1994.

McKnight JL: Hospitals and the health of their communities. *Hosp Health Netw* 68:40–41, January 1994.

Packard NJ: The price of choice: Managed care in America. *Nurs Adm Q* 17: 8–15, Spring 1993.

Riesch SK: Nursing centers: An analysis of the anecdotal literature. *J Prof Nurs* 8:16–25, January–February 1992.

Rosenberg D: General hospital: One-stop shopping. *Newsweek* 122:106, December 1993.

Sharp N: Recognizing APNs: It's now or never! *Nurs Mgt* 25:14–16, February 1994.

Taylor KS: Fighting AIDS at home: Hospitals, physicians seek community AIDS strategies. *Hosp Health Netw* 68:52–53, January 1994.

Woolhandler S, Himmelstein D: The deteriorating administration efficiency of the U.S. health care system. *N Engl J Med* 1253–1258, May 1992.

Good reference sources for current issues, problems, and trends in organized settings for care are *Hospital and Health Network*, the AHA journal, *Health Progress*, the Catholic Hospital Association journal, and the publications of the Group Health Association of America, which represents managed care (GHAA). There are additionally journals from every segment of the industry, including home health, occupational health, hospice, and rehabilitation, to name a few. All include nontechnical articles. The journal *Family and Community Health* puts great emphasis on innovative health care delivery. Almost every issue has several pertinent articles.

The best source of current, comprehensive data on health resources, although usually several years old, is the U.S. Department of Health and Human Services.

Chapter 8

Health Care Delivery: Who?

Barter M et al: Use of unlicensed assistive personnel by hospitals. *Nurs Econ* 12:82–87, March–April 1994.

Chaistakes P, Feudtner C: Ethics in a short coat: The ethical dilemmas that medical students confront. *Acad Med* 68:249–254, July 1993.

Foreman S: Graduate medical education: Focus for change. *Acad Med* 65:77–84, February 1990.

Ginzberg E: *The medical triangle: Physicians, politi-*

cians and the Public. Cambridge, MA: Harvard University Press, 1990.

The increasing role of the pharmacist in home care. *Caring* 13:42–46, April 1994.

Johnson S: GME financing: A well kept secret. *Nurs Mgt* 25:43–46, April 1994.

Jones PE et al: Physician assistants and health system reform: Clinical capabilities, practice activities, and potential roles. *JAMA* 271:1266–1272, April 27, 1994.

Klitzman R: *A Year Long Night: Tales of a Medical Internship.* New York: Penguin Books, 1990.

Phelps G: Adaptability or extinction: Trends in generalist and subspecialty medicine. *Am Fam Physician* 49:1055–1058, April 1994.

Stanfield P: *Introduction to the Health Professions.* Boston: Jones and Bartlett, 1990.

For more information about trends in the health professions, the journals of each occupation and profession and general hospital, home care, and long-term care facilities are the best sources. They are usually available in health professions libraries.

Section Two
NURSING IN THE HEALTH CARE SCENE

Chapter 9
Nursing as a Profession

Barnum B: *Nursing theory: Analysis, Appliation, Evaluation,* 4th ed. Philadelphia: Lippincott, 1994.

Benner PE: *From Novice to Expert.* Menlo Park, CA: Addison-Wesley, 1984.

Benner P, Wrubel J: *The Primacy of Caring.* Menlo Park, CA: Addison-Wesley, 1989.

Benner, P, Tanner C: Clinical Judgment: How expert nurses use intuition. *Am J Nurs* 87:23–31, January 1987.

Fagin C, Diers D: Nursing as metaphor. *Am J Nurs* 83:1362, September 1983.

Gortner S: Nursing values and science: Toward a science philosophy. *Image* 22:101–105, Summer 1990.

Henderson V: The essence of nursing in high technology. *Nurs Adm Q* 9:1–9, 1985.

Kalisch PA, Kalisch BJ: *The Advance of American Nursing,* 3d ed. Philadelphia: Lippincott, 1995.

Koch B, McGovern J: EXTEND: A prototype expert system for teaching nurse diagnoses. *Comput Nurs* 11:35–41, January–February 1993.

Marriner-Tomey A: *Nursing Theorists and Their Work,* 2d ed. St Louis, MO: Mosby, 1989.

McCloskey JC, Bulechek GM: Standardizing the language for nursing treatments: An overview of the issues. *Nurs Outlook* 42:56–63, March–April 1994.

Miller BK et al: A behavioral inventory for professionalism in nursing. *J Prof Nurs* 9:290–295, September–October 1993.

National League for Nursing: *Patterns of Nursing Theories in Practice.* New York: The League, 1993.

Newman MA: Prevailing paradigms in nursing. *Nurs Outlook* 40:10–12, January–February 1992.

Packard SA, Polifroni EC: The dilemma of nursing science: Current quandaries and lack of direction. *Nurs Sci Q* 4: 7–13, Spring 1991.

Pinkley CL: Exploring NANDA's definition of nursing diagnoses: Linking diagnostic judgments with the selection of outcomes and interventions. *Nursing Diagnoses* 2:26–32, January–March 1991.

Reverby S: *Ordered to Care: The Dilemma of American Nursing.* New York: Basic Books, 1987.

Twardon C et al: A competency achievement orientation program: Professional development of the home health care nurse. *J Nurs Adm* 23:20–25, July–August 1993.

Upvall MJ: Therapeutic syncretism: A conceptual framework of persistence and change for international nursing. *J Prof Nurs* 9:56–61, January–February 1993.

Wiens AG: Patient autonomy in care: A theoretical framework for nursing. *J Prof Nurs* 9:95–103, March–April 1993.

Chapter 10
Professional Ethics and the Nurse

Aroskar MA: Incompetent, unethical, or illegal practice—teaching students to cope. *J Prof Nurs* 9:130, May–June 1993.

Carter M: Ethical framework for care of the chronically ill. *Holistic Nurs Pract* 8:67–77, October 1993.

Carroll, P, Maher V: Legal aspects of a code. *AD Nurs* 4:8, March–April 1989.

Cassel C, Meier D: Morals and moralism in the debate over euthanasia and assisted suicide. *N Eng J Med* 323:750–752, Sept 13, 1990.

Curtin L: DNR in the OR: Ethical concerns and hospital policies. *Nurs Mgt* 25:29–31, February 1994.

Curtin L: Ethical concerns of nutritional support. *Nurs Mgt* 25:14–16, January 1994.

Curtin L: Ethics and economic pressure: Case in point. *Nurs Mgt* 24:17–20, November 1993.

Edwards B: When the physician won't give up. *Am J Nurs* 93:34–37, September 1993.

Eliason M: Ethics and transcultural nursing care.

Nurs Outlook 41:225–228, September–October 1993.

Elsea S, Miya P: Refusal of blood——An ethical issue. *MCM* 6:379–387, November–December 1991.

Ensor J, Giovinco G: Ethical issues related to chemical dependency. *Imprint* 38:85–87, November–December 1991.

Erlen J: Ethical dielmmas in the high-risk nursery: Wilderness experiences. *J Pediatr Nurs* 9:21–25, February 1994.

Hamblet J: Ethics and pediatric perioperative nurse. *Today's OR Nurse* 16:15–21, March–April 1994.

Holly C: The ethical quandaries of acute care nursing practice. *J Prof Nurs* 9:110–115, March–April 1993.

Hoyer P et al: Clinical cheating and moral development. *Nurs Outlook* 39:170–173, July–August 1994.

Jones S, Clark V: Do's and Don't's of a code: Dealing with a cardiac arrest. *AD Nurs* 4:10–15, March–April 1989.

Kleck G: Collegial support for the addicted nurse. *Imprint* 38:76–81, November–December 1991.

Macklin R: Women's health: An ethical perspective. *J Law Med Ethics* 21:23–29, Spring 1993.

Marsh F, Yarborough M: *Medicine and Money: A Study of the Role of Beneficence in Health Care Cost Containment.* Westport, CT: Greenwood Press, 1990.

Miller H: Addiction in a co-worker: Getting past the denial. *Am J Nurs* 90:72–75, May 1990.

Milner S: An ethical nursing practice model. *J Nurs Adm* 23:22–25, March 1993.

Monagle J, Thomasma D: *Health Care Ethics: Critical Issues.* Rockville, MD: Aspen, 1994.

Morreim E: Profoundly diminished life: The casualties of coercion. *Hastings Ctr Rep* 24:33–42, January–February 1994.

O'Quinn J, Hulme P: After HIV testing: What's next? *Nurs Health Care* 14:92–94, February 1993.

Pearson C: Facing ethical dilemmas in the neonatal intensive care unit. *J Pediatr Nurs* 9:131–132, April 1994.

Pence T: *Ethics in Nursing: An Annotated Bibliography,* 3d ed. New York: National League for Nursing, 1994.

Purtilo R: *Ethical Dilemmas in the Health Professions,* 2d ed. Philadelphia: Saunders, 1993.

Some states are creating a new document called "nonhospital DNR order." Here's why. *Choice in Dying News* 2:1–5, Spring 1993.

Swenson I, Foster B: Nursing administrators' responses to physically, mentally and substance-impaired nurses. *Hosp Topics* 71:38–44, Spring 1993.

Windle P, Wintersgill C: The chemically impaired nurse's reentry to practice. *AORN J* 59:1266–1273, June 1994.

Zimbleman J: Good Life, good death, and the right to die: Ethical considerations for decisions at the end of life. *J Prof Nurs* 10:22–37, January–February 1994.

See also references and bibliography of Chap. 22 since the topics are closely related. Many nursing journals have columns on ethics, and the Hastings Center Report focuses on ethics. Choice for Dying, based in New York, provides a newsletter, living wills, and many publications on right to die issues.

Almost the entire issue of the *ANNA J*, October 1993, is devoted to ethical dilemmas in nephrology.

Chapter 11

Profile of the Modern Nurse

Baruch E et al: *Embryos, Ethics and Women's Rights: Exploring the New Reproductive Technologies.* New York: Haworth Press, 1988.

Chinn PL: Diversity: What does it mean? *Nurs Outlook* 40:54, March–April 1992.

Eddy D et al: Importance of professional nursing values: A national study of baccalaureate programs. *J Nurs Educ* 33:257–262, June 1994.

Fong CM: Nursing needs minorities. *Adv Clin Care* 6:19–21, January–February 1991.

Hendrickx L, Finke L: High school guidance counselor's attitudes toward nursing as a career. *J Nurs Educ* 33:87–88, February 1994.

Hine D: *Black Women in White: Racial Conflict and Cooperation in the Nursing Profession. 1890–1950.* Indianapolis, IN: Indiana University Press, 1989.

Kalisch P, Kalisch BJ: *The Changing Image of the Nurse.* Palo Alto, CA: Addison-Wesley, 1987.

Kohler P, Edwards T: High school student's perception of nursing as a career choice. *J Nurs Educ* 29:26–30, January 1990.

Kraegel J, Kachoyeanos M: *Just a Nurse.* New York: Dutton, 1989.

Lewis J et al: Men in nursing: Some disturbing data. *Am J Nurs* 90:30, August 1990.

Messner RL et al: Chemical abuse in nurses. *Adv Clin Care* 6:6–8, November–December 1991.

Pillitteri A: A contrast in images: Nursing and non-nursing college students. *J Nurs Educ* 33:132–133, March 1994.

Rosella JD et al: The need for multicultural diversity among health professionals. *Nurs Health Care* 15:242–246, May 1994.

Ryan S, Porter S: Men in nursing: A cautionary comparative critique. *Nurs Outlook* 41:262–267, November–December 1993.

The Kalisches have written many interesting articles, over the years, on nursing's image in the literature, press, movies, and television. A number of additional works are listed in the bibliography of the fifth edition of this book. Surveys in various journals such as the *American Journal of Nursing, Nursing*, and *RN* often present provocative, although limited, looks at nurses' views on various topics.

Section Three

NURSING EDUCATION AND RESEARCH

Various nursing journals carry a large number aof articles on nursing education and research: *Journal of Nursing Education, Nurse Educator, Journal of Continuing Education, Journal of Professional Nursing, Nursing Outlook*, and *Nursing and Health Care. The Chronicle of Higher Education* is an excellent weekly publication that carries both articles and news items related to education. ANA, NLN, and AACN have extensive publication lists that include books, proceedings, reports, and position papers on nursing education. *The American Nurse* also carries news items, as well as editorials and articles on the subject.

Chapter 12

Major Issues and Trends in Nursing Education

Bednash G: The changing pool of students, in McCloskey J, Grace HK (eds): *Current Issues in Nursing*. St Louis, MO: Mosby, 1994, pp 163–169.

Berbiglia V et al: The honors program: Pathway to excellence. *J Nurs Educ* 8:379–380, October 1993.

Bergman K, Gaitskill T: Faculty and student perceptions of effective clinical teachers: An extension study. *J Prof Nurs* 6:33–44, January–February 1990.

Billings D et al: Collaboration in distance education between nursing schools and hospitals. *Holistic Nurs Prac* 8:64–70, April 1994..

Dailey MA: The lived experience of nurses enrolled in the Regents College nursing program. *J Prof Nurs* 10:244–254, July–August 1994.

Donley R: Health care reform: Implications for staff development. *Nurs Econ* 12:71–74, March–April 1994.

Donnelly G et al: A faculty-practice program: Three

perspectives. *Holistic Nurs Pract* 8:71–80, April 1994.

Fagin CM, Lynaugh JE: Reaping the rewards of radical change: A new agenda for nursing education. *Nurs Outlook* 40:213–220, September–October 1992.

Germain CP et al: Evaluation of a PhD program: Paving the way. *Nurs Outlook* 42: 117–119, May–June 1994.

Hart S: Single purpose institutions for nursing programs: To be or not to be. *J Prof Nurs* 6:55–58, January–February 1990.

Hegyvary ST: Nursing education for health care reform. *J Prof Nurs* 8, March 1992.

Kersten J et al: Motivating factors in a student's choice of nursing as a career. *J Nurs Educ* 30:30–33, January 1991.

Leininger M: Trancultural nursing education: A worldwide imperative. *Nurs Health Care* 15:254–257, May 1994.

Lenburg C: Do external degree programs really work? *Nurs Outlook* 38:234–238, September–October 1990.

Lipman TH, Deatrick JA: Enhancing specialist preparation for the next century. *J Nurs Educ* 33:53–58, February 1994.

Nugent KE et al: Facilitators and inhibitors of practice: A faculty perspective . . . The role of faculty practice. *J Nurs Educ* 32:293–300, September 1993.

Oermann M: Professional nursing education in the future: Changes and challenges. *JOGNN* 23:153–159, February 1994.

Oermann M: Reforming nursing education for future practice. *J Nurs Educ* 33:215–218, May 1994.

Okrainec G: Perceptions of nursing education held by male nursing students. *West J Nurs Res* 16:94–107, February 1994.

Rothert ML et al: Partnerships in nursing education: Expanding boundaries, in McCloskey J, Grace HK (eds): *Current Issues in Nursing*. St Louis, MO: Mosby, 1994, pp 170–176.

Ryan M, Irvine P: Nursing profession in America: Projected retirements and replacements. *J Nurs Educ* 33:67–73, February 1994.

Sanford K: Future education: What do nurse executives need? *Nurs Econ* 12: 126–130, May–June 1994.

Seidle A, Sauter D: The new non-traditional student in nursing. *J Nurs Educ* 29:13–19, January 1990.

Sheehe J, Schoener L: Risk and reality for nurse educators. *Holistic Nurs Pract* 8:53–58, January 1994.

Sheil E, Wassem R: Thoughts of college graduates in nursing bacalaureate program. *J Nurs Educ* 33:91–92, February 1994.

Sherman S, Waters V: Community college-nursing home partnerships, in McCloskey J, Grace HK (eds): *Current Issues in Nursing.* St Louis, MO: Mosby, 1994, pp 177–181.

Sparks SM: The educational technology network. *Nurs Health Care* 15:134–141, March 1994.

Starck PL et al: Developing a nursing doctorate for the 21st century. *J Prof Nurs* 9:212–219, July–August 1993.

Wassem R, Sheil E: National survey of nursing program options designed for the second degree student. *J Nurs Educ* 33:29–30, January 1994.

Weeks WB: A comparison of the educational costs and incomes of physicians and other professionals. *N Engl J Med* 330:1280–1286, May 1994.

Chapter 13
Programs in Nursing Education

Barger SE, Kline PM: Community health service programs in academe: Unique learning opportunities for students. *Nurs Educ* 18:22–26, November–December 1993.

Downs F: Differences between the professional doctorate and the academic/research doctorate. *J Prof Nurs* 5: 261–265, September–October 1989.

Dvorak EM et al: A survey of BSN curricula: Research content. *J Nurs Educ* 32:265–269, June 1993.

Gay JT et al: Graduate education for nursing students who have English as a second language. *J Prof Nurs* 9:104–109, March–April 1993.

Grant P: Formative evaluation of a nursing orientation program: Self-pace vs. lecture-discussion. *J Contin Educ Nurs* 24:245–248, November–December 1993.

Helms LB et al: Funding for nursing education under Medicare: A window of opportunity. *Nurs Health Care* 15:344–349, October 1994.

Herbener DJ, Watson JE: Models for evaluating nursing education programs. *Nurs Outlook* 40:27–32, January–February 1992.

Hiestand WC, O'Day VC: Access to graduate education for registered nurses with non-nursing baccalaureate degrees. *J Prof Nurs* 9:220–227, July–August 1993.

Hoeffer B: Geropsychiatric nursing: Essential curriculum content. *J Psychosoc Nurs Ment Health Serv* 32:33–38, 40–41, April 1994.

Ihlenfeld JT: Teaching computerized data analysis in the classroom. *Comput Nurs* 11:269–270, November–December 1993.

Jewell ML: Partnerships in learning: Education as liberation. *Nurs Health Care* 15:360–364, September 1994.

Kramer MK: Concept clarification and critical thinking: Integrated processes. *J Nurs Educ* 32:406–414, November 1993.

Lawless KA: Nursing informatics as a needed emphasis in graduate nursing administration education: The student perspective. *Comput Nurs* 11:263–268, November–December 1993.

Lipman TH, Deatrick JA: Enhancing specialist preparation for the next century. *J Nurs Educ* 33:53–58, February 1994.

Minnick A: MSN in nursing administration and the dual degree. *Nurs Health Care* 14:22–26, January 1993.

Murphy MA: Integrating nursing informatics into a graduate research course. *J Nurs Educ* 32:332–334, September 1993.

Sherer J: Will college nursing education include managed care? *Hosp Health Netw* 67:47, July 1993.

Tschikota S: The clincal decision-making processes of student nurses. *J Nurs Educ* 32:389–398, November 1993.

Waddel DL: Why do nurses participate in continuing education? A meta-analysis. *J Contin Educ Nurs* 24:52–56, March–April 1993.

Watson J, Phillips S: Colorado nursing doctorate model as exemplar. *Nurs Outlook* 40:20–26, January–February 1992.

Weis D et al: Professional values in bacalaureate nursing education. *J Prof Nurs* 9:336–342, November–December 1993.

Chapter 14
Nursing Research: Status, Problems, Issues

Albrecht M: Research priorities for home health nursing. *Nurs Health Care* 13:538–541, December 1992.

Betz C et al: Nursing research productivity in clinical settings. *Nurs Outlook* 38:180–183, July–August 1990.

Kessenick C: Nursing research: Challenge to excellence. *Imprint* 39:84–85, September–October 1992.

Kjervick D, Penticuff J: The future of nursing research in ethics and law. *J Prof Nurs* 8:141, May–June 1992.

Larson E: Nursing research and societal needs: Political, corporate, and international perspectives. *J Prof Nurs* 9:73–77, March–April 1993.

Laske J et al: Using clinical innovations for research-based practice. *AACN Clin Issues* 5:103–113, May 1994.

Nokes K, Dolan M: Experience of nurse-researchers in gaining access to subjects for clinical nursing research. *J Prof Nurs* 8:115–119, March–April 1992.

Pettingil M et al: Factors encouraging and discouraging the use of nursing research findings. *Image* 26:143–148, Summer 1994.

Polit D, Hunsler B: *Nursing Research: Principles and Methods.* Philadelphia, PA: Lippincott, 1991.

Porter C, Villarruel A: Nursing research with African-American and Hispanic people: Guidelines for action. *Nurs Outlook* 41:59–67, March–April 1993.

Reilly D: Research in nursing education: Yesterday, today, tomorrow. *Nurs Health Care* 11:138–143, March 1990.

Selby ML et al: Building administrative support for your research: A neglected key for turning a research plan into a funded project. *Nurs Outlook* 40:73–77, March–April 1992.

Turner B, Weiss M: How to make research happen: Working with staff. *JOGNN* 23:345–349, May 1994.

It is useful to become acquainted with the books on nursing research and all the nursing research journals. The latter frequently have abstracts of research as well as detailed articles.

Section Four
THE PRACTICE OF NURSING

Chapter 15
Opportunities in Modern Nursing

Aiken L: Charting the future of hospital nursing. *Image* 22:72–78, Summer 1990.

Alward RR, Monk TH: *The Nurses' Shift Work Handbook.* Washington, DC: American Nurses Publishing, 1993.

American Nurses Association: *Registered Professional Nurses and Unlicensed Assistive Personnel.* Washington; DC: American Nurses Publishing, 1994.

Armstrong JR: Operation Desert Storm: Nursing in a combat zone fleet hospital. *Emerg Care Q* 7:70–78, January 1992.

Barter M et al: The use of unlicensed personnel by hospitals. *Nurs Econ* 12:82–87, March–April 1994.

Batra C: Socializing nurses for nursing entrepreneurship roles. *Nurs Health Care* 11:34–37, January 1990.

Bower KA: *Case Management by Nurses.* Washington, DC: American Nurses Publishing, 1992.

Brett JL, Tonges MC: Restructured patient care delivery: Evaluation of the ProAct model. *Nurs Econ* 8:36–44, January 1990.

Brider P: The move to patient focused care. *Am J Nurs* 92:26–33, September 1992.

Brush BG: Shortage as shorthand for the crisis in caring. *Nurs Health Care* 13:480–485, November 1992.

Bullough B: Alternative models for specialty nursing practice. *Nurs Health Care* 13:254–259, May 1992.

Carty B: The protean nature of the nurse informaticist. *Nurs Health Care* 15:174–178, April 1994.

Cassey MC, Savalle-Dunn J: Sketching the future: Trends influencing nursing informatics. *JOGNN* 23:175–181, February 1994.

Corley NC et al: The clinical ladder: Impact on nurse satisfaction and turnover. *J Nurs Adm* 24:42–48, February 1994.

deSavorgnani AA et al: Recruiting and retaining registered nurses in home health care. *J Nurs Adm* 23:42–46, June 1993.

Edwards GB et al: Unit-based shared governance can work! *Nurs Mgt* 25:74–77, April 1994.

Fagin C: Collaboration between nurses and physicians: No longer a choice. *Acad Med* 67:295–303, May 1992.

Fiesta J: Legal update, part II: assigning, delegating and staffing: *Nurs Manage* 24:14–15, February 1993.

Fiesta J: Staff implications: A legal update. *Nurs Manage* 25:34–35, June 1994.

Finkler S et al: Innovation in nursing: A benefit/cost analysis. *Nurs Econ* 12:18–37, January–February 1994.

Flanagan L: *Self-Employment in Nursing.* Washington, DC: American Nurses Publishing, 1993.

Forbes KE et al: Clinical nurse specialist and nurse practitioner care curricula survey results. *Nurse Pract* 15:43, 46–48, April 1990.

Friss L: The nursing shortage: Do we dislike it enough to cure it? *Inquiry* 25:232–242, Summer 1988.

Ginzberg E: What physcians should know about the nursing shortage. *Ann Intern Med* 112:319–320, March 1990.

Giorella EC: Education: Culturally competent care and the school environment. *J Prof Nurs* 10:6, January–February 1994.

Hayes PM: Non-nursing functions: Time for them to go. *Nurs Econ* 12:120–125, May–June 1994.

Hovis B: *Station Hospital Saigon: A Navy Nurse in Vietnam, 1963-1964.* Annapolis, MD: United States Naval Institute, 1991.

Huber D et al: Use of nursing assistants: Staff nurse opinions. *Nurs Mgt* 25:64, May 1994.

Keane A, Richmond T: Tertiary nurse practitioners. *Image* 25:281–284, Winter 1993.

Keyes MA: Recognition and reward: A unit-based program. *Nurs Mgt* 25:52–54, February 1994.

Klinefelter G: Role efficacy and job satisfaction of hospital nurses. *J Nurs Staff Dev* 9:179–183, July–August 1993.

Koerner JG et al: Implementing differentiated practice: The Sioux Valley Hospital experience: *J Nurs Adm* 19:13–20, February 1989.

Kramer M: Trends to watch at the magnet hospitals. *Nurs 90* 20:67–74, June 1990.

Lengacher C: Redesigning nursing practice: The partners in patient care model. *J Nurs Adm* 23:31–37, December 1993.

Madden MJ, Ponte PR: Advanced practice roles in the managed care environment. *J Nurs Adm* 24:56–62, January 1994.

Mallach KM et al: A model for differentiated nursing practice. *J Nurs Adm* 20:20–26, February 1990.

Manthey M: Staffing and productivity. *Nurs Mgt* 22:20–21, 1991.

Masters F et al: Role development: The nursing quality assurance coordinator. *J Nurs Qual Assur* 4:51–62, February 1990.

McCloskey JC et al: Who helps you with your work? *Am J Nurs* 4:43–46, 1991.

McHenry L: Implementing self-directed teams. *Nurs Mgt* 25:801–805, March 1994.

Meyer C: The richness of oncology nursing. *Am J Nurs* 92:71, 72, 74, 76, 78, May 1992.

Mullinix CF: Regulation of temporary nursing services—what does it mean? *J Prof Nurs* 7:263, September–October 1991.

National Council of State Boards of Nursing: *Concept Paper on Delegation.* Chicago: The Council, 1990.

National Council of State Boards of Nursing: *Position Paper on the Licensure of Advanced Nursing Practice.* Chicago: The Council, 1992.

Orchard MCH, Nelson Swenson G: Enhancing professional communication: A formal computerized nurse-to-nurse consultation system. *Nurs Adm Q* 18:66–79, Fall 1993.

Patton S, Stanley J: Bridging quality assurance and continuous quality improvement. *J Nurs Care Qual* 7:15–23, January 1993.

Peplau H: Future directions in psychiatric nursing from the perspective of history. *J Psychosoc Nurs* 27:18–21, 25–28, February 1988.

Phillips CY et al: Case manager/nurse manager: A blending of roles. *Nurs Mgt* 24:26–28, October 1993.

Prescott PC et al: Changing how nurses spend their time. *Image* 23:23–28, January 1991.

Prescott P: Nursing: An important component of hospital survival under a reformed health care system. *Nurs Econ* 11:192–199, 1993.

Robertson JF, Cummings CC: What makes long term care nursing attractive? *Am J Nurs* 91:41–46, November 1991.

Saba V et al: *Computers in Nursing Management.* Washington, DC: American Nurses Publishing, 1994.

Sawyers SE: Defining your role in ambulatory care: Clinical nurse specialist or nurse practitioners. *Clin Nurs Spec* 7:4–7, January 1993.

Stratton TD et al: How states respond to the rural nursing shortage. *Nur Health Care* 14:238–243, May 1993.

Villaire M: Marie Manthey on the evolution of primary nursing. *Crit Care Nurs* 13:100–107, December 1993.

Walton MK et al: A collaborative practice model for the clinical nurse specialist. *J Nurs Adm* 23:55–59, February 1993.

Possibly hundreds of articles on NPs have appeared since 1967 in nursing, medical, hospital, and public health journals, including information on education and practice, and evaluation research. In addition, the NP and specialty journals, such as the *Journal of Nurse Midwifery*, carry articles on the role of their constituency. For those who are interested in the variety of careers available to nurses, almost all the nursing journals publish articles on careers periodically. *Career Guide* is published annually by the *American Journal of Nursing*.

Chapter 16

Leadership for an Era of Change

Baker ER: Use of diffusion of innovation model for agency consultation. *Clin Nurs Spec* 4:163–166, Fall 1990.

Boyd MA et al: Creating organizational change in an inpatient long-term care facility. *Psychosoc Rehabil J* 15:47–54, January 1994.

Bushy A: Managing change: Strategies for continuing education. *J Contin Educ Nurs* 23:197–200, May 1992.

Cauthorne-Lindstrom C: Organizational change from the "mom and pop" perspective. *J Nurs Adm* 22:61–64, July–August 1992.

Clinton HR: Nurses in the front lines. *Nurs Health Care* 14:286–288, June 1993.

Crawford DI: The glass ceiling in nursing management. *Nurs Econ* 11:333–341, November–December 1993.

Dixon IL: Continuous quality improvement in shared leadership. *Nurs Mgt* 24:40–41, 44–45, January 1993.

Gardner JW: *On Leadership*. The Free Press, 1993.

Goodroe J, Beres M: Network leadership and today's nurse. *Nurs Mgt* 22:56–62, June 1991.

Hein EC, Nicholson MJ: *Contemporary Leadership Behavior*, 4th ed, Philadelphia: Lippincott, 1994.

Keller B: Nurse empowerment: Increasing the nurse manager's ability to delegate authority. *Recruit Reten Rep* 7:1–4, March 1994.

Mason D et al: *Policy and Politics for Nurses*. Philadelphia: Saunders, 1993.

McDaniel C, Wolf JA: Transformational leadership in nursing service. *J Nurs Adm* 22:60–65, February 1992.

McHenry L: Implementing self-directed teams. *Nurs Manage: Crit Care Manage Ed* 25:80I–J, 80L, March 1994.

Meyer C: Nurses on the political front. *Am J Nurs* 92:56–64, October 1992.

Mitchell MK: CHAP: Nursing's legacy of leadership. *Nurs Health Care* 13:296–302, June 1992.

Murphy NJ: Nursing leadership in health policy decision making. *Nurs Outlook* 40:158–161, July–August 1992.

Peck SL: Leadership strategies for organizational change: Applications in community nursing centers. *Nurs Adm Quart* 17:60–68, Fall 1992.

Sagrestano LM: The use of power and influence in a gendered world. *Psych Women Q* 16:439–447, Spring 1992.

Schoolfield M, Orduna A: Understanding staff nurse responses to change. *Clin Nurs Spec* 8: 57–62, January 1994.

Sims HP, Lorenz P: *The New Leadership Paradigm*. Newbury Park, CA: Sage Publications, 1992.

Olson R, Vance C: *Mentorship in Nursing: A Collection of Research Abstracts 1977–1992*. Houston: University of Texas Printing Services, 1993.

Valadez AM, Lund CA: Mentorship: Maslow and me. *J Contin Educ Nurs* 24:259–263, November–December 1993.

Wolf GA et al: A transformational model for the practice of professional nursing. *J Nurs Adm* 24:51–57, April 1994.

Yoder JD, Kahn AS: Toward a feminist understanding of women and power. *Psych Women Quart* 16:381–388, Winter 1992.

Biographies or interviews of living nursing leaders and their perceptions of nursing appear periodically in a number of nursing journals. See various issues of *Nursing and Health Care, Nursing Outlook, The American Journal of Nursing, Nursing Economics*, and *The American Nurse*. Books about nursing leaders are cited in this chapter's reference list. Videotapes of some nursing leaders are available from Sigma Theta Tau, Teachers College Columbia University, the Mugar Library in Boston, and the University of Pennsylvania Center for Nursing Research. Some other nursing libraries contain archives of nursing leaders, and videotaped interviews.

Section 5
LEGAL RIGHTS AND RESPONSIBILITIES

Listed in each chapter are a number of books on health and/or nursing law that are valuable. The styles and formats vary, but the basic information on law is the same. Later editions and the tremendous number of new books on nursing law are more current and therefore more accurate, but some earlier works are included because of the clarity of information on basic principles of law. To keep up to date on legal decisions and legislation concerning women's and children's rights or on changes in basic principles of law, read major newspapers, news and business magazines, women's magazines, some health professional journals, and law journals. Especially useful is the *Journal of Law Medicine and Ethics*. See also columns on legal aspects of nursing in various journals such as *RN, Nursing Management*, and the journals of specialty organizations. Also useful are the legislative bulletins of ANA and NLN. Many references and the bibliography in the sixth edition of this book are also still useful.

Chapter 17
An Introduction to Law

Aburdene P, Naisbett J: *Megatrends for Women*. New York: Villard Books, 1992.

Freda M: Childbearing, reproductive control, aging women, and health care: The projected ethical debates. *JOGNN* 23:144–151, February 1994.

Goldstein J et al: *In the Best Interests of the Child*. New York: Free Press, 1986.

Goodner E et al: Sexual harassment: Perspectives

from the past, present policy, and prevention. *J Cont Ed Nurs* 24:57–60, March–April 1994.

Hornsby J: Don't tolerate sexual harassment at work. *RN* 53:69–73, January 1990.

Jenkins J et al: Early childhood intervention: The law. *MCN,* 19:135–142, May–June 1994.

Outwater L: Sexual harassment issues in home care: What employers should do about it. *Caring* 13:54–60, May 1994.

Ross M, Ross J: *Handbook of Everyday Law.* New York: Gramercy, 1986.

Schreiber R: Pay equity and North American nurses. *Nurs Health Care* 14:28–33, January 1993.

Statham A et al: *The Worth of Women's Work: A Qualitative Synthesis.* Albany, NY: State University of New York Press, 1988.

Weiss J, Hansell MJ: Substance abuse during pregnancy: Legal and health policy issues. *Nurs Health Care* 13:472–479, November 1992.

Most nursing law books have a section on basic law and legislation.

Chapter 18
The Legislative Process

Congress and health: An introduction to the legislative process and its key participants. New York: National Health Council, revised periodically, sometimes with each congress.

DeVries CM, Vanderbilt MW: *The Grassroots Lobbying Handbook: Empowering Nurses through Legislative and Political Action.* Washington, DC: American Nurses Publishing 1993.

DeVries CM, Vanderbilt MW: Grassroots lobbying: Influencing the legislative process. *Am Nurse* 25, April 1993.

Goldwater M, Zusy MJL: *Prescription for Nurses: Effective Political Action.* St Louis: Mosby 1990.

Harrington C, Estes CL: *Health Policy and Nursing: Crisis and Reform in the U.S. Health Care Delivery System.* Boston: Jones and Bartlett, 1994.

Kayuha AA: Demystifying the legislative process. *Health Care Trends Transit* 1:20–21, March 1990.

Mason D et al: *Policy and Politics for Nurses, 2d ed.* Philadelphia: Saunders, 1993.

Positioned for Power: Obtaining Government Appointments for Nurses. Washington, DC: American Nurses Publishing, 1993.

Wakefield MK: Perspectives on health policy: Influencing the legislative process. *Nurs Econ* 8:188–190, May–June 1990.

Many publications of ANA and NLN relate to legislation and politics, as do those of most other large health associations and the National Health Council. Useful government publications include *Congressional Record* (verbatim transcript of the preceedings of the Senate and House, *Congressional Record* Office, H-112, Capitol, Washington, DC 20515) and annual subscription from the Superintendent of Documents, Government Printing Office, Washington, DC 20401; *Digest of Public General Bills*, also from the Superintendent of Documents; *Committee Prints and Hearing Records,* available about two months after the close of hearings, is free but requires a self-addressed label sent to the publications clerk of the committee from which the document is issued; and a *Catalogue of Washington Health Newsletters*, developed by some congressional staffs, available from the Health Policy Center, The Graduate School, Georgetown University, Washington, DC 20057. Major newspapers and news magazines always carry political-legislative news, with or without editorials.

Chapter 19
Major Legislation Affecting Nursing

Benjamin A: A historical perspective on home care policy. *Milbank Q* 71(1):129–166, 1993.

Brown L: *Health Policy in the United States: Issues and Options.* New York: Ford Foundation, 1988.

Cassetta R: FMLA: A first step toward equitable leave policies. *Am Nurs* 25:21, September 1993.

Dinn V: Commentary: Women, research, and the National Institutes of Health. *Am J Prev Med* 8:324–327, September–October 1992.

Donley S: Ethics in the age of health care reform. *Nurs Econ* 11:19–24, January–February 1993.

Estes C, Harrington C, Davis S: *Health Policy and Nursing: Crisis and Reform in the U.S. Health Care Delivery System.* Boston: Jones and Bartlett, 1994.

Helms L, Anderson M: Medicare and the financing of nursing education: Implications of Board of Trustees v. Sullivan. *J Prof Nurs* 9:139–147, May–June 1993.

Kirschstein, R: Research on women's health. *Am J Public Health* 81:291–293, March 1991.

LaRosa J: Gender bias in biomedical research. *J Am Med Wom Assoc* 48:145–151, September–October 1993.

Michels K: HCFA issues final rule on "Medicare payment; fee schedule for physicians' services." *AANA* 59:508–515, December 1991.

Natapoff J, Weiczorek R (eds): *Maternal-Child Health Policy.* New York: Springer, 1990.

Wold J: Worker's compensation and the occupational health nurse. *AAOHN J* 8:385–387, August 1990.

The American Nurse, The American Journal of Nursing, Nursing in Health Care, and most of the clinical specialty and management journals present monthly or periodic updates on national legislation and pertinent state legislation. Popular news magazines and major newspapers also report on legislation.

Chapter 20
Licensure and Health Manpower Credentialing

Affara FA, Styles MM: *Nursing Regulation Guidebook: From Principle to Power*. Geneva: International Council of Nurses, 1993.

Carson WY: Regulatory findings on states granting second licensure (for advanced practice nurses). Unpublished report. Washington DC: American Nurses' Association, 1993.

Credentialing in Nursing. A series of monographs dealing with a variety of aspects of the topic: Specialization, A world view on credentialing, Internal versus external regulation, Certification. Kansas City, MO: American Nurses Association, 1986.

Hurley ML: The push for specialty certification. *RN* 36–44, June 1994.

National Council of State Boards of Nursing: *Position Paper on the Licensure of Advanced Nursing Practice*. Chicago: The Council, 1992.

Safriet B: Health care dollars and regulatory sense: The role of advanced practice nursing. *Yale Journal on Regulation* 9:419–486, Summer 1992.

States with Some Form of Nurse privileging, Unpublished report. Washington, DC: American Nurses Association, 1993.

See also the references and bibliography of Chaps. 9, 13, 15, and 16. News items on changes in licensure and appropriate articles appear in almost all nursing journals. ANA, NLN, and the National Council of State Boards of Nursing (NCSBN) all have materials about licensure in their publications lists. *Issues*, a NCSBN news publication, is very useful.

Unpublished ANA reports on current credentialing issues are often available through your state nurses association.

Chapter 21
Nursing Practice and the Law

Betta P: Documenting to stay out of the courtroom. *Imprint* 38:39–40, April–May 1991.

Blackwell M: Documentation serves as invaluable defense tool. *Am Nurse* 25:40–41, July–August 1993.

Carroll P, Maher V: Legal issues in the care of patients with sickle cell disease. *AD Clin Care* 5:6, 19, September–October 1990.

Carson W: AIDS and the nurse—A legal update. *Am Nurse* 25:18, March 1993.

Cohn S: *Malpratice and Liability in Clinical Obstetrical Nursing*. Rockville, MD: Aspen, 1990.

Fiesta J: Agency nurses: Whose liability? *Nurs Mgt* 21:16–17, March 1990.

Fiesta J: Duty to communicate—"doctor notified" *Nurs Mgt* 25:24–25, January 1994.

Fiesta J: *The Law and Liability: A Guide for Nurses*. Albany, NY: Delmar, 1988.

Fiesta J: Legal update for nurses—1992: Part III. *Nurs Mgt* 24:16–17, March 1993.

Fiesta J: Malpractice and the federal employee. *Nurs Mgt* 25:22–23, May 1994.

Fiesta J: Nursing torts: From plaintiff to defendant. *Nurs Mgt* 25:17–18, February 1994.

Kadzielski M: Exploring the legal aspects of quality improvement. *Am Nurse* 25:7, January 1993.

Koehler C: Lawsuit demands coping skills. *Am Nurse* 24:33, June 1992.

Koehler C: The nurse as defendant. *Am Nurse* 24:17, April 1992.

Maher V: AIDS—the legal issues. *AD Clin Care* 6:28–30, March–April 1991.

Mahoney D: Under oath: Testifying against a physician. *Am J Nurs* 90:23, 26, February 1990.

Mandell M: What you don't say can hurt you. *Am J Nurs* 93:15–16, August 1993.

Pozgar G: *Legal Aspects of Health Care Administration*, 5th ed. Rockville, MD: Aspen, 1993.

Pozgar G et al: *Long-Term Care and the Law*. Rockville, MD: Aspen, 1992.

Quigley F: Responsibilities of the consultant and expert witness. *Focus Crit Care* 18:238–239, July 1991.

Rhodes AM: Locating case law. *MCN* 19:107, March–April 1994.

Scott R: *Legal Aspects of Documenting Patient Care*. Rockville, MD: Aspen, 1994.

Turley J: A framework for the transition from nursing records to a nursing information system. *Nurs Outlook* 40:177–191, July–August 1992.

Articles on nursing law are found periodically, sometimes monthly, in almost all nursing journals. Books on nursing law usually cover every topic in this chapter; books on medical and health care law also have pertinent information. *Health Law Reporter,* published by the Bureau of National Affairs in Washington, DC is a weekly review of legislative, regulatory, and legal developments. At times there are also special publications by HHS, such as *Issues in Medical Liability: A Working Conference,* 1991, based on conferences.

Chapter 22
Health Care and the Rights of People

Alpert S: Smart cards, smarter policy: Medical records, privacy, and health care reform. *Hastings Center Rep* 23:13–23, November–December 1993.

Boisaubin E: Legal decisions affecting the limitation of nutritional support. *Hospice J* 9:131–147, 2, 1993.

Carrol P, Maher V: Feeding tubes: Maintaining life or stalling death? The nurses' role. *AD Clin Care* 5:6, March–April 1990.

Carrol P, Maher V: Legal aspects of contagious infectious diseases. *Ad Clin Care* 5:6, May–June 1990.

Carrol P, Maher V: Legal issues in experimental investigations of medications. *AD Clin Care* 5:6, May–June 1990.

Carrol P, Maher V: The patient in pain: Legal issues in competency assessment. *AD Clin Care* 4:6, September–October 1989.

Chabalewski F, Norris G: The gift of life: Talking to families about organ and tissue donation. *Am J Nurs* 94:29–33, June 1994.

Charo R: Life after *Casey:* The view from Rehnquist's Potemkin Village. *J Law Med Ethics* 21:59–66, Spring 1993.

Celo Cruz M: Aid-in-dying: Should we decriminalize physician-assisted suicide and physician-committed euthanasia? *Am J Law Med* 18:369–394, April 1992.

Curtin L: Abortion: A tangle of rights. *Nurs Mgt* 24:26–31, June 1993.

Curtin L: Patient privacy in a public institution. *Nurs Mgt* 24:26–27, June 1993.

Euthanasia in the Netherlands. *Int Nurs Rev* 41:63–64, March–April 1994.

Frawley K: Confidentiality in the computer age. *RN* 57:59–60, July 1994.

Goodner E, Kolenick D: Sexual harassment in nursing school. *Imprint* 41:54–55, 58, 63, January 1994.

Gostin L: Drawing a line between killing and letting die: The law and law reform, on medically assisted dying. *J Law Med Ethics* 21:94–101, Spring 1993.

Greve P: Has the PSDA made a difference? *RN* 57:59–64, February 1994.

Hague S, Moody L: A study of the public's knowl-

edge regarding advance directions. *Nurs Econ* 11:303–307, September–October 1993.

Jones S: Genetic-based and assisted reproductive technology of the 21st century. *JOGNN* 23:106–169, February 1994.

Ketter J: Sex discrimination targets men in some hospitals. *Am Nurse* 26:3, April 1994.

Meisal A: Legal myths about terminating life support. *Arch Intern Med* 151:1497–1501, August 1991.

Mezey M et al: The Patient Self-determination Act: Sources of concern for nurses. *Nurs Outlook* 42:30–38, January –February 1994.

Milholland K: Privacy and confidentiality of patient information: Challenges for nursing. *J Nurs Adm* 24:19–24, February 1994.

Mosely C, Beard M: Norplant: Nursing's responsibility in procreative rights. *Nurs Health Care* 15:294–297, June 1994.

Philipsen N, McMullen P: Medical records: Promoting patient confidentiality. *Nurs Connect* 6:48–50, Winter 1993.

Quill T et al: *N Eng J Med* 327:1380–1387, Nov 5, 1992.

Ramsey M: Patient rights and obligations. *AD Clin Care* 5:29–30, January–February 1990.

Rinas J, Chyne-Jackson S: *Professional Conduct and Legal Concerns in Mental Health Practice.* Norwalk, CT: Appleton and Lange, 1988.

Ross L: Moral grounding for the participation of children as organ donors. *J Law Med Ethics* 21:251–257, Spring 1993.

Rost A: Anencephalic infants and organ procurement. *Imprint* 37:61–62, September–October 1990.

Scanlon C: Safeguarding a patient's right to self-determination. *Am Nurse* 25:20–21, November–December 1993.

Schwarz J: Living wills and health care proxies. *Nurs Health Care* 13:92–96, February 1992.

Thurkauf G: Understanding the beliefs of Jehovah's Witnesses. *Focus Crit Care* 16:199–204, June 1989.

Weber G: Tips on implementing the Patient Self-determination Act. *Nurs Health Care* 14:86–91, February 1993.

Wendling E: Anencephalics as organ donors. *Imprint* 37:47–48, April–May 1990.

Wolf S et al: Sources of concern about the Patient Self-determination Act. *N Engl J Med* 325:1666–1667, December 5, 1991.

See also references and bibliography of Chaps. 6, 10, 17, and 24 for related topics. Journals such as the *Hastings Center Report* and *Health Care, Law and*

Ethics periodically have special issues on certain topics such as physician-assisted dying (*Health Care, Law and Ethics*, Winter 1992).

PART III
PROFESSIONAL COMPONENTS AND CAREER DEVELOPMENT

Section One
ORGANIZATIONS AND PUBLICATIONS

Chapter 23
Organizational Procedures and Issues

LaBranche GA: Enlisting the baby boomers: Generational differences to attract today's volunteers. *Leadership* L 37–39, L 42, 1992.

Association Management, the monthly magazine of the Society of Association Executives, contains excellent articles on organizational issues, as well as articles geared to association staff. The society has also published a series of booklets to help volunteers function more effectively in associations (for example, "Getting Involved: The Challenge of Committee Participation" and "Moving Forward: Providing Leadership as the Chief Elected Officer").

Chapter 24
National Student Nurses Association

Beck CT: How students perceive faculty caring: A phenomenological study. *Nurs Educ* 16:18–22, 1991.
Polk D et al: The chemically dependent student nurse: Guidelines for policy development. *Nurs Outlook* 41:166–170, July–August 1993.
Williams RP: The concerns of beginning nursing students. *Nurs Health Care* 14:178–184, April 1993.

The *American Journal of Nursing* usually reports on the annual NSNA conventions, in addition to providing news items and pertinent articles to serve a student audience. Various publications of NSNA may be requested from its headquarters. *Imprint*, the NSNA journal, is the best reference.

Chapter 25
American Nurses' Association

Information about the activities of ANA is found most extensively in the ANA publications described in Chap. 25 and the ANA publications list. In addition, ANA conventions are reported in the *American Journal of Nursing, Nursing Outlook*, and *American Nurse*. A useful reference about the American Acad-

emy of Nursing is Rosemary McCarthy, *History of the American Academy of Nursing 1973–1982*, Kansas City, MO: American Academy of Nursing, 1985.

Chapter 26
National League for Nursing

The best source of current information about NLN can be found in the NLN publications noted in Chap. 26 and the NLN publications list. This includes information about position papers, and conference proceedings. NLN conventions and meetings are reported in some depth in *Nursing and Health Care*.

Chapter 27
Other Nursing and Related Organizations in the United States

Kalisch B, Kalisch P: *Nurturer of Nurses: A History of the Division of Nursing of the U.S. Public Health Service and Its Antecedents, 1798–1977*. Summary report of a study for the Division of Nursing, March 1977.
Mullen F: Plague and politics: *The Story of the U.S. Public Health Service*. New York: Basic Books, 1989.

All of the included organizations have journals, newsletters, and other published material that are identified in the chapter. *AJN* reports on the meetings and positions of a broad range of organizations.

Chapter 28
Major International Organizations

Reports of ICN congresses are usually found in the *American Journal of Nursing, Nursing Outlook*, and other nursing journals that carry news items about ICN activities. Other news is carried in the *International Nursing Review*. The World Health Organization has a number of publications that report on its activities. Sigma Theta Tau International publications, particularly *Reflections*, update STTI activities.

Section Two
TRANSITION INTO PRACTICE

Nursing journals and the yearly *Career Guide*, published by some of them, periodically carry articles on career guidance and employment guidelines. (Some are in the reference lists and bibliography.) Business journals, and especially career women's magazines, have also been emphasizing these topics. Any bookstore has a section devoted to career development; some of the books are best-sellers and may be found in paperback.

Chapter 29
Making Choices: Job Selection

Bleich M, Sullivan J: How to make informed employment decisions. *AD Clin Care* 4:18–21, September–October 1989.

Davidhizar F: Feeling like a nurse. *Imprint* 41:53–54, April–May 1994.

Davidhizar R: Is this job for you? *Imprint* 40:11–15, January 1993.

Ketter J: Surviving layouffs. *Am Nurs* 26:25, July–August 1994.

Mullin M: Where in the world are the new grad jobs? *Imprint* 41:6, 8 January 1994.

Netherton H: Tips on successful interviewing. *Imprint* 39:27, 29, January 1992.

Nowak J, Grindel C: *Career Planning in Nursing.* Philadelphia, Lippincott, 1984.

Rhores J, Young M: Surviving your first job. *Healthcare Trends Transit* 3:24–27, May 1992.

Rodriguez K: Avoid interview turn-off to ensure success. *Am Nurse* 24:19, September 1992.

Sills F: Five strategies to survive your first interview. *Imprint* 40:31–32, January 1993.

Stein A, Licht B: Questions and answers on the computerized NCLEX exam. *Imprint* 41:9–11, January 1994.

Stille P: Life insurance: An important part of the benefit pie. *Healthcare Trends Transit* 3:54, March 1992.

Study explores nurses' attitudes about career issues. *Am Nurse* 25:12, October 1993.

Washington R: A practical guide to interviewing. *Imprint* 37:38–39, December 1990–January 1991.

Wheeler I: Success in your first interview. *Imprint* 41:20, 37, January 1994.

See also references and bibliography of Chaps. 11, 15, 16, 19, 20, 22, and 30. The November–December 1991 issue of *Healthcare Trends and Transition* is almost entirely devoted to job search.

For more information about trends in the health professions, the journals of each occupation and profession and general hospital, home care, and long-term care facilities are the best source. They are usually available in health professions libraries.

Chapter 30
Career Management

Barter M et al: Use of unlicensed assistive personnel by hospitals. *Nurs Econ* 12:82–84, May–June 1994.

Benner P: *From Novice to Expert.* Menlo Park, CA: Addison-Wesley, 1984.

Bradley-Springer L: Anticipating care for HIV-infected clients: Nurses' reactions. *J Assoc Nurses AIDS Care* 5:29–38, January–February 1994.

Brewington JG: The AIDS epidemic: Caring for caregivers. *Nurs Adm Q* 18:22–29, Winter 1994.

Christman L: Perspectives on role socialization of nurses. *Nurs Outlook* 39:209–212, September–October 1991.

Cooney AT: An orientation program for new graduate nurses: The basis of staff development and retention. *J Contin Educ Nurs* 23:216–219, September–October 1992.

Dienemann J: *Continuous Quality Improvement in Nursing.* Washington, DC: American Nurses Publishing, 1992.

The dual epidemics of tuberculosis and AIDS [entire issue]. *J Law Med Ethics* 21:277–393, Fall–Winter 1993.

Dubbert PM et al: Development of a measure of willingness to provide nursing care to AIDS patients. *Nurs Adm Q* 18:16–21, Winter 1994.

Fiesta J: Whistleblowers: Heros or stool pigeons? Part I. *Nurs Mgt* 21:16–17, June 1990.

Fiesta J: Whistleblowers: Retaliation or protection? Part II. *Nurs Mgt* 21:38, July 1990.

Fighting staff cuts: California RNs push for enforceable patient ratios. *Am J Nurs* 93:81, 84, January 1993.

Finnis SJ, Robbins I: Sexual harassment of nurses: An occupational hazard? *J Clin Nurs* 3:87–85, March 1994.

Flarey DL et al: Collaboration in labor relations: A model for success. *J Nurs Adm* 22:15–22, September 1992.

Gardner DL: Conflict and retention of new graduate nurses. *West J Nurs Res* 14:76–85, February 1994.

Gowell YM, Boverie PE: Stress and satisfaction as a result of shift and number of hours worked. *Nurs Adm Q* 16:14–19, Summer 1992.

Grainger R: Anxiety interrupters. *Am J Nurs* 90:14, February 1990.

Grainger R: Managing fatigue. *Am J Nurs* 90:13, March 1990.

Hood JN, Smith HL: Quality of work life, in home care: The contribution of leaders' personal concern for staff. *J Nurs Adm* 24:40–47, January 1994.

Jolma DJ: Relationship between nursing workload and turnover. *Nurs Econ* 8:110–114, February 1990.

Kane D: Invest in yourself. Coping with multiple roles: Mother/wife/nurse. *Nurs Forum* 28:17–21, October–December 1993.

Kennedy P: Burn-out: Can we risk ignoring it? *Nurs Mgt* 1:185–188, July 1993.

Klemm R, Schreiber EJ: Paid and unpaid benefits: Strategies for nurse recruitment and retention. *J Nurs Adm* 22:52–56, March 1992.

Klinefelter G: Role efficiency and job satisfaction of hospital nurses. *J Nurs Staff Dev* 9:179–183, 1993.

Kramer M, Schmalenberg C: Job satisfaction and retention: Insights for the 90's, part 2. *Nurse* 21:51–55, April 1991.

Kruger P: Superwoman's daughters. *Working Woman* 19:60–67, May 1994.

Lengacher CA: Development of a predictive model for role strain in registered nurses returning to school. *J Nurs Educ* 32:301–308, September 1993.

Lewis J et al: Preventing AIDS: Knowledge, attitudes and practices. *J Gerontol Nurs* 20:21–28, February 1994.

Marquis BL, Huston CJ: Motivation to join or reject unions. *J Nurs Adm* 24:4, February 1994.

McEachen I: Promoting retention strategies in a unionized environment. *Recruit Reten Rep* 6:4–7, November 1993.

Moreau D: Implementing an expanded role: Rewarding experienced nurses. *Recruit Reten Rep* 5:1–3, June 1992.

Murphy E: Professional autonomy v "At Will" employee status. *Nurs Outlook* 38:248, September–October 1990.

Nayak S: Strategies to support the new nurse in practice. *J Nurs Staff Dev* 7:64–66, March–April 1991.

Northrop C: Refusing unsafe assignments. *Imprint* 36:20, February–March 1989.

Plawecki HM: Write right. *J Holistic Nurs* 12:135–137, June 1994.

Poteet GW et al: Graduate education: Making the right choice. *Medsurg Nurs* 2:216–217, June 1993.

Quimby CH: Women and the family of the future. *JOGNN* 23:115–119, February 1994.

Ramiriz D: Culture in a nursing service organization. *Nurs Mgt* 21:14–15, 17, January 1990.

Ricci ES: Reproductive hazards in the workplace. *Clin Issues Perinat Wom Health Nurs* 1:226–239, February 1990.

Schmieding NJ: Nurse empowerment through context, structure, and process. *J Prof Nurs* 9:239–245, July–August 1993.

Schroeder I: Private lives. *Nurs Times* 89:81–83, September 1993.

Scott VL, Totten NW: Giving the dream: Shared governance in the role of nurse executive. *J Nurs Adm* 23:44–48, December 1993.

Serow WJ et al: Health care corporatization and the employment conditions of nurses. *Nurs Econ* 11:279–291, September–October 1993.

Sherer JL: Can hospitals and organized labor be partners in redesign? *Hosp Health Netw* 68:56, 58, March 1994.

Snow C, Willard D: *I'm Dying to Take Care of You: Nurses and Co-Dependence: Breaking the Cycle.* Redmond, WA: Professional Counselor Books, 1990.

Spechko PL: Bloodborne pathogens. Can you become infected from your older patient? *J Gerontol Nurs* 19:12–15, July 1993.

Staff cuts are sparking unionizing drives. *Am J Nurs* 93:9, September 1993.

Van Servellen G, Leake B: Burn-out in hospital nurses: A comparison of acquired immune deficiency syndrome, oncology, general medical, and intensive care unit nurses. *J Prof Nurs* 9:169–177, May–June 1993.

Vosel L: *Mothers on the Job.* New Brunswick, NJ: Rutgers University Press, 1993.

Wicker CP: AIDS and HIV: The dilemma of the health care worker. *Today's OR Nurse* 15:1422, March–April 1993.

Worthington K: Workplace hazards: The effect on nurses as women. *Am Nurs* 26:15, February 1994.

Author Index*

*Authors listed here are those in chapter references. The page noted is the location of the documented material. The complete citation appears at the end of each chapter.

Subject Index

Page numbers in italics refer to figures; page numbers followed by t or E refer to tables or exhibits, respectively.

ISBN 0-07-105477-4

9 780071 054775

KELLY/DIMEN PROF NURS